Blackwell's Five-Minute
Veterinary Consult
Clinical Companion

Small Animal Gastrointestinal Diseases

T0325459

Blackwell's Five-Minute
Veterinary Consult
Clinical Companion

Small Animal Gastrointestinal Diseases

Edited by

Jocelyn Mott, DVM, DACVIM (SAIM)
Jo Ann Morrison, DVM, MS, DACVIM (SAIM)

WILEY Blackwell

This edition first published 2019
© 2019 John Wiley & Sons, Inc.

All rights reserved. No part of this publication may be reproduced, stored in a retrieval system, or transmitted, in any form or by any means, electronic, mechanical, photocopying, recording or otherwise, except as permitted by law. Advice on how to obtain permission to reuse material from this title is available at http://www.wiley.com/go/permissions.

The right of Jocelyn Mott and Jo Ann Morrison to be identified as the authors of the editorial material in this work has been asserted in accordance with law.

Registered Office
John Wiley & Sons, Inc., 111 River Street, Hoboken, NJ 07030, USA

Editorial Office
111 River Street, Hoboken, NJ 07030, USA

For details of our global editorial offices, customer services, and more information about Wiley products visit us at www.wiley.com.

Wiley also publishes its books in a variety of electronic formats and by print-on-demand. Some content that appears in standard print versions of this book may not be available in other formats.

Limit of Liability/Disclaimer of Warranty
While the publisher and authors have used their best efforts in preparing this work, they make no representations or warranties with respect to the accuracy or completeness of the contents of this work and specifically disclaim all warranties, including without limitation any implied warranties of merchantability or fitness for a particular purpose. No warranty may be created or extended by sales representatives, written sales materials or promotional statements for this work. The fact that an organization, website, or product is referred to in this work as a citation and/or potential source of further information does not mean that the publisher and authors endorse the information or services the organization, website, or product may provide or recommendations it may make. This work is sold with the understanding that the publisher is not engaged in rendering professional services. The advice and strategies contained herein may not be suitable for your situation. You should consult with a specialist where appropriate. Further, readers should be aware that websites listed in this work may have changed or disappeared between when this work was written and when it is read. Neither the publisher nor authors shall be liable for any loss of profit or any other commercial damages, including but not limited to special, incidental, consequential, or other damages.

Library of Congress Cataloging-in-Publication Data

Names: Mott, Jocelyn, editor. | Morrison, Jo Ann, editor.
Title: Blackwell's five-minute veterinary consult clinical companion. Small
   animal gastrointestinal diseases / edited by Jocelyn Mott, Jo Ann Morrison.
Other titles: Five-minute veterinary consult clinical companion | Small
   animal gastrointestinal diseases
Description: Hoboken, NJ : Wiley-Blackwell, [2019] | Includes bibliographical
   references and index. |
Identifiers: LCCN 2018051892 (print) | LCCN 2018052959 (ebook) | ISBN
   9781119376330 (Adobe PDF) | ISBN 9781119376323 (ePub) | ISBN 9781119376347
   (pbk.)
Subjects: | MESH: Gastrointestinal Diseases–veterinary | Animal
   Diseases–therapy | Pets | Handbooks
Classification: LCC SF992.G38 (ebook) | LCC SF992.G38 (print) | NLM SF 981 |
   DDC 636.089/633–dc23
LC record available at https://lccn.loc.gov/2018051892

Cover design: Wiley
Cover images: © Jocelyn Mott, © Jim Hoskinson

Set in 10/12.5pts Berkeley by SPi Global, Pondicherry, India
Printed in Singapore by Markono Print Media Pte. Ltd.

10 9 8 7 6 5 4 3 2 1

Contents

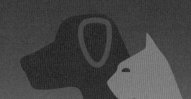

Contributors xiii
About the Companion Website xix

Section I	Clinical Signs of Gastrointestinal Disease

Chapter **1** — Acute Abdomen 3
Steven L. Marks

Chapter **2** — Constipation and Obstipation 10
Albert E. Jergens

Chapter **3** — Diarrhea, Acute 15
Erin Portillo

Chapter **4** — Diarrhea, Chronic – Canine 20
Jocelyn Mott

Chapter **5** — Diarrhea, Chronic – Feline 28
Sina Marsilio

Chapter **6** — Dyschezia and Tenesmus 45
Alana Redfern

Chapter **7** — Dysphagia 51
Alana Redfern

Chapter **8** — Flatulence 58
Gavin Olsen

Chapter **9** — Hematemesis 63
Jocelyn Mott

Chapter **10** — Hematochezia 70
Julie Stegeman

Chapter **11** — Melena 76
Julie Stegeman

Chapter **12** — Nutritional Approach to Acute Vomiting and Diarrhea 84
Caitlin Grant, Sarah Dodd and Adronie Verbrugghe

Chapter **13** — Ptyalism 88
Valerie J. Parker

Chapter **14** — Rectal and Anal Prolapse 95
Eric R. Pope

Chapter **15** — Regurgitation 103
Rhonda L. Schulman

Chapter **16**   Vomiting, Acute 110
Erin Portillo

Chapter **17**   Vomiting, Chronic 116
John M. Crandell

Section II   Diseases of the Oral Cavity

Chapter **18**   Craniomandibular Osteopathy 127
Nina R. Kieves, Amy N. Zide, Kathleen L. Ham and James Howard

Chapter **19**   Feline Eosinophilic Dermatitis 134
Alexander H. Werner Resnick and Karen Helton-Rhodes

Chapter **20**   Oral Neoplasia, Benign 141
Heidi B. Lobprise and Jason W. Soukup

Chapter **21**   Oral Neoplasia, Malignant 147
Heidi B. Lobprise and Jason W. Soukup

Chapter **22**   Phenobarbital-Responsive Sialadenosis 155
Vivian K. Yau

Chapter **23**   Sialadenitis 159
Jo Ann Morrison

Chapter **24**   Salivary Mucocele 164
Amy N. Zide, Nina R. Kieves, Kathleen L. Ham and James Howard

Chapter **25**   Stomatitis 172
Larry Baker

Chapter **26**   Stomatitis, Caudal – Feline 179
Jan Bellows

Section III   Diseases of the Esophagus

Chapter **27**   Cricopharyngeal Achalasia 189
Romy M. Heilmann and Stanley L. Marks

Chapter **28**   Gastroesophageal Diverticula 195
Albert E. Jergens

Chapter **29**   Esophageal Fistula 198
Louisa Ho-Eckart and Eric Zellner

Chapter **30**   Esophageal Foreign Bodies 205
Albert E. Jergens

Chapter **31**   Esophageal Neoplasia 209
Marlene L. Hauck

Chapter **32**   Esophageal Stricture 214
Michael D. Willard

Chapter **33**   Esophagitis 220
Steve Hill

Chapter **34**   Hiatal Hernia 231
Kathryn A. Pitt, Philipp D. Mayhew and Stanley L. Marks

Chapter **35**   Megaesophagus. 238
Emilie Chaplow

Chapter **36**   Nutritional Approach to Gastroesophageal Reflux Disease and
Megaesophagus. 247
Caitlin Grant, Sarah Dodd and Adronie Verbrugghe

Chapter **37**   *Spirocerca lupi* 251
Jocelyn Mott

Section **IV**   Diseases of the Stomach

Chapter **38**   Gastric and Intestinal Motility Disorders .259
Jo Ann Morrison

Chapter **39**   Gastric Dilation-Volvulus. 266
April Blong

Chapter **40**   Gastric Neoplasia, Benign. 273
Jennifer A. Mahoney

Chapter **41**   Gastric Neoplasia, Malignant 278
Jennifer A. Mahoney

Chapter **42**   Gastric Parasites. 285
Jeba Jesudoss Chelladurai and Matt T. Brewer

Chapter **43**   Gastritis, Acute. 289
Romy M. Heilmann

Chapter **44**   Gastritis, Atrophic 296
Jessica M. Clemans

Chapter **45**   Gastritis, Chronic 300
Michelle Pressel

Chapter **46**   Gastroduodenal Ulceration/Erosion. 306
Michael D. Willard

Chapter **47**   Gastroesophageal Reflux 313
Albert E. Jergens

Chapter **48**   *Helicobacter*-Associated Gastritis 317
Jan S. Suchodolski

Chapter **49**   Hypertrophic Pyloric Gastropathy, Chronic 324
Steven L. Marks

Section **V**   Diseases of the Intestines

Chapter **50**   Bilious Vomiting Syndrome. 331
Romy M. Heilmann and David C. Twedt

Chapter **51**   Canine Parvovirus Infection 337
Willem J. Botha and Johan P. Schoeman

Chapter **52**   Cobalamin Deficiency. 345
Jörg M. Steiner

Chapter **53**	Cryptosporidiosis	350
	Jeba Jesudoss Chelladurai and Matt T. Brewer	
Chapter **54**	Diarrhea, Antibiotic Responsive	354
	Karin Allenspach	
Chapter **55**	Enteritis, Bacterial.	360
	Krysta Deitz	
Chapter **56**	Enterocolitis, Granulomatous	370
	Sina Marsilio	
Chapter **57**	Feline Viral Enterides	378
	Jennifer E. Slovak	
Chapter **58**	Food Reactions (Gastrointestinal), Adverse	384
	Laura Van Vertloo and Albert E. Jergens	
Chapter **59**	Fungal Enteritides.	389
	Jean-Sébastien Palerme	
Chapter **60**	Gastroenteritis, Eosinophilic	396
	Michelle Pressel	
Chapter **61**	Gastroenteritis, Hemorrhagic	402
	Michael Curtis	
Chapter **62**	Gastroenteritis, Lymphocytic-Plasmacytic	409
	John M. Crandell	
Chapter **63**	Gastrointestinal Obstruction.	418
	Jean-Sébastien Palerme and Albert E. Jergens	
Chapter **64**	Gastrointestinal Lymphoma, Canine	425
	Steven E. Suter	
Chapter **65**	Gastrointestinal Lymphoma, Feline	431
	Jennifer A. Mahoney	
Chapter **66**	Giardiasis	438
	Jeba Jesudoss Chelladurai and Matt T. Brewer	
Chapter **67**	Gluten-Sensitive Enteropathy in Irish Setters	441
	Krysta Deitz	
Chapter **68**	Immunoproliferative Enteropathy of Basenjis	444
	Gavin Olsen	
Chapter **69**	Inflammatory Bowel Disease.	449
	Albert E. Jergens	
Chapter **70**	Intestinal Dysbiosis	454
	Jan S. Suchodolski and Jörg M. Steiner	
Chapter **71**	Intestinal Neoplasia, Benign	460
	Carrie A. Wood	
Chapter **72**	Intestinal Neoplasia, Malignant.	464
	Carrie A. Wood	

Chapter **73**   Intussusception 470
Louisa Ho-Eckart and Eric Zellner

Chapter **74**   Irritable Bowel Syndrome 478
Alana Redfern

Chapter **75**   Lymphangiectasia. 484
Michael D. Willard

Chapter **76**   Nutritional Approach to Chronic Enteropathies. 490
Sarah Dodd, Caitlin Grant and Adronie Verbrugghe

Chapter **77**   Parasites, Gastrointestinal. 506
Jeba Jesudoss Chelladurai and Matt T. Brewer

Chapter **78**   Protein-Losing Enteropathy. 513
Jörg M. Steiner

Chapter **79**   Salmon Poisoning Disease 521
Jennifer E. Slovak

Chapter **80**   Short Bowel Syndrome. 526
Krysta Deitz

Section **VI**   Diseases of the Colon

Chapter **81**   Atresia Ani. 533
Eric Zellner and Louisa Ho-Eckart

Chapter **82**   Clostridial Enterotoxicosis. 539
Jennifer E. Slovak

Chapter **83**   Colitis and Proctitis. 546
Jo Ann Morrison

Chapter **84**   Colitis, Histiocytic Ulcerative 554
Jo Ann Morrison

Chapter **85**   Colonic Neoplasia, Benign 559
Carrie A. Wood

Chapter **86**   Colonic Neoplasia, Malignant. 564
Marlene L. Hauck

Chapter **87**   Fiber-Responsive Large Bowel Diarrhea. 568
Michael S. Leib

Chapter **88**   Megacolon. 573
Laura Van Vertloo and Albert E. Jergens

Chapter **89**   Perianal Fistula 581
Eric R. Pope

Chapter **90**   Perineal Hernia. 588
Fiona M. Little

Chapter **91**   Rectal Stricture 593
Eric R. Pope

Chapter **92**   Rectoanal Polyps 601
Eric R. Pope

Chapter **93**   *Trichomoniasis* 608
Jeba Jesudoss Chelladurai and Matt T. Brewer

Section VII   Diseases of the Pancreas

Chapter **94**   Nutritional Approach to Exocrine Pancreas Disease 613
Caitlin Grant, Sarah Dodd and Adronie Verbrugghe

Chapter **95**   Exocrine Pancreatic Insufficiency 621
Jörg M. Steiner

Chapter **96**   Pancreatic Abscess 628
Panagiotis G. Xenoulis

Chapter **97**   Pancreatic Neoplasia 632
Nick Dervisis

Chapter **98**   Pancreatic Nodular Hyperplasia 637
Kate Holan

Chapter **99**   Pancreatic Parasites 640
Jessica C. Pritchard

Chapter **100**   Pancreatic Pseudocyst 645
Panagiotis G. Xenoulis

Chapter **101**   Pancreatitis, Canine 649
Jean-Sébastien Palerme and Albert E. Jergens

Chapter **102**   Pancreatitis, Feline 656
Albert E. Jergens

Section VIII   Clinical Signs of Hepatobiliary Disease

Chapter **103**   Icterus 665
Jean-Sébastien Palerme

Chapter **104**   Coagulopathy of Liver Disease 673
Peter J. Fernandes

Section IX   Diseases of the Liver

Chapter **105**   Arteriovenous Malformation of the Liver .681
Ashleigh Seigneur

Chapter **106**   Cholangitis/Cholangiohepatitis Syndrome .687
Jo Ann Morrison

Chapter **107**   Cholangitis, Destructive 697
Jonathan A. Lidbury

Chapter **108**   Cirrhosis and Fibrosis of the Liver 702
Jo Ann Morrison

Chapter **109**   Copper-Associated Hepatopathy 711
Jo Ann Morrison

Chapter **110**   Ductal Plate Malformation 721
Jo Ann Morrison

Chapter **111**   Glycogen Storage Disease 729
Jessica C. Pritchard and Sharon A. Center

Chapter **112**   Glycogen-Type Vacuolar Hepatopathy. 734
Ashleigh Seigneur

Chapter **113**   Hepatic Amyloid. 742
Kate Holan

Chapter **114**   Hepatic Encephalopathy. 748
Manolis K. Chatzis and Panagiotis G. Xenoulis

Chapter **115**   Hepatic Failure, Acute 755
Yuri A. Lawrence

Chapter **116**   Hepatic Lipidosis. 763
Panagiotis G. Xenoulis

Chapter **117**   Hepatic Neoplasia, Benign 771
Nick Dervisis

Chapter **118**   Hepatic Neoplasia, Malignant. 775
Nick Dervisis

Chapter **119**   Hepatic Nodular Hyperplasia and Dysplastic Hyperplasia 781
Sean P. McDonough and Sharon A. Center

Chapter **120**   Hepatitis, Chronic. 786
Sean P. McDonough and Sharon A. Center

Chapter **121**   Hepatitis, Granulomatous. 796
Jocelyn Mott

Chapter **122**   Hepatitis, Infectious (Viral) Canine 801
Kate Holan

Chapter **123**   Hepatitis, Lobular Dissecting. 807
Jonathan A. Lidbury

Chapter **124**   Hepatitis, Nonspecific, Reactive 813
Jonathan A. Lidbury

Chapter **125**   Hepatitis, Suppurative and Hepatic Abscess 817
Ashleigh Seigneur

Chapter **126**   Hepatopathy, Hyperthyroidism – Feline. 823
Jonathan A. Lidbury

Chapter **127**   Hepatopathy, Infectious 828
Yuri A. Lawrence and Randi Gold

Chapter **128**   Hepatoportal Microvascular Dysplasia. 836
Sean P. McDonough and Sharon A. Center

Chapter **129**   Hepatotoxins 843
Michael D. Willard

Chapter **130**   Hypertension, Portal. 850
Jo Ann Morrison

Chapter **131**   Leptospirosis 858
Mathios E. Mylonakis

Chapter **132**   Nutritional Approach to Hepatobiliary Diseases. 866
Sarah Dodd, Caitlin Grant and Adronie Verbrugghe

Chapter **133**   Portosystemic Shunting, Acquired 878
Julie Stegeman

Chapter **134**   Portosystemic Vascular Anomaly, Congenital .885
Kathleen L. Ham, James Howard, Amy N. Zide and Nina R. Kieves

Section **X**	**Diseases of the Biliary Tract**

Chapter **135**   Bile Duct Obstruction (Extrahepatic) 901
Jocelyn Mott

Chapter **136**   Biliary Duct or Gallbladder Rupture and Bile Peritonitis 910
Rebecca A.L. Walton

Chapter **137**   Biliary Neoplasia. 918
Christine Mullin and Craig A. Clifford

Chapter **138**   Cholecystitis and Choledochitis 925
Yuri A. Lawrence

Chapter **139**   Cholecystitis, Emphysematous 932
Vivian K. Yau

Chapter **140**   Cholelithiasis 937
Jocelyn Mott

Chapter **141**   Gallbladder Mucocele. 943
James Howard, Kathleen L. Ham, Amy N. Zide and Nina R. Kieves

Index 953

Contributors

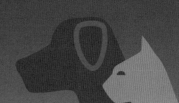

Karin Allenspach, Dr.med.vet., DECVIM, PhD
Department of Veterinary Clinical Sciences
College of Veterinary Medicine
Iowa State University
Ames, Iowa, USA

Larry Baker, DVM, FAVD, DAVDC
Northgate Pet Clinic
Decatur, Illinois, USA

Jan Bellows, DVM, DAVDC, ABVP
All Pet Dental
Weston, Florida, USA

April Blong, DVM, DACVECC
Lloyd Veterinary Medical Center
College of Veterinary Medicine
Iowa State University
Ames, Iowa, USA

Willem J. Botha, BSc, BVSc (Hons)
Department of Companion Animal Clinical
   Studies, Faculty of Veterinary Science
University of Pretoria
Onderstepoort, South Africa

Matt T. Brewer, DVM, PhD, DACVM
College of Veterinary Medicine
Iowa State University
Ames, Iowa, USA

Sharon A. Center, DVM, DACVIM
Department of Clinical Sciences
Cornell University College of Veterinary
   Medicine
Ithaca, New York, USA

Emilie Chaplow, VMD, DACVIM
VCA Animal Specialty Group
Los Angeles, California, USA

Manolis K. Chatzis, DVM, PhD
Clinic of Medicine
Faculty of Veterinary Medicine
University of Thessaly
Karditsa, Greece

Jeba Jesudoss Chelladurai, BVSc & AH,
   MS, DACVM
College of Veterinary Medicine
Iowa State University
Ames, Iowa, USA

Jessica M. Clemans, DVM, DACVIM
VCA MidWest Veterinary Referral &
   Emergency Center
Council Bluffs, Iowa, USA

Craig A. Clifford, DVM, MS, DACVIM
   (Oncology)
Hope Veterinary Specialists
Malvern, Pennsyslvania, USA

John M. Crandell, DVM, DACVIM
MedVet Akron
Akron, Ohio, USA

Michael Curtis, DVM, PhD, DACVA
Lloyd Veterinary Medical Center
College of Veterinary Medicine
Iowa State University
Ames, Iowa, USA

Krysta Deitz, DVM, MS, DACVIM
Southeast Veterinary Oncology and
  Internal Medicine
Jacksonville, Florida, USA

**Nick Dervisis, DVM, PhD, DACVIM
  (Oncology)**
Department of Small Animal Clinical
  Sciences
Virginia-Maryland Regional College of
  Veterinary Medicine
Blacksburg, Virginia, USA

Sarah Dodd, DVM, BSc
Ontario Veterinary College
University of Guelph
Guelph, Ontario, Canada

Peter J. Fernandes, DVM, DACVP
IDEXX Laboratories
Irvine, California, USA

Randi Gold, VMD, PhD
Department of Veterinary Pathobiology
Texas A&M College of Veterinary Medicine
College Station, Texas, USA

Caitlin Grant, DVM, BSc
Ontario Veterinary College
University of Guelph
Guelph, Ontario, Canada

Kathleen L. Ham, DVM, MS, DACVS-SA
Michigan State University
East Lansing, Michigan, USA

**Marlene L. Hauck, DVM, PhD, DACVIM
  (Oncology)**
Bear Creek Veterinary Services
Victor, Montana, USA

**Romy M. Heilmann, med.vet., Dr.med.vet.,
  DACVIM (SAIM), DECVIM-CA, PhD**
Small Animal Veterinary Teaching Hospital
College of Veterinary Medicine
University of Leipzig
Leipzig, Germany

Karen Helton-Rhodes, DVM, DACVD
Ceffyl Consulting
Edisto Island, South Carolina, USA

**Steve Hill, DVM, MS, DACVIM
  (SAIM)**
Veterinary Specialty Hospital by Ethos
  Veterinary Health
San Diego, California, USA

**Louisa Ho-Eckart, BVSc Hons, MS,
  DACVS-SA**
Lloyd Veterinary Medical Center
College of Veterinary Medicine
Iowa State University
Ames, Iowa, USA

Kate Holan, DVM, DACVIM
Department of Small Animal Clinical
  Sciences
Veterinary Medical Center
Michigan State University
East Lansing, Michigan, USA

James Howard, DVM, MS
The Ohio State University
Columbus, Ohio, USA

Albert E. Jergens, DVM, PhD, DACVIM
Department of Veterinary Clinical
  Sciences
College of Veterinary Medicine
Iowa State University
Ames, Iowa, USA

**Nina R. Kieves, DVM, DACVS-SA,
  DACVSMR**
The Ohio State University
Columbus, Ohio, USA

**Yuri A. Lawrence, DVM, MS, MA, PhD,
  DACVIM (SAIM)**
Department of Small Animal Clinical
  Sciences
College of Veterinary Medicine
Texas A&M University
College Station, Texas, USA

Michael S. Leib, DVM, MS, DACVIM
Virginia Maryland College of Veterinary
    Medicine
Virginia Tech
Blacksburg, Virginia, USA

Jonathan A. Lidbury, BVMS, MRCVS, PhD,
    DACVIM, DECVIM-CA
Department of Small Animal Clinical
    Sciences
College of Veterinary Medicine
Texas A&M University
College Station, Texas, USA

Fiona M. Little, VMD, DACVS
Pasadena Veterinary Specialists
South Pasadena, California, USA

Heidi B. Lobprise, DVM, DAVDC
Main Street Veterinary Hospital
Haslet, Texas, USA

Jennifer A. Mahoney, DVM, DACVIM
    (Oncology)
Ryan Veterinary Hospital
University of Pennsylvania School of
    Veterinary Medicine
Philadelphia, Pennsylvania, USA

Stanley L. Marks, BVSc, DACVIM (SAIM,
    Oncology), DACVN, PhD
University of California Davis School of
    Veterinary Medicine
Davis, California, USA

Steven L. Marks, BVSc, MS, MRCVS,
    DACVIM (SAIM)
North Carolina State University
College of Veterinary Medicine
Raleigh, North Carolina, USA

Sina Marsilio, Dr.med.vet., DVM, DACVIM
    (SAIM), DECVIM-CA
Department of Small Animal Clinical
    Science
Texas A&M University
College Station, Texas, USA

Philipp D. Mayhew, BVM&S, DACVS
University of California Davis School of
    Veterinary Medicine
Davis, California, USA

Sean P. McDonough, DVM, PhD, DACVP
College of Veterinary Medicine
Cornell University
Ithaca, New York, USA

Jo Ann Morrison, DVM, MS, DACVIM
Banfield Pet Hospital
Vancouver, Washington, USA

Jocelyn Mott, DVM, DACVIM (SAIM)
Pasadena Veterinary Specialists
South Pasadena, California, USA

Christine Mullin, VMD, DACVIM
    (Oncology)
Hope Veterinary Specialists
Malvern, Pennsylvania, USA

Mathios E. Mylonakis, DVM, PhD
Companion Animal Clinic
School of Veterinary Medicine
Aristotle University of Thessaloniki
Thessaloniki, Greece

Gavin Olsen, DVM, DACVIM (SAIM)
Carolina Veterinary Specialists
Greensboro, North Carolina, USA

Jean-Sébastien Palerme, DVM, MSc, DACVIM
College of Veterinary Medicine
Iowa State University
Ames, Iowa, USA

Valerie J. Parker, DVM, DACVIM, DACVN
College of Veterinary Medicine
The Ohio State University
Columbus, Ohio, USA

Kathryn A. Pitt, DVM, MS
College of Veterinary Medicine
Michigan State University
East Lansing, Michigan, USA

Eric R. Pope, DVM, MS, DACVS
School of Veterinary Medicine
Ross University
St Kitts, West Indies

Erin Portillo, MS, DVM, DACVIM
Valley Oak Veterinary Center
Chico, California, USA

Michelle Pressel, DVM, MS, DACVIM
Pacific Veterinary Specialists + Emergency
    Service
Santa Cruz, California, USA

Jessica C. Pritchard, VMD, MS, DACVIM
    (SAIM)
University of Wisconsin-Madison School of
    Veterinary Medicine
Madison, Wisconsin, USA

Alana Redfern, DVM, MSc, DACVIM
Blue Pearl Specialty + Emergency Pet
    Hospital
Long Island City, New York, USA

Johan P. Schoeman, BVSc, MMedVet (Med),
    PhD, DECVIM
Department of Companion Animal Clinical
    Studies, Faculty of Veterinary Science
University of Pretoria
Onderstepoort, South Africa

Rhonda L. Schulman, DVM, DACVIM
    (SAIM)
Animal Specialty Group
Los Angeles, California, USA

Ashleigh Seigneur, DVM, MVSc, DACVIM
South Carolina Veterinary Specialists and
    Emergency Care
Columbia, South Carolina, USA

Jennifer E. Slovak, DVM, MS, DACVIM
Veterinary Clinical Services
College of Veterinary Medicine
Washington State University
Pullman, Washington, USA

Jason W. Soukup, DVM, DAVDC
School of Veterinary Medicine
University of Wisconsin-Madison
Madison, Wisconsin, USA

Julie Stegeman, DVM, DACVIM (SAIM)
Southern California Veterinary Specialty
    Hospital
Irvine, California, USA

Jörg M. Steiner, med.vet., Dr.med.vet.,
    PhD, DACVIM, DECVIM-CA, AGAF
Department of Small Animal Clinical
    Sciences
College of Veterinary Medicine and
    Biomedical Sciences
Texas A&M University
College Station, Texas, USA

Jan S. Suchodolski, Dr.med.vet., PhD,
    DACVM
Department of Small Animal Clinical
    Sciences
College of Veterinary Medicine and
    Biomedical Sciences
Texas A&M University
College Station, Texas, USA

Steven E. Suter, VMD, MS, PhD, DACVIM
    (Oncology)
North Carolina State University
College of Veterinary Medicine
Raleigh, North Carolina, USA

David C. Twedt, DVM, DACVIM (SAIM)
Colorado State University
Veterinary Teaching Hospital
Fort Collins, Colorado, USA

Laura Van Vertloo, DVM, MS, DACVIM
Department of Veterinary Clinical Sciences
College of Veterinary Medicine
Iowa State University
Ames, Iowa, USA

Adronie Verbrugghe, DVM, PhD, Dip ECVCN
Ontario Veterinary College
University of Guelph
Guelph, Ontario, Canada

Rebecca A.L. Walton, DVM, DACVECC
Lloyd Veterinary Medical Center
College of Veterinary Medicine
Iowa State University
Ames, Iowa, USA

Alexander H. Werner Resnick, VMD,
  DACVD
Animal Dermatology Center
Studio City, California, USA

Michael D. Willard, DVM, MS, DACVIM
College of Veterinary Medicine and
  Biomedical Sciences
Texas A&M University
College Station, Texas, USA

Carrie A. Wood, DVM, DACVIM (Oncology)
Tufts University
Cummings School of Veterinary Medicine
North Grafton, Massachusetts, USA

Panagiotis G. Xenoulis, DVM, Dr.med.vet.,
  PhD
Clinic of Medicine
Faculty of Veterinary Medicine
University of Thessaly
Karditsa, Greece

Vivian K. Yau, DVM, DACVIM (SAIM)
Veterinary Specialty Group of Glendora
Glendora, California, USA

Eric Zellner, DVM, DACVS-SA
Lloyd Veterinary Medical Center
College of Veterinary Medicine
Iowa State University
Ames, Iowa, USA

Amy N. Zide, DVM
The Ohio State University
Columbus, Ohio, USA

About the Companion Website

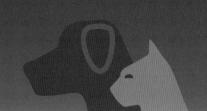

This book is accompanied by a companion website:

www.fiveminutevet.com/gastrointestinal

The website includes:
- Client education handouts.

Clinical Signs of Gastrointestinal Disease

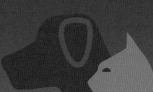

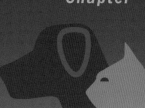

Acute Abdomen

DEFINITION/OVERVIEW

Acute abdomen is an emergency condition characterized by historical and physical examination findings of a tense, painful abdomen. May be due to a life-threatening condition.

ETIOLOGY/PATHOPHYSIOLOGY

- A patient with abdominal pain has pain associated with distension of an organ, inflammation, traction on the mesentery or peritoneum, or ischemia.
- The abdominal viscera are sparsely innervated, and diffuse involvement is often necessary to elicit pain; nerve endings also exist in the submucosa-muscularis layers of the intestinal wall.
- Any process that causes fluid or gaseous distension (i.e., intestinal obstruction, gastric dilation-volvulus, ileus) may produce pain.
- Inflammation produces abdominal pain by releasing vasoactive substances that directly stimulate nerve endings.
- Many nerves in the peritoneum are sensitive to a diffuse inflammatory response.

Systems Affected

Systems affected may depend on severity of pain and underlying disorder.
- Behavioral – trembling, inappetence, vocalizing, lethargy, depression, and abnormal postural changes such as the praying position to achieve comfort.
- Cardiovascular – severe inflammation, ischemia, systemic inflammatory response syndrome (SIRS), and sepsis may lead to acute circulatory collapse (shock). In addition, tachycardia or other arrhythmias may affect capillary refill time and mucous membrane color. Pain may lead to arrhythmias on its own.
- Gastrointestinal – vomiting, diarrhea, inappetence, generalized functional ileus; pancreatic inflammation, necrosis, and abscesses may lead to cranial abdominal pain, vomiting, and ileus.
- Hepatobiliary – jaundice associated with extrahepatic cholestasis from biliary obstruction (including pancreatitis) and bile peritonitis.
- Renal/urologic – azotemia can be due to prerenal causes (dehydration, hypovolemia, and shock), renal causes (acute pyelonephritis and acute kidney injury), and postrenal causes (urethral obstruction and uroperitoneum from bladder rupture).
- Respiratory – increased respiratory rate due to pain or metabolic disturbances.

Blackwell's Five-Minute Veterinary Consult Clinical Companion: Small Animal Gastrointestinal Diseases, First Edition. Edited by Jocelyn Mott and Jo Ann Morrison.
© 2019 John Wiley & Sons, Inc. Published 2019 by John Wiley & Sons, Inc.
Companion website: www.fiveminutevet.com/gastrointestinal

SIGNALMENT/HISTORY

- Dog and cat.
  - Dogs more commonly but can be challenging to identify abdominal pain in feline patients.
- Younger animals tend to have a higher incidence of trauma-related problems, intussusceptions, and acquired diet- and infection-related diseases; older animals have a greater frequency of malignancies.
- Male cats and dogs are at higher risk for urethral obstruction.
- Male Dalmatians in particular have a higher risk of urethral obstruction because of the high incidence of urate urinary calculi.
- German shepherds with pancreatic atrophy have a higher risk of mesenteric volvulus.
- Patients treated with corticosteroids and nonsteroidal antiinflammatory drugs (NSAIDs) are at higher risk for gastrointestinal (GI) ulceration and perforation.

Risk Factors

- Exposure to NSAIDs or corticosteroid treatment – gastric, duodenal, or colonic ulcers.
- Garbage or inappropriate food ingestion – pancreatitis or intestinal obstruction.
- Foreign body ingestion – intestinal obstructions.
- Abdominal trauma – hollow viscus rupture.
- Hernia-intestinal obstruction/strangulation.

Historical Findings

- Trembling, reluctance to move, inappetence, vomiting, diarrhea, vocalizing, and abnormal postures (tucked up or praying position) – signs that the owner may notice.
- Question owner carefully to ascertain what system is affected; for example, hematemesis with a history of NSAID treatment suggests GI mucosal disruption.

CLINICAL FEATURES

- Abnormalities include abdominal pain, splinting of the abdominal musculature, gas- or fluid-filled abdominal organs, abdominal mass, ascites, pyrexia or hypothermia, tachycardia, and tachypnea.
- Once abdominal pain is confirmed, attempt to localize the pain to cranial, middle, or caudal abdomen.
- Perform a rectal examination to evaluate the colon, pelvic bones, urethra, and prostate, as well as the presence of melena, fresh blood or mucus.
- Rule out extraabdominal causes of pain by careful palpation of the kidneys, sublumbar muscles, and thoracolumbar and lumbar vertebrae.
- Pain associated with intervertebral disk disease often causes referred abdominal guarding and is often mistaken for true abdominal pain. Renal pain can be associated with pyelonephritis.

DIFFERENTIAL DIAGNOSIS

- Renal-associated pain, retroperitoneal pain, spinal or paraspinal pain, and disorders causing diffuse muscle pain may mimic abdominal pain; careful history and physical examination are essential in pursuing the appropriate problem.
- Parvoviral enteritis can present similarly to intestinal obstructive disease; fecal parvoviral antigen assay and complete blood cell count (leukopenia) are helpful differentiating diagnostic tests.

Gastrointestinal

- Stomach – gastritis, ulcers, perforation, foreign bodies, gastric dilation-volvulus.
- Intestine – obstruction (foreign bodies, intussusception, hernias), enteritis, ulcers, perforations.
- Rupture after obstruction, ulceration, or blunt or penetrating trauma, or due to tumor growth.
- Vascular compromise from infarction, mesenteric volvulus, or torsion.

Pancreas

- Pain associated with inflammation, abscess, ischemia.
- Pancreatic masses or inflammation obstructing the biliary duct/papilla will cause jaundice.

Hepatic and Biliary System

- Rapid distension of the liver and its capsule can cause pain.
- Gallbladder obstruction, rupture, or necrosis may lead to bile leakage and peritonitis.
- Hepatic abscess.

Spleen

- Splenic torsion, splenic masses, splenic thrombus, splenic abscess.

Urinary Tract

- Distension is the main cause of pain in the urinary tract.
- Lower urinary tract obstruction can be due to tumors of the trigone area of the bladder or urethra, urinary calculi, or granulomatous urethritis.
- Traumatic rupture of the ureters or bladder is associated with blunt trauma and increased intraabdominal pressure.
- Urethral tears can be associated with pelvic fractures from acute trauma.
- Free urine in the peritoneal cavity leads to a chemical peritonitis.
- Acute pyelonephritis, acute renal failure, nephroliths, and ureteroliths are uncommon causes of acute abdomen.

Genital Tract

- Prostatitis and prostatic abscess, pyometra; ruptured pyometra or prostatic abscess can cause endotoxemia, sepsis, and cardiovascular collapse.
- Infrequent causes include rupture of the gravid uterus after blunt abdominal trauma, uterine torsion, ovarian tumor or torsion, and intraabdominal testicular torsion (cryptorchid).

Abdominal Wall/Diaphragm

- Umbilical, inguinal, scrotal, abdominal, or peritoneal hernias with strangulated viscera.
- Trauma or congenital defects leading to organ displacement or entrapment in the hernia will lead to abdominal pain if the vascular supply of the organs involved becomes impaired or ischemic.
- Hernias – intestinal obstruction/strangulation.

 DIAGNOSTICS

Complete Blood Cell Count/Biochemistry/Urinalysis

- Inflammation or infection may be associated with leukocytosis or leukopenia.
- Active inflammation will be characterized by a neutrophilic left shift.
- Anemia may be seen with blood loss associated with GI ulceration.

- Azotemia is associated with prerenal, renal, and postrenal causes.
- Electrolyte abnormalities can help to evaluate GI disease (i.e., hypochloremic metabolic alkalosis with gastric outflow obstruction) and renal disease (i.e., hyperkalemia with acute renal failure or postrenal obstruction).
- Hyperbilirubinemia and elevated hepatic enzymes help localize a problem to the liver or biliary tract. These changes may also be seen when associated with sepsis.
- Urine specific gravity (before fluid therapy) is needed to differentiate prerenal, renal, and postrenal problems.
- Urine sediment may be helpful in acute renal failure, ethylene glycol intoxication, and pyelonephritis.

Other Laboratory Tests

- Venous blood gas analysis including lactate concentration may indicate acid–base abnormalities, and increased lactate may be associated with hypoperfusion.
- Canine and feline pancreatic lipase immunoreactivity can be useful in evaluating pancreatitis.

Imaging

Abdominal Radiography

- May see abdominal masses or changes in shape or shifting of abdominal organs.
- Loss of abdominal detail with abdominal fluid accumulation is an indication for abdominocentesis.
- Free abdominal gas is consistent with a ruptured GI viscus or infection with gas-producing bacteria and is an indication for emergency surgery. Use caution when interpreting radiographs following abdominocentesis with an open needle. Free gas may be introduced with this technique.
- Use caution when evaluating postoperative radiographs; free gas is a normal postoperative finding.
- Ileus is a consistent finding with peritonitis.
- Characterize ileus as functional (due to metabolic or infectious causes) or mechanical (due to obstruction).
- Foreign bodies may be radiopaque.
- Upper GI barium contrast radiographs are useful in evaluating the GI tract, particularly for determination of GI obstruction.
- Loss of contrast and detail in the area of the pancreas can be observed with pancreatic inflammation.

Abdominal Ultrasound

- A sensitive diagnostic tool for the detection of abdominal masses, abdominal fluid, abscesses, cysts, lymphadenopathy, and biliary or urinary calculi.
- FAST (focused assessment with sonography in trauma) may be used for rapid assessment.

Abdominal Computed Tomography (CT)

- Very sensitive diagnostic tool that may be utilized especially when surgeon requires additional information preoperatively.

Diagnostic Procedures

Abdominocentesis/Abdominal Fluid Analysis

- Perform abdominocentesis on all patients presenting with acute abdomen. Using a four-quadrant approach my improve yield. Fluid can often be obtained for diagnostic evaluation even when only a small amount of free abdominal fluid exists, well before detectable radiographic sensitivity. Ultrasound is much more sensitive than radiography for the detection of fluid and can be used to direct abdominocentesis. Abdominal fluid analysis with elevated white blood cell count, degenerate neutrophils, and intracellular bacteria is consistent with septic peritonitis and is an indication for immediate surgery.

- Diagnostic peritoneal lavage can be performed by introducing sterile saline (10–20 mL/kg, warmed to approach body temperature) and performing abdominocentesis.
- Measurement of glucose concentration in abdominal effusion may aid in the diagnosis of septic abdomen.
- Pancreatitis patients may have an abdominal effusion characterized as a nonseptic (sterile) peritonitis.
- Creatinine concentration higher in abdominal fluid than in serum indicates urinary tract leakage.
- Similarly, higher bilirubin concentration in abdominal fluid than in serum indicates bile peritonitis.

Sedation and Abdominal Palpation
- Because of abdominal splinting associated with pain, a thorough abdominal palpation is often not possible without sedation; this is particularly useful for detecting intestinal foreign bodies that do not appear on survey radiographs.

Exploratory Laparotomy
- Surgery may be useful diagnostically (as well as therapeutically) when ultrasonography is not available or when no definitive cause of the acute abdomen has been established with appropriate diagnostics.

 THERAPEUTICS

- Inpatient management with supportive care until decision about whether the problem is to be treated medically or surgically. Early intervention with surgery is important when indicated.
- Aggressive therapy and prompt identification of the underlying cause are very important.
- Many causes of acute abdominal pain require emergency surgical intervention.

Drugs of Choice
- Pain medication may be indicated for control of abdominal discomfort and provide some sedation.

Opioids
- Fentanyl: 2–5 µg/kg as initial IV bolus, 2–10 µg/kg/h as constant rate infusion (CRI).
- Hydromorphone: 0.05–0.2 mg/kg SQ, IM, IV q 4–6 h.
- Morphine: 0.5–2 mg/kg SQ, IM, q 4–6 h.
- Buprenorphine: 0.01–0.02 mg/kg SQ, IM, IV q 4–6 h.
- Methadone: 0.1–0.4 mg/kg SQ, IM, IV q 6 h.

Histamine H2 Antagonists
- Reduce gastric acid production.
- Famotidine: 0.1–0.2 mg/kg IV, SQ or IM q 12 h.
- Ranitidine: 2 mg/kg IV q 8 h.

Proton Pump Inhibitor (PPI)
- Pantoprazole: 0.5–1 mg/kg IV as a CRI over 12–24 h.

Protectants
- Sucralfate: 0.25–1 g PO q 8 h.

Antiemetics
- Metoclopramide: 0.2–0.4 mg/kg IV q 6–8 h (or 24-hour CRI).
- Maropitant: 1 mg/kg SQ q 24 h dogs, 0.5 mg/kg SQ q 2 4 h cats.
- Ondansetron: 0.5–1 mg/kg IV slowly q 6–12 h.
- Dolasetron: 1 mg/kg IV qd.

Antibiotics
- Antibiotics may be indicated if signs of infection (fever, elevated white blood cell count, positive culture) are seen.
- Broad spectrum for gram positive, gram negative, and anaerobic bacteria.
- Gram stain and cultures prior to treatment if possible.

Precautions/Interactions
- Gentamicin and most NSAIDs can be nephrotoxic and should be used with caution in hypovolemic patients and those with renal impairment.
- Do not use metoclopramide if GI obstruction is suspected.

Appropriate Health Care
- Keep patient NPO if vomiting, until a definitive cause is determined and addressed.
- Intravenous fluid therapy is usually required because of the large fluid loss associated with an acute abdomen; the goal is to restore the normal circulating blood volume.
- If severe circulatory compromise (shock) exists, supplement initially with isotonic crystalloid fluids (90 mL/kg dogs; 45–60 mL/kg cats) over 1–2 h; hypertonic fluids or colloids may also be beneficial.
- Evaluate hydration and electrolytes (with appropriate treatment adjustments) frequently after commencement of treatment.

Nursing Care
- Patients usually require intensive medical care and frequent evaluation of vital signs and laboratory parameters.

Diet
- Most patients will be NPO during assessment until a diagnosis can be made. Dietary decisions should be made with consideration of the underlying disease and required therapy. Diets designed for tube feeding may also be required.

Activity
- Activity levels will be dictated by underlying disease and required procedures.

Surgical Considerations
- Many different causes of an acute abdomen (with both medical and surgical treatments) exist; make a definitive diagnosis whenever possible prior to surgical intervention.
- This can prevent both potentially unnecessary and expensive surgical procedures and associated morbidity and mortality.
- It will also allow the surgeon to prepare for the task and to educate the owner on the prognosis and costs involved.

COMMENTS

Client Education

- Discussions with client should be based on presenting problem and differential diagnoses as well as diagnostic and therapeutic plan.
- Financial investment and prognosis are based on underlying disease, signalment, and required therapeutic interventions.

Patient Monitoring

- Dependent on underlying disease.
- Dependent on required therapeutic interventions.
- Dependent on in patient or out patient monitoring.

Expected Course and Prognosis

Prognosis is based on underlying disease, signalment and required therapeutic interventions.

Synonyms

Colic, but not commonly used in small animal patients.

Abbreviations

- CRI = constant rate infusion
- FAST = focused assessment with sonography in trauma
- GDV = gastric dilation-volvulus
- GI = gastrointestinal
- NSAID = nonsteroidal antiinflammatory drugs
- PPI = proton pump inhibitor
- SIRS = systemic inflammatory response syndrome

See Also

- Biliary Duct or Gallbladder Rupture and Bile Peritonitis
- Gastric Dilation and Volvulus Syndrome
- Gastroduodenal Ulceration/Erosion
- Gastrointestinal Obstruction
- Intussusception
- Pancreatitis, Canine
- Pancreatitis, Feline

Internet Resources

Google Search:
- Acute abdomen in dogs and cats.
- Abdominal pain in dogs and cats.

Suggested Reading

Beal MW. Approach to the acute abdomen. Vet Clin North Am Small Anim Pract 2005;35:375–396.
Heeren V, Edwards L, Mazzaferro EM. Acute abdomen: diagnosis. Compend Contin Educ Pract Vet 2004;26:350–363.
Heeren V, Edwards L, Mazzaferro EM. Acute abdomen: treatment: Compend Contin Educ Pract Vet 2004;26:3566–3673.
Mazzaferro EM. Triage and approach to the acute abdomen: Clin Tech Small Anim Pract 2003;18:1–6.
Strombeck DR, Guilford WG. Small Animal Gastroenterology, 2nd ed. Davis: Stonegate Publishing, 1990:81–86.

Acknowledgments: The author and editors acknowledge the prior contributions of Dr Juan Carlos Sardinas, Dr Albert E. Jergens, and Elizabeth M. Streeter.

Author: Steven L. Marks BVSc, MS, MRCVS, DACVIM (SAIM)

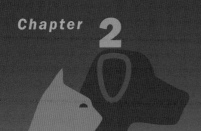

Chapter 2

Constipation and Obstipation

DEFINITION/OVERVIEW

- Constipation is defined as infrequent, incomplete, or difficult defecation with passage of hard or dry feces. This does not imply abnormal motility or loss of function.
- Obstipation denotes intractable constipation caused by prolonged retention of hard, dry feces; defecation is impossible in the obstipated patient.

ETIOLOGY/PATHOPHYSIOLOGY

- Constipation can develop with any disease that impairs the passage of feces through the colon. Potential causes include congenital vertebral malformation, spinal cord disease, pelvic canal narrowing (trauma), rectal mass lesions causing obstruction, and perianal disease causing painful defecation. Often in cats, no underlying etiology can be identified.
- Delayed fecal transit allows removal of additional salt and water, producing drier feces. Clinical signs are attributable to dehydration and potential toxemia resulting from fecal retention.
- Peristaltic contractions may increase during constipation, but eventually motility diminishes because of smooth muscle degeneration secondary to chronic overdistension.
- Prolonged colonic distension can result in permanent damage to colonic smooth muscle and innervation.

Systems Affected

- Gastrointestinal.

SIGNALMENT/HISTORY

- Dog and cat.
- More common in cat.

Risk Factors

- Manx cats may be predisposed due to vertebral (sacral) abnormalities.
- Drug therapy – anticholinergics, narcotics, barium sulfate.
- Metabolic disease causing dehydration.
- Intact male – perineal hernia, benign or infectious prostatic disease.
- Castrated male – prostatic neoplasia.
- Perianal fistula.

Blackwell's Five-Minute Veterinary Consult Clinical Companion: Small Animal Gastrointestinal Diseases, First Edition. Edited by Jocelyn Mott and Jo Ann Morrison.
© 2019 John Wiley & Sons, Inc. Published 2019 by John Wiley & Sons, Inc.
Companion website: www.fiveminutevet.com/gastrointestinal

- Pica – foreign material.
- Excessive grooming – hair ingestion.
- Decreased grooming/inability to groom – long-haired cats, pseudocoprostasis.
- Pelvic fracture.

Historical Findings

- Reduced, absent, or painful defecation.
- Hard, dry feces.
- Small amount of liquid, mucoid stool, sometimes with blood present produced after prolonged tenesmus.
- Occasional vomiting, inappetence, and/or lethargy.

 CLINICAL FEATURES

- Colon filled with hard feces. Severe impaction may cause abdominal distension +/– pain.
- Other findings depend on the underlying cause.
- Rectal examination may reveal mass, stricture, perineal hernia, anal sac disease, foreign body or material (hair), prostatic enlargement, and/or narrowed pelvic canal.

 DIFFERENTIAL DIAGNOSIS

- Dyschezia and tenesmus (e.g., caused by colitis or proctitis) – unlike constipation, associated with increased frequency of attempts to defecate and frequent production of small amounts of liquid feces containing blood and/or mucus; rectal examination reveals diarrhea and lack of hard stool.
- Stranguria (e.g., caused by cystitis/urethritis) – unlike constipation, can be associated with hematuria and abnormal findings on urinalysis (pyuria, crystalluria, bacteriuria).

Dietary

- Bones.
- Hair.
- Foreign material.
- Excessive fiber.
- Inadequate water intake.

Environmental

- Lack of exercise.
- Change of environment – hospitalization, dirty litter box.
- Inability to ambulate.

Drugs

- Anticholinergics.
- Antihistamines.
- Opioids.
- Barium sulfate.
- Sucralfate.
- Antacids.
- Kaopectolin.
- Iron supplements.
- Diuretics.

Painful Defecation (Dyschezia)

- Anorectal disease – anal sacculitis, anal sac abscess, perianal fistula, anal stricture, anal spasm, rectal foreign body, rectal prolapse, proctitis.
- Trauma – fractured pelvis, fractured limb, dislocated hip, perianal bite wound or laceration, perineal abscess.

Mechanical Obstruction

- Extraluminal – healed pelvic fracture with narrowed pelvic canal, prostatic hypertrophy, prostatitis, prostatic neoplasia, intrapelvic neoplasia, sublumbar lymphadenopathy.
- Intraluminal and intramural – colonic or rectal neoplasia or polyp, rectal stricture, rectal foreign body, rectal diverticulum, perineal hernia, rectal prolapse, and congenital defect (atresia ani).

Neuromuscular Disease

- Central nervous system – paraplegia, spinal cord disease, intervertebral disk disease, cerebral disease (lead toxicity, rabies).
- Peripheral nervous system – dysautonomia, sacral nerve disease, sacral nerve trauma (e.g., tail fracture/pull injury).
- Colonic smooth muscle dysfunction – idiopathic megacolon in cats.

Metabolic and Endocrine Disease

- Impaired colonic smooth muscle function – hyperparathyroidism, hypothyroidism, hypokalemia (chronic renal failure), hypercalcemia.
- Debility – general muscle weakness, dehydration, neoplasia.

 # DIAGNOSTICS

Complete Blood Count/Biochemistry/Urinalysis

- Usually unremarkable.
- May detect hypokalemia, hypercalcemia.
- High packed cell volume and total protein found in dehydrated patients.
- High white blood cell count in patients with severe obstipation secondary to bacterial or endotoxin translocation, abscess, perianal fistula, prostatic disease.
- Pyuria and hematuria with prostatitis.

Other Laboratory Tests

- If patient (dog) is hypercholesterolemic, consider a thyroid panel to rule out hypothyroidism.
- If patient is hypercalcemic, consider parathyroid hormone assay.

Imaging

- Abdominal radiography documents severity of colonic impaction. Other findings may include colonic or rectal foreign body, colonic or rectal mass, prostatic enlargement, fractured pelvis, dislocated hip, or perineal hernias.
- Pneumocolon radiography (after enemas to clean colon) may better define an intraluminal mass or stricture.
- Ultrasonography may help define extraluminal mass and prostatic disease.

Other Diagnostic Procedures

- Colonoscopy may be needed to identify a mass, stricture, or other colonic or rectal lesion; rectal/colonic mucosal biopsy specimens should always be obtained.

 ## THERAPEUTICS

Drug(s) of Choice

- Emollient laxatives – docusate sodium or docusate calcium (dogs 50–100 mg PO q 12–24 h; cats 50 mg PO q 12–24 h).
- Stimulant laxatives – bisacodyl (5 mg/animal PO q 8–24 h). Ensure that animal is not obstructed prior to use of stimulant laxatives.
- Saline laxatives – isosmotic mixture of polyethylene glycol and poorly absorbed salts; usually administered as a trickle amount via nasoesophageal tube over 6–12 h. Polyethylene glycol 3350 is a palatable oral laxative powder that can be mixed into food. Dose should be titrated to effect.
- Disaccharide laxative – lactulose (1 mL/4.5 kg PO q 8–12 h to effect).
- Warm water enemas may be needed; a small amount of mild soap or docusate sodium can be added but is usually not needed; sodium phosphate retention enemas (e.g., Fleet; C.B. Fleet Co.) are contraindicated because of their association with severe hypocalcemia.
- Suppositories can be used as a replacement for enemas; use glycerol, bisocodyl, or docusate sodium products.
- Motility modifiers can be administered – cisapride (dogs 0.1–0.5 mg/kg PO q 8–12 h; cats 2.5–7.5 mg/cat PO q 8–12 h) may stimulate colonic motility. For both species, best if given 30 minutes prior to feeding.

Precautions/Interactions

- Lubricants such as mineral oil and white petrolatum are NOT recommended because of the danger of fatal lipid aspiration pneumonia due to their lack of taste.
- Fleet enemas.
- Anticholinergics.
- Diuretics.
- Cisapride and cholinergics can be used with caution; contraindicated in obstructive processes.
- Avoid the use of metoclopramide because it does not affect the colon.

Appropriate Health Care

- Remove or ameliorate any underlying cause if possible.
- Discontinue any medications that may cause constipation.
- May need to treat as inpatient if obstipation and/or dehydration present.

Nursing Care

- Dehydrated patients should receive intravenous (preferably) or subcutaneous balanced electrolyte solutions (with potassium supplementation if indicated).

Diet

- Dietary supplementation with a bulk-forming agent (bran, methylcellulose, canned pumpkin, psyllium) is often helpful, though they can sometimes worsen colonic fecal distension; in this instance, feed a low-residue diet.

Activity

- Encourage activity.

Surgical Considerations

- Manual removal of feces with the animal under general anesthesia (after rehydration) may be required if enemas and medications are unsuccessful.
- Subtotal colectomy may be required with recurring obstipation that responds poorly to assertive medical therapy.

 COMMENTS

Client Education

Feed appropriate diet and encourage activity.

Patient Monitoring

Monitor frequency of defecation and stool consistency at least twice a week initially, then weekly or biweekly in response to dietary and/or drug therapy.

Prevention/Avoidance

Keep pet active and feed appropriate diet. Subcutaneous fluids to ensure hydration can help reduce the frequency of constipation, particularly in cats.

Possible Complications

- Chronic constipation or recurrent obstipation can lead to acquired megacolon.
- Overuse of laxatives and enemas can cause diarrhea.
- Colonic mucosa can be damaged by improper enema technique, repeated rough mechanical breakdown of feces, or ischemic necrosis secondary to pressure of hard feces.
- Perineal irritation and ulceration can lead to fecal incontinence.

Expected Course and Prognosis

- Fair to good prognosis with early diagnosis and intervention.
- Recurring bouts of constipation/obstipation may occur dependent on underlying cause.

Synonyms

- Colonic impaction
- Fecal impaction

See Also

- Megacolon
- Nutritional Approach to Chronic Enteropathies

Suggested Reading

Chandler M. Focus on nutrition: dietary management of gastrointestinal disease. Compend Contin Educ Vet 2013;35(6):E1–3.
Tam FM, Carr AP, Myers SL. Safety and palatability of polyethylene glycol 3350 as an oral laxative in cats. J Feline Med Surg 2011;13(10):694–697.

Author: Albert E. Jergens DVM, PhD, DACVIM

Chapter 3

Diarrhea, Acute

DEFINITION/OVERVIEW

- Abrupt or recent onset of abnormally increased fecal water and/or solid content.

ETIOLOGY/PATHOPHYSIOLOGY

- Caused by imbalance in the absorptive, secretory, and/or motility actions of the intestines.
- Mechanisms of diarrhea: (1) Osmotic – excess molecules in the intestinal lumen draw in water, overwhelming the intestinal absorptive capacity (e.g., diet changes, malabsorption or overeating). (2) Secretory – stimulation of small intestinal secretion that overwhelms the intestinal absorptive capacity (e.g., toxins). Stimulation of the parasympathetic nervous system or exposure to a variety of secretagogues can increase intestinal secretion. (3) Exudative/permeability – leakage of tissue fluid, serum proteins, blood, or mucus from sites of infiltration or ulceration. (4) Dysmotility – hypomotility (ileus) is more common than hypermotility. Hypermotility can be primary (irritable bowel syndrome) or secondary (obstruction, malabsorption leading to intestinal distention). (5) Mixed.

Systems Affected

- Cardiovascular – hypovolemia, tachycardia, pale mucous membranes, prolonged capillary refill time (CRT) and weak pulses; hypokalemia can cause cardiac arrhythmias.
- Endocrine/metabolic – electrolyte and acid–base abnormalities, dehydration, and prerenal azotemia.
- Gastrointestinal – abdominal pain, hypokalemia can lead to decreased motility.
- Musculoskeletal – hypokalemia can lead to muscle weakness.

SIGNALMENT/HISTORY

- Dogs and cats.
- Any animal can suffer from acute diarrhea; kittens and puppies are most frequently affected.

Risk Factors

- Systemic illness may also result in diarrhea as a secondary event.
- Dietary indiscretion – ingestion of garbage, nonfood material, or spoiled food.
- Dietary changes – abrupt changes in amount or type of foodstuffs.
- Dietary intolerance – malassimilation of food, dietary hypersensitivity.
- Metabolic diseases – hypoadrenocorticism, liver disease, renal disease, and pancreatic disease can cause acute or chronic diarrhea.

Blackwell's Five-Minute Veterinary Consult Clinical Companion: Small Animal Gastrointestinal Diseases, First Edition. Edited by Jocelyn Mott and Jo Ann Morrison.
© 2019 John Wiley & Sons, Inc. Published 2019 by John Wiley & Sons, Inc.
Companion website: www.fiveminutevet.com/gastrointestinal

- Obstruction – foreign bodies, intussusception, or intestinal/mesenteric volvulus.
- Idiopathic – hemorrhagic gastroenteritis.
- Viral – parvovirus, coronavirus, rotavirus, canine distemper virus.
- Bacterial – *Salmonella, Campylobacter, Clostridium* spp., *Escherichia coli*, etc.
- Parasitic – verminous (hookworms, ascarids, whipworms, and cestodes) or protozoal (*Giardia,* coccidia, *Trichomonas,* and *Entamoeba*).
- Rickettsial – salmon poisoning (*Neorickettsia*).
- Fungal – histoplasmosis.
- Drugs and toxins – heavy metals (e.g., lead), organophosphates, nonsteroidal antiinflammatories, steroids, antimicrobials, antineoplastic agents, chocolate, etc.

Historical Findings

- Increased fecal fluidity and/or volume and/or frequency of short duration.
- Owner may report fecal accidents, changes in fecal consistency and volume, blood or mucus in the feces, or straining to defecate.
- Owners may be able to report exposure to toxins, dietary changes, or dietary indiscretion.

 # CLINICAL FEATURES

- Varies with the disease severity.
- Dehydration or lethargy often present.
- Abdominal pain or discomfort, fever, signs of hypotension, nausea, and weakness may occur in more severely affected individuals.
- Rectal exam may reveal blood, mucus or altered consistency of stool.

 # DIFFERENTIAL DIAGNOSIS

- Patients should have a complete physical examination, fecal flotation, and assessment of their hydration status.
- Further diagnostic tests depend on the extent of illness and other clinical signs.

 # DIAGNOSTICS

Complete Blood Cell Count/Biochemistry/Urinalysis

- Generally normal; not necessary unless systemic involvement.
- Can see neutropenia with parvoviral enteritis and marked hemoconcentration with a discordant normal or low-normal plasma protein concentration with *C. perfringens* and *C. difficile*-associated hemorrhagic diarrhea.
- Electrolytes are commonly abnormal because of intestinal losses (hypokalemia, hypochloremia, hyponatremia).

Other Laboratory Tests

- Canine pancreas specific lipase (spec cPL) for pancreatitis, trypsin-like immunoreactivity (TLI) for exocrine pancreatic insufficiency (EPI), cobalamin, and folate (altered absorption) – the latter are more commonly performed with chronic diarrhea.
- Enzyme-linked immunosorbent assay (ELISA) and indirect fluorescent antibody (IFA) fecal testing are available for *Giardia* and *Cryptosporidium* spp.
- Diarrhea polymerase chain reaction (PCR) panel – to evaluate for common specific infectious diseases (e.g., *Salmonella*, parvovirus)

Imaging

- Radiographs – generally not necessary in patients with mild illness.
- Abdominal radiographs can help identify or rule out masses, intestinal foreign bodies or obstruction.
- More severe signs (e.g., abdominal pain or persistent vomiting) may increase the likely diagnostic benefit of abdominal imaging.
- Contrast abdominal radiography and ultrasonography may be useful with some patients, especially looking for lymphadenopathy or an intestinal obstruction.

Diagnostic Procedures

- Perform fecal flotation for parasites on all patients.
- Because helminth ova and *Giardia* cysts can be shed in low numbers or intermittently, multiple fecal analyses are recommended, and empiric treatment is advisable. The *Giardia* ELISA is a sensitive assay and should be combined with fecal flotation to increase the diagnostic yield of *Giardia* spp.
- Can perform fecal ELISA tests for parvovirus antigen in dogs.
- Endoscopy and biopsy – useful in selected cases; more commonly needed in chronic diarrhea.

Pathologic Findings

Dependent on etiology.

 THERAPEUTICS

Drug(s) of Choice

- Antidiarrheal drugs can be classified as motility-modifying drugs, antisecretory drugs, or intestinal protectants.
- Motility-modifying drugs generally operate by increasing segmental motility and thus increasing transit time (i.e., narcotics such as loperamide; 0.1 mg/kg PO q 8–12 h in dogs; 0.08 mg/kg PO q 12 h in cats) or by decreasing forward motility (i.e., anticholinergics); these medications are not necessary in mild disease, as it is generally self-limiting. Do not use these medications longer than 1–2 days because of adverse effects.
- Acute diarrhea that does not resolve with antidiarrheal drugs merits further investigation.
- Anthelmintics (e.g., fenbendazole 50 mg/kg PO q 24 h for 5 days) and antiprotozoal drugs (e.g., metronidazole 10–20 mg/kg PO q 12 h for 5 days) are recommended as empiric treatment for patients with acute diarrhea or those with positive fecal analyses. Coccidiostatic (e.g., sulfadimethoxine, ponazuril) drugs can be used if fecal analysis warrants.
- Antibiotic therapy is unnecessary for most cases of mild illness and may actually exacerbate the diarrhea.
- Patients with bacterial enteritis, severe illness, concomitant leukopenia, or suspected breakdown of the gastrointestinal mucosal barrier (as evidenced by blood in the feces) may be treated with antimicrobial agents. Recent studies suggest antimicrobial agents may not be indicated in all cases of hemorrhagic gastroenteritis (HGE).
- Probiotics may also be useful (*Lactobacillus*, *Enterococcus*). Probiotics have been shown to shorten the duration of acute, nonspecific diarrhea in some studies. Use probiotics from premium pet food companies in light of studies showing suboptimal quality of probiotics that have not undergone rigorous testing. VSL#3 at 10–20 billion/kg has been shown to be effective.

Precautions/Interactions

- Most cases of acute mild diarrhea resolve with minimal treatment (low-fat diet and time); be cautious of excessive diagnostics and overtreating.
- Almost any drug can produce adverse effects (often including diarrhea and vomiting); these may be more severe than the initial problem.
- Cats can be sensitive to subsalicylates and should not be given high or frequent doses.
- Long-term use of metronidazole can lead to neurologic complications.
- Some animals are sensitive to sulfa-containing mediations used for treatment of coccidia.
- Anticholinergics in patients with suspected intestinal obstruction, glaucoma, or intestinal ileus – use with caution or do not use.
- Narcotic analgesics – can cause central nervous system (CNS) depression; undesirable in patients with more severe illness that are already depressed or lethargic – use with caution or do not use.
- Narcotic analgesics in patients with liver disease and bacterial or toxic enteritis – use with caution or do not use.

Alternative Drug(s)

Kaolin pectin.

Appropriate Health Care

Depends largely on the severity of illness; patients with mild illness can often be handled as outpatients with symptomatic therapy; patients with more severe illness or that fail to respond to therapy should be treated more aggressively.

Nursing Care

- Fluid therapy and correction of electrolyte imbalances is the mainstay of treatment in most cases.
- Can give crystalloid fluid therapy (PO, SQ or IV) as required.
- Aim to return the patient to proper hydration status (over 12–24 h) and replace ongoing losses.
- Severe volume depletion can occur with acute diarrhea; aggressive fluid therapy may be necessary.
- Use of potassium supplementation is based on severity (potassium chloride 20–40 mEq/L) in most patients, but not during shock fluid therapy. Hypokalemia can worsen ileus.

Diet

Patients with mild illness that are not vomiting can be managed with a fat-restricted, digestible intestinal diet, either home-cooked (boiled rice and chicken in 4:1 ratio) or low-fat cottage cheese (1%) and rice or a commercial prescription intestinal diet. This should be fed for a few days then slowly transitioned back to the normal diet.

Activity

Animals should have limited activity until the diarrhea has stopped.

Surgical Considerations

Patients with obstructions may require surgery to evaluate the intestine and remove the foreign objects.

COMMENTS

Client Education

- Limiting exposure to garbage, foods other than the patient's normal diet, and potential foreign bodies.
- Proper puppy and kitten vaccination and deworming schedules.

Patient Monitoring

- Most acute diarrhea resolves within a few days.
- If clinical signs persist, additional diagnostics and treatments may be necessary.
- Upon completion of medication, recheck patients that exhibited parasites by fecal analysis.

Prevention/Avoidance

- Animals should be fed a consistent high-quality diet.
- Owners should attempt to control indiscriminate eating and monitor for foreign body ingestion.

Possible Complications

- Intussusception is thought to be associated with increased intestinal motility (e.g., parvoviral enteritis and parasitism).

Expected Course and Prognosis

Most cases of acute diarrhea resolve spontaneously without treatment or with minimal treatment.

Abbreviations

- CNS = central nervous system
- CPV = canine parvovirus
- CRT = capillary refill time
- ELISA = enzyme-linked immunosorbent assay
- EPI = exocrine pancreatic insufficiency
- HGE = hemorrhagic gastroenteritis
- IFA = indirect fluorescent antibody
- Spec cPL = canine pancreas specific lipase
- TLI = trypsin-like immunoreactivity

See Also

- Diarrhea, Antibiotic Responsive
- Nutritional Approach to Acute Vomiting and Diarrhea
- Vomiting, Acute

Suggested Reading

Hall EJ, German AJ. Diseases of the small intestine. In: Ettinger SJ, Feldman EC, eds. Textbook of Veterinary Internal Medicine, 7th ed. St Louis: Elsevier, 2010:1526–1572.
Scorza V, Lappin MR, Greene CE, Chapman S, Gookin JL. In: Greene CE, ed. Infectious Diseases of the Dog and Cat, 4th ed. St Louis: Saunders Elsevier, 2012:785–801.
Willard MD. Diarrhea. In: Ettinger SJ, Feldman EC, eds. Textbook of Veterinary Internal Medicine, 7th ed. St Louis: Elsevier, 2010:201–203.

Author: Erin Portillo MS, DVM, DACVIM

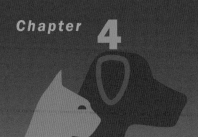

Chapter 4

Diarrhea,
Chronic – Canine

DEFINITION/OVERVIEW

- Chronic or chronic intermittent diarrhea of at least 3 weeks' duration.

ETIOLOGY/PATHOPHYSIOLOGY

- Secretory diarrhea – results from increased water excretion into the intestinal lumen, commonly as a result of toxic or infectious etiologies.
- Osmotic diarrhea – increased water is pulled into the intestinal lumen, due to excessive luminal contents, maldigestion or malabsorption.
- Increased permeability – physical changes to the intestinal wall decrease the integrity of the intestinal barrier, allowing leakage into the lumen.
- Abnormal gastrointestinal (GI) motility – e.g., hyperperistalsis.
- Many cases involve combinations of these pathophysiologic mechanisms.
- Chronic diarrhea can be a manifestation of primary gastrointestinal disease (primary enteropathy) or extragastrointestinal diseases (secondary enteropathy) (Box 4.1).
- Primary enteropathy is the most common cause of chronic diarrhea. Primary enteropathy can be divided into chronic inflammatory enteropathies, infectious, neoplastic, and mechanical disorders. Chronic inflammatory enteropathies are the most common cause of chronic diarrhea, with a frequency of 71%.

BOX 4.1. Causes of chronic diarrhea in dogs.

Primary enteropathy	Secondary enteropathy
• Chronic inflammatory enteropathy (71%)	• Exocrine pancreatic disease
○ Food-responsive enteropathy (66%)	• Renal disease
○ Antibiotic-responsive enteropathy	• Liver disease
○ Steroid-responsive enteropathy	• Endocrine disease
• Infectious disease	• Congestive heart failure
• Neoplasia	
• Mechanical	
• Toxic	

Blackwell's Five-Minute Veterinary Consult Clinical Companion: Small Animal Gastrointestinal Diseases,
First Edition. Edited by Jocelyn Mott and Jo Ann Morrison.
© 2019 John Wiley & Sons, Inc. Published 2019 by John Wiley & Sons, Inc.
Companion website: www.fiveminutevet.com/gastrointestinal

- Chronic inflammatory enteropathies can be further classified as food-responsive enteropathy, antibiotic-responsive enteropathy or immunosuppressive or steroid-responsive enteropathy. Food-responsive enteropathy accounts for 66% of dogs with chronic inflammatory enteropathies.
- Second leading cause of chronic diarrhea is infectious (ex. *Giardia, Coccidia, Toxocara, Leishmania*).

Systems Affected

- Gastrointestinal.
- Musculoskeletal-weight loss.

SIGNALMENT/HISTORY

- Male dogs are overrepresented.
- Middle-aged dogs most common.

Risk Factors

- Dietary changes, feeding poorly digestible or high-fat diets, stress or psychological factors.
- Large-breed dogs, especially German shepherds, have the highest incidence of antibiotic-responsive diarrhea.
- Large-breed dogs have a higher risk of intestinal volvulus/torsion; may be seen in association with exocrine pancreatic insufficiency (EPI).
- Pythiosis occurs most often in young, large-breed dogs living in rural areas, with a higher incidence bordering the Gulf of Mexico.
- Histiocytic ulcerative colitis (invasive adherent *Escherichia coli* associated) – boxers, French bulldogs <3 years old.

Historical Findings

- Diarrhea – large bowel diarrhea (increased frequency of defecation, excess mucus, tenesmus, and hematochezia), small bowel diarrhea (normal to mildly increased frequency of defecation, normal to increased amount of fecal volume, weight loss +/– vomiting, +/– melena) or mixed bowel diarrhea.
- Lethargy.
- Weight loss.
- Flatulence.
- Abdominal pain.
- Vomiting.
- Borborygmi.
- Melena/hematochezia.
- Polyphagia to anorexia.
- Pruritus.

CLINICAL FEATURES

- Weight loss.
- Abdominal distension.
- Borborygmi.
- Dehydration.
- Hematochezia on glove from rectal palpation.

- Rectal palpation may reveal irregularity of the colorectal mucosa, intraluminal or extraluminal rectal masses, rectal stricture, or sublumbar lymphadenopathy.
- Palpable thickened loops of bowel.
- Abdominal effusion.

DIFFERENTIAL DIAGNOSIS

- Primary enteropathy.
    - Diet-responsive enteropathy.
    - Antibiotic-responsive enteropathy.
    - Infectious causes such as *Giardia*, histoplasmosis, feline leukemia virus, feline immunodeficiency virus, *Pythium*, helminths.
    - Neoplasia such as lymphoma, carcinoma, leiomyosarcomas, mast cell tumors.
    - Inflammatory bowel disease (IBD).
    - Lymphangiectasia.
    - Mechanical obstruction.
    - Irritable bowel disease.
- Secondary enteropathy.
    - Most common is exocrine pancreatic insufficiency.
    - Others include pancreatitis, atypical Addison's, hypothyroidism, hyperthyroidism, renal disease, liver disease (portosystemic shunt) or congestive heart failure.

DIAGNOSTICS

Figure 4.1 is an algorithm for the diagnostic approach to canine chronic diarrhea.

Complete Blood Cell Count/Biochemistry/Urinalysis

- Anemia.
- Severe hypoalbuminemia (<2 g/dL) associated with poor outcome. Panhypoproteinemia can be associated with protein-losing enteropathy (PLE).

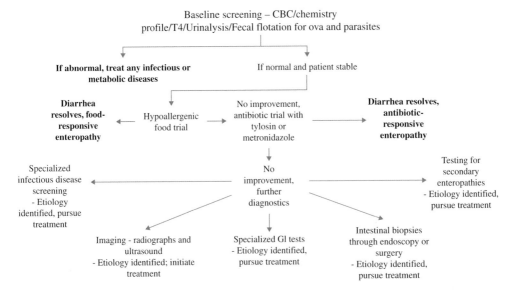

■ **Fig. 4.1.** Diagnostic approach to canine chronic diarrhea.

- Mild to moderate increases in liver enzymes (alanine aminotransferase (ALT), alkaline phosphatase (ALP)) can occur secondary to reactive hepatopathy.
- Hypocholesterolemia can be seen in dogs with lymphangiectasia because cholesterol is lost in lymphatic fluid and malabsorption occurs.

Other Laboratory Tests

- Infectious causes.
    - Fecal floatation with centrifugation to identify ova and parasites.
    - Fecal floatation with $ZnSO_4$ with centrifugation is recommended to identify *Giardia* cysts. Three separate fecal samples collected 3 days apart should be evaluated to increase sensitivity of the test. Direct immunofluorescence assays or SNAP® tests may increase diagnostic yield.
    - Fecal polymerase chain reaction (PCR) assay can be used to detect eggs of *Heterobilharzia americana*, *Cryptosporidia*, and other infectious diseases.
    - An enzyme immunoassay is available for *Histoplasma* antigen detection in serum or urine.
    - *Pythium* can be diagnosed with two serological tests (immunoblot assay and enzyme linked immunosorbent assay – ELISA). The organism can also be cultured from intestinal tissue or PCR assay on infected tissues.
    - Feline leukemia virus and feline immunodeficiency virus serologic screening to rule out virus associated enteritis.
- Specialized gastrointestinal tests.
    - Cobalamin may be measured and if subnormal can indicate exocrine pancreatic insufficiency, severe disease of ileal mucosa, and intestinal dysbiosis. Severe hypocobalaminemia (<200 pg/mL) is associated with poor outcome.
    - Trypsin-like immunoreactivity (TLI) is decreased with exocrine pancreatic insufficiency.
    - Canine pancreatic lipase immunoreactivity (spec cPL) can be elevated with pancreatitis. Dogs with IBD and elevated spec cPL have poor response to steroids and outcome.
    - Fecal alpha-1-proteinase inhibitor assay is a diagnostic test for protein-losing enteropathy. Three separate fecal samples need to be collected and frozen prior to shipping.
    - Canine microbiota dysbiosis index can be measured on feces by PCR. This can also help to predict the ability for the pet to convert fecal bile acids.
    - Assay for canine calprotectin in serum and feces may be a useful biomarker for dogs with chronic diarrhea. Fecal calprotectin may be able to distinguish between food-responsive, antibiotic-responsive, and steroid-responsive enteropathies.
    - Presence of perinuclear antineutrophil cytoplasmic antibody (pANCA) titers has been associated with chronic enteropathies and more specifically food-responsive enteropathies.
- Testing for causes of secondary enteropathies.
    - Atypical Addison's can cause chronic waxing and waning GI signs. A resting cortisol >2 µg/dL rules out hypoadrenocorticism. If resting cortisol is <2 µg/dL, an ACTH stimulation should be performed to assess the adrenal glands' ability to respond appropriately to stimulation.
    - Thyroid testing to evaluate for hyperthyroidism in cats and hypothyroidism in dogs.
    - Bile acids to detect hepatobiliary disease.

Imaging

- Abdominal radiographs may be unremarkable or be consistent with pancreatitis, partial intestinal obstruction, masses, foreign bodies, organomegaly, hepatobiliary disease, and/or effusion.

- Thoracic radiographs are often unremarkable but may reveal metastatic disease or pleural effusion with PLE.
- Abdominal ultrasound allows assessment of all abdominal organs. Extraintestinal causes for diarrhea may be identified. Intestinal wall thickness is an insensitive and nonspecific indicator of chronic enteropathies. Echogenicity of the bowel wall mucosa is a more specific indicator of inflammatory disease. Presence of hyperechoic striations in duodenum or jejunum is suggestive of protein-losing enteropathy. Presence of hyperechoic speckles in duodenum or jejunum can indicate inflammatory disease.

Additional Diagnostic Tests

- Ultrasound-guided fine needle aspiration of gastrointestinal mass lesions can be helpful for diagnosing mast cell tumors, carcinomas, and large cell lymphoma.
- Seeding of neoplastic cells is a concern.
- Intestinal biopsies may be required for diagnosis – either full thickness through exploratory laparotomy or partial thickness through endoscopy. When large and small bowel diarrhea are present, collection of ileal and duodenal biopsies is warranted.
- Therapeutic trials.
  - Diet trial for food-responsive enteropathy. If maldigestive (EPI), metabolic, parasitic, dietary, and infectious causes have been excluded, then consider a dietary trial using an elimination diet (novel, single protein source) for 2 weeks in stable dogs prior to performing advanced diagnostics (endoscopy or laparotomy and biopsy).
  - Antibiotic trial for antibiotic-responsive enteropathy – trial of tylan or metronidazole for 10 days.

Pathologic Findings

- Gastrointestinal and colonic biopsies may be unremarkable or display inflammation (lymphocytic plasmacytic, eosinophilic or mixed cell).

 # THERAPEUTICS

- Chronic diarrhea secondary to infectious diseases or secondary enteropathies should be addressed appropriately medically.
- A diet trial can be used to diagnose food-responsive enteropathy.
- Antibiotic trial can be used to diagnose antibiotic-responsive enteropathy.
- Steroid- or immunosuppressive-responsive enteropathy may respond to prednisolone or immunosuppressive drugs. Further diagnostics including gastrointestinal biopsies are often required at this stage.

Drug(s) of Choice

- Antibiotic-responsive enteropathy.
  - Therapeutic trial with metronidazole (10–15 mg/kg PO q 12 h) or tylosin (25 mg/kg PO q 12 h) for at least 10 days.
- Immunosuppressive- or steroid-responsive enteropathy.
  - Prednisolone or prednisone (0.5–1 mg/kg PO q 12–24 h) or cyclosporine (5 mg/kg PO q 24 h).
- Fiber supplementation has shown to modify the fecal microbiota of dogs with chronic diarrhea to more closely resemble that of healthy dogs.

Precautions/Interactions

Anticholinergics can exacerbate the situation with many causes of chronic diarrhea; they are sometimes used to relieve cramping associated with irritable bowel syndrome.

Alternative Drugs

Preliminary studies indicate that infusions of allogenic adipose tissue-derived mesenchymal stem cells may have a future place in treating chronic enteropathies.

Appropriate Health Care

- Dogs with chronic diarrhea can usually be treated as outpatients.
- Patients with dehydration may require hospitalization and intravenous fluid supportive care.

Nursing Care

- It is important to keep the perianal area clean and dry. Sanitary clipping of this area may help with hygiene and comfort.

Diet

- Cats with chronic diarrhea may respond to diet change within 1–3 weeks; however, dietary fat content does not appear to be a factor.
- Dogs with inflammatory bowel disease show improved clinical response and reduced relapses with hydrolyzed protein diets than novel protein diets. Dogs with IBD requiring drugs responded better with a hydrolyzed protein diet than with drugs alone.
- Dogs with chronic idiopathic large bowel diarrhea often respond to a highly digestible diet with addition of soluble fiber (Metamucil® 2 tablespoons/day or 1.33 g of psyllium/kg/day).

Activity

Low-intensity to moderate-intensity interval exercise in sedentary dogs improved symptoms of chronic diarrhea.

Surgical Considerations

- Full-thickness biopsies can be obtained from clearly visualized segments/locations of the intestinal tract.
- A surgical approach can be the most advantageous/pragmatic approach if biopsies of multiple organs (e.g., small intestine, lymph nodes, stomach, pancreas, liver) are desired with the ability to correct abnormal findings.
- Other indications for a surgical approach include evidence of obstruction, intestinal mass, or mid-small bowel disease unreachable via ultrasound-guided procedure or if a diagnosis based on endoscopic biopsy or ultrasound-guided procedure is questioned because of poor response to therapy.

 COMMENTS

Client Education

- Avoid abrupt diet changes, table scraps, and dietary indiscretion.
- Chronic diarrhea may or may not require extensive work-up for definitive diagnosis.
- Chronic diarrhea in some cases may not resolve completely with treatment.

Patient Monitoring

- Frequency and consistency of the stool, appetite, and body weight.
- In dogs with PLE – serum proteins, cholesterol, and clinical signs (ascites, subcutaneous edema, pleural effusion).
- Resolution of diarrhea is usually gradual with treatment; if it does not resolve, reevaluate the diagnosis.

Prevention/Avoidance

- Avoid dietary indiscretion.
- Feed easily digestible high-quality diet.

Possible Complications

- Dehydration.
- Lowered body condition.
- Abdominal effusions as related to specific cause of chronic diarrhea.
- Ascites, subcutaneous edema, and/or pleural effusion with hypoalbuminemia from PLEs.

Expected Course and Prognosis

- Prognosis is variable with underlying disease process.
- Anemia, severe hypoalbuminemia, and hypocobalaminemia are associated with poor prognosis.
- Young dogs with large bowel signs are more likely to have food-responsive enteropathy and good prognosis.

Synonyms

- Idiopathic chronic diarrhea

Abbreviations

- EPI = exocrine pancreatic insufficiency
- GI = gastrointestinal
- IBD = inflammatory bowel disease
- PCR = polymerase chain reaction
- PLE = protein-losing enteropathy
- Spec cPL = canine specific pancreatic lipase immunoreactivity

See Also

- Cobalamin Deficiency
- Colitis, Histiocytic Ulcerative
- Diarrhea, Antibiotic Responsive
- Fiber-Responsive Large Bowel Diarrhea
- Food Reactions (Gastrointestinal), Adverse
- Exocrine Pancreatic Insufficiency
- Gastroenteritis, Lymphocytic-Plasmacytic
- Gastrointestinal Lymphoma, Canine
- Giardiasis
- Inflammatory Bowel Disease
- Intestinal Dysbiosis
- Intestinal Neoplasia, Malignant
- Irritable Bowel Syndrome
- Nutritional Approach to Chronic Enteropathies
- Parasites, Gastrointestinal
- Protein-Losing Enteropathy

Suggested Reading

Berghoff N, Steiner JM. Laboratory tests for the diagnosis and management of chronic canine and feline enteropathies. Vet Clin Small Anim 2011;41:311–328.

Casamian-Sorrosal D, Willard MD, Murray JK, et al. Comparison of histopathologic findings in biopsies from the duodenum and ileum of dogs with enteropathy. J Vet Intern Med 2010;24:80–83.

Florey J, Viall A, Streu S, et al. Use of granulocyte immunofluorescence assay designed for humanes for detection of antineutrophil cytoplasmic antibodies in dogs with chronic enteropathies. J Vet Intern Med 2017;31:1062–1066.

Gaschen L, Kircher P, Stussi A, et al. Comparison of ultrasonographic findings with clinical activity index (CIBDAI) and diagnosis in dogs with chronic enteropathies. Vet Radiol Ultrasound 2008;49(1):56–64.

Huang HP, Lien YH. Effects of a structured exercise programme in sedentary dogs with chronic diarrhea. Vet Rec 2017;180(9):224.

Laflamme DP, Xu H, Long GM. Effects of diets differing in fat content on chronic diarrhea in cats. J Vet Intern Med 2011;25:230–235.

Leib MS. Treatment of chronic idiopathic large bowel diarrhea in dogs with a highly digestible diet and soluble fiber: a retrospective review of 37 cases. J Vet Intern Med 2000;14:27–32.

Marchesi MC, Timpano CC, Busechian S, et al. The role of diet in managing inflammatory bowel disease affected dogs: a retrospective cohort study on 76 cases. Veterin Ital 2017;53(4):297–302.

Perez-Merino EM, Uson-Casaus JM, Zaragoza-Bayle C, et al. Safety and efficacy of allogeneic adipose tissue-derived mesenchymal stem cells for treatment of dogs with inflammatory bowel disease: clinical and laboratory outcomes. Vet J 2015;206:385–390.

Volkmann M, Steiner JM, Fosgate GT, et al. Chronic diarrhea in dogs – retrospective study in 136 cases. J Vet Intern Med ;31(4):1043–1055.

Acknowledgments: The author and editors acknowledge the prior contribution of Dr Mark Hitt.

Author: Jocelyn Mott DVM, DACVIM (SAIM)

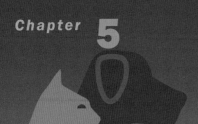
Diarrhea, Chronic – Feline

DEFINITION/OVERVIEW

- Decreased fecal consistency, increased stool frequency or volume for more than three weeks.
- Might be stable or progressive; persistent or intermittently recurrent (waxing and waning).
- Small bowel, large bowel, or mixed in origin.

ETIOLOGY/PATHOPHYSIOLOGY

Chronic diarrhea is almost always the result of a combination of the following factors.
- Osmotic diarrhea – excess of osmotically active particles in the intestinal lumen causing water to be drawn passively into the lumen.
  - Ingestion of solutes that cannot be absorbed (e.g., lactulose, excess of soluble and insoluble fiber).
  - Malabsorption of solutes (e.g., lactose, overfeeding, malabsorptive/maldigestive disease).
- Secretory diarrhea – excessive secretion of water into the lumen.
  - Infection (bacterial or viral toxins, usually associated with acute diarrhea).
  - Drugs.
  - Vasculitis.
  - Bile acid malabsorption (usually associated with chronic infiltrative gastrointestinal (GI) disease or dysbiosis).
- Malabsorption/maldigestion.
  - Exocrine pancreatic insufficiency (EPI).
  - Reduced luminal bile acids (e.g., due to EPI).
  - Short bowel syndrome.
  - Dysbiosis.
  - Mucosal disease (e.g., infiltration of the mucosa with inflammatory or neoplastic cells or with infectious agents such as fungi or algae).
- Inflammatory/neoplastic.
  - Inflammatory bowel disease (IBD).
  - Alimentary lymphoma.
- Dysmotility.
  - Hypermotility – increased forward motility propelling food distally.
  - Hypomotility – decreased segmental motility leading to decreased mucosal contact with food and malabsorption. May lead to constipation or diarrhea.

Blackwell's Five-Minute Veterinary Consult Clinical Companion: Small Animal Gastrointestinal Diseases,
First Edition. Edited by Jocelyn Mott and Jo Ann Morrison.
© 2019 John Wiley & Sons, Inc. Published 2019 by John Wiley & Sons, Inc.
Companion website: www.fiveminutevet.com/gastrointestinal

- Pancreatitis.
- Peritonitis.
- Abdominal surgery.
- Drugs.
- Hyperthyroidism.
- Irritable bowel syndrome (IBS).

Systems Affected

- Endocrine/metabolic – catabolic state, malnutrition, acid–base, electrolyte, fluid, possible underlying endocrinopathy.
- Gastrointestinal – primary inflammation causing diarrhea, secondary inflammation, and dysbiosis due to infection or extraintestinal cause of diarrhea.

SIGNALMENT /HISTORY

- Chronic diarrhea tends to occur more frequently in older cats.
- Kittens can suffer from chronic diarrhea (mostly intermittent, recurrent) due to infectious causes and/or possibly incompletely developed GI immunity.
- Food-responsive enteropathy tends to occur in young to middle-aged cats.
- IBD commonly occurs in middle-aged cats; Siamese and other Asian breeds may be predisposed.
- Alimentary small cell lymphoma tends to occur in older cats.
- Certain historical, physical exam, and laboratory findings (e.g., lethargy, moderate to severe weight loss, low body condition score (BCS), hypocobalaminemia, etc.) indicate the need for a more aggressive and faster work-up.
- Diarrhea should be identified as either small or large bowel in origin (Table 5.1); mixed diarrhea will have characteristics of both.

TABLE 5.1. **Differentiation between small and large bowel diarrhea.**			
	Clinical sign	Small bowel	Large bowel
Feces	Mucus	Rare	Common
	Blood	Melena	Hematochezia
	Volume	Large	Small
	Fat	Possible	Absent
Defecation	Frequency	Normal to slightly increased (2–3/d)	Increased (>3/d)
	Tenesmus	Rare	Common
	Urgency	Rare	Common
	Dyschezia (pain)	Absent	Possible
Other findings	Weight loss	Common	Rare
	Vomiting	Common	Rare
	Fecal incontinence	Absent	Possible
	Serum cobalamin ↓	Possible	Absent
	Serum folate ↓↑	Possible	Absent

Risk Factors

- Age.
- Dietary changes.
- Poorly digestible or high-fat diets.
- Underlying GI disease should be suspected in cats with chronic/intermittent diarrhea that are adult, healthy, and living in an environment with a low infectious pressure/stress, but test repeatedly positive for facultative infectious agents such as *Giardia*, *Cryptosporidium* spp., *Cystoisospora* spp., etc.
- IBD may progress over time to low-grade alimentary lymphoma.

Historical Findings

- Diarrhea might be the only clinical sign or can occur with other signs of gastrointestinal disease. Owners tend to underestimate/ under-recognize GI signs others than diarrhea; always ask specifically about weight loss, vomiting, hyporexia or polyphagia.
- Weight loss is common and often overlooked; always try to get former weight measurements for comparison.
- Clinical signs are often intermittent with spontaneous remissions. Triggers may be dietary indiscretion/ change, change of daily routine, drugs, etc., but often remain unknown.
- Chronic diarrhea can be classified as small bowel, large bowel or mixed diarrhea (see Table 5.1).

 CLINICAL FEATURES

- Vary with duration, severity, and location (mostly small vs mostly large bowel diarrhea) of disease.
- Poor body condition or selective muscle wastage (abdominal fat pad is often preserved).
- Poor or unkempt hair coat.
- Abdominal palpation may reveal generalized thickened small bowel loops ("ropy" loops), masses (neoplasia, mesenteric lymphadenopathy, foreign body, intussusception) or abdominal effusion (fluid wave).
- Rectal palpation may reveal melena (dark brown to black feces), hematochezia, masses, strictures or sublumbar lymphadenopathy.
- Dehydration is uncommon in stable patients.
- Some cats have concurrent cutaneous disease with pruritus.

 DIFFERENTIAL DIAGNOSIS

Extraintestinal Disease

Metabolic
- Renal disease.
- Hepatopathy.
- Hepatobiliary disease – often concurrent with chronic enteropathy ± pancreatitis = triaditis.
- Portosystemic shunt.
- Pancreatic disorders (pancreatitis often concurrent with chronic enteropathy ± hepatobiliary disease, EPI).
- Adverse drug reaction.

Endocrine
- Hyperthyroidism.
- Hypoadrenocorticism (very rare).

Systemic disease
- Infection – feline immunodeficiency virus (FIV) (rarely associated with diarrhea), feline leukemia virus (FeLV), feline infectious peritonitis (FIP).
- Neoplasia.

Gastrointestinal Disease

Dietary
- Dietary indiscretion (usually acute diarrhea).
- Dietary changes (usually acute diarrhea).
- Dietary intolerance (e.g., to lactose, gluten, etc.) – no direct immune response involved, often dose dependent.
- Dietary hypersensitivity (active primary immune response, dose independent).

Inflammatory – Infectious
- Parasites (e.g., *Tritrichomonas foetus*, *Giardia*, *Toxocara* spp., *Ancylostoma*, *Toxascaris leonina*, *Cryptosporidium* spp., *Cystoisospora* spp., etc.).
- Mycotic (e.g., histoplasmosis).
- Viral – uncommon cause of chronic diarrhea (e.g., enteric coronavirus, FIP, FeLV associated, FIV associated (rare)).
- Bacterial (e.g., *Salmonella* spp., *Campylobacter jejuni*, etc.) – usually acute diarrhea.
- Other (e.g., prototothecosis, pythiosis) (rare).

Inflammatory – Noninfectious
- Chronic enteropathy (CE).
  - Dietary-responsive enteropathy (very common).
  - Fiber-responsive enteropathy (large bowel diarrhea).
  - Antibiotic-responsive enteropathy.
  - Steroid-responsive enteropathy – IBD (e.g., most commonly lymphoplasmacytic enteritis, eosinophilic enteritis (rare), granulomatous enteritis (very rare)).

Neoplastic
- Alimentary lymphoma (e.g., small cell lymphoma, large granular lymphocyte lymphoma).
- Adenocarcinoma.
- Mast cell tumor (intestinal or systemic).

Miscellaneous
- Dysmotility (pancreatitis, abdominal surgery, peritonitis, FIP, idiopathic).
- Dysbiosis (usually associated with CE or EPI).
- Short bowel syndrome.
- Partial obstruction (e.g., foreign body, intussusception, neoplasia).
- Duodenal ulcers.

 DIAGNOSTICS

- In cats that are stable, without history of significant weight loss and normal body condition, no abnormal findings on physical exam, and no signs of systemic disease, a "diagnostic treatment trial" can be performed (see "Therapeutics" and Figure 5.1).
- Fecal flotation and testing for *Giardia* should be performed and the cat should be dewormed with broad-spectrum anthelmintics.
- If the patient does not respond, a hypoallergenic diet can be fed for 1–2 weeks. It is important to choose a high-quality diet (see section on "Diet"). Cats with exclusively large bowel

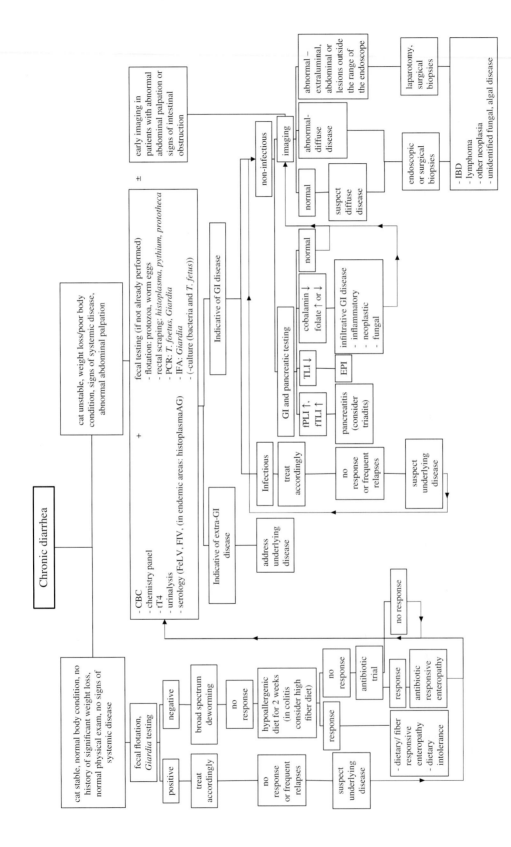

■ **Fig. 5.1.** Algorithm showing the approach to cats with chronic diarrhea.

diarrhea may respond to a high-fiber diet and/or the addition of fiber to a (hypoallergenic) diet (see section on "Prebiotics"). In addition, or before treatment with antibiotics, probiotics can be considered, usually in combination with a diet change. If no response is noted after two weeks (usually less), an antibiotic trial with tylosin or metronidazole may be considered.

■ Cats that are unstable, and cats with a history of significant weight loss, a poor body condition, abnormal findings on physical exam or signs of systemic disease should undergo a more extensive work-up including fecal testing, complete blood cell count, chemistry panel, total T4, urinalysis, and possibly imaging. Serologic testing for FeLV, FIV, and fungal diseases might be considered if appropriate. The same applies for cats that have undergone unsuccessful symptomatic treatment (see Figure 5.1).

Complete Blood Cell Count/Chemistry Panel/Urinalysis

■ Complete blood cell count.
  • Stress leukogram is common in any disease process including chronic diarrhea.
  • Leukocytosis with neutrophilia and bands may indicate severe systemic inflammation, e.g., due to bacterial translocation (leaky gut, rupture, foreign body, etc.), fungal disease, etc.
  • Leukopenia – excessive consumption in systemic inflammatory responses, FeLV, FIV.
  • Eosinophilia – common in cats with chronic diarrhea due to parasitism or allergic diseases. Rarely, eosinophilic enteritis, hypereosinophilic syndrome or hypoadrenocorticism can cause eosinophilia and chronic diarrhea.
  • Anemia – FeLV infection or hyperthyroidism can cause diarrhea and macrocytic anemia. Chronic GI bleeding and (subsequent) iron deficiency causes microcytic nonregenerative anemia. Dependent on duration of GI bleeding, anemia may be regenerative or nonregenerative.
  • Thrombocytopenia – can be seen in cats with FeLV infection (platelet clumping should always be excluded as the most common cause for a low platelet count).
  • Thrombocytosis – can indicate chronic GI bleeding.
■ Chemistry panel.
  • Blood urea nitrogen (BUN) – can be increased in cats with chronic diarrhea and renal disease, GI bleeding, dehydration or postprandially. Decreased BUN may be associated with liver failure or portosystemic shunts.
  • Creatinine – advanced chronic kidney disease (CKD) may cause GI signs, dehydration (interpret with urine specific gravity – USG).
  • Cholesterol – hepatobiliary disease can cause increased serum cholesterol and chronic diarrhea. Maldigestion, malabsorption, and hyporexia can cause serum cholesterol to decrease.
  • Phosphorus – hyperthyroidism and renal disease are disorders causing chronic diarrhea and increased phosphorus concentration, while maldigestion and malabsorption may cause serum phosphorus levels to decrease.
  • Total protein – often increased in cats with chronic diarrhea due to dehydration (increase of albumin and globulin) or hyperglobulinemia due to chronic antigenic stimulation or (rarely) neoplasia. Protein-losing enteropathy is rare in cats, but can cause decreased total protein concentrations.
  • ALT/ALP – increased liver enzyme activities are commonly seen in cats with chronic diarrhea and can indicate concurrent hepatobiliary disease. Chronic enteropathy, hepatobiliary disease, and pancreatitis often occur together in cats, a combination often referred to as triaditis.
  • Bilirubin – an increase may indicate hepatobiliary disease and/or triaditis.

- Urinalysis.
  - USG – should be part of every minimal database and needs to be interpreted with BUN, creatinine, albumin, and total protein to rule out renal disease.

Other Laboratory Testing

- Histoplasma antigen testing – should be performed on urine or serum samples from cats from or with a travel history to endemic areas. This test cross-reacts with *Blastomyces* antigens, and thus a positive test may indicate histoplasmosis or blastomycosis.
- Thyroid testing.
  - Total T4 (tT4) – is the test of choice for hyperthyroidism. Occasionally, total T4 might be normal in cats with hyperthyroidism and other tests need to be pursued. Alternatively, the cat can be retested in 1–3 months. Hyperthyroidism is not likely to be the cause of chronic diarrhea in cats with a normal tT4.
  - Free T4 (fT4) – is a very sensitive test for the diagnosis of hyperthyroidism in cats. However, fT4 lacks specificity (high rate of false-positive results) and can be increased in many other disease processes.
  - T3 suppression test – can be used to confirm or exclude hyperthyroidism in cats with a strong clinical suspicion but normal tT4 and increased fT4.
  - Thyroid scintigraphy – can be used to confirm or exclude hyperthyroidism in cats with a strong clinical suspicion but normal tT4 and increased fT4.
- Serologic testing.
  - FeLV enzyme linked immunosorbent assay (ELISA) – during the initial stage of acute viral replication, diarrhea is common. However, progressive FeLV infection is more commonly associated with other signs such as weight loss, fever, and bone marrow disorders (cytopenias) than with chronic diarrhea. A positive ELISA in low-risk or asymptomatic cats should be confirmed with an indirect fluorescent antibody (IFA) test.
  - FIV ELISA – FIV is rarely, if ever, the primary cause of chronic diarrhea.
- Fecal testing.
  - Direct smear – protozoal trophozoites (e.g., *Cystisospora* sp., *Giardia*, *Toxoplasma*) may be identified.
  - Fecal flotation or zinc sulfate flotation – protozoal trophozoites (e.g., *Cystisospora* sp., *Giardia*, *Toxoplasma*) and worm eggs may be identified.
  - *Giardia* – besides fecal flotation (zinc sulfate), ELISA, polymerase chain reaction (PCR) or IFA testing is available.
  - *T. foetus* – PCR testing or in-house culture using the commercially available culture system In Pouch™ TF.
  - Bacterial culture – bacteria (e.g., *Salmonella* spp., enterotoxic *E. coli*, other Enterobacteriaceae species, *Clostridium* spp.) can be cultured. Usually bacterial infections are not the primary cause of chronic diarrhea and an underlying GI disease should be suspected in recurring bacterial infections.
- GI tests.
  - Cobalamin – is bound to intrinsic factor (IF), secreted by the pancreas and absorbed in the ileum. Mucosal infiltration with cells (inflammatory or neoplastic) or with fungal organisms (e.g., histoplasmosis) can disrupt absorption of cobalamin. EPI can lead to decreased secretion of IF and dysbiosis, which can both cause decreased serum cobalamin concentrations. In cats with chronic diarrhea and hypocobalaminemia that eventually undergo biopsy sampling of the intestinal tract, an effort should be made to also collect ileal samples (e.g., ileocolonoscopy or surgically). Important findings can be missed if tissue samples are exclusively collected from the upper small intestinal tract. Some cats with hyperthyroidism show low serum cobalamin concentrations and thus a tT4 should be measured prior to any invasive diagnostics.

- Folate – is absorbed in the small intestine and can be decreased due to infiltrative mucosal disease (inflammatory, neoplastic, fungal). On the other hand, dysbiosis may also lead to increased serum folate concentrations due to bacterial folate synthesis.
- Pancreatic tests.
  - Feline pancreatic lipase immunoreactivity (fPLI) – increased in pancreatitis. Chronic pancreatitis, enteropathy, and hepatobiliary disease often occur together in cats, a combination often referred to as triaditis.
  - Feline trypsin-like immunoreactivity (fTLI) – decreased in patients with EPI. It should be noted that patients should be fasted for 12–18 h prior to blood draw, as food may falsely increase TLI. TLI may be increased in pancreatitis.
  - Table 5.2 provides a summary of diagnostic testing for cats with chronic diarrhea.

Imaging

- Abdominal ultrasonography may demonstrate bowel wall thickening, abnormal bowel wall layering, GI or extra-GI masses, intussusception, foreign body, ileus, abdominal effusion, hepatobiliary disease, renal disease, or mesenteric lymphadenopathy.
- Survey abdominal radiography may indicate intestinal obstruction, abnormal intestinal pattern, organomegaly, mass, foreign body, pancreatic disease, hepatobiliary disease, urinary disease, or abdominal effusion. Usually very low yield in chronic diarrhea.
- Abdominal radiographs and ultrasound might be normal despite significant diffuse GI disease. If abnormal findings are present, ultrasound can help to determine the best way to proceed. If diffuse mucosal disease is suspected, endoscopy might be the best option to further determine the nature of the disease. Extraluminal lesions, abdominal masses or lesions outside the range of the endoscope warrant surgical biopsies.

Other Diagnostic Tests

Endoscopy

- GI flexible endoscopy allows visualization and biopsy of the intestinal mucosa.
- A flexible endoscope can usually be advanced into the proximal jejunum in cats.
- Targeted biopsies can be taken from normal and abnormal areas.
- Always obtain multiple (8–15) mucosal specimens from each segment/area.
- Minimal recovery time.
- In cases where mixed small and large bowel diarrhea are present, gastroduodenoscopy and ileocolonoscopy should be performed if possible, especially if hypocobalaminemia is present (see section on "Diagnostics – Cobalamin").
- If large bowel signs are exclusively present, limited lower GI scoping might be justified.
- Earlier studies implied that full-thickness biopsies were generally superior to endoscopically derived specimens. However, with the recent advancements in diagnostics, including immunohistochemistry and PCR for receptor rearrangement (PARR), these advantages are no longer evident.

Surgical Biopsy

- A surgical approach is beneficial if:
  - Biopsies of multiple organs (small intestine, lymph nodes, stomach, pancreas, liver) are warranted.
  - Extramural lesions or lesions outside the range of the endoscope (usually mid to distal jejunal) are present.
  - The cat shows signs of intestinal obstruction.
- Full-thickness biopsies of the large intestine are considered to carry a significant risk for dehiscence of the incisional biopsy sites and septic peritonitis.

TABLE 5.2. Testing for cats with chronic diarrhea.

Tests	Parameter	Results that can be seen in cats with chronic diarrhea	Common underlying GI or extra-GI diseases that cause chronic diarrhea associated with this result
CBC	WBC	Stress leukogram	Common due to any disease process including GI disease
		Leukocytosis +/– bands	Systemic infection; bacterial translocation (leaky gut, rupture, foreign body), fungal disease, etc.
		Leukopenia	FeLV, FIV
		Eosinophilia	Parasitism, allergic diseases, eosinophilic enteritis, hypereosinophilic syndrome, hypoadrenocorticism (very rare in cats)
	RBC	Anemia	
		Macrocytic	Hyperthyroidism, FeLV
		Microcytic	GI bleeding, iron deficiency
		Regenerative	GI bleeding
		Nonregenerative	Any chronic disease including GI disease, GI bleeding
	PLT	Thrombocytopenia	FeLV, platelet clumping
		Thrombocytosis	GI bleeding
Chemistry panel	BUN	Increased	Postprandial, GI bleeding
		Decreased	Hepatopathy (shunt)
	Creatinine	Increased	Renal disease – in CKD GI signs usually occur late in the disease process from IRIS stage III upwards with creatinine ≥2.9 mg/dL
		Decreased	Weight/muscle mass loss
	Cholesterol	Increased	Hepatobiliary disease
		Decreased	Maldigestion/malabsorption, hyporexia
	Phosphorus	Increased	Renal disease, hyperthyroidism
		Decreased	Maldigestion/malabsorption
	TP	Increased	Dehydration (albumin and globulin), hyperglobulinemia due to any inflammatory disease and rarely neoplasia
		Decreased	Protein-losing enteropathy (uncommon in cats)
	ALT/ALP	Increased	Primary GI disease, concurrent hepatobiliary disease
	Bilirubin	Increased	Hepatobiliary disease (often concurrent with CE)

TABLE 5.2. *Continued*

Tests	Parameter	Results that can be seen in cats with chronic diarrhea	Common underlying GI or extra-GI diseases that cause chronic diarrhea associated with this result
Urinary tests	USG	<1.020	Renal disease (interpret with BUN, creatinine to evaluate if renal disease is likely to be cause for chronic diarrhea)
	Histoplasma AG test	Positive	Histoplasmosis, blastomycosis
Thyroid tests	Total T4	Increased	Hyperthyroidim
Serologic tests	FeLV ELISA	Positive	Confirm with IFA in low-risk cats
	FIV ELISA	Positive	FIV is rarely the primary cause of chronic diarrhea
	Histoplasma AG test	Positive	Histoplasmosis, blastomycosis
Fecal tests	Direct smear	Protozoal trophozoites	*Cystisospora* sp., *Giardia*, *Toxoplasma*
	Fecal flotation/zinc sulfate flotation (feces collected on three days)	Protozoal trophozoites	*Cystisospora* sp., *Giardia*, *Toxoplasma*, worm eggs
	Rectal scraping	Fungal organisms, algae	*Histoplasma*, *Pythium* (rare), *Prototheca* (rare)
	Giardia (ELISA, PCR, IFA)		*Giardia*
	T. foetus (PCR, culture)		*T. foetus*
	Culture		Bacteria (e.g., *Salmonella* spp., enterotoxic *E. coli*, other Enterobacteriaceae species, *Clostridia* spp.). Usually not the primary cause of chronic diarrhea
GI tests	Cobalamin	Decreased	Infiltrative GI (ileal) disease (inflammatory, neoplastic, fungal), hyperthyroidism, EPI
	Folate	Decreased	Infiltrative GI disease (inflammatory, neoplastic, fungal)
		Increased	Dysbiosis, EPI
Pancreatic tests	fPLI	Increased	Pancreatitis (often concurrent with primary GI ± hepatobiliary disease = triaditis)
	TLI	Increased	Pancreatitis
		Decreased	EPI

AG, antigen; ALP, alkaline phosphatase; ALT, alanine aminotransferase; BUN, blood urea nitrogen; CBC, complete blood count; CE, chronic enteropathy; CKD, chronic kidney disease; ELISA, enzyme-linked immunosorbent assay; EPI, exocrine pancreatic insufficiency; FeLV, feline leukemia virus; FIV, feline immunodeficiency virus; fPLI, feline pancreatic lipase immunoreactivity; GI, gastrointestinal; IFA, indirect fluorescent antibody; IRIS, International Renal Interest Society; PCR, polymerase chain reaction; PLT, platelets; RBC, red blood cells; T3, triiodothyronine; T4, thyroxine; TLI, trypsin-like immunoreactivity; TP, total protein; USG, urine specific gravity; WBC, white blood cells.

Ultrasound-Guided GI Aspiration or Biopsy

- Ultrasound-guided fine-needle aspiration (FNA) can be attempted on some GI lesions (e.g., distinct masses, severely thickened bowel loops, mesenteric lymph nodes, etc.). Cytologic interpretation accuracy is subject to sample quality, expertise, and limitations of the technique.
- Neoplasia or infectious diseases might be diagnosed via FNA. However, the two most common forms of chronic enteropathies, lymphoplasmacytic IBD and small cell lymphoma, cannot be distinguished based on cytology as both diseases encompass mature lymphocytes which might be inflammatory (i.e., polyclonal) or neoplastic (i.e., clonal).
- Ultrasound-guided microcore (true-cut) biopsies on noncavitated lesions (>2 cm in diameter) are performed less frequently.
- Paracentesis of peritoneal fluid for fluid analysis, cytology ± culture is recommended.

Pathologic Findings

- Pathologic findings vary, dependent on the underlying disease and duration. Inflammation in the GI tract can be seen due to various inciting causes within and even outside the GI tract. Generally, biopsies should only be taken after a diligent work-up ruling out extraintestinal and infectious GI diseases as well as diet- and antibiotic-responsive enteropathy. This usually narrows the differential diagnoses down to IBD and neoplastic diseases by the time biopsies are collected. Depending on the extent, duration, and location of the inflammation, mesenteric and abdominal lymphadenopathy may be present. In cats with concurrent hepatobiliary disease and/or pancreatitis, pathologic changes will be present in the liver and pancreas as well.
- IBD – the most common form of IBD is lymphoplasmacytic inflammation, followed by eosinophilic, neutrophilic, and granulomatous IBD (all rare).
- Lymphoplasmacytic enteritis – small, mature lymphocytes and plasma cells dominate the mucosal cellular infiltrate. A diagnosis of lymphoplasmacytic IBD is established if all extraintestinal diseases and intestinal diseases such as infection, diet-responsive and antibiotic-responsive enteropathy as well as alimentary small cell lymphoma have been excluded.
- Eosinophilic enteritis – if eosinophilic enteritis is found, parasitic and allergic disease should again be ruled out before a diagnosis of eosinophilic IBD is made. Rarely, cats suffer from hypereosinophilic syndrome, characterized by severe eosinophilic inflammation of the intestinal mucosa and submucosa, lymph nodes, and sometimes other organs.
- Neutrophilic and granulomatous enteritis – neutrophils and macrophages are usually a negligible component of the inflammatory cell population in IBD. Suppurative colitis is sometimes found in kittens, which is suspected to result from a bacterial infection. Macrophages dominate the picture in granulomatous inflammation and may indicate bacterial (e.g., Mycobacteria) or fungal infection or a reaction to foreign material (foreign body). Suppurative or granulomatous IBD are very rare and a bacterial or fungal cause should always be ruled out again using culture, special stains, and/or fluorescence *in situ* hybridization (FISH).
- Alimentary small cell lymphoma (SCL) – SCL is a common cause of chronic diarrhea in older cats. Small, mature lymphocytes dominate the mucosal cellular infiltrate (epithelium and/or lamina propria) and may extend into the submucosa or even transmurally. However, concurrent inflammation is often present and IBD might progress to lymphoma. This illustrates why it can be difficult for the pathologist to distinguish lymphoplasmacytic enteritis from SCL based on hematoxylin and eosin (H&E) staining alone. In ambiguous cases, advanced diagnostics including immunohistochemistry and PARR should be performed. It also shows why SCL cannot be diagnosed using fine needle aspirates. Small mature lymphocytes ± other inflammatory cells can indicate a reactive or neoplastic process, and thus cannot be distinguished by cytology.

THERAPEUTICS

- The objective of treatment is in most cases to eliminate diarrhea and, if present, other signs of GI disease. Treatment and prognosis are dependent on the underlying disease.
- If no definitive diagnosis is possible, empirical treatment ("diagnostic treatment trial") with diet, pro- and prebiotics, antibiotics, and immunosuppressive drugs in ascending and subsequent order can be performed (see "Diagnostics" and Figure 5.1).
- To establish which treatment worked, do not change more than one treatment at a time.
- In cats with IBD, lymphoma or other neoplastic disease, complete remission and sustained remission may not be possible and flare-ups may occur.

Drug(s) of Choice

Broad-Spectrum Anthelmintics and Antiprotozoal Treatments

- Cats should be dewormed with broad-spectrum anthelmintics regardless of the fecal results, since this technique lacks sensitivity and shedding may be intermittent (Tables 5.3 and 5.4).
- In cases with persistent giardiasis, a combination of fenbendazole at 50 mg/kg once daily with metronidazole at 25 mg/kg BID for five days can be used. If giardiasis persists or relapses, an underlying GI disease should be suspected.

TABLE 5.3. Anthelmintics for cats.

Drug(s)	Target parasites	Route	Veterinary formulation
Emodepside/praziquantel	Roundworms, hookworms, tapeworms	Topical	Profender®
Epsiprantel	Tapeworms	Oral	Cestex®
Imidacloprid/moxidectin	Roundworms, hookworms, *Diroflaria immitis* prevention	Topical	Advantage Multi®
Milbemycin oxime	Roundworms, hookworms, *Dirofilaria immitis* prevention	Oral	Sentinel® (with lufenoron), Trifexis® (with spinosad)
Praziquantel	Tapeworms	Oral	Droncit®
Praziquantel/pyrantel pamoate	Roundworms, hookworms, tapeworms	Oral	Drontal® and generic formulations
Selamectin	Roundworms, hookworms, *Dirofilaria immitis* prevention	Topical	Revolution®

TABLE 5.4. Treatment of protozoan parasites.

Drug*	Dosage	Indication	Administration
Fenbendazole	50 mg/kg PO q 24 h	*Giardia*	5 days
Metronidazole	25 mg/kg PO q 12 h	*Giardia*	7 days
Sulfadimethoxine	50 mg/kg PO q 24 h	*Cystoisospora*	10–14 days
Toltrazuril	15 mg/kg PO q 24 h	*Cystoisospora*	3 days
Ponazuril	30 mg/kg PO	*Cystoisospora*	Single dose
Ronidazole	30 mg/kg PO q 24 h	*T. Foetus*	14 days

*Drugs are not approved for use in cats and/or for the indication.
PO, by mouth (*per os*).

Probiotics

- Scientific studies are lacking but experience shows that probiotics can be very effective in treating chronic diarrhea.
- High-dose, multistrain products seem to have better efficacy.
- Veterinary formulation: Proviable® (combination of pro- and prebiotics; capsules or paste) and others.
- Human formulation with anecdotal efficacy in cats: Visbiome® Vet 1-2 capsules per day. Capsules can be opened and given with food.

Prebiotics

- Substances that induce the growth or activity of microorganisms (e.g., bacteria and fungi) that contribute to the well-being of their host.
- Soluble and insoluble fibers (fructooligosaccharides (FOS), mannan-oligosaccharides (MOS) etc.), often included in high-fiber diets.
- Fiber is fermented by microbiota into different products such as short-chain fatty acids (especially butyrate) with beneficial effects of colonocytes. In addition, fibers induce antiinflammatory cytokines and regulatory T cells that can ameliorate an inflammatory response.
- Psyllium – insoluble fiber source that also forms soluble fiber (gel) in the GI tract. Dose: ¼ teaspoon to a meal, titrate up dependent on response.
- Excessive fiber may induce diarrhea.

Vitamin B Deficiency

- Risk of toxicity is very low as both vitamin B12 and B9 are water-soluble.
- Vitamin B12 – cobalamin.
    - Parenteral: cyanocobalamin 250 µg/cat SQ; weekly injections for six weeks, then one dose a month later, and retesting cobalamin levels one month after the last dose.
    - Oral: 250 µg/cat PO q 24 h for 12 weeks.
    - Concentrations should be supranormal at time of recheck. Most cats need indefinite treatment (serum concentrations will fall without supplementation in most cats).
- Vitamin B9 – folate/folic acid: 200–400 µg/cat q 24 h.

Appetite Stimulants and Antiemetics

- May be tried in cats with concurrent hypo- to anorexia as a short-term solution; exclude intestinal obstruction first.
- Mirtazapine (atypical antidepressant, appetite stimulant) – 3.75 mg/cat (¼ of a 15 mg tablet) PO every three days, or ¼ of a 7.5 mg tablet every 24–48 h.
- Maropitant (neurokinin-1 (NK-1) receptor antagonist, antiemetic) – 1 mg/kg SQ or PO q 24 h.

Antibiotics

- After extraintestinal and parasitic causes for chronic diarrhea have been excluded, an antibiotic trial may be performed with the following drugs.
    - Metronidazole 10–15 mg/kg q 12 h.
    - Tylosin 10–40 mg/kg (~1/16 tsp/cat) q 12 h.
- If the patient responds, administer until clinical signs resolve, then taper to lowest effective dose.
- Cats that respond initially and relapse should receive further work-up for other causes of chronic diarrhea.

Immunosuppressive Therapy

- May be used if a definitive diagnosis cannot be established (Table 5.5).
- Owners should be informed that interpretation of intestinal biopsies can be challenging or precluded once steroids or other immunosuppressive drugs have been used empirically.
- Discontinue treatment at least two weeks prior to biopsy sampling.

TABLE 5.5. Immunosuppressive therapy for cats with chronic diarrhea.

Drug*	Dosage	Common side effects
Prednisolone	1–2 mg/kg q 12 h, taper to lowest effective dose	Polyuria, polydipsia, diabetes mellitus, urinary tract infection
Budesonide	1 mg/cat PO q 24 h, taper to lowest effective dose	Same as prednisolone; considered to have fewer systemic effects
Cyclosporine	1–4 mg/kg PO q 12–24 h	Nausea, vomiting, anorexia
Chlorambucil	For refractory IBD ± steroids: >4 kg: start at 2 mg/cat q 48 h <4 kg: start at 2 mg/cat q 72 h For SCL different regimes described ± steroids: - high-pulse dose: 15 mg/m² PO q 24 h for 4 days, repeat every 3 weeks - lower pulse dose: 20 mg/ m² PO once every 2 weeks - 2 mg/cat q 48–72 h	Myelosuppression

*Drugs are not approved for use in cats.
IBD, inflammatory bowel disease; PO, by mouth (*per os*); SCL, small cell lymphoma.

Precautions/Interactions

- Anticholinergics exacerbate most types of chronic diarrhea and should not be used for empiric treatment.
- Opiate antidiarrheals such as diphenoxylate and loperamide can cause hyperactivity and respiratory depression in cats and should not be used for more than three days.

 # THERAPEUTICS

Nursing Care

- Most cats with chronic diarrhea do not require fluid therapy unless they experience an acute exacerbation or are systemically affected.
- Hyporectic cats that do not respond to antiemetics and appetite stimulants, are anorectic for more than three days or that are systemically ill need an (esophageal) feeding tube (Figure 5.2).
- Hyporectic cats should never be force fed. Force feeding can result in long-term food aversion.

Diet

- A diet trial with a hypoallergenic diet should be performed before antibiotics or immunosuppressive drugs are used or more invasive tests are performed. The diet is chosen based on the previous dietary history and should not contain a meat and carbohydrate source that have been fed previously (Table 5.6).
- Prefer prescription diets to over-the-counter (OTC) hypoallergenic diets, as the latter have been shown to contain meat sources other than those on the label.
- Choose a diet that has a high owner and cat compliance (i.e., that is consistently fed by the owner and consumed by the cat).

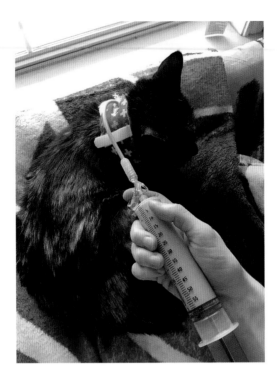

■ **Fig. 5.2.** Cat with an esophageal feeding tube that is fed in the home environment.Placing a feeding tube is easy with minimal surgical equipment and skills required. Owners usually learn how to handle the feeding tube very quickly and cats can be fed comfortably at home. Tube feeding ensures supplementation of required calories, allows for time to investigate the underlying cause of GI signs, allows for treatment to start working, and prevents complications such as hepatic lipidosis. In addition, new diet and medication can be given through the tube without further stressing the cat. Source: Courtesy of Dr Kimberly Anderson.

TABLE 5.6. Hypoallergenic diets for treatment of cats with chronic diarrhea.		
Diet type	**Pros**	**Cons**
Hydrolyzed	Can be used in patients with an extensive dietary history	Possibility of persistent immunogenicity
	Can be used as a second or third choice after failure of other diet trials	Limited availability of treats
Novel protein	Better acceptance in some cats Treats can be bought or home-made (venison, rabbit, etc.)	As commercial cat food increasingly contains "exotic meats" (e.g., duck, venison, etc.), it might be difficult to find a meat source the cat has not had contact with

■ High-fiber diet and/or the addition of fiber might be beneficial in cats with exclusively large bowel diarrhea.
■ In cats with fixed food preferences, try to introduce hypoallergenic diet gradually over 3–4 weeks by replacing 25% of the current diet with the hypoallergenic diet each week. If food intake drops below 70%, slow the transition or choose a different diet.

COMMENTS

Client Education

Clients with cats on a dietary trial should be instructed to exclusively feed this diet and prevent the cat from accessing food from other cats in the household or the neighborhood. Appropriate treats may be given (see section on "Diet").

Patient Monitoring

- Assess changes in frequency and severity of diarrhea and body weight.
- Resolution usually occurs within 2–3 weeks following successful implementation of dietary therapy; consider reevaluating the diagnosis if diarrhea does not resolve.

Prevention/Avoidance

- Regular deworming of outdoor cats.
- Feeding a balanced, high-quality diet.
- Appropriate hygiene (e.g., number of litter boxes = number of cats/household +1).

Possible Complications

The classification of enteropathies into diet-responsive, antibiotic-responsive, and steroid/immunosuppressive-responsive enteropathy (IBD) is an attempt to classify diseases and understand underlying mechanisms scientifically. However, the disease course is often progressive and can transition from one category to another. In addition, IBD might progress into SCL. Therefore, patients that relapse after an initial response may need to be assessed again.

Expected Course and Prognosis

The prognosis is mostly dependent on the underlying disease. The median survival time for cats with IBD is not well documented. In contrast, the median survival for cats with alimentary SCL is reported to be between three and almost four years and most cats have a very good quality of life. Considering that SCL mostly occurs in older cats, the overall prognosis for SCL is very good.

Synonyms

The terms IBD and steroid-responsive enteropathy are often used interchangeably.

Abbreviations

- BCS = body condition score
- CE = chronic enteropathy
- CKD = chronic kidney disease
- ELISA = enzyme-linked immunosorbent assay
- EPI = exocrine pancreatic insufficiency
- FeLV = feline leukemia virus.
- FIP = feline infectious peritonitis
- FISH = fluorescence *in situ* hybridization
- FIV = feline immunodeficiency virus
- FNA = fine needle aspirate
- FOS = fructooligosaccharides
- fPLI = feline pancreatic lipase immunoreactivity
- fT4 = free T4

- fTLI = feline trypsin-like immunoreactivity
- GI = gastrointestinal
- H&E – hematoxylin and eosin stain
- IBD = inflammatory bowel disease
- IBS = irritable bowel syndrome
- IFA = indirect fluorescent antibody
- IRIS = International Renal Interest Society
- MOS = mannan-oligosaccharides
- OTC = over the counter
- PARR = PCR for receptor rearrangement
- PCR = polymerase chain reaction
- SCL = small cell lymphoma
- T3 = triiodothyronine
- tT4 = total T4 (thyroxine)
- USG = urine specific gravity

See Also

- Cobalamin Deficiency
- Diarrhea, Antibiotic Responsive
- Food Reactions (Gastrointestinal), Adverse
- Gastroenteritis, Eosinophilic
- Gastroenteritis, Lymphocytic-Plasmacytic
- Gastrointestinal Lymphoma – Feline
- Inflammatory Bowel Disease
- Fiber-Responsive Large Bowel Diarrhea
- Nutritional Approach to Chronic Enteropathies
- Pancreatitis – Feline

Suggested Reading

Jergens AE. Feline idiopathic inflammatory bowel disease: what we know and what remains to be unraveled. J Feline Med Surg 2012;14:445–458.

Jergens AE. Current veterinary therapy: antibiotic responsive enteropathy. In: Current Veterinary Therapy XV. St Louis: Elsevier Saunders, 2013.

Pope KV, Tun AE, McNeill CJ. Outcome and toxicity assessment of feline small cell lymphoma: 56 cases (2000–2010). J Vet Med Sci 2015;1(2):51–62.

Willard MD, Mansell J, Fosgate GT, et al. Effect of sample quality on the sensitivity of endoscopic biopsy for detecting gastric and duodenal lesions in dogs and cats. J Vet Intern Med 2008;22(5):1084–1089.

Author: Sina Marsilio Dr.med.vet., DVM, DACVIM (SAIM), DECVIM-CA

Chapter 6

Dyschezia and Tenesmus

DEFINITION/OVERVIEW

- **Dyschezia** – difficulty or pain while defecating.
- **Tenesmus** – recurrent inclination to defecate seen as straining to defecate.
- **Hematochezia** – fresh undigested blood in or on the stool originating from the colon, rectum or anus.

ETIOLOGY/PATHOPHYSIOLOGY

Any disease affecting the health of the colon, rectum, anus, and anal sacs has the potential to cause dyschezia and tenesmus. These diseases include (but are not limited to) inflammation, neoplasia, infection, foreign body, etc. (Figures 6.1 and 6.2).

Systems Affected

- Gastrointestinal.
- Hematologic – chronic blood loss from hematochezia may lead to a microcytic, hypochromic, nonregenerative anemia.

SIGNALMENT/HISTORY

- Any dog or cat of any age or breed may be affected.
- Perianal fistulae – German shepherd.
- Histiocytic ulcerative colitis – boxers, French bulldogs, and other associated breeds.

Risk Factors

- Ingestion of hair, bone, foreign material may contribute to constipation and subsequent dyschezia.
- Environmental factors such as a dirty litter pan, infrequent outside walks may contribute to constipation and subsequent dyschezia.

Historical Findings

- Tenesmus – straining to defecate with repeated attempts at defecation.
- Increased frequency with a decreased stool volume. Cats may be noted going in and out of the litter box frequently.
- Vocalizing while defecating.
- Avoidance or decreased frequency of defecation due to pain which may lead to constipation.

Blackwell's Five-Minute Veterinary Consult Clinical Companion: Small Animal Gastrointestinal Diseases,
First Edition. Edited by Jocelyn Mott and Jo Ann Morrison.
© 2019 John Wiley & Sons, Inc. Published 2019 by John Wiley & Sons, Inc.
Companion website: www.fiveminutevet.com/gastrointestinal

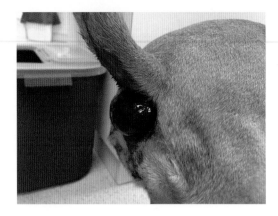

■ **Fig. 6.1.** Rectal prolapse secondary to rectal adenocarcinoma.

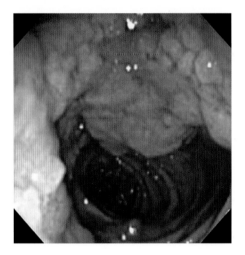

■ **Fig. 6.2.** Endoscopic view of rectal adenocarcinoma causing tenesmus in a dog.

■ Mucoid, bloody diarrhea with a marked increase in frequency and scant fecal volume in patients with colitis.
■ Scooting may be associated with anal sac disease.
■ It is important to inquire about urination. Stranguria can be easily confused with tenesmus.

 CLINICAL FEATURES

■ Rectal exam – palpating for lymphadenopathy, strictures, masses/polyps, foreign bodies, prostatomegaly, perineal hernias.
  • Anal sacs should be expressed so they can be fully evaluated.
  • Evaluate for the presence of melena, hematochezia, hard stool (constipation), mucus, etc.
■ Perianal fistulas may be visualized as bloody or painful fistulous tracts around the anus.
■ Anal occlusion with matted hair and feces occurs with pseudocoprostasis.

DIFFERENTIAL DIAGNOSIS

- Rectal/anal disease.
  - Perianal fistulas.
  - Rectal prolapse.
  - Perianal hernia.
  - Rectal stricture.
  - Benign rectal polyps.
  - Proctitis.
  - Neoplasia (lymphoma, adenocarcinoma, etc.).
  - Pelvic fractures.
  - Anal sacculitis.
  - Anal sac neoplasia.
  - Pseudocoprostasis.
- Colonic disease.
  - Infection/parasitism.
    - Bacterial – *Campylobacter*, *Clostridium perfringens*, *Salmonella*, etc.
    - Parasitic – whipworm, hookworm, coccidia.
    - Fungal (and other) – *Histoplasma*, pythiosis, parvovirus.
  - Inflammation.
    - Inflammatory bowel disease.
    - Stress colitis.
    - Food-responsive enteropathy.
  - Neoplasia.
    - Adenocarcinoma.
    - Lymphoma.
    - Other.
  - Idiopathic megacolon.
  - Histiocytic ulcerative colitis.
  - Chronic idiopathic large bowel diarrhea (CILBD).
- Trauma (pelvic fracture, bite wounds, etc.).
- Prostatic disease.
- Dysuria, stranguria, or hematuria.
- Dystocia – differentiate with history and imaging.

 DIAGNOSTICS

- When working up dyschezia, it is imperative to first differentiate stranguria from tenesmus. Owners see straining and frequently assume that animals are straining to defecate.
- Focal and diffuse disease may cause similar clinical signs. Rectal exam may help to localize focal rectal or anal disease whereas increased frequency and change in consistency of stool may indicate colonic disease.
- Stool that is thin or ribbon-like in shape may indicate prostatic disease or neoplasms that may be intraluminal or extraluminal, reducing the rectal diameter.

Complete Blood Count/Biochemistry/Urinalysis

- Frequently unremarkable.
- Acute blood loss may be appreciated as a regenerative anemia while varying degrees of chronicity may be associated with iron deficiency and a microcytic, hypochromic, nonregenerative anemia.

- Inflammatory leukogram (neutrophilia, etc.) may be appreciated with inflammatory or infectious disease.
- Urinalysis – helps rule out urinary disease leading to stranguria and hematuria.

Other Laboratory Testing

- Fecal flotation/additional testing such as wet mounts, antigen testing, polymerase chain reaction (PCR), etc. – rule out gastrointestinal parasitism.

Imaging

- Abdominal/pelvic radiographs – identify possible masses, pelvic fractures, foreign body, megacolon, etc.
- Ultrasonography may further characterize prostatic disease or caudal abdominal masses; pelvic masses and distal colon may not be visible due to fecal material and the bony structures of the pelvis. In these cases, abdominal computed tomography may be beneficial.

Other Diagnostic Procedures

- Colonoscopy/proctoscopy with biopsies to evaluate for inflammatory or neoplastic disease. Lesions may be localized; evaluation of the entire large intestine, including the cecum, is important to help determine the source of bleeding.
- Representative biopsies should be taken endoscopically of the colon. This is vital in a macroscopically normal colon.

Pathologic Findings

Gross and microscopic findings will be dependent upon the underlying etiology for the clinical signs.

 ## THERAPEUTICS

- Determined by the underlying cause.
- Colonic strictures secondary to unknown trauma, foreign bodies, and neoplasms can be managed via surgical excision or balloon catheter dilation.
- Consider laxatives (lactulose, polyethylene glycol) to ease defecation and discomfort in animals with colorectal strictures or masses.
- Colorectal masses are best removed surgically or via endoscopy (snare and cauterization for polyps).

Drugs of Choice

- Antibiotics – bacterial infection (e.g., anal sac abscess).
  - Amoxicillin/clavulanic acid: 15 mg/kg PO q 12 h for 7–10 days for anal sacculitis.
  - Metronidazole: 10–15 mg/kg q 12 h is commonly used with hematochezia to fight against bacterial translocation.
  - Enrofloxacin: 5–10 mg/kg q 24 h for 6–8 weeks for histiocytic ulcerative colitis.
- Antiinflammatory drugs – sulfasalazine or prednisone (dogs) and prednisolone (cats) if colitis, eosinophilic or inflammatory bowel disease is present.
- Immune modulation – cyclosporine (5 mg/kg q 12 h for 3–4 months with gradual taper thereafter) for dogs with perianal fistulas.
- Laxatives – lactulose, 1 mL/4.5 kg PO q 8–12 h to effect.
  - Docusate sodium or docusate calcium – dogs 50–100 mg PO q 12–24 h; cats 50 mg PO q 12–24 h.
  - Polyethylene glycol – 2.5–5 mL per cat PO q 8–12 h to effect (soft, regular stool).

- Prokinetic – indicated for megacolon in cats. Typically used in conjunction with lactulose and dietary therapy. Obstructive disease should be ruled out prior to use; cisapride – 5 mg/cat PO q 12 h.

Precautions/Interactions

- In dogs with perianal fistulas, combination medication therapy (e.g., cyclosporine and ketoconazole) has been described. Due to involvement of the cytochrome p450 enzyme system, numerous drug interactions are possible.
- Aggressive therapy with laxatives may result in profound diarrhea, with resultant dehydration and electrolyte imbalances.

Alternative Drugs

Some patients will respond to empiric deworming or a dietary trial. In cases of more severe immune-mediated disease, additional immunosuppressives may be warranted.

Appropriate Health Care

If hemorrhage associated with dyschezia/tenesmus is profound, anemia may be severe and warrant aggressive supportive measures. Patients that are prescribed immune-suppressive medication may be at risk for opportunistic infections. Clients should be counseled in ways to minimize risk.

Nursing Care

- Depending on the etiology, some patients may be in significant discomfort/pain and may warrant targeted analgesic therapy. Caution should always be exercised when handling painful patients.
- If dyschezia/tenesmus has resulted in constipation/obstipation, hospitalization for fluid therapy and electrolyte support, and more aggressive measures to reinstate normal colonic function may be necessary.

Diet

- Dyschezia due to constipation, luminal narrowing – diets high in soluble fiber are preferred to help soften stool. Avoid agents that cause increased fecal bulk (insoluble fiber).
- Diarrhea associated with colitis – insoluble fiber may help increase bulk to stool.

Activity

Activity does not need to be restricted in most cases. Note that analgesic therapy should not be withheld in an effort to restrict activity.

Surgical Considerations

Surgery may be recommended in cases of neoplasia or colorectal stricture (from any etiology). Note that surgical manipulation of the colon/rectum may be complicated, has a higher risk of infection/contamination, and may be associated with fecal incontinence. Consultation with a board-certified veterinary surgeon is recommended.

 COMMENTS

Client Education

Ensure clients understand the difference between tenesmus and stranguria. Patients showing clinical signs should be evaluated as soon as possible. Patients with surgical disease may be at risk for fecal incontinence which may be permanent.

Patient Monitoring

Dependent upon underlying etiology and medical therapy prescribed. Patients showing clinical signs of tenesmus/dyschezia should be evaluated as quickly as possible.

Prevention/Avoidance

Minimize parasitism and foreign body ingestions.

Possible Complications

- Surgical resection of colorectal tumors, stricture, and anal sacs may lead to lifelong fecal incontinence.
- Secondary megacolon may occur if obstipation is severe and long term.
- Obstipation may become life threatening. If severe constipation/obstipation is prolonged, the integrity of the colon becomes impaired which may result in peritonitis and sepsis.

Expected Course and Prognosis

Depend upon etiology and individual patient response to therapy and medications.

Abbreviations

- CILBD = chronic idiopathic large bowel diarrhea
- PCR = polymerase chain reaction

See Also

- Inflammatory Bowel Disease
- Colitis/Proctitis
- Colitis, Histiocytic Ulcerative
- Colonic Neoplasia, Benign
- Colonic Neoplasia, Malignant
- Constipation and Obstipation
- Fiber-Responsive Large Bowel Diarrhea
- Megacolon
- Nutritional Approach to Chronic Enteropathies
- Rectal Stricture
- Rectoanal Polyps

Suggested Reading

Case VL. Melena and hematochezia. In: Textbook of Veterinary Internal Medicine, 7th edn. St Louis: Elsevier, 2010, pp. 203–206.

Foley P. Constipation, tenesmus, dyschezia and fecal incontinence. In: Textbook of Veterinary Internal Medicine, 7th edn. St Louis: Elsevier, 2010, pp. 206–209.

Webb CB. Anal-rectal disease. In: Bonagura JD, Twedt DC, eds. Current Veterinary Therapy XIV. St Louis: Elsevier, 2009, pp. 527–531.

Acknowledgments: The author and editors acknowledge the previous contribution of Dr Stanley L. Marks.

Author: Alana Redfern DVM, MSc, DACVIM

Chapter 7

Dysphagia

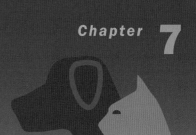

DEFINITION/OVERVIEW

- Dysphagia refers to difficulty swallowing which may elicit clinical signs such as dropping food or water, gagging, regurgitation, coughing, etc.
- Dysphagia is classified based on its anatomic origin: oral, pharyngeal, cricopharyngeal, and esophageal.
- Pharyngeal and cricopharyngeal dysphagia are the most common areas of dysphagia but up to one-third of dysphagic patients may have more than one area affected.
- Odynophagia refers to painful swallowing and is most commonly seen in association with esophageal disease (foreign bodies, severe esophagitis, etc.).
- Esophageal dysphagia is discussed in the chapters on Megaesophagus and Regurgitation.
- Morphologic/structural (foreign bodies, strictures, masses, etc.) and functional (incoordination, weakness due to neuromuscular disease, etc.) problems can cause dysphagia.

ETIOLOGY/PATHOPHYSIOLOGY

- The *oral preparatory phase* is voluntary and begins with the prehension and maceration of food and the formation of a bolus with the teeth and tongue. Abnormalities of the oral preparatory phase usually are associated with dental disease, xerostomia, weakness of diseases of the lips (cranial nerves V and VII), tongue (cranial nerve XII), and cheeks (cranial nerves V and VII).
- Oral dysphagia is typically diagnosed by physical examination and watching the patient eat.
- The *pharyngeal phase* begins as the bolus reaches the base of the tongue and pharynx. The bolus mechanically stimulates the caudal pharynx. Rostral to caudal pharyngeal contractions propel the bolus caudally.
- Abnormalities of the pharyngeal phase of swallowing are associated with pharyngeal weakness secondary to neuropathies or myopathies, pharyngeal tumors or foreign bodies, or cricopharyngeus muscle disorders.
- The *cricopharyngeal phase* is defined by the passage of the bolus through the upper esophageal sphincter (UES). It involves synchrony of the relaxation of the cricopharyngeus muscle and contraction of the pharyngeal musculature that allow bolus passage through the UES.
- Elevation of the soft palate and larynx and retroflexion of the epiglottis protect the nasal passages, vocal folds, and airways respectively.
- There are two forms of disease.
  - Deficits of opening or closure of the cricopharyngeus (achalasia).
  - Incoordination between cricopharyngeal relation and pharyngeal contraction.

Blackwell's Five-Minute Veterinary Consult Clinical Companion: Small Animal Gastrointestinal Diseases,
First Edition. Edited by Jocelyn Mott and Jo Ann Morrison.
© 2019 John Wiley & Sons, Inc. Published 2019 by John Wiley & Sons, Inc.
Companion website: www.fiveminutevet.com/gastrointestinal

- The oropharyngeal phase repeats several times, causing successive swallows.
- The *esophageal phase* is involuntary and begins with relaxation of the UES and movement of the bolus into the esophagus down and through the lower esophageal sphincter (LES).

Systems Affected

- Gastrointestinal.
- Nervous.
- Neuromuscular.
- Respiratory.

SIGNALMENT/HISTORY

- Dog and cat (rare).
- Congenital disorders that cause dysphagia (e.g., cricopharyngeal achalasia, cleft palate, hiatal hernia) are usually diagnosed in animals <1 year old.
- Puppies are more likely to have congenital abnormalities such as cricopharyngeal achalasia, congenital megaesophagus, vascular ring anomalies, and cleft palates.
- Vascular ring anomalies are likely to present with regurgitation when weaned onto solid food at 6–8 weeks.
- Puppies with cleft palates are frequently diagnosed while nursing as milk is refluxed through the nose.
- Puppies with cricopharyngeal achalasia typically present for repeated swallowing, gagging, and retching during swallowing. May have nasal reflux of water, milk or food.
- Acquired esophageal dysmotility and pharyngeal weakness is more common in older patients.
- Older dogs, in particular Labrador retrievers, are more likely to have esophageal dysmotility secondary to a polyneuropathy, etc.
- Oral neoplasia (male>female) – cocker spaniel, boxer, Weimaraner, golden retriever, German shepherd, German shorthair, Gordon setter, miniature poodle, chow chow.
- Oropharyngeal dysphagia – bouvier des Flandres, golden retriever, Labrador retriever.
- Oral eosinophilic granuloma – Siberian husky.
- Incidence is variable depending on underlying etiology.
- Up to one-third of dogs with dysphagia have multiple areas of dysfunction on videofluoroscopy.
- Esophageal dysmotility accounts for nearly half of dysphagic patients. Megaesophagus is one of the most common causes of dysphagia in dogs.
- Cats – oral dysphagia is common secondary to tumors, dental disease, etc. Oropharyngeal dysfunction in cats is rarely diagnosed.

Historical Findings

- Drooling (due to pain or inability to swallow saliva), gagging, ravenous appetite, repeated or exaggerated attempts at swallowing, swallowing with the head in an abnormal position (neck extended, bent, etc), excessive mandibular movement, nasal discharge (due to nasal reflux of food and liquids into the nasopharynx), coughing (due to aspiration), regurgitation, painful swallowing, and occasionally reluctance to eat and weight loss are all possible. If the tongue is not functioning normally, problems with prehension and mastication may be seen such as food dropping, etc.
- Determine onset and progression. Foreign bodies cause acute dysphagia; pharyngeal dysphagia may be chronic and insidious in onset.

CLINICAL FEATURES

- A complete physical exam, neurologic exam, sedated oropharyngeal exam and observing the patient eating and drinking are necessary when diagnosing dysphagia.
  - Physical exam – evaluate for signs of a generalized neuromuscular disorder. Muscle weakness, atrophy, stiffness.
  - Neurologic exam – cranial nerves; assess tongue and jaw tone and function. Identify any signs of neuromuscular disease, decreased or absent spinal reflexes. Gag reflex – presence or absence does not correlate with the ability to swallow.
  - Oropharyngeal exam – evaluate laryngeal function. Rule out morphologic abnormalities such as dental disease, foreign bodies, inflammatory lesions, cleft palate, glossal abnormalities, and oropharyngeal tumors.
  - Observation of eating (canned and kibble) – helps to localize the problem to oral, pharyngeal, or esophageal dysphagia.
- Oral dysphagia – modified eating behavior (e.g., dropping food, tilting head, difficulty opening or closing mouth). Difficulty with prehension and bolus formation. Pain and food packed in the buccal folds suggest oral dysphagia.
- Pharyngeal dysphagia.
  - Prehension of food is normal.
  - Repeated swallowing is typical of pharyngeal dysphagia. Excessive gagging and food falling out of the mouth may occur.
- Cricopharyngeal dysphagia.
  - Repetitive nonproductive swallowing is common. Patients frequently regurgitate or spit out food.
  - Gag reflex and prehension are normal.
  - Nasal reflux is commonly observed when food hits the closed UES.
- Esophageal dysphagia.
  - Most common causes include esophageal dysmotility secondary to megaesophagus, esophagitis, esophageal stricture, esophageal foreign bodies.
  - Diagnosis made with survey radiographs of the thorax and neck followed by videofluoroscopy.
- Gastroesophageal dysphagia – most common cause is a sliding hiatal hernia that is often associated with gastroesophageal reflux and subsequent esophagitis.

 ## DIFFERENTIAL DIAGNOSIS

Oral Dysphagia

- Mechanical abnormalities may be associated with dental disease, neoplasia, masticatory muscle myositis, mandibular fractures, temporomandibular joint disorders.
- Inflammatory diseases (ulceration, stomatitis, glossitis, eosinophilic granuloma, severe lymphadenopathy, sialoadenitis, oral abscess, etc.) may be associated with pain causing reluctance to chew, form a bolus or swallow.
- Neurologic abnormalities may be associated with cranial nerve disorders affecting CN V (trigeminal neuritis etc.) or CN VII. Myasthenia gravis and other acquired diseases may affect neurologic function.

Cricopharyngeal Dysphagia

- Mechanical abnormalities associated with pharyngeal neoplasia, foreign body, etc.
- Inflammatory disease causing pharyngeal weakness: inflammation, immune-mediated polymyositis, infectious myositis (*Toxoplasma, Neospora*, viral papillomatosis, etc.).

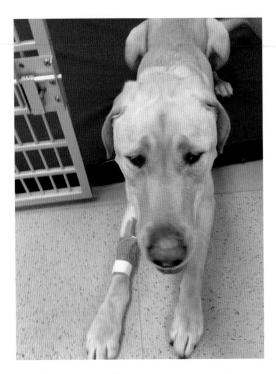

■ **Fig. 7.1.** Risus sardonicus – the characteristic facial appearance in a dog with tetanus causing severe dysphagia.

- Neurologic/neuromuscular – polymyositis, polyneuropathies, neuromuscular junctionopathies (myasthenia gravis, botulism, tetanus, tick bite paralysis), muscular dystrophy, rabies, hypothyroidism. Other central nervous system (CNS) diseases affecting brainstem or peripheral nerves (Figure 7.1).
- Cricopharyngeal achalasia – unknown etiology; neuromuscular disorder in young dogs where there is asynchrony of UES relaxation during pharyngeal contraction.

Esophageal Dysphagia

- Must differentiate regurgitation (passive) from vomiting (active).
- Mechanical abnormalities may lead to obstruction or dysmotility: megaesophagus, neoplasia, foreign body, stricture, vascular ring anomalies, parasitic nodules (*Spirocerca lupi*).
- Inflammatory disease – esophagitis is a common cause of dysmotility. Esophagitis can be a consequence of vomiting, gastroesophageal reflux (primary and secondary to general anesthesia).

DIAGNOSTICS

Complete Blood Count/Biochemistry/Urinalysis

- May be within normal limits.
- Inflammatory conditions – may cause a leukocytosis.
- Myopathy may be evident with increased creatinine kinase.

Other Laboratory Testing

- Acetylcholine receptor antibody serology – myasthenia gravis.
- Type 2M muscle antibody serology – masticatory muscle myositis.

- T4, free T4, TSH, antithyroglobulin antibodies – hypothyroidism.
- Feline immunodeficiency virus/feline leukemia virus (FIV/FeLV).

Imaging

- Survey radiographs of neck and thorax in all dysphagic animals once oral dysphagia has been ruled out. Beneficial in establishing aspiration pneumonia.
- Barium esophagram (liquid barium administered orally followed by immediate thoracic radiographs) may be beneficial in diagnosing esophageal disease (mass, stricture, etc.). A normal esophagram does not exclude esophageal dysmotility.
- Videofluoroscopy with barium is necessary to fully evaluate pharyngeal, cricopharyngeal, and esophageal function and proper coordination of the upper and lower esophageal sphincters.
- Computed tomography (CT) and/or magnetic resonance imaging (MRI) may be necessary to further evaluate suspected masses.

Other Diagnostic Procedures

- Endoscopy of the pharynx, esophagus, upper and lower esophageal sphincter – retroflexion of the endoscope over the soft palate to evaluate the nasopharynx.
- Electromyography – to determine presence of a myopathy.
- Repetitive nerve stimulation/Tensilon test (edrophonium chloride 0.1–0.2 mg/kg IV) for suspected myasthenia gravis.
- Cerebrospinal fluid analysis in patients with a CNS disorder.

Zoonotic Potential

Rabies – if a dysphagic animal dies of rapidly progressive neurologic disease, submit the head to a qualified laboratory designated by the local or state health department for rabies examination.

 THERAPEUTICS

- When possible, treating the underlying cause of the dysphagia is central to the successful management and resolution of signs.
- Cricopharyngeal myotomy appears to be beneficial for cricopharyngeal achalasia.

Drug(s) of Choice

Treatment for dysphagia is directed at the underlying cause.

Precautions/Interactions

Use barium sulfate for radiographs/videofluoroscopy with caution as patients with dysphagia are at higher risk of aspiration.

Nursing Care

- Most patients can be managed on an outpatient basis if clinically appropriate.
- Complicating factors such as aspiration pneumonia, CNS disease, generalized severe weakness, etc. may warrant hospitalization, supportive care, and targeted therapies.
- Supportive modalities may be necessary in the case of aspiration pneumonia (oxygen, coupage, etc.).
- Appropriate nursing care is imperative, particularly for patients with generalized weakness due to myopathies, neuromuscular junctionopathies: rotating position, good padding, and physical therapy.

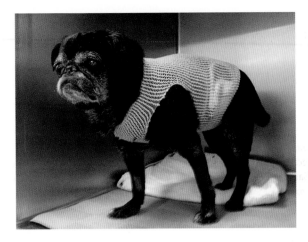

■ **Fig. 7.2.** A percutaneous endoscopic gastrotomy tube (PEG) tube in a dog with cricopharyngeal dysphagia.

Diet

- Developing an appropriate and complete nutritional strategy for all dysphagic patients should be a priority.
- Elevated feedings and maintaining the pet in an upright and elevated (vertical) position during and for 10–15 mins post feeding may be beneficial; however, the long-term benefits are questionable.
- When oral feedings are not tolerated, a feeding tube (gastrotomy/percutaneous endoscopic gastrotomy (PEG) tube) should be placed to maintain adequate hydration, nutrition, and medication administration (Figure 7.2).
- Cricopharyngeal dysphagia patients may tolerate dry kibble over canned/moist foods.

Surgical Considerations

Cricopharyngeal myotomy may benefit patients with cricopharyngeal dysphagia/achalasia; a correct diagnosis is essential, using videofluoroscopy before surgery.

 COMMENTS

Client Education

Clients should be taught to monitor for signs of possible aspiration pneumonia (mucopurulent nasal discharge, respiratory rate, coughing, dyspnea, tachypnea).

Possible Complications

- Aspiration pneumonia – daily monitoring of respiratory rate and effort is recommended.
- Malnutrition/dehydration – frequent reassessment of nutrition plan and hydration status.

Expected Course and Prognosis

Variable, dependent on the cause.

Abbreviations

- CN = cranial nerve
- CNS = central nervous system
- CT = computed tomography
- FeLV = feline leukemia virus
- FIV = feline immunodeficiency virus
- LES = lower esophageal sphincter
- MRI = magnetic resonance imaging
- PEG = percutaneous endoscopic gastrotomy
- UES = upper esophageal sphincter

See Also

- Cricopharyngeal Achalasia
- Megaesophagus
- Regurgitation
- Nutritional Approach to Gastroesophageal Reflux Disease and Megaesophagus
- Phenobarbital Responsive Sialadenosis
- Sialadenitis

Suggested Reading

Kook PH. Gastroesophageal reflux. In: Bonagura JD, Twedt DC, eds. Kirk's Current Veterinary Therapy XV. St Louis: Elsevier Saunders, 2014, pp. 501–504.

Marks SL. Oropharyngeal dysphagia. In: Bonagura JD, Twedt DC, eds. Kirk's Current Veterinary Therapy XV. St Louis: Elsevier Saunders, 2014, pp. 495–500.

Washabau, Robert J., and Michael J. Day. Dysphagia and gagging. In: Canine & Feline Gastroenterology. St. Louis: Elsevier Saunders, 2013, pp. 114–117.

Acknowledgments: The author and editors acknowledge the previous contribution of Dr Stanley L. Marks.

Author: Alana Redfern DVM, MSc, DACVIM

Flatulence

 ## DEFINITION/OVERVIEW

- Excessive formation of gases in the stomach or intestinal tract. Eructation is the passage of gas from the stomach through the mouth, while flatus refers to the gas released through the anus.

 ## ETIOLOGY/PATHOPHYSIOLOGY

- Often results from a diet change or indiscretion but may herald a more serious gastrointestinal (GI) disease.
- Swallowed air (aerophagia) and the bacterial fermentation of nutrients are the main sources of gastrointestinal gas; less significant sources include the interaction of gastric acid and pancreatic/salivary bicarbonate and diffusion of gases from the blood.
- Poorly digestible diets that escape intestinal assimilation, and are therefore available for colonic fermentation, and diets that liberate odiferous gases are associated with flatulence; these include slowly absorbed or nonabsorbable oligosaccharides (wholegrains, soybeans, beans, and peas), spoiled food, high-fat diets, milk products, and spices.
- Fiber-containing foods contribute to flatus indirectly through reduced dry matter digestibility and directly by fermentation of the fiber in the colon.
- Dogs and cats are lactose intolerant; a dietary lactose concentration of 1.5 g/kg/day (11 g lactose in 1 cup of milk) may produce flatus and diarrhea.
- A rapid change in diet or an increase in the concentration of a dietary component, especially carbohydrate or fiber, may cause flatus during a period of intestinal adaptation.
- Protein maldigestion is often responsible for production of malodorous gases.
- Disease states causing malassimilation of nutrients (such as protein-losing enteropathies in dogs or inflammatory bowel disease), making them available for colonic fermentation, can cause flatus.

Systems Affected

Gastrointestinal.

 ## SIGNALMENT/HISTORY

- Common complaint in dogs; rare in cats.
- Excessive aerophagia is seen in brachycephalic breeds, sporting dogs, and those with gluttonous/competitive eating behavior.
- Can occur at any age.

Blackwell's Five-Minute Veterinary Consult Clinical Companion: Small Animal Gastrointestinal Diseases,
First Edition. Edited by Jocelyn Mott and Jo Ann Morrison.
© 2019 John Wiley & Sons, Inc. Published 2019 by John Wiley & Sons, Inc.
Companion website: www.fiveminutevet.com/gastrointestinal

- No sex predilection.
- No known genetic basis, although brachycephalic breeds are overrepresented.

Risk Factors

- Increased aerophagia.
  - Gluttony or competitive eating.
  - Respiratory disease or any cause of increased respiratory rate.
  - Feeding shortly after exercise.
  - Brachycephalic breeds.
- Diet related.
  - Diets high in nonabsorbable oligosaccharides – soybeans, peas, beans.
  - Diets high in fermentable fiber – lactose, pectin, inulin, psyllium, oat bran. Diets high in complex starches (e.g., wholegrains) that are slowly digested.
  - Spoiled diets.
  - Milk products.
  - Abrupt changes in diet.
  - Spices and food additives/supplements.
- Disease conditions.
  - Acute and chronic intestinal disease – including protein-losing enteropathies (PLE); inflammatory bowel disease; intestinal dysbiosis; neoplasia; irritable bowel syndrome; parasitism; bacterial, protozoal, or viral enteritis; and food allergy or intolerance.
  - Exocrine pancreatic insufficiency.
- Miscellaneous.
  - Nervous, gluttonous, or competitive eating.
  - Eating soon after exercise.
  - Brachycephalic breeds.
  - Abrupt dietary changes.
  - Inappropriate (feeding table food that is likely to be fermented) or spoiled foods.
  - Sedentary lifestyle – a 1998 study reported that 43% of randomly chosen dog owners detected flatulence, most commonly in sedentary pets, with no association to a particular diet.

Historical Findings

Increased frequency and possibly volume of flatus detected by the pet owner.

 ## CLINICAL FEATURES

- Mild abdominal discomfort caused by gastrointestinal distension possible – mild discomfort can be difficult to recognize but may be reported by owner as a pet that has repeated swallowing efforts, restlessness, or lethargy.
- When flatus is due to gastrointestinal disease, concurrent gastrointestinal signs such as diarrhea, vomiting, borborygmus, changes in appetite, and weight loss may be present.

 ## DIFFERENTIAL DIAGNOSIS

- Distinguish dietary and behavioral causes of flatus from gastrointestinal disease by thorough evaluation of the patient history; this allows the clinician to ascertain the type of diet, amount fed, frequency of feeding, frequency of dietary changes or additions, and the environment in which the patient is fed.

- Investigate feeding method – frequency, amount, relationship to exercise, how offered, and incidence of competitive eating. Observation of the patient while eating may be required to identify gluttony.
- Perform a complete physical examination with a focus on gastrointestinal evaluation. Palpate the abdomen for gassy bowel loops, pain and distension; auscultate the abdomen for bowel sounds, the absence of which indicates ileus. Rectal examination for evaluation of rectal and pelvic anatomy.
- Assess body condition score; if low, this may indicate concurrent gastrointestinal disease or inadequate food intake. Obesity may be associated with a sedentary lifestyle that may be a risk factor.

 ## DIAGNOSTICS

Complete Blood Cell Count/Biochemistry/Urinalysis

Usually normal minimum database unless significant bowel disease is present (e.g., hypoalbuminemia in PLE).

Other Laboratory Tests

- Rectal cytology to evaluate for presence of neoplasia, parasites, fungal organisms.
- Zinc sulfate flotation tests or fecal enzyme-linked immunosorbent assay (ELISA)/ polymerase chain reaction (PCR) to evaluate for giardiasis.
- Fecal PCR for *Tritrichomonas* in young cats or kittens.
- Fecal cultures or PCR to evaluate for salmonellosis or campylobacteriosis.
- Serum trypsin-like immunoreactivity to evaluate for exocrine pancreatic insufficiency.
- Serum cobalamin and folate concentrations to test for severe small intestinal disease.

Imaging

- Abdominal radiographs may be unremarkable or reveal gas-distended small intestines (Figure 8.1).

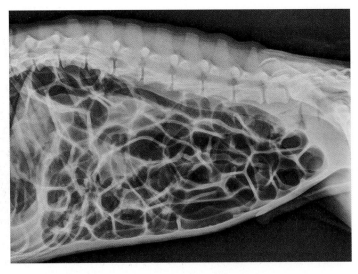

■ **Fig. 8.1.** Right lateral radiograph of an adult male Labrador retriever with excessive gas production. Gas-distended small intestines were concerning for an underlying condition (such as foreign body or torsion), but all diagnostics, including histopathology of intestines, were normal/negative.

- Abdominal ultrasonography to diagnose gastrointestinal masses or mural thickening.
- Contrast studies may be needed in some cases to detect an obstructive pattern.
- Assessment of gut motility is difficult at best, but scintigraphic markers can be used in some referral facilities. Upper GI series using barium can be used to detect delayed gastric or intestinal emptying; however, the study can be extremely variable secondary to stress.

Additional Diagnostic Tests

Gastrointestinal biopsy specimens obtained at surgery or via endoscopy to detect infiltrative gastrointestinal disease.

 # THERAPEUTICS

Goal of therapy is to reduce the flatulence and make the patient more comfortable, understanding that complete elimination of flatulence may not be possible.

Drug(s) of Choice

- Carminatives are medications that relieve flatulence – there are no studies to show safety or benefit of these drugs in dogs or cats.
- Zinc acetate binds sulfhydryl compounds.
- *Yucca schidigera* binds ammonia and is added to pet foods as a flavoring agent.
- Dry activated charcoal absorbs virtually all odiferous gases when mixed directly with human feces and flatus; however, the number of flatus events, gas volume, or odor were not decreased in people.
- Inclusion of activated charcoal, *Y. schidigera,* and zinc acetate in a treat reduced the frequency of highly odiferous episodes in dogs.
- Bismuth subsalicylate (dogs 1 mL/kg PO initially then 0.25 mL/kg q 6 h) adsorbs hydrogen sulfide and has antibacterial properties; however, long-term, multiple daily dosing precludes its practicality. Not recommended for use in cats due to potential for salicylate toxicity.
- Simethicone is an antifoaming agent that reduces the surface tension of gas bubbles, allowing easier coalescence and release of intestinal gas; however, gas production is unaltered.
- Pancreatic enzyme supplements may reduce flatulence in some patients with reduced pancreatic enzyme production.

Precautions/Interactions

Avoid bismuth subsalicylate in cats and in dogs with gastroduodenal ulceration and bleeding disorders.

Alternative Drug(s)

- More than 30 herbal and botanical preparations are available; however, the dosage, safety, and efficacy are unknown.
- Use of probiotics to normalize or stabilize the intestinal microenvironment has been advocated and would be safe to try; however, no studies of the efficacy of this approach have been completed.

Appropriate Health Care

Outpatient – treat any underlying gastrointestinal disease.

Diet

- Feed smaller meals more frequently in an isolated, quiet environment.

- Change diet to one that is highly digestible, with low fiber and fat concentrations (e.g., intestinal or hypoallergenic diets formulated for prescription purposes are all reasonable choices), or feed home-made diets containing boiled chicken and white rice (dogs) or whole chicken with skin (fat) balanced with vitamins and minerals. (Note: cats should not be fed a carbohydrate source, to eliminate carbohydrate intolerance as part of this issue.)
- A change in the protein or carbohydrate source, or removing the additives, benefits some individuals.

Activity

Encourage an active lifestyle – exercise increases GI motility, which will help expel flatus and increase regularity of defecation.

 COMMENTS

Client Education

Discourage dietary indiscretion (e.g., garbage ingestion or coprophagia).

Patient Monitoring

Response to therapy.

Prevention/Avoidance

- Avoid diets high in nonabsorbable oligosaccharides and high in fermentable or nonfermentable fibers.
- Avoid milk products, spoiled diets, and abrupt changes in diet.
- Do not feed shortly after exercise.
- Use of probiotics to improve the commensal bacterial flora may be beneficial if bacterial disruption is the primary cause of flatulence.

Abbreviations

- ELISA = enzyme-linked immunosorbent assay
- GI = gastrointestinal
- PCR = polymerase chain reaction
- PLE = protein-losing enteropathy

See Also

- Enteritis, Bacterial
- Exocrine Pancreatic Insufficiency
- Inflammatory Bowel Disease
- Intestinal Dysbiosis
- Irritable Bowel Syndrome

Suggested Reading

Davenport DJ, Remillard RL, Simpson KW, et al. Gastrointestinal and exocrine pancreatic disease. In: Hand MS, Thatcher CD, Remillard RL, et al., eds. Small Animal Clinical Nutrition, 5th ed. Topeka: Mark Morris Institute, 2010, pp. 725–810.

Giffard CJ, Collins SB, Stoodley N, et al. Ability of an antiflatulence treat to reduce the hydrogen sulfide content of canine flatulence. Proceedings of the 18th ACVIM Meeting, 2000, p. 726.

Matz ME. Flatulence. In: Ettinger SJ, Feldman EC, eds. Textbook of Veterinary Internal Medicine, 7th ed. St. Louis: Elsevier, 2010, pp. 148–149.

Roudebush P. Flatulence: what do we know about intestinal gas? Proceedings of the 19th ACVIM Meeting, 2001, pp. 592–594.

Acknowledgments: The author and editors acknowledge the prior contribution of Dr Debra L. Zoran and Dr Stanley L. Marks.

Author: Gavin Olsen DVM, DACVIM (SAIM)

Chapter 9

Hematemesis

DEFINITION/OVERVIEW

The vomiting of blood (Figure 9.1).

ETIOLOGY/PATHOPHYSIOLOGY

A disruption in the gastric or upper small intestinal mucosal barrier leading to inflammation and bleeding. Coagulopathies can also present with hematemesis. An animal may also vomit blood that originated in the oral cavity or respiratory system and was swallowed.

Systems Affected

- Gastrointestinal – inflammation, trauma, ulceration, neoplasia, and/or foreign body in the oral cavity, pharyngeal area, esophagus, stomach, and/or duodenum.
- Cardiovascular – acute, severe hemorrhage may result in tachycardia, systolic heart murmur, and/or hypotension.
- Hematologic – coagulopathy with gastrointestinal hemorrhage can lead to hematemesis.
- Respiratory – respiratory hemorrhage with subsequent ingestion can lead to hematemesis.

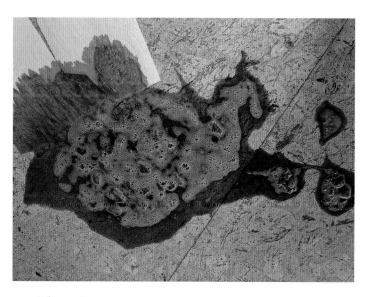

■ **Fig. 9.1.** Hematemesis from a dog.

Blackwell's Five-Minute Veterinary Consult Clinical Companion: Small Animal Gastrointestinal Diseases,
First Edition. Edited by Jocelyn Mott and Jo Ann Morrison.
© 2019 John Wiley & Sons, Inc. Published 2019 by John Wiley & Sons, Inc.
Companion website: www.fiveminutevet.com/gastrointestinal

SIGNALMENT/HISTORY

- Dog and, less commonly, cat.
- There appears to be an overrepresentation of chow chows and Siamese cats with gastric adenocarcinoma.
- All ages can be affected.
- Male dogs have increased incidence of gastric carcinoma.

Risk Factors

- Administration of ulcerogenic drugs – nonsteroidal antiinflammatory drugs (NSAIDs), glucocorticoids, toceranib phosphate.
- Critically ill patients.
- Hypovolemic or septic shock.
- Thrombocytopenia.
- Concurrent administration of NSAIDs and glucocorticoids.

Causes

Coagulopathies

- Thrombocytopenia.
- Thrombocytopathia – von Willebrand's disease, NSAIDs, drugs, uremia.
- Hyperviscosity syndrome.
- Disseminated intravascular coagulopathy.
- Anticoagulant rodenticide toxicity.
- Coagulation factor deficiency.
- Liver failure.
- Polycythemia.

Drugs

NSAIDs, glucocorticoids, toceranib phosphate.

Gastrointestinal Diseases

- Inflammatory bowel disease.
- Gastric or duodenal neoplasia.
- Gastric or duodenal foreign body.
- Gastric or intestinal volvulus or torsion.
- Hemorrhagic gastroenteritis.
- Gastroduodenal ulcers.
- Gastroesophageal intussusception.

Toxicity

- Heavy metal poisoning (arsenic, zinc, thallium, iron, or lead).
- Plant intoxication (dieffenbachia, sago palm, mushroom, castor bean).
- Chemical intoxication (phenol, ethylene glycol, corrosive agents, psoriasis creams – vitamin D analogs).
- Pesticide/rodenticide toxicity (cholecalciferol).
- Snake bite.
- Aflatoxins.
- Bee sting.

Infectious Diseases

- Gastrointestinal parasitism.
- Pythiosis (fungal oomycete).
- Viral, fungal, or bacterial gastroenteritis.

- Virulent systemic feline calicivirus.
- Rickettsial infections.

Metabolic Diseases
- Renal failure.
- Liver disease.
- Intrahepatic shunts.
- Hypoadrenocorticism.
- Pancreatitis.

Neoplasia
- Mastocytosis.
- Gastrinoma.
- Oral, nasal, respiratory (blood is swallowed and subsequently vomited), or gastrointestinal tumors.
- Tumors of the amine precursor uptake decarboxylase cells (APUDomas).

Neurologic Diseases
- Head trauma.
- Spinal cord disease.

Respiratory Diseases
- Nasal disease – neoplasia, fungal infection.
- Pulmonary and airway disease – neoplasia, severe pneumonia, fungal infection, foreign body, heartworm disease.
- Mediastinal neoplasia.

Stress/Major Medical Illness
- Stress-related mucosal disease.
- Hospitalization for nongastrointestinal diseases.
- Septic or hypovolemic shock.
- Severe illness.
- Burns.
- Heat stroke.
- Major surgery.
- Sustained strenuous exercise.
- Trauma.
- Systemic hypertension.
- Thromboembolic disease.
- Hypotension.

Historical Findings
- Vomiting with blood – blood in the vomitus may appear as fresh flecks of blood, blood clots, or digested blood, which looks like coffee grounds.
- Melena can be observed.
- Anorexia.
- Abdominal pain (may assume the praying position).

 ## CLINICAL FEATURES

- Abdominal pain.
- Melena.
- If patient is anemic – tachycardia, heart murmur, pallor, weakness, and/or collapse.

DIFFERENTIAL DIAGNOSIS

- Hemoptysis – thoracic radiographs may reveal presence of airway or pulmonary disease.
- Regurgitation or vomiting of swallowed blood from extragastrointestinal diseases (e.g., oropharyngeal, nasopharyngeal, and cutaneous diseases).
- Ingestion and vomiting of foreign materials or foods that look like fresh or digested blood (e.g., oral iron).

DIAGNOSTICS

Complete Blood Count/Biochemistry/Urinalysis

- If acute (3–5 days) blood loss – nonregenerative anemia (normocytic, normochromic, minimal reticulocytosis).
- If blood loss >5–7 days in duration – regenerative anemia (macrocytic, reticulocytosis).
- If chronic blood loss – iron deficiency anemia (microcytic, hypochromic, variable reticulocytosis, with or without thrombocytosis).
- ± Thrombocytopenia.
- ± Panhypoproteinemia with alimentary hemorrhage.
- May have mature neutrophilia or left shift neutrophilia with sepsis and/or gastroduodenal ulcer perforation.
- BUN: creatinine ratio may be elevated with gastrointestinal hemorrhage, but will also be increased with dehydration.

Other Laboratory Tests

- Fecal occult blood test may be false positive if dog is not on a nonmeat diet for three days prior to test.
- Fecal flotation – to screen for gastrointestinal parasitism.
- Coagulation profile – if a coagulopathy is suspected.
- Bile acids – if liver disease is suspected.
- Adrenocorticotropic hormone (ACTH) stimulation – if hypoadrenocorticism is suspected.

Imaging

- Abdominal radiography may identify a gastric or duodenal foreign body or mass, pancreatitis, pneumoperitoneum, effusion or changes consistent with kidney, pancreas, or liver disease.
- Thoracic radiographs may reveal esophageal foreign body or mass, gastroesophageal intussusception, mediastinal mass, pulmonary or airway disease, and/or pulmonary metastasis.
- Abdominal ultrasonography may identify a gastric or duodenal mass, gastric or duodenal wall thickening or altered layering, gastric ulcer, and/or abdominal lymphadenopathy.
- Abdominal ultrasound can also screen for abnormalities in the pancreas, liver, kidneys, and other abdominal organs as source of hematemesis.
- Gastrointestinal scintigraphy may be used to localize gastrointestinal blood loss.

Diagnostic Procedures

- Endoscopy to evaluate the mucosal appearance of the esophagus, stomach, and upper small intestinal tract once extragastrointestinal causes of hematemesis are ruled out.
- Biopsy mucosal lesions and submit for histopathology to determine the nature of the underlying gastrointestinal disease. Use caution when obtaining biopsies of lesions with damaged mucosa.

- Ambulatory light-based imaging (ALICAM) is swallowed by the dog and then can provide images of the entire gastrointestinal tract.
- Abdominocentesis may identify septic peritonitis.
- Obtain fine needle aspirates or biopsy specimens of cutaneous or intraabdominal masses to identify neoplasia/disease.

Pathologic Findings

- Gastroduodenal inflammation and hemorrhage.
- Ulcers may have more necrosis, microthrombi, and hemorrhage, and deeper tissue penetration than erosions.

 # THERAPEUTICS

Drug(s) of Choice

- Proton pump inhibitors (PPI) (omeprazole 1 mg/kg PO q 12 h, dog and cat; pantoprazole 1 mg/kg IV q 12 h, dog) – omeprazole is the most potent inhibitor of gastric acid secretion and treatment of choice (including gastrinomas with evidence of metastasis or nonresectable disease).
- Less desirable are histamine (H_2) receptor antagonists which competitively inhibit gastric acid secretion and can be given with or without food (famotidine 0.5–1 mg/kg PO, IV q 12–24 h, dog and cat; nizatidine 5 mg/kg PO q 24 h, dog). H2 receptor antagonists differ in potency and duration of action. Famotidine is the most potent. Treat for at least 6–8 weeks. Rebound gastric acid hypersecretion may occur when H_2 blockers are discontinued but can be minimized by tapering the dose as it is discontinued.
- H2-receptor antagonists are less potent than proton pump inhibitors.
- Antacids neutralize gastric acid and some induce local synthesis of mucosal protectants but must be given at least 4–6 times/day to be effective. Owner compliance with this regimen is often poor.
- Sucralfate suspension (0.5–1 g PO q 6–8 h) protects ulcerated tissue (cytoprotection) by binding to ulcer sites, adsorbing pepsin and bile salts, and stimulating prostaglandin synthesis. Binding is greater in duodenal than gastric ulcers.
- Antibiotic(s) with activity against enteric gram-negative bacteria and anaerobes should be given parenterally if a break in gastrointestinal mucosal barrier is suspected or aspiration pneumonia is present.
- Antiemetics (chlorpromazine 0.5 mg/kg q 6–8 h SQ, IM, IV, dog and cat; prochlorperazine 0.1–0.5 mg/kg q 6–8 h SQ, IM, dog and cat; ondansetron 0.5 mg/kg IV q 12 h, dog; 0.2 mg/kg IV q 12 h, cat; metoclopramide 1–2 mg/kg/24 h CRI, dog and cat; maropitant 1 mg/kg SQ or IV q 24 h, dog and cat; 2 mg/kg PO q 24 h, dog) are administered if vomiting occurs frequently or results in significant fluid losses.
- Antifibrinolytic drugs may show promise in treatment of bleeding disorders in dogs.

Precautions/Interactions

- H2 blockers prevent uptake of omeprazole by oxyntic cells.
- Sucralfate may alter absorption of other drugs. Thus, it should be given on an empty stomach 2 h before or after other oral drugs.
- Antacids may alter oral absorption and renal elimination of other drugs.
- Avoid drugs that might damage the gastroduodenal mucosal barrier (e.g., NSAIDs and corticosteroids).
- Continued famotidine therapy can lead to tachyphylaxis.

Alternative Drugs

Misoprostol, synthetic prostaglandin analog (3 µg/kg PO q 8–12 h) with antisecretory and cyto protective actions helps prevent NSAID-induced ulcers. There may be some efficacy in treating gastroduodenal ulcerations from other causes.

Appropriate Health Care

- Treat any underlying causes.
- Treat on an outpatient basis if the cause is identified and removed, vomiting is not excessive, and gastroduodenal bleeding is minimal.
- Inpatients – those with severe gastroduodenal bleeding, ulcer perforation, excessive vomiting, and/or shock.

Nursing Care

- Intravenous fluids to maintain hydration.
- May need aggressive intravenous fluid treatment for shock – crystalloids and/or colloids.
- Severely hypoproteinemic patients may require colloids and/or plasma to increase vascular oncotic pressure.
- May need transfusions (whole blood or packed red blood cells) in patients with severe gastroduodenal hemorrhage.
- Patients with underlying coagulopathies may need whole blood or fresh frozen plasma to replace clotting factors.
- In severe cases of hematemesis – to stop the gastrointestinal bleeding, ice water lavage (10–20 mL/kg remaining in stomach for 15–30 min) or lavage with norepinephrine (8 mg/500 mL) diluted in ice water can be attempted.

Diet

- Discontinue oral intake if vomiting.
- When feeding is resumed, feed small amounts in multiple feedings.

Surgical Considerations

Surgical treatment is indicated if medical treatment fails after 5–7 days, hemorrhage is uncontrolled, gastroduodenal ulcer perforates, and/or potentially resectable tumor is identified.

    COMMENTS

Client Education

- NSAIDs should be administered to pets only under the guidance of a veterinarian.
- Administration of NSAIDs (including cyclooxygenase-2 (COX-2) inhibitors) can result in gastroduodenal ulcerations and perforations.
- Adverse effects of NSAIDs can be reduced by giving drug with food and concurrent administration of a synthetic prostaglandin E1 analog (e.g., misoprostol).

Patient Monitoring

- Improvement in some cases may be assessed on resolution of clinical signs; packed cell volume, total protein, fecal occult blood, and BUN may help to detect continued blood loss.
- Depending on the underlying cause of the hematemesis, specific laboratory or imaging tests may be necessary to monitor response to therapy.

Prevention/Avoidance

- Avoid gastric irritants (e.g., NSAIDs, corticosteroids).
- Concurrent use of misoprostol or PPI with NSAIDs; PPI may be preferable because they are therapeutic as well.
- Administer NSAIDs with food.
- COX-2 selective or dual lipoxygenase (LOX)/COX inhibitors may have less adverse gastrointestinal effects than nonselective NSAIDs.

Possible Complications

- Severe blood loss.
- Sepsis.
- Ulcer perforation.

Expected Course and Prognosis

- Varies with underlying causes.
- Patients with malignant gastric neoplasia, renal failure, liver failure, pythiosis, systemic mastocytosis, sepsis, and/or gastric perforation – guarded to poor prognosis.
- Hematemesis secondary to NSAID administration, coagulopathies, inflammatory bowel disease, or hypoadrenocorticism – prognosis may be good to excellent, depending on severity of disease.
- Hematemesis secondary to heat stroke, toxicities, and snake bites can have variable prognoses.

Abbreviations

- ACTH = adrenocorticotropic hormone
- ALICAM = ambulatory light-based imaging
- APUDoma = amine precursor uptake decarboxylase cells
- COX = cyclooxygenase
- LOX = lipoxygenase
- NSAID = nonsteroidal antiinflammatory drug
- PPI = proton pump inhibitor

See Also

- Gastroduodenal Ulcer Disease
- Melena

Suggested Reading

Case V. Melena and hematochezia. In: Ettinger SJ, Feldman EC, eds. Textbook of Veterinary Internal Medicine Diseases of the Dog and Cat, 7th ed. St Louis: Saunders Elsevier, 2010, pp. 203–206.

Neiger R. Gastric ulceration. In: Bongura JD, Twedt DC, eds. Kirk's Current Veterinary Therapy XV. St Louis: Elsevier Saunders, 2014, pp. e251–e255.

Tolbert K, Bissett S, King A, et al. Efficacy of oral famotidine and 2 omeprazole formulations for the control of intragastric pH in dogs. J Vet Intern Med 2011;25:47–54.

Tolbert K, Odunayo A, Howell RS, et al. Efficacy of intravenous administration of combined acid suppressants in healthy dogs. J Vet Intern Med 2015;29:556–560.

Author: Jocelyn Mott DVM, DACVIM (SAIM)

Chapter 10

Hematochezia

DEFINITION/OVERVIEW

Frank (red) blood on or in the feces, whether feces are formed or not.

ETIOLOGY/PATHOPHYSIOLOGY

- Hematochezia with formed feces.
    - Constipation and/or feces which are too firm and dry.
    - Passage of foreign material in the feces.
    - Rectal polyps, other rectal or anal growths.
    - Perianal fistulas.
    - Anal sac disease (infection or impaction).
    - Primary coagulation disorders (thrombocytopenia and thrombocytopathia).
- Soft or diarrheic feces +/− mucus.
    - Parasitism (*Giardia*, cocccidia,whipworms, hookworms, etc.).
    - Bacterial colitis (*Clostridium perfringens*, *C. difficile*, *Salmonella*, *Campylobacter*).
    - Histiocytic ulcerative colitis (invasive *E. coli* in susceptible dogs: boxers, French bulldogs, others).
    - Inflammatory bowel disease.
    - Fungal or algal colitis (histoplasmosis, *Pythium*, *Prototheca*, etc.).
    - Colitis associated with pancreatitis.
    - Infiltrative neoplasia (primarily lymphoma).

Hematochezia is common in clinical practice due to the many underlying causes.

Systems Affected

- Gastrointestinal.
- Hemic/lymphatic/immune.

SIGNALMENT/HISTORY

Any age, dog or cat, no sex predilection.

Risk Factors

- For constipation – increased risk with dehydration, chronic renal disease, increasing age, cats (megacolon).
- For parasitic causes of colitis – younger animals.

Blackwell's Five-Minute Veterinary Consult Clinical Companion: Small Animal Gastrointestinal Diseases, First Edition. Edited by Jocelyn Mott and Jo Ann Morrison.
© 2019 John Wiley & Sons, Inc. Published 2019 by John Wiley & Sons, Inc.
Companion website: www.fiveminutevet.com/gastrointestinal

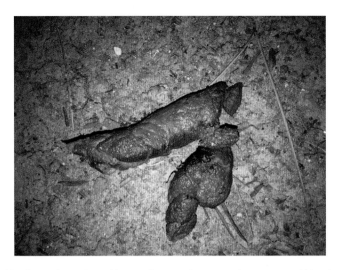

■ **Fig. 10.1.** Frank blood on a formed stool from a dog one day post colonoscopy and biopsies.

■ Perianal fistula – increased risk for German shepherd dogs.
■ Histiocytic ulcerative colitis – boxers, French bulldogs, others.

Historical Findings

■ Holding defecation posture for a long period of time while producing a bowel movement, or repeatedly making efforts to defecate, whether productive or not.
■ Vocalization when defecating or reluctance to defecate.
■ Frank blood on the outside of excessively firm feces.
■ Streaks of blood on normally formed stool (Figure 10.1).
■ Frank blood mixed in with loose stools, with excessive mucus and increased frequency of defecation (signs consistent with colitis).
■ Scooting on bottom or excessively licking anal region, especially with anal gland disease.
■ Vomiting or inappetence occur infrequently with colonic or rectal disease.
■ Blood in the urine or bruising on skin or mucosal surfaces if systemic coagulopathy.

 CLINICAL FEATURES

■ Rectal exam – imperative for diagnosis.
  • Oozing fistulous tracts around anus and perineum = perianal fistulas.
  • Anal or rectal stricture – benign stricture versus malignant neoplasia.
  • Rectal mass – polyp versus malignancy (adenocarcinoma, lymphoma, other) (Figure 10.2).
  • Fecal consistency hard/firm – constipation, obstipation.
  • Fecal consistency soft or mucoid – colitis.
  • Fecal consistency normal but blood present – likely a polyp or a partially occlusive mass; rule out coagulopathy, colonic vascular ectasia.
  • Foreign material – foreign body.
■ Check for bleeding from any other surfaces – petechiae or ecchymoses of the skin, gingiva, sclera which can indicate platelet disorders.

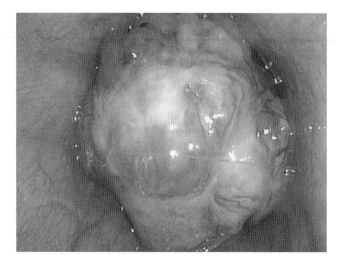

■ **Fig. 10.2.** Rectal adenocarcinoma in a dog who had a two-year history of hematochezia.

- Abdomen – palpate for caudal or dorsal abdominal masses or discomfort.
- Assess hydration – dehydration can cause constipation.

 ## DIFFERENTIAL DIAGNOSIS

- Hematochezia could be confused with hematuria, hemorrhagic vaginal discharge, or bleeding from perianal structures.
- Physical examination and history will quickly differentiate in most cases.

 ## DIAGNOSTICS

Complete Blood Cell Count/Biochemical Panel/Urinalysis

- Complete blood cell count – usually normal unless thrombocytopenic.
- Serum biochemistry panel – usually normal unless azotemia is causing constipation.
- Urinalysis – usually normal unless renal azotemia is causing constipation.

Additional Laboratory Tests

- Fecal floatation, enzyme-linked immunosorbent assay, and/or polymerase chain reaction tests for infectious causes of colitis.
- Pancreas-specific lipase testing (Spec cPL, Spec fPL, Precision SPL) – may be elevated if pancreatitis is causing colitis.

Imaging

- Abdominal radiographs – may show accumulation of solid fecal material, abrupt narrowing of fecal material if mass or stricture is present. Rarely can see colonic masses.
- Abdominal ultrasound – may show thickened colonic wall, colonic masses, lymphadenopathy. Intrapelvic structures cannot be easily visualized with this technique due to bone of pelvis blocking the view.

Other Diagnostic Tests

- Colonoscopy/proctoscopy – often the only way to fully assess rectal and colonic disease; allows visualization of the mucosal surface and acquisition of mucosal biopsies. If there is a mass, histopathology will differentiate benign (polyp) from malignant (carcinoma *in situ*, carcinoma, other).

Pathologic Findings

- Grossly and upon histopathology – may appear normal except for the colonic or rectal mucosa, which may demonstrate erythema, blood, a polyp, mass, stricture, or vascular ectasia (dilated blood vessels with submucosal hemorrhage).
- Colonic mucosa may contain lymphoplasmacytic, neutrophilic or histiocytic inflammation.
- Anal glands and anal mucosa may have areas of swelling or erosion if infected or involved in a fistula.

 THERAPEUTICS

Drug(s) of Choice

- Parasitic colitis (*Giardia*, *Tritrichomonas*, coccidia, etc.) – per usual therapy for each (fenbendazole, ronidazole, sulfonamides, etc.).
- Nonspecific colitis.
  - Metronidazole 10–15 mg/kg PO q 12 h for 5–10 days (dogs and cats), or chronic if needed.
  - Tylosin 10–20 mg/kg PO q 12 h for 5–10 days (dogs and cats), or chronic if needed.
  - Sulfasalazine or mesalazine may be used short term in dogs.
- Histiocytic ulcerative colitis – enrofloxacin 10 mg/kg PO q 24 h (dogs) for one month.
- Perianal fistulas – cyclosporine A modified 5 mg/kg PO q 12 h (dogs), hypoallergenic diet, topical tacrolimus ointment.
- Anal sac abscess – amoxicillin/clavulanic acid 13.5 mg/kg PO q 12 h for 7–10 days (after lavage of the abscess site).
- Constipation/stool softeners
  - Lactulose 1 mL/4.5 kg PO q 6–24 h to effect.
  - Docusate sodium 50–100 mg PO q 12–24 h daily depending on pet size.
  - Miralax® ¼ to 1 tsp PO q 8–12 h with food.
  - Canned pumpkin ½ to 2 tsp PO q 12 h with food.
- Obstipation without physical obstruction – laxatives as above plus cisapride 0.1–0.5 mg/kg PO q 8–12 h.
- Fungal or algal colitis – amphotericin B, oral azole antifungals, lifelong.
- Thrombocytopenia – immune suppression or doxycycline as indicated by primary cause.
- Vascular ectasia (rare) – may respond to estrogens.

Precautions/Interactions

- Cisapride should not be used if there is a physical obstruction to passage of feces such as an occlusive mass or a stricture. Cisapride has many p450 hepatic enzyme interactions; check formulary for interactions before adding to regimen.
- Metronidazole is associated with idiosyncratic neurologic side effects (typically vestibular symptoms) when used at high doses, or sometimes with long-term use at normal doses. Signs resolve after stopping the drug.
- Sulfasalazine is associated with keratoconjunctivitis sicca and other immune-mediated side effects, especially with chronic use. It is not recommended for use in cats.

Alternative Drugs

If cisapride is not available, ranitidine at a dose of 1–2 mg/kg PO q 8–12 h (dogs) and 3.5 mg/kg PO q 12 h (cats) may offer some prokinetic effects.

Appropriate Health Care

- Monitor comfort of defecation, frequency of defecation, and stool consistency.
- Maintain optimal hydration (canned foods, extra water dishes, water fountains).

Nursing Care

- Pet may need more frequent opportunities to defecate if colitis is present.
- Perineal sanitary shaving may be needed periodically.

Diet

- For chronic colitis or constipation – increased fiber, both insoluble and soluble.
- Perianal fistula – hypoallergenic diet.

Activity

No restriction unless thrombocytopenia.

Surgical Considerations

- Patients with rectal polyp can be treated by sharp excision with mucosal oversew, or via endoscopic polypectomy snare. Rectal carcinoma or carcinoma *in situ* may require colonic resection and anastomosis, via either pelvic split approach or rectal pull-through.
- Benign rectal stricture may be treated with endoscopic balloon dilation procedure.

 COMMENTS

Client Education

- Depends on the underlying disease condition.
- Most conditions can be resolved or managed, and the client is asked to communicate any lack of success or any relapse of signs to optimize outcomes.

Patient Monitoring

- Depends on cause.
- Client observation may be enough monitoring for outcome for simple colitis or constipation. Hematochezia should resolve with surgical resection of polyps or masses, unless there is recurrence.
- Rectal exam is recommended on polypectomy patients 1–2 weeks postoperatively, then at one month and then every three months for life.
- Abdominal ultrasound may be indicated for some more aggressive lesions.
- Thrombocytopenic patients need frequent complete blood cell count monitoring.

Prevention/Avoidance

- Only relevant with parasitism (fecal screening and preemptive deworming).
- Constipation can be avoided in at-risk patients by maintaining proper hydration and a moist diet +/– laxatives.
- Recurrence of rectal polyps may be reduced with administration of piroxicam 0.3 mg/kg PO once daily (dogs).

Possible Complications

- May include obstipation and associated risk for bacterial translocation, sepsis, and even death in advanced cases.
- Fecal scalding of the perineal skin can occur with chronic colitis.
- Anal stricture can occur from chronic perianal fistulas, and can also result from exuberant scarring from rectal mass resection.
- Severe hemorrhage can occur if hematochezia is due to thrombocytopenia or colonic vascular ectasia.
- Fecal incontinence is a risk of extensive rectal and colonic resection, as well as extensive perianal or anal surgery.

Expected Course and Prognosis

- Acute colitis is short-lived and typically easily controlled.
- Chronic colitis or chronic constipation are usually manageable, but diet/medications may need to be lifelong.
- Histiocytic ulcerative colitis usually responds well to antibiotic therapy, but bacterial resistance can occur.
- Fungal or algal colitis generally has a guarded to poor prognosis.
- Rectal polyps have a good prognosis if removed early, but can progress to carcinoma *in situ* or carcinoma if untreated, which could become fatal (due to obstructive effects if they regrow or due to metastatic disease).
- Rectal strictures are sometimes challenging to dilate effectively and safely.
- Perianal fistulas have a variable but typically good response to therapy, but therapy may be expensive and is usually lifelong.
- Immune-mediated thrombocytopenia has generally good outcome if the patient survives the first two weeks, but may relapse.

See Also

- Clostridial Enterotoxicosis
- Colitis and Proctitis
- Colitis, Histiocytic Ulcerative
- Colonic Neoplasia, Benign
- Colonic Neoplasia, Malignant
- Constipation and Obstipation
- Dyschezia and Tenesmus
- Enteritis, Bacterial
- Fiber-Responsive Large Bowel Diarrhea
- Giardiasis
- Melena
- Parasites, Gastrointestinal
- Perianal Fistula
- Perianal Hernia
- Rectal Stricture
- Rectoanal Polyps
- Trichomoniasis

Suggested Reading

Adamovich-Ripper KN, Mayhew PD, Marks SL, et al. Colonoscopic and histologic features of rectal masses in dogs: 82 cases (1995–2012). J Am Vet Med Assoc 2017;250(4):424–430.

Foley P. Constipation, tenesmus, dyschezia and fecal incontinence. In: Ettinger S, Feldman E, eds. Textbook of Veterinary Internal Medicine, 7th ed. Philadelphia: WB Saunders, 2010, pp 206–209.

Nucci DJ, Liptak JM, Selmic LE, et al. Complications + outcomes following rectal pull-through surgery in dogs with rectal masses: 74 cases (2000–2013). J Am Vet Med Assoc 2014;245(6):684–695.

Pieper J, McKay L. Perianal fistulas. Compend Contin Educ Vet 2011;33 9):E4.

Simpson KW. Canine ulcerative colitis. In: Bonagura J, Twedt DC, eds. Kirk's Veterinary Therapy XIV. Philadelphia: Saunders/Elsevier, 2009, pp. 521–523.

Acknowledgments: The author and editors acknowledge the prior contribution of Dr Stanley L. Marks.

Author: Julie Stegeman DVM, DACVIM (SAIM)

Chapter 11

Melena

DEFINITION/OVERVIEW

Melena is the presence of digested blood in the feces (Figure 11.1).

ETIOLOGY/PATHOPHYSIOLOGY

- Melena is the result of blood passing through the upper gastrointestinal (GI) tract and being digested, then being passed out in the feces. Melena appears as a dark brown to black, sticky or "tarry" substance in the stool.
- Underlying causes include the following.
  - The oral cavity (Figure 11.2), esophagus, stomach, small intestines, nasal cavity or expectorated from the lungs.
  - Foreign object, ulcerated tumor, gastritis, inflammatory bowel disease, pancreatitis, fungal or atypical bacterial infection, parasitism, ulceration from medications (non-steroidal antiinflammatory medication (NSAIDs), corticosteroids, etc.), uremia, liver failure, or gastrinoma.
  - Decreased mucosal blood flow, including systemic hypotension, hypoadrenocorticism, GI torsion, or thrombosis.
  - Thrombocytopenia.
- Melena is relatively common in hospitalized ill pets, and is an indicator of significant blood loss into the GI tract.

Systems Affected

- Gastrointestinal – bleeding from the oral cavity to the distal small intestine.
- Hemic/lymphatic/immune system – melena can cause regenerative anemia, mild thrombocytopenia if acute, and thrombocytosis if bleeding is chronic. Thrombocytopenia can cause gastrointestinal bleeding.
- Respiratory – rarely a severe bleed originating in the sinus cavity, nose, or lungs will lead to swallowing of blood and thus melena.

SIGNALMENT/HISTORY

- There is no breed or sex predilection.
- More commonly reported in dogs than cats, possibly due to cats burying their feces in the litter box.

Blackwell's Five-Minute Veterinary Consult Clinical Companion: Small Animal Gastrointestinal Diseases, First Edition. Edited by Jocelyn Mott and Jo Ann Morrison.
© 2019 John Wiley & Sons, Inc. Published 2019 by John Wiley & Sons, Inc.
Companion website: www.fiveminutevet.com/gastrointestinal

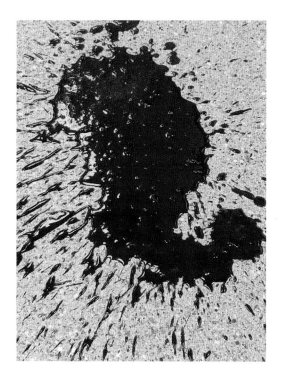

■ **Fig. 11.1.** Melena.

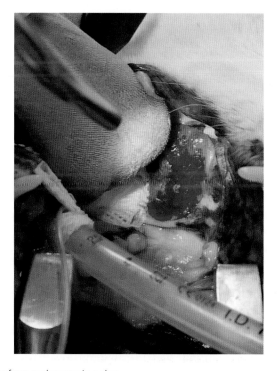

■ **Fig. 11.2.** Oral bleeding from melanoma in a dog.

Risk Factors

- Thrombocytopenia.
- NSAIDs or glucocorticoid administration.
- Gastrointestinal, nasal or pulmonary neoplasia.
- Gastric dilation-volvulus, intestinal torsion, intestinal intussusception.
- Recent gastrointestinal surgery.
- Hypoadrenocorticism.
- Gastrointestinal foreign body.

Historical Findings

- Stools appear black and tarry, or darker than normal.
- +/– Poor appetite.
- +/– Vomiting, diarrhea, lethargy.
- +/– Weakness, collapse, or pallor.
- If thrombocytopenia – bruising of the skin, oral cavity or sclera.
- If oral lesion – blood in the pet's food or water dishes.
- If respiratory origin – epistaxis, noisy respiration, or hemoptysis.

CLINICAL FEATURES

- Rectal exam is the only way to confirm the presence of melena. The feces will be dark reddish brown to black, or may have normal color mixed with reddish brown to black fecal material.
- +/– Blood in the oral cavity or nostrils.
- Possible abdominal discomfort or mass effect.
- Pale gums or petechiation.
- +/– Tachycardia and weak pulse.

DIFFERENTIAL DIAGNOSIS

- Charcoal or Pepto-Bismol in the stool.
- Differentiated from hematochezia, which is frank blood from bleeding in the colon or distally.

DIAGNOSTICS

Complete Blood Cell Count/Biochemistry Panel/Urinalysis

- Complete blood cell count.
    - Regenerative anemia.
    - Microcytosis, hypochromasia, thrombocytosis consistent with iron deficiency.
    - Thrombocytopenia (platelet count <50 000/μL) can cause melena.
- Serum biochemistry panel.
    - Blood urea nitrogen (BUN) may be elevated from the "high protein meal" of digested blood.
    - Hypoalbuminemia – loss from bleeding.
    - If hypoadrenocorticism – hyperkalemia, hyponatremia, hypoalbuminemia, and/or hypocholesterolemia.
    - If uremic ulceration – severe azotemia (BUN, creatinine, SDMA elevations).
    - If liver failure – +/– severely elevated alanine aminotransferase (ALT), alkaline phosphatase (ALKP), total bilirubin, very low albumin, low BUN, +/– hypocholesterolemia +/– hypoglycemia.
- Urinalysis – usually normal.

Other Laboratory Tests

- Resting cortisol or adrenocorticotropic hormone (ACTH) stimulation test – screen for hypoadrenocorticism.
- Pancreas-specific lipase testing (spec cPL, spec fPL, Precision PSL) – screen for pancreatitis.
- Fecal examination – check for parasitism (hookworms, whipworms).
- Coagulation studies (prothrombin time and partial thromboplastin time) – usually normal, unless liver failure.
- Buccal mucosal bleeding time – prolonged in thrombocytopathic patients (do not undertake if thrombocytopenic).
- Serum gastrin level.
  - Significantly increased with gastrinoma.
  - Check with laboratory regarding withdrawal of antacids prior to sampling.

Imaging

- Thoracic radiographs.
  - Esophageal foreign body.
  - Pulmonary nodules/masses if expectoration of blood from the lungs.
  - Metastatic lesions from GI neoplasia.
- Abdominal radiographs.
  - Mass or foreign body in the GI tract.
  - Torsion of the stomach or intestine.
- Barium series (abdominal radiographs) – gastrointestinal ulceration, foreign material, obstruction, or masses.
- Abdominal ultrasound.
  - Gastrointestinal masses, ulceration, obstruction, or intussusception.
  - Free fluid.
  - Lymphadenopathy or concurrent disease.
  - Kidneys, liver, and portal vein can also be assessed.
  - Helpful in deciding whether to pursue surgery or endoscopy next.

Other Diagnostic Tests

- Capsule endoscopy.
  - Locates the site of gastrointestinal ulceration and bleeding.
  - May help plan further diagnostics or therapeutics such as endoscopy versus surgical exploratory.
  - No sedation.
- Endoscopy of the upper GI tract.
  - The key in most cases to diagnosis unless lesion is beyond the reach of the endoscope (jejunum).
  - Preceded by other imaging (radiographs, ultrasound, capsule endoscope, etc.).
  - The only way to assess the mucosal surface of the gastrointestinal tract.
  - Allows biopsy of the lesion.
  - Bleeding polyp can be removed endoscopically (Figure 11.3).
- Exploratory surgery.
  - If a lesion is identified in the small intestines beyond the reach of an endoscope, or if imaging and endoscopy have failed to identify a source for melena.
  - Benefit – ability to excise a mass.
  - Disadvantage – inability to view the mucosal surface.
- Nasal evaluation (computed tomography magnetic resonance imaging, rhinoscopy) – if epistaxis observed.
- Bronchoscopy – if hemoptysis observed or suspected.

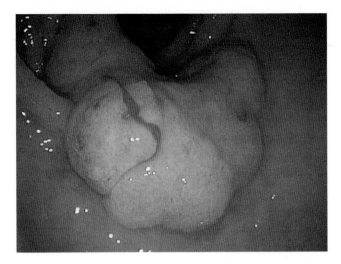

■ **Fig. 11.3.** Benign polyp located at the gastroduodenal junction in a cat with severe regenerative anemia and melena. The lesion was removed endoscopically. Concurrent epitheliotropic small cell lymphoma was diagnosed.

Pathologic Findings

■ Gross pathologic findings might be normal (aside from generalized pallor) if a pet has diffuse GI bleeding. Pathologic findings may be consistent with underlying etiology (inflammatory, infectious, drug induced, neoplastic diseases).
■ Thickening of the intestines or stomach, or a mass in the GI.
■ +/– Free fluid in the abdomen and/or adhesion of the mesentery to a site of GI perforation.
■ Gastrinoma – tiny nodule in pancreas, cluster of atypical neuroendocrine cells.
■ Neoplasms or vascular anomalies of the nasal passages and pulmonary tissue.

 # THERAPEUTICS

Objectives

■ Replenish red blood cell volume.
■ Stop ongoing hemorrhage.
■ Prevent future bleeding.

Drug(s) of Choice

■ Blood transfusion – if clinical signs related to anemia (weakness, tachycardia, tachypnea).
■ Whole blood, packed red blood cells or blood component therapy.
■ Cross-match advised but not required in first transfusion for a dog.
■ ALL cats blood typed and cross-matched prior to transfusion.
■ Intravenous crystalloid and colloid fluid therapy – patients may be volume depleted, dehydrated.
■ Sucralfate.
  • Essential in any patient with GI ulceration. It binds to mucosal ulcers and forms a barrier.
  • Most effective in the acidic stomach; can be effective in the esophagus and the small intestine.

- Dose 100 mg PO q 12 h to 2000 mg PO q 6 h (dogs and cats).
- Give at least 60 min apart from food and other medication.
- Proton pump inhibitors (PPI) (omeprazole, pantoprazole, esomeprazole, etc.).
  - Essential in the treatment of gastrointestinal ulceration.
  - Dose 0.5–1 mg/kg q 12–24 h (dogs and cats).
- Misoprostol.
  - Of greatest benefit in preventing GI ulceration from NSAID therapy, but also used in therapy of ulcers which have been induced by NSAIDs.
  - Synthetic prostaglandin E1 analog – increases gastrointestinal mucosal blood flow and bicarbonate and mucus secretion. Dose 2–5 μg/kg PO q 8–12 h (dogs).
- H2 blockers (famotidine, ranitidine, etc.).
  - Less effective in control of gastric pH, but are commonly also used in this situation.
  - Dose 1 mg/kg q 12 h (dogs and cats) for famotidine, the most effective of this group.
  - No benefit to using these together with a PPI; PPI alone is effective without the H2 blocker.
- Immune suppressant therapy or doxycycline for thrombocytopenia as indicated by cause.
- Antibiotics, often metronidazole +/– a second agent, are often used to reduce bacterial colonization and translocation from ulcerated GI mucosa.
- Other supportive care/medications/nutritional support as needed.

Precautions/Interactions

- Blood transfusions may cause transfusion reactions. Ensure the product is not expired, is stored and warmed properly, cross-match where applicable, and monitor the patient closely for signs of a reaction.
- Sucralfate – given separately from meals and other medications; may interfere with absorption of other meds. Long-term use in chronic renal failure could cause aluminum toxicity. Can cause constipation.
- Proton pump inhibitors may have p450 hepatic enzyme drug interactions; caution should be used in drug combinations. May affect the absorption of some medications that depend on an acidic gastric environment. May cause small intestinal bacterial overgrowth and diarrhea.
- Misoprostol – potential abortifacient, should not be handled by women who are pregnant or wishing to become pregnant.
- H2 blockers can have p450 hepatic enzyme drug interactions, especially cimetidine.

Alternative Drugs

Barium may adhere to ulcerated mucosal surfaces and form a barrier.

Appropriate Health Care

- Avoid NSAIDS. If NSAID is required, then give with misoprostol to try to prevent GI ulceration. NSAID dose should begin at half the usual dose and increase if needed.
- Any special dietary needs should be followed closely, and any melena or even darker stool than normal should be reported to the veterinarian immediately.
- High-dose steroid therapy should also be avoided if possible.

Nursing Care

Patients with severe GI bleeding may need frequent cleaning of the perineum to prevent fecal scalding, and recumbent care if they are in critical condition.

Diet

- A bland, easily digested, soft diet may be needed initially.
- If food allergy or inflammatory bowel disease, feed novel protein or hydrolyzed protein diet.
- If kidney failure or liver failure, feed a diet formulated for the needs of those patients.

Activity

Activity should slowly be increased over several days to weeks as the patient's condition allows.

Surgical Consideration

- Surgical excision of a large gastric ulcer, or ulcerated gastric or intestinal mass, may be necessary.
- Some patients will not stabilize until a bleeding lesion is excised surgically.

 COMMENTS

Client Education

- Monitor pet's stools daily for recurrence of melena.
- Report loss of appetite or any signs of GI upset to veterinarian.
- Consult with your veterinarian before starting any new medications.

Patient Monitoring

- The packed cell volume (PCV) may need to be checked every few hours initially. Once bleeding stabilizes, PCV is checked daily to every 3–4 days. Frequency determined by severity and cause of the bleed.
- Complete blood cell count should be monitored every 2–3 days to weekly, then monthly or less for thrombocytopenic patients on immune suppressive or other therapy.

Prevention/Avoidance

- Avoid NSAIDs and glucocorticoid therapy or use with close monitoring
- Avoid chew toys which could become lodged in the GI tract.
- If immune-mediated thrombocytopenia, limit exposure to certain antibiotics (sulfonamides, beta-lactams) and limit vaccinations and other immune stimulants.

Possible Complications

- Fatal hemorrhage if source is not identified and bleeding stopped.
- GI resection and anastomosis sites might not heal properly, leading to peritonitis or stricture.
- If a malignant neoplasm is the cause of the bleeding, even with surgery, recurrence or metastasis may occur, so follow-up chemotherapy or surveillance will be indicated.
- Arrhythmias may develop secondary to anemia; usually transient idioventricular rhythm but can develop ventricular tachycardia.
- Transfusion reactions may occur (consisting of possible fever, vomiting, diarrhea, anaphylaxis, even death).
- Disseminated intravascular coagulation can occur with massive blood loss.
- Immune-mediated thrombocytopenia – complications occur from immune suppressive therapy (opportunistic infection, hepatic damage, etc.).

Expected Course and Prognosis

- If melena is due to immune-mediated thrombocytopenia, prognosis is fair to good in general; most patients that survive the initial two weeks will live long term.
- If due to focal bleeding, GI lesion which was excised, prognosis is excellent if the cause was a benign mass (leiomyoma, etc.) but guarded if it was a malignancy (adenocarcinoma, etc.).
- Gastrinoma-associated ulceration can be very difficult to control, prognosis is poor.
- NSAID or steroid-associated ulceration most often is successfully resolved medically.

Abbreviations

- ACTH = adrenocorticotropic hormone
- ALKP = alkaline phosphatase
- ALT = alanine aminotransferase
- BUN = blood urea nitrogen
- GI = gastrointestinal
- NSAID = nonsteroidal antiinflammatory drug
- PCV = packed cell volume

See Also

- Gastroenteritis
- Gastric Neoplasia, Benign
- Gastric Neoplasia, Malignant
- Gastroduodenal Ulceration/Erosion
- Gastroenteritis, Eosinophilic
- Hematemesis
- Intestinal Neoplasia, Benign
- Intestinal Neoplasia, Malignant
- Parasites, Gastrointestinal

Suggested Reading

Davignon DL, Lee AC, Johnston AN, et al. Evaluation of capsule endoscopy to detect mucosal lesions associated with gastrointestinal bleeding in dogs. J Small Anim Pract 2016;57:148–158.

Sutaro S, Ruetten M, Hartnack, et al. The effect of orally administered ranitidine and once-daily or twice-daily orally administered omeprazole on intragastric pH in cats. J Vet Intern Med 2015;29:840–846.

Tolbert K, Bissett A, King A, et al. Efficacy of oral famotidine and two omeprazole formulations for the control of intragastric pH in dogs. J Vet Intern Med 2011;25;47–54.

Unterer S, Busch K, Leipig M, et al, Endoscopically visualized lesions, histologic findings, and bacterial invasion in the gastrointestinal mucosa of dogs with acute hemorrhagic diarrhea syndrome "AHDS". J Vet Intern Med 2014;28:52–58.

Waldrop JE, Rozanski EA, Freeman LM, et al. Packed red blood cell transfusion in dogs with gastrointestinal hemorrhage: 55 cases (1999–2001). J Am Anim Hosp Assoc 2003;39:523–527.

Acknowledgments: The author and editors acknowledge the prior contribution of Dr Lisa E. Moore.

Author: Julie Stegeman DVM, DACVIM (SAIM)

Chapter 12

Nutritional Approach to Acute Vomiting and Diarrhea

The gastrointestinal (GI) system is perhaps the organ system that can be most affected directly by nutritional management. It plays a vital role in nutrient digestion and absorption and therefore nutritional management is an important part of the treatment for acute gastroenteritis. Signs of acute gastroenteritis such as vomiting, diarrhea, abdominal pain, and anorexia or hyporexia are some of the most common complaints for dogs and cats presented for a veterinary visit.

There are two methods to classify acute gastroenteritis, one based on severity and the second based on region affected. Categories for levels of severity of acute gastroenteritis range from mild self-limiting gastroenteritis that is not life-threatening, usually caused by dietary indiscretion, adverse food reaction or a parasite, to very severe and potentially fatal acute gastroenteritis. Causes for this level of gastroenteritis can be intestinal obstruction or a severe enteric infection such as salmonellosis. The category in the middle consists of causes of moderately severe gastroenteritis, usually an underlying disease resulting in secondary gastroenteritis such as hypoadrenocorticism. Alternatively, causes of acute gastroenteritis can be classified based on region affected: the stomach (gastritis), small intestine (enteritis), or large intestine (colitis).

If possible, the underlying condition causing the acute gastroenteritis should be determined, but the reality is that the cause of the majority of cases usually remains unknown; standard therapy is initiated and animals are treated symptomatically.

OVERALL NUTRITIONAL CONSIDERATIONS

Historically, the standard recommendation for dogs and cats presenting with acute gastroenteritis was to provide "gut rest" (Guilford and Matz 2003). This was a period of 24–48 hours during which food and sometimes water would be withheld from the animal. This was then usually followed with feeding a bland diet in small volumes, multiple times per day for a few days, and then slow reintroduction of the patient's regular diet once GI signs were improving. It was thought that by fasting, GI signs such as vomiting and diarrhea would subside due to decreased motility and reduced stimulation of the gut mucosa. More recent research has found this not to be true and has in fact supported the idea of feeding through the diarrhea and providing early enteral nutrition (Mohr et al. 2003). Decreased motility and even ileus can be seen with most cases of enteritis but oral feeding can actually prevent ileus by promoting normal motility. Oral feeding also can have a prokinetic effect. Therefore, a reduction in vomiting and increased forward motility of the GI tract can sometimes be achieved simply through feeding.

Blackwell's Five-Minute Veterinary Consult Clinical Companion: Small Animal Gastrointestinal Diseases,
First Edition. Edited by Jocelyn Mott and Jo Ann Morrison.
© 2019 John Wiley & Sons, Inc. Published 2019 by John Wiley & Sons, Inc.
Companion website: www.fiveminutevet.com/gastrointestinal

TABLE 12.1. Recommended components for nutritional support in acute vomiting/diarrhea.

Key nutritional factor	Requirement	Cats (DM basis)	Dogs (DM basis)
Energy density	High	4–4.5 kcal/g	4–4.5 kcal/g
Protein	>87% digestible*	30–40%	25–30%
Carbohydrate	>90% digestible	>90%	>90%
Crude fiber	Low	>5%	>5%
	Moderate**	7–15%	7–15%
Fat	Moderate	15–22%	12–15%
Sodium		0.3–0.5%	0.3–0.5%
Chloride		0.5–1.3%	0.5–1.3%
Potassium		0.8–1.1%	0.8–1.1%

*Hydrolyzed proteins are highly digestible and are particularly indicated in cases of hypersensitivity.
**Fiber-enhanced diets may not meet >4000 kcal/kg recommendation due to decreased energy density.
DM, dry matter.

The current nutritional therapy for managing an acute gastroenteritis case is therefore focused on the type of food offered as well as amounts and frequency that the animals are fed (Table 12.1). Gastric retention time is an important factor to consider and this can be influenced by a number of variables. Increased dry matter content, large meal volume and diets high in fat, soluble fiber or starch can all prolong gastric retention time and therefore can lead to vomiting. The main goal for nutritional management of acute gastroenteritis, regardless of underlying cause, is to maintain delivery of nutrients and prevent nutritional deficiencies and malnutrition.

Water

Patients that present with acute vomiting and/or diarrhea are at risk for potentially life-threatening dehydration. This is due to excessive fluid loss as well as the inability of the animal to replace those losses. Therefore, water is the most important nutrient for these patients and hydration status must be assessed and addressed first before further nutritional considerations. If the patient is moderately to severely dehydrated, correction of the dehydration with parenteral fluid therapy is indicated.

Along with correcting dehydration, fluid therapy is also used to treat electrolyte disorders, which can result from gastric and intestinal secretion loss in acute vomiting and/or diarrhea. Serum electrolyte concentrations can be used to modify the fluid therapy. The most common electrolyte abnormalities seen with acute vomiting and diarrhea patients are a mild hypokalemia, hypochloremia, and either hypernatremia or hyponatremia. Acidemia is also commonly seen in animals with diarrhea due to the high concentration of bicarbonate and sodium ions in the fluid that is secreted in the caudal small intestine and large intestine. The patient must be hemodynamically stable and have acid–base disturbances corrected before further nutritional management can begin.

Protein

A diet moderate to high in a highly digestible protein source should be selected. Protein is important as an energy source and also prevents animals from losing muscle condition when the body is in a catabolic state. If an adverse reaction to food is suspected as the underlying cause of the acute gastroenteritis, either a diet with a novel protein source or a hydrolyzed diet can be considered.

Fat

Fat is very energy dense, so when we feed a higher fat food, we can feed less volume and are still able to meet an animal's energy and nutrient requirements. This is beneficial in a hospital setting when animals may be inappetant and will not eat a large volume of food. It is also important in patients with GI disease because it limits how much food enters the GI tract, which can have an effect on clinical signs. Another important characteristic of fat is that it is very palatable, so there may be a better chance of encouraging an otherwise inappetant animal to eat if we offer a diet higher in fat. Fat is also essential for proper absorption of the fat-soluble vitamins (A, D, E, and K) and for essential fatty acids.

As mentioned above, however, diets higher in fat tend to increase gastric retention time as well as total GI transit time. Undigested fat can cause secretory diarrhea due to the presence of hydroxy fatty acids and unconjugated bile acids. These negative effects of fat could therefore increase nausea, abdominal pain, vomiting, and diarrhea. In general, a diet with moderate fat is selected initially for nutritional management of an acute gastroenteritis case in order to achieve a balance between the positive and negative effects of fat content in the diet.

Fiber

Dietary fiber has many effects on the GI system, which can be beneficial or not when managing a case of acute gastroenteritis. Digestibility is an important factor to consider when selecting an appropriate diet for an animal suffering from acute vomiting and/or diarrhea. Normal digestion and absorption of nutrients will be impaired in animals with acute GI disease and therefore one approach is to feed a highly digestible diet. In order to achieve this, the accepted fiber level to recommend is <5% crude fiber on a dry matter basis.

However, some cases of acute gastroenteritis may respond to the positive effects of higher fiber. Therefore, a second approach is to add a source of fiber to the diet. One way to achieve this would be to consider adding a source of soluble fiber, such as pectins, gums, or psyllium husk (1 tsp per 5–10 kg body weight daily titrated to effect). Soluble fibers can act to form a gel-like substance which can aid in improving fecal consistency by binding excess water in cases of diarrhea. These soluble fibers have more beneficial effects including normalization of intestinal motility and transport rate, binding toxins and bile acids, and fermentation via bacteria in the colon to short chain fatty acids, which can be used as energy for the enterocytes and colonocytes. Insoluble fiber, such as cellulose and peanut hulls, is usually reserved for cases of large bowel diarrhea or constipation where an increase in fecal bulk is desired. Therefore, insoluble fiber is usually contraindicated in cases of acute gastroenteritis.

FEEDING RECOMMENDATIONS

After rehydration and normalization of any acid–base or electrolyte disturbances, immediately begin oral feeding. Calculate the animal's resting energy requirement (RER) based on its ideal body weight. For animals that have been inappetant for an extended period, the goal is to feed one-third of the animal's RER on day 1, two-thirds RER on day 2, and full RER on day 3. The feedings should be split into multiple (6–8) small meals fed throughout the day. A highly digestible, energy-dense diet that is palatable should be selected first in an effort to ensure the animal is eating voluntarily and to ensure that energy sources, especially fat and protein, are provided from exogenous sources. For cases with suspected adverse reaction to food, a hydrolyzed protein diet can be given. *Novel protein sources, however, should not be introduced in the hospital setting.* Inflammation of the gastric mucosa in acute gastroenteritis results in increased mucosal wall permeability, meaning that animals will be at risk of developing new dietary hypersensitivities during this time. Therefore, novel protein sources should be reserved for later, once the animal has recovered.

For animals that remain anorexic in the hospital, placement of a feeding tube may be warranted to deliver appropriate nutrition, in which case options may be limited as to what diet can be fed. If the patient is willing to eat voluntarily, one approach could be to select a highly digestible, low-fiber, moderate-fat diet. If the GI signs do not improve in 24 h, a diet higher in fiber could be selected to see if the patient responds to the higher levels of fiber. The patient should be sent home with the selected diet upon discharge from the hospital and maintained on that diet until fully recovered.

Once recovered, the patient can be gradually transitioned back to their regular diet, or an appropriate diet if the underlying cause of the acute gastroenteritis was identified, over a period of 7–10 days (or longer if needed). If an adverse reaction to food was suspected as the cause of the acute gastroenteritis, a hydrolyzed diet can be fed, or continue to be fed if that was the diet fed in hospital, or novel protein sources can be chosen. An elimination challenge trial should be performed in order to confirm the diagnosis of an adverse food reaction.

KEY POINTS

- First correct hydration, acid–base, and electrolyte abnormalities.
- Small frequent meals.
- High energy density.
- Highly digestible, high-quality protein source. Hydrolyzed or novel protein source if hypersensitivity is suspected.
- Moderate fat.

References

Guilford WG, Matz ME. The nutritional management of gastrointestinal tract disorders in companion animals. NZ Vet J 2003;51(6):284–291.

Mohr AJ, Leisewitz AL, Jacobson LS, Steiner JM, Ruaux CG, Williams DA. Effect of early enteral nutrition on intestinal permeability, intestinal protein loss, and outcome in dogs with severe parvoviral enteritis. J Vet Intern Med 2003;17:791–798.

Suggested Reading

Cave N. Nutritional management of gastrointestinal diseases. In: Fascetti AJ, Delaney SJ, eds. Applied Veterinary Clinical Nutrition. Chichester: Wiley-Blackwell, 2012.

Mansfield CS, James FE, Steiner JM, et al. A pilot study to assess tolerability of early enteral nutrition via esophagostomy tube feeding in dogs with severe acute pancreatitis. J Vet Intern Med 2011;25:419–425.

Authors: Caitlin Grant DVM, BSc, Sarah Dodd DVM, BSc, Adronie Verbrugghe DVM, PhD, Dip ECVCN

Chapter 13

Ptyalism

DEFINITION/OVERVIEW

- Excessive production and secretion of saliva (Figure 13.1).
- Pseudoptyalism is the excessive release of saliva that has accumulated in the oral cavity due to the inability to swallow.

ETIOLOGY/PATHOPHYSIOLOGY

- Saliva is constantly produced and secreted into the oral cavity from the salivary glands (parotid, sublingual, mandibular, zygomatic).
- Saliva production increases when salivary nuclei in the brainstem are stimulated.
- Higher centers in the CNS can also excite or inhibit the salivary nuclei.
- Taste and tactile stimuli in the oral cavity increase saliva production.
- Normal physiologic hypersalivation may occur with anticipation of eating, hyperthermia, and purring (cats).
- Saliva production may be increased with gastrointestinal or CNS disorders.

Systems Affected

- Gastrointestinal.
- Hepatic.
- Nervous/neuromuscular.
- Renal/urologic.

Causes

Conformational Disorder of the Lips

Most common in giant-breed dogs.

Oral and Pharyngeal Diseases

- Oral trauma.
- Foreign body (e.g., stick, foxtail, sewing needle).
- Neoplasm.
- Abscess.
- Gingivitis or stomatitis – secondary to periodontal disease, bacterial, viral (e.g., FeLV or FIV) or fungal infection, immune-mediated disease (e.g., lymphoplasmacytic stomatitis, pemphigus vulgaris), uremia, ingestion of a caustic agent, poisonous plants, effects of radiation therapy to the oral cavity or burns (e.g., biting on an electrical cord).

Blackwell's Five-Minute Veterinary Consult Clinical Companion: Small Animal Gastrointestinal Diseases,
First Edition. Edited by Jocelyn Mott and Jo Ann Morrison.
© 2019 John Wiley & Sons, Inc. Published 2019 by John Wiley & Sons, Inc.
Companion website: www.fiveminutevet.com/gastrointestinal

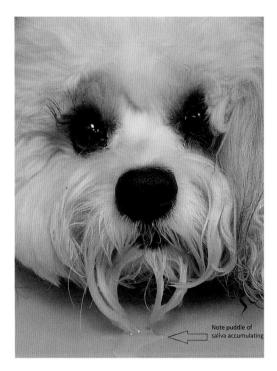

■ **Fig. 13.1.** A dog with ptyalism.

■ Neurologic or functional disorders affecting the swallowing center or oropharyngeal structural disease.

Salivary Gland Diseases

■ Sialoadenitis.
■ Sialolithiasis.
■ Sialedenosis (idiopathic enlargement).
■ Salivary mucocele.
■ Salivary gland fistula.
■ Foreign body.
■ Neoplasm.
■ Infarction.
■ Immune-mediated disease (rare).

Esophageal or Gastrointestinal Disorders

■ Esophageal foreign body.
■ Esophageal neoplasm.
■ Esophagitis.
■ Gastroesophageal reflux.
■ Infection (e.g., spirocercosis, pythosis).
■ Hiatal hernia.
■ Megaesophagus.
■ Esophageal dysmotility.
■ Gastric distension-volvulus.
■ Gastric ulcer.
■ Gastroenteritis.

Metabolic Disorders

- Hepatoencephalopathy (especially in cats) – caused by congenital or acquired portosystemic shunt or hepatic failure.
- Hyperthermia.
- Uremia.

Neurologic Disorders

- Rabies – decreased swallowing causes increased drooling.
- Pseudorabies in dogs.
- Botulism.
- Tetanus.
- Dysautonomia.
- Disorders that cause dysphagia.
- Disorders that cause facial nerve palsy or a dropped jaw (e.g., trigeminal neuritis).
- Disorders that cause seizures – during a seizure, ptyalism may occur because of autonomic discharge or reduced swallowing of saliva, and may be exacerbated by chomping of the jaws.
- Nausea associated with vestibular disease.
- Anxiety.

Drugs and Toxins

- Items that are caustic (e.g., household cleaning products and some common house plants).
- Anesthesia may induce reflux esophagitis. Drugs used for premedication may induce nausea, vomiting or ptyalism.
- Oral, otic or ophthalmic medications that are poorly palatable (especially in cats).
- Drugs that induce hypersalivation, including organophosphate compounds, cholinergic drugs, insecticides containing boric acid, pyrethrin and pyrethroid insecticides, ivermectin (dogs), fluids containing benzoic acid derivatives (cats), clozapine (a tricyclic dibenzodiazepine), caffeine, and illicit drugs such as amphetamines, cocaine, and opiates.
- Animal venom (e.g., black widow spider, Gila monster, and North American scorpion).
- Toad and newt secretions.
- Plant consumption or prehension (e.g., poinsettia, Christmas trees, *Amanita* mushrooms) may cause increased salivation.

 # SIGNALMENT/HISTORY

Species

Dog and cat.

Breed Predilections

- Breeds with a relatively higher incidence of congenital portosystemic shunts include Yorkshire terrier, Maltese terrier, Australian cattle dog, miniature schnauzer, and Irish wolfhound.
- Megaesophagus is hereditary in wire-haired fox terrier and miniature schnauzer; familial predispositions have been reported in German shepherd, Newfoundland, Great Dane, Irish setter, Chinese shar-pei, greyhound, and retriever breeds, as well as in Siamese cats.
- Congenital hiatal hernia has been recognized in the Chinese shar-pei.
- Giant breeds, such as St Bernard, Great Dane, and mastiff, typically exhibit excessive drooling due to lower lip conformation.

Mean Age and Range

- Congenital abnormalities (e.g., portosystemic shunt) are more likely to be diagnosed in younger animals.
- Young animals may also be more likely to have ingested toxic or caustic agents or a foreign body.

Genetics

Megaesophagus is hereditary in wire-haired fox terrier and miniature schnauzer.

Risk Factors

Certain drugs and toxins.

Historical Findings

- Anorexia – seen most often in patients with oral lesions, gastrointestinal disease, and systemic disease.
- Eating behavior changes – patients with oral disease or cranial nerve dysfunction may refuse to eat hard food, chew only on the unaffected side (if unilateral lesion), maintain an unusual head/neck position, or drop prehended food.
- Other behavioral changes – irritability, aggressiveness, and reclusiveness are common, especially in patients with a painful conditions.
- Dysphagia – may be seen with inability to swallow.
- Nausea – may present as increased swallowing.
- Regurgitation – in patients with esophageal disease.
- Vomiting – secondary to gastrointestinal or systemic disease.
- Weight loss – as a consequence of many of the above findings.
- Pawing at the face or muzzle – patients with oral discomfort or pain.
- Neurologic signs – patients that have been exposed to caustic drugs or toxins, those with hepatic encephalopathy, patients with seizure disorders or other intracranial disease.

 CLINICAL FEATURES

Physical Examination Findings

- Periodontal disease.
- Gingivitis/stomatitis caused by toxins, infection, immune-mediated disease, or nutritional deficiency.
- Oral mass – neoplasia or granuloma.
- Glossitis caused by ulceration, mass, or foreign body.
- Lesions of the oropharynx may be due to inflammation, ulceration, mass, or foreign body.
- Blood in the saliva suggests bleeding from the oral cavity, pharynx, or esophagus.
- Halitosis is usually caused by oral disease, but may also be the result of esophageal and/or gastric disease.
- Facial pain may be seen with oral or pharyngeal disease.
- Dysphagia may be caused by oral, pharyngeal, pharyngoesophageal, and esophageal causes, and can be precipitated by anatomic or structural causes or underlying neuropathic, myopathic, or junctionopathic causes.
- Cranial nerve deficits – trigeminal nerve (CN V) lesions can cause drooling due to inability to close the mouth; facial nerve palsy (CN VII) can cause drooling from the affected side; glossopharyngeal (CN IX), vagus (CN X), and hypoglossal (CN XII) nerve lesions can cause a loss of the gag reflex or inability to swallow.
- Cheilitis or acne – persistent drooling can lead to dermatologic lesions.

DIFFERENTIAL DIAGNOSIS

- Differentiating causes of ptyalism and pseudoptyalism requires a thorough history, including vaccination status, current medications, possible toxin exposure, and duration of ptyalism.
- May be able to distinguish salivation associated with nausea (signs of depression, lip smacking, and retching) from dysphagia by observing the patient.
- Complete physical examination (with special attention to the oral cavity and neck) and neurologic examination are critical; wear examination gloves when rabies exposure is possible.

 DIAGNOSTICS

- CBC – often unremarkable; leukocytosis in patients with immune-mediated, inflammatory, or infectious disease.
- Stress leukogram – common in animals that have ingested a caustic agent or organophosphate.
- FeLV-infected cats may have leukopenia and nonregenerative anemia.
- Serum creatine kinase (CK) activity should be evaluated in all dysphagic patients for evidence of underlying myopathic condition.
- Possible microcytosis with portosystemic shunts.
- Biochemical analysis – usually unremarkable except in patients with renal disease (azotemia, hyperphosphatemia) and hepatoencephalopathy (possibly elevated hepatic enzyme activities, decreased BUN, hypoalbuminemia, hypocholesterolemia, hyperbilirubinemia, and hypoglycemia).
- Marked ptyalism can result in hypokalemia and acidosis from the loss of potassium and bicarbonate-rich saliva.
- Urinalysis – often normal; decreased urine specific gravity with renal or hepatic disease.
- Urate urolithiasis may be noted in patients with portosystemic shunts.

Other Laboratory Tests

- Fasting and postprandial bile acids and/or fasting ammonia when hepatoencephalopathy is suspected.
- Serologic FeLV and FIV testing in cats with oral lesions.
- Acetylcholine receptor antibody titer if focal myasthenia gravis is suspected as the cause of megaesophagus.
- Serum cholinesterase level if organophosphate toxicosis is suspected.
- Postmortem fluorescent antibody testing of brain tissue if rabies is suspected.

Imaging

- Survey radiography of the oral cavity, neck, and thorax when foreign body, structural abnormality, or neoplasm is suspected.
- Abdominal radiographs ± abdominal ultrasound may help diagnose cause of vomiting; may also help diagnose hepatic or renal disease.
- Ultrasonographic evaluation, portal venography, or portal scintigraphy may help diagnose a portosystemic shunt.
- Fluoroscopic evaluation of swallowing may be useful in dysphagic patients to evaluate esophageal function and motility; use caution during barium administration in animals that are dysphagic. Liquid barium swallow should be assessed first. Animals that have trouble with swallowing solid food may then be evaluated with barium-coated food.

- MRI or CT for suspected intracranial lesions.
- CT of skull may be more sensitive than radiographs, especially when foreign body or neoplasia is suspected.

Diagnostic Procedures

- Biopsy and histopathology of mucocutaneous lesions – possibly including immunofluorescence testing when immune-mediated disease (e.g., pemphigus vulgaris) is suspected.
- Fine-needle aspiration of oral lesions and regional lymph nodes.
- Biopsy and histopathology of oral lesion, salivary gland, or mass.
- Consider esophagoscopy or gastroscopy if lesions distal to the oral cavity are suspected; endoscopic removal of foreign bodies may be possible.

 # THERAPEUTICS

- Treat the underlying cause (refer to sections pertaining to specific conditions).
- Symptomatic treatment to reduce the flow of saliva – generally unnecessary, may be of little value to the patient, and may mask other signs of the underlying cause and thus delay diagnosis; only recommended when hypersalivation is prolonged and severe and, if possible, after the underlying condition has been diagnosed.

Drug(s) of Choice

- Anticholinergic medications may be given symptomatically to reduce the flow of saliva; atropine (0.05 mg/kg SQ PRN) or glycopyrrolate (0.01 mg/kg SQ PRN).
- Antiemetics given in conjunction with opioid premedication have variable effects on nausea, vomiting, and ptyalism (see Chapter 16 for list of antiemetics and dosages).
- Crystalloid fluids may be given IV or SQ to treat dehydration caused by prolonged or severe ptyalism.
- Phenobarbital (2 mg/kg PO q 12 h) has been effective in treating idiopathic hypersialosis.
- Anticonvulsant therapy is indicated for seizure activity.

Appropriate Health Care

Depending on underlying cause, hospitalization with intravenous fluids and nutritional support may be necessary.

Nursing Care

- Petroleum jelly can be applied to areas of the face constantly wet from saliva to help prevent moist dermatitis.
- Astringent solutions applied for 10 min q 8–12 h can be used to treat areas of moist dermatitis.

Diet

- Enteral nutritional support (esophagostomy, gastrostomy tubes, etc.) may be needed in patients with ptyalism and anorexia secondary to severe oral, gastrointestinal, or metabolic causes.
- Reduced protein diets may be recommended for patients with hepatic encephalopathy or renal disease, but are not necessarily warranted in animals with portosystemic shunts that are not encephalopathic.

Surgical Considerations

Surgical attenuation or ligation of portosystemic shunt may be recommended.

COMMENTS

Rabies has zoonotic potential.

Client Education

- Nutritional support and maintaining hydration status are necessary.
- Clients may need to be instructed on using feeding tubes at home.
- Ptyalism requires veterinary attention for diagnosis of underlying cause and treatment.

Patient Monitoring

- Depends on the underlying cause (see "Causes").
- Continually monitor hydration, body weight, serum electrolytes, and nutritional status, especially in dysphagic or anorexic animals.

Possible Complications

- Metabolic acidosis.
- Dehydration.
- Hypokalemia.
- Moist dermatitis.
- Aspiration pneumonia.

Synonyms

- Drooling
- Hypersalivation
- Sialism
- Sialorrhea
- Sialosis

Abbreviations

- CN = cranial nerve
- CNS = central nervous system
- CT = computed tomography
- FeLV = feline leukemia virus
- FIV = feline immunodeficiency virus
- MRI = magnetic resonance imaging

See also

- Dysphagia
- Esophagitis
- Hepatic Encephalopathy
- Megaesophagus
- Stomatitis

Suggested Reading

Claude AK, Dedeaux A, Chiavaccini L, Hinz S. Effects of maropitant citrate or acepromazine on the incidence of adverse effects associated with hydromorphone premedication in dogs. J Vet Intern Med 2014;8:1414–1417.

Niemiec BA. Ptyalism. In: Ettinger SJ, Feldman EC, eds. Textbook of Veterinary Internal Medicine, 7th ed. St Louis: Elsevier, 2010, pp. 185–188.

Van der Merwe LL, Christie J, Clift SJ, Dvir E. Salivary gland enlargement and sialorrhoea in dogs with spirocercosis: a retrospective and prospective study of 298 cases. J S Afr Vet Assoc 2012;83(1):920.

Author: Valerie J. Parker DVM, DACVIM, DACVN

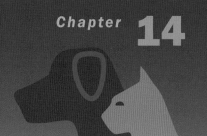

Chapter 14

Rectal and Anal Prolapse

DEFINITION/OVERVIEW

Rectal and anal prolapse are differentiated by the tissue layers affected. An anal prolapse (incomplete prolapse) is a protrusion of anorectal mucosa through the external anal orifice.

Rectal prolapse (complete prolapse) is a double-layer invagination of the full thickness of the rectal tube through the anal orifice.

ETIOLOGY/PATHOPHYSIOLOGY

Prolapse of the anal mucosa may occur during defecation, especially if the feces are hard and dry, but usually reduces spontaneously. If the prolapse is persistent, the anal mucosa can become red and swollen and require treatment. Rectal prolapse can occur with any condition that causes prolonged tenesmus. Once the prolapse is initiated, continued straining results in eversion of more tissue appearing as an elongated mass. The everted tissue becomes edematous and with continued exposure, the mucosa may be appear dark red or black and become ulcerated or necrotic.

Systems Affected

Gastrointestinal.

SIGNALMENT/HISTORY

- Dog and cat of any age, sex or breed.
- Manx cat – the genetic mutation which causes taillessness can also cause sacral, vertebral, and spinal cord malformations resulting in anal laxity.
- Higher prevalence for young, parasitized dogs or cats with diarrhea.

Risk Factors

- Gastrointestinal disorders that cause diarrhea and tenesmus, such as parasitism, colitis/enteritis, constipation/obstipation, rectal foreign body, rectal deviation and diverticulum, proctitis, and rectal or anal tumors.
- Urogenital disorders, such as cystitis, urolithiasis, prostatitis, prostatic hypertrophy, and dystocia.
- Tenesmus following perineal, rectal, or urogenital surgery (e.g., perineal herniorrhaphy).

Blackwell's Five-Minute Veterinary Consult Clinical Companion: Small Animal Gastrointestinal Diseases, First Edition. Edited by Jocelyn Mott and Jo Ann Morrison.
© 2019 John Wiley & Sons, Inc. Published 2019 by John Wiley & Sons, Inc.
Companion website: www.fiveminutevet.com/gastrointestinal

Historical Findings

- Straining to defecate – some owners interpret as being due to constipation.
- Diarrhea.
- Visible mass protruding from the anus.
- Recent perineal surgery.

 # CLINICAL FEATURES

- Anal prolapse – a doughnut of anal mucosa protruding through the anal orifice after defecation.
- Rectal prolapse – elongated cylindrical tube of rectal tissue protruding through the anal orifice (Figure 14.1).

 # DIFFERENTIAL DIAGNOSIS

- Prolapsed intussusception – rule out by (1) passing a finger or blunt probe between the mass and the anus (Figures 14.2 and 14.3) (the probe should not penetrate more than 1–2 cm before contacting the fornix; if the probe easily passes 5–6 cm, then suspect prolapsed intussusception) or (2) abdominal ultrasonography (look for increased intestinal layering).
- Neoplasia – rule out by palpation, fine-needle aspiration and cytology, and/or biopsy and histopathology.

 # DIAGNOSTICS

Rectal palpation.

Complete Blood Cell Count/Biochemistry/Urinalysis

Often unremarkable.

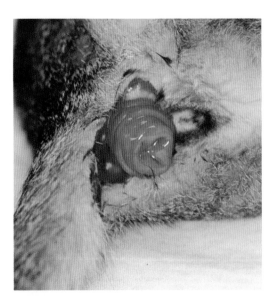

■ **Fig. 14.1.** Rectal prolapse in young cat.

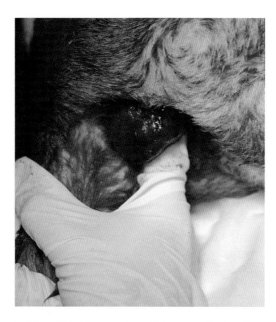

■ **Fig. 14.2.** Rectal prolapse is differentiated from prolapsed intussusception by attempting to insert finger between the anus and prolapsed tissue. A finger could be inserted almost 10 cm in this case, confirming prolapsed intussusception.

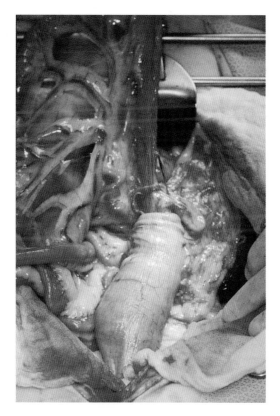

■ **Fig. 14.3.** Intraoperative photograph of the intussusception.

Other Laboratory Tests

- Fecal examination may confirm parasitism.

Imaging

- Abdominal radiography – may demonstrate foreign body, prostatomegaly, cystic calculi, or colonic fecal distension.
- Abdominal ultrasonography – may demonstrate prostatomegaly, cystic calculi, bladder wall thickening, or intussusception.

Other Diagnostic Procedures

Colonoscopy may help evaluate recurrent prolapse for an underlying cause.

Pathologic Findings

Assess viability of the prolapsed tissue by surface appearance and tissue temperature. Vital tissue appears swollen and hyperemic, and red blood exudes from the cut surface; devitalized tissue appears dark purple or black, and dark cyanotic blood exudes from the cut surface. Ulcerations may be present.

 THERAPEUTICS

- Most prolapses can be successfully treated with a purse-string suture following reduction (Figure 14.4).
- Resection and anastomosis is necessary with devitalized prolapses or when the prolapse cannot be reduced.
- Colopexy is indicated for recurrent prolapses.

Drug(s) of Choice

- Anthelmintic based on fecal examination.
- Stool softeners – docusate sodium (dogs, 50–200 mg PO q 8–12 h; cats, 50 mg PO q 12–24 h) or lactulose (10 g/15 mL solution or syrup, 1 mL/4.5 kg q 8–1 2 h to effect); continue for 2–3 weeks after removal of the purse-string suture.

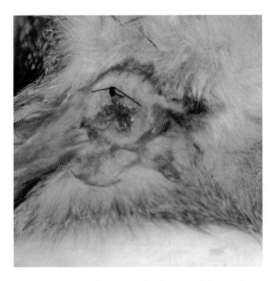

■ **Fig. 14.4.** A loose purse-string was placed after manual reduction of the prolapse. A rectal examination should be performed to confirm that the prolapse has been completely reduced.

Nursing Care

Keep perineal area clean.

Diet

Feed a low-residue diet until purse-string suture is removed.

Surgical Considerations

- Conservative management.
  - General anesthesia facilitates manipulation of the tissue back into the rectum.
  - Gently replace prolapsed tissue through the anus with the use of lubricants and gentle massage; topical osmotic agents may help if severe swelling exists.
  - Place a purse-string suture at the mucocutaneous junction using monofilament nonabsorbable suture material to aid retention and prevent acute recurrence; place the suture loose enough to allow room for defecation. A syringe case or other blunt object can be inserted into the rectum to avoid overtightening the purse-string suture.
  - The purse-string suture is usually removed in 3–5 days but can be maintained longer if necessary.
  - Placing local anesthetic (e.g., 1% dibucaine) into the rectum periodically has been recommended to prevent straining.
- Rectal resection and anastomosis.
  - Indicated when the prolapse cannot be reduced or the prolapsed tissue is nonviable.
  - Anesthetize the patient and place in ventral recumbency with rear legs over the end of the padded surgery table with the tail tied over the back.
  - Use of an epidural facilitates treatment and relieves discomfort.
  - Administer prophylactic antibiotics (e.g., cefazolin 22 mg/kg IV or cefoxitin 30 mg/kg IV).
  - Aseptically prep and drape the perineal area.
  - Place a well-lubricated probe (e.g., syringe barrel or case) into the rectum to facilitate stay suture placement (Figure 14.5).
  - Place 3–4 full-thickness stay sutures incorporating both layers of the intussusception.
  - Resect the prolapsed rectal tissue 1–2 cm from the anus. It may be easier to cut and suture the rectal tissue sequentially in each segment between the stay sutures, especially if tension is present (Figure 14.6).

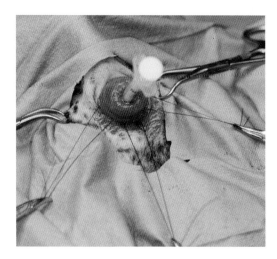

■ **Fig. 14.5.** Nonreducible prolapse in a young dog. A syringe was placed in the prolapsed segment and then 3 stay sutures were placed through both layers of the prolapse to prevent retraction of the proximal segment as the prolapse was resected.

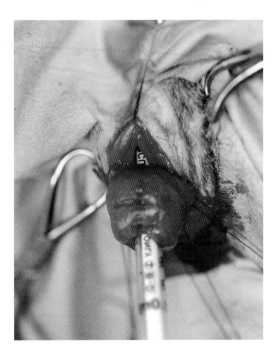

■ **Fig. 14.6.** After incising through all layers the anastomosis was begun on the dorsal midline using simple interrupted sutures. Be sure to incorporate the submucosa of each layer segment.

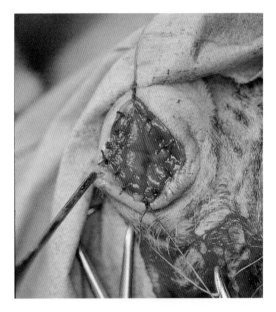

■ **Fig. 14.7.** The completed rectal anastomosis. The dorsal and ventral suture tags were kept long to prevent retraction into the pelvic canal until the anastomosis was completed.

- Suture the two ends with 3-0 or 4-0 synthetic absorbable suture material. The sutures must engage the submucosa of both segments (Figure 14.7).
- Remove the stay sutures and reduce the prolapse.
- A purse-string can be placed in case tenesmus persists immediately after surgery.

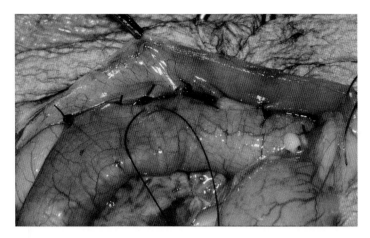

■ **Fig. 14.8.** Colopexy for a recurrent rectal prolapse. Two rows of interrupted sutures were placed between the ventrolateral body wall and descending colon while maintaining cranial traction on the colon.

■ Colopexy.
  • Colopexy is indicated when rectal prolapse recurs after multiple attempts at conservative management. Colopexy is preferred over rectal resection and anastomosis for recurrent prolapses.
  • Anesthetize the patient and clip and prep the ventral abdomen.
  • Place the patient in dorsal recumbency and perform a ventral midline celiotomy.
  • Expose the colon and apply cranial traction on the descending colon close to the pelvis. A nonsterile assistant can assist with the reduction back through the anus and verify that the reduction is complete by visual inspection and rectal palpation.
  • Both incisional and nonincisional colopexies have been described and are equally effective. The author typically performs nonincisional colopexies in rectal prolapse cases.
  • While maintaining cranial traction on the descending colon, place a row of 5–6 interrupted sutures between the antimesenteric border of the descending colon and left abdominal wall approximately 2.5–3 cm lateral to the midline using 2-0 or 3-0 monofilament absorbable (e.g., polydioxanone or polyglyconate) or nonabsorbable (e.g., nylon or polypropylene) suture material (Figure 14.8).
  • Roll the colon toward the midline and place a second row of sutures.
  • The sutures in the colon must engage the submucosa but penetration of the lumen should be avoided.
  • Scarifying the serosa of the colon and body wall with a scalpel blade or dry sponge has been recommended by some veterinary surgeons but the efficacy of this in enhancing adhesion formation has not been evaluated.
  • Close the abdominal incision.

 COMMENTS

Client Education
■ Observe for recurrence or persistent straining.
■ Repeat anthelmintic treatment at appropriate intervals.

Patient Monitoring

Examine for rectal stricture if straining persists following rectal resection and anastomosis. This is more common in cats.

Prevention/Avoidance

Treat underlying/predisposing causes.

Possible Complications

- Recurrence – most likely following manual reduction and purse-string placement.
- Rectal stricture following resection of the prolapse and rectal anastomosis, especially in cats.
- Infection.
- Dehiscence of anastomosis.

Expected Course and Prognosis

- Identification and treatment of the underlying cause is important.
- The long-term prognosis is excellent, especially if rectal resection can be avoided.

See Also

- Colitis and Proctitis
- Dyschezia
- Hematochezia
- Intussusception

Suggested Reading

Aronson LR. Rectum, anus, perineum. In: Tobias KM, Johnston SA, eds, Veterinary Small Animal Surgery. St Louis: Elsevier Saunders, 2012, pp. 1564–1600.

Engen MH. Management of rectal prolapse. In: Bojrab MJ, Waldron D, Toombs JR, eds. Current Techniques in Small Animal Surgery, 5th ed. Jackson: Teton NewMedia, 2014, pp. 303–306.

Radlinsky MG. Rectal prolapse. In: Fossum TW, ed. Small Animal Surgery, 4th ed. St Louis: Elsevier Mosby, 2013, pp. 577–580.

Author: Eric R. Pope DVM, MS, DACVS

Chapter 15

Regurgitation

DEFINITION/OVERVIEW

- Passive expulsion of ingesta or fluid from the esophagus or stomach.
- Regurgitation is passive, unlike vomiting which is a centrally mediated forceful expulsion of ingesta and/or fluid.

ETIOLOGY/PATHOPHYSIOLOGY

- Any disease which affects the motility of the esophagus or prevents passage of ingesta through the esophagus or stomach may lead to regurgitation.
- Regurgitation can be distinguished from vomiting by the lack of associated signs of nausea, lack of hypersalivation preceding the event as well as the absence of retching or other evidence of active expulsion.
- The timing of the event in relationship to eating does *not* distinguish between vomiting and regurgitation.

Systems Affected

Underlying diseases and disorders which may cause regurgitation include the following.
- Esophageal.
  - Megaesophagus, both primary and secondary.
  - Esophagitis.
  - Obstruction: foreign body, stricture, neoplasia, vascular ring anomalies, other.
  - Infectious: *Spirocerca, Pythium.*
- Gastrointestinal (GI).
  - Gastric dilation-volvulus.
  - Pyloric outflow obstruction.
  - Hiatal hernia.
- Neuromuscular.
  - Myasthenia gravis.
  - Polymyositis,
  - Dermatomyositis.
  - Dysautonomia.
  - Tetanus.
  - Botulism.
  - Distemper.

Blackwell's Five-Minute Veterinary Consult Clinical Companion: Small Animal Gastrointestinal Diseases, First Edition. Edited by Jocelyn Mott and Jo Ann Morrison.
© 2019 John Wiley & Sons, Inc. Published 2019 by John Wiley & Sons, Inc.
Companion website: www.fiveminutevet.com/gastrointestinal

- Endocrine.
    - Hypoadrenocorticism.
    - Hypothyroidism.
- Respiratory – aspiration pneumonia; nasal discharge.
- Immune mediated.
    - Thymoma.
    - Systemic lupus erythematosus.
- Toxic.
    - Lead.
    - Acetylcholinesterase.

 ## SIGNALMENT/HISTORY

- Regurgitation may be seen due to congenital diseases including primary megaesophagus. More common in dogs than cats. Suggested breed predispositions include Irish setter, Great Dane, German shepherd, Labrador retriever, Chinese shar-pei, Newfoundland, miniature schnauzer, fox terrier dogs, and Siamese cats.
- Vascular ring anomalies typically become evident at weaning, with affected patients regurgitating solid food (Figure 15.1).
- Hiatal hernias are typically congenital and may be more common in males and Chinese shar-peis.

Risk Factors

- General anesthesia may allow for esophageal reflux which in turn can lead to both esophagitis and/or esophageal stricture, both of which may cause regurgitation.
- Esophageal foreign bodies may cause regurgitation, both at the time of obstruction and a few weeks later if an esophageal stricture develops secondary to the previously lodged foreign body.

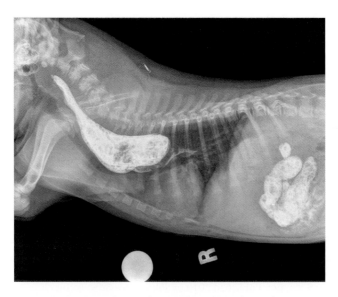

■ **Fig. 15.1.** Lateral radiograph of a dog with a persistent right aortic arch.

Historical Findings

- In addition to regurgitation, owners may also note weight loss and general lack of health.
- Other signs of the underlying systemic disease may be noted.

 ## CLINICAL FEATURES

- Physical examination may be normal.
- Cachexia may be present.
- Increased respiratory rate, effort, and bronchovesicular sounds if aspiration pneumonia is present.

 ## DIFFERENTIAL DIAGNOSIS

- Regurgitation needs to be distinguished from vomiting. Lack of clinical aspects associated with vomiting (salivation, nausea, retching) suggests regurgitation.
- Animals may also have signs suggestive of concurrent aspiration pneumonia (fever, coughing).

 ## DIAGNOSTICS

The approach to the diagnosis of underlying etiology of regurgitation may be multifaceted (Figure 15.2).

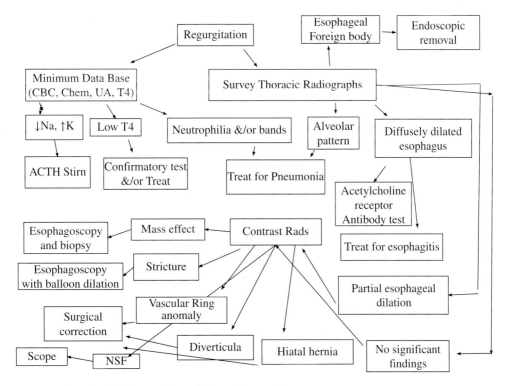

■ **Fig. 15.2.** Flowchart for diagnostic investigation of regurgitation.

Complete Blood Cell Count/Biochemistry Panel/Urinalysis

Minimum database consisting of a complete blood cell count, chemistry profile, urinalysis, and T4 should be obtained to look for underlying diseases and complications.

Other Laboratory Tests

- In cases where megaesophagus is found, further diagnostics looking for an underlying cause should be performed. Potential testing to be considered includes the following.
  - Acetylcholine receptor antibody titers.
  - Adrenocorticotropic hormone (ACTH) stimulation test (looking for hypoadrenocorticism).
  - Additional thyroid testing.
  - Lead levels.

Imaging

- Thoracic radiographs are a crucial diagnostic for regurgitating patients. Radiographs may demonstrate an enlarged, air- or food-filled esophagus suggestive of megaesophagus. In dyspneic patients, being able to repeatedly find a dilated esophagus may be necessary to rule out transient aerophagia. Partial dilation found only orad to the heart base is consistent with a vascular ring anomaly or other obstruction. Thoracic radiographs may also reveal esophageal foreign bodies (Figure 15.3) or neoplasia. Small amounts of fluid or air in the esophagus suggest esophagitis. Thoracic radiographs may show aspiration pneumonia.
- An esophagram may be helpful in equivocal cases of megaesophagus. Caution must be exercised to avoid the patient aspirating the contrast material. Esophagrams are often useful in diagnosing esophageal strictures as well as tumors.

Other Diagnostic Tests

Where available, esophagoscopy is warranted to look for strictures and masses. Endoscopy also allows examination of the stomach and small intestine.

(a)

(b)

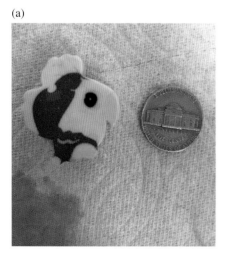
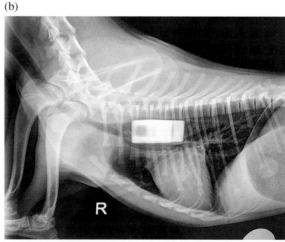

■ **Fig. 15.3.** (a) Lateral radiograph of a dog with an esophageal foreign body. (b) The foreign body is shown next to a nickel for size comparison.

THERAPEUTICS

The primary goal is to prevent further regurgitation. Controlling regurgitation is crucial to avoid aspiration pneumonia. Underlying conditions should be treated appropriately.

Drug(s) of Choice

- Many regurgitating patients suffer from esophagitis, either as the primary cause for the regurgitation or secondary to esophageal exposure to gastric acid. Gastroprotectants including sucralfate 0.5–1 g dissolved in 5–10 cc of water to make a slurry PO q 8 h and omeprazole 0.5–1 mg/kg PO q 12–24 h should be administered.
- The ability of promotility drugs to affect the esophageal motility is questionable. Cisapride 1.25–2.5 mg/cat PO q 8–12 h may be helpful in cats as their esophagus contains smooth muscle. For dogs, metoclopramide 0.2–0.5 mg/kg PO q 8–12 h may be beneficial in tightening the lower esophageal sphincter, thus preventing some reflux.
- The COX-2 inhibitor celecoxib may also increase lower esophageal pressure in dogs. In humans, COX-2 inhibitors inhibit esophageal cancers.
- Underlying conditions should be treated as appropriate.
- Judicious use of antibiotics is warranted for aspiration pneumonia.

Alternative Drugs

A new study suggests that sildenafil 1 mg/kg PO q 12 h may reduce regurgitation in dogs with congenital idiopathic megaesophagus.

Appropriate Health Care

- Regurgitation makes patients very susceptible to developing aspiration pneumonia. Owners should be cautioned to monitor their pet's respiration.
- Some patients with persistent regurgitation cannot consume sufficient calories. The patient's weight should be carefully monitored. In certain cases, gastric feeding tubes may be necessary to provide sufficient nutritional support.

Diet

- Feeding considerations are very important for dogs with regurgitation.
- Patients should be fed in an upright position and maintained upright for approximately 15 min after eating. Patients can be trained to eat off a counter or some other surface or a "Bailey chair," which holds the dog upright, can be used.
- Patients should receive small, frequent meals.
- Different food consistencies should be tried to see what is best tolerated. Many patients do best with either a gruel consistency or small meatballs of canned food.
- Feeding tubes should be considered for patients with persistent weight loss and a noncorrectable underlying condition.

Surgical Considerations

- Endoscopic techniques may be ideal in some cases of regurgitation.
  - Esophageal foreign bodies can often be removed endoscopically.
  - Esophageal strictures can be dilated using a balloon catheter endoscopically.
- Certain underlying conditions leading to regurgitation may be surgically correctable.
  - Vascular ring anomalies.
  - Esophageal diverticula.
  - Some esophageal neoplasias.
  - Large hiatal hernias.

COMMENTS

Client Education

- Client education will obviously be dictated by what disease or condition is leading to regurgitation.
- Many of the underlying conditions such as megaesophagus and myasthenia gravis can be medically managed but not cured. Owners need to be cautioned as to the lifelong care these patients will require.
- Clients need to be educated about aspiration pneumonia and to monitor their pets for any respiratory difficulties.
- In cases of esophageal foreign bodies and esophagitis, clients should be warned of the potential for esophageal strictures forming a few weeks later.

Patient Monitoring

- Regardless of the underlying disease or condition, thoracic radiographs should be obtained whenever aspiration pneumonia is suspected (Figure 15.4).
- Patient's weight and body condition should be monitored to ensure they are receiving adequate caloric intake.
- Underlying systemic conditions such as hypoadrenocorticism and myasthenia gravis will need to be monitored.

Possible Complications

- As previously stated, aspiration pneumonia frequently develops in patients with persistent regurgitation.
- Bacterial resistance is a concern for patients who need to receive multiple courses of antibiotics. In certain cases of repeat pneumonia, it may be advisable to determine antibiotic selection based upon culture of tracheal wash or bronchoalveolar lavage.
- Some patients with severe, persistent regurgitation cannot ingest sufficient calories to meet physiologic demands and will need feeding tubes.

(a)

(b)

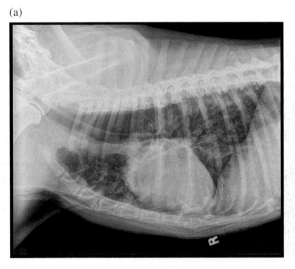 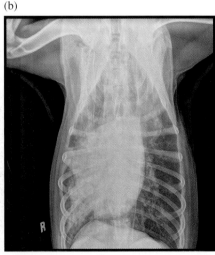

■ **Fig. 15.4.** (a) Lateral and (b) dorsoventral radiographs of a dog with aspiration pneumonia and megaesophagus.

Expected Course and Prognosis

- Prognosis varies with underlying cause for regurgitation.
- Idiopathic megaesophagus carries a poor prognosis as most patients will develop aspiration pneumonia.

Abbreviations

- ACTH = adrenocorticotropic hormone

See Also

- Cricopharyngeal Achalasia
- Dysphagia
- Esophageal Foreign Bodies
- Esophageal Neoplasia
- Esophageal Stricture
- Esophagitis

- Hiatal Hernia
- Megaesophagus
- Nutritional Approach to Gastroesophageal Reflux Disease and Megaesophagus
- *Spirocerca lupi*

Suggested Reading

De la Fuente SG, McMahon RL, Clary EM, et al. Celecoxib (Celebrex) increases canine lower esophageal sphincter pressure. J Surg Res 2002;107:154–158.

Jergens AE. Diseases of the esophagus. In: Ettinger SE, Feldman EC, eds. Textbook of Veterinary Internal Medicine, 7th ed. St Louis: Saunders Elsevier, 2010.

Woolley CS. Dysphagia and regurgitation. In: Ettinger SE, Feldman EC, eds. Textbook of Veterinary Internal Medicine, 7th ed. St Louis: Saunders Elsevier, 2010.

Acknowledgments: The author and editors acknowledge the prior contribution of Dr Stanley L. Marks.

Author: Rhonda L. Schulman DVM, DACVIM (SAIM)

Chapter 16

Vomiting, Acute

DEFINITION/OVERVIEW

- Forceful, neurologically mediated reflex expulsion of gastric contents from the oral cavity.
- Acute vomiting is defined as vomiting of short duration (<5–7 days) and variable frequency.

ETIOLOGY/PATHOPHYSIOLOGY

- A complex set of reflex activities under central neurologic and hormonal control involving the coordination of gastrointestinal (GI), abdominal, and respiratory musculature.
- Often preceded by prodromal signs of nausea.
- In the first stage (stage 1), there is increased saliva production with bicarbonate to lubricate the esophagus and neutralize gastric acid.
- This is followed by decreased gastric and esophageal motility and increased retrograde motility of the proximal small intestine.
- Stage 2 consists of retching, which is forceful contractions of the abdominal muscles and diaphragm with a resultant negative intrathoracic pressure and positive intraabdominal pressure to facilitate moving gastric contents orally.
- In stage 3 the gastric contents are expelled. There is a change in the intrathoracic pressure from negative to positive via the force generated by the abdominal and diaphragm muscles. Concurrently, respiration is inhibited and the nasopharynx and glottis close to prevent aspiration.
- Neural activation causing vomiting may occur with stimulation of stretch receptors, chemoreceptors, and osmoreceptors. These are located throughout the GI tract, hepatobiliary system, genitourinary system, peritoneum, and the pancreas. (The duodenum has the most receptors.)
- The humoral stimuli are mediated through the chemoreceptor trigger zone (CTZ), with a more permeable blood–brain barrier.
- Cats have poorly developed CTZ dopaminergic receptors and therefore respond poorly to apomorphine or D2 dopaminergic receptor antagonists such as metoclopramide.
- Higher centers can lead to psychogenic vomiting, and input from the vestibular apparatus (e.g. motion sickness, vestibular disease) can stimulate the emetic center.

Systems Affected

- Cardiovascular – hypovolemia causing tachycardia, pale mucous membranes, and weak pulses; hypokalemia can cause cardiac arrhythmias.

Blackwell's Five-Minute Veterinary Consult Clinical Companion: Small Animal Gastrointestinal Diseases, First Edition. Edited by Jocelyn Mott and Jo Ann Morrison.
© 2019 John Wiley & Sons, Inc. Published 2019 by John Wiley & Sons, Inc.
Companion website: www.fiveminutevet.com/gastrointestinal

- Gastrointestinal – reflux esophagitis.
- Metabolic – electrolyte and acid–base abnormalities (e.g. hypokalemia, hyponatremia, hypochloremia, metabolic alkalosis), prerenal azotemia, and dehydration.
- Nervous – lethargy.
- Respiratory – aspiration pneumonia, rhinitis from vomitus refluxed into the nasopharynx.

 ## SIGNALMENT/HISTORY

No age, breed, or sex predisposition.

Risk Factors

- Adverse food reactions – most frequent cause of acute vomiting; indiscretions (eating rapidly, ingestion of foreign material); intolerances (e.g., sudden diet change, allergies).
- Drugs – antibiotics, antiinflammatory drugs (corticosteroids, nonsteroidal antiinflammatory drugs (NSAIDs)), chemotherapeutics, digitalis, narcotics, xylazine.
- GI inflammation – infectious enteritis: viruses (parvovirus, distemper, coronavirus), bacteria (*Salmonella, Campylobacter, Helicobacter* spp.), rickettsial (salmon poisoning); hemorrhagic gastroenteritis.
- Gastroduodenal ulcers.
- GI obstruction – foreign bodies, intussusception, neoplasia, volvulus, ileus, constipation, mucosal hypertrophy.
- Systemic disease – uremia, hepatic failure, sepsis, acidosis, electrolyte imbalance (hypokalemia, hypocalcemia, hypercalcemia).
- Abdominal disorders – pancreatitis, peritonitis, pyometra.
- Endocrine disease – hypoadrenocorticism, diabetic ketoacidosis.
- Neurologic disease – vestibular disturbances, meningitis, encephalitis, central nervous system (CNS) trauma.
- Parasitism – ascarids, *Giardia, Physaloptera, Ollulanus tricuspis* (cats).
- Toxins – lead, ethylene glycol, zinc, mycotoxins, house plants.
- Miscellaneous – anaphylaxis, heat stroke, motion sickness, pain, fear.

Historical Findings

- Variable vomiting of food and/or fluid. It is essential to differentiate between vomiting and regurgitation when obtaining the history.
- Ingestion of foreign material.
- Variable lethargy and appetite loss; may see diarrhea and/or melena

 ## CLINICAL FEATURES

- May include dehydration (e.g., dry mucous membranes, reduced skin turgor, sunken eyes, pale mucous membranes, tachycardia, weak pulses), fluid-filled bowel loops, excessive gut sounds, abdominal pain (localized, e.g., foreign body, pancreatitis, pyelonephritis, hepatic disease, vs diffuse, e.g., peritonitis, severe enteritis), or abdominal mass (e.g., foreign body, intussusception, torsed viscus).
- May note diarrhea or melena on rectal examination.
- May see fever with infectious and inflammatory causes.
- May be unremarkable.

DIFFERENTIAL DIAGNOSIS

Differentiating Similar Signs

- Vomiting usually includes hypersalivation, retching, and forceful contractions of the abdominal muscles and diaphragm.
- Must always be differentiated from regurgitation, which is the passive expulsion of fluid or food from the esophagus or pharyngeal cavity, and dysphagia (difficulty in swallowing), which is observed during eating or drinking.
- Animals that are vomiting may have disorders that additionally cause regurgitation, and frequent vomiting can lead to reflux esophagitis and regurgitation.

Differentiating Causes

- If no signs of serious vomiting (e.g., dehydration, lethargy, fever, anorexia, or abdominal pain), can assess with a thorough history and physical examination alone.
- When indications of serious vomiting exist, when frequency intensifies, or when signs do not resolve over 2–3 days, obtain a minimum database (including complete blood count (CBC), biochemical analysis, urinalysis, and survey abdominal radiographs) in an attempt to find the primary cause.

 DIAGNOSTICS

Complete Blood Count/Biochemistry Panel/Urinalysis

- In nonsevere vomiting, the hemogram, biochemical profile, and urinalysis are typically unremarkable unless the animal is dehydrated.
- Anemia with panhypoproteinemia seen with severe gastric ulceration and bleeding.
- Dehydration – may see hemoconcentration (high packed cell volume (PCV) and total protein).
- May see a stress leukogram.
- Infectious or inflammatory causes – may see an inflammatory leukogram.
- Acute hepatopathies – may see elevated liver enzymes and serum bilirubin.
- Pancreatitis – may see elevated lipase, amylase, and liver enzymes.
- Hyponatremia, hyperkalemia, hypoglycemia, and azotemia suggest hypoadrenocorticism.
- Hyperglycemia with glucosuria and ketonuria indicates ketoacidotic diabetes mellitus.
- Hypochloremic metabolic acidosis suggests gastric outflow obstruction.

Other Laboratory Tests

Additional blood tests for specific diseases when indicated (e.g., blood lead level, ethylene glycol assay, adrenocorticotropic hormone (ACTH) stimulation testing for hypoadrenocorticism, and canine pancreatic lipase immunoreactivity (cPL) or feline pancreatic lipase immunoreactivity (fPL) testing for pancreatitis).

Imaging

- Survey abdominal radiographs are often unremarkable, but radiodense foreign bodies, segmental ileus, or gastric distension indicating volvulus or outflow obstruction may be observed; serosal detail may be lost ("ground glass" appearance) with pancreatitis or peritonitis; a mass effect or haziness in the right cranial quadrant or persistent gas in the descending duodenum may indicate pancreatitis.

- Can use contrast radiography to evaluate for radiolucent foreign bodies, obstruction, intussusception, or volvulus.
- Can use abdominal ultrasonography to visualize an obstruction, an intussusception, lymphadenopathy, masses or pancreatitis.

Diagnostic Procedures

Endoscopy may be useful to assess for gastroduodenal ulceration and gastric and proximal duodenal foreign bodies.

Pathologic Findings

Dependent on etiology.

 THERAPEUTICS

Drug(s) of Choice

- May use antiemetics in patients with severe vomiting causing electrolyte and/or acid–base disturbances or reflux esophagitis.
- Several antiemetics are available for both dogs and cats – phenothiazine derivatives that act at the CTZ and emetic center include chlorpromazine (0.5 mg/kg SQ q 8 h, dogs and cats) and metoclopramide, a dopamine antagonist and motility modifier that acts at the CTZ and on local receptors in the gut (0.2–0.5 mg/kg PO or SQ q 6–8 h, or 1–2 mg/kg/day as a constant rate infusion (CRI)); H1-receptor antagonists acting on the CTZ can be used in motion sickness (e.g., diphenhydramine 2–4 mg/kg PO, IM q 6–8 h, dogs only); maropitant, a neurokinin-1 antagonist (1 mg/kg SQ or IV q 24 h or 2 mg/kg PO q 24 h, dogs and cats).
- Patients with ulceration – can use H2-receptor antagonists such as ranitidine (1–2 mg/kg PO, SQ, IV q 12 h, dogs) and famotidine (0.5–1 mg/kg PO, SQ, IV q 12 h, dogs and cats), proton pump inhibitors such as omeprazole (0.7–1 mg/kg PO q 12–24 h, dogs and cats), and/or gastric mucosal protectants such as sucralfate (250 mg/cat PO q 6–12 h, 250–1000 mg/dog PO q 6–12 h) dissolved into a slurry and given on an empty stomach.
- Fever or mucosal injury (hematemesis, melena) – antibiotics may be indicated (e.g., ampicillin, enrofloxacin).

Precautions/Interactions

- Use phenothiazines with caution in dehydrated patients because of possible hypotension from their alpha-receptor antagonist effect.
- Do not use anticholinergics; they can cause gastric atony and intestinal ileus, which could exacerbate vomiting.
- Do not use prokinetics such as metoclopramide and cisapride in patients with GI obstruction.
- Maropitant should be used with caution in patients with hepatic disease.
- Use antiemetics cautiously; they may suppress vomiting and mask progressive disease or hamper an important means of monitoring response to primary therapy.
- Anticholinergics and opioids may negate the effect of metoclopramide.

Alternative Drug(s)

- Cisapride.
- Famotidine.
- Dolasetron.
- Pantoprazole.

Appropriate Health Care

- Outpatient if vomiting nonserious.
- Hospitalize if severe vomiting.

Nursing Care

- Fasting the animal is not warranted unless the vomiting is intractable and the risk of aspiration pneumonia is increased.
- Patients with frequent episodes of vomiting should be treated initially by keeping the animal NPO and administering intravenous crystalloid fluids.

Diet

- If vomiting resolves, initially offer small amounts of water or ice cubes, and if vomiting does not recur, follow with an easily digestible, low-fat, intestinal diet or single protein and single carbohydrate-source diet such as nonfat cottage cheese or skinless white chicken and rice in a 1:4 ratio. Offer small frequent meals to assess tolerance.
- If vomiting does not recur, wean the patient back onto the normal diet over 4–5 days.

Activity

Animals should have limited activity until the vomiting has stopped.

Surgical Considerations

Surgery should be considered for obstructions of any kind as well as for peritonitis or volvulus.

 ## COMMENTS

Client Education

Owners should be educated on the risks of giving their pet table scraps and to refrain from feeding high-fat treats. They should limit the pet's access to the trash and monitor the pet while it plays with toys to prevent ingestion of foreign bodies.

Patient Monitoring

- If frequency of vomiting increases or the animal has systemic evidence of disease, hospitalize for treatment and obtain appropriate diagnostics.
- If vomiting persists beyond seven days despite conservative therapy, pursue appropriate testing for chronic vomiting.

Prevention/Avoidance

- Animals should be fed a highly digestible fat-restricted diet.
- Owners should attempt to control indiscriminate eating and monitor for foreign body ingestion.

Possible Complications

- Aspiration pneumonia.
- Esophagitis.
- Dehydration.
- See "Systems Affected."

Expected Course and Prognosis

- Recovery from nonserious vomiting is usually rapid and spontaneous.
- Feeding of a highly digestible, fat-restricted diet will frequently control nonserious vomiting.
- GI foreign bodies have a good prognosis after endoscopic retrieval or surgical removal.

Synonym

- Emesis.

Abbreviations

- ACTH = adrenocorticotropic hormone
- CNS = central nervous system
- cPL = canine pancreatic lipase immunoreactivity
- CRI = constant rate infusion
- CTZ = chemoreceptor trigger zone
- fPL = feline pancreatic lipase immunoreactivity
- GI = gastrointestinal
- NSAID = nonsteroidal antiinflammatory drug
- PCV = packed cell volume
- Spec cpl = canine pancreas specific lipase

See Also

- Diarrhea, Acute
- Gastroduodenal Ulceration/Erosion

Suggested Reading

Simpson KW. Diseases of the stomach. In: Ettinger SJ, Feldman EC, eds. Textbook of Veterinary Internal Medicine, 7th ed. St Louis: Elsevier, 2010, pp. 1504–1526.

Twedt DC. Vomiting. In: Ettinger SJ, Feldman EC, eds. Textbook of Veterinary Internal Medicine, 7th ed. St Louis: Elsevier, 2010, pp. 195–200.

Author: Erin Portillo MS, DVM, DACVIM

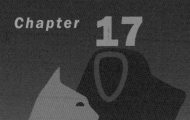

Chapter 17

Vomiting, Chronic

DEFINITION/OVERVIEW

- Persistent vomiting lasting longer than 5–7 days or vomiting that occurs intermittently several days/week.
- This condition is usually nonresponsive to symptomatic treatment.

ETIOLOGY/PATHOPHYSIOLOGY

- Vomiting occurs when the vomiting center, located within the medulla oblongata, is activated by the humoral or neural pathway.
- There are four main components to the vomiting reflex: (1) visceral receptors within the gastrointestinal (GI) tract; (2) vagal and sympathetic afferent neurons; (3) chemoreceptor trigger zone (CRTZ); and (4) vomiting center.
- The humoral pathway is mediated via activation of the CRTZ and is affected by uremic toxins, liver disease, digoxin toxicity, endotoxemia, apomorphine, and other blood-borne triggers.
- The neural pathway is mediated via activation of the vomiting center and is affected by disorders associated with obstruction, distension, or inflammation of the gastrointestinal tract.
- All causes of vomiting (including the vestibular apparatus and cerebrum) are ultimately mediated via the vomiting center.

Systems Affected

- Endocrine/metabolic – dehydration, electrolyte, and acid–base imbalances.
- Cardiovascular – hypovolemia or electrolyte and acid–base imbalances can cause arrhythmias.
- Gastrointestinal – gastroesophageal reflux, esophagitis, and subsequent esophageal stricture.
- Respiratory – aspiration pneumonia.
- Neurologic – altered mentation.

SIGNALMENT/HISTORY

- Dog and cat.
- Young animals are more likely to ingest foreign bodies; linear foreign bodies are more common in cats.

Blackwell's Five-Minute Veterinary Consult Clinical Companion: Small Animal Gastrointestinal Diseases, First Edition. Edited by Jocelyn Mott and Jo Ann Morrison.
© 2019 John Wiley & Sons, Inc. Published 2019 by John Wiley & Sons, Inc.
Companion website: www.fiveminutevet.com/gastrointestinal

- Confirmed or suspected breed predispositions – brachycephalic breeds are prone to pyloric outflow obstruction secondary to mucosal hypertrophy; basenjis, German shepherds, and shar-peis are prone to inflammatory bowel disease; rottweilers are prone to eosinophilic IBD; Airedale terriers are prone to pancreatic carcinoma; beagles, Bedlington terriers, cocker spaniels, Doberman pinschers, Labrador retrievers, Skye terriers, and standard poodles are prone to chronic hepatitis. Yorkshire terriers are predisposed to intestinal lymphangiectasia.

Historical Findings

- Vomiting of food, clear or bile-stained fluid, hematemesis, decreased appetite or anorexia, pica, melena, polydipsia, and abdominal distension are typical of gastric disease.
- Diarrhea and profound weight loss are more characteristic of intestinal disease.
- Signs such as weakness, polyuria, or jaundice relate to other underlying metabolic diseases.

 # CLINICAL FEATURES

- Weight loss and poor hair coat may indicate chronic malnutrition.
- Abdominal palpation may reveal abdominal distension, pain, thickened bowel loops, lymphadenopathy, or mass effects.
- Tacky mucous membranes and prolonged skin tenting if dehydration is present; pale membranes if patient is anemic.
- Oral examination may reveal uremic ulcerations or sublingual string foreign bodies.
- Rectal examination may detect diarrhea, hematochezia, or melena.

 # DIFFERENTIAL DIAGNOSIS

- Vomiting must first be differentiated from regurgitation.
- Regurgitation is a passive retrograde movement of fluid or undigested food that has not yet reached the stomach into the oronasal cavity and occurs without an abdominal component, thus localizing disease to the esophagus.
- Vomiting is a centrally mediated reflex often preceded by prodromal signs of restlessness, nausea, salivation, and repeated swallowing.
- Vomiting patients may also regurgitate because of secondary esophagitis.
- Vomitus of food or partially digested food is more common with primary gastric disease, while vomitus of bile is more likely intestinal in origin.

Causes

Esophageal Disease

- Hiatal hernia (more commonly associated with regurgitation).
- Gastroesophageal reflux (more commonly associated with regurgitation).

Infectious Disease

- *Helicobacter*-related gastritis.
- Histoplasmosis.
- Pythiosis.
- Small intestinal bacterial overgrowth.
- Gastric parasites – *Physaloptera* spp. (Figure 17.1).
- Intestinal parasitism.

Metabolic Diseases

- Renal disease.
- Hepatobiliary disease.
- Hypoadrenocorticism.
- Chronic pancreatitis.
- Diabetic ketoacidosis (DKA).
- Metabolic acidosis.
- Electrolyte abnormalities – hypo/hyperkalemia, hyponatremia, hypercalcemia.

Inflammatory Bowel Disease

- Lymphocytic, plasmacytic, eosinophilic, or granulomatous (Figure 17.2).
- Gastritis, enteritis, or colitis.

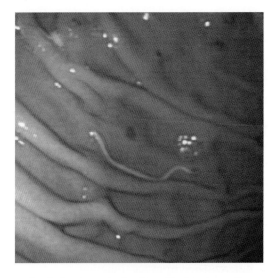

■ **Fig. 17.1.** *Physaloptera* organism in the stomach of a dog with chronic vomiting.

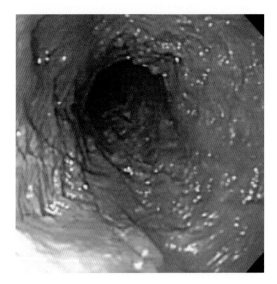

■ **Fig. 17.2.** Moderate lymphocytic-plasmacytic enteritis in the duodenum of a dog with chronic vomiting, diarrhea, and weight loss.

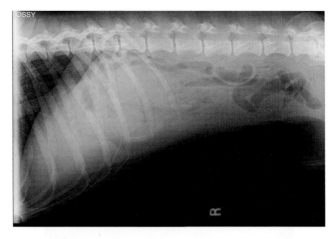

■ **Fig. 17.3.** Midjejunal foreign body in a dog with chronic intermittent vomiting of over six months' duration. Foreign body was part of a ball. Surgical removal resulted in resolution of all vomiting.

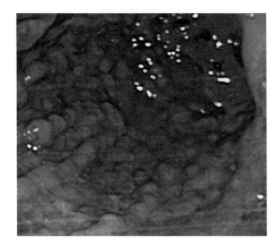

■ **Fig. 17.4.** Severe gastric wall thickening and erythema associated with gastric lymphoma.

Obstructive GI Disease
- Foreign body (Figure 17.3).
- Congenital pyloric stenosis.
- Chronic pyloric hypertrophic gastropathy.
- Intussusception.

Neoplastic Disease
- GI lymphoma (Figure 17.4), adenocarcinoma (Figure 17.5), fibrosarcoma, gastrointestinal stromal cell tumor.
- Pancreatic adenocarcinoma.
- Gastrin-secreting tumor (gastrinoma).
- Systemic mastocytosis.

Neurologic
- Cerebral edema.
- CNS tumors.

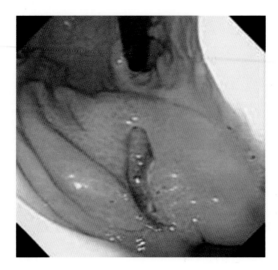

■ **Fig. 17.5.** Ulcerated gastric mass in the incisura angularis of a dog. Note the endoscope and gastric fundus in the background as the picture was taken during retroflexion in the stomach.

- Encephalitis/meningoencephalitis.
- Vestibular disease.

Motility Disorders
- Postgastric dilation.
- Postsurgical – gastric, duodenal.
- Electrolyte imbalances.
- Ileus (see Chapter 38 for underlying causes).

Miscellaneous
- Drug induced (e.g., NSAIDs, glucocorticoids, chemotherapeutics, antibiotics, antifungals).
- Food intolerance/allergy.
- Toxicity.

Additional Causes in Cats
- Parasitic – dirofilariasis, *Ollulanus tricuspis*.
- Inflammatory – cholecystitis, cholangiohepatitis.
- Metabolic – hyperthyroidism.
- Functional – constipation/obstipation.

DIAGNOSTICS

Complete Blood Count/Biochemistry Panel/Urinalysis
- CBCs are often unremarkable with primary gastric disease.
- Chronic GI bleeding can cause a nonregenerative anemia, often with characteristics of iron deficiency (microcytosis, hypochromasia, thrombocytosis).
- Acute GI bleeding can cause either regenerative or nonregenerative anemia, depending on severity and duration.
- Nonregenerative anemia may also occur secondary to chronic metabolic or inflammatory diseases.

- IBD, chronic pancreatitis, cholangiohepatitis, and cholecystitis may cause neutrophilic leukocytosis and monocytosis.
- Eosinophilia can occur from eosinophilic gastroenteritis, adrenocortical insufficiency, and GI parasitism.
- Thrombocytopenia has been reported with IBD.
- Dehydration increases the packed cell volume and albumin/total protein.
- Biochemistry provides diagnostic and therapeutic information; normal results rule out metabolic disease as the underlying etiology with the exception of atypical hypoadrenocorticism, which can have normal electrolytes.
- Electrolyte and acid–base imbalances reflect severity of losses and can help to localize disease.
- Hypochloremic metabolic alkalosis, often with hypokalemia, indicates substantial loss of gastric content, most consistent with a gastric outflow obstruction.
- Hyperkalemia in the vomiting patient suggests hypoadrenocorticism or oliguric/anuric renal failure; occasionally, enteritis caused by trichuriasis or bacterial infection (salmonellosis) mimics hypoadrenocorticism.
- Metabolic acidosis is common in patients with dehydration, renal failure, DKA, and severe gastroenteritis with diarrhea.
- Increased liver enzyme activity, hypoalbuminemia, hyperbilirubinemia, hypoglycemia, or low urea nitrogen concentration indicates hepatic disease.
- Persistent hyperglycemia and glucosuria are consistent with diabetes mellitus.
- Hyperglobulinemia may indicate chronic inflammation, neoplasia, or infection.
- Hypoalbuminemia, lymphopenia, and hypomagnesemia occur secondary to a protein-losing enteropathy caused by infiltrative intestinal diseases such as lymphocytic plasmacytic gastroenteritis, neoplasia, histoplasmosis, or primary intestinal lymphangiectasia.
- Hypocholesterolemia may also be seen with lymphangiectasia.
- Urinalysis is used to rule out non-GI causes of chronic vomiting such as renal failure and DKA.
- Acidic urine in the hypokalemic, hypochloremic, alkalotic patient indicates substantial loss of gastric content as would occur with gastric outflow obstruction.

Other Laboratory Tests

- ACTH stimulation test is used to confirm hypoadrenocorticism. A resting cortisol test <2 µg/dL should be followed with an ACTH stimulation test to confirm hypoadrenocorticism.
- Pancreatic lipase immunoreactivity assay may help confirm pancreatitis together with supportive history and physical exam and ultrasound findings.
- Bile acid concentration (pre- and postprandial) is used to help confirm hepatobiliary dysfunction.
- Fecal testing for gastrointestinal parasitism.

Imaging

- Survey radiographs of the abdomen may help identify foreign bodies, GI distension with fluid or gas, and displacement, malposition, shape, and/or size changes of abdominal organs.
- Survey radiographs of the thorax are used to evaluate for pulmonary metastases, gross esophageal abnormalities, or infectious disease.
- A gastrogram or upper GI series can be used to identify foreign bodies, GI wall masses or infiltrative disease, mucosal ulceration, delayed gastric emptying, and motility disorders; however, the procedure is relatively insensitive for detection of mucosal ulceration.
- Abdominal ultrasonography helps identify parenchymal abnormalities of the liver, gallbladder, kidneys, pancreas, GI tract, and mesenteric lymph nodes.
- CT and MRI further evaluate for parenchymal abnormalities of abdominal organs.

Diagnostic Procedures

- Gastroduodenoscopy – allows direct inspection of the gastric and intestinal lumen to identify gross mucosal lesions and foreign bodies and provides a minimally invasive method of biopsy to evaluate for microscopic disease. Limitations of endoscopy include the working length of the endoscope (unable to access the jejunum in large-breed dogs) and depth of the biopsies.
- Laparoscopy or exploratory laparotomy is used for more extensive diagnostic and therapeutic procedures.

 # THERAPEUTICS

- Specific treatment should be aimed at eliminating the underlying cause in conjunction with supportive therapy.
- If vomiting is intractable, stop oral intake of food and water for 12–24 hours or until the vomiting episodes are better controlled with antiemetics.
- Use crystalloid fluid therapy to replace deficits and to provide for maintenance and ongoing losses.
- If acid–base status is unknown or if hypochloremic metabolic alkalosis is present, use 0.9% sodium chloride.
- If metabolic acidosis is present, use lactated Ringer's (or similar) solution.
- Supplement potassium if hypokalemia is present; 20 mEq of KCl/L of fluid can be safely added for replacement and maintenance; use higher concentrations if severe hypokalemia is present.
- Debilitated patients and those in poor nutritional condition may need supplemental parenteral or enteral nutrition.
- Blood transfusion in severely anemic patients with evidence of active GI bleeding.
- Use surgical treatment if uncontrolled hemorrhage, obstruction, or perforation is suspected.

Drugs of Choice

- Antisecretory drugs such as H2-receptor blockers (e.g., famotidine, ranitidine) or proton pump inhibitors such as omeprazole (more potent) – famotidine 0.5–1 mg/kg PO, IV, or SQ q 12 h; ranitidine 1–2 mg/kg PO, IV q 12 h; omeprazole 0.7–1.5 mg/kg PO q 12–24 h; pantoprazole 0.7–1 mg/kg IV q 12 h.
- Protectants such as sucralfate (0.5–1 g/dog PO q 8–12 h; 0.25 g/cat PO q 8–12 h) to accelerate gastric mucosal healing; can be used with antisecretory drugs for patients with evidence of upper GI bleeding (e.g., hematemesis or melena).
- Antibiotics – indicated for treatment of *Helicobacter*-associated gastritis, intestinal dysbiosis, and as an adjunct to corticosteroids in the treatment of IBD.
- Suggested treatment of *Helicobacter*-associated gastritis – amoxicillin 20 mg/kg PO q 8 h plus omeprazole 0.7–1.5 mg/kg PO q 24 h and metronidazole 10 mg/kg PO q 12 h for 21 days; clarithromycin 7.5 mg/kg PO q 12 h can be used with amoxicillin and metronidazole (as above) as an alternative therapy for cats.
- Metronidazole – may be used at 10 mg/kg PO q 12 h in conjunction with corticosteroids to treat IBD, although evidence of direct benefit of this approach is currently lacking.
- Antibiotic-responsive enteropathy (tylosin-responsive enteropathy) – tylosin is the drug of choice administered at 25 mg/kg PO q 12 h for 6–8 weeks. Alternative option is metronidazole (10 mg/kg q 12 h for 8–12 weeks) although tylosin is felt to be superior for this disorder.

- Use corticosteroids in conjunction with dietary changes to treat biopsy-confirmed IBD; azathioprine, chlorambucil, or cyclosporine can also be used in patients with poor response to corticosteroids alone or to decrease the dosage of steroids required to control symptoms. Avoid the use of more than two immunomodulatory drugs given concurrently.
- Prokinetic drugs (e.g., metoclopramide, cisapride or erythromycin) are used to treat delayed gastric emptying not associated with obstructive disease.
- Pyrantel pamoate is effective for *Physaloptera*; fenbendazole is effective for *Ollulanus*.
- Iron supplementation for animals with chronic GI bleeding that develop microcytic hypochromic anemia.
- Surgery and/or chemotherapy for neoplasia, depending on the tumor type and location.
- Paraneoplastic hypersecretion of gastric acid, as occurs with mastocytosis and gastrin-secreting pancreatic tumors, is best treated with antisecretory drugs (e.g., omeprazole) to diminish gastritis, gastric ulcer, and chronic vomiting.
- Reserve antiemetics for patients with persistent vomiting unresponsive to treatment of the underlying disease. Maropitant is a neurokinin-1 receptor antagonist suppressing vomiting at the CRTZ, vomiting center, and vagal afferents: maropitant 1 mg/kg IV, SQ q 24 h, 2 mg/kg PO q 24 h. Phenothiazines (e.g., chlorpromazine) work at both the CRTZ and vomiting center: chlorpromazine 0.5 mg/kg SQ, IM q 6–8 h.
- Prokinetic drugs (e.g., metoclopramide) – metoclopramide also blocks the dopaminergic 2 receptors at the CRTZ, but this effect is far weaker in cats compared to dogs; metoclopramide 0.2–0.5 mg/kg IV, IM, PO q 6–8 h; metoclopramide can also be administered as a continuous rate infusion of 1–2 mg/kg/24 h in hospitalized patients.
- Vomiting caused by chemotherapy is best treated with ondansetron 0.5–1 mg/kg IV, PO given 30 min before chemotherapy.

Precautions/Interactions

- Do not give alpha-adrenergic blockers such as chlorpromazine to dehydrated patients as they can cause hypotension.
- Use antiemetics with caution, as they can mask the underlying problem.
- Metoclopramide can cause lethargy, restlessness, agitation, and other behavioral changes, particularly in cats.
- Corticosteroids are immunosuppressive and are a risk factor for development of GI ulceration; use caution when treating IBD with corticosteroids at high dosages or for long periods.
- Azathioprine and chlorambucil are myelotoxic; monitor CBCs for neutropenia and thrombocytopenia every two weeks for the first month of treatment and monthly thereafter.
- Cyclosporine can exacerbate vomiting and diarrhea when used at high dosages; use with caution in patients with renal disease.
- Do not use anticholinergics as antiemetics, as they can exacerbate vomiting by causing gastric atony and gastric retention.
- Metoclopramide and cisapride are contraindicated in patients with GI obstruction.
- Ranitidine interferes with hepatic metabolism of theophylline, phenytoin, and warfarin, and should not be used concurrently with these drugs.
- Avoid use of cimetidine because it is a weak H2-receptor antagonist and is a potent inhibitor of the cytochrome p450 enzyme pathway.

Diet

- Small frequent meals of an easily digestible or bland diet are ideal if tolerated. Prolonged fasting should be avoided as this may compromise enterocyte health.
- Dietary therapy for patients with suspected food allergy or IBD should use an elimination diet containing a single, novel protein source or a hydrolyzed diet.

COMMENTS

Client Education

Helicobacter heilmanii and *H. felis* may have zoonotic potential; they have been isolated from humans with chronic gastritis, most of whom have had close contact with dogs or cats.

Expected Course and Prognosis

Prognosis depends on the underlying etiology of the chronic vomiting.

Abbreviations

- ACTH = adrenocorticotropic hormone
- CNS = central nervous system
- CRTZ = chemoreceptor trigger zone
- CT = computed tomography
- DKA = diabetic ketoacidosis
- GI = gastrointestinal
- IBD = inflammatory bowel disease
- MRI = magnetic resonance imaging
- NSAID = nonsteroidal antiinflammatory drug

See Also

- Gastritis, Chronic
- Inflammatory Bowel Disease
- Nutritional Approach to Acute Vomiting and Diarrhea
- Nutritional Approach to Chronic Enteropathies

Suggested Reading

Gallagher A. Vomiting and regurgitation. In: Ettinger SJ, Feldman EC, Cote E, eds. Textbook of Veterinary Internal Medicine, 8th ed. St Louis: Elsevier, 2017, pp. 158–167.

Guilford WG, Center SA, Williams DA, Meyer DJ. Chronic gastric diseases. In: Strombeck's Small Animal Gastroenterology, 3rd ed. Philadelphia: Saunders, 1996, pp. 275–302.

Simpson K. Diseases of the stomach. In: Ettinger SJ, Feldman EC, Cote E, eds. Textbook of Veterinary Internal Medicine, 8th ed. St Louis: Elsevier, 2017, pp. 1495–1516.

Author: John M. Crandell DVM, DACVIM

Diseases of the Oral Cavity

Chapter 18

Craniomandibular Osteopathy

DEFINITION/OVERVIEW

- Affects musculoskeletal system.
- A nonneoplastic, noninflammatory proliferative bone disease.
- Mandibular rami and tympanic bullae most commonly affected (can be isolated to only mandible or tympanic bullae); occipital and parietal zygomatic portion of the temporal can also be affected.
- Bilateral symmetric involvement most common.

ETIOLOGY/PATHOPHYSIOLOGY

- Incidence of 1.4 per 100 000 cases.
- Incidence higher in Western region and in Southern plains of United States.
- Possible viral involvement.

Systems Affected

- Musculoskeletal.
- Gastrointestinal – secondary to inadequate nutrition.

SIGNALMENT/HISTORY

- Males and females equally affected.
- Most patients affected are younger than 12 months of age.
- Cairn terriers, West Highland white terriers, Scottish terriers are at increased risk.
- Boxers, Labrador retrievers, Great Danes, Boston terriers, Shetland sheepdogs, German wire-haired pointers, German shepherd dogs, Doberman pinschers, English bulldogs, Pyrenean Mountain dogs, bullmastiffs, basset hounds, Catahoulas, Weimaraners, Irish setters also reported.
- Breed predisposition suggests a heritable etiology – autosomal recessive mode of inheritance in West Highland white terriers.

Risk Factors

Neutering may increase incidence.

Blackwell's Five-Minute Veterinary Consult Clinical Companion: Small Animal Gastrointestinal Diseases,
First Edition. Edited by Jocelyn Mott and Jo Ann Morrison.
© 2019 John Wiley & Sons, Inc. Published 2019 by John Wiley & Sons, Inc.
Companion website: www.fiveminutevet.com/gastrointestinal

Historical Findings

- Usually related to persistent or intermittent pain around the mouth in young growing animals.
- Difficulty with opening the mouth, prehension, and mastication.

CLINICAL FEATURES

- Difficulty eating, drinking.
- Temporal and masseter muscle atrophy is common.
- Palpable irregular thickening of the mandibular rami +/– temporomandibular joint (TMJ) region (Figure 18.1).
- Inability to fully open jaw, even under general anesthesia.
- Intermittent pyrexia.
- Bilateral exophthalmos can occur.

DIFFERENTIAL DIAGNOSIS

- Metabolic bone disease – often long bones affected as well; can have systemic illness.
- Osteomyelitis – bones not symmetrically affected; generally not as extensive; lysis; lack of breed predilection; history of penetrating wound.
- Neoplasia – mature patient; not symmetrically affected; more lytic bone reaction; metastatic disease.
- Calvarial hyperostosis – young patient involves frontal, parietal, and occipital bones; does not involve mandible; may have long bone involvement.

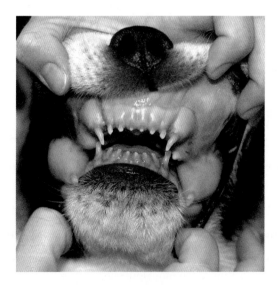

■ **Fig. 18.1.** Antemortem photo of a dog with confirmed craniomandibular osteopathy (CMO) showing palpable thickening of the maxilla. Source: Image courtesy of Dr Mathieu Glassman.

DIAGNOSTICS

Complete Blood Cell Count/Biochemistry Panel/Urinalysis

- Serum alkaline phosphatase (ALP) and inorganic phosphate may be high
- May note hypogammaglobulinemia or alpha-2-hyperglobulinemia.

Imaging

- Radiographs – irregular, bead-like osseous proliferations most commonly of mandibles +/– tympanic bullae; periosteal new bone formation (exostoses) affecting one or more bones around the TMJ; temporal bones and other cranial or long bones can also be affected; teeth are unaffected; later in disease exostoses stop proliferating and regress (Figures 18.2–18.4).
- Computed tomography – may identify lesions sooner than radiographs (Figure 18.5).
- Diagnosis made based on history, clinical findings, and radiographs.

Other Diagnostic Procedures

Biopsy of bone with culture can be performed in atypical cases to rule out neoplasia and osteomyelitis.

Pathologic Findings

- Histology shows normal lamellar bone being replaced via osteoclastic resorption followed by presence of primitive bone expanding beyond the periosteum.
- Normal bone marrow is replaced by highly vascular fibrous-type stroma.
- Adjacent connective tissue and muscle fibers are destroyed.

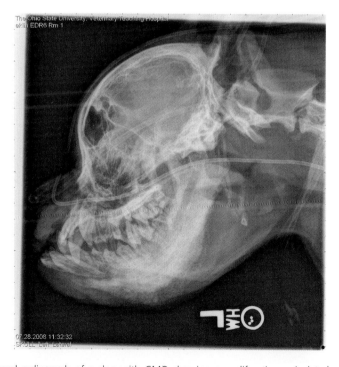

■ **Fig. 18.2.** A lateral radiograph of a dog with CMO showing a proliferative, spiculated, periosteal response present along both bodies of the mandible, extending proximally to the level of the temporomandibular joints. A nasoesophageal tube is present.

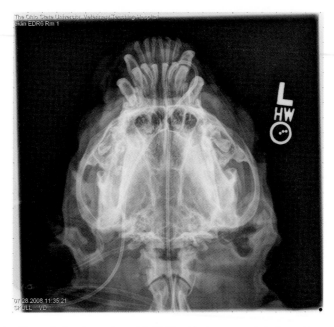

■ **Fig. 18.3.** Lateral radiograph showing a dog with CMO with the tympanic bulla and temporomandibular joint affected rather than the mandible as seen in Figure 18.2.

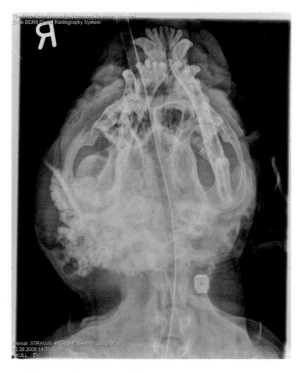

■ **Fig. 18.4.** Ventrodorsal radiograph of the skull affecting primarily the right tympanic bulla and temporomandibular joint.

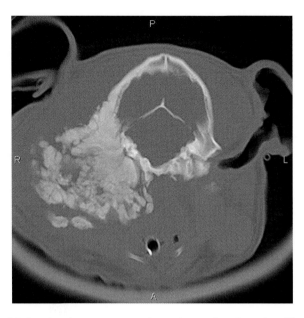

■ **Fig. 18.5.** CT scan axial slice showing severe expansion and smooth periosteal proliferation of the ramus and angle of the right hemimandible, the right squamous temporal bone with filling of the right tympanic bulla with smooth expansile bone and obliteration of the ear canal.

THERAPEUTICS

Treatment is aimed at supportive care to decrease pain and inflammation and provide nutritional support.

Drug(s) of Choice

- Analgesics and antiinflammatories are warranted.
- Nonsteroidal antiinflammatory drugs (NSAIDs) inhibit cyclooxygenase enzymes.
  - Carprofen (2.2 mg/kg PO q 12 h or 4.4 mg/kg q24h, chewable).
  - Deracoxib (1–2 mg/kg PO q 24 h, chewable).
  - Meloxicam (0.1 mg/kg PO q 24 h – liquid).
  - Firocoxib (5 mg/kg PO q 24 h).

Precautions/Interactions

NSAIDs should not be given concurrently with steroids.

Alternative Drugs

If an FDA veterinary-approved prescription NSAID cannot be afforded, aspirin may be used.

Appropriate Health Care

Supportive care.

Nursing Care

Supportive care consisting of pain management and nutritional support is warranted.

Diet

High-calorie, high-protein gruel is recommended.

Activity

Activity does not need to be modified.

Surgical Considerations

- Surgical placement of a pharyngostomy, esophagostomy, or gastrostomy tube to provide nutritional support may be needed.
- Surgical excision of exostoses is not recommended as they regrow within weeks.

 COMMENTS

Client Education

Client education regarding supportive care.

Patient Monitoring

Frequent reexamination to monitor nutritional status is recommended.

Prevention/Avoidance

- Do not repeat dam–sire breedings that resulted in affected offspring.
- Discourage breeding of affected animals.

Possible Complications

- In severe cases dogs may have difficulty eating, which can lead to severe malnutrition.
- In such cases, if appropriate supportive care cannot be provided, humane euthanasia should be discussed.

Expected Course and Prognosis

- Disease may be self-limiting between approximately 11–13 months of age with regression of exostoses.
- Patients with involvement of the bullae are typically more severely affected as this interferes with the articulation of the TMJ.
- Extensive involvement of the TMJ may necessitate humane euthanasia.

Synonyms

- Craniomandibular osteoarthropathy
- Craniomandibular osteodystrophy
- Lion jaw
- Mandibular periostitis
- Scotty jaw
- Westie jaw

Abbreviations

- ALP = alkaline phosphatase
- NSAID = nonsteroidal antiinflammatory drugs
- TMJ = temporomandibular joint

Suggested Reading

DeCamp CE, Johnston SA, Dejardin LM, et al. Disease conditions in small animals. In: Brinker, Piermattei, and Flo's Handbook of Small Animal Orthopedics and Fracture Repair, 5th ed. St Louis: Elsevier, 2016, pp. 821–837.

Ratterree WO, Glassman MM, Driskell EA, et al. Craniomandibular osteopathy with a unique neurological manifestation in a young Akita. J Am Anim Hosp 2011;47(1):e7–12.

Towle HA, Breur GJ. Miscellaneous orthopedic conditions. In: Tobias KM, Johnston SA, eds. Veterinary Surgery: Small Animal. St Louis: Elsevier, 2011, pp. 1112–1126.

Watson ADJ, Adams WM, Thomas CB. Craniomandibular osteopathy in dogs. Compend Contin Educ Pract Vet 1995;17:911–921.

Acknowledgments: The authors and editors acknowledge the prior contribution of Dr Steven Cogar.

Authors: Nina R. Kieves DVM, DACVS-SA, DACVSMR, Amy N. Zide DVM, Kathleen L. Ham DVM, MS, DACVS-SA, James Howard DVM, MS

Feline Eosinophilic Dermatitis

DEFINITION/OVERVIEW

- Feline eosinophilic dermatitis or eosinophilic granuloma complex (EGC) is often a confusing term for four distinct syndromes grouped primarily according to their clinical similarities as a disease complex, their frequent concurrent (and recurrent) development, and their positive response to antiinflammatory therapeutics. EGC is a description, not a diagnosis.
- Eosinophilic plaque.
- Eosinophilic granuloma.
- Indolent ulcer.
- Allergic miliary dermatitis.

ETIOLOGY/PATHOPHYSIOLOGY

- Eosinophilic plaque: hypersensitivity reaction, most often to insects (fleas, mosquitos), food or environmental allergens; exacerbated by mechanical trauma.
- Eosinophilic granuloma: multiple causes; idiopathic, genetic predisposition, and hypersensitivity.
- Indolent ulcer: may have both hypersensitivity and genetic causes.
- Allergic miliary dermatitis: not always included within the EGC; very common hypersensitivity reaction, most often to fleas.
- Eosinophil: major infiltrative cell for eosinophilic granuloma, eosinophilic plaque, and allergic miliary dermatitis, but not indolent ulcers.
- Indolent ulcers are most often associated with allergic or parasitic conditions, as well as a more general role in the inflammatory reaction.
- Several reports of related affected individuals and a study of disease development in a colony of specific pathogen-free cats indicate that genetic predisposition may be a significant component for development of eosinophilic granuloma and indolent ulcer.
- A heritable dysfunction of eosinophil regulation has been proposed.

Systems Affected
- Skin/exocrine.
- Gastrointestinal – oral cavity.

Blackwell's Five-Minute Veterinary Consult Clinical Companion: Small Animal Gastrointestinal Diseases,
First Edition. Edited by Jocelyn Mott and Jo Ann Morrison.
© 2019 John Wiley & Sons, Inc. Published 2019 by John Wiley & Sons, Inc.
Companion website: www.fiveminutevet.com/gastrointestinal

SIGNALMENT/HISTORY

- No breed predilection.
- Eosinophilic plaque: 2–6 years of age.
- Genetic/idiopathic eosinophilic granuloma: less than one year of age.
- Allergic disorder: often greater than one year of age.
- Indolent ulcer: no age predisposition.
- Predilection for females reported.
- Lesions of all four syndromes may develop spontaneously and acutely; lesions of more than one syndrome may occur simultaneously.
- Development of eosinophilic plaques may be preceded by periods of lethargy.
- Waxing and waning of clinical signs is common.
- Seasonal incidence in some geographic locations may indicate insect or environmental allergen exposure.
- Distinguishing among the syndromes depends on both clinical signs and dermatohistopathologic findings.

 ## CLINICAL FEATURES

- Eosinophilic plaque: alopecic, erythematous, erosive patches or well-demarcated, steep-walled plaques; usually occur in the inguinal, perineal, lateral thigh, ventral abdomen, and axillary regions; frequently moist or glistening; regional lymphadenopathy common; secondary infection common (Figure 19.1).

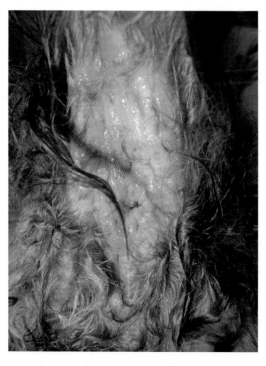

■ **Fig. 19.1.** Perianal lesions of eosinophilic dermatitis in an 8-year-old female-spayed DLH. Secondary bacterial infection and self-trauma were noted in this patient.

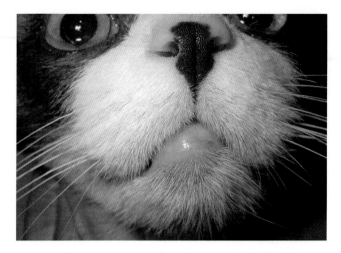

■ **Fig. 19.2.** Swelling on the rostral chin in a 7-year-old female-spayed DSH. This appearance of a "pouty chin" is characteristic of eosinophilic granuloma.

- Eosinophilic granuloma: five, occasionally overlapping, presentations.
  - Distinctly linear orientation (linear granuloma) along the caudal thigh; lesions more often palpated than visualized.
  - Individual or coalescing plaques located anywhere on the body; ulcerated with a "cobblestone" or coarse pattern; white or yellow, possibly representing collagen degeneration.
  - Lip margin and chin swelling ("pouting") (Figure 19.2).
  - Footpad swelling, pain, and lameness (most common in cats under two years of age).
  - Oral cavity ulcerations (especially on the tongue, palate, and palatine arches); cats with oral lesions may be dysphagic, have halitosis, and drool.
- Indolent ulcer (rodent ulcer): classically concave and indurated ulcerations with a granular, orange-yellow color, confined to the upper lips adjacent to the philtrum; secondary infection common (Figure 19.3).
- Allergic miliary dermatitis: multiple brown/black crusted and erythematous papules; lesions more often palpated than visualized; may be associated with alopecia; usually associated with pruritus; frequently affects the dorsum; may be associated with secondary bacterial folliculitis.

 DIFFERENTIAL DIAGNOSIS

- Includes the other diseases in the complex.
- Herpesvirus dermatitis.
- Feline leukemia virus (FeLV)- or feline immunodeficiency virus (FIV)-associated dermatitis.
- Unresponsive lesions.
  - Pemphigus foliaceus.
  - Dermatophytosis or deep fungal infection.
  - Demodicosis.
  - Bacterial folliculitis.
  - Neoplasia (especially metastatic adenocarcinoma, squamous cell carcinoma, and cutaneous lymphosarcoma).

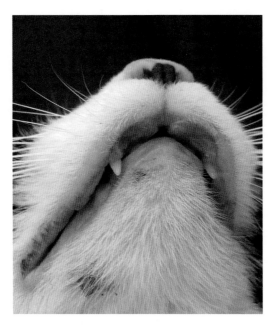

■ **Fig. 19.3.** Indolent or "rodent" ulcer on the lip margins of a 6-year-old male-castrate DSH. The lip margins are thickened and eroded. Exposed surfaces near the philtrum have the orange-yellow hue seen with collagen degeneration.

 DIAGNOSTICS

- Complete blood count (CBC): mild to moderate eosinophilia; serum chemistries and urinalysis usually normal; FeLV and FIV serum testing usually negative.

Diagnostic Procedures

- Impression smears from lesions: large numbers of eosinophils; bacteria commonly found with eosinophilic plaques and indolent ulcers (Figure 19.4).
- Insect hypersensitivity: parasite control (especially flea) to assist in excluding flea or mosquito bite hypersensitivity.
- Cutaneous adverse reaction to food: restricted-ingredient food trial: dechallenge/challenge to induce development of new lesions.
- Atopy: intradermal testing (preferred) or serum testing followed by allergen-specific immunotherapy.
- Dermatohistopathologic diagnosis: required for definitive diagnosis and distinguishing the EGC syndromes.

Pathologic Findings

- Eosinophilic plaque: severe epidermal and follicular spongiosis and mucinosis with eosinophilic exocytosis; intense perivascular to diffuse dermal eosinophilic infiltrate; eroded or ulcerated epidermis.
- Eosinophilic granuloma: epidermal acanthosis with scattered apoptotic keratinocytes; distinct foci of eosinophilic degranulation and collagen degeneration ("flame figures"); nodular to diffuse granulomatous inflammation; eosinophilic and giant cell infiltrate.

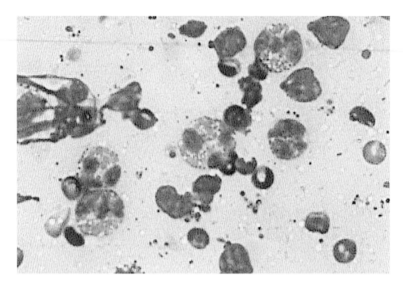

■ **Fig. 19.4.** Cytology from a touch-prep of a lesion of eosinophilic granuloma demonstrating large numbers of eosinophils with intracytoplasmic granules, as well as many free granules in the surrounding fluid from disrupted cells.

- Indolent ulcer: severe ulceration of the epidermis or mucosa with fibrosing dermatitis and neutrophilic inflammation; degree of eosinophilia varies, but significant eosinophilic infiltration unusual.
- Allergic miliary dermatitis: discrete foci of epidermal erosion and necrosis with brightly eosinophilic crusts; dermal perivascular to interstitial eosinophil-rich infiltrate.

 THERAPEUTICS

- Adequate flea control measures paramount to manage a majority of cases.
- Outpatient unless severe oral disease prevents adequate fluid intake.
- Identify and eliminate offending allergen(s) in addition to providing medical intervention.
- Allergen-specific immunotherapy in cats with atopic dermatitis; successful in a majority of cases; preferable to long-term corticosteroid administration.
- Deter patient from damaging lesions by excessive grooming with behavior modification techniques and/or distraction.

Drugs of Choice

- Eosinophilic plaque and indolent ulcer: may improve with antibiotics: amoxicillin trihydrate-clavulanate 12.5 mg/kg bid, clindamycin 5.5 mg/kg bid, cephalexin 22 mg/kg bid, trimethoprim-sulfadiazine 10–15 mg/kg bid.
- Injectable methylprednisolone: 20 mg/cat, repeat in two weeks (if needed); tachyphylaxis common with repeated administration; not advised for long-term therapy; increased risk for diabetes mellitus with repeated administration.
- Prednisolone (2–4 mg/kg), dexamethasone (0.1–0.2 mg/kg) or triamcinolone (0.1–0.2 mg/kg); initial daily dosage tapered to minimal dose and frequency required to control lesions; tachyphylaxis may occur and may be specific to the drug administered.
- Cyclosporine 7.3 mg/kg initial daily dosage tapered to minimal dose and frequency required to control lesions.

- Topical: fluocinolone/dimethyl sulfoxide (DMSO) (Synotic® lotion) to individual lesions; not practical and/or may cause systemic effects in patients with large numbers of lesions.

Alternative Drugs

- Chlorambucil 0.1–0.2 mg/kg PO q 48–72 h.
- Indolent ulcer: alpha-interferon 300–1000 iu daily PO in cycles of seven days on, seven days off; limited success; side effects rare; no specific treatment monitoring required.
- Doxycycline 5–10 mg/kg PO q 24 h.
- Megestrol acetate 2.5–5 mg PO every 2–7 days; significant incidence of side effects (diabetes, mammary cancer, epidermal atrophy) preclude use in all but severe, recalcitrant cases.

Nursing Care

Cats with oral eosinophilic granuloma complex may need pain medications and encouragement to eat.

Diet

Hypoallergenic diets may be useful in cats with allergic component to their disease.
    Soft, canned food may be better tolerated in cats with oral lesions.

 COMMENTS

Patient Monitoring

- Treatment monitoring is based on medications prescribed (e.g., CBC, serum chemistry profile, and urinalysis with culture recommended frequently during treatment induction and then every 6–12 months for patients on chronic immunomodulatory therapy).
- Cats: cyclosporine blood level should be measured when on maintenance dosage to prevent immunosuppression; patients must be FeLV/FIV negative; initial exposure to toxoplasmosis during treatment may be fatal.

Prevention/Avoidance

- Adequate flea prevention may be necessary to help prevent reoccurrence in some cases.

Possible Complications

- Complications from treatment are dependent on drug used.
- Prednisolone can be associated with development of diabetes mellitus or congestive heart failure.
- Chlorambucil can be associated with bone marrow suppression, vomiting and/or diarrhea, and rarely neurotoxicity.
- Side effects of megestrol acetate therapy may include diabetes, mammary cancer, and/or epidermal atrophy.

Expected Course and Prognosis

- Lesions should resolve permanently if a primary cause can be identified and controlled.
- Most lesions wax and wane, with or without therapy; an unpredictable schedule of recurrence should be anticipated.
- Drug dosages should be tapered to the lowest possible level (or discontinued, if possible) once the lesions have resolved.
- Lesions in cats with the inheritable disease may resolve spontaneously after several months to years.

Abbreviations

- CBC = complete blood count
- CEG = canine eosinophilic granuloma
- DMSO = dimethyl sulfoxide
- EGC = eosinophilic granuloma complex
- FeLV = feline leukemia virus
- FIV = feline immunodeficiency virus

See Also

- Dysphagia
- Ptyalism

Suggested Reading

King S, Favrot C, Messinger L, et al. A randomized double-blinded placebo-controlled study to evaluate an effective ciclosporin dose for the treatment of feline hypersensitivity dermatitis. Vet Derm 2012;23:440–e84.

Miller WH, Griffin CE, Campbell KL. Muller & Kirk's Small Animal Dermatology, 7th ed. St Louis: Elsevier Mosby, 2013.

Power HT, Ihrke PJ. Selected feline eosinophilic skin diseases (eosinophilic granuloma complex). Vet Clin North Am Small Anim Pract 1995;25:833–850.

Rosenkrantz WS. Feline eosinophilic granuloma complex. In: Griffin CE, Kwochka KW, MacDonald JM, eds. Current Veterinary Dermatology: The Science and Art of Therapy. St Louis: Mosby, 1993.

Authors: Alexander H. Werner Resnick VMD, DACVD, Karen Helton-Rhodes DVM, DACVD

Chapter 20

Oral Neoplasia, Benign

DEFINITION/OVERVIEW

- Benign tumors may be locally invasive but do not metastasize to distant sites.
- Odontogenic tumors are lesions derived from epithelial, ectomesenchymal, and/or mesenchymal elements that still are, or have been, part of the tooth-forming apparatus.
- Any tumor that does not arise from odontogenic tissues is considered to be nonodontogenic.
- Hamartomas are disorganized accumulations of histologically normal tissues (odontomas).
- Cysts are epithelium-lined potential spaces, generally of odontogenic origin. Although solitary cysts are not considered tumors, many of the odontogenic tumors have the potential to produce cysts.
- Epulis is a general term referring to a gingival mass of any type; in general, the term may be best avoided in favor of more specific nomenclature.

ETIOLOGY/PATHOPHYSIOLOGY

- Odontogenic tumors comprise a large portion of oral tumors seen in dogs, and are less common in cats than nonodontogenic tumors.
  - Epithelial nests that remain after eruption are usually quiescent, but carcinogenic stimulation can result in transformation into odontogenic tumors or cysts.
  - The reciprocal inductive interaction between ectomesenchymal cells and the oral epithelium may determine the type of odontogenic tumor (ameloblastic fibroma subtypes).
- Peripheral odontogenic fibroma (POF) (formerly known as fibrous or ossifying epulides).
  - Originally thought to arise from the periodontal ligament (PDL).
  - Base is often anchored to the periosteal surface of alveolar crestal bone with no definitive PDL involvement.

Systems Affected

- Gastrointestinal.
- Oral cavity.

SIGNALMENT/HISTORY

- Odontomas and papillomas are usually identified in younger dogs.
- Feline inductive odontogenic tumor (FIOT) usually identified in younger cats.

Blackwell's Five-Minute Veterinary Consult Clinical Companion: Small Animal Gastrointestinal Diseases, First Edition. Edited by Jocelyn Mott and Jo Ann Morrison.
© 2019 John Wiley & Sons, Inc. Published 2019 by John Wiley & Sons, Inc.
Companion website: www.fiveminutevet.com/gastrointestinal

Historical Findings

- Swelling or deformity of facial/oral structures.
- Excessive drooling or bleeding from mouth, halitosis.
- Missing teeth or teeth that have moved.
- Difficulty eating or grooming (cats).

 CLINICAL FEATURES

Nonodontogenic Benign Tumors

- Oral melanocytoma – benign variant of melanoma. Very well circumscribed, less than 1 cm in diameter (Figure 20.1).
- Osteoma.
  - Benign, well circumscribed in dog or cat.
  - Hard palate, zygomatic arch, caudal mandible.
- Plasmacytoma.
  - Well-circumscribed dark pink to red mass <1 cm.
  - Dorsal surface of tongue, lip, gingiva, mucosa.
- Papilloma.
  - Multiple verrucous lesions.
  - Often regress on their own.
  - Severe refractory cases in older dogs due to immunocompromised disease, lymphoma.
- Ossifying (cementifying) fibroma.
  - Local asymptomatic swelling of the mandible with distinct margins.
  - Complete or mixed radiolucent center.
  - Ossifying fibroma may have some bone lysis.

Odontogenic Benign Tumors

- Ameloblastoma.
  - Slowly growing, locally invasive.
  - Expansile with minimal gingival involvement.
  - Also known as solid – multicystic.
  - Uni- to multilocular radiolucency.

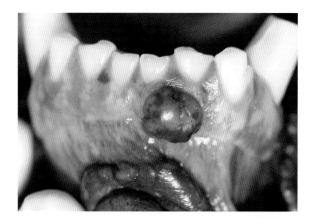

■ **Fig. 20.1.** Although slightly over 1 cm, this well-circumscribed melanocytoma was completely excised.

- Canine acanthomatous ameloblastoma (CAA).
  - 45% of all odontogenic tumors in dogs.
  - Most are extraosseous (peripheral); some intraosseous in dogs.
  - Irregular surface arises in the gingiva, can be locally aggressive.
  - More common in the rostral mandible.
  - Middle-aged dogs.
  - Possibly Golden retriever overrepresented.
- Amyloid-producing odontogenic tumor (APOT), calcifying epithelial odontogenic tumor (CEOT).
  - Slow-growing, expansile mass, locally invasive.
  - Uni- to multilocular radiolucency (APOT), then mixed lucency-opacity when mineralized (CEOT).
  - Middle-aged to older dogs.
- Ameloblastic fibroma (-dentinoma; -odontoma).
  - Slow growing.
  - Unilocular expansile lesion with central radiolucency.
  - May eventually contain small densities (dentin/enamel) depending on degree of odontogenic differentiation (-dentinoma; -odontoma).
- Feline inductive odontogenic tumor (FIOT) – inductive fibroameloblastoma.
  - Large swelling of rostral maxilla in young cats.
  - Expansile osteolytic lesion with variable amounts of periosteal proliferation, typically with impacted canine tooth.
  - Locally infiltrative, no metastatic potential.
- Odontomas, hamartomas: high degree of odontogenic differentiation and morphogenesis.
- Complex odontoma – more amorphous.
- Compound odontoma – discrete tooth-like denticles.
  - Asymptomatic alveolar swelling in maxilla or mandible of young dog; potentially expand to a large size.
  - Abnormal number of teeth – either some "missing" or supernumerary teeth.
  - Invasive, osteolytic, expansile lesion.
  - Mixed central opacity with corticated border next to a thin radiolucent margin.
  - Presence of denticles – pathognomonic.
- Peripheral odontogenic fibroma (POF) (Figure 20.2).
  - Firm, sessile to pedunculated, nonulcerated mass associated with the free gingiva and sometimes the attached gingiva, though some with a broader base across several teeth.
  - Not invasive, but if large, can impact periodontal health.
  - Mineralization within the mass may be in contact with alveolar bone, but no direct osseous impact.
  - Fibrous and ossifying type (previously termed fibrous epulis and ossifying epulis).
- Feline "epulides."
  - May be analogous to POF in dogs.
  - Can have fibromatous, ossifying, and acanthomatous features in the same lesion.
  - Usually multifocal sites.
- Odontogenic myxoma/myxofibroma – rare.
  - Slow-growing mandibular swelling, highly infiltrative.
  - Uni- to multilocular radiolucency – honeycomb.
  - Displacement or resorption of roots, cortical expansion.

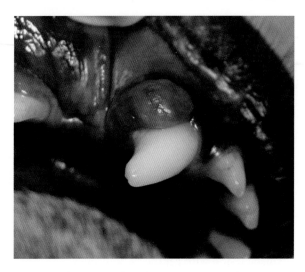

■ **Fig. 20.2.** Peripheral odontogenic fibroma (POF) at the gingival margin of 104.

DIFFERENTIAL DIAGNOSIS

- Focal fibrous hyperplasia (FFH).
- Pyogenic granuloma.
- Peripheral cell giant granuloma.
- Fibrous dysplasia (bone replaced by connective tissue).
- Cysts – developmental, inflammatory.

DIAGNOSTICS

Complete Blood Cell Count/Biochemistry/Urinalysis

Often unremarkable.

Imaging

- Radiographs (see individual descriptions).
  - May show no lysis or central mineralization (POF), or focal lysis (CAA).
  - Little or no periosteal proliferation.
  - Displacement of teeth more common than root resorption, seen with malignant tumors.
- Advanced imaging – computed tomography (CT): assess extent more accurately, better for surgical planning.

Pathologic Findings

- Histopathological assessment, including border readout, on excisional biopsies are critical.
- If possible, utilize a facility that specializes in oral maxillofacial pathology.
- Specific descriptions of each tumor type are beyond the scope of this chapter.

THERAPEUTICS

Appropriate Health Care

- Depends on the tumor type.
- Benign tumors are treatable with long-term success via surgery and sometimes with radiation therapy.

Nursing Care

- Pain control.
- Supportive care.

Surgical Considerations

- Melanocytoma – marginal or wide excision.
- Plasmacytoma – 1 cm margins usually curative.
- Osteoma – debulking or resective procedure.
- Ossifying fibromas.
  - Enucleation of well-defined lesions.
  - Wide 1 cm margins of less defined, invasive or recurrent lesions.
  - Good to excellent prognosis.
- Ameloblastoma.
  - Complete wide surgical margins.
  - Good to excellent with clean margins on rostral lesions.
  - Radiation therapy – variable results.
  - Intraosseous types more radio-resistant. CAA – classified as benign but can be locally aggressive (Figure 20.3).
  - May need 1–2 cm margins to completely excise.
  - Intralesional bleomycin.
- APOT/CEOT – 1 cm margins, less likely to locally recur.
- Ameloblastic fibroma – *en bloc* resection or surgical enucleation if well differentiated.
- FIOT.
  - Not radioresponsive.
  - If removed in its entirety, not likely to recur, with good to excellent prognosis.
- Odontoma – conservative enucleation and curettage; excellent prognosis.
- POF.
  - Tooth extraction or *en bloc* resection historically recommended.
  - Local conservative excision with attention to removing the entire lesion, down to and including the affected periosteum, should be curative.
  - Gingiva may have to be reconstructed – if recurrent or broad-based, more aggressive removal needed.
- Feline epulides.
  - Multiple extractions and gingivectomy often needed to manage multifocal lesions.
  - May have higher recurrence rate.
- Odontogenic myxomas – 1 cm margins needed.

COMMENTS

Client Education

Early detection is important; regular oral examinations and home care can be helpful.

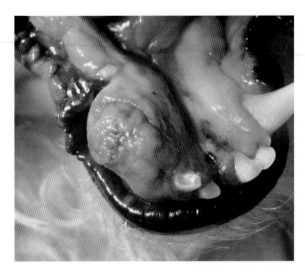

■ **Fig. 20.3.** Although considered benign, this canine acanthomatous ameloblastoma required 2 cm margins for mandibulectomy.

Patient Monitoring

Varies with the type of mass and treatment selected.

Possible Complications

Resection with removal of teeth may allow apposing teeth to traumatize the healing area.

Expected Course and Prognosis

See surgical recommendation above for individual tumor type prognosis.

Synonyms

- Pindborg tumor – CEOT
- Epulis

Abbreviations

- APOT = amyloid-producing odontogenic tumor
- CAA = canine acanthomatous ameloblastoma
- CEOT = calcifying epithelial odontogenic ameloblastoma

- CT = computed tomography
- FFH = focal fibrous hyperplasia
- FIOT = feline inductive odontogenic tumor
- PDL = periodontal ligament
- POF = peripheral odontogenic fibroma

See Also

- Oral Neoplasia, Malignant

- Ptyalism

Suggested Reading

Ettinger SJ, Feldman EC, eds. Textbook of Veterinary Internal Medicine, 7th ed. St Louis: Saunders Elsevier, 2010.
Fosum T. Small Animal Surgery, 3rd ed. St Louis: Mosby Elsevier, 2007.
Harvey CE, Emily PP. Small Animal Dentistry. Philadelphia: Mosby, 1993.
Lobprise HB, Dodd JR. Wigg's Veterinary Dentistry: Principles and Practice. Hoboken: Wiley, 2019.
Meuten DJ. Tumors in Domestic Animals. Ames: Iowa State University Press, 2002.
Nelson RW, Couto CG. Small Animal Internal Medicine, 3rd ed. St Louis: Mosby, 2003.
Wiggs RB, Lobprise HB. Veterinary Dentistry: Principles and Practice. Philadelphia: Lippincott-Raven, 1997.

Authors: Heidi B. Lobprise DVM, DAVDC, Jason W. Soukup DVM, DAVDC

Chapter 21

Oral Neoplasia, Malignant

DEFINITION/OVERVIEW

- Oral mass that has the potential to metastasize to other sites in the body.
- Oral masses comprise 5% of all canine tumors, and 6–10% of all feline tumors.
- In dogs, the oral cavity is the fourth most common site of neoplasia.

ETIOLOGY/PATHOPHYSIOLOGY

Dog – the most common malignant oral tumor in the dog is malignant melanoma (MM), followed by squamous cell carcinoma (SCC) and fibrosarcoma (FSA).

- Cat – SCC is the most common oral tumor, accounting for 60–70% of cases, followed by FSA.

Systems Affected

- Gastrointestinal.
- Oral cavity.

SIGNALMENT/HISTORY

- Increased prevalence with age with most malignant tumors.
  - Cats: SCC mean age 12.5 years, fibrosarcoma 10.3 years.
  - Papillary SCC often seen in younger dogs (<1 year), but also in mature dogs.
- Increased prevalence of MM and FSA in male dogs.
- Increased prevalence of MM in dogs with pigmented oral mucosa.
- Increased prevalence of FSA in large-breed dogs.

Risk Factors

Environmental risk factors of second-hand smoke, flea collars, and canned foods for feline SCC, and urban environments for dogs with tonsillar SCC.

Historical Findings

- Excessive drooling or bleeding from mouth, halitosis.
- Loose teeth.
- Difficulty eating or grooming (cats).

Blackwell's Five-Minute Veterinary Consult Clinical Companion: Small Animal Gastrointestinal Diseases, First Edition. Edited by Jocelyn Mott and Jo Ann Morrison.
© 2019 John Wiley & Sons, Inc. Published 2019 by John Wiley & Sons, Inc.
Companion website: www.fiveminutevet.com/gastrointestinal

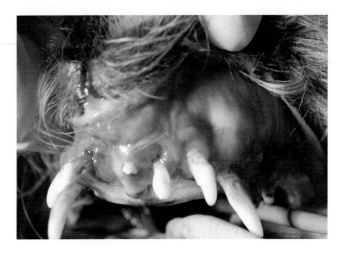

■ **Fig. 21.1.** Malignant tumors are generally locally more aggressive, and will displace teeth and deform maxillofacial bones.

- Swelling or deformity of facial/oral structures, including exophthalmos.
- Weight loss.
- Nasal deformity or discharge/bleeding (advanced maxillary tumor) (Figure 21.1).

CLINICAL FEATURES

- Malignant melanoma (MM).
  - Ulcerated, friable, readily bleeding and often pigmented, but up to 40% are amelanotic.
  - Tongue, gingiva, mucosa.
  - Necrosis common.
  - Great degree of variation in aggressiveness, metastatic rate, and mean survival time (MST); tumor size is prognostic factor.
- Squamous cell carcinoma (SCC).
  - Pink or red, verrucous, ulcerated, may bleed; loose teeth.
  - In cats – infiltrates bone rapidly, up to 30% rate of metastasis.
  - In dogs – rostral mass has a low rate of metastasis, but higher rate for tonsillar SCC or lingual SCC (Figure 21.2).
- Fibrosarcoma (FSA).
  - Raised, broad-based maxillary mass (palate, lateral muzzle).
  - Histologically low-grade, biologically high-grade FSA (high-low FSA).
  - Infiltrative – challenging to determine extent.
  - High-low FSA – 12% pulmonary metastasis, 20% lymph node metastasis.
- Osteosarcoma (OSA) – better prognosis than appendicular OSA. Soft tissue mass, red and friable, with bone lysis.
- Mast cell tumor (MCT) – near adjacent skin, seldom in gingiva; wax and wane.
- Malignant peripheral nerve sheath tumor – diffuse, poorly delineated mass involving a large portion of mandible or maxilla; local recurrence can track along a nerve sheath.
- Multilobular tumor of bone – osteochondrosarcoma.
  - Hard, well circumscribed, nonulcerated.
  - Caudal mandible, hard palate, base of skull, cranium.
  - Combination of well-circumscribed areas and nonmineralized tissue (typical "popcorn ball" description of appearance).

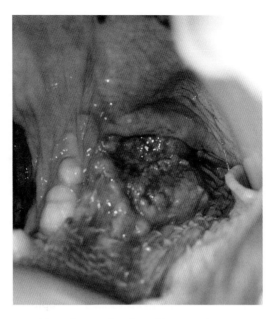

■ **Fig. 21.2.** Tonsillar squamous cell carcinoma of a dog with aggressive tumor growth expanding outside the tonsillar crypt.

■ Lymphosarcoma – diffuse epitheliotropic lymphoma, cutaneous T-cell lymphoma.
  • Depigmented oral mucosa and adjacent skin.
  • Gingiva diffusely red with punctate areas of redness and petechiation.
  • Low MST, even with chemotherapy.

 DIFFERENTIAL DIAGNOSIS

■ Infection – viral/bacterial/fungal. Periodontal disease – loose or missing teeth.
■ Inflammation.
  • Stomatitis.
  • Pyogenic granuloma.
■ Cystic structures (dentigerous, periapical).
■ Eosinophilic granuloma.
■ Calcinosis circumscripta.
■ Gingival enlargement (hyperplasia).
■ Oral ulceration (uremic ulcers, autoimmune disease, gum-chewer syndrome).
■ Sialocele.

 DIAGNOSTICS

■ Every tumor should be assessed using the TNM (Tumor-Node-Metastasis) system.
  • Size in three dimensions should be recorded, as well as attachment (pedunculated or broad based).
  • Regional lymph nodes should be assessed; mandibular lymph nodes can be easily accessed, but medial retropharyngeal nodes are more challenging to examine.
  • Evidence of lymph or pulmonary metastasis should be determined.

Complete Blood Cell Count/Biochemistry/Urinalysis

Used to rule out other primary or secondary complications, e.g., anemia, uremia.

Imaging

- Radiographically, malignant tumors often show a combination of bone lysis and periosteal proliferation, with evidence of root resorption.
- Advanced imaging (computed tomography – CT) is more helpful to assess the extent of tumors for surgical planning and in lymph node evaluation.
- Magnetic resonance imaging (MRI) provides more accurate information regarding the size of the masses and invasion of adjacent structures. Since melanomas have a hyperintense signal on T1-weighted images and a hypointense signal on T2-weighted images, it facilitates identification of the extent of the local growth.
- CT provides better images of calcification and cortical bone erosion. CT images can be enhanced with the use of contrast medium (e.g., iohexol) to delineate the tumor.

Other Diagnostic Tests

- Immunohistochemical tests may be required to specifically identify some tumor types.
- Aspirate, biopsy, or surgically remove enlarged regional lymph nodes for cytology and/or histology to evaluate for metastasis.

Pathologic Findings

- Histopathological assessment, including border readout on excisional biopsies, is critical.
- If possible, utilize a facility that specializes in oral maxillofacial pathology.
- Specific descriptions of each tumor type are beyond the scope of this chapter.

 # THERAPEUTICS

Drug(s) of Choice

- Very few oral malignancies have recommended chemotherapeutic protocols.
- Feline tonsillar SCC – see below.
- Palliative piroxicam (0.3 mg/kg PO q 24 h dogs) may be used in cases that are not amenable to surgical or other therapy.

Appropriate Health Care

- Depends on the tumor type.
- Malignant tumors are treated surgically with varying success depending on tumor type, location, and metastasis at presentation.
- In advanced circumstances, combined therapy (surgery, chemotherapy, and radiation) may provide the best outcome.
- Molecularly targeted therapies provide oncologists with tools to treat cancers with greater specificity. These modalities can be used further to classify tumors, aid in predicting the prognosis, and help determine the exact treatment plan.

Nursing Care

- Pain control.
- Supportive care.

Diet

Providing adequate nutrition can be challenging postoperatively, so feeding tubes may be necessary.

Surgical Considerations

- Early diagnosis and treatment offer the best chance for a successful outcome.
- The first surgical resection offers the best chance for complete resection.
- Complete *en bloc* excision is the treatment of choice, with surgical margins ranging from 1 to 2 cm dependent on the tumor type.
- Radiation therapy should be offered in cases where complete excision is not possible and/or the mass is located in the caudal aspect of the oral cavity and precludes complete surgical excision.
- Megavoltage radiation therapy is presently considered the standard of care for treatment of oral tumors; however, intensity-modulated radiation therapy (IMRT) is a relatively new technology that is quickly being adopted.
- Malignant melanoma.
  - Prognosis improves if the tumor is small and located in the rostral mandible.
  - If surgery is chosen for therapy, it should be aggressive (2 cm clean surgical margins); typically mandibulectomy or maxillectomy.
  - Median survival times average eight months.
  - Combination of surgery, radiation, and chemotherapy (low-dose cisplatin) yielded a median survival of 14 months in one study.
  - Pigmentation does not affect the prognosis.
  - Relatively radioresistant; one study showed a median survival time of 14 months after radiation only.
  - The problem with melanoma is not local disease management but metastasis.
  - A conditionally licensed vaccine may be administered by oncologists (four vaccinations two weeks apart, then every six months) after locoregional disease control.
  - Single-agent platinum analogs used alone or with piroxicam have been shown to have antitumor activity for malignant melanoma.
- Squamous cell carcinoma.
  - Better long-term prognosis than MM or FSA in the dog.
  - May be widely surgically excised or irradiated in the dog, especially if the lesion is rostral (better prognosis than those located caudally).
  - Perform a maxillectomy or mandibulectomy with a 2 cm clean surgical margin as a goal (Figure 21.3).
  - In dogs, radiation alone delivers a median survival rate of 15–17 months.
  - In dogs, prognosis for survival following treatment of lingual involvement is poor.
  - Dogs tolerate partial glossectomy involving 40–60% of the tongue.
  - For tumors larger than 2 cm or those with incomplete resections, surgery, radiation, and chemotherapy (mitoxantrone or cisplatin with piroxicam) may be the best options.
  - In cats, surgical resection gives a mean survival rate of one year for resectable tumors.
  - One can use carboplatin or mitoxantrone for palliative treatment.
  - Radiation locally along with aminobisphosphonate is considered a good palliative treatment for cats with SCC.
  - A recent study looked at combining accelerated radiation therapy and carboplatin with better results, particularly with tonsillar SCC in cats.

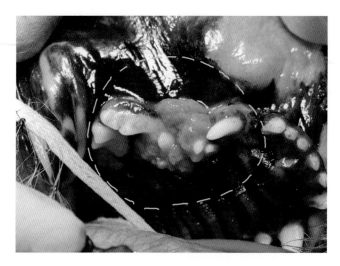

■ **Fig. 21.3.** While an incisional biopsy returned a presumptive diagnosis of papillary oral squamous cell carcinoma, the 1 cm planned margins for the maxillectomy were sufficient to provide tumor-free margins for this squamous cell carcinoma.

- Fibrosarcoma.
  - Surgical excision with at least 2 cm margins usually results in a 12-month median survival rate.
  - Usually requires a maxillectomy or mandibulectomy.
  - Surgical excision in combination with radiation therapy and chemotherapy offers the best prognosis.
  - Radiation or chemotherapy alone offers a poorer median survival rate than surgery alone.
  - Palatine FSA carries the poorest prognosis because of the inability to surgically resect.
  - Radiation therapy can be useful after surgical removal.
- Osteosarcoma.
  - Wide surgical removal with 2 cm margins is ideal.
  - Recurrence can occur at metastatic sites.
  - Radiation therapy should be considered post surgery for microscopic disease.
  - Palliative radiation therapy can be used alone.

 COMMENTS

Client Education

Early detection is important; regular oral examinations and home care can be helpful.

Patient Monitoring

Varies with the type of mass and treatment selected.

Prevention/Avoidance

Minimize environmental factors when possible (second-hand smoke, flea collars).

Possible Complications

- Surgical removal of part of the tongue may result in avascular necrosis if the tongue is transected just caudal to the origin of dorsal branches of the lingual arteries.
- Postoperative complications of mandibulectomy include wound dehiscence, prehension dysfunction, tongue lag, medial drift (orthodontic buttons with elastics can minimize this), excessive drooling, palatal ulceration secondary to malocclusion, and pressure necrosis.
- Mandibulectomies can be performed in cats, but they result in greater complications (tongue swelling, ranula formation) than in dogs. Surgery can result in esthetic complications.
- Low-dose radiation can cause diarrhea, nausea, vomiting, and hair loss (regrowth of hair is usually white) within the first few weeks.
- High-dose radiation has the above effects as well as oral ulceration/necrosis, mucositis, cataracts (these lesions occur in almost all cases and are self-limiting with supportive care), and radiation-induced tumors (mainly in young dogs that underwent radiation therapy for radioresponsive tumors).
- Late radiation effects can occur with bone and muscle necrosis but are unlikely.
- Nonhealing surgical sites may occur in an area previously irradiated.
- IMRT offers a more accurate dose distribution and is rapidly being accepted as the best form of radiation therapy with fewer side effects.
- Complications of chemotherapy are varied depending on the drug used.
- The use of bisphosphonates has been associated with osteonecrosis of the jaw in humans.

Expected Course and Prognosis

- Dogs with inadequate tumor-free surgical margins were 2.5 times more likely to die of the tumor than those with complete histological excision.
- Some surgical patients need gastrostomy tubes to facilitate nutritional supplementation during the treatment period.
- Dogs with tumors located caudal to the first premolar had three times greater risk of dying from the disease than those with tumors located rostral to the first premolar.
- Staging of oral tumors using the TNM (primary Tumor, regional distant lymph Nodes (cervical, submandibular, and parotid nodes), and Metastasis) classification system allows for a more accurate prognosis; the higher the stage (I–IV), the worse the prognosis.
- High-grade (biologically)/low-grade (histologically) fibrosarcomas that are reported in large-breed dogs (mainly golden retrievers) offer a poor prognosis due to rapid growth and metastasis.
- Locoregional disease control of MM followed by vaccine in a timely manner resulted in longer MST than historical controls.

Abbreviations

- CT = computed tomography
- FSA = fibrosarcoma
- IMRT = intensity-modulated radiation therapy
- MCT = mast cell tumor
- MM = malignant melanoma
- MRI = magnetic resonance imaging
- MST = mean survival time
- OSA = osteosarcoma
- SCC = squamous cell carcinoma
- TNM = Tumor-Node-Metastasis.

See Also

- Oral Neoplasia, Benign
- Ptyalism

Suggested Reading

Ettinger SJ, Feldman FC, eds. Textbook of Veterinary Internal Medicine, 7th ed. St Louis: Saunders Elsevier, 2010.

Fidel J, Lyons J, Tripp C, et al. Treatment of oral squamous cell carcinoma with accelerated radiation therapy and concomitant carboplantin in cats. J Vet Intern Med 2011;25(3):504–510.

Fosum T. Small Animal Surgery, 3rd ed. St Louis: Mosby Elsevier, 2007.

Harvey CE, Emily PP. Small Animal Dentistry. Philadelphia: Mosby, 1993.

Lobprise HB, Dodd JR. Wigg's Veterinary Dentistry: Principles and Practice. Hoboken: Wiley, 2019.

Meuten DJ. Tumors in Domestic Animals. Ames: Iowa State University Press, 2002.

Nelson RW, Couto CG. Small Animal Internal Medicine, 3rd ed. St Louis: Mosby, 2003.

Wiggs RB, Lobprise HB. Veterinary Dentistry: Principles and Practice. Philadelphia: Lippincott-Raven, 1997.

Authors: Heidi B. Lobprise DVM, DAVDC, Jason W. Soukup DVM, DAVDC

Chapter 22

Phenobarbital-Responsive Sialadenosis

DEFINITION/OVERVIEW

- Bilateral, painless, noninflammatory, uniform, nonneoplastic enlargement of salivary glands.
- Also known as idiopathic sialadenosis.
- Diagnosis involves exclusion of other diseases with similar signs as there is no specific test for definitive diagnosis.
- Diagnosis of phenobarbital-responsive sialadenosis (PRS) is confirmed by rapid improvement of clinical signs after phenobarbital treatment.

ETIOLOGY/PATHOPHYSIOLOGY

The etiology of this condition remains unclear but it has been associated with an unusual form of limbic epilepsy.

Systems Affected

- Gastrointestinal – gagging, ptyalism, nausea, lip smacking, regurgitation, vomiting, weight loss, hyporexia, and anorexia.
- Neurological – dysphagia.

SIGNALMENT/HISTORY

- Rare in dogs.
- One presumptive case in a cat.
- Due to the paucity of reported cases, risk factors for developing PRS and gender or breed predisposition have not been identified.

CLINICAL FEATURES

- Bilateral salivary gland enlargement.
- Exophthalmos (if enlarged zygomatic salivary gland).
- Retching or gulping.
- Lip smacking.
- Ptyalism.
- Dysphagia.

Blackwell's Five-Minute Veterinary Consult Clinical Companion: Small Animal Gastrointestinal Diseases,
First Edition. Edited by Jocelyn Mott and Jo Ann Morrison.
© 2019 John Wiley & Sons, Inc. Published 2019 by John Wiley & Sons, Inc.
Companion website: www.fiveminutevet.com/gastrointestinal

- Regurgitation.
- Vomiting.
- Snorting.
- Sensitivity to gentle external palpation of throat.
- Hyporexia.
- Anorexia.
- Weight loss.

 DIFFERENTIAL DIAGNOSIS

- Salivary gland neoplasm.
- Sialadenitis.
- Sialoceles.
- Salivary gland infarction.
- Sialolithiasis.
- Esophagitis.
- Esophageal foreign body.
- Atypical hypoadrenocorticism.
- Inflammatory bowel disease.
- Gastrointestinal neoplasm.
- Pancreatitis.
- Trauma to the hyoid apparatus.
- Hiatal hernia.

 DIAGNOSTICS

Complete Blood Cell Count/Biochemistry/Urinalysis

- Complete blood cell count may be unremarkable.
- Neutrophilic leukocytosis.
- Hemoconcentration.
- Hyperalbuminemia.
- Hypokalemia.

Imaging

- Abdominal radiography – unremarkable.
- Thoracic radiography – unremarkable. Hiatal hernia may be visualized.
- Ultrasonography – unremarkable.

Other Laboratory Tests

- Esophagogastroduodenoscopy.
  - Esophagitis.
  - Gastritis.
  - Enteritis.
- Cytology of salivary gland.
  - Normal.
  - May confirm salivary origin.
- Histopathology of salivary glands – normal.

THERAPEUTICS

- May require inpatient treatments for stabilization and diagnostic testing if profuse vomiting and prolonged anorexia.
- Intravenous fluid therapy to restore fluid and electrolytes imbalance.

Drug(s) of Choice

Phenobarbital: 1–2 mg/kg PO q 12 h.

Precautions/Interactions

Phenobarbital – monitor liver enzymes.

Nursing Care

- Monitor caloric intake through enteral nutrition.
- Feeding tube may be necessary during treatment if prolonged anorexia or dysphagia.

Diet

No specific diet to treat this particular disease.

Activity

Normal.

Surgical Considerations

Incisional versus excisional biopsy of the salivary gland is performed to exclude other diseases.

 # COMMENTS

Client Education

- Monitor size of salivary gland.
- Monitor caloric intake.
- Report any diarrhea and/or vomiting.

Patient Monitoring

- Physical examination with follow-up complete blood count and chemistry panel is recommended every 2–4 weeks until all abnormalities are resolved.
- Routine recheck is recommended every 3–4 months once patient fully recovered.
- May be able to taper off phenobarbital after three months in some patients.
- Some patients may need long-term treatment to prevent recurrence.

Prevention/Avoidance

Early diagnosis and medical treatment is the key for recovery.

Possible Complications

- Long-term vomiting can lead to esophagitis and/or hiatal hernia.
- Malnutrition from prolonged anorexia.

Expected Course and Prognosis

Prognosis is good if positive response to phenobarbital treatment.

Abbreviations

- PRS = phenobarbital-responsive sialadenosis

See Also

- Dysphagia
- Salivary mucocele
- Salivary neoplasia
- Sialadenitis

Suggested Reading

Alcoverro E, Tabar MD, Lloret A, et al. Phenobarbital-responsive sialadenosis in dogs: case series. Topics Compan Anim Med 2014;29:109–112.

Boydell P, Pike R, Crossley D, Whitbread T. Sialadenosis in dogs. J Am Vet Med Assoc 2000;216:872–874.

Boydell P, Pike R, Crossley D. Presumptive sialadenosis in a cat. J Small Anim Pract 2000;41:573–574.

Dagan A. Sialadenosis in a dog. Isr J Vet Med 2011;66:32–35.

Sozmen M, Brown PJ, Whitbread TJ. Idiopathic salivary gland enlargement (sialadenosis) in dogs: a microscopic study. J Small Anim Pract 2000;41:243–247.

Author: Vivian K. Yau DVM, DACVIM (SAIM)

Chapter 23

Sialadenitis

DEFINITION/OVERVIEW

- Sialadenitis is defined as inflammation of the salivary gland; it is common to name the affected gland (e.g., zygomatic, submandibular, etc.).

ETIOLOGY/PATHOPHYSIOLOGY

- The condition is rare and the precise pathophysiology is unknown.
- Potential etiologies that have been described include trauma, local or systemic infection, immune-mediated conditions, and extension from regional (e.g., periorbital) disease or inflammation.

Systems Affected

- Gastrointestinal – dysphagia, ptyalism, inappetence, pain on opening the mouth.
- Hemic/lymphatic/immune – fever, inflammatory cell infiltrates into affected glands.
- Musculoskeletal – pain on opening the mouth. Involvement of the medial pterygoid muscle has been described, especially with zygomatic sialadenitis.
- Ophthalmic – swelling and/or pain with retrobulbar involvement, exophthalmos, chemosis. Severely affected patients may present with blindness, especially if the zygomatic gland is affected.

SIGNALMENT/HISTORY

- True breed or sex predilections are difficult to assess, due to the rare nature of the condition.
- One report of 11 dogs indicated a male predisposition (10/11 cases).
- Most dogs in that study were middle-aged to older (mean eight years with a range of 3–12 years) and were medium or large breeds (mean body weight 23.4 kg with a range of 8.7–45 kg).

Risk Factors

None known.

Historical Findings

- Lethargy/malaise.
- Fever.

Blackwell's Five-Minute Veterinary Consult Clinical Companion: Small Animal Gastrointestinal Diseases, First Edition. Edited by Jocelyn Mott and Jo Ann Morrison.
© 2019 John Wiley & Sons, Inc. Published 2019 by John Wiley & Sons, Inc.
Companion website: www.fiveminutevet.com/gastrointestinal

- Pain.
- Inappetence/anorexia.
- Ptyalism.
- Dysphagia.
- Difficult prehension.
- Ocular signs include:
  - Third eyelid (nictitating membrane) protrusion.
  - Ocular discharge.
  - Periocular swelling.
  - Blindness.

 ## CLINICAL FEATURES

- Salivary gland (e.g., zygomatic) papilla swelling.
- Pain on opening the mouth.
- Pain on retropulsion.
- Decreased or absent retropulsion.
- Ocular signs include:
  - Conjunctival hyperemia.
  - Chemosis.
  - Blepharospasm and episcleral injection.
  - Exophthalmos or enophthalmos.
  - Strabismus.
  - Epiphora.
  - Exposure keratitis.
  - Lagophthalmos.
  - Ptosis and eyelid erythema.

 ## DIFFERENTIAL DIAGNOSIS

- Etiologies for swellings/pain in the region of a salivary gland include:
  - Hematoma.
  - Neoplasia.
  - Abscess.
  - Granuloma.
  - Traumatic injury.
- Etiologies of salivary pathology include:
  - Sialodenosis.
  - Sialocele formation.
  - Salivary neoplasia.
  - Sialolithiasis.

 ## DIAGNOSTICS

Complete Blood Cell Count/Biochemistry/Urinalysis

- An inflammatory leukogram (leukocytosis, neutrophilia) may be seen.
- The remainder of the minimum database tends to be within normal limits.

Other Laboratory Tests

- Cytology – cytologic evaluation of the affected glands reveals a mucinous background due to thick, tenacious salivary fluid, which may be blood-tinged. Primary cell types include neutrophils (nondegenerate) and large, foamy macrophages. Ductal epithelial cells, plasma cells, lymphocytes, and multinucleated cells may also be seen. Cytology of regional lymph nodes may be performed if neoplasia is suspected.
- Microbiology – samples submitted for aerobic and anaerobic culture are negative for the majority of cases in the small numbers of samples reported.
- Special stains – background staining of cytology samples with periodic acid–Schiff and/or toluidine blue are strongly positive for mucin.

Imaging

Radiographs
- Radiographs of the affected region may show sialoliths and associated soft tissue swelling.
- Three-view thoracic films may be obtained when neoplasia is suspected.

Ultrasonography
- Ultrasound of the periorbital tissues and retrobulbar space may show a retrobulbar mass of variable echogenicity.
- Ultrasonography may also facilitate fine needle aspiration of lesions.

Computed Tomography (CT) and Magnetic Resonance Imaging (MRI)
- CT and MRI may be performed to elucidate affected tissues, rule out other differential diagnoses, and evaluate tissue intensity (MRI) or contrast enhancement (CT).
- The optic nerve, medial pterygoid muscle, globe position, and periorbital tissues may be evaluated. Additional salivary pathology (e.g., sialoliths, sialocele) may be discovered.
- Advanced imaging assists with potential surgical planning or histopathology sample collection.

Pathologic Findings
- Gross – as described above in "Clinical Findings."
- Histopathology – provides a definitive diagnosis. Findings include an inflammatory infiltrate of mixed inflammatory cells. Necrosis and lobular degeneration may be seen.

 # THERAPEUTICS

Upon diagnosis, the objective of treatment is primarily to control inflammation in the affected gland and surrounding tissues.

Drug(s) of Choice

Systemic Medications
- Nonsteroidal antiinflammatory drugs (NASIDs – multiple medications have been described) at label dosages, for example carprofen (4.4 mg/kg PO q 24 h or divided q 12 h).
- Corticosteroids at antiinflammatory dosages, for example prednisone or prednisolone (0.5–1 mg/kg PO q 12–24 h for seven days then tapering dosages).
- Analgesic medication (multiple options exist): tramadol (4–10 mg/kg PO q 8 h prn for pain).
- Antibiotics – when indicated (rarely), should be based on culture and sensitivity results from salivary gland samples.

Topical (Ocular) Medications

- Neomycin/polymyxin/dexamethasone (ointment or solution) when corneal ulceration has been ruled out.
- Artificial tears if exposure keratitis is noted.
- Neomycin/polymyxin/bacitracin (ointment or solution) if corneal trauma/ulceration is present.

Precautions/Interactions

- Concurrent use of NSAIDs and steroids is contraindicated due to increased risk of side effects, especially gastrointestinal (GI). Risk of GI side effects is possible with therapy of either drug class as monotherapy so potential addition of GI medications (e.g., H2-blockers) and monitoring for side effects may be warranted.
- Clinicians should remember that corticosteroids have numerous side effects and multiple drug interactions are possible.
- Changing therapy from one NSAID to another should be done cautiously and only after following recommendations for NSAID-specific "wash-out" periods prior to administration.

Appropriate Health Care

Affected patients may present with dehydration and may potentially be undernourished, especially if clinical signs have been severe/chronic.

Nursing Care

Dogs may present with blindness or impaired vision. Cautious movement of these patients through the environment is recommended.

Diet

Patients may benefit from soft/moistened/canned food while symptomatic. Long-term dietary therapy changes should not be necessary.

Surgical Considerations

Histopathology sample collection may be obtained via needle or incisional biopsy. Severely affected dogs may require excision of the affected gland (s) and/or temporary tarsorrhaphy.

 COMMENTS

Due to the anatomic location of select salivary glands, surgical approach for biopsy or removal may be complicated and referral to a board-certified surgeon should be considered.

Client Education

In patients with vision impairment, take appropriate safety measures at home (e.g., furniture, stairs, etc.). Ensure affected patients are able to meet hydration and caloric needs.

Patient Monitoring

- Resolution of inflammation should be verified with improvement in clinical signs (e.g., return of vision, reduction of ptyalism, reduction of fever, improved attitude, improved prehension and swallowing).
- Depending on the medication prescribed, monitoring should be tailored to the individual patient (e.g., follow-up serum biochemical evaluation for patients on NSAIDs).

Possible Complications

- Dehydration.
- Loss of vision.
- Ocular lesions.
- Xerostomia.

Expected Course and Prognosis

- Due to the rare nature of this condition, prognosis should be considered guarded.
- The majority of cases identified in the literature have had overall good prognoses with resolution of clinical signs and no reports of recurrence.

Abbreviations

- CT = computed tomography
- GI = gastrointestinal
- MRI = magnetic resonance imaging
- NSAID = nonsteroidal antiinflammatory drug

See Also

- Dysphagia
- Phenobarbital-Responsive Sialodenosis
- Ptyalism
- Salivary Mucocele
- Salivary Neoplasia

Suggested Reading

Cannon MS, Paglia D, Zwingenberger AL, et al. Clinical and diagnostic imaging findings in dogs with zygomatic sialadenitis: 11 cases (1990–2009). J Am Vet Med Assoc 2011;239(9):1211–1218.

McGill S, Lester N, McLachlan A, et al. Concurrent sialocoele and necrotising sialadenitis in a dog. J Small Anim Pract 2009;50:151–156.

Perez-Ecija A, Estepa JC, Mendoza FJ. Granulomatous giant cell submandibular sialadenitis in a dog. Can Vet J 2012;53:1211–1213.

Reiter AM, Soltero-Rivera MM. Oral and salivary gland disorders. In: Ettinger SJ, Feldman EC, Cote E, eds. Textbook of Veterinary Internal Medicine, 8th ed. St Louis: Elsevier, 2017.

Simison WG. Sialadenitis associated with periorbital disease in a dog. J Am Vet Med Assoc 1993;202(12):1983–1985.

Author: Jo Ann Morrison DVM, MS, DACVIM

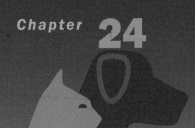

Chapter 24

Salivary Mucocele

DEFINITION/OVERVIEW

A salivary mucocele, also known as a sialocele, is a collection of saliva outside the salivary gland or salivary duct, within the subcutaneous tissues. The four most common types of sialoceles are cervical, sublingual (ranula), pharyngeal, and zygomatic.

ETIOLOGY/PATHOPHYSIOLOGY

- A salivary mucocele results when saliva escapes from the salivary gland or ducts. Saliva collects in the subcutaneous tissue and granulation tissues form around the collection of saliva. These swellings are not true cysts, as they are not lined with epithelium.
- The salivary glands are normal on palpation with salivary mucoceles.
- There are two types of salivary glands: major and minor. Major glands: parotid, zygomatic, mandibular, and sublingual salivary glands. There are many minor salivary glands, but disease is rarely seen in these tissues.
- The mandibular and sublingual salivary glands are closely associated and share a capsule.
  - The mandibular is the larger of the two and is located caudomedially to the ramus of the mandible.
  - The sublingual gland lies at the cranial aspect of the mandibular gland and has monostomatic and polystomatic portions. The monostomatic portion is caudal to the lingual nerve and drains into the sublingual duct. The polystomatic portion is rostral to the lingual nerve and is organized as small clusters that empty directly into the oral cavity.
- The zygomatic gland is located medial to the zygomatic arch and rostrolateral to the globe.
- The parotid gland is located lateral to the vertical ear canal.
- Most commonly, saliva leaks from the sublingual salivary gland or duct, resulting in a cervical sialocele. Leakage from the mandibular complex can also result in a cervical mucocele.
- Damage in this complex can also result in a sublingual or pharyngeal sialocele.
- Zygomatic sialoceles result from damaged zygomatic salivary tissue.
- Parotid mucoceles are uncommon and are related to the parotid salivary gland and duct.

Systems Affected

- Skin – most commonly, sialoceles result in subcutaneous, soft swellings.
- Gastrointestinal – dysphagia may occur due to sublingual and pharyngeal sialoceles.
- Ophthalmic – exophthalmos is the most common clinical sign noted with zygomatic sialoceles. Additionally, third eyelid protrusion and orbital swelling can occur.
- Respiratory – pharyngeal sialoceles can result in dyspnea if airway obstruction occurs.

Blackwell's Five-Minute Veterinary Consult Clinical Companion: Small Animal Gastrointestinal Diseases, First Edition. Edited by Jocelyn Mott and Jo Ann Morrison.
© 2019 John Wiley & Sons, Inc. Published 2019 by John Wiley & Sons, Inc.
Companion website: www.fiveminutevet.com/gastrointestinal

SIGNALMENT/HISTORY

- No consistent sex or age predilection.
- Poodles, German shepherd dogs, Australian silky terriers, and dachshunds may be predisposed, but all breeds can be affected.
- Salivary mucoceles are rare in cats.

Risk Factors

- Trauma (such as choke collars/chains, bite wounds, or chewing on foreign material).
- Neoplasia, sialoliths, and glandular foreign bodies have also been reported.
- There are case reports of tooth extraction, hemimaxillectomy, and dirofilariasis infection being associated with sialocele formation.

Historical Findings

- Cervical – acute onset of swelling in the intermandibular region or ventral cervical region. The swelling may be noted to change in size. May be lateralized, especially initially.
- Sublingual – tongue deviation to one side, difficulty prehending food, swallowing or chewing. Additionally, hemorrhagic oral discharge may be noted secondary to trauma.
- Zygomatic – exophthalmos.
- Pharyngeal – respiratory distress, dysphagia or stridor. Less common clinical signs include gagging, hypersalivation, and stertor.
- Parotid – swelling ventral to the ear.

CLINICAL FEATURES

- Cervical – the intermandibular subcutaneous swelling is usually fluctuant and nonpainful. It may be unilateral or central. These swelling can be very large.
- Sublingual – a swelling on the ventrolateral aspect of the tongue is noted (Figure 24.1).
- Zygomatic – exophthalmos, third eyelid protrusion, and periorbital swelling are noted. On oral exam, a ventral deviation of mucosa may be noted in the region of the upper last molar.

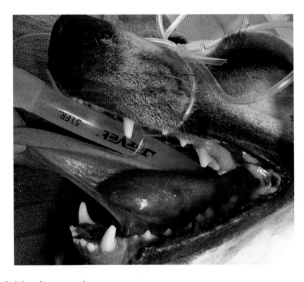

■ **Fig. 24.1.** Sublingual sialocele or ranula.

- Pharyngeal – pharyngeal mucoceles may be an incidental finding during an oral examination. A soft swelling within the wall of the pharynx will be noted. Often sedation and oropharyngeal exam are required to observe and diagnose.
- Parotid – soft swelling ventral to the ear.

 ## DIFFERENTIAL DIAGNOSIS

- Sialadenosis – bilateral nonpainful swelling of the salivary glands, most commonly the mandibular glands. Often associated with underlying esophageal disease. Clinical signs include retching, gulping, lip smacking, hypersalivation, and weight loss. This condition has also been reported in cats. Unusual form of limbic epilepsy. Diagnosis of exclusion. Reported to be responsive to phenobarbital therapy (1–2 mg/kg PO q 12 h).
- Sialoadenitis – inflammation of salivary glands which may progress to glandular necrosis. Terrier breeds are predisposed. Clinical signs similar to sialadenosis, but salivary glands are painful on palpation and vomiting may be seen. Diagnosis based on histopathology. Reported to be responsive to phenobarbital therapy (1–2 mg/kg PO q 12 h).
- Necrotizing sialometaplasia (NSM) – sialoadenitis progressing to necrosis of the seromucinous glands and squamous metaplasia of the acini and ducts.
- Salivary neoplasia – uncommon. Mandibular and parotid glands are most frequently affected. Regional lymph node and/or distant metastasis can occur. Clinical signs include unilateral, nonpainful, firm, often fixed, swelling of the affected gland, halitosis, exophthalmos, and dysphagia. Fine needle aspiration of the mass can aid in diagnosis of neoplasia.
- Sialoliths – most often associated with the parotid duct, but also reported in the mandibular-sublingual complex. Clinical signs include swelling which may be painful or occur then regress. Diagnostics include palpation, radiographs or computed tomography (CT) +/– sialography.
- Cervical abscess – swelling that is firm, warm to the touch, and painful. Aspirate commonly reveals signs of inflammation and/or intracellular bacteria.
- Foreign body – often associated with abscessation. Diagnosis often made based on history, followed by CT or surgical explore with foreign body removal and abscess debridement.
- Hematoma – swelling of variable size. Aspirate will reveal blood.
- Cystic or neoplastic lymph nodes – firm swelling. Aspirate will reveal lymph node tissue or neoplastic cells if the lymph node has been effaced.
- Skin or subcutaneous neoplasm – examples include myxoma, myxosarcoma, lipoma, etc. Mass lesion possibly associated with a sialocele-like component. CT and biopsy are required for differentiation.
- Tonsil cysts – cyst arising from the tonsil or tonsillar crypt.
- Thyroglossal cysts (rare) – swelling anywhere in the neck. Serosanguinous, noninflammatory fluid consistent with a cyst on cytology. True cyst with epithelial lining will be noted on histopathology.

 ## DIAGNOSTICS

- Physical exam – palpation of mass as nonpainful, soft, and fluctuant in a location consistent with a mucocele.
- In order to determine the affected side in patients with large or central cervical mucoceles, the patient may be positioned in dorsal and the mucocele will generally move toward the affected side.

Complete Blood Cell Count/Biochemistry/Urinalysis

Usually unremarkable.

Other Diagnostic Tests

Fine needle aspiration – aseptic paracentesis using a 20 gauge needle.

Imaging

- Sialography - retrograde sialography can be performed with traditional radiography or CT. Findings of these studies may highlight a defect within the duct of the examined salivary gland which can confirm the gland that needs to be removed prior to surgery.
- CT +/– sialography – CT or CT sialography can be performed in the dog in order to image the salivary glands and their ducts.

Pathologic Findings

- Fine needle aspiration – fluid aspirated from the swelling (not the salivary gland) is generally clear, yellow or serosanguinous. A thick, ropey, mucinous fluid will be aspirated.
- When analyzed cytologically, a low cellularity consisting of nondegenerate, nucleated cells will be noted. Increased presence of white blood cells may be more consistent with infection or abscess.
- Periodic acid–Schiff (PAS) staining will confirm the presence of mucus.
- Histopathology – histopathology of the lining of the mucocele will be consistent with granulation tissue.

 # THERAPEUTICS

Treatment of salivary mucoceles involves surgical removal of the affected salivary gland and associated salivary duct. Removal of the granulation-lined mucocele is not necessary.

Drug(s) of Choice

- Salivary mucoceles do not warrant medical treatment unless an associated infection is identified.
- If concurrent infection is diagnosed, treatment can be initiated with a broad-spectrum antibiotic (amoxicillin and clavulanic acid, 13.75–20 mg/kg PO q 12 h) until culture and sensitivity results are obtained.

Appropriate Health Care

No specific requirements.

Nursing Care

Nursing care is generally unnecessary.

Diet

Dietary modification is generally unnecessary, with the exception of ranulas. Soft food should be offered for 2–3 weeks following surgery.

Activity

Activity restriction should be suggested for 2–3 weeks following surgery. Activities which promote head shaking (chew toys, tug of war) should be discontinued for the same time period.

Surgical Considerations

- Sublingual and mandibular sialadenectomy for cervical, sublingual, and pharyngeal mucoceles. A lateral or ventral approach to the glands can be performed.
  - Ventral – an incision is made just caudal to the ramus and extended rostrally toward the mandibular symphysis. The jugular bifurcation is identified and the salivary gland complex should be located cranial to the bifurcation (Figure 24.2). An incision is made into the capsule, ensuring that the salivary gland is identified rather than the mandibular lymph node. The gland is removed from the capsule. The duct is followed rostrally to the digastricus. The salivary glands are excised and the duct is pulled dorsal to the digastricus. The dissection is continued rostrally, to the level of the lingual nerve (Figure 24.3), where the duct is ligated and transected as rostrally as possible.
  - If a ranula is present, the dissection should continue rostrally (dorsal to the mylohyoideus) to remove all of the glandular tissue to the level of the sublingual caruncle.
  - The sialocele can be resected if it is large, but this may result in more tissue trauma and hemorrhage. Alternatively, incisional drainage can be performed. Both procedures are followed with placement of a ventrally dependent Penrose drain or active suction drain (Figures 24.4, 24.5).
  - Lateral – a horizontal incision is made over the jugular bifurcation. The sialocele may need to be incised and drained prior to dissection of the glands. The glands are dissected free from surrounding tissue as previously described. Dissection is continued rostrally, parallel to the duct. A hemostat is placed distally across the duct and used to provide caudal traction to aid in dissection. Once all the duct is dissected, it can be ligated. Alternatively, traction may be placed on the hemostat at the level of desired transection and used to separate the duct from the oral cavity.
- Ranula or pharyngeal mucocele marsupialization.
  - Combined with the previously described mandibular and sublingual sialadenectomy.
  - Marsupialization is performed by excising a large, full-thickness section of tissue overlying the sialocele. Then, the oral mucosa is sutured to the sialocele lining, granulation tissue.

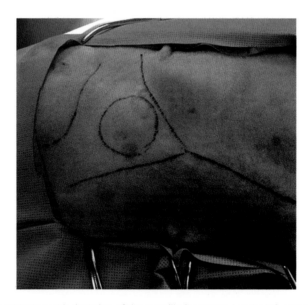

■ **Fig. 24.2.** Patient positioning with depiction of the mandibular ramus, jugular bifurcation, and relative location of the sublingual and mandibular salivary gland complex.

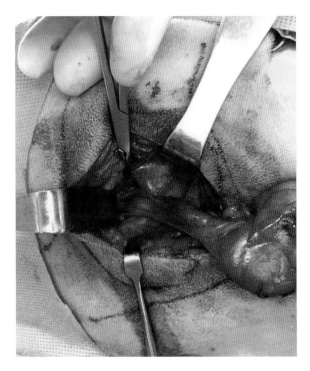

■ **Fig. 24.3.** Dissection of the duct to the level of the lingual nerve.

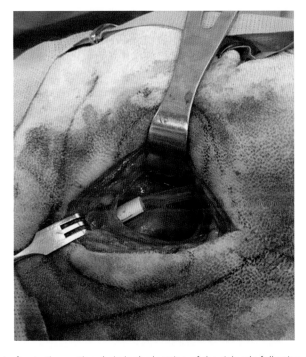

■ **Fig. 24.4.** Placement of an active suction drain in the location of the sialocele following surgery.

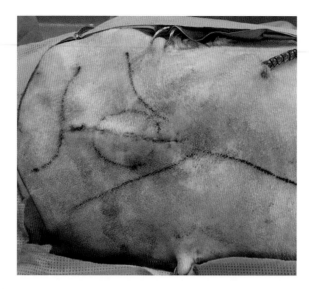

■ **Fig. 24.5.** Closure following sublingual and mandibular sialadenectomy with drain placement.

■ Zygomatic sialadenectomy – an incision is made on the dorsal aspect of the zygomatic arch. The masseter muscle is dissected free. In order to access the gland, a portion of the rostral and lateral arch must be removed with a saw or rongeurs as the gland is located medial to the arch. The gland is dissected from the surrounding tissue, taking careful note of the malar artery and vein which are closely associated with the gland.

■ Parotid sialadenectomy – an incision is made from the ventral aspect of the external acoustic meatus and extended ventrally to the angle of the mandible. The gland is bluntly dissected free from its attachments. The facial nerve is in close proximity and care should be taken to not damage the nerve.

■ Bilateral sialadenectomy – when bilateral swellings are present, or the side of origin cannot be determined, such as in the case of a large cervical mucocele, bilateral sialadenectomy of inciting glands can be performed. Additionally, patients can develop mucoceles on the contralateral side, at which time the gland should be removed.

 COMMENTS

Client Education

■ Patients should be monitored for signs of respiratory distress which can be associated with sublingual or pharyngeal mucoceles.

■ Owners should also note if patients are painful, as this could be a sign of developing infection.

■ Following surgery, patients should be monitored for recurrence.

■ If lingual or hypoglossal nerve damage occurs, patients may experience loss of sensation and motor of the tongue, lower jaw, lip, cheek, and oral mucosa. This could result in dysphagia or self-trauma following surgery.

Patient Monitoring

Patients should be monitored for new swellings on the same or contralateral side.

Prevention/Avoidance

There are no recommended prevention strategies.

Possible Complications

- The most common complication following sialadenectomy is seroma formation.
- Other complications include infection and incision dehiscence.
- Recurrence rates are generally very low following surgery, but development of a contralateral mucocele, or one at another location, is possible.

Expected Course and Prognosis

The prognosis for cure following surgery is excellent provided the correct salivary gland and associated duct are removed.

Synonyms

- Ranula – sublingual salivary mucocele
- Sialocele
- Mandibular mucocele
- Cervical mucocele
- Pharyngeal mucocele
- Zygomatic mucocele
- Sublingual mucocele
- Salivary or honey cyst

Abbreviations

- CT = computed tomography
- NSM = necrotizing sialometaplasia
- PAS = periodic acid–Schiff

See Also

- Phenobarbital-Responsive Sialadenosis
- Sialadenitis

Suggested Reading

Benjamino KP, Birchard SJ. Pharyngeal mucoceles in dogs: 14 cases. J Am Anim Hosp Assoc 2012;48:31–35.

Hamaide A, Griffon D. *Complications in Small Animal Surgery*. Chichester: Wiley-Blackwell, 2016.

Radlinsky MG. Surgery of the digestive system. In: Fossum TW, ed. Small Animal Surgery, 4th ed. St Louis: Elsevier, 2012, pp. 417–422.

Ritter MJ Stanley BJ. Salivary glands. In: Johnston SA, Tobias KM, eds. Veterinary Surgery: Small Animal, 2nd ed. St Louis: Elsevier, 2017, pp. 1653–1663.

Ritter MJ, von Pfeil DJ, Stanley BJ, et al. Mandibular and sublingual sialocoeles in the dog: a retrospective evaluation of 41 cases, using the ventral approach for treatment. N Z Vet J 2006;54(6):333–337.

Spangler WL, Culbertson MR. Salivary gland disease in dogs and cats: 245 cases (1985–1988). J Am Vet Med Assoc 1991;198(3):465–469.

Acknowledgments: The authors and editors acknowledge the prior contribution of Dr Susanne Lauer.

Authors: Amy N. Zide DVM, Nina R. Kieves DVM, DACVS-SA, DACVSMR, Kathleen L. Ham DVM, MS, DACVS-SA, James Howard DVM, MS

Chapter 25

Stomatitis

DEFINITION/OVERVIEW

Inflammation of the mucous lining of any of the structures in the mouth. Inn clinical use, the term may be reserved to describe widespread oral inflammation (beyond gingivitis and periodontitis) that may also extend into submucosal tissues.

ETIOLOGY/PATHOPHYSIOLOGY

- Inflammation and other changes may develop in the normal oral mucosa because of the tremendous amount of vasculature in the area and its proximity to the external environment.
- Can also affect behavior due to discomfort and difficulties in eating; ophthalmic conditions due to proximity of some oral structures to ocular structures; and skin may be involved if inflammation extends to the perioral area.
- Can be due to viral or bacterial infections, toxins, secondary to systemic disease, or a combination of any of these. Etiology is unknown in feline chronic gingivostomatitis (FCGS), chronic ulcerative paradental stomatitis (CUPS), and resorptive lesions (Figure 25.1) in teeth that often present with an associated local gingivitis.

Systems Affected

- Gastrointestinal – mouth, by definition, is affected. Remainder of gastrointestinal tract is normal unless other disease is present that affects more than the oral cavity.
- Musculoskeletal – may be affected due to pain when eating. Animal may not eat enough to maintain a healthy body weight.
- Skin often affected in cats with stomatitis due to their reluctance to groom.
- Immune system is likely involved with FCGS, CUPS, and periodontitis.

SIGNALMENT/HISTORY

- Ulcerative stomatitis in Maltese terriers – higher incidence in males.
- Oral eosinophilic granuloma – most commonly in Siberian husky (may be hereditary).
- Gingival hyperplasia in large breeds – breed predilection for boxers and collies.
- Rapidly progressive periodontitis seen mostly in young adult animals, such as in the greyhound and the shih tzu.
- Localized juvenile periodontitis in the maxillary or mandibular incisor region – especially common in the miniature schnauzer.

Blackwell's Five-Minute Veterinary Consult Clinical Companion: Small Animal Gastrointestinal Diseases, First Edition. Edited by Jocelyn Mott and Jo Ann Morrison.
© 2019 John Wiley & Sons, Inc. Published 2019 by John Wiley & Sons, Inc.
Companion website: www.fiveminutevet.com/gastrointestinal

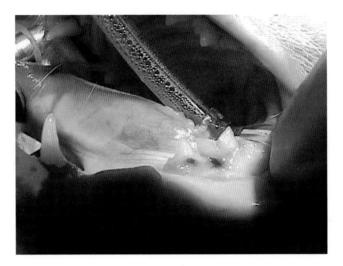

■ **Fig. 25.1.** Resorptive lesions.

- Juvenile-onset periodontitis in young cats. Can appear similar to FCGS.
- Periodontal disease associated with calculus is seen most often in older dogs and cats and in susceptible breeds. Smaller breeds are generally more susceptible.

Risk Factors

- Poor oral health due to gingivitis, plaque, calculus, or periodontitis.
- Stress may be a factor in caudal stomatitis in cats.
- May be environmental factors in some cases.

 CLINICAL FEATURES

- Erythema of oral mucous membranes.
- Pain – often exacerbated by touching suspect lesions and/or by opening the mouth.
- Halitosis.
- Dysphagia – if chronic, may be accompanied by weight loss.
- Extensive plaque and calculus.
- Roughened hair coat in cats due to lack of grooming.
- Caudal mucositis is often present with FCGS (Figure 25.2).
- Calculus frequently seen with periodontitis.
- Inflamed gingival tissue adjacent to teeth that have little or no calculus frequently seen with juvenile periodontitis and FCGS.
- Ulceration and inflammation on buccal mucous membranes directly adjacent to cheek teeth is often diagnostic of "kissing ulcers" (Figure 25.3).
- Severely inflamed gingival tissues seen in dogs with CUPS (Figure 25.4). May resemble chronic periodontitis, but frequently seen in younger dogs.
- Ptyalism.
- Gingival hyperplasia with gingival tissue around and sometimes over the entire tooth or teeth. Especially noted adjacent to and around incisors.
- Edema.
- Periocular inflammation possible due to proximity to oral cavity.
- Overcrowding of teeth can contribute to periodontal disease.

- A tight lip frenulum attachment can contribute to inflammation of the lip.
- Tight lip syndrome in shar-peis.
- Malocclusions can contribute to periodontal disease.
- Malocclusions may cause mandibular teeth to contact palate.
- Uremia which may induce high ammonia levels in saliva.
- Vasculitis and xerostomia seen with diabetes mellitus.
- Macroglossia and puffy lips as seen with hypothyroidism.

 # DIFFERENTIAL DIAGNOSIS

Immune Mediated

- Pemphigus foliaceus.
- Pemphigus vulgaris.
- Bullous pemphigoid.
- Systemic lupus erythematosus and discoid lupus erythematosus in the dog.
- Acute hypersensitivity to drugs.

Infectious

- Opportunistic oral flora secondary to oral lesions.
- Mycotic stomatitis.
- Systemic infections.
- Leptospirosis: petechiae.
- Feline leprosy (mycobacterium): raised plaques.
- Calicivirus or herpesvirus infections – cat.
- Canine distemper.
- Viral papillomatosis – dogs.

Trauma

- Irritation from calculus and plaque.
- Foreign objects – gum-chewer's syndrome.
- Electrical cord shock.

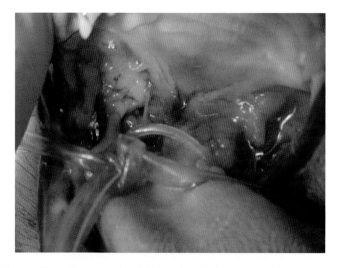

■ **Fig. 25.2.** Caudal mucositis is often present with feline chronic gingivostomatitis.

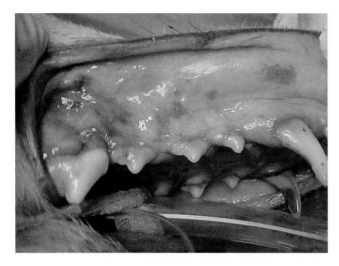

■ **Fig. 25.3.** Ulceration and inflammation on buccal mucous membranes directly adjacent to cheek teeth or "kissing ulcers."

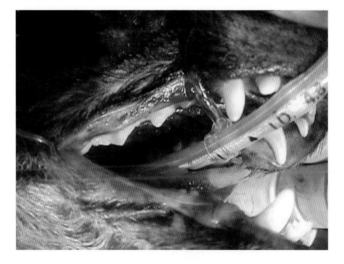

■ **Fig. 25.4.** Chronic ulcerative paradental stomatitis with cheilitis.

- Chemical burns.
- Lacerations.
- Snake bite.
- Trauma.

Toxic

- Certain plants causing irritation when contacting oral mucous membranes.
- Chemotherapy.
- Radiotherapy.
- Chemical irritants.

Other Differentials

- Eosinophilic plaques.
- Oral tumors.
- Gingival hyperplasia due to side effects of certain drugs (cyclosporine, amlodipine) has been reported.
- Dental resorptive lesions.
- Oral ulceration secondary to uremia.
- CUPS.
- Idiopathic osteomyelitis.
- Lymphoma – can affect palate and/or tongue.
- Chronic periodontitis.
- Toxins.
- FCGS in cats.
- Trauma.
- Foreign bodies (sometimes from plants).

DIAGNOSTICS

- Biopsy may be helpful for FCGS, but lymphoplasmocytic infiltrate is not diagnostic, and simply may indicate chronicity. Biopsy is necessary to ascertain oral tumor types or other conditions.
- Dental imaging to observe periodontal bone loss associated with periodontitis (Figure 25.5).
- Complete blood count (CBC) and metabolic profile helpful to rule out systemic disease.
- Cultures are often not helpful due to the normally large numbers of oral bacteria present.
- Immunologic testing.
- Mycotic cultures.
- Virus isolation.
- Toxicologic studies.
- Serum protein electrophoresis.
- Endocrine tests.

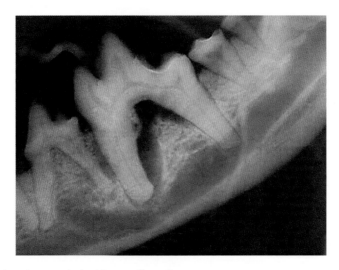

■ **Fig. 25.5.** Bone loss due to periodontitis on radiographs.

THERAPEUTICS

Drug(s) of Choice

- Antimicrobials – broad-spectrum antibiotics; amoxicillin-clavulanate; clindamycin; metronidazole (10 mg/kg PO q 12 h or 40–50 mg/kg as a loading dose on the first day, followed by 20–25 mg/kg q 8 h for seven days or less); doxycycline (5 mg/kg PO loading dose, 2.5 mg/kg PO 12 h later, and 2.5 mg/kg PO once daily thereafter); chlorhexidine solution or gel (CHX, VRx Products, Harbor City, CA) – plaque retardant; and Maxi/Guard (Addison Biological, Fayette, MO) – zinc-organic acid solutions and gels to promote tissue healing and retard plaque accumulation.
- Antiinflammatory drugs – prednisolone or prednisone; for eosinophilic plaques (2–4.4 mg/kg PO once a day; for chronic cases use 0.5–1 mg/kg PO every other day); for adjunctive therapy of feline plasma cell gingivitis–pharyngitis – may improve inflammation and appetite.
- Immunosuppressive drugs if secondary to autoimmune disease (cyclosporine has been reported to cause gingival hyperplasia on occasion).
- Chemotherapy if secondary to lymphoma.
- Omega interferon (recombinant feline interferon) – submucosal infiltrations: 1–2 MU/buccal cavity, repeated three times at two-week intervals if necessary, or 1 MU/kg SQ q 48 h for five injections (this treatment has been found to be ineffective on many occasions).
- Feline chronic gingivostomatitis has frequently been treated with corticosteroids, but this only produces temporary improvement.

Appropriate Health Care

- Correct nutritional or hydration deficiencies as needed, on an inpatient or outpatient basis.
- Dental disease or periodontal disease present should be treated. Dental scaling and/or extractions are helpful with periodontitis.
- Full-mouth extractions are frequently required to treat FCGS. Imaging is necessary to ensure that all roots and root fragments are removed.
- Extractions usually required for CUPS. Resorptive dental lesions can only be treated successfully by extractions.
- Esophageal tube after surgery may be helpful in some cases until healing occurs.
- Dietary adjustments may need to be made depending on the patient's ability to eat if painful.

Diet

- Consider using a hypoallergenic diet to reduce the antigen load that accumulates on the tooth surfaces in plaque.
- Dietary adjustments may need to be made depending on the patient's ability to eat if painful.

COMMENTS

Client Education

- Clients must be aware that some cases are multifactorial, and may be a chronic condition that will require constant management, with variable responses from patients.
- Brushing teeth and oral rinses are helpful in prevention of periodontitis and oral ulcers resulting from dental calculus.
- Dry kibble is preferred to canned food in preventing dental calculus.

Patient Monitoring

Evaluate oral cavity periodically to monitor for resolution or recurrence of oral lesions.

Possible Complications

Studies have shown an association between bacteremia from periodontal disease and renal, cardiac, hepatic, and pulmonary disease.

Expected Course and Prognosis

Varies with underlying cause.

Abbreviations

- CUPS = chronic ulcerative paradental stomatitis
- FCGS = feline chronic gingivostomatitis
- MU = million units

Suggested Reading

Bellows J. Small Animal Dental Equipment, Materials and Techniques. Oxford: Blackwell, 2004.

Harvey CE, Emily PP. Oral lesions of soft tissues and bone: differential diagnosis. In: Harvey CE, Emily PP, eds. Small Animal Dentistry. St Louis: Mosby, 1993, pp. 42–88.

Holmstrom S, Frost PF, Eisner E. Veterinary Dental Techniques, 3rd ed. Philadelphia: Saunders, 2004.

Wiggs RB, Lobprise HB. Veterinary Dentistry: Principles and Practice. Philadelphia: Lippincott-Raven, 1997, pp. 104–139.

Author: Larry Baker DVM, FAVD, DAVDC

Chapter 26

Stomatitis, Caudal – Feline

DEFINITION/OVERVIEW

- Inflammatory response affecting the oral cavity in cats.
- Oral and oropharyngeal inflammation is classified by location as follows.
  - Gingivitis – inflammation of gingiva.
  - Periodontitis – inflammation of nongingival periodontal tissues (i.e., the periodontal ligament and alveolar bone).
  - Alveolar mucositis – inflammation of alveolar mucosa (i.e., mucosa overlying the alveolar process and extending from the mucogingival junction without obvious demarcation to the vestibular sulcus and to the floor of the mouth).
  - Sublingual mucositis – inflammation of mucosa on the floor of the mouth.
  - Labial/buccal mucositis – inflammation of lip and cheek mucosa respectively.
  - Caudal mucositis – inflammation of mucosa of the caudal oral cavity, bordered medially by the palatoglossal folds and fauces, dorsally by the hard and soft palate, and rostrally by alveolar and buccal mucosa.
  - Palatitis – inflammation of mucosa or covering the hard and/or soft palate.
  - Glossitis – inflammation of mucosa of the dorsal and/or ventral surface of the tongue.
  - Cheilitis – inflammation of the lip (including the mucocutaneous junction area and skin of the lip).
  - Osteomyelitis – inflammation of jaw bone and bone marrow.
  - Stomatitis – inflammation of the mucous lining of any of the structures in the mouth; in clinical use, the term should be reserved to describe widespread oral inflammation (beyond gingivitis and periodontitis) that may also extend into submucosal tissues.
  - Tonsillitis – inflammation of the palatine tonsil.
  - Pharyngitis – inflammation of the pharynx.

ETIOLOGY/PATHOPHYSIOLOGY

- The specific etiology of stomatitis is unknown.
- Bacteria, oral food antigens, environmental antigens, and viruses have all been suggested as inciting causes. Many cats with stomatitis test positive for feline calicivirus, herpesvirus, and/or *Bartonella* species. Definitive studies are still needed to prove a causative relationship. More commonly, it is believed that stomatitis is secondary plaque stimulation on a disregulated immune system.
- Approximately 0.7% of cats in British general practice were reported to have stomatitis in one report.

Blackwell's Five-Minute Veterinary Consult Clinical Companion: Small Animal Gastrointestinal Diseases,
First Edition. Edited by Jocelyn Mott and Jo Ann Morrison.
© 2019 John Wiley & Sons, Inc. Published 2019 by John Wiley & Sons, Inc.
Companion website: www.fiveminutevet.com/gastrointestinal

Systems Affected

- Gastrointestinal – oral cavity is affected.
- Musculoskeletal – weight loss.

SIGNALMENT/HISTORY

- Cats.
- Purebred breeds predisposed – Abyssinian, Persian, Himalayan, Burmese, Siamese, and Somali.

Risk Factors

- Immunosuppression from FeLV or FIV can also lead to poorly responsive infections; most affected cats are negative for FeLV and FIV.
- Associated with calicivirus.

Historical Findings

Clinical signs associated with stomatitis can include halitosis, dysphagia, preference for soft food, ptyalism, anorexia, weight loss, and a scruffy hair coat from lack of grooming.

CLINICAL FEATURES

- Physical examination findings may vary dependent on severity of disease.
- Erythematous, ulcerative, proliferative lesions affecting the gingiva, glossopalatine arches, tongue, lips, buccal mucosa, and/or hard palate.
- Gingival inflammation commonly surrounds the tooth, compared with gingivitis, which usually occurs on the buccal and labial surfaces.
- May extend to the glossopharyngeal arches as well as the palate (Figure 26.1).

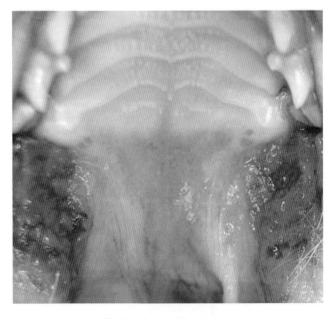

■ **Fig. 26.1.** Moderate stomatitis lesions affecting the caudal oral cavity.

DIFFERENTIAL DIAGNOSIS

- Periodontal disease.
- Oral malignancy.
- Eosinophilic granuloma complex.

DIAGNOSTICS

- Stomatitis is primarily diagnosed visually as widespread mucosal inflammation which is more extensive than periodontal disease. Most cases include caudal stomatitis affecting the glossopalatine arches.
- T lymphocyte subset ratios (CD4+/CD8+) are generally low due to high numbers of CD8+ (suppressor-cytotoxic T cells). CD4+ (Th-1 and Th-2 helper induced T cells) recognize MHC II on surface antigen-presenting cells, other T-cells, --cells, some mesenchymal cells, and osteoblasts whereas CD8+ cells recognize MHC I universally exhibited on all cell types.
- The levels of salivary IgA are low and IgG and IgM are high in stomatitis patients.

Complete Blood Count/Biochemistry/Urinalysis

- Elevated globulin; polyclonal gammopathy secondary to antibody production following bacterial invasion into periodontal tissues.
- Leukocytosis and eosinophilia may be present.

Imaging

Intraoral radiographs to evaluate periodontal disease and tooth resorption.

Additional Diagnostic Procedures

Biopsy (especially unilateral lesions) to rule out malignant neoplasia, primarily squamous cell carcinoma.

Pathologic findings

Dermal-epidermal inflammatory reaction of predominantly plasma cells and lymphocytes suggestive of an immunoreactive condition.

THERAPEUTICS

- Initial therapy for early mucositis (vs stomatitis) involves dental scaling above and below the gingiva and treatment (extraction) for teeth affected with grades 3 and 4 periodontal disease and/or tooth resorption. For mild cases, the elimination of bacteria/plaque from the teeth, sulci, and periodontal ligament space followed by daily plaque control is the treatment of choice.
- For cases of focal vestibular and alveolar mucositis, extraction of the locally affected teeth in proximity to the lesions usually results in resolution.
- In a study of 30 cats with caudal stomatitis, extraction of the maxillary and mandibular teeth caudal to the canines, or extraction of all the teeth, resulted in resolution of inflammation in 60% of cases without further need for medication, 20% of cases required control with medication, and 20% did not resolve (Figure 26.2).
- To aid full mouth extractions, create a gingival flap in all quadrants for exposure. After completely extracting all the teeth, use a high-speed drill with water spray to create a trough of

(a)   (b)

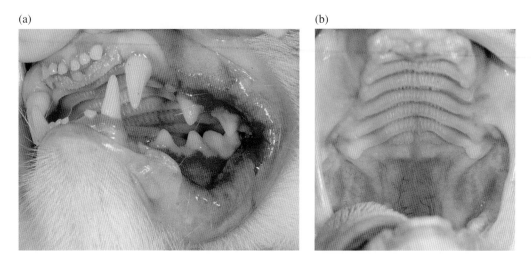

■ **Fig. 26.2.** Marked stomatitis before (a) and after (b) full mouth extractions.

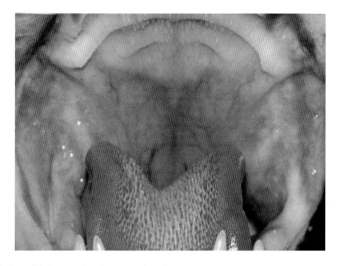

■ **Fig. 26.3.** Resolution of inflammation four months after treatment.

bone where the roots were, removing most of the keratinized gingiva, periodontal ligament, and periradicular alveolar bone. Before suturing, "smooth down" the alveolar margin to remove sharp edges with a round or football-shaped diamond bur.

- If patients do not respond to extraction of the teeth distal to the canines, consider a trial of prednisolone 2 mg/kg every other day to control the inflammation, or remove all teeth. When extracting the teeth, pay meticulous attention to removing all dental hard tissue; take intraoral radiographs before and after surgery; postoperative application of fluocinonide 0.05% (Lidex Gel) to the gingival margin may help healing (Figure 26.3).

- Refractory cases with extensive proliferative lesion in the caudal oral cavity and pharynx warrant a more guarded prognosis.

- CO_2 laser energy is often effective in decreasing or eliminating caudal stomatitis after full mouth extraction. The laser decreases the physical amount of inflamed tissue. Monthly (1–3×) laser energy is applied at 2–4 watts in continuous mode to the inflamed caudal oral

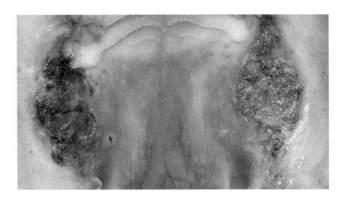

■ **Fig. 26.4.** Laser rastering of inflamed tissue with extraction.

cavity tissues after precautions are in place to avoid lasering teeth and the endotracheal tube. After an application, the char is removed with a saline-moistened gauze sponge to allow another laser application (Figure 26.4).

Drug(s) of Choice

- Medication and other therapies have been used with limited long-term success; lack of permanent response to conventional oral hygiene, antimicrobials, antiinflammatory drugs, and immunosuppressive drugs is typical. Medications should not be regarded as the primary method to control oropharyngeal inflammation.
- Corticosteroids – prednisolone (2 mg/kg orally initially daily, followed by every other day); methylprednisolone acetate (2 mg/kg orally q 7–30 days) may also help control inflammation.
- Interferon-alpha or -omega – 30 IU/day orally, seven days on, seven days off, indefinitely.
- Cyclosporine – 2 mg/kg orally bid.

Precautions/Interactions

Repeated doses of repositol steroids (Depomedrol®, Zoetis) should be avoided. Cyclosporine should also be used with caution; anecdotal cases of cancer have been reported with chronic use.

Appropriate Health Care

Some cats may need hospitalization for intravenous fluids to support hydration and continued nutritional support.

Nursing Care

Some cats may not be able to eat immediately after dental extractions and will require feeding tubes (nasoesophageal, esophagostomy or percutaneous gastrostomy tube).

Diet

Soft canned foods should be offered.

Surgical Considerations

Often patients presented for surgical care are too painful to eat, resulting in a negative nitrogen balance. For these patients, placement of an esophagostomy tube for nutritional support is recommended which continues until the cat eats normally.

COMMENTS

Stomatitis is a painful syndrome that is commonly resolved by removing plaqu- retentive surfaces (all the teeth). Those cats that present without caudal stomatitis carry a better prognosis for complete cure.

Client Education

- Home care after full mouth extractions is minimal other than making sure the cat is getting needed nutrition.
- An internet resource is www.avdc.org.

Patient Monitoring

Weekly oral cavity examinations should be conducted to monitor healing. Complete healing should occur within six weeks.

Prevention/Avoidance

For those cases where teeth still remain after primary care, stringent plaque control (daily application of a Q-tip to the gingival margins to remove plaque and Veterinary Oral Health Council (www.vohc.org)-accepted plaque-retardant products are recommended.

Possible Complications

In untreated cases, the inflammation can increase with resultant morbidity.

Expected Course and Prognosis

- Most cats will be cured within months after full mouth extractions are performed. For those refractory cases where stomatitis persists despite full mouth extractions and follow-up laser rastering, every other day prednisolone (1 mg/kg) generally results in a functional outcome.
- The course of disease is dependent on comorbidity factors where the presence of FIV, FeLV, or diabetes decreases the prognosis for a complete cure.

Synonyms

- Lymphocytic plasmacytic stomatitis
- Stomatitis
- Gingivostomatitis

Abbreviations

- FeLV = feline leukemia virus
- FIV = feline immunodeficiency virus

See Also

- Feline Eosinophilic Dermatitis
- Oral Neoplasia, Benign
- Oral Neoplasia, Malignant
- Ptyalism
- Stomatitis

Suggested Reading

Bellows JE. Feline Dentistry. Oxford: Wiley Blackwell, 2010.

Jennings MW, Lewis JR, Soltero-Rivera MM, Brown DC, Reiter AM. Effect of tooth extraction on stomatitis in cats: 95 cases (2000–2013). J Am Vet Med Assoc 2015;246(6):654–660.

Wiggs RB, Lobprise HB. Veterinary Dentistry: Principles and Practice. Philadelphia: Lippincott-Raven, 1997.

 Client Education Handout available online

Author: Jan Bellows DVM, DAVDC, ABVP

Diseases of the Esophagus

Chapter 27

Cricopharyngeal Achalasia

DEFINITION/OVERVIEW

- Cricopharyngeal achalasia (CPA) is a common cause of oropharyngeal dysphagia that is characterized by diminished compliance of the cricopharyngeus muscle resulting in an incomplete relaxation of the proximal esophageal sphincter and causing difficulties with the transsphincteric movement of food and/or liquids.
- Cricopharyngeal achalasia must be distinguished from an intermittent failure of the cricopharyngeus muscle to relax, known as cricopharyngeal dyssynchrony.

ETIOLOGY/PATHOPHYSIOLOGY

- Swallowing (deglutition) is orchestrated by a complex reflex arch involving sensory receptors, visceral afferents, and motor efferent neurons. The *oral preparatory phase* is voluntary and begins with liquid or solids entering the mouth, which then undergo mastication and lubrication. During the *oral phase* of swallowing, the bolus is moved from the tongue to the pharynx, which is facilitated by tongue, jaw, and hyoid muscle movements. The *pharyngeal phase* begins as the bolus reaches the oropharynx and is characterized by elevation of the soft palate to protect the nasopharynx, elevation and forward movement of the larynx and hyoid, retroflexion of the epiglottis and closure of the vocal folds to seal the laryngeal opening, contraction of the pharyngeal muscles and relaxation of the cricopharyngeus muscle (major contributor to the upper or proximal esophageal sphincter), resulting in passage of the bolus into the proximal esophagus. Respiration is briefly halted during this phase of swallowing. During the *esophageal phase* (involuntary), the bolus is moved aborad towards the gastroesophageal junction (lower or distal esophageal sphincter) to then enter the stomach.
- Cricopharyngeal achalasia is a disorder of the cricopharyngeus muscle that causes a relative inability of the proximal esophageal sphincter to relax and compromises the passage of a food or liquid bolus into the esophagus during the pharyngeal phase of swallowing.
- Cricopharyngeal dyssynchrony (CPD) is characterized by incoordination between relaxation of the cricopharyngeus muscle and contraction of the pharyngeal muscles.

Systems Affected

- Gastrointestinal – some patients have concurrent esophageal hypomotility or megaesophagus.
- Respiratory – patients with cricopharyngeal dysphagia are at risk for development of aspiration pneumonia.

Blackwell's Five-Minute Veterinary Consult Clinical Companion: Small Animal Gastrointestinal Diseases, First Edition. Edited by Jocelyn Mott and Jo Ann Morrison.
© 2019 John Wiley & Sons, Inc. Published 2019 by John Wiley & Sons, Inc.
Companion website: www.fiveminutevet.com/gastrointestinal

SIGNALMENT/HISTORY

- Predominantly a disease in dogs, presumed to be very rare in cats.
- Most dogs are diagnosed at a young age (<1 year old), particularly after weaning; uncommon diagnosis in older patients.
- Overrepresented breeds include dachshund, Maltese, springer spaniel, and cocker spaniel (about 90%) for cricopharyngeal achalasia, golden retriever for cricopharyngeal dyssynchrony.
- No sex predisposition.

Risk Factors

- Hypothyroidism has been linked to cricopharyngeal dysphagia.
- Myasthenia gravis has been associated with cricopharyngeal achalasia.

Historical Findings

- Chronic and often insidious onset of dysphagia, including difficulty swallowing, usually with multiple chewing and swallowing attempts, repeated prehension of food fallen from the mouth, excessive salivation, extension of the neck after food intake, often followed by gagging, regurgitation, and coughing.
- Differentiation of vomiting (with abdominal contractions, sometimes presence of prodromal signs) from regurgitation (no abdominal contractions, no prodromal signs) is important.
- Nasal discharge of food or water is a hallmark sign of cricopharyngeal achalasia and occurs due to pharyngeal contractions forcing the food or liquid bolus against an incompletely relaxed proximal esophageal sphincter and resulting in a reflux of food and liquids into the nasopharynx.
- Despite having a ravenous appetite, affected patients are often small for their breed and age.

 CLINICAL FEATURES

- A thorough patient history and careful observation of the dysphagic patient eating (both kibble and canned food) and drinking are pivotal aspects of the diagnostic evaluation and are essential for localizing the problem to the pharynx.
- Results of the physical examination are usually unremarkable.
- A complete neurologic examination is important, with particular emphasis on evaluation of the cranial nerves. The neurologic examination is usually unremarkable in patients with cricopharyngeal dysphagia. Findings that support a generalized neuromuscular disorder may be present with cricopharyngeal dysphagia associated with myasthenia gravis.
- A thorough examination of the oropharynx of the sedated or anesthetized patient is necessary to rule out important differentials (e.g., foreign bodies, cleft palate, oropharyngeal neoplasia, laryngeal paralysis).

 DIFFERENTIAL DIAGNOSIS

- Differential diagnoses include pharyngeal weakness secondary to neuropathies or myopathies (e.g., muscular dystrophy, inflammatory myopathy), pharyngeal tumors, penetrating foreign bodies, or trauma.
- Other causes of dysphagia include cleft palate, iatrogenic shortening of the soft palate (pharyngeal dysphagia), esophageal hypomotility, or megaesophagus (esophageal dysphagia).

DIAGNOSTICS

Complete Blood Cell Count/Biochemistry/Urinalysis

- Results are usually unremarkable.
- Complete blood cell count abnormalities (e.g., leukocytosis) may be consistent with aspiration pneumonia.
- An increased serum creatine kinase (CK) activity may suggest an underlying myopathy.

Other Laboratory Tests

- A thyroid panel (consisting of total thyroxine (tT4), free thyroxine (fT4), thyroid-stimulating hormone (TSH), and antithyroglobulin antibodies) should be performed as CPA can be associated with hypothyroidism and will respond to L-thyroxine supplementation.
- Serology for acetylcholinesterase receptor (AChR) antibodies or type 2M muscle autoantibodies can help diagnose an underlying acquired myasthenia gravis or primary myositis (associated with masticatory muscle myositis).

Imaging

- Plain cervical and thoracic radiographs are usually unremarkable, but are important to rule out other causes of dysphagia (e.g., foreign bodies) or complications of cricopharyngeal dysphagia (i.e., aspiration pneumonia).
- Ultrasonographic evaluation of the pharynx is of limited utility but may be useful in patients with mass lesions and for obtaining ultrasound-guided fine needle aspirates or biopsy specimens.
- Computed tomography and magnetic resonance imaging are also not useful to document cricopharyngeal dysphagia but can help rule out other differentials (e.g., myositis, neoplasia).

Other Diagnostic Tests

- Videofluoroscopic swallowing studies (with a minimum 1/5 sec frame rate) using liquid barium and different types of food (canned, kibble) mixed with barium are necessary to document cricopharyngeal dysphagia, differentiate it from pharyngeal dysphagia (for which treatment options to correct cricopharyngeal dysphagia would be contraindicated), and to distinguish cricopharyngeal achalasia (lack of opening of the proximal esophageal sphincter) from cricopharyngeal dyssynchrony (delayed opening of the proximal esophageal sphincter) based on the shape of the cricopharyngeal region. The swallow study should be performed in the nonsedated patient and in a standing position, with 3–5 swallows for each type of food or liquid. Contrast videofluoroscopy typically reveals restricted transsphincteric movement of the bolus, distension of the pharynx with food or liquid, and repeated pharyngeal contractions that will result in a small stream of barium entering the esophagus (Figure 27.1). The calculated pharyngeal constriction ratio and the time to proximal esophageal sphincter opening are the most useful indices in clinical practice. Finding the shape of the cricopharyngeal region to be distorted during these pharyngeal contractions is the hallmark in patients with cricopharyngeal achalasia.
- Repetitive nerve stimulation and edrophonium chloride (0.1–0.2 mg/kg IV) can be used to test for suspected myasthenia gravis. Electromyography (EMG) of skeletal musculature may help to document the presence of a myopathy.

Pathologic Findings

Neuromuscular defects that are suspected to be congenital (myofiber degeneration, denervation atrophy, hypertrophy, necrosis, and fibrosis) or acquired (idiopathic inflammation).

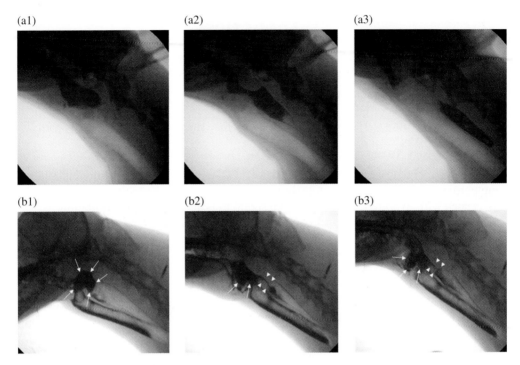

■ **Fig. 27.1.** Videofluoroscopic evaluation (single frame images) of the pharynx and proximal esophagus in a healthy dog (a1–3) and in a dog with cricopharyngeal achalasia (b1–3). Arrows indicate the bolus pooling within the oropharynx, arrowheads indicate the cricopharyngeal bar (noncompliant cricopharyngeal muscle). Notice also a small amount of contrast along the lining of the proximal trachea resulting from mild aspiration. Source: Image courtesy of Dr Ingmar Kiefer, College of Veterinary Medicine, University of Leipzig, Germany.

 # THERAPEUTICS

Drug(s) of Choice

- Injection of botulinum toxin (Botox®) into the cricopharyngeus muscle (using a total of 40 IU, divided in three different spots) can be considered for temporary relief.
- L-thyroxine should be supplemented in patients diagnosed with hypothyroidism.

Precautions/Interactions

Sildenafil (Viagra®) has been recommended for achalasia of the distal esophageal sphincter (smooth muscle) but will not be effective at the proximal esophageal sphincter (striated muscle).

Appropriate Health Care

- Patients with cricopharyngeal achalasia or dyssynchrony can usually be managed on an outpatient basis. Hospitalization will be necessary with complicating factors (e.g., aspiration pneumonia, dehydration).
- Permanent relief of cricopharyngeal achalasia can only be achieved with surgical correction.
- Temporary treatment options may be considered prior to surgery.

Nursing Care

- Supportive treatment is recommended in patients with dehydration (intravenous fluids) or aspiration pneumonia (oxygen therapy, nebulization, coupage, appropriate antibiotics).
- Patients with generalized weakness (e.g., due to myasthenia gravis) require good nursing care (soft padding, rotating patient position, patient hygiene, physical therapy).

Diet

- Malnutrition needs to be avoided as it has prognostic significance.
- Alterations in feeding practices (e.g., feeding with the food bowl elevated or using a Bailey chair, adding water to the diet or making the diet into a slurry) are usually not effective, although dogs with cricopharyngeal dysphagia will often handle kibble better than canned food or water.
- Tube feeding may be considered as an option to manage patients with concurrent esophageal stricture or megaesophagus (e.g., via percutaneous gastrostomy tube) or that have failed surgical correction.

Activity

Patients with CPA or CPD can resume their normal level of activity.

Surgical Considerations

- Patients should be carefully selected for surgical correction as the failure rate can be high if malnutrition or concurrent aspiration pneumonia are not addressed prior to the procedure. Surgical correction is also contraindicated in patients with concurrent mechanical (e.g., esophageal stricture) or functional disorders (e.g., myasthenia gravis, laryngeal paralysis, pharyngeal dysphagia).
- Traditional surgical treatment comprises a transcervical cricopharyngeal myectomy or myotomy with or without a partial or complete thyropharyngeal myotomy using either a ventral or a lateral approach.
- Transcervical cricopharyngeal myotomy to relieve the constriction has been reported to have a success rate of 40–100%, and a bilateral approach is needed in individual dogs.
- Endoscopic laser myotomy is a less invasive alternative treatment option.
- Potential complications of surgery include recurrent laryngeal paralysis, esophageal perforation, development of a pharyngocutaneous fistula, postprocedural fibrosis leading to treatment failure with recurrence of dysphagia.

 COMMENTS

Client Education

- Educate the client that not all dogs undergoing surgical correction will be cured.
- Educate the client that careful patient management and monitoring will be long term in dogs that are not good candidates for surgery or have failed surgical correction (see above). In particular, owners need to be advised to monitor for signs of possible aspiration pneumonia.

Patient Monitoring

- Clinical signs of possible aspiration pneumonia (most common complication): dyspnea, tachypnea, coughing, fever, lethargy.
- Nutritional and hydration status also need to be carefully monitored.

Possible Complications

- Aspiration pneumonia is the most common complication and some patients may first present with respiratory signs or even as respiratory emergencies.
- Emaciation is another complication if the condition is left untreated.

Expected Course and Prognosis

- Cricopharyngeal achalasia carries a good prognosis for cure with successful surgical correction. Patients that are not good candidates for surgery, or that have failed surgical correction, have a guarded prognosis.
- Temporary treatment options have a good chance for transient relief.

Abbreviations

- AChR = acetylcholinesterase receptor
- CPA = cricopharyngeal achalasia
- CPD = cricopharyngeal dyssynchrony
- CK = serum creatine kinase
- EMG = electromyography
- fT4 = free thyroxine
- TSH = thyroid-stimulating hormone
- tT4 = total thyroxine

See Also

- Dysphagia
- Esophagitis
- Megaesophagus
- Regurgitation

Suggested Reading

Bruchim Y, Kushnir A, Shamir MH. L-thyroxine responsive cricopharyngeal achalasia associated with hypothyroidism in a dog. J Small Anim Pract 2005;46(11):553–554.

Elliott RC. An anatomical and clinical review of cricopharyngeal achalasia in the dog. J S Afr Vet Assoc 2010;81(2):75–79.

Niles JD, Williams JM, Sullivan M, et al. Resolution of dysphagia following cricopharyngeal myectomy in six young dogs. J Small Anim Pract 2001;42:32–35.

Pollard RE, Marks SL, Davidson A, et al. Quantitative videofluoroscopic evaluation of pharyngeal function in the dog. Vet Radiol Ultrasound 2000;41(5):409–412.

Steiner JM. Small Animal Gastroenterology. Hannover: Schlütersche, 2008.

Warnoch JJ, Marks SL, Pollard RE, et al. Surgical management of cricopharyngeal dysphagia in dogs: 14 cases (1989–2001). J Am Vet Med Assoc 2003;223:1462–1468.

Washabau RJ, Day MJ. Canine and Feline Gastroenterology. St Louis: Elsevier, 2013.

Authors: Romy M. Heilmann med.vet., Dr.med.vet., DACVIM (SAIM), DECVIM-CA, PhD, Stanley L. Marks BVSc, DACVIM (SAIM, Oncology), DACVN, PhD

Chapter 28

Gastroesophageal Diverticula

DEFINITION/OVERVIEW

- Pouch-like sacculations of the esophageal wall that accumulate fluids and ingesta.
- Diverticula may occur as either congenital or acquired lesions.

ETIOLOGY/PATHOPHYSIOLOGY

- Two forms of diverticula are recognized: pulsion and traction types.
  - Pulsion diverticula occur secondary to increased intraluminal pressure. Seen with esophageal obstructive disorders such as foreign body.
  - Traction diverticula occur secondary to periesophageal inflammation where fibrosis and contraction pull out the wall of the esophagus into a pouch.
- Diverticuli most commonly occur at the thoracic inlet or near the hiatus.

Systems Affected

- Gastrointestinal (regurgitation).
- Musculoskeletal (weight loss).
- Respiratory (aspiration pneumonia).

SIGNALMENT/HISTORY

- Rare; more common in dog than cat.
- No genetic basis proven.
- No important breed or sex predisposition.

Risk Factors

Pulsion Diverticulum

- Embryonic developmental disorders of the esophageal wall.
- Esophageal foreign body, mass or focal motility disturbances (uncommon).

Traction Diverticulum

- Inflammatory processes associated with the trachea, lungs, hilar lymph nodes, or pericardium; resultant fibrous connective tissue adheres to the esophageal wall.

Historical Findings

Clinical signs of esophageal dysfunction – postprandial regurgitation, dysphagia, anorexia, weight loss with chronicity.

Blackwell's Five-Minute Veterinary Consult Clinical Companion: Small Animal Gastrointestinal Diseases, First Edition. Edited by Jocelyn Mott and Jo Ann Morrison.
© 2019 John Wiley & Sons, Inc. Published 2019 by John Wiley & Sons, Inc.
Companion website: www.fiveminutevet.com/gastrointestinal

CLINICAL FEATURES

- Coughing.
- Tachypnea.
- Respiratory distress.

DIFFERENTIAL DIAGNOSIS

Esophageal Redundancy

- Barium contrast accumulation in the region of the thoracic inlet can occur normally in young dogs (especially brachycephalic breeds and Chinese shar-pei).

Periesophageal Mass

- Esophagram or esophagoscopy should differentiate the presence of a mass causing luminal narrowing.
- Esophagitis.
- Esophageal foreign body.

DIAGNOSTICS

Complete Blood Count/Biochemistry/Urinalysis

Usually within normal limits.

Imaging

- Thoracic radiography – may show air or soft tissue opacity cranial to the diaphragm or cranial to the thoracic inlet.
- Positive contrast esophagram – shows contrast accumulation within the diverticulum.
- Videofluoroscopy – useful to evaluate for disturbances in esophageal motility.

Diagnostic Procedures

- Esophagoscopy confirms ingesta/debris within outpouchings of the esophagus.
- Esophagoscopy or esophagram will confirm mass lesion causing obstruction.

THERAPEUTICS

If the diverticulum is small and not causing significant clinical signs, treat conservatively with elevated feedings of a soft, bland diet followed by copious liquids.

Drug(s) of Choice

- Drug therapy for esophagitis, if present.
- Proton pump inhibitors such as omeprazole are more potent and effective antacids than the H2 histamine antagonists for management (0.7–1.5 mg/kg PO q 12 h) of severe esophagitis.
- Use broad-spectrum antibiotics if the patient has concurrent aspiration pneumonia; if severe pneumonia is present, base antibiotic selection on culture and sensitivity of samples obtained by transtracheal wash or bronchoalveolar lavage.
- If there is significant mucosal injury, treatment is recommended: sucralfate slurry (0.5–1 g/dog PO q 8 h) for mucosal cytoprotection and healing.

Nursing Care

- Fluid therapy, antibiotics, and aggressive nursing, if concurrent aspiration pneumonia is present.
- Enteral nutrition via gastrostomy tube may be necessary in patients with aspiration pneumonia.

Surgical Considerations

If the diverticulum is large or is associated with significant clinical signs, surgical resection is recommended.

 COMMENTS

Client Education

Client education should include the importance of dietary management and the potential for aspiration pneumonia.

Patient Monitoring

- Evaluate for evidence of infection or aspiration pneumonia.
- Maintain positive nutritional balance throughout disease process.

Possible Complications

Patients with diverticula and impaction are predisposed to perforation, fistula, stricture, and postoperative incisional dehiscence.

Expected Course and Prognosis

Prognosis is guarded in patients with large diverticula and overt clinical signs.

See Also

- Esophageal Fistula
- Esophageal Foreign Bodies
- Esophageal Stricture
- Esophagitis
- Nutritional Approach to Gastroesophageal Reflux Disease and Megaesophagus

Suggested Reading

Jergens AE. Diseases of the esophagus. In: Ettinger SJ, Feldman EC, eds. Textbook of Veterinary Internal Medicine, 7th ed. Philadelphia: Saunders, 2009.

Sherding RG, Johnson SE. Esophagoscopy. In: Tams TR, Rawlings CA, eds. Small Animal Endoscopy, 3rd ed. Philadelphia: Mosby, 2011, pp. 41–95.

Author: Albert E. Jergens DVM, PhD, DACVIM

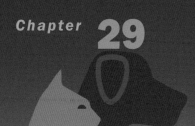
Esophageal Fistula

DEFINITION/OVERVIEW

- Esophageal fistula is an abnormal communication between the esophagus and trachea, bronchus, pulmonary parenchyma, aorta or skin.
- It is classified based on localization of the communicating tract.
- Bronchoesophageal (BEF) and tracheoesophageal (TEF) fistula are the most commonly reported types of esophageal fistula.
- It is commonly associated with an esophageal diverticula, a circumscribed outpouching of the lining of the mucosa through a defect in the esophageal wall. Esophageal diverticulum may be present before an acquired bronchoesophageal fistula forms. Clinical signs, case presentation, and diagnostic procedures are similar to esophageal fistula.

ETIOLOGY/PATHOPHYSIOLOGY

- The congenital form has been associated with incomplete separation of the esophagus from the respiratory tract during embryologic development.
- The acquired form is a common sequela of esophageal perforation from foreign bodies, chronic irritation, infection, pulmonary abscessation, neoplasia, periesophageal inflammation or trauma.
- The pathogenesis is believed to begin with esophageal wall inflammation, leading to necrosis and perforation, with leakage of esophageal contents into adjacent tissues. Healing of this area leads to the development of a communicating tract and continuous airway contamination with esophageal contents.
- This can progress to an esophageal traction diverticulum from the inflammatory reaction between the esophagus and bronchi.
- Most bronchoesophageal fistulas occur from obstructions of the thoracic esophagus caudal to the heart, commonly with the right caudal or middle lung lobe.
- Secondary complications with bronchoesophageal fistulas include focal pneumonia, pulmonary abscessation, and pleuritis.

Systems Affected

- Respiratory – can lead to pneumonia, bronchitis, lung lobe abscessation, pleuritis.
- Gastrointestinal – can lead to esophageal irritation, stricture, chronic regurgitation, or esophageal diverticula.

Blackwell's Five-Minute Veterinary Consult Clinical Companion: Small Animal Gastrointestinal Diseases, First Edition. Edited by Jocelyn Mott and Jo Ann Morrison.
© 2019 John Wiley & Sons, Inc. Published 2019 by John Wiley & Sons, Inc.
Companion website: www.fiveminutevet.com/gastrointestinal

SIGNALMENT/HISTORY

- Esophageal fistulas have been reported in dogs and cats.
- Toy and small terrier type dogs are more commonly reported, with the Cairn terrier and miniature poodle being overrepresented.
- Acquired esophageal fistula can occur at any age, with reported ages between six months and seven years.
- Congenital esophageal fistula tends to show clinical symptoms at a younger age.

Risk Factors

- History of esophageal foreign body.
- Previous esophageal surgery.
- Chronic esophageal irritation.
- Esophageal diverticula.
- Megaesophagus.

Historical Findings

- Coughing, especially after eating, drinking.
- Lethargy.
- Dyspnea.
- Weight loss.
- Regurgitation.
- Anorexia.
- Nasal discharge.
- Dysphagia.

 # CLINICAL FEATURES

- Coughing is the most common clinical sign.
- Any young animal with recurrent aspiration pneumonia or localized pneumonia associated with coughing after eating or drinking should raise suspicion of an esophageal fistula.
- May display ill-thrift, listlessness, emaciation depending on severity.
- May have oculonasal discharge.
- Respiratory crackles heard over affected lung regions or dyspnea are common findings.

 # DIFFERENTIAL DIAGNOSIS

- Esophageal diverticulum, esophageal foreign body, esophageal neoplasia, megaesophagus, esophageal stricture.
- Aspiration pneumonia, chronic bronchitis, lung lobe abscess, lung lobe neoplasia, heart disease, mediastinal masses.

 # DIAGNOSTICS

Complete Blood Count/Biochemistry/Urinalysis

- Leukogram – can range from normal to leukocytosis, depending on severity of disease.
- Biochemistry – generally within normal limits, can show electrolyte derangements and hypoalbuminemia.

Other Laboratory Tests

Blood gas evaluation may reveal acidosis and hypoxemia, depending on degree of respiratory compromise.

Imaging

- Survey thoracic radiographs may reveal radiopaque esophageal foreign bodies; esophageal dilation; pulmonary consolidation; pulmonary abscessation: paraesophageal anomalies; pleural effusion; focal interstitial, alveolar or bronchial lung patterns (Figure 29.1).
- Survey abdominal radiographs may detect gas passage from lungs to the esophagus with gastric dilation.
- Contrast esophagram is gold standard (Figure 29.2).
  - Iodinated contrast agents should be avoided – they are hyperosmolar and can result in pulmonary edema.
  - Low osmolarity, nonionic, water-soluble contrast media such as iohexol are preferred.
  - Diluted barium solution is an alternative – this is nonreactive, inert, and rapidly cleared by mucociliary apparatus. A thin mixture of 20–30% weight/volume can fill a small fistula more efficiently than thick barium with food. However, barium has been reported to induce a granulomatous mediastinitis or pneumonitis.
- Esophagoscopy and bronchoscopy – can directly visualize and localize the origin of the fistula. Repeat examinations may be necessary as false negatives can be possible if a small fistula opening exists. A transtracheal wash or bronchoalveolar lavage can be concurrently performed. Transtracheal wash may show suppurative inflammatory response.
- Computed tomography – provides good anatomic delineation (Figure 29.3).

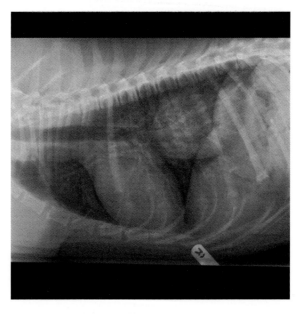

■ **Fig. 29.1.** A right lateral radiograph of the thorax. Note the soft tissue opacity caudal to the heart, suspected to be an esophageal or paraesophageal abscess or diverticulum as the most likely differential diagnoses. Source: Courtesy of Veterinary Specialist Services, QLD, Australia.

(a)   (b)

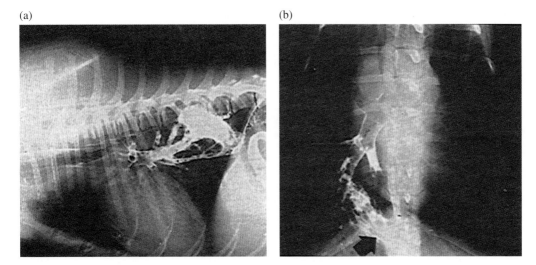

■ **Fig. 29.2.** Lateral (a) and dorsoventral (b) radiographs of the thorax postesophageal contrast study. There is contrast material in the bronchi. The arrow in (b) indicates the location of the bronchoesophageal fistula. Source: Courtesy of Iowa State University, USA.

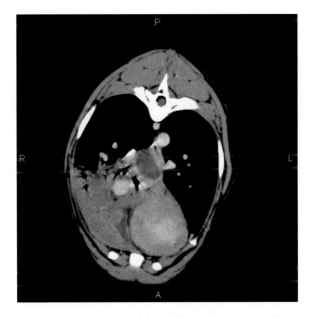

■ **Fig. 29.3.** A transverse (cross-section) CT image of the midthorax (same case as Figure 29.1). There is consolidation of the right middle lung lobe and ventral aspect of the right caudal lung lobe, likely aspiration pneumonia. The esophagus at this level appears fluid-filled and mildly dilated. Source: Courtesy of Veterinary Specialist Services, QLD, Australia.

Pathologic Findings

- Histologic sections of the fistula reveal stratified squamous epithelial lining to cuboidal respiratory epithelium.
- Congenital fistula is lined with squamous epithelium or columnar epithelium (ciliated or nonciliated); a lack of inflammatory process supports a congenital nature.

- Resected lung lobe may show thick fibrous pleura, interstitial fibrosis, atelectasis, with possible fragment of foreign material along with suppurative inflammation within the bronchi or alveoli. Culture and sensitivity is recommended.
- Necropsy may reveal a transmural perforation from the esophagus communicating with the adhered lung lobe.

 # THERAPEUTICS

Drug(s) of Choice

- Prophylactic use of broad-spectrum antibiotics with good respiratory tissue penetration is recommended, such as amoxicillin-clavulanic acid (13.75^mg/kg PO q 12 h), fluoroquinolones (enrofloxacin 10–20^mg/kg PO q 24 h), doxycycline (5^mg/kg PO q 12 h).
- Antibiotic treatment based on culture and sensitivity results of transtracheal wash or bronchoalveolar lavage is preferred.
- Long-term antibiotic administration may be required for 4–6 weeks or until two weeks post radiographic resolution of pneumonia.

Precautions/Interactions

Fluoroquinolones should be avoided in young animals affected by congenital form to prevent cartilaginous lesions during development.

Appropriate Health Care

Patient stabilization is initially required if there are signs of dyspnea or systemic illness such as septicemia.

Nursing Care

If pneumonia is present, supportive care with nebulization, coupage, and oxygen supplementation may be necessary.

Diet

- If chronic regurgitation exists, consider total or parenteral nutrition until surgical intervention.
- Placement of a gastrostomy feeding tube may be necessary to bypass esophageal fistula or postoperative significant esophageal resection.
- Most patients can be fed within 24 hours of surgical correction.
- Soft food is recommended post surgery to assist with peristalsis.
- Avoidance of rawhides, sticks or other hard food material should be instituted for two weeks.

Activity

Recommend controlled activity for 10–14 days postoperatively.

Surgical Considerations

- Surgical correction should be performed when patient is stable to undergo anesthesia and surgery.
- Anesthesia will be complicated with compromised pulmonary function.
- Surgery consists of dissection, ligation, and excision of the fistula, with reconstruction of the tracheal, bronchial or esophageal walls.
- A lung lobectomy is often performed due to extensive pathology in the communicating lung lobe.

- A lateral thoracotomy is usually performed at the level and side of the fistula and affected lung lobe.
- A delayed closure may be indicated if esophageal tissues are necrotic or edematous, and may require patching with local muscle flaps. Concurrent endoscopy during exploratory thoracotomy is preferred to facilitate identification of the fistula using guidewire.
- Correction of esophageal diverticula can be attempted concurrently at the time of fistula removal.

 ## COMMENTS

Client Education

- Surgical intervention is recommended. Conservative management can lead to worsening of condition and eventual death by pulmonary compromise.
- Patients with esophageal diverticulum may need a second procedure to be attempted at a later time, or can be corrected concurrently.
- Patients with megaesophagus can have continued regurgitation.

Patient Monitoring

- Monitor for aspiration pneumonia in the perioperative phase. Prokinetics and prokinetic agents should be instituted perioperatively.
- Postoperative monitoring of thoracostomy tube for fluid and/or air, with oxygen supplementation provided as needed.
- Feeding may need to be in an upright position, with gruel-like food given, if megaesophagus or a severely dilated esophageal diverticula exists.
- Repeat thoracic radiographs, contrast study or fluoroscopy performed at two weeks postoperatively can assess progression of pulmonary changes, resolution of fistula, and esophageal motility.

Prevention/Avoidance

Limiting situations in which patients can be exposed to dietary indiscretion or foreign body ingestion. Avoid rawhides and bones as treats.

Possible Complications

- Aspiration pneumonia can occur during anesthesia or postrecovery stage.
- Chronic regurgitation can persist.
- Recurrence is possible if the fistula tract is not removed, or if the communication remains patent. Ligation, rather than complete division of the fistula, increases the incidence of recurrence.
- Esophageal dehiscence and stricture formation from surgical correction can occur due to a lack of serosa or omentum, constant peristaltic motion, and segmental blood supply.

Expected Course and Prognosis

Prognosis ranges from good to guarded, depending on preoperative condition, ability to resolve pulmonary infection, success of surgery, and other complications such as esophageal trauma, pyothorax, septicemia, dehiscence, and esophageal stricture.

Abbreviations

- BEF = bronchoesophageal fistula
- TEF = tracheoesophageal fistula

See Also

- Esophageal Diverticula
- Esophageal Foreign Bodies
- Esophageal Neoplasia

- Esophageal Stricture
- Megaesophagus
- Regurgitation

Suggested Reading

Charoonrut P, Riengvirodkij N, Kamta C. Case report: bronchoesophageal fistula in mixed breed dog. J Appl Anim Sci 2015;8(1):37–46.

Della Ripa MA, Gaschen F, Gaschen L, et al. Canine bronchoesophageal fistulas: case report and literature review. Compend Contin Educ Pract Vet 2010;32(4):E1–E10.

Kaminen PS, Vitanen SJ, Lappalainen AK, et al. Management of a congenital tracheoesophageal fistula in a young Spanish water dog. BMC Vet Res 2014;10:16.

Nawrocki MA, Mackin AJ, McLaughlin R, et al. Fluoroscopic and endoscopic localization of an esophagobronchial fistula in a dog. J Am Anim Hosp Assoc 2003;39:257–261.

Park RD. Bronchoesophageal fistula in the dog: literature survey, case presentations and radiographic manifestations. Compend Contin Educ 1984;6(7):669–676.

Authors: Louisa Ho-Eckart BVSc Hons, MS, DACVS-SA, Eric Zellner DVM, DACVS-SA

Chapter 30

Esophageal Foreign Bodies

DEFINITION/OVERVIEW

- Ingestion of foreign material or foodstuffs too large to pass through the esophagus, causing partial or complete luminal obstruction.
- Occurs most often with an object whose size, shape, or texture does not allow free movement through the esophagus, causing it to become lodged before it can pass.

ETIOLOGY/PATHOPHYSIOLOGY

- Esophageal foreign bodies cause mechanical obstruction, mucosal inflammation with edema, and possibly ischemic necrosis and esophageal stricture formation.
- Bones, coins, and clothing are ingested by dogs; cats may consume linear foreign bodies.

Systems Affected

- Gastrointestinal.
- Respiratory – if aspiration pneumonia.

SIGNALMENT/HISTORY

- Dogs have a higher incidence than cats due to their indiscriminate eating habits.
- The pet may have been observed ingesting a foreign body.

Risk Factors

- More common in small-breed dogs; terrier breeds often overrepresented.
- More common in young to middle-aged animals.

Historical Findings

Most common client complaints include retching, gagging, lethargy, anorexia, ptyalism, regurgitation, restlessness, dysphagia, odynophagia, and persistent gulping.

CLINICAL FEATURES

- Retching/gagging.
- Ptyalism +/– repeated swallowing attempts.
- Occasional discomfort when palpating the neck or cranial abdomen
- Tachypnea and/or labored breathing if aspiration pneumonia.

Blackwell's Five-Minute Veterinary Consult Clinical Companion: Small Animal Gastrointestinal Diseases, First Edition. Edited by Jocelyn Mott and Jo Ann Morrison.
© 2019 John Wiley & Sons, Inc. Published 2019 by John Wiley & Sons, Inc.
Companion website: www.fiveminutevet.com/gastrointestinal

DIFFERENTIAL DIAGNOSIS

- Esophagitis.
- Esophageal stricture.
- Esophageal neoplasia.
- Megaesophagus.
- Other esophageal disorders.

DIAGNOSTICS

Complete Blood Count/Biochemistry/Urinalysis

- Usually unremarkable.
- Occasionally, electrolyte abnormalities, an inflammatory leukogram, and/or hemoconcentration, depending upon the severity of signs and duration of dehydration.

Imaging

- Most esophageal foreign bodies are radiodense and are readily visualized on thoracic radiographs. These objects most commonly lodge at points of minimal esophageal distension, including the thoracic inlet, base of the heart, and esophageal hiatus.
- Esophageal distension with air may be visualized cranial to the foreign body. Retained air in the esophagus is not always associated with esophageal foreign bodies and may be seen with aerophagia.
- A contrast esophagram or videofluoroscopy is required to identify radiolucent objects. If perforation is suspected, use an aqueous organic iodide contrast agent for imaging studies.
- Air and/or fluid in the mediastinum or pleural space suggests esophageal perforation; depending on severity, this can be an indication for surgery instead of esophagoscopy.
- Pulmonary infiltrates suggest aspiration pneumonia.

Diagnostic Procedures

- Options for foreign body removal include endoscopic extraction or surgery.
- Esophagoscopy affords direct visualization of both the foreign object and the esophageal mucosa, allowing assessment of the extent of esophageal injury (Figure 30.1).

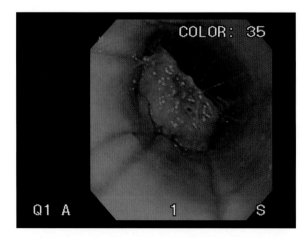

■ **Fig. 30.1.** Endoscopic visualization of an esophageal foreign body. Source: Courtesy of Dr Mike Willard.

- Esophagoscopy allows removal of most foreign bodies using retrieval instruments. It also allows for visual inspection of the mucosa for trauma after foreign body removal.

 # THERAPEUTICS

Drug(s) of Choice

- If there is significant mucosal injury, treatment for esophagitis is recommended: sucralfate slurry (0.5–1 g/dog PO q 8 h) for mucosal cytoprotection and healing.
- Proton pump inhibitor (omeprazole or pantoprazole at 1 mg/kg q 12 h) for robust suppression of gastric secretions which may contribute to reflux esophagitis.
- Broad-spectrum antibiotics (amoxicillin or Clavamox™) are *only* administered to animals with mucosal perforation.
- Metoclopramide (0.2–0.5 mg/kg IV, SQ, PO q 8 h) or cisapride (0.5 mg/kg q 8–12 h PO for dogs; 2.5 mg/cats) is administered to stimulate gastric motility and minimize reflux esophagitis.
- Gastrostomy tube placement for enteral nutrition may be indicated in animals with severe mucosal trauma.
- Viscous lidocaine gel administered with water and given 2–3 times daily can help reduce esophageal pain, if warranted.

Appropriate Health Care

- Emergencies – due to the risk of esophageal perforation and subsequent patient morbidity/mortality, treat as an emergency and perform endoscopy as soon as possible after diagnosis.
- If endoscopic retrieval of the foreign body succeeds and esophageal damage is minimal, the patient may be discharged the same day.

Nursing Care

- If the procedure to remove the foreign body is atraumatic and the esophagus has sustained minimal damage, no special aftercare is needed, beyond patient monitoring.
- Severe mucosal trauma may require placing a gastrostomy tube for enteral nutritional support during esophageal healing. Fluid therapy may also be required to maintain normal hydration status during periods of prolonged esophageal rest.

Diet

No change needed other than, perhaps, altering the food to a more liquid consistency.

Activity

The patient may resume normal activity after a foreign body has been routinely removed.

Surgical Considerations

- Surgery is indicated when endoscopy fails to retrieve the foreign body; when endoscopy enables advancement of the object into the gastric lumen but it is too large to pass through the gastrointestinal tract; or when a large esophageal perforation or area of necrosis requires resection.
- It is often less traumatic to advance a bone foreign body into the stomach than to attempt retrieval transorally via endoscopy. Gastrostomy, if required, may then be performed.
- Most bone foreign bodies can be safely left to dissolve in the stomach without need for surgical removal. Nondigestible foreign objects (wood, metal, plastic) passed into the stomach may need to be removed surgically.

COMMENTS

Client Education

Discuss the possibility of complications and repeat offenders.

Patient Monitoring

- Examine the esophagus closely via endoscopy for mucosal damage after foreign body removal.
- Mild erythema/erosions are not uncommon and often heal uneventfully.
- Perform postprocedural thoracic radiographs to assess for pneumomediastinum and/or pneumothorax. Small esophageal defects may be difficult to visualize from the mucosal surface.
- Monitor over 2–3 weeks for stricture formation. The most common clinical sign is regurgitation with evidence of odynophagia in many animals; esophagram or videofluoroscopy and/or esophagoscopy may be indicated to confirm stricture.

Prevention/Avoidance

Carefully monitor the environment and what is fed to the pet. Ensure that toys and items for chewing are of an appropriate size for the pet.

Possible Complications

- Approximately 25% of patients with foreign bodies develop complications.
- Complications most frequently encountered include esophageal perforation, esophageal strictures, esophageal fistulas, and severe esophagitis. Focal, transient esophageal motility disturbances can occur secondary to esophageal trauma.
- Pneumomediastinum, pneumothorax, pneumonia, pleuritis, mediastinitis, and bronchoesophageal fistulas can all occur secondarily to perforation.

Expected Course and Prognosis

- Most patients do well and recover uneventfully.
- With complications, the prognosis is more guarded.

See Also

- Esophageal Diverticula
- Esophageal Fistula
- Esophageal Stricture
- Esophagitis

Suggested Reading

Deroy C, Corcuff JB, Billen F, et al. Removal of oesophageal foreign bodies: comparison between oesophagoscopy and oesophagotomy in 39 dogs. J Small Anim Pract 2015;56:613–617.

Pratt CL, Reineke EL, Drobatz KJ. Sewing needle foreign body ingestion in dogs and cats: 65 cases (2000–2012). J Am Vet Med Assoc 2014;245:302–308.

Tams TR. Endoscopic removal of gastrointestinal foreign bodies. In: Tams TR, Rawlings CA, eds. Small Animal Endoscopy, 3rd ed. Philadelphia: Mosby, 2011, pp. 247–295.

Author: Albert E. Jergens DVM, PhD, DACVIM

Chapter 31

Esophageal Neoplasia

DEFINITION/OVERVIEW

- Malignant neoplasia includes any tumor with the ability to metastasize.
- Even tumors with low metastatic potential can cause esophageal stricture or obstruction and result in the death of a patient.

ETIOLOGY/PATHOPHYSIOLOGY

- *Spirocerca lupi* (SL) are found in the southern regions of the United States and tropical or subtropical areas of the world.
- Infection with SL can lead to the development of sarcomas of the distal esophagus in dogs.
- SL infections can result in (among other lesions) esophageal fibrous nodules that can undergo neoplastic transformation to sarcomas.
- Fibrosarcomas, osteosarcomas, and undifferentiated sarcomas have been reported from SL infection.
- Metastasis from SL-induced sarcomas is common.
- Esophageal leiomyomas and leiomyosarcomas are also found in the esophagus with no known risk factors for development.
- Metastasis from leiomyosarcomas appears to be uncommon.
- No known causes of esophageal carcinomas in dogs and cats.
- Metastasis from esophageal carcinomas appears to be uncommon, but animals are often euthanized due to local disease.

Systems Affected

Gastrointestinal – esophagus: strictures or obstructive lesions.

SIGNALMENT/HISTORY

- Sarcomas secondary to SL occur in dogs with a median age of 6–7 years, but can occur over a wide age range.
- Most SL-induced sarcomas are in large dog breeds.
- There may be an increased incidence of SL sarcomas in spayed females, and a decreased incidence in castrated males.
- Leiomyosarcomas tend to occur in older dogs (range of 9–14 reported).
- No sex predilection for sarcomas noted.
- Epithelial esophageal neoplasms also appear to occur in older dogs (9–11 years).
- Epithelial neoplasia in cats does not appear to have a sex predilection.

Blackwell's Five-Minute Veterinary Consult Clinical Companion: Small Animal Gastrointestinal Diseases, First Edition. Edited by Jocelyn Mott and Jo Ann Morrison.
© 2019 John Wiley & Sons, Inc. Published 2019 by John Wiley & Sons, Inc.
Companion website: www.fiveminutevet.com/gastrointestinal

- Age range reported for cats with epithelial/neuroendocrine tumors is 8–10 years.
- The single case report of an esophageal sarcoma in a cat involved a three year old.
- There is no evidence for a genetic basis of this disease in dogs or cats.

Clinical Signs

- Vomiting/regurgitation.
- Weight loss.
- Dysphagia.
- Lethargy/depression.
- Pyrexia.
- Coughing.
- Salivation.
- Bruxism.

Additional Clinical Signs in Dogs with SL Sarcomas

- Respiratory signs.
- Lameness.
- These signs may occur as a result of pneumonia, pleurisy, mediastinitis, bronchial displacement, metastasis or hypertrophic osteopathy.

Risk Factors

Living in an SL endemic area is a risk factor for SL-induced sarcomas.

 # CLINICAL FEATURES

- Weight loss.
- Bruxism reported in a cat.

 # DIFFERENTIAL DIAGNOSIS

- Esophageal stricture.
- Esophagitis.
- Gastroesophageal reflux disease.
- Megaesophagus.
- SL-induced fibromas.

 # DIAGNOSTICS

Complete Blood Count/Biochemistry/Urinalysis

- Leukocytosis, microcytic hypochromic anemia.
- Biochemistry panel is often unremarkable.

Additional Laboratory Tests

Fecal float (diagnose SL infection if a differential).

Imaging

- Thoracic radiographs, +/– computed tomography scan (evaluate esophageal structure, may see mass).

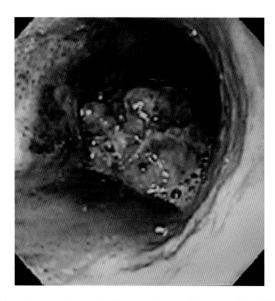

■ **Fig. 31.1.** Endoscopic view of an esophageal melanoma. Source: Courtesy of Dr Mike Willard.

- SL-induced fibromas/sarcomas are typically in the caudal esophagus, but may occur in the hilar region.
- Contrast esophagram +/– fluoroscopy (demonstrate stricture/obstruction, overall esophageal function).

Other Diagnostic Tests

Esophageal endoscopy to visualize mass/potential biopsy (Figure 31.1).

Pathologic Findings

- Due to the overlying mucosa, endoscopic biopsies of sarcomas can be nondiagnostic.
- Endoscopic biopsies of carcinomas can also miss a diagnosis due to secondary ulceration/ infection/necrosis.
- Pathology of a representative sample of the mass is consistent with the tumor type. Tumors reported in the esophagus include fibrosarcoma, osteosarcoma, undifferentiated sarcoma, leiomyosarcoma, leiomyoma, angioleiomyosarcoma, squamous cell carcinoma, adenosquamous carcinoma, melanoma, and neuroendocrine carcinoma.

 # THERAPEUTICS

Given the difficulty of antemortem differentiation between SL-induced fibromas and sarcomas, it may be worth treating the SL infection and watching for resolution of the lesions if the presenting mass is small. However, if the mass does not respond and clinical signs do not improve, surgical options should be considered in a timely fashion as a sarcoma will not decrease in size following treatment for SL.

Drug(s) of Choice

- SL infection is treated with avermectins or milbemycin-oxime: doramectin 200 µg/kg SQ every 14 days for three treatments.

- SL-induced sarcomas have received adjuvant chemotherapy (efficacy unknown): doxorubicin 30 mg/m² IV every three weeks for 5–6 treatments.

Nursing Care

Patients often develop megaesophagus secondary to esophageal neoplasms, and so should be cared for in an appropriate manner (e.g., frequent small feedings, elevated feedings).

Diet

Patients with partially obstructive lesions may benefit from a liquid diet.

Surgical Considerations

- Surgical excision is the treatment of choice for esophageal neoplasia.
- Gastric advancement has been used successfully for caudal esophageal tumors.
- Esophageal leiomyomas or low-grade leiomyosarcomas may be treated effectively with marginal excision (survivals >1 year).
- Pre- and postoperative management of megaesophagus is important for the survival of the patient.
- Palliative transesophageal debulking of SL-induced sarcomas was reported to have a median survival of 202 days in nine dogs.

 COMMENTS

Client Education

Clients should be informed on the care of a dog with abnormal esophageal function (e.g., megaesophagus).

Patient Monitoring

Patients with SL-induced sarcomas should be monitored with thoracic radiographs every 2–3 months for the occurrence of metastasis.

Prevention/Avoidance

Preventive treatment for SL in endemic areas has been shown to decrease the incidence of infection and severity of lesions which develop in the treated dogs.

Possible Complications

Surgical complications may include dehiscence, perforation, esophagitis, megaesophagus, aspiration pneumonia, and death.

Expected Course and Prognosis

- SL-induced sarcomas appear highly malignant, which warrants a guarded prognosis.
- Not all dogs with SL-induced sarcomas develop metastasis, however.
- Esophageal leiomyomas and low-grade leiomyosarcomas have a good prognosis, even with incomplete excision.
- Esophageal carcinomas in cats warrant a guarded prognosis; sarcomas may have a better prognosis.

Abbreviations

- SL = *Spirocerca lupi*

See Also

- Dysphagia
- Esophageal Stricture
- Megaesophagus
- Regurgitation

Suggested Reading

Farese JP, Bacon NJ, Ehrhart NP, et al. Oesophageal leiomyosarcoma in dogs: surgical management and clinical outcome of four cases. Vet Comp Oncol 2008;6:1:31–38.

Gualtiermi, M, Monzeglaniod, MG, di Giancamillo, M. Oesophageal squamous cell carcinoma in two cats. J Small Anim Pract 1999;40:79–83.

Ranen E, Lavy E, Aizenberg I, Perl S, Harrus S. Spirocercosis-associated esophageal sarcomas in dogs. A retrospective study of 17 cases (1997–2003). Vet Parasitolol 2004;119:209–221.

Shipov A, Kelmer G, Lavy E, Milgram J, Aroch I, Segev G. Long-term outcome of transendoscopic oesophageal mass ablation in dogs with Spirocerca lupi-associated oesophageal sarcoma. Vet Rec 2015;177;14:365–369.

Author: Marlene L. Hauck DVM, PhD, DACVIM (Oncology)

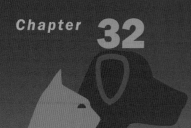

Chapter 32

Esophageal Stricture

DEFINITION/OVERVIEW

A fixed narrowing of the esophagus due to scar tissue, resulting in partial or complete obstruction.

ETIOLOGY/PATHOPHYSIOLOGY

- Benign strictures typically occur when there is severe esophagitis, encompassing greater than 270° of the esophageal circumference. Regardless of the initiating event, if severe esophagitis develops, there can be a decrease in lower esophageal sphincter (LES) tone which can result in more acid reflux and subsequent worsening of the esophagitis. Once severe esophagitis is present, it can extend into the lamina propria and muscularis layers. This incites a fibroblastic proliferation and contraction, leading to stricture formation.
- Malignant strictures from direct tumor invasion occur rarely in dogs and cats.

Causes

- Reflux during anesthesia is a common cause of benign esophageal stricture, accounting for about ~65% of cases. Decreased LES tone occurring during anesthesia allows gastroesophageal reflux and subsequent acid injury to the esophageal mucosa.
- Severe esophageal foreign bodies (if >270° mucosal damage occurs).
- Tablets and capsules lodging in the esophagus can induce esophagitis leading to stricture. The most commonly incriminated drugs are doxycycline, clindamycin and aspirin.
- Gastroesophageal reflux independent of anesthesia.
- Prolonged vomiting of gastric contents.
- Swallowing of caustic substances.
- Esophageal neoplasia (squamous cell carcinoma and lymphoma most common).
- Vascular ring anomaly (congenital).
- *Spirocerca lupi* granuloma – rare in the US.

Systems Affected

- Gastrointestinal – in the case of strictures due to acid reflux, the esophagus may have one or multiple strictures present.
- Respiratory – in some cases, strictures may also be present in the nasopharynx or nasal choanae. Regurgitation is common with strictures, which sometimes cause secondary aspiration pneumonia.

Blackwell's Five-Minute Veterinary Consult Clinical Companion: Small Animal Gastrointestinal Diseases,
First Edition. Edited by Jocelyn Mott and Jo Ann Morrison.
© 2019 John Wiley & Sons, Inc. Published 2019 by John Wiley & Sons, Inc.
Companion website: www.fiveminutevet.com/gastrointestinal

SIGNALMENT/HISTORY

- Dog and cat.
- No known breed or sex predilections for acquired, benign stricture.
- Puppies and kittens with vascular ring anomaly classically become symptomatic at weaning although some are first diagnosed in later life due to foreign body obstruction at the site of the stricture.
- No predominant sex.

Risk Factors

- General anesthesia, especially with drugs that decrease LES tone or when the table is tilted head down.
- Oral medications given with a dry swallow (60–80% of capsules do not pass into the stomach after five minutes following a dry swallow).
- Foreign body ingestion.
- Great Danes, Irish setters, and German shepherds are genetically predisposed to congenital vascular ring anomalies.

Historical Findings

- Pain during swallowing (odynophagia).
- Dysphagia.
- Increased salivation.
- Regurgitation.
- Hyporexia.
- Weight loss.
- If regurgitation leads to aspiration pneumonia, cough and dyspnea can develop.

 # CLINICAL FEATURES

- Regurgitation (especially solid food).
- Pain when swallowing.
- Weight loss.

 # DIFFERENTIAL DIAGNOSIS

- Megaesophagus.
- Esophageal foreign body.
- Esophageal neoplasia.
- Extrinsic esophageal compression (mass, abscess).
- Gastroesophageal reflux.
- Vomiting (any cause).
- Oropharyngeal dysphagia.

 # DIAGNOSTICS

Complete Blood Count/Biochemistry/Urinalysis

- Usually unremarkable.
- May have neutrophilic leukocytosis if secondary aspiration pneumonia develops.

Other Laboratory Tests

Usually unremarkable.

Imaging

- Thoracic radiographs – usually unremarkable, unless secondary aspiration pneumonia develops. Occasionally gas-filled dilation or foreign body material cranial to the stricture may be seen.
- Videofluoroscopic barium swallow – procedure of choice. Use of barium mixed with food makes procedure more sensitive. If videofluoroscopy is unavailable, administer liquid barium mixed with food followed immediately by radiography. Peristalsis proximal to the stricture site can be abnormal with concurrent esophagitis. Usually recognize an abrupt narrowing of the esophageal lumen at the stricture site. Most reliably demonstrated with canned food or kibble mixed with barium. May demonstrate more than one stricture. Many cases of reflux-induced strictures are between the heart base and diaphragm. Many cases of pill-induced strictures are near the thoracic inlet (especially cats).

Other Diagnostic Tests

- Endoscopy – there is usually an abrupt decrease in luminal diameter at the stricture site (Figure 32.1). The mucosa may appear normal (smooth and pink) or can appear hyperemic and ulcerated if esophagitis is present. Scar tissue may/may not be obvious.
- Often the scope cannot be advanced beyond the stricture without balloon dilation. However, large dogs may have strictures that decrease luminal diameter >50% but may be missed by novice endoscopists, especially when using small-diameter endoscopes. Strictures right at the LES may be missed by novice endoscopists who think that they have just passed the scope through the LES and do not recognize that a stricture is also present.
- The location of the stricture should be measured from the upper canine teeth.

Pathologic Findings

If an esophageal mass is present, biopsy with histopathology is warranted. Otherwise, benign strictures do not need to be biopsied (it is almost impossible to biopsy nonneoplastic esophageal tissue with flexible endoscopic forceps). Variable degree of esophagitis may be seen.

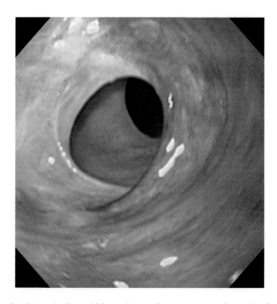

■ **Fig. 32.1.** An esophageal stricture in the midthoracic esophagus seen endoscopically.

THERAPEUTICS

Drug(s) of Choice

- Following dilation, medications for esophagitis are used, including cisapride (0.5–0.75 mg/kg PO q 8 h) to increase LES tone and enhance gastric emptying, and omeprazole (1–2 mg/kg PO q 12 h) to decrease gastric acid. Pain can be partially alleviated with sucralfate suspension (0.5–1 g/patient PO q 6–12 h as needed).
- Broad-spectrum antibiotics are used if aspiration pneumonia is present.

Precautions/Interactions

Esophageal perforation can occur with overzealous balloon dilation of the stricture. Overzealous dilation can also cause excessive trauma resulting in rapid reformation of the stricture. Therefore, it is sometimes appropriate to sequentially increase diameter of balloons.

Alternative Drugs

- Erythromycin, metoclopramide or ranitidine can be used to increase LES tone (although cisapride is superior).
- Histamine H2-receptor blockers are poorly effective for alleviating esophagitis and should not be used.

Appropriate Health Care

- Outpatient medical management can sometimes be transiently successful for mild strictures, but failure to resolve the stricture puts the patient at risk for future esophageal foreign bodies.
- More severe strictures will lead to progressive malnutrition and possible aspiration pneumonia, and require inpatient intervention. If there are complications (esophageal perforation, aspiration pneumonia), then inpatient care is required.

Nursing Care

- With mild strictures, feeding gruel from an elevated platform might be successful but this is not recommended due to risk of future esophageal foreign bodies.
- With more severe strictures, oral alimentation will not be successful. Intravenous fluids may be necessary if the animal is dehydrated.
- Other medications depend on the presence of esophagitis, complications, and results of dilation.

Diet

- With mild strictures, gruel feeding (ideally partially elevated) may be successful.
- Recommend feeding a fat-restricted diet to enhance gastric emptying.
- Canned food can be fed in small frequent amounts following dilation, even when severe esophageal tearing occurs.
- In some cases, persistent restricturing occurs, necessitating percutaneous endoscopic gastrostomy (PEG) tube feeding while multiple dilations are employed.

Activity

If pneumonia is present, the degree of hypoxia will determine appropriate activity level.

Surgical Considerations

- The first-line treatment of benign esophageal strictures is mechanical dilation of the stricture. Techniques include bougienage and balloon dilation. Both can be effective. Neither should be attempted unless the clinician has received specific training in their use. Both require either endoscopic or fluoroscopic guidance.

- Esophageal dilation balloons are elongated (i.e. not circular) and are made of special plastic that makes the balloon extremely rigid when maximally inflated, generally up to 45 psi. The balloon is inflated until it reaches the manufacturer's rated pressure or until the stricture is dilated sufficiently. Sequentially larger balloons are used until the clinician subjectively judges the degree of mucosal tearing to be acceptable
- The technique is very subjective in veterinary medicine, with many variables not defined by controlled studies. Typically, an initial balloon diameter is selected that is up to 50–100% larger than the estimated stricture diameter. If there is doubt, selection of a smaller balloon with gradually larger subsequent dilations is safest. The sequence of subsequent larger dilations is then determined by the degree of mucosal tearing. The final dilation diameter is usually based upon the degree of mucosal tearing and the size of the patient. The goal is not anatomic normalcy – the goal is functionality. However, remember that if any stricture remains, the patient may be at increased risk for future esophageal foreign body obstruction.
- Injection of intralesional submucosal triamcinolone in a four-quadrant pattern either before or after dilation and/or nicking the stricture at three or four equidistant spots with either electrosurgery or laser prior to dilation might reduce the frequency of restricture. Similarly, topical application of mitomycin-C to the torn mucosa after dilation may also reduce the frequency of restricture.
- Some authors recommend sequential dilations at intervals ranging from every three days to weekly to decrease the likelihood of restricture formation.
- If multiple dilations have been performed with subsequent stricture recurrence, or if the stricture is longer than a few centimeters, then more advanced techniques such as a self-expanding covered stent or a BE tube can be employed. It is important that a stent be secured with sutures to prevent stent migration. It is important that clients be screened to be sure that they can manage a patient with a BE tube.
- Surgical management (resection and anastomosis) is only performed as a last resort because it has a high failure rate.

COMMENTS

Client Education

- With mild strictures, gruel feeding (ideally partially elevated) may be possible. However, dilation is recommended.
- Owners should be aware that dilation procedures are not always successful, and that multiple attempts are required in some patients. It is important that medical management for esophagitis be diligently employed following dilation procedures to help reduce the risk of restricture.
- Many cases have a successful outcome.
- If there is failure after several attempts, or if the stricture is longer than a few centimeters, then advanced techniques (e.g., intralesional steroid injections, nicking the stricture at 3–4 sites, painting the torn mucosa with mitomycin-C, stent placement, use of a BE tube) should be considered.
- Patients with esophageal neoplasia have a poor prognosis.

Patient Monitoring

- Clinical signs are monitored for stricture recurrence (mainly regurgitation). An appropriate consistency food should be fed. Repeat stricture dilation may be considered based on recurrence of clinical signs.
- Aspiration pneumonia is monitored by clinical signs and radiographic resolution.

Prevention/Avoidance

- Preanesthetic administration of a proton pump inhibitor (e.g., omeprazole) +/– a prokinetic such as cisapride decreases the number of reflux events in anesthetized dogs, but the cost-effectiveness of this pretreatment is controversial.
- Medications with ulcerogenic potential (e.g., doxycycline, clindamycin, ciprofloxacin, aspirin) should be given with at least 6 mL of water or food (a "wet swallow").

Possible Complications

- Complications of balloon dilation include perforation, severe mucosal tearing and esophagitis, excessive bleeding, and restricture.
- Aspiration pneumonia secondary to regurgitation.
- Complications of stent placement include stent migration, tissue ingrowth into the stent resulting in stent occlusion, food obstruction, hemorrhage, perforation, airway compression, pressure necrosis/fistula formation, dysphagia, and pain.

Expected Course and Prognosis

- The overall successful treatment rate of balloon dilation is reported to be between 70% and 88% in dogs and cats. The median number of dilations required for successful treatment is two, but it can require several (>5–8).
- Prognosis is poorer with longer strictures and those which have recurred repeatedly after dilation. It is important to note that some patients fail therapy with all techniques.
- The prognosis for esophageal neoplasia is poor.

Synonyms

- Esophageal narrowing
- Esophageal blockage or obstruction

Abbreviations

- BE = balloon esophagostomy
- LES = lower esophageal sphincter
- PEG = percutaneous endoscopic gastrostomy

Suggested Reading

Bissett SA, Davis J, Subler K, et al. Risk factors and outcome of bougienage for treatment of benign esophageal strictures in dogs and cats: 28 cases (1995–2004). J Am Vet Med Assoc 2009;235(7):844–850.

Lam N, Weisse C, Berent A, et al. Esophageal stenting for treatment of refractory benign esophgeal strictures in dogs. J Vet Intern Med 2013;27(5):1064–1070.

Zacuto AC, Marks SL, Osborn J, et al. The influence of esomeprazole and cisapride on gastroesophageal reflux during anesthesia in dogs. J Vet Intern Med 2012;26(3):518–525.

Acknowledgments: The author and editors acknowledge the prior contribution of Dr Keith Richter.

Client Education Handout available online

Author: Michael D. Willard DVM, MS, DACVIM

Chapter 33

Esophagitis

DEFINITION/OVERVIEW

- Inflammation of the esophagus typically affecting the esophageal body and gastroesophageal sphincter or lower esophageal sphincter (LES). Esophagitis is most commonly due to gastroesophageal reflux (GER) or secondary to vomiting. The cricopharyngeal sphincter or upper esophageal sphincter is less commonly affected.
- Esophagitis will vary from a mild self-limiting condition to severe ulcerative esophagitis involving the submucosa and muscularis which can result in stricture formation, which is one of the most severe complications.

ETIOLOGY/PATHOPHYSIOLOGY

Pathophysiology

- Physiologic defense mechanisms protecting the esophagus from inflammation are the esophageal mucosal barrier (stratified squamous epithelium, intracellular tight junctions, mucus gel, surface bicarbonate), the LES, clearance by esophageal motility, and the neutralizing effect of alkaline saliva.
- Disruption of these esophageal defense mechanisms can result in esophageal inflammation with erosion and/or ulceration.
- Esophagitis can result in impaired esophageal motility and LES incompetence which may lead to further GER, perpetuating esophagitis and esophageal damage.

Etiology

- Commonly due to GER secondary to general anesthesia (Figures 33.1 and 33.2), hiatal hernia (Figures 33.3 and 33.4), persistent or chronic vomiting and gastrointestinal (GI) disease resulting in delayed gastric emptying.
- Gastroesophageal reflux disease (GERD) secondary to a primary LES abnormality is poorly understood in veterinary patients.
- Esophageal retention of tablets or capsules (doxycycline most common in cats, clindamycin, nonsteroidal antiinflammatory drugs (NSAIDs)).
- Esophageal foreign body (Figure 33.5).
- Infectious agents – pythiosis, *Spirocerca lupi*, *Candida* infection secondary to immune suppression.
- Other causes of esophagitis include esophageal tumors, radiation injury, megaesophagus, vascular ring anomalies, gastrinoma (Zollinger–Ellison syndrome), and malpositioned esophageal tubes.

Blackwell's Five-Minute Veterinary Consult Clinical Companion: Small Animal Gastrointestinal Diseases, First Edition. Edited by Jocelyn Mott and Jo Ann Morrison.
© 2019 John Wiley & Sons, Inc. Published 2019 by John Wiley & Sons, Inc.
Companion website: www.fiveminutevet.com/gastrointestinal

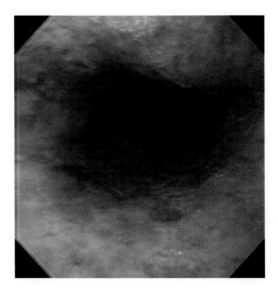

■ **Fig. 33.1.** Postanesthetic reflux esophagitis which progressed to a stricture.

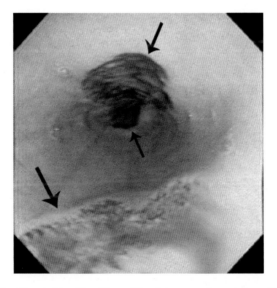

■ **Fig. 33.2.** Postanesthetic reflux esophagitis with multifocal deep esophageal ulcers (*black arrows*).

- Eosinophilic esophagitis is one of the most common causes of esophagitis in humans and has been reported in veterinary patients but is rare.
- Idiopathic.

Incidence/Prevalence/Geographic Distribution

- Esophagitis is a common clinical diagnosis based on the history or clinical circumstances. The truce incidence of esophagitis is probably underestimated, as most cases are not definitively diagnosed endoscopically or histologically. In human medicine, GERD is the most common outpatient diagnoses made by gastroenterologists in the USA which affects about 20% of the adult population weekly and 7% daily. This disorder significantly affects the well-being and quality of life of human patients.

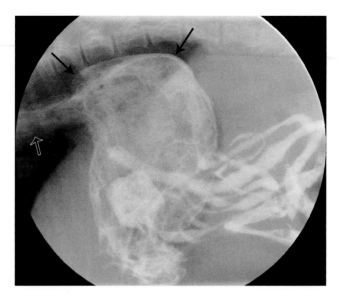

■ **Fig. 33.3.** Hiatal hernia (*black arrows*) and associated GER (*black arrow with white border*) diagnosed with barium contrast esophagram with fluoroscopy in a dog.

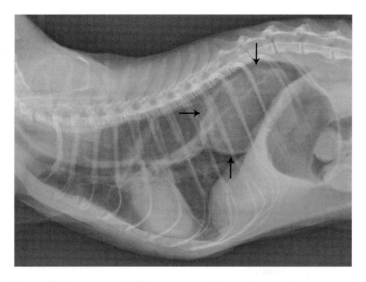

■ **Fig. 33.4.** Hiatal hernia (*black arrows*) with diffuse esophageal dilation diagnosed on survey radiography in a cat.

- Esophagitis caused by *Pythium* spp. (typically in states that border the Gulf of Mexico) and rarely *Spirocerca lupi* (southern states).

Systems Affected

- Gastrointestinal – esophagus (esophageal body and LES most commonly affected) and in the vomiting patient primary or secondary GI disease.
- Respiratory – with regurgitation and GER, aspiration pneumonia may develop as well as reflux laryngitis, pharyngitis, and/or rhinitis. Clinicians should be aware of these extraesophageal respiratory signs which may be a covert presentation for GER.

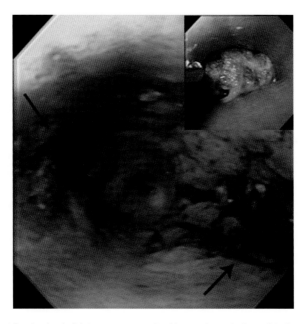

■ **Fig. 33.5.** Esophageal foreign body (*right upper corner*) with esophageal ulcers (*black arrows*) post foreign body removal.

 # SIGNALMENT/HISTORY

- Reflux esophagitis resulting from upper airway obstruction in brachycephalic breeds occurs due to increased negative intrathoracic pressure upon inspiration increasing the tendency for GER and possibly hiatal hernia (HH).
- Animals of any age can be affected.
- Young animals with congenital esophageal HH and older animals that are anesthetized are at greater risk of developing GER and reflux esophagitis.

Risk Factors

- Anesthetic premedications, induction agents, and maintenance drugs including all opioid class drugs, glycopyrrolate, atropine, acepromazine, diazepam, xylaxine, propofol, and halogenated anesthetic agents have all been associated with decreased LES tone and GER.
- Hiatal hernia – increases risk for gastroesophageal reflux.
- Preanesthetic fasting for prolonged periods (≥24 h) puts a patient at greater risk for gastroesophageal reflux and increased gastric acidity.

Historical Findings

- Regurgitation.
- Ptyalism.
- Dysphagia (difficulty swallowing, gagging, retching).
- Odynophagia (pain when swallowing, repeated swallowing efforts, and extension of the head and neck during swallowing).
- Hyporexia or anorexia.
- Weight loss.
- Coughing and/or nasal discharge if there are extraesophageal manifestations (aspiration pneumonia and reflux laryngitis, pharyngitis, and/or rhinitis).

CLINICAL FEATURES

- Often normal physical examination.
- Oral and pharyngeal inflammation and/or ulceration if caustic or irritating substances have been ingested or with severe extraesophageal (oropharyngeal) reflux of acidic gastric contents.
- Fever and pain in some patients with severe ulcerative esophagitis or aspiration pneumonia.
- Halitosis, ptyalism, and possibly pain on palpation of neck and esophagus.
- Cachexia and weight loss with chronic esophagitis or esophageal stricture.
- Respiratory signs including nasal discharge and congestion with reflux rhinitis and cough, increased bronchovesicular sounds, pulmonary crackles and dyspnea as well as systemic signs including lethargy and fever in patients with aspiration pneumonia.

 ## DIFFERENTIAL DIAGNOSIS

- Esophageal foreign body – usually detected by survey radiography or esophagoscopy.
- Esophageal stricture – segmental narrowing revealed by barium contrast radiography or esophagoscopy.
- Oropharyngeal dysphagia – diagnosed by evaluating swallowing with a videofluoroscopic swallow study.
- Hiatal hernia – usually recognized as a gas or fluid-filled opacity in the caudodorsal thorax at the level of the esophageal hiatus; a contrast esophagram with fluoroscopy may be required to document a HH (see Figures 33.3 and 33.4).
- Megaesophagus – survey radiography usually reveals diffuse dilation of the esophageal body.
- Esophageal diverticula – focal pouches detected by survey or contrast radiography or esophagoscopy.
- Vascular ring anomaly – usually revealed by contrast radiography as a focal dilation of the proximal esophageal body.
- Esophageal neoplasia – esophageal mass effect with possible esophageal dilation diagnosed with survey or contrast radiography, thoracic computed tomography (CT) or esophagoscopy.

Brachycephalic Dogs

Observations show a correlation between upper respiratory and gastrointestinal tract disease in brachycephalic breeds. Hiatal hernia, GER, and esophagitis as well as other GI lesions have been reported. Surgical treatment of upper respiratory disease improves GI clinical signs and medical management of gastroesophageal disease improves the outcome for surgically treated brachycephalic dogs.

 ## DIAGNOSTICS

Complete Blood Count/Biochemistry/Urinalysis

Usually unremarkable although patients with ulcerative esophagitis or aspiration pneumonia may have a leukocytosis and neutrophilia.

Imaging

- Survey thoracic radiography – often unremarkable but may reveal mild esophageal dilation or fluid accumulation in the distal esophagus; aspiration pneumonia may be evident in the dependent portions of the lung; potentially dilation of the esophagus cranial to a stricture, an esophageal foreign body, hiatal hernia (see Figure 33.4) or an intraluminal or extraluminal mass may be detected.

- Barium contrast esophagram (static images and/or fluoroscopic) – may reveal esophageal dilation with retention of barium in esophagus, strictures, foreign bodies or masses; fluoroscopic studies allow for evaluation of swallowing, esophageal motility, strictures which may not be apparent on a static esophagram, sliding HH (see Figure 33.3) and GER (the latter two conditions may require abdominal compressions to demonstrate).
- Thoracic CT is now more routinely being used and can be helpful especially for esophageal masses, foreign bodies, and HHs.

Diagnostic Procedures

- Endoscopy and biopsy – most reliable means of diagnosis (see Figures 33.1, 33.2, and 33.5). Mild cases of esophagitis may be endoscopically normal. Visual findings of mucosal hyperemia and edema are common and, in more severe cases, ulceration and active bleeding. In patients with GER, changes are usually most apparent in the caudal third of the esophagus. If esophagoscopy is performed in a patient with concurrent GI signs, gastroduodenoscopy should also be performed to evaluate for GI causes of vomiting which can result in esophagitis.
- Diagnostic-quality esophageal biopsies are difficult to obtain endoscopically due to the composition of the esophageal mucosa which has a tough stratified squamous epithelium. Histopathology provides the most definitive evidence of esophagitis although endoscopy and biopsies are usually reserved for cases unresponsive to therapy.
- Most cases of aspiration pneumonia will resolve when treated with supportive care and broad-spectrum antibiotics. Endotracheal or transtracheal aspiration, or bronchoscopy with bronchoalveolar lavage with samples collected for cytology, and for culture and sensitivity testing may be performed in patients not responding to empirical therapy.
- Esophageal manometry and ambulatory pH monitoring, which are performed in humans to document GERD, are not currently utilized in clinical veterinary medicine.

Pathologic Findings

- Mucosal squamous hyperplasia or dysplasia with erosions and ulcers and lymphocytic plasmacytic and neutrophilic inflammation.
- Barrett's esophagus is esophageal squamous metaplasia associated with chronic GERD that can lead to epithelial dysplasia and esophageal cancer in humans; it has been reported in cats but is rare.

 # THERAPEUTICS

Successful treatment of esophagitis involves: (1) addressing underlying risk factors and predisposing conditions when possible; (2) gastric acid suppression to reduce esophageal mucosal injury; (3) increasing LES pressure and promoting gastric emptying to reduce GER, and (4) protecting the esophageal mucosa from further injury.

Drug (s) of Choice

Acid Suppression

- The most important therapeutic strategy for the treatment of GERD and associated esophagitis is gastric acid suppression. H2-receptor antagonists (H_2RAs) and proton pump inhibitors (PPIs) are the two main classes of acids suppressors. PPIs provide superior gastric acid suppression compared to H_2RAs in humans, dogs, and cats. Of the routinely used gastric acid suppressors, PPIs are most often prescribed and are the most effective.

- In humans, optimal treatment of GERD occurs at a target intragastric pH of >4 for ≥67% of the day. It's been established in healthy dogs and cats that to achieve the target intragastric pH for the treatment for GERD in humans, a PPI should be used at a dosage of 1 mg/kg PO q 12 h. The most commonly used PPIs for the treatment of GER and esophagitis in dogs and cats are omeprazole 1 mg/kg PO q 12 h, optimally given 30 min before a meal, and pantoprazole 1.0 mg/kg IV or PO q 12 h. Lansoprazole or esomeprazole 1 mg/kg PO q 12 h are other available PPIs. Esomeprazole given as a single dose at 1 mg/kg was shown to significantly increase intragastric pH after IV, PO, and SQ administration.

- Fractionated enteric-coated omeprazole tablets remain effective despite disruption of the enteric coating. Tablets need to be cleanly split and they cannot be crushed.

- In humans there has been widespread media attention in recent years concerning potential adverse effects of PPIs, including dementia, vitamin and mineral imbalances, bone fracture risk, renal insufficiency, and increased risk of infection. The current evidence is inadequate to establish causal relationships between PPI therapy and these proposed associations. Patients with a clinical indication for a PPI should continue to receive it at the lowest effective dose for the shortest period of time, and when possible stop the drug and switch the patient to on-demand PPI use. A human study found that a longer duration of PPI use is associated with a progressive increase in risk of death, so the length of PPI treatment should be minimized when medically appropriate. Caution should be exercised when prescribing gastric acid suppressors as they are among the most overprescribed drugs in both human and veterinary medicine.

- The other major class of commonly prescribed acid suppressors are the H_2RAs. Famotidine is the most effective and commonly recommended H_2RA and is given at a dose of 0.5–1.0 mg/kg PO, SQ, IV q 12 h. Famotidine is inferior to PPIs in suppressing gastric acid even at the dose of 1 mg/kg PO q 12 h. The target pH for managing GERD in humans is not achieved even at a famotidine dose of 1 mg/kg q 12 h in dogs. In addition, famotidine has been shown to have a diminished effect over time with repeated administration. Dogs treated with famotidine had a significantly lower pH on days 13 and 14 when compared to days 1 and 2. Famotidine is appropriate for short-term gastric acid suppression but caution is advised when recommending long-term administration in dogs. The H_2RA ranitidine given at 2.0 mg/kg PO, SQ, IV q 8–12 h is less effective than famotidine for acid suppression but does have prokinetic activity. Cimetidine and nizatidine are uncommonly prescribed.

- Combined acid suppressants –because PPIs may take time to accumulate and H_2RAs have a more immediate action, it has been recommended to combine an H_2RA with a PPI when initiating PPI therapy. A study in dogs found that short-term combination treatment with famotidine and pantoprazole was not superior to pantoprazole alone for increasing intragastric pH in dogs, so when prescribing a PPI overlap with an H_2RA during initial dosing is unnecessary.

- When discontinuing a PPI after > 3–4 weeks of therapy the PPI should be gradually tapered by 50% increments over 2 to 3 weeks to avoid rebound gastric hypersecretion.

- Dosing for metabolic disease (renal failure and liver failure) has not been established so a lower dose or longer dose interval may be appropriate for these conditions.

- Vonoprazan, a novel potassium-competitive acid blocker undergoing evaluation in humans, may provide clinical benefit in acid-related disorders. This class of drugs has not been evaluated in veterinary medicine.

GI Prokinetics

- The second most common class of drugs used to treat GER and esophagitis are the GI prokinetics. Gastrointestinal prokinetic drugs increase LES pressure which reduces GER and promotes gastric emptying. The most effective prokinetic is cisapride at a dose of 0.5–1.0 mg/kg PO q 8 h. Cisapride has been withdrawn as a human pharmaceutical due to its association with serious cardiac arrhythmias. This association has not been recognized in veterinary patients and cisapride is readily available in compounding pharmacies. Cisapride is only administered PO.

- Metoclopramide is another commonly prescribed GI prokinetic drug that also has antiemetic effects in dogs. Metoclopramide is dosed at 0.2–1.0 mg/kg PO, SQ q 8 h or 1.0–3.0 mg/kg/day as a constant rate infusion (CRI). The higher end of the dose range may be necessary depending on the response. Metoclopramide tends to be most effective as a GI prokinetic when given as a CRI.

Mucosal Protectants
- Sucralfate 0.5–1.0 g PO q 8 h is given as a suspension mixed into a slurry with water and administered on an empty stomach. Sucralfate is a mucosal protectant that forms an insoluble complex that binds to inflamed tissue, creating a protective barrier and preventing further damage caused by pepsin, acid, and bile as well as inactivating pepsin and binding bile acids. Another effect is an increase in mucosal defense and repair mechanisms through stimulation of bicarbonate and prostaglandin E production and binding of epidermal growth factor, which occurs at a neutral pH. Additionally, sucralfate has been reported to relieve symptoms in humans.
- In humans, a new drug called Essox® (hyaluronic acid-chondroitin sulfate-based bioadhesive formulation) for mucosal protection with acid suppression was shown to improve symptoms and quality of life in patients with nonerosive reflux disease. This drug has not been evaluated in veterinary patients.

Additional Drugs and Other Therapies
- Antibiotics are indicated with aspiration pneumonia, to prevent bacterial colonization with severe esophageal ulceration, and with esophageal perforation.
- Analgesics may be needed to manage esophageal pain, especially in more severe cases. Lidocaine solution (2.0 mg/kg PO q 4–6 h) can be used for local analgesia and tramadol 2–5 mg/kg PO q 8–12 h as an oral analgesic.
- Antiinflammatory dosage of corticosteroids (e.g., prednisone 0.5–1 mg/kg PO per day or divided q 12 h) may decrease fibrosis and esophageal stricture formation in severe cases, although this is controversial and efficacy has not been supported by the literature. Avoid corticosteroids when there is evidence of aspiration pneumonia. Budesonide oral suspension has been reported to be effective in humans with eosinophilic esophagitis and results in improvement in symptomatic, endoscopic, and histologic parameters. Budesonide has not been evaluated for the treatment of esophagitis in veterinary patients.
- Intravenous fluids to maintain hydration in more severe cases.
- Medications may need to be given parenterally during hospitalization.
- Oxygen therapy may be necessary in patients with severe aspiration pneumonia.

Precautions/Interactions
Sucralfate may interfere with gastrointestinal absorption of other drugs so it should be given separately from other medications by 2 h if possible.

Alternative Drug(s)
- Narcotic analgesics including buprenorphine, methadone, and fentanyl may be necessary in severe cases of painful esophagitis.
- Ranitidine 2.0 mg/kg PO q 12 h, nizatidine 2.5–5.0 mg/kg PO q 24 h and erythromycin 0.5–1.0 mg/kg PO, IV have GI prokinetic effects and may be alternative or additive drugs.

Appropriate Health Care

Mildly affected animals can be managed as outpatients while those with more severe esophagitis (persistent regurgitation, dehydration) and complications (aspiration pneumonia) may require hospitalization.

Nursing Care

- Upright or elevated feeding will be of benefit when there is regurgitation associated with abnormal esophageal motility secondary to esophagitis.
- Coupage and nebulization are provided for patients with aspiration pneumonia.

Diet

- With severe esophagitis, food and water are withheld until regurgitation is resolved and severe cases may require gastrostomy tube feedings or, rarely, total parenteral nutrition.
- Feed multiple small meals of a highly digestible, low-residue diet with a soft or gruel consistency. Hill's Prescription Diet i/d™, Purina EN Gastroenteric®, and Royal Canin Gastrointestinal Moderate Calorie® are good choices.

Surgical Considerations

- Percutaneous endoscopic gastrostomy (PEG) tube or surgical gastrostomy tube placement is indicated in severe cases.
- Surgical correction for HH is pursued when medical management for GER is not effective.
- Esophageal surgery poses challenges due to anatomic location and healing potential and is not commonly performed. Surgery may be necessary for large perforations, some difficult esophageal foreign bodies, esophageal neoplasia or stricture resection.

    COMMENTS

Client Education

- Discuss the need to restrict food intake in patients with severe esophagitis. Advise upright or elevated feeding when there is esophageal dysmotility.
- Discuss potential complications, including aspiration pneumonia, esophageal stricture, esophageal dysmotility, and, rarely, esophageal perforation.

Patient Monitoring

- Patients with mild esophagitis usually do not require follow-up and tracking of clinical signs is sufficient.
- Consider follow-up endoscopy in patients with ulcerative esophagitis and those at risk for esophageal stricture.

Prevention/Avoidance

- Consider two doses of omeprazole 1 mg/kg PO or famotidine 1 mg/kg PO given 12–24 h and 1–4 h prior to anesthesia and surgery, especially in patients at higher risk (those with GI disease, brachycephalic breeds or patients with known GER) to reduce gastric acidity.
- Giving a prokinetic drug (cisapride 1 mg/kg; metoclopramide 0.2–1.0 mg/kg PO, SQ) with an acid suppressor may also help reduce GER during anesthesia and surgery.
- Maropitant citrate is shown to reduce nausea and vomiting post hydromorphone administration and is useful to prevent vomiting and regurgitation associated with opioid premedications and anesthesia.

- If GER is the cause of esophagitis, owners should avoid late-night feedings which tend to diminish LES pressure during sleep.
- Proper patient preanesthetic fasting decreases the risk of GER. Withholding of water for 4–8 h and food for 8–12 h prior to anesthesia is recommended.
- Follow oral administration of capsules and tablets with a 5–10 mL bolus of water (especially for doxycycline) or give with a meal or treat such as a pill pocket to hasten esophageal transit of pills to the stomach. Coating pills with butter or applying Nutri-Cal® to the nose to stimulate licking after administration of tablets may also be effective.

Possible Complications

- Esophageal stricture formation.
- Aspiration pneumonia.
- Chronic reflux esophagitis.
- Permanent esophageal dysmotility.
- Chronic cough due to laryngopharyngeal aspiration or tracheal microaspiration.
- Esophageal perforation (rare).
- Barrett's esophagus (rare complication of chronic reflux esophagitis reported in cats).
- H_2RAs, PPIs, and glucocorticoids should all be used with caution during pregnancy.

Expected Course and Prognosis

- Best results when treated with gastric acid suppression, a GI prokinetic, and possibly a mucosal protectant.
- Mild esophagitis – good to excellent prognosis.
- Severe or ulcerative esophagitis – greater potential for complications which warrants a more guarded to poor prognosis.
- Complete recovery can be expected especially when treated before serious complications develop.

Abbreviations

- CRI = constant rate infusion
- CT = computed tomography
- GER = gastroesophageal reflux
- GERD = gastroesophageal reflux disease
- GI = gastrointestinal
- HH = hiatal hernia
- H_2RA = H2-receptor antagonist

- LES = lower esophageal sphincter
- NSAID = nonsteroidal antiinflammatory drug
- PEG = percutaneous endoscopic gastrostomy
- PO = *per os*, by mouth or orally
- PPI = proton pump inhibitor

See Also

- Esophageal Diverticula
- Esophageal Foreign Bodies
- Esophageal Stricture
- Hiatal Hernia
- Megaesophagus

- Nutritional Approach to Gastroesophageal Reflux and Megaesophagus
- Ptyalism
- Regurgitation

Suggested Reading

Garcia RS, Belafsky PC, DellaMaggiore A, et al. Prevalence of gastroesophageal reflux in cats during anesthesia and effect of omeprazole on gastric pH. J Vet Intern Med 2017;31(3):734–742.

Glazer A, Walters PC. Esophagitis and esophageal strictures. Compend Contin Educ Pract Vet 2008;30(5):281–292.

Hay Kraus BL. Effect of dosing interval on efficacy of maropitant for prevention of hydromorphone-induced vomiting and signs of nausea in dogs. J Am Vet Med Assoc 2014;245(9):1015–1020.

Hwang JH, Jeong J-W, Song G-H, Koo TS, et al. Pharmacokinetics and acid suppressant efficacy of esomeprazole after intravenous, oral, and subcutaneous administration to healthy beagle dogs. J Vet Intern Med 2017;31(3):743–750.

Jergens AE. Diseases of the esophagus. In: Ettinger SJ, Feldman EC, eds. Textbook of Veterinary Internal Medicine, 7th ed. St Louis: Elsevier, 2010, pp. 1487–1499.

Kempf J, Lewis F, Reusch CE, Kook PH. High-resolution manometric evaluation of the effects of cisapride and metoclopramide hydrochloride administered orally on lower esophageal sphincter pressure in awake dogs. Am J Vet Res 2014;75(4):361–366.

Kook PH. Gastroesophageal reflux. In: Bonagura JD, Twedt DC, eds. Current Veterinary Therapy XV, 15th ed. St Louis: Elsevier, 2014, pp. 501–504.

Marks SL, Kook PH, Papich MG, et al. ACVIM consensus statement: Support for rational administration of gastrointestinal protectants to dogs and cats. J Vet Intern Med 2018;32:1823–1840.

Parkinson S, Tolbert K, Messenger K, et al. Evaluation of the effect of orally administered acid suppressants on intragastric pH in cats. J Vet Intern Med 2015;29:104–112.

Poncet CM, Dupre GP, Freiche VG, et al. Prevalence of gastrointestinal tract lesions in 73 brachycephalic dogs with upper respiratory syndrome. J Small Anim Pract 2005;46(6): 273–279.

Poncet CM, Dupre GP, Freiche VG, et al. Long-term results of upper respiratory syndrome surgery and gastrointestinal tract medical treatment in 51 brachycephalic dogs. J Small Anim Pract 2006;47(3):137–142.

Tolbert K, Bissett S, King A, et al. Efficacy of oral famotidine and 2 omeprazole formulations for the control of intragastric pH in dogs. J Vet Intern Med 2011;25:47–54.

Tolbert K, Graham A, Odunayo A, et al. Repeated famotidine administration results in a diminished effect on intragastric pH in dogs. J Vet Intern Med 2016;31(1):117–123.

Tolbert K, Odunayo A, Howell RS, et al. Efficacy of intravenous administration of combined acid suppressants in healthy dogs. J Vet Intern Med 2015;29:556–560.

Willard MD, Carsten E. Esophagitis. In: Bonagura JD, Twedt DC, eds. Current Veterinary Therapy XIV, 14th ed. St Louis: Elsevier, 2009, pp. 482–486.

Zacuto AC, Marks SL, Osborn J, et al. The influence of esomeprazole and cisapride on gastroesophageal reflux during anesthesia in dogs. J Vet Intern Med 2012;26:518–525.

Author: Steve Hill DVM, MS, DACVIM (SAIM)

Chapter 34

Hiatal Hernia

DEFINITION/OVERVIEW

- Hiatal herniation – when abdominal contents (most commonly the stomach) herniate cranial to the diaphragm into the thorax through the esophageal hiatus.

ETIOLOGY/PATHOPHYSIOLOGY

- Generally caused by congenital abnormalities of the esophageal hiatus.
- The esophageal hiatus is formed by musculature of the medial portion of the lumbar crus of the diaphragm.
- Four types of hernia have been described (Figure 34.1).
  - Type I (sliding hiatal hernia (SHH); most common).
  - Type II (paraesophageal hiatal hernia).
  - Type III (includes elements of both types I and II).
  - Type IV (herniation of organs other than the stomach).
- Acquired hiatal hernias have also been reported, and are most commonly associated with severe upper respiratory disease (brachycephalic syndrome, laryngeal paralysis).
- Dogs with upper airway obstructive disease are hypothesized to experience a decrease in intrapleural and intraesophageal pressure, causing the distal esophagus and parts of the stomach to be pulled into the thorax during inspiration.

Systems Affected

- Gastrointestinal.
- Pulmonary – with aspiration pneumonia.

SIGNALMENT/HISTORY

- Mainly occurs in dogs but has been reported in cats.
- English bulldogs and shar-peis appear to be predisposed.
- Type I HH is commonly congenital and therefore seen in younger animals.
- Most symptomatic animals will have clinical signs present before they reach one year of age.

Clinical Signs

- Regurgitation.
- Inability to gain weight.
- Weight loss.
- Vomiting.

Blackwell's Five-Minute Veterinary Consult Clinical Companion: Small Animal Gastrointestinal Diseases, First Edition. Edited by Jocelyn Mott and Jo Ann Morrison.
© 2019 John Wiley & Sons, Inc. Published 2019 by John Wiley & Sons, Inc.
Companion website: www.fiveminutevet.com/gastrointestinal

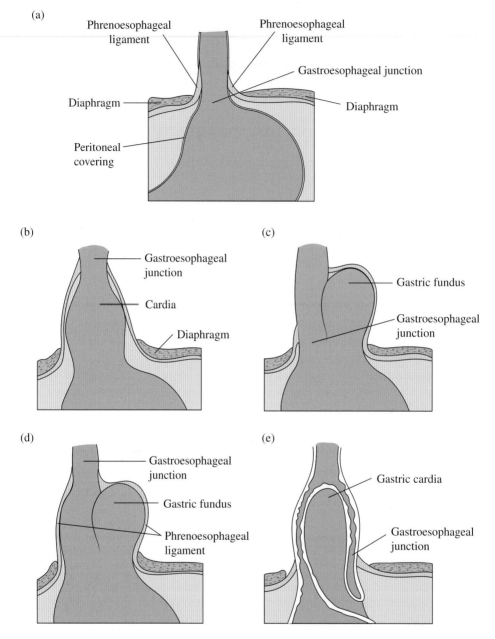

Fig. 34.1. (a) Normal anatomy. (b) Type I sliding hiatal hernia (most common). (c) Type II paraesophageal hiatal hernia. (d) Type III: combination of types I and II. (e) Gastroesophageal intussusception. Source: Fossum T. Small Animal Surgery, 3rd ed. © 2007 Mosby/Elsevier.

- Respiratory distress.
- Dysphagia.
- Hypersalivation.
- Anorexia.
- Most clinical signs are secondary to esophagitis and subsequent esophageal dysmotility.
- In very young animals (between two and four months), clinical signs often coincide with weaning.

Risk Factors

- Congenital – breed predisposition; brachycephalic breeds, shar-pei.
- Acquired – generally type I HH are described as a result of severe upper respiratory disease: brachycephalic airway syndrome, laryngeal paralysis.

Historical Findings

- Many cases are asymptomatic.
- Most reported clinical signs are related to esophagitis.
- Owners may report frequent regurgitation which is often misinterpreted as vomiting, hence the importance of a comprehensive history.
- Some dogs present with recurrent episodes of aspiration pneumonia.

 # CLINICAL FEATURES

- Physical exams are generally unremarkable unless the patient has developed aspiration pneumonia. In dogs with aspiration pneumonia, lung sounds can vary from being unremarkable to harsh or loud. Adventitious lung sounds (crackles or wheezes) or quieter lung sounds can be detected in approximately 25% and 12% of affected dogs, respectively.
- Weight loss can be noted in chronic or severe cases.

 # DIFFERENTIAL DIAGNOSIS

- Must distinguish from other causes of regurgitation. Esophageal neoplasia, extraluminal masses, vascular ring anomalies, esophageal intussusception, esophageal diverticulum, esophageal foreign body, and megaesophagus are all possible causes of regurgitation.
- Do not confuse hiatal hernias with peritoneopericardial or traumatic diaphragmatic hernias despite occasionally having similar appearances on thoracic radiographs.

 # DIAGNOSTICS

Complete Blood Count/Biochemistry/Urinalysis

- Generally unremarkable; survey of overall patient health may find inflammatory leukogram secondary to aspiration pneumonia, if present.

Imaging

Thoracic Radiography (Figure 34.2)

- May note cranial displacement of stomach, soft tissue mass in the caudal thorax adjacent to diaphragm, and/or gas-filled viscera in thorax.
- Hiatal hernia is infrequently diagnosed on survey thoracic radiographs alone.

Positive Contrast Esophagram

- Preferably performed using videofluoroscopy.
- Helps to confirm the diagnosis and differentiate between types I and II hiatal hernias.
- Can also diagnose associated gastroesophageal reflux (GER) and esophageal dysmotility.
- False-negative studies are common due to the highly intermittent and dynamic nature of hiatal herniation. Repeating the videofluoroscopic swallow study several days later can be helpful in cases in which the initial study was negative for SHH.

Fluoroscopy

- Beneficial when the displacement is intermittent.
- Can also demonstrate esophageal dysmotility and GER.
- Compression of the abdomen during fluoroscopy may help to identify a hernia, although this procedure is generally unrewarding.

Diagnostic Procedures

- Esophagoscopy – can document mild to severe reflux esophagitis, GER, and the presence of strictures.
- Herniation can occasionally be seen during esophagoscopy facilitated by completion of a J-maneuver to directly visualize the lower esophageal sphincter (LES) and gastroesophageal juncture (GEJ).

 # THERAPEUTICS

- Not all dogs that have radiographic evidence require treatment. Conservative therapy with a fat-restricted diet to facilitate enhanced gastric emptying can be successful in controlling clinical signs in dogs with mild hiatal herniation.
- Not all patients require surgical intervention.
- Dogs with mild or infrequent herniation can often be managed as an outpatient unless the animal has severe aspiration pneumonia.
- Goals.
    - Reduce gastric acid secretion (proton pump inhibitors are vastly superior to H2-receptor antagonists).
    - Increase rate of gastric emptying and increase LES sphincter tone (prokinetic agents such as cisapride are superior to metoclopramide).
    - Provide esophageal mucosal protection (sucralfate).

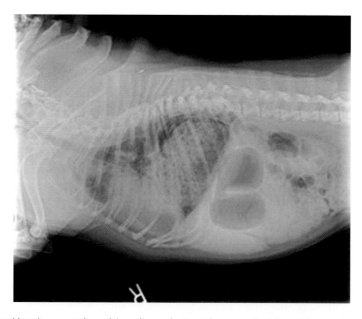

■ **Fig. 34.2.** Hiatal hernia captured on plain radiograph. Note the stomach visible within the thoracic cavity

- Feed a fat-restricted diet in an elevated position in small frequent portions (3–4 times daily).
- Thirty-day trial of medical management (see drug options below) before surgery often recommended; not all patients require surgery.

Drug(s) of Choice

- Acid suppressants help to neutralize gastric pH and therefore reduce esophagitis secondary to strong acid reflux events (pH <4.0). Avoid use of H2-receptor antagonists due to their inferior acid suppression effects compared to proton pump inhibitors (PPIs), and their decreased efficacy in dogs following repeated administration over several weeks due to tolerance. PPIs should be administered every 12 h instead of every 24 h in dogs and cats to maximize the effect of the drug.

Proton Pump Inhibitors

- Omeprazole 1.0–1.5 mg/kg q 12 h PO (dogs and cats).
- Pantoprazole 1.0–1.5 mg/kg q 12 h IV.
- The PPIs should be administered 30–60 min before a meal, and should be gradually tapered over 3–4 weeks when discontinued to avoid an acid rebound hypersecretion phenomenon.

Prokinetics

- Increase gastric emptying and increase LES sphincter tone.
- Cisapride 0.5–1.0 mg/kg q 8–12 h PO (dogs). Cisapride is vastly superior to metoclopramide for enhancing gastric emptying and increasing LES sphincter tone.
- Metoclopramide 0.2–0.5 mg/kg q 6–8 h PO, SQ, or IV (bolus injection) or 1–2 mg/kg/24 h as a CRI (the CRI administration method is superior to other administration options due to the short half-life of the drug in dogs – 90 min).

Mucosal Protectants

Sucralfate suspension (1 g/10 mL) or tablets (1 g). Dose for small dogs and cats: 0.25–0.5 g PO q 6–8 h; dose for medium to large dogs: 0.5–1.0 g PO q 6–8 h.

Precautions/Interactions

- Drugs that increase gastric pH can interfere with absorption of azole antifungal drugs (ketoconazole, itraconazole, posaconazole).
- Di- and trivalent cations ($AlOH_3$, $MgOH_3$) can interfere with drug absorption (fluoroquinolones, tetracyclines).
- Sucralfate suspension (but not sucralfate tablets) can decrease absorption of orally administered doxycycline in dogs.
- Long-term administration of PPIs (>1 year) in humans has been associated with several adverse effects, including altered bone metabolism and pathologic fractures, hyomagnesemia and B12 deficiency, increased risk of *C. difficile* infection, and intestinal dysbiosis. No studies have been published assessing the long-term (>60 days) consequences of acid suppressant administration in dogs and cats to date.
- Sucralfate administration can be associated with constipation.
- Prokinetics can cause diarrhea.

Nursing Care

- If severe esophageal dysmotility is present, feeding the patient in an upright position to enhance gravity-assisted feeding may help reduce regurgitation.

Diet

Feed a highly digestible, fat-restricted diet.

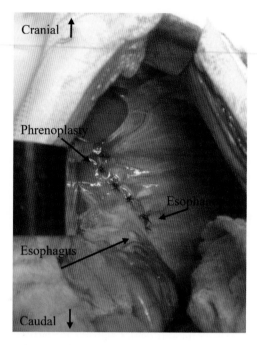

Cranial ↑

Phrenoplasty

Esoph

Esophagus

Caudal ↓

■ **Fig. 34.3.** Surgical image of an esophagopexy. The hiatus has been closed (phrenoplasty) and an esophagopexy performed.

Activity

No specific recommendations for activity alteration for patients with this condition.

Surgical Considerations

- Patients nonresponsive to medical therapy.
- Treat with acid suppressants, sucralfate suspension, and prokinetics prior to surgery.
- Surgical procedures (used alone or in combination).
  - Phrenoplasty – diaphragmatic hiatal reduction.
  - Esophagopexy – attachment of the distal esophagus to the left diaphragmatic crus and crural muscle with absorbable or nonabsorbable suture (Figure 34.3).
  - Left-sided incisional gastropexy (Figure 34.4).

COMMENTS

Patient Monitoring

- Long-term medical therapy may be indicated in both surgically and conservatively managed patients.
- Postoperative – monitor for dyspnea, worsening regurgitation (may require second surgery), abdominal distension that could result from overtightening of the hiatus resulting in an inability to eructate.

Prevention/Avoidance

- Standard postoperative instructions are warranted for these patients.
- There are no actions that the owner can take to prevent or avoid recurrence of the condition.

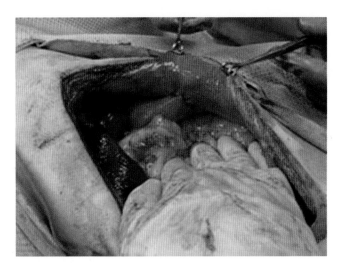

■ **Fig. 34.4.** Surgical image of left-sided gastropexy.

Possible Complications

- Persistent regurgitation, even with surgical correction.
- Worsening regurgitation from surgical overcorrection.
- Episodes of bloat (from overreduction of the hiatus).
- Initial improvements after surgical therapy are sometimes not durable, presumably associated with loosening of hiatal reconstruction over time.

Expected Course and Prognosis

- Overall prognosis is generally good.
- In many cases medical management is sufficient, and surgical intervention is not required.
- When medical management fails, surgical correction leads to a positive outcome in the majority of cases.

Abbreviations

- GEJ = gastroesophageal juncture
- GER = gastroesophageal reflux
- LES = lower esophageal sphincter
- PPI = proton pump inhibitors
- SHH = sliding hiatal hernia

Suggested Reading

Callan MB, Washabau RJ, Saunders HM, et al. Medical treatment versus surgery for hiatal hernias. J Am Vet Med Assoc 1998;213:800.

Guiot LP, Lansdowne JL, Rouppert P, et al. Hiatal hernia in the dog: a clinical report of four Chinese Shar-Peis. J Am Anim Hosp Assoc 2008;44:335–341.

Kogan DA, Johnson LR, Jandrey KE, et al. Clinical, clinicopathologic, and radiographic findings in dogs with aspiration pneumonia: 88 cases (2004–2006). J Am Vet Med Assoc 2008;233:1742–1747.

Lorinson D, Bright RM. Long-term outcome of medical and surgical treatment of hiatal hernias in dogs and cats: 27 cases (1978–1996). J Am Vet Med Assoc 1998;213:381–384.

Sivacolundhu RK, Read RA, Marchevsky AM. Hiatal hernia controversies: a review of pathophysiology and treatment options. Aust Vet J 2002;80:48–53.

Authors: Kathryn A. Pitt DVM, MS, Philipp D. Mayhew BVM&S, DACVS, Stanley L. Marks BVSc, DACVIM (SAIM, Oncology), DACVN, PhD

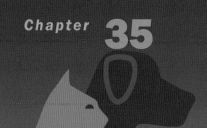
Megaesophagus

DEFINITION/OVERVIEW

Megaesophagus (ME) is a diffuse dilation, focal or generalized, of the esophagus characterized by decreased or absent motility of the esophagus.

ETIOLOGY/PATHOPHYSIOLOGY

- Esophageal contraction occurs in response to swallowing and esophageal dilation.
- Presence of food in the esophagus initiates primary peristalsis by stimulating afferent vagal receptors in the pharynx and proximal esophagus. These impulses are transmitted centrally to the nucleus ambiguous in the brainstem. Motor impulses then travel down the efferent neurons of the vagal nerve to stimulate striated muscle (canine) and smooth muscle (feline). Relaxation of the lower esophageal sphincter (LES) in advance allows passage of food into the stomach. The LES then closes to avoid reflux of gastric contents back into the esophagus.
- Congenital ME etiology.
  - Idiopathic.
  - Pathogenesis unclear but suspected to be due to defects in the vagal afferent innervation of the esophagus which fails to respond to the mechanical stimulus of introducing food, thus resulting in ineffective peristalsis.
- Acquired ME etiology.
  - Idiopathic (most common).
  - Neuromuscular disease.
    - Myasthenia gravis (MG) – MG (focal or generalized) is the most common (25% of all acquired ME cases).
    - Systemic lupus erythematosus, myopathy/myositis, dysautonomia (more common in cats), polyneuropathy (affecting the vagus nerve), botulism, glycogen storage diseases, muscular dystrophy, tetanus.
  - May be an association with laryngeal paralysis due to both diseases having a common pathogenesis involving the vagus nerve.
  - Gastrointestinal (GI).
    - Esophageal obstruction – neoplasia, parasitic granuloma (*Spirocerca lupi*), vascular ring anomaly, stricture, esophageal foreign body.
    - Esophagitis.
  - Endocrine – hypoadrenocorticism, hypothyroidism.
  - Hiatal disorders – hiatal hernia, gastroesophageal intussusception (more often a consequence of megaesophagus than a cause).

Blackwell's Five-Minute Veterinary Consult Clinical Companion: Small Animal Gastrointestinal Diseases,
First Edition. Edited by Jocelyn Mott and Jo Ann Morrison.
© 2019 John Wiley & Sons, Inc. Published 2019 by John Wiley & Sons, Inc.
Companion website: www.fiveminutevet.com/gastrointestinal

- Toxicity – lead, organophosphate.
- Distemper – due to demyelination.
- Thymoma is associated with megaesophagus in approximately 25% of cats.
- LES achalasia-like syndrome – the LES remains closed when swallowing is triggered.

Systems Affected

- Gastrointestinal – regurgitation, weight loss, dysphagia.
- Musculoskeletal – weakness, exercise intolerance.
- Neuromuscular – manifestations of systemic neuromuscular disease.
- Respiratory – aspiration pneumonia, coughing.

 ## SIGNALMENT/HISTORY

- Congenital.
  - Inherited in Parson Russell terriers, springer spaniels, and smooth fox terriers (autosomal recessive trait) which results in a deficiency or functional abnormality of acetylcholine receptors (AchRs) at the neuromuscular junction.
  - Inherited in the miniature schnauzer (autosomal dominant or autosomal recessive with partial penetrance).
  - Increased prevalence in Great Danes, German shepherds, Labrador retrievers, Newfoundlands, Irish setters, Irish wolfhounds and Chinese shar-peis, and Siamese cats.
  - Congenital MG in Jack Russell terriers.
- Acquired.
  - Idiopathic ME appears spontaneously in large-breed dogs 5–12 years old (no breed predisposition).
  - Many other systemic diseases may cause acquired megaesophagus which individually may have breed predispositions or genetic causes.

Risk Factors

- Gastroesophageal reflux may predispose to esophagitis.
- Esophageal foreign bodies may lead to esophageal strictures.
- Access to toxins (lead, thallium, anticholinesterase drugs, acrylamide).
- Parasitic infection (*Spirocerca lupi*) causing an esophageal granuloma and thus esophageal dilation proximal to the granuloma.

Historical Findings

- Regurgitation (vs vomiting from owner's perspective) – it is important to differentiate between regurgitation and vomiting.
- Ptyalism, dysphagia.
- Coughing and nasal discharge (with aspiration pneumonia).
- Musculoskeletal weakness (with neuromuscular disease).
- Weight loss despite a good appetite.

 ## CLINICAL FEATURES

- Physical exam may be normal.
- Coughing and nasal discharge with aspiration pneumonia.

- +/− Poor body condition with severe regurgitation.
- Occasionally ventral cervical swelling if distended esophagus is filled with ingesta.

 DIFFERENTIAL DIAGNOSIS

- Vomiting versus regurgitation.
  - Regurgitation typically has no or minimal abdominal component. Regurgitated material may be undigested food, foam, or mucus or a combination of all. No relation to time of eating is necessary.
  - Vomiting has an active abdominal effort. There may be digested ingesta as well as the presence of bile.
- Aerophagia from dyspnea or panting can lead to transient air-filled esophagus. In a patient with pneumonia, the esophageal dilation can be secondary to aerophagia. True megaesophagus is persistent despite resolution of the aerophagia. Demonstrating megaesophagus on repeat radiographs is required.

 DIAGNOSTICS

Complete Blood Count/Biochemistry/Urinalysis

- Often normal.
- May see a leukocytosis +/− left shift if aspiration pneumonia is present.
- Elevated creatine kinase (CK) may indicate myopathy.
- Electrolyte disturbances may be seen with Addison's disease.
- Changes in the red blood cells such as basophilic stippling could increase suspicion for lead poisoning.

Other Laboratory Tests

- Acetylcholine receptor antibody titer for MG. A negative titer does not rule out MG. The titer can be negative early on in the disease and thus testing should be repeated in 2–3 months.
- Baseline cortisol (adrenocorticotropic hormone (ACTH) stimulation if cortisol is <2 μg/dL) for Addison's disease.
- T4, free T4, TSH for hypothyroidism.
- Lead levels (blood and urine).
- Blood cholinesterase levels for organophosphate toxicity.
- Distemper titers.

Imaging

- Thoracic radiographs. Diffuse dilation of the esophagus.
- The esophagus can be filled with air, fluid, or ingesta.
- Serial radiographs are helpful in differentiating aerophagia from megaesophagus.
  - Focal dilation of the esophagus may be seen proximal to an esophageal stricture or mass.
  - Pulmonary infiltrates if aspiration pneumonia is present (Figures 35.1 and 35.2).
  - Tracheal deviation may be seen (ventral deviation on the lateral views and lateral deviation on the ventrodorsal view).
  - Presence of a mediastinal mass should increase suspicion for MG associated with a thymoma (Figure 35.3).
  - Hiatal hernias and esophageal masses may be seen.

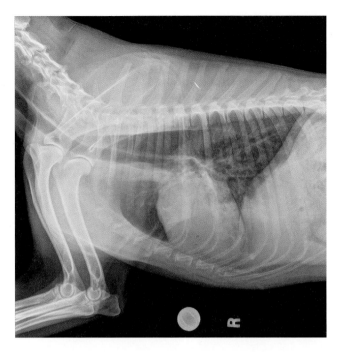

■ **Fig. 35.1.** Lateral thoracic radiograph showing megaesophagus and aspiration pneumonia.

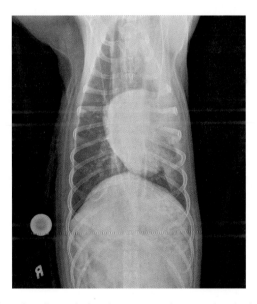

■ **Fig. 35.2.** Ventrodorsal thoracic radiograph showing megaesophagus and aspiration pneumonia.

■ Barium swallow/contrast esophagram.
  • Barium liquid or barium-soaked food may be fed to an animal to assess for esophageal dilation, decreased motility, and structural abnormalities (e.g., stricture or mass).
  • Videofluoroscopic swallow studies can be used to assess formation of a bolus and passage into the esophagus (dysphagia) and transit through the esophagus (assess for primary and secondary peristalsis).

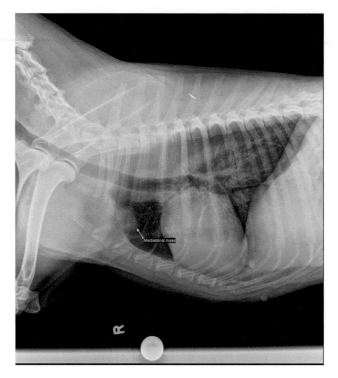

■ **Fig. 35.3.** Lateral thoracic radiograph showing a mediastinal mass and megaesophagus.

■ Newer work is being done with the development of trapezoidal holding chambers or kennels (patented) where the dogs are funneled into the narrow end of an enclosure. This allows the videofluouroscopic study to assess swallowing in an animal which is upright and minimally restrained to allow for assessment of normal swallowing behavior.

■ Dogs with megaesophagus are at high risk for aspiration pneumonia so any barium contrast study should be attempted with caution and animals should be closely monitored after the procedure.

Other Diagnostic Tests

■ Esophagoscopy.
  • Used to evaluate for strictures, masses, or other obstructive lesions.
  • Care should be taken during recovery from anesthesia due to increased risk of aspiration pneumonia.
■ Additional tests.
  • Electrophysiology in cases of suspected neuromuscular disease.
  • Muscle and nerve biopsy.
  • Magnetic resonance imaging for cases of suspected intracranial disease (+/− cerebrospinal fluid tap).
  • Fecal exam − *Spirocerca lupi*.

Pathologic Findings

■ No pathognomonic pathologic findings.
■ Secondary to any underlying etiology or the presence of complicating factors.

THERAPEUTICS

There are two main goals in management of megaesophagus dogs. The first is to identify and treat any underlying causes. Treatment of the underlying cause may resolve the megaesophagus but it is most likely that the megaesophagus will not resolve. The second is to try to decrease the amount of regurgitation and thus hope to decrease the incidence of aspiration pneumonia and allow appropriate nutritional intake.

Drug(s) of Choice

- Antibiotics if aspiration pneumonia is present.
  - Ideally, the choice of antibiotic should be made based on culture and sensitivity of a transtracheal wash or bronchoalveolar lavage.
  - After repeated episodes of aspiration pneumonia, the risk of antibiotic-resistant organisms increases.
- Acid blockers to treat or reduce the incidence of esophagitis. Omeprazole is a proton pump inhibitor which has been shown to have superior acid blocking in comparison to H2-blockers (famotidine, raniditine, cimetidine). 1 mg/kg PO orally q 12 h.
- Prokinetic use is controversial.
  - Pro – tightens lower esophageal sphincter to help reduce gastroesophageal reflux and thus esophagitis.
  - Con – tightens lower esophageal sphincter which could possibly increase the risk of aspiration pneumonia.
  - Metoclopramide 0.2–0.4 mg PO q 3 h 30 minutes before meals.
  - Cisapride (0.1 mg/kg PO q 8–12 h).
  - May also help in cats with dysmotility affecting the smooth muscle in the distal third of the esophagus.
- LES achalasia-like syndrome – current research into the use of ballooning catheters and botox therapy at the LES.
- Therapy for underlying etiology.
  - Pyridostigmine.
  - Immunosuppression (mycophenylate, prednisone).
  - Myasthenia gravis, which is an immune-mediated disease, and the use of immunosuppressives is indicated for cases of MG without megaesophagus. In MG dogs with megaesophagus, the use of immunosuppressives can be problematic due to the increased risk of aspiration pneumonia.
- Hypothyroidism – levothyroxine.
- Addison's disease – prednisone, +/– desoxycorticosterone pivalate (DOCP) or fludricortisone.
- Congenital idiopathic megaesophagus – sildenafil use has been shown to improve clinical signs and radiographic features. Sildenafil is a phosphodiesterase-type 5 (PDE-5) inhibitor which relaxes smooth muscle. Its use is based on the premise that a decreased LES tone would facilitate the entry of ingesta into the stomach.

Precautions/Interactions

- Oral medications may not be consistently well absorbed if regurgitation prevents their entry into the stomach.
- Injectable forms may be preferable in cases of severe regurgitation.
- Use caution with immunosuppression due to risk of aspiration pneumonia.

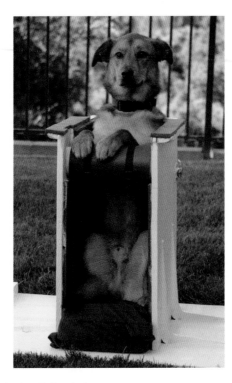

■ **Fig. 35.4.** Photograph of a dog in a Bailey chair.

Appropriate Health Care

- Treatment of underlying etiology when applicable.
- Feeding techniques to help decrease regurgitation which will help decrease the incidence of aspiration pneumonia and allow the animal to receive adequate nutrition.
- Feeding and drinking should be done in an elevated position (45–90° from the floor) and the animals should remain upright for 15–20 minutes after feeding.
- A Bailey chair may be constructed which can help the animal to comfortably remain upright (Figure 35.4).
- If adequate nutrition cannot be attained through upright feedings, placement of a gastrostomy tube should be considered. It is important to educate clients that this will not remove the risk of aspiration pneumonia as these dogs will still regurgitate foam and saliva.
- Placement of esophagoscopy tubes for suction of esophageal contents may also be helpful for dogs with persistent regurgitation.

Nursing Care

- Oxygen supplementation, IV)fluids, and IV antibiotics may be required for dogs with aspiration pneumonia.
- Recumbent care for animals which are not mobile. Maintaining these animals in sternal recumbency can help decrease aspiration.

Diet

- Liquid vs "meatballs" vs slurries. Different megaesophagus dogs respond to different consistencies. Owners should be encouraged to experiment.

- Calculate the nutritional requirement to make sure that the diet fed contains an adequate caloric content.

Surgical Considerations

- Surgery is indicated for thymomas, vascular ring anomalies, and some obstructive lesions or foreign bodies.
- Balloon dilation or stent placement can be attempted for esophageal strictures.

 COMMENTS

Megaesophagus is most commonly not a condition which is cured. It requires much time and patience on the owner's part and recurrent episodes of aspiration pneumonia are mentally and fiscally challenging.

Client Education

- Clients should be educated on the importance of upright feedings regardless of whether or not they are witnessing regurgitation. Some regurgitation is immediately swallowed and not perceived by the owner.
- There is a Yahoo list serve which can be very helpful in providing clients with emotional support from other megaesophagus owners.
- Bailey chair – can be built (better to be fit to the dog) or can be purchased prebuilt.

Patient Monitoring

- Repeat thoracic radiographs if clinical signs or auscultation raise suspicion for aspiration pneumonia.
- Repeat acetylcholine receptor antibody titers to monitor treatment of myasthenia. Spontaneous remission may occur in MG, usually within the first six months. Megaesophagus may persist despite achievement of remission.
- Congenital megaesophagus may have spontaneous remission so serial thoracic radiographs should be performed.
- Patients should be seen regularly to check their weight. Weight loss due to inadequate nutritional intake is a concern in regurgitating patients.
- Weight loss secondary to inadequate nutritional intake.
- Owners need to be educated on the amount of work required to take care of a megaesophagus dog and the potential financial investment.
- While the prognosis is generally reported to be poor, many dogs can be maintained and have a good quality of life with proper home care.

Prevention/Avoidance

- The use of bully sticks, rawhides, and other chewing items should be avoided as they are common causes of esophageal foreign bodies.
- Rapid removal of an esophageal foreign body can help to decrease the incidence of esophageal stricture.
- Preventive deworming to avoid *Spirocerca lupi* in endemic areas.

Possible Complications

- Aspiration pneumonia.
- Weight loss.
- Others will depend on etiology.

Expected Course and Prognosis

- Congenital cases have a guarded prognosis.
- Prognosis for acquired megaesophagus depends on underlying etiology.
- Prognosis for adult-onset, idiopathic megaesophagus is poor.
- Repeated episodes of aspiration pneumonia.

Synonyms

- Esophageal dilation
- Esophageal aperistalsis

Abbreviations

- AchR = acetylcholine receptor
- ACTH = adrenocorticotropic hormone
- ALP = alkaline phosphatase
- ALT = alanine aminotransferase
- AP = aspiration pneumonia
- CNS = central nervous system
- DOCP = desoxycorticosterone pivalate
- GI = gastrointestinal
- IV = intravenous
- LES = lower esophageal sphincter
- ME = megaesophagus
- MG = myasthenia gravis
- PDE-5 = phosphodiesterase type 5.

See Also

- Cricopharyngeal Achalasia
- Dysphagia
- Esophageal Foreign Bodies
- Esophageal Neoplasia
- Esophageal Stricture
- Esophagitis
- Hiatal Hernia
- Regurgitation
- Nutritional Approach to Gastroesophageal Reflux Disease
- *Spirocerca lupi*

Suggested Reading

Johnson B, Denovo R, Mears E. Canine megaesophagus. In: Bonagura JD, Twedt DC, eds. Current Veterinary Therapy XV, 15th ed. St Louis: Elsevier, 2014, web chapter 47.

Mace S, Shelton GD, Eddlestone S. Megaesophagus. Compend Contin Educ Vet 2012;34 (2):E1.

McBrearty A, Ramsey I, Courcier E, Mellor D. Clinical factors associated with death before discharge and overall survival time in dogs with generalized megaesophagus. JAVMA 2011;238(12):1622–1628.

Acknowledgments: The author and editors acknowledge the prior contribution of Dr Marguerite F. Knipe and Dr Stanley L. Marks

Author: Emilie Chaplow VMD, DACVIM

Nutritional Approach to Gastroesophageal Reflux Disease and Megaesophagus

Chapter **36**

Gastroesophageal reflux disease (GERD) is a condition in which there is reflux of gastric or intestinal fluid into the lumen of the esophagus. Gastroesophageal reflux (GER) occurs as a result of relaxation or decreased pressure of the lower esophageal sphincter (LES), which lies at the level of the diaphragm. The LES, in a healthy normal animal, maintains an area of high pressure between the stomach and esophagus which aids in unidirectional flow of food material and liquid from the esophagus into the stomach.

There are a number of factors that can contribute to impaired function of the LES including anesthetic agents, prolonged fasting, intraabdominal surgical procedures, as well as structural abnormalities such as a hiatal hernia. The fluid that is regurgitated can contain gastric acid, pepsin, bicarbonate, trypsin, and bile salts which can damage the mucosa of the esophagus with prolonged or repetitive contact, potentially leading to esophagitis. In severe cases, this can lead to severe ulceration or esophageal stricture. Another common medical complication that is secondary to GER is aspiration pneumonia. Treatment of this condition is therefore important to minimize damage to the esophageal mucosa and to minimize the risk of aspiration pneumonia.

Nutritional management of GERD is an integral part of the treatment plan. Animals with this condition can be malnourished and polyphagic because they are not passing enough food material through the stomach, and thus not digesting and absorbing sufficient nutrients to meet their nutritional requirements. The goals of nutritional management are to minimize regurgitation episodes, avoid secondary pneumonia and provide adequate nutrition to regain or maintain ideal body weight and condition. Treatment of GERD can also involve antacid therapy and use of prokinetic agents.

MAIN CONSIDERATIONS

Animals with GERD require a complete and balanced diet and benefit from energy-dense foods (Table 36.1). Feeding animals with GERD can be challenging and the goals of dietary management are to provide them with their nutritional requirements, which will allow them to maintain ideal body condition or regain body condition if malnourished, as well as to minimize frequency of regurgitation. An energy-dense diet allows for the animal to receive its total daily caloric requirement in a smaller volume of food, resulting in fewer total episodes and smaller volumes of regurgitation.

Protein

Dietary protein has a stimulatory effect on gastrin and gastric acid secretion. This effect causes an increase in lower esophageal sphincter pressure and this increase in pressure can reduce incidences of reflux. It is therefore recommended to feed a diet adequate in protein (>25% for dogs and >35% for cats) to animals with GERD.

Blackwell's Five-Minute Veterinary Consult Clinical Companion: Small Animal Gastrointestinal Diseases, First Edition. Edited by Jocelyn Mott and Jo Ann Morrison.
© 2019 John Wiley & Sons, Inc. Published 2019 by John Wiley & Sons, Inc.
Companion website: www.fiveminutevet.com/gastrointestinal

TABLE 36.1. Recommended components for nutritional support in GERD/megaesophagus.

Key nutritional factor	Requirement	Cats (DM basis)	Dogs (DM basis)
Energy density	High	>4200 kcal/kg	>4000 kcal/kg
Protein	Adequate	>35%	>25%
Fat*	High	>20%	>15%
Crude fiber	Low	<5%	<5%

*Moderate fat is recommended if regurgitation persists: dog <15%, cat <20%.
DM, dry matter.

Fat

The ideal dietary fat levels to feed an animal with GERD vary with the individual. Research showed that high dietary fat delays gastric emptying and reduces LES pressure which promotes gastroesophageal reflux (Davenport et al. 2010). Therefore, historically, moderate-fat diets, <20% for cats and <15% for dogs, have been recommended for animals with GERD for this reason. However, Pehl et al. (1999, 2001), demonstrated that in human patients fed either a high-fat, calorie-dense meal or a low-fat, low-calorie meal, there was no difference in changes to LES pressure or to the frequency of regurgitation episodes. This supports the idea that the fat content of the diet is not a primary factor that should be considered when initially assessing the diet and making recommendations for animal patients with GERD.

Factors that contribute to loss of LES pressure more significantly appear to be volume and rate of food intake. Therefore, if a smaller volume is fed slowly, a reduction in frequency and volume of regurgitation can be noted. The volume of food fed can be decreased by increasing the energy density of the diet, which is directly correlated with dietary fat content. Smaller volumes of a high-fat diet could be fed to meet the total daily caloric requirement of an animal with GERD, minimizing regurgitation episodes. Again, there may be individual variation to the dietary fat content that is best tolerated by each animal so a period of trial and error may be involved to find the most suitable dietary fat level. Initiating a trial with a high-fat diet to allow for smaller total volumes of food may be ideal and if regurgitation remains uncontrolled, switching to a moderate-fat diet may be indicated, bearing in mind that this will change the energy density of the diet and therefore the amount to be fed.

Fiber

Diets with very little fiber should be selected for animals with GERD in order to maximize energy density. Crude fiber content should be 5% or less on a dry matter basis.

FEEDING RECOMMENDATIONS

Assess the food the animal is currently being fed and compare digestibility and nutrient levels to the recommended levels described above. If nutritional factors in the current food do not match the recommended levels, changing to a more appropriate food is indicated. Feeding an energy-dense, highly digestible, high-protein veterinary therapeutic diet will provide the animal with the nutrients it needs while minimizing frequency and amount of reflux. As discussed above, ideally a diet also high in fat is fed to increase energy density unless the high level of fat is not tolerated by the animal.

Along with selecting a diet with appropriate nutrient levels, it is important to consider the consistency of the food fed to animals with GERD. There is variation seen with respect to what consistency and texture type is best tolerated by the animal, so a period of trial and error may be involved in order to determine what is best for the individual animal. Gruel-type foods tend to be most tolerated overall due to gravity fill of the stomach caused by the liquid form of the food.

Animals with GERD need to be fed small volumes of food multiple times per day. Maintenance energy requirement should be calculated for each animal to determine daily volume of food to be fed. This amount should then be split into 3–4 meals per day, or more if the patient does not tolerate the volume. If the animal has an episode of regurgitation, the amount should be measured, recorded, and subtracted from the total calories fed to the animal to determine the amount that was actually ingested.

The animal should be fed in an upright position if possible and remain in that position for 20–30 minutes post-feeding to allow for flow of food from the esophagus to the stomach, using gravity as an aid. Examples of ways to achieve this include elevated food bowls, holding smaller animals after eating, or hand-feeding animals while they are sitting upright. If feeding the animal in this manner is not possible, or is not sufficiently controlling the reflux, placement of a gastrostomy or enterostomy tube can be considered. This will allow for bypass of the esophagus; regurgitation is still possible with this method of feeding but the chances of aspiration are reduced.

Animals should be closely monitored and adjustments may be made on amount, type, and consistency of food fed based on the animal's body weight and condition as well as frequency and volume of reflux.

MEGAESOPHAGUS

Megaesophagus is a motility disorder of the esophagus and can result from either sensory or motor pathway dysfunction. If the sensory pathway is affected, there will be no initiation of esophageal peristalsis in the presence of a food bolus. In contrast, when the motor pathway is affected, the presence of a food bolus is sensed but muscular contraction necessary for the peristaltic waves is prevented.

There are many causes of megaesophagus which can be either idiopathic, such as congenital megaesophagus or acquired megaesophagus caused by myasthenia gravis, or secondary to other neurologic disorders, endocrine disorders, or a toxicity. Clinical signs are usually regurgitation and a dilated cervical esophagus seen on radiographs. Other common signs include dyspnea, pyrexia, weight loss, and coughing. An important clinical sequela to megaesophagus is aspiration pneumonia, as with GERD.

Other than correction of the underlying cause, if one is present, there is no successful medical or surgical treatment for megaesophagus. Management of the condition is similar to the nutritional management of GERD. A highly energy-dense diet should be selected and the animal should be in an upright position while eating, and remain in that position for 15 minutes after eating. It is best to experiment with food consistency (liquid, gruel, canned food rolled into meatballs, kibble) to determine what is best tolerated by the individual animal because as with animals afflicted with GERD, this may differ between patients.

KEY POINTS

- Feed a diet with high energy density.
- Moderate dietary fat levels.
- High dietary protein levels.
- Multiple small meals.
- Patient kept upright for 20–30 minutes post-feeding.
- Placement of gastrostomy or enterostomy tube if unable to control regurgitation.

References

Davenport DJ, Leib MS, Remillard, RL. Pharyngeal and esophageal disorders. In: Hand MS, Thatcher CD, Remillard RL, Roudebush P, Novotny BJ, eds. Small Animal Clinical Nutrition, 5th ed. Topeka: Mark Morris Institute, 2010.

Pehl C, Waizenhoefer A, Wendl B, et al. Effect of low and high fat meals on lower esophageal sphincter motility and gastroesophageal reflux in healthy subjects. Am J Gastroenterol 1999;94(5):1192–1196.

Pehl C, Pfeiffer A, Waizenhoefer A, Wendl B, Schepp W. Effect of caloric density of a meal on lower oesophageal sphincter motility and gastro-oesophageal reflux in healthy subjects. Aliment Pharmacol Therapeut 2001;15(2):233–239.

Suggested Reading

Cave N. Nutritional management of gastrointestinal diseases. In: Fascetti, AJ, Delaney SJ, eds. Applied Veterinary Clinical Nutrition. Chichester: Wiley-Blackwell, 2012.

German A, Zentek J. The most common digestive diseases: the role of nutrition. In: Pibot P, Biourge, V, Elliot D, eds. Encyclopedia of Canine Clinical Nutrition. Paris: Aniwa SAS/Royal Canin, 2006.

Han E. Diagnosis and management of reflux esophagitis, Clin Techn Small Anim Pract 2003;18:231–238.

Jergens AE. Gastroesophageal reflux. In: Smith FWK, Tilley LP, eds. Blackwell's Five-Minute Veterinary Consult: Canine and Feline, 6th ed. Ames: Wiley-Blackwell, 2016.

Knipe MF, Marks SL. Megaesophagus. In: Smith FWK, Tilley LP, eds. Blackwell's Five-Minute Veterinary Consult: Canine and Feline, 6th ed. Ames: Wiley-Blackwell, 2016.

Authors: Caitlin Grant DVM, BSc, Sarah Dodd DVM, BSc, Adronie Verbrugghe DVM, PhD, Dip ECVCN

Chapter 37

Spirocerca lupi

DEFINITION/OVERVIEW

Spirocerca lupi (*S. lupi*) is a parasitic nematode in dogs distributed worldwide although most common in tropical and subtropical regions.

ETIOLOGY/PATHOPHYSIOLOGY

- Dogs ingest stage 3 larvae (L3) of *S. lupi* through consumption of intermediate hosts (coprophagous beetles) or paratenic hosts (wild birds, lizards, rodents, poultry, rabbits).
- The L3 larvae excyst and migrate from the stomach via the celiac artery to the abdominal aorta and then thoracic aorta where they mature to young adults (approximately three months).
- Migration causes scarring of artery walls which can lead to aneurysms, rupture, and death.
- The young adults then migrate to the esophagus, penetrate the esophagus and form nodules (visible 3–9 months after larval ingestion).
- Approximately 26% of these esophageal nodules can transform to neoplasia (sarcomas) with or without metastasis. Spirocercosis is a major cause of esophageal neoplasia in dogs.
- Lesions associated with *S. lupi* are due to migration (including aberrant migration) and persistence of larvae or adult worms in tissues.
- Migration to lungs, aorta, trachea, mediastinum, pleura, lymphatics, vertebral bodies, rectum, skin, heart, spinal cord, stomach, small intestines, and urinary system has been reported.
- *S. lupi* eggs with L1 larvae leave the nodules via an opercule and are shed in the feces or vomit of dogs.
- *S. lupi* eggs are ingested by intermediate hosts (coprophagous beetles) where they encyst in tissues to infective stage L3.
- Beetles are then ingested by dogs or paratenic hosts.

Systems Affected

- Gastrointestinal – esophageal nodules +/– neoplasia; secondary megaesophagus; nodules in cardia.
- Cardiovascular – aortic mineralization and aneurysms; thrombosis; aberrant migration to heart.
- Musculoskeletal – spondylitis of thoracic vertebrae. Hypertrophic osteopathy associated with esophageal sarcomas.
- Respiratory – aberrant migration to lungs and mediastinum. Cases of pyothorax related to *S. lupi* have been reported.

Blackwell's Five-Minute Veterinary Consult Clinical Companion: Small Animal Gastrointestinal Diseases,
First Edition. Edited by Jocelyn Mott and Jo Ann Morrison.
© 2019 John Wiley & Sons, Inc. Published 2019 by John Wiley & Sons, Inc.
Companion website: www.fiveminutevet.com/gastrointestinal

- Nervous – extraskeletal osteosarcoma metastasis to brain and spinal cord have been reported in a dog. Extradural and intradural spinal aberrant migration can occur.
- Renal/urologic – aberrant migration to kidneys and urinary bladder.
- Skin/exocrine – aberrant migration to skin.

 # SIGNALMENT/HISTORY

- Large breeds have been reported in some studies to be at higher risk of infection.
- No age or sex predilection.
- Spayed females with *S. lupi* may be predisposed to malignant transformation of esophageal nodules.

Risk Factors

- Tropical or subtropical endemic regions.
- Proximity to dung beetles and paratenic hosts.

Historical Findings

- Regurgitation.
- Pyrexia.
- Weakness.
- Cough/respiratory abnormalities/dyspnea.
- Anorexia.
- Weight loss.
- Dysphagia.
- Ptyalism.
- Odynophagia.
- Paraparesis.
- Melena.
- Sudden death.

 # CLINICAL FEATURES

- Cachexia/emaciation.
- Back pain.
- Sialoadenosis.
- Mild peripheral lymphadenopathy.
- Dyspnea.
- Paraparesis.

 # DIFFERENTIAL DIAGNOSIS

- Other diseases which cause regurgitation, including esophagitis, megaesophagus, and esophageal neoplasia.
- Respiratory diseases (can occur in conjunction with *S. lupi* or mimic the infection in the respiratory tract) such as pneumonia, pyothorax, mediastinitis, and neoplasia.
- Nervous system diseases such as intervertebral disc disease, discospondylitis, trauma or neoplasia.
- Cardiac disease, neoplasia, renal disease, hyperadrenocorticism, hypothyroidism, and gastric dilation-volvulus are other diseases that can cause aortic thromboembolism.

DIAGNOSTICS

Complete Blood Count/Biochemistry/Urinalysis

- Normocytic (+/− hypochromic) anemia.
- Leukocytosis often characterized by neutrophilia and monocytosis.
- Hypoalbuminemia +/− elevated creatine kinase (CK) may be present.

Other Laboratory Tests

- Fecal – *S. lupi* eggs are heavier than other helminths so flotation fluid should be a higher specific gravity and require special laboratory techniques. Shedding of eggs in feces may be intermittent and unpredictable.
- There are no currently available serological tests for *S. lupi*. There is serological cross-reactivity between *Dirofilaria immitis* (*D. immitis*) and *S. lupi*. This should be taken into consideration in regions where both parasites are prevalent.
- Molecular assays such as polymerase chain reaction on feces may increase ability to diagnose *S. lupi* cases earlier and monitor therapy in the future.

Imaging

Radiographs

- Caudal esophageal mass(es), scarring of caudal thoracic aorta with mineralization and aneurysms and spondylitis of the 6th–12th thoracic vertebrae.
- Silhouetting of thoracic aorta was found in 100% of dogs in one study in St Kitts.
- Hypertrophic osteopathy can be present with *S. lupi*-induced esophageal sarcomas.

Computed Tomography

- Aortic mineralization and aneurysms (often in caudal thorax); aortic thrombi; esophageal mass.

Additional Diagnostic Tests

- Visualization of esophageal nodules/masses by endoscopy is most sensitive test (Figure 37.1).
- Endoscopy biopsies often are mucosal and may or may not differentiate granuloma from neoplasia.

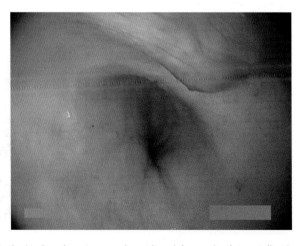

■ **Fig. 37.1.** *Spirocerca lupi*-induced canine esophageal nodule proximal to cardia. Source: Image courtesy of Dr Mike Willard.

- The use of fine needle aspirates of esophageal nodules to detect *S. lupi* eggs has been reported.

Pathologic Findings

- Gross – benign esophageal nodules are often small and smooth with nipple-like orifices; malignant esophageal nodules are often large, lobulated, cauliflower-like, ulcerated, and necrotic.
- Histopathology – lymphoplasmacytic inflammation characterizes the nodules with pockets of neutrophils around the eggs, worms, and migratory paths.

 THERAPEUTICS

Drug(s) of Choice

- Doramectin 0.5 mg/kg PO q 24 h for total of 42–126 days eliminates *S. lupi* nodules.
- Doramectin 400 μg/kg SQ q 14 days for six treatments and then q 30 days until resolution of esophageal nodules has also been reported.
- Imidacloprid 10%/moxidectin 2.5% weekly topical treatments for 19 weeks.

Precautions/Interactions

- Doramectin and ivermectin can be toxic in collies and other herding dogs. Toxicity is associated with mutation in multidrug-resistant (MDR)I gene. Dogs should be tested for the MDRI (also known as the ABCB1) gene mutation prior to treatment with doramectin.
- Doramectin use is off-label.
- Medetomidine should be avoided as it has been associated with a case of aortic rupture thought to be precipitated by the increase in peripheral vascular tone.

Alternative Drugs

- Ivermectin 600 μg/kg SQ twice a week combined with oral prednisone 0.25 mg/kg q 12 h then lowering dose every two weeks.
- Milbemycin oxime 0.5 mg/kg PO days 0, 7, and 28 then monthly (total of six times).

Appropriate Health Care

- Dehydrated patients may need to be hospitalized and treated with intravenous fluids.
- Secondary diseases such as esophagitis and aspiration pneumonia may need to be addressed as well.

Diet

- Regurgitation may limit the amount of nutrition the patient can retain.
- Gruel-like consistency diets may be better tolerated than dry kibble or canned diets.

Surgical Considerations

- Preferred approach for *S. lupi*-induced esophageal sarcomas is thoracotomy with partial esophagectomy.
- Transendoscopic esophageal mass ablation may be an alternative therapy in some cases .

 COMMENTS

The antemortem differentiation of benign and malignant *S. lupi*-induced esophageal tumors can be difficult.

Client Education

- Pets living in areas endemic for *S. lupi* should be on preventive medication.
- Benign canine spirocercosis can transform into malignancy.

Prevention/Avoidance

- Milbemycin oxime 0.5 mg/kg at 14–28-day intervals prevents establishment of *S. lupi* in esophagus; however, damage to the aorta is not prevented once L1 migration has occurred.
- Imidacloprid 10%/moxidectin 2.5% monthly for prevention.
- Remove dog feces.
- Prevent feco-oral transmission and preying on paratenic hosts.
- Control beetle population.

Possible Complications

- Esophageal neoplasia.
- Metastatic disease.
- Hypertrophic osteopathy.
- Aberrant migration to other organs.
- Acute hemothorax or hemoabdomen due to rupture of aortic aneurysms.
- Sudden death.

Expected Course and Prognosis

- Esophageal granulomas caused by *S. lupi* can be successfully treated.
- Esophageal nodules that have transformed to neoplasia carry a grave prognosis. Metastasis may occur.

Synonyms

- Dog esophageal worm

Abbreviations

- CK = creatine kinase
- MDR = multidrug resistant

See Also

- Dysphagia
- Esophageal Neoplasia
- Ptyalism
- Regurgitation

Suggested Reading

Aroch I, Rojas A, Slon P, et al. Serological cross-reactivity of three commercial in-house immunoassays for detection of *Dirofilaria immitis* antigens with *Spirocerca lupi* in dogs with benign esophageal spirocercosis. Vet Parasitol 2015 ;211:303–305.

Austin CM, Kok DJ, Crafford D, et al. The efficacy of a topically applied imidacloprid 10%/moxidectin 2.5% formulation (advocate®, Advantage® Multi, Bayer) against immature and adult *Spirocerca lupi* worms in experimentally infected dogs. Parasitol Res 2013;112:s91–s108.

Berry WL. *Spirocerca lupi* esophageal granulomas in 7 dogs: resolution after treatment with doramectin. J Vet Intern Med 2000;14:609–612.

Dvir E, Kirberger RM, Mukorera V, et al. Clinical differentiation between dogs with benign and malignant spirocercosis. Vet Parasitol 2008;155(1-2):80–88.

Kok, DJ, Schenker R, Archer NJ, et al. The efficacy of milbemycin oxime against pre adult *Spriocerca lupi* in experimentally infected dogs. Vet Parasitol 2011;177:111–118.

Le Sueur C, Bour S, Schaper R. Efficacy of a combination of imidacloprid 10%/moxidectin 2.5% spot on (Advocate® for dogs) in the prevention of canine spirocercosis (*Spirocerca lupi*). Parasitol Res 2010;107:1463–1469.

Lobetti R. Successful resolution of oesophageal spirocercosis in 20 dogs following daily treatment with oral doramectin. Vet J 2012;193(1):277–278.

Lobetti R. Follow-up survey of the prevalence, diagnosis, clinical manifestations and treatment of *Spirocerca lupi* in South Africa. J S Afr Vet Assoc 2014;85(1):e1–e7.

Mazaki-Tovi M, Baneth G, Aroch I, et al. Canine spirocercosis: clinical, diagnostic, pathologic, and epidemiologic characteristics. Vet Parasitol 2002;107(3):235–250.

Psader R, Balogh M, Papa K, et al. Occurrence of *Spirocerca lupi* infection in Hungarian dogs referred for gastroscopy. Parasitol Res 2017;116:s99–s108.

Van der Merwe LL, Kirberger RM, Clift S, et al. *Spirocerca lupi* infection in the dog: a review. Vet J 2008;176(3):294–309.

Author: Jocelyn Mott DVM, DACVIM (SAIM)

Chapter 38

Gastric and Intestinal Motility Disorders

DEFINITION/OVERVIEW

- Disruption of normal gastric and/or intestinal peristalsis leading to abnormal gastrointestinal (GI) retention or distension. Dysmotility may be primary or secondary in etiology (see below).
- Peristalsis may be defined as the involuntary, coordinated system of alternating GI wall contraction and relaxation resulting in the controlled, unidirectional movement of ingesta through the GI system, allowing for normal digestion and absorption of nutrients.

ETIOLOGY/PATHOPHYSIOLOGY

Normal GI Motility

- Normal GI motility occurs as a result of:
  - Neuronal and hormonal stimulations onto GI smooth muscle.
  - Osmoreceptors and chemoreceptors.
- Characteristics of ingesta:
  - Fats.
  - Proteins.
  - Carbohydrates.
  - Water.
  - Size.
  - Saliva and other gastric/intestinal secretions.
- Large, strong peristaltic contractions (sometimes referred to as "housekeeping contractions") called migrating myoelectric complexes (MMC) periodically travel through the GI tract. These MMCs function to prepare the GI tract for the next meal and occur primarily in the fasted state.
- The gastrocolic reflex begins with the oral intake of a meal and causes contraction of the large intestine to propel ingesta into the rectum, in anticipation of defecation. Allowing patients the opportunity to eliminate after eating helps facilitate normal GI motility.

Secondary GI Dysmotility

- Secondary dysmotility is the result of mechanical or functional lesions and represent the majority of cases.
  - Mechanical.
    - Obstructive lesions – foreign bodies, intussusceptions, neoplasia, etc.

Blackwell's Five-Minute Veterinary Consult Clinical Companion: Small Animal Gastrointestinal Diseases, First Edition. Edited by Jocelyn Mott and Jo Ann Morrison.
© 2019 John Wiley & Sons, Inc. Published 2019 by John Wiley & Sons, Inc.
Companion website: www.fiveminutevet.com/gastrointestinal

- Functional.
  - ○ Hypoadrenocorticism.
  - ○ Esophagitis.
  - ○ Acquired megaesophagus.
  - ○ Dysautonomia.

Primary GI Motility Disorders

Primary dysmotility is poorly understood and incompletely described. Most cases are idiopathic as an underlying etiology cannot be identified.

Systems Affected

- Gastrointestinal – depending on the etiology, differing portions of the GI tract may be affected.
  - Primary gastric lesions may predispose to gastroesophageal reflux disease (GERD).
  - Duodenal disease may lead to duodenogastric (biliary) reflux.
- Hemic/lymphatic/immune – prolonged dysmotility may lead to enterocyte atrophy and subsequent risk of bacterial translocation.
- Musculoskeletal – depending on the etiology, generalized weakness and loss of normal body condition and lean muscle mass may be seen.
- Nervous – with prolonged obstruction (e.g., constipation/obstipation), normal motility may be lost even with successful relief of obstruction.
- Renal/urologic – severe cases may have components of prerenal azotemia.

SIGNALMENT/HISTORY

- No breed or sex predilections are identified for primary motility disorders. Congenital diseases (e.g., congenital megaesophagus) are expected to be identified in younger patients and certain breeds are predisposed (e.g., wire-haired fox terrier).
- Most cases of primary GI dysmotility are expected to be found in older patients.

Risk Factors

Underlying genetic predispositions for primary disease have not been identified. Certain etiologies (i.e., dysautonomia) may have a toxic, infectious, or geographic etiology that has not been totally defined.

Historical Findings

- Owners may report changes in appetite, flatulence, and chronic vomiting (especially after eating), and may mistake regurgitation for vomiting.
- Additional signs may include tenesmus and constipation if the large intestine/colon is affected.
- Astute owners may notice nausea (ptyalism), pica, and borborygmus.

CLINICAL FEATURES

- Physical examination findings will depend upon the underlying etiology (if a secondary motility disorder is present) and severity and chronicity of disease.
- Abdominal distension and pain on abdominal palpation may be present.
- Decreased gut sounds on peritoneal auscultation.
- If motility disorder is due to intestinal mucosal disease, abnormal mucosa may be palpable on rectal examination.

- Loss of body condition and decreased muscle mass.
- Dehydration.
- Signs of aspiration pneumonia may be present in cases with protracted or severe vomiting or regurgitation.

 DIFFERENTIAL DIAGNOSIS

The differential list for any patient presenting with primarily GI signs may be extensive. Initial differentials should be listed as GI or extra-GI in origin.

- GI.
  - Gastric atrophy.
  - Intestinal lymphoma.
  - Histoplasmosis.
  - *Physaloptera* sp.
  - Salt water ingestion.
- Extra-GI.
  - Azotemia.
  - Vascular ring anomaly.
  - Hypoadrenocorticism.
  - Paraneoplastic.
- Extra-GI differentials may in large part be excluded with evaluation of signalment, history, physical examination, minimum database (complete blood count, serum biochemistry, urinalysis) and plain radiography (thorax and/or abdomen depending on presentation).
- Once extra-GI causes have been excluded, further investigation into the GI tract may be pursued (see diagnostic evaluation below).
- Owners should be warned that primary GI motility disorders are primarily a diagnosis of exclusion, after other differentials have been ruled out. The diagnostic work-up may be extensive.

 DIAGNOSTICS

Complete Blood Count/Biochemistry/Urinalysis

- May indicate the presence of primary disease resulting in a secondary GI dysmotility (e.g., hypoadrenocorticism).
- Indicators of GI dysmotility may include electrolyte abnormalities and acid–base disorders.
- Conversely, the minimum database may be within normal limits.

Other Laboratory Tests

Depending upon the presentation, additional laboratory tests may be warranted for metabolic disease (e.g., adrenocorticotropic (ACTH) stimulation testing) or GI disease (e.g., cobalamin and folate concentrations).

Imaging

Radiographs

- Primary GI motility disorders may show radiographic signs of ileus, focal or generalized, on survey abdominal films.
- Gastrointestinal distension may be due to retained food, water, or air and findings may be concerning for GI obstruction.

Ultrasound
- May be used to evaluate for intestinal wall lesions or peristalsis.
- Note that the presence of air within the GI tract may make ultrasonographic imaging difficult.

Contrast Radiography
- Note that the assessment of GI motility in the hospital setting may be problematic.
- The stress of being in the hospital may negatively impact peristalsis (reduced peristalsis, slowed GI transit time), even in the normal animal. Therefore, strict adherence to GI motility or gastric emptying times may lead to difficulties in interpretation.
- Options for contrast radiography include barium swallow studies – liquid, semi-solid, and solid states. If fluoroscopic equipment is available, fluoroscopy evaluation of motility may be performed.
- Barium-impregnated polyethylene spheres (BIPS) are available in small and large sizes to help facilitate imaging studies. The use of BIPS may be safer compared to syringe feeding liquid barium in patients with a history of vomiting/regurgitation.
- Options exist for radionuclide imaging studies, but this equipment is generally limited to specialty centers. Use of this imaging modality may require specialized housing/isolation facilities due to the radioactive nature of the study.
- Wireless capsules that patients can swallow may also be used to transmit information remotely via radio sensor. Information on temperature, pH, time, and pressures may be collected.

Additional Diagnostic Tests

Depending upon the presentation, additional diagnostics consisting of gastroduodenoscopy, colonoscopy, and abdominal exploratory may be indicated. Representative samples of the GI tract or any abnormal-appearing tissues (e.g., lymph nodes) should be obtained.

Pathologic Findings

Pathologic findings will depend upon the underlying etiology for the presenting signs. In cases of idiopathic/primary GI motility disorders, pathology may be unremarkable.

 # THERAPEUTICS

- When a motility disorder is the result of an underlying etiology, therapy should be directed at the primary disease. Examples include the following.
  - Endoscopic removal of an obstructive gastric foreign body.
  - Steroid supplementation for patients with glucocorticoid-deficient hypoadrenocorticism.
  - Surgical correction of a persistent right aortic arch.
- In the rare cases where a primary GI motility disorder is diagnosed, therapy is supportive and symptomatic, primarily directed at improving peristalsis.

Drug(s) of Choice
Promotility Agents
Medications that increase GI motility may have different mechanisms of action and primary sites of action (Tables 38.1, 38.2). These agents should not be used in cases of mechanical obstruction and usage of most is contraindicated in cases of GI hemorrhage.

Precautions/Interactions
- Do not use prokinetic agents in cases of mechanical GI obstruction as GI perforation could result. Most prokinetic agents are contraindicated in cases of GI hemorrhage due to potential exacerbation of blood loss.

TABLE 38.1. Promotility agents.

Medication	Mechanism of action	Primary activity	Notes
Metoclopramide	Dopamine receptor antagonist	Increases contractions of gastric and proximal small intestine	Weak prokinetic activity; more effective as antiemetic
Cisapride	5-HT$_4$ agonist	Increases lower esophageal sphincter pressure; increases gastric emptying and small and large intestinal motility	Available as compounded medication; human product has been removed from market
Ranitidine (and other related medications)	H2-receptor antagonist	Increases lower esophageal sphincter pressure and may stimulate motility	Effects appear weak and evidence to support usage is questionable
Erythromycin (and other related medications)	Motilin receptor agonist	Promotes gastric emptying	Doses are subantimicrobial

TABLE 38.2. Promotility agents: dosage regimes.

Medication	Dose	Route	Interval
Metoclopramide	0.2–0.5 mg/kg 0.01–0.1 mg/kg/h	PO, SQ, IM IV	q 6–8 h Constant rate infusion (CRI)
Cisapride	0.1–0.5 mg/kg	PO	q 8–12 h
Ranitidine	1–2 mg/kg	PO, SQ, IM or slow IV	q 8–12 h
Erythromycin	0.5–1 mg/kg	PO	q 8–12 h

IM, intramuscular; IV, intravenous; PO, by mouth (*per os*); SQ, subcutaneous.

- Metoclopramide may have centrally mediated effects in some patients and has many potential drug interactions.
- Cisapride was removed from the human market due to potential cardiovascular side effects (prolonged QT interval) but this has not been clinically identified in veterinary patients.

Alternative Drugs

In lieu of identification of an underlying disorder, in cases of gastric distension (without volvulus), placement of a feeding tube (e.g., percutaneous endoscopic gastrotomy (PEG) tube) may facilitate removal of excess gastric juices or gas.

Appropriate Health Care

- Abdominal cramping, pain or discomfort may be experienced by some patients. Consider analgesic medications, including the potential impacts of analgesics (e.g., opiates) on GI motility.
- Routine controlled exercise may help maintain GI motility and improve postoperative ileus.
- Monitor patients for signs of malnutrition/malabsorption.

Nursing Care

Depending upon the etiology, associated vomiting or regurgitation may predispose to aspiration pneumonia. As some episodes of aspiration may be occult, monitor for signs such as tachypnea, dyspnea, coughing or fever.

Diet

- Dietary therapy should be tailored to the individual patient needs and response to therapy. General recommendations include the following.
  - Smaller, more frequent meals.
  - Consider a late night small meal/snack to help avoid potential bilious vomiting.
  - Increasing energy density (i.e., dietary fat) may reduce the volume of food needed but may also increase digestive and absorptive complexity. Tailor to patient.
  - Dietary fiber (soluble and insoluble) should be modified based on patient response. In general, increasing soluble fiber is recommended; however, increases in insoluble fiber may assist with peristalsis in some patients.
- See Chapter 76 for more information.

Activity

Regular, controlled (nonstrenuous) exercise may assist with normal GI motility and elimination.

Surgical Considerations

- Surgical indications may exist for underlying diseases that affect GI motility (e.g., gastric dilation-volvulus, mechanical obstruction from neoplastic disease, etc.).
- Primary GI dysmotility is managed medically.

 COMMENTS

Primary gastric and/or intestinal motility disorders are rare. In the majority of cases, a complete diagnostic work-up will reveal an underlying etiology and motility disorders are secondary in nature.

Client Education

Medical and dietary manipulations may change over time. Monitor for signs of changes in GI motility (e.g., changes in elimination or appetite, evidence of abdominal discomfort, etc.) and alert the veterinarian about any changes noted. Subsequent adjustments to medical/dietary therapy may improve clinical signs.

Patient Monitoring

- Monitor the following to assess treatment effectiveness.
  - Appetite.
  - Presence of vomiting or regurgitation.
  - Defecation frequency and effort.
  - Body condition score and body weight.
  - Presence of abdominal distension, borborygmus, flatulence.

Possible Complications

- Lack of response to treatment.
- Patient pain or discomfort.
- Concerns for quality of life.

Expected Course and Prognosis

- If a treatable/curable underlying etiology is discovered, GI motility may return to normal. However, it may take several days to weeks for normal peristalsis to fully return. Some primary etiologies (e.g., canine dysautonomia) have a guarded to grave prognosis.

- If the motility disorder is primary in origin, prognosis is guarded, pending evaluation of initial response to treatment.

Synonyms

- Gastric atony
- Atrophic gastritis
- Ileus

Abbreviations

- ACTH = adrenocorticotropic hormone
- BIPS = barium-impregnated polyethylene spheres
- CRI = constant rate infusion
- GI = gastrointestinal
- MMC = migrating myoelectric complex

See Also

- Constipation and Obstipation
- Dysphagia
- Gastritis, Atrophic
- Gastroesophageal Reflux
- Megacolon
- Megaesophagus
- Nutritional Approach to Chronic Enteropathies
- Regurgitation

Suggested Reading

Boscan P, Cochran S, Monnet E, et al. Effect of prolonged general anesthesia with sevoflurane and laparoscopic surgery on gastric and small bowel propulsive motility and pH in dogs. Vet Anaesth Analg 2014;41(1):73–81.

Gaschen FP. Gastric and intestinal motility disorders. In: Bonagura JB, Twedt DC, eds. Current Veterinary Therapy XV. St Louis: Elsevier, 2014, pp. 513–518.

Sanderson JJ, Boysen SR, McMurray JM, et al. The effect of fasting on gastrointestinal motility in healthy dogs as assessed by sonography. J Vet Emerg Crit Care 2017;27(6):645–650.

Simpson KW. Stomach. In: Washabau RJ, Day MJ, eds. Canine and Feline Gastroenterology. St. Louis: Elsevier, 2013, pp. 606–650.

Warrit K, Boscan P, Ferguson LE, et al. Minimally invasive wireless motility capsule to study canine gastrointestinal motility and pH. Vet J 2017;227:36–41.

Washabau RJ. Prokinetic agents. In: Washabau RJ, Day MJ, eds. Canine and Feline Gastroenterology. St. Louis: Elsevier, 2013, pp. 530–536.

Acknowledgments: The author and editors acknowledge the contribution of David C. Twedt, DVM.

Author: Jo Ann Morrison DVM, MS, DACVIM

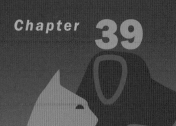

Chapter 39

Gastric Dilation-Volvulus

DEFINITION/OVERVIEW

- Gastric dilation-volvulus (GDV) occurs when the stomach rotates on its mesenteric (short) axis.
- The vast majority of cases present with a peracute onset, but chronic gastric volvulus and intermittent GDV that periodically occur and spontaneously resolve have been reported.
- Simple gastric dilation (GD) occurs when the stomach becomes overly distended with gas, fluid, or ingesta but does not rotate out of its normal position.
- The symptoms of GDV and GD are identical.
- The terms *bloat* and *gastric torsion* may also be used describe GDV.

ETIOLOGY/PATHOPHYSIOLOGY

- Volvulus can occur in any orientation and to varying degrees, but the majority are a clockwise approximately three-quarter turn with the pylorus being trapped dorsally and to the left of the esophagus.
- Either gastric dilation or volvulus can occur first, but once volvulus occurs, dilation is progressive due to gas and fluid accumulation within the stomach.
- The combination of gastric dilation and volvulus rapidly results in cardiovascular compromise and shock.
- Obstructive shock occurs when progressive gastric dilation compresses the surrounding low-pressure veins, preventing blood caudal to the diaphragm from returning to the heart.
- Shock and tissue compromise result in most patients having systemic inflammatory response syndrome (SIRS). This can lead to failure of almost any organ system and, rarely, multiorgan dysfunction syndrome (MODS).

Systems Affected

- Cardiovascular – obstructive shock results in weakness, depressed mentation, pale gums, prolonged capillary refill time (CRT), poor pulse quality, and cool extremities. Reduced coronary blood flow secondary to shock and cardioactive cytokines can predispose to ventricular arrhythmias. Arrhythmias may occur pre-, intra-, or postoperatively and can further decrease systemic perfusion.
- Gastrointestinal – gastric overdistension, in conjunction with malpositioning, and shock can result in gastric ulceration and necrosis. Preoperatively, this can culminate in gastric rupture, while postoperatively, necrosis can lead to septic peritonitis.
- Hemic/lymphatic/immune – splenic congestion typically occurs, but infarction or torsion may also occur. Most patients with GDV will meet the criteria for SIRS which can lead to

Blackwell's Five-Minute Veterinary Consult Clinical Companion: Small Animal Gastrointestinal Diseases,
First Edition. Edited by Jocelyn Mott and Jo Ann Morrison.
© 2019 John Wiley & Sons, Inc. Published 2019 by John Wiley & Sons, Inc.
Companion website: www.fiveminutevet.com/gastrointestinal

dysfunction of a variety of organ systems and MODS. Dysfunction of the coagulation system can manifest as disseminated intravascular coagulation (DIC) and subsequent coagulopathy.

- Hepatobiliary – elevation of alanine aminotransferase (ALT) can occur secondary to liver hypoperfuson and shock. Hyperbilirubinemia secondary to SIRS and hepatic dysfunction can also occur.
- Musculoskeletal – weakness and collapse may be seen secondary to shock.
- Renal/urologic – although uncommon, shock and SIRS can both result in acute kidney injury.
- Respiratory – abdominal distension and tympany can prevent adequate ventilation and result in respiratory distress. Aspiration pneumonia is also relatively common in dogs with GDV and can worsen respiratory compromise as well as contributing to systemic inflammation.

 # SIGNALMENT/HISTORY

- Gastric dilation-volvulus occurs most often in large- and giant-breed dogs such as Great Danes, Weimaraners, St Bernards, Gordon setters, Irish setters, and standard poodles.
- It has been rarely reported in small-breed dogs such as miniature dachshunds, cats, and other mammals.
- Adult and geriatric animals are typically affected.
- No genetic cause identified but suspected based on the association between an individual's risk and having a family history of GDV being positively correlated.

Risk Factors

- Having a first-order relative (dam, sire, sibling) who has had GDV is a significant risk factor.
- Military working dogs, such as German shepherds, are at increased risk.
- Older dogs are at higher risk than younger dogs.
- Dogs with deeper chest conformations (higher thoracic depth-to-width ratio) are at higher risk.
- Being exposed to stressful events, particularly around the time of feeding.
- Having a more stress-prone temperament; being fearful, aggressive, or nervous.
- Being fed from an elevated food bowl.

Historical Findings

- Vomiting and/or unproductive retching.
- Ptyalism.
- Anxiety and restlessness.
- Abdominal distension.
- Abdominal pain – stretching or hunched posture.
- Collapse.

 # CLINICAL FEATURES

- Signs of shock and hypoperfusion – poor pulse quality, tachycardia, pale mucous membranes, prolonged CRT, cool extremities.
- Abdominal distension is typically present, but is harder to assess in obese or heavily muscled dogs. Additionally, the stomach can remain cranially positioned under the ribcage, making gastric distension more difficult to assess.

- A firm, tympanic structure (stomach) may be present in the cranial abdomen.
- Ptyalism.
- Tachypnea and increased respiratory effort may be noted due to respiratory compromise.
- Irregular cardiac rhythm, possibly with pulse deficits, may be present.
- Splenomegaly may be palpable.

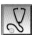

DIFFERENTIAL DIAGNOSIS

- Gastric dilation.
- Hemoabdomen.
- Septic abdomen.
- Intestinal volvulus.
- Acute portal thromboembolism.

DIAGNOSTICS

Complete Blood Count/Biochemistry/Urinalysis

- Complete blood count is typically not useful. In rare cases where disseminated intravascular coagulation (DIC) is also present, thrombocytopenia may be noted.
- Biochemistry – electrolyte abnormalities are common. Azotemia may be present.
- Urinalysis – may see increased specific gravity with dehydration.

Other Laboratory Tests

- Blood lactate level is typically elevated.
- Venous blood gas will typically reveal metabolic acidosis of varying degree with hyperlactatemia.
  - Some studies have suggested that a lactate level >6.0 mmol/L is associated with an increased risk of mortality and gastric necrosis, while other studies have not demonstrated a decrease in survival until the lactate is >9.0 mmol/L
  - Other studies have suggested that the change in lactate, or delta-lactate, is more predictive. In these studies, a poststabilization decrease in lactate (compared to pretreatment levels) of at least 42% was more likely to be associated with survival.
  - It is *important to note* that these values are associated with increased or decreased rate of survival and are *not* meant to be used as absolute indicators of mortality or gastric necrosis. While they may predict a population of dogs well, there is often much poorer performance in the ability to predict the outcome of a single individual.
- Prothrombin time/partial thromboplastin time may be prolonged in rare cases where DIC is present.

Imaging

- Abdominal radiograph.
  - Right lateral view typically shows a gas/fluid-distended stomach with compartmentalization (also called the reverse C, double bubble, or "Popeye" sign) (Figure 39.1).
  - Orthogonal or other views may be needed if the degree of rotation is atypical.
- Thoracic radiographs may be used to detect the presence of aspiration pneumonia.

Pathologic Findings

- Gross pathology reveals an abnormally positioned stomach. The pylorus is typically displaced dorsally and to the left of the midline to varying degrees.

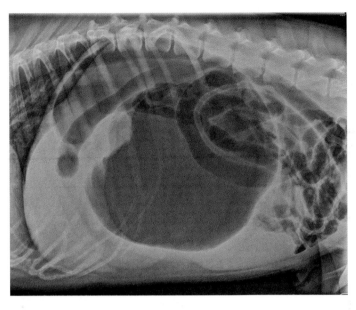

■ **Fig. 39.1.** Right lateral abdominal radiographs of dog with GDV.

■ Evidence of gastric venous congestion and/or necrosis is present (red to black colored tissue).
■ In severe cases, rupture of the stomach with free ingesta in the abdomen.

 # THERAPEUTICS

Successfully treating dogs with GDV includes treating their shock state with intravenous (IV) fluids and gastric decompression (trocar or orogastric tube) followed by prompt surgical intervention to derotate the stomach and restore normal anatomy and blood flow. Failure to aggressively treat shock and cardiovascular instability results in poor outcomes and death.

Drug(s) of Choice

■ Intravenous fluids are necessary to alleviate the symptoms of shock seen in patients with gastric dilation with or without volvulus. Fluids should be administered incrementally until desired hemodynamic goals are met.
  • Isotonic crystalloids (lactated Ringer's solution, Norm-R, 0.9% NaCl, PlasmaLyte A) 20–30 mL/kg over 15 minutes.
  • Hypertonic saline 5 mL/kg over 10–15 minutes.
  • Synthetic colloids 5–10 mL/kg over 15 minutes – synthetic colloids may be associated with an increased risk of acute kidney injury and death.
■ Analgesia is necessary to improve patient comfort and will help address tachycardia since distension of visceral organs is typically very painful.
  • Full mu-opioids are preferred because of their minimal cardiorespiratory effects, quick onset of action, potency, and ability to be reversed.
  • Hydromorphone 0.05–0.1 mg/kg IV or IM.
  • Methadone 0.1–0.3 mg/kg IV or IM.
  • Fentanyl 2–5 μg/kg IV followed by a constant rate infusion (CRI) of 2–5 μg/kg/h.

- Lidocaine may be necessary if significant ventricular arrhythmias are present (ventricular tachycardia >160–180 bpm, multiform ventricular premature complexes, or cardiovascular instability due to the ventricular arrhythmia).
  - Dogs should be given lidocaine at 2 mg/kg IV as a slow bolus over a couple minutes. The bolus dose can be repeated up to a total of three times.
  - If bolus dosing is effective, a CRI should be started at 50–80 µg/kg/min to maintain a normal rhythm.
- Gastric acid reduction medications can be considered.
  - Pantoprazole 1 mg/kg IV q 12–24 h.
  - Omeprazole 1 mg/kg PO q 12–24 h.
  - Famotidine 1–2 mg/kg IV, SQ, PO q 12–24 h.
- Perioperative antibiotics can be used during the time of surgery. Ongoing antibiotic therapy is not necessary unless aspiration pneumonia is present or abdominal contamination occurs during surgery.
  - Cefazolin 22 mg/kg IV at induction and every 90 minutes until surgery is complete.
  - If aspiration pneumonia is present, consider broader spectrum coverage.

Precautions/Interactions

- Heavy sedation prior to medical and surgical stabilization may be detrimental as these patients typically have a significant degree of cardiovascular compromise, making them high risk for heavy sedation (i.e., dexmedetomidine) prior to stabilization.
- Cimetidine may increase the risk of lidocaine toxicity when given concurrently.

Alternative Drugs

- Antiarrhythmics – in cases where lidocaine is not effective or is not available, the following antiarrhythmic drugs can be considered.
  - Magnesium sulfate or magnesium chloride 0.3 mEq/kg IV over 20 minutes.
  - Procainamide 10 mg/kg IV followed by a CRI at 20–50 µg/kg/min.
  - Sotalol 1–2 mg/kg PO.

Appropriate Health Care

Gastric dilation-volvulus is a medical and surgical emergency. Animals must be aggressively and emergently stabilized using IV fluids and gastric decompression before being taken for surgical correction as expediently as possible.

Gastric decompression methods include the following.

Trocarization

- The area of greatest tympany, typically just caudal to the ribs on the right or left abdomen, is chosen as the site for trocarization.
- The area should be clipped and surgically prepared.
- A short, large-gauge (14–16 gauge) needle should be inserted perpendicular to the abdominal wall.
- Gas from the stomach should exit the needle hub if successful. Once gas is no longer coming out, the needle should be removed.
- This process can be repeated as needed until other decompression or surgical derotation is performed.

Orogastric Intubation

- The patient is rapidly induced under general anesthesia and an endotracheal tube is placed and appropriately cuffed.

- A smooth orogastric tube is then measured from the nose to the last rib and marked accordingly.
- Lubrication is applied to the tube and it is passed orally into the stomach.
- The stomach is then decompressed and lavaged.
- If the tube cannot be easily passed then trocarization or elevating the front half of the patient should be performed to try and facilitate passage.
- It is important not to force the orogastric tube as rupture of the esophagus or stomach can occur.

Nursing Care

Postoperatively, the patient should have close hemodynamic monitoring. Continuous electrocardiogram monitoring is recommended due to the risk of arrhythmias developing or persisting postoperatively.

Diet

After the patient is recovered from anesthesia, small frequent meals of a bland diet can be offered. It is not thought that any long-term dietary modification is necessary.

Activity

After the surgical site is healed, no long-term activity modification is necessary.

Surgical Considerations

- Gastropexy is recommended for all patients experiencing GDV as derotating the stomach is necessary to restore normal stomach function and blood flow.
- In patients with known or suspected GDV that spontaneously derotate, gastropexy as soon as possible is still recommended as these patients have a high rate of recurrence.
- In patients with recurrent or severe gastric dilation without volvulus, gastropexy should be considered to prevent volvulus occurring in the future.
- After derotation, the gastric mucosa should be allowed time to restore normal perfusion and then it should be assessed for viability. Invagination or partial gastrectomy should be performed in areas where the mucosal integrity is suspect.
- Splenectomy may be necessary if the spleen has been damaged or thrombosed as a result of the GDV.
- A variety of gastropexy techniques can be used, but they all have the goal of creating an adhesion between the pyloric antrum and the right body wall.
- The gastropexy site should *not* be incorporated into the ventral midline abdominal incision as this can result in complications if future abdominal surgery is necessary.

 COMMENTS

Client Education

- Standard postoperative care and exercise restriction should be implemented until the abdominal incision is fully healed.
- Clients who own first-order relatives of affected dogs should be encouraged to seek prophylactic gastropexy.

Patient Monitoring

It is important to note that dogs who have previously been gastropexied can still experience bloat (which can rarely be life-threatening) without torsion.

Prevention/Avoidance

Gastropexy may be performed prophylactically in any deep-chested dog. This may be of particular benefit in dogs who are known to have a first-order relative that has been affected with GDV.

Expected Course and Prognosis

With aggressive stabilization, surgical intervention, and supportive care, the prognosis is good, with about 85% of dogs surviving.

Synonyms

- Bloat
- Gastric torsion

Abbreviations

- ALT = alanine aminotransferase
- CRI = constant rate infusion
- CRT = capillary refill time
- DIC = disseminated intravascular coagulation
- GD = gastric dilation
- GDV = gastric dilation-volvulus
- MODS = multiorgan dysfunction syndrome
- SIRS = systemic inflammatory response syndrome

Suggested Reading

Radlinsky MG. Surgery of the digestive system. In: Fossum TW, ed. Small Animal Surgery, 4th ed. St Louis: Elsevier, 2013.

Sharp CR. Gastric dilatation-volvulus. In: Silverstein DC, Hopper K, eds. Small Animal Critical Care Medicine, 2nd ed. St Louis: Elsevier, 2015.

Acknowledgments: The authors and editors acknowledge the prior contribution of Dr S. Brent Reimer.

Author: April Blong DVM, DACVECC

Chapter 40

Gastric Neoplasia, Benign

DEFINITION/OVERVIEW

- Uncommon benign tumors arising from the smooth muscle (leiomyoma) or epithelial lining (adenoma/adenomatous polyps) of the stomach.
- Other benign gastric lesions include hypertrophic gastropathy and hamartoma. Some gastrointestinal stromal tumors (GISTs) may also exhibit benign behavior, although these are relatively uncommon in the stomach.
- Prognosis is usually good.

ETIOLOGY/PATHOPHYSIOLOGY

- Unknown.
- *Helicobacter* spp. have been identified in gastric polyps, but unlike in humans, it is unknown if *Helicobacter* infection leads to polyp formation.
- Incidence/prevalence – uncommon in dogs and rare in cats.

Systems Affected

- Gastrointestinal.

SIGNALMENT/HISTORY

- No known breed predilection.
- Older dogs (median age 11 years for leiomyomas).
- One study showed an increased incidence of leiomyomas in male dogs (82%).

Historical Findings

- Related to mass effect in the stomach.
- Anorexia.
- Vomiting, particularly if causing outflow obstruction.
- +/– Hematemesis.
- Weight loss.
- Leiomyoma: signs related to hypoglycemia, a possible paraneoplastic condition.
  - Seizures.
  - Weakness, ataxia.
  - Lethargy.
  - Polyuria/polydipsia.

Blackwell's Five-Minute Veterinary Consult Clinical Companion: Small Animal Gastrointestinal Diseases, First Edition. Edited by Jocelyn Mott and Jo Ann Morrison.
© 2019 John Wiley & Sons, Inc. Published 2019 by John Wiley & Sons, Inc.
Companion website: www.fiveminutevet.com/gastrointestinal

CLINICAL FEATURES

- Weight loss.
- Palpable abdominal mass (uncommon).
- Abdominal discomfort.
- Gastric polyps are often incidental findings on endoscopy or necropsy.

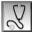

DIFFERENTIAL DIAGNOSIS

- Foreign body.
- Inflammatory bowel disease.
- Parasites.
- Pancreatitis.
- GIST.
- Adenocarcinoma.
- Leiomyosarcoma.

DIAGNOSTICS

Complete Blood Count/Biochemistry/Urinalysis

- Labwork is usually normal.
- Hypoglycemia – may be seen as a paraneoplastic syndrome in dogs with leiomyoma, leiomyosarcoma, or GIST, usually associated with larger tumors. Possibly caused by tumor secretion of active insulin-like growth factor 2 (IGF-2).
- Anemia – may be normocytic, normochromic (chronic disease) or microcytic, hypochromic (iron deficiency anemia) if blood loss from an ulcerated tumor.
- Mild and persistent elevations in blood urea nitrogen in the face of normal creatinine can support blood loss from a gastric tumor.

Imaging

- Abdominal ultrasonography – may reveal a thickened wall of the stomach or a luminal mass, as well as evaluate for abnormalities in other abdominal organs. In general, benign tumors are usually pedunculated and well circumscribed.
- Leiomyomas are most commonly found as discrete, smooth masses near the cardia (Figure 40.1).
- Polyps may be sessile or pedunculated, and solitary or cauliflower-like lesions. Most appear echogenic and confined to the mucosa, with no involvement of the submucosa.
- Lymph node enlargement is rare in cases of benign gastric masses.
- Positive contrast radiography – may see a luminal mass that causes a filling defect if there is a corresponding outflow obstruction. May also see delayed gastric emptying and decreased motility.
- Thoracic radiographs – consider as part of staging or preanesthetic evaluation.

Other Diagnostic Procedures

- Fine needle aspirates (FNA) – leiomyomas and other benign lesions often exfoliate poorly, limiting the usefulness of FNA.
- Endoscopic biopsy may be performed, but is often nondiagnostic if tumors are deep to the mucosal surface, or if the mass is beyond the reach of the endoscope. May be useful for

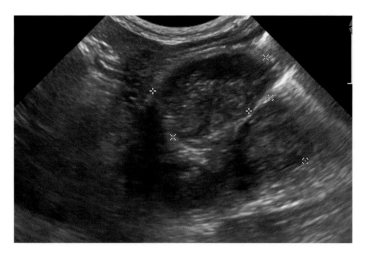

■ **Fig. 40.1.** Ultrasonographic image from a gastric mass in a dog who presented with a history of vomiting and hypoglycemia. There is a lobular, bilobed mass extending from the cardia to the fundus along the lesser curvature, measuring approximately 2.2 × 3.5 cm. There is a small cystic region within the mass. The stomach is distended with a large amount of gas and rounded hyperechoic shadowing structures consistent with food ingesta. Source: Courtesy of Dr Wilfried Mai, University of Pennsylvania School of Veterinary Medicine.

visualizing masses and collecting biopsies; can also evaluate the overlying mucosa. Leiomyomas are usually submucosal with normal overlying mucosa.
■ Open surgical biopsy with exploratory laparotomy is the gold standard, often required to confirm a diagnosis.

Pathologic Findings

■ Leiomyoma.
  - Gross – firm, submucosal masses with normal overlying mucosa.
  - Cytologic – tend to exfoliate poorly.
  - Histopathologic – submucosal lesion that expands the muscular layer; neoplastic cells resemble well-differentiated smooth muscle cells, arranged in long, interlacing fascicles (Figure 40.2).
  - May need immunohistochemistry (IHC) to differentiate from a GIST.
    ○ Leiomyoma: IHC positive for smooth muscle actin, +/– desmin.
    ○ GIST: IHC positive for KIT (c-kit or CD117), +/– CD34.
■ Adenoma.
  - Gross – luminal lesions that project above the plane of the mucosal surface.
  - Cytologic – tend to exfoliate poorly.
  - Histopathologic – normal epithelium covering a fibrovascular core infiltrated by a variety of inflammatory cells. Usually minimal anisocytosis/anisokaryosis with no mitotic figures.
  - World Health Organization classification scheme: hyperplastic (regenerative) or inflammatory (benign lymphoid).

 ## THERAPEUTICS

Drug(s) of Choice

Chemotherapy is not required for benign tumors.

(a) (b)

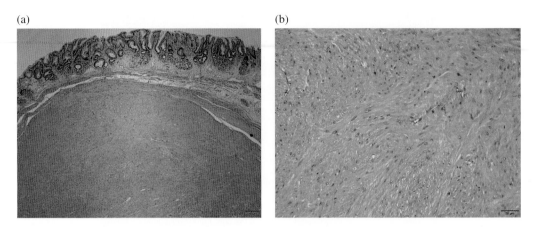

■ **Fig. 40.2.** (a) Histopathology specimen (4× magnification) from the gastric mass in Figure 40.1. The intramural neoplasm expands the muscularis layer and is well demarcated from the adjacent smooth muscle wall. (b) 20× magnification of the specimen in Figure 40.2a. The neoplastic cells are arranged in long interlacing fascicles and have a moderate amount of eosinophilic fibrillar cytoplasm and oval to fusiform, blunt-ended nuclei with coarsely stippled chromatin and one to two nucleoli. The final histopathologic diagnosis was consistent with a gastric leiomyoma. Blood glucose concentration normalized after surgery. Source: Courtesy of Dr Amy Durham, University of Pennsylvania School of Veterinary Medicine.

Nursing Care

■ Consider small, frequent meals during surgical recovery.
■ Consider feeding tube placement if necessary.
■ Antiemetics, antacids, analgesics for supportive care.
■ Blood glucose monitoring in hypoglycemic patients, along with appropriate treatment (dextrose supplementation).

Surgical Considerations

■ Surgical resection is the treatment of choice, and can be curative if the tumor is resectable.
■ Even large leiomyomas can often be removed successfully via gastrotomy and removal of the submucosa.

 COMMENTS

Client Education

Leiomyomas with paraneoplastic hypoglycemia – monitor for clinical signs of hypoglycemia until the time of surgery and in the immediate postoperative period.

Patient Monitoring

■ In cases of complete resection, no additional follow-up is necessary apart from normal postoperative rechecks.
■ Monitor for return of clinical signs as an indication of recurrence or new gastrointestinal lesions.
■ If tumors are incompletely excised – regular rechecks for palliative care of clinical signs, and for leiomyomas with hypoglycemia, blood glucose monitoring.

Possible Complications

Gastric perforation and sepsis, secondary to tumor growth or dehiscence of surgical site.

Expected Course and Prognosis

- Excellent long-term prognosis following complete excision.
- Leiomyoma – median survival time two years.
- Currently unknown if canine gastric polyps can undergo malignant transformation, as has been reported with hyperplastic polyps in humans.

Abbreviations

- FNA = fine-needle aspirate
- GIST = gastrointestinal stromal tumor
- IGF-2 = insulin-like growth factor 2
- IHC = immunohistochemistry

See Also

- Gastric Neoplasia, Malignant

Suggested Reading

Amorim I, Taulescu MA, Ferreira A, et al. An immunohistochemical study of canine spontaneous gastric polyps. Diagn Pathol 2014;9:166.

Beaudry D, Knapp DW, Montgomery T, et al. Hypoglycemia in four dogs with smooth muscle tumors. J Vet Intern Med 1995;9(6):415–418.

Diana A, Penninck DG, Keating JH. Ultrasonographic appearance of canine gastric polyps. Vet Radiol Ultrasound 2009;50(2):201–204.

Frost D, Lasota J, Miettinen M. Gastrointestinal stromal tumors and leiomyomas in the dog: a histopathologic, immunohistochemical, and molecular genetic study of 50 cases. Vet Pathol 2003;40:42–54.

Taulescu MA, Valentine BA, Amorim I, et al. Histopathological features of canine spontaneous non-neoplastic gastric polyps – a retrospective study of 15 cases. Histol Histopathol 2014;29(1):65–75.

Acknowledgment: The author and editors acknowledge the prior contributions of Dr Laura D. Garrett.

Author: Jennifer A. Mahoney DVM, DACVIM (Oncology)

Chapter 41

Gastric Neoplasia, Malignant

DEFINITION/OVERVIEW

- Uncommon malignant tumors arising from the epithelial lining (adenocarcinoma) or smooth muscle (leiomyosarcoma) of the stomach, or from the interstitial cells of Cajal (gastrointestinal stromal tumors).
- Other malignant gastric tumors include lymphoma (most common gastric tumor in cats; less common in dogs), extramedullary plasma cell tumors, mast cell tumors, fibrosarcoma.

ETIOLOGY/PATHOPHYSIOLOGY

- Overall unknown.
- Genetic and environmental factors suspected.
- Uncontrolled activity of KIT in the gastrointestinal tract suspected to be linked to development of gastrointestinal stromal tumors (GISTs).
- Adenocarcinoma.
    - Dogs – one report of increased incidence in laboratory dogs with long-term nitrosamine administration; clinical relevance unknown.
    - Dogs and cats – chronic gastritis suspected as a possible cause, particularly in Norwegian Lundehunds with a history of atrophic gastritis.
    - *Helicobacter pylori* infection is a risk factor in humans, but this is uncommon in dogs. Dogs do have other, similar gastrointestinal bacteria, but the association with gastric neoplasia is unknown.
- Overall incidence – gastric tumors comprise less than 1% of malignant tumors.
- Dogs – adenocarcinoma is the most common (70–80%), followed by leiomyosarcoma, GIST, and lymphoma. Leiomyosarcomas are more commonly found in the stomach compared to GISTs.
- Cats – lymphoma is the most common gastric tumor, followed by adenocarcinoma (more commonly found in the intestine) and mast cell tumors.

Systems Affected

- Gastrointestinal.
- Possible metastatic sites.
    - Hemic/lymphatic/immune (regional lymph nodes, less commonly spleen).
    - Hepatobiliary.
    - Respiratory.
    - Reproductive (testes are a possible metastatic site of adenocarcinoma in dogs).

Blackwell's Five-Minute Veterinary Consult Clinical Companion: Small Animal Gastrointestinal Diseases, First Edition. Edited by Jocelyn Mott and Jo Ann Morrison.
© 2019 John Wiley & Sons, Inc. Published 2019 by John Wiley & Sons, Inc.
Companion website: www.fiveminutevet.com/gastrointestinal

SIGNALMENT/HISTORY

- Mostly middle-aged to older (>6 years) dogs and cats.
- Adenocarcinoma.
  - Dogs – median age 8–10 years, more common in males.
  - Predisposed breeds – Belgian shepherds, Chow Chows, German shepherd dogs, Norwegian Lundehunds, Dutch Tervueren shepherds, Staffordshire bull terrier, Rough collies, Groenendael, Bouvier des Flandres, Standard Poodle.
  - Cats – Siamese cats are predisposed; one report of two related Persian cats with gastric adenocarcinoma.
- Leiomyosarcoma/GIST.
  - Median age 10–11 years.
  - No breed or sex predilection.

Historical Findings

- Signs may occur over weeks to months, and typically appear late in the course of disease, unless the lesion is at the pylorus and causing an outflow obstruction.
- Anorexia.
- Vomiting, possibly with hematemesis or "coffee grounds."
- Weight loss.
- Lethargy.
- Leiomyosarcoma/GIST – signs related to hypoglycemia (seizures, weakness, etc.).

 CLINICAL FEATURES

- Weight loss.
- Palpable abdominal mass (uncommon).
- Abdominal discomfort.

 DIFFERENTIAL DIAGNOSIS

- Leiomyoma.
- Adenoma.
- Foreign body.
- Pancreatitis.
- Parasites.

 DIAGNOSTICS

Complete Blood Count/Biochemistry/Urinalysis

- Labwork is usually normal.
- Anemia – may be normocytic, normochromic (chronic disease) or microcytic, hypochromic (iron deficiency anemia) if severe blood loss from an ulcerated tumor.
- Leukocytosis, usually neutrophilic.
- Mild and persistent elevations in blood urea nitrogen in the face of normal creatinine can support blood loss from a gastric tumor.
- Elevated hepatic enzymes in cases of hepatic metastasis or common bile duct obstruction.

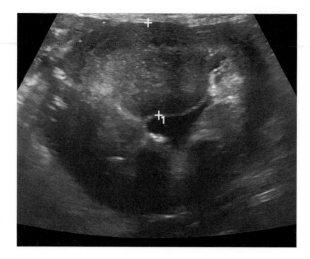

■ **Fig. 41.1.** Ultrasonographic image of a gastric adenocarcinoma mass in the antrum of the stomach. In the gastric antrum, immediately orad to the pylorus, arising from the mucosa, there is an approximately 2 × 3 cm tubular mass that is markedly hyperechoic with hypoechoic mottling. Source: Courtesy of Dr Wilfried Mai, University of Pennsylvania School of Veterinary Medicine.

- Hypoalbuminemia.
- Leiomyosarcoma/GIST – may see hypoglycemia as a paraneoplastic syndrome.

Additional Laboratory Tests

- Fecal occult blood may be positive.
- Adenocarcinoma – gastrin levels may be elevated.

Imaging

- Abdominal ultrasonography – may see gastric wall thickening or a luminal mass, and can also identify enlarged lymph nodes or abnormalities in other organs. Adenocarcinomas are often fixed and located along the lesser curvature in the pyloric antrum, involving all layers of the stomach wall (Figure 41.1). Leiomyosarcomas are usually submucosal and more commonly found near the cardia.
- Positive contrast radiography – may see a luminal mass that causes a filling defect if there is a corresponding outflow obstruction. May also see delayed gastric emptying and decreased motility.
- Advanced imaging with contrast computed tomography or magnetic resonance imaging can provide highest quality images of gastrointestinal tract, with increased sensitivity for identification of gastric masses.
- Abdominal radiographs – may see loss of serosal detail, thickening of the gastric wall, and/or a mass effect, but usually difficult to identify a gastric mass.
- Thoracic radiographs – should be performed for complete staging, although pulmonary metastases are rarely seen at the time of initial diagnosis.

Other Diagnostic Procedures

- Fine needle aspirates (FNA) – if a gastric mass, thickening, or enlarged lymph node is seen with ultrasound, FNA with cytology may show epithelial or mesenchymal cells with features of malignancy, supportive of either a carcinoma or sarcoma, respectively. This can also be useful to rule out lymphoma. However, mesenchymal tumors may not exfoliate well.
- Endoscopy – useful for visualizing masses and collecting biopsies; can also evaluate the overlying mucosa.

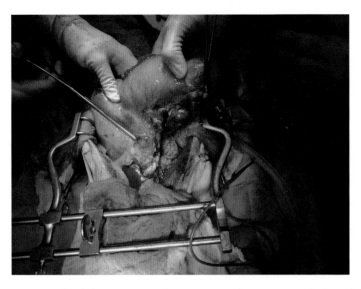

■ **Fig. 41.2.** Intraoperative view of the gastric mass in Figure 41.1. The tumor extends along the lesser curvature from the pyloric antrum to the body of the stomach, as outlined by the surgeons' thumbs. The Doyen forceps represent the extent of gastric resection, while the hemostats are used for vessel ligation. Note the discoloration of the left limb of the pancreas, which was removed during this procedure. Source: Courtesy of Dr Joel Takacs.

- Endoscopic biopsy may be performed but is often nondiagnostic if tumors are deep to the mucosal surface, or if the mass is beyond the reach of the endoscope. Adenocarcinomas in particular often contain areas of necrosis and inflammation, making false-negative histopathology results common.
- Open surgical biopsy with exploratory laparotomy is the gold standard, often required to confirm a diagnosis (Figures 41.2, 41.3).

Pathologic Findings

- Adenocarcinoma.
  - Gross – usually scirrhous (firm, white serosal surface) and nondistensible, an appearance referred to as *linitis plastica*. Often ulcerated with a central necrotic crater.
  - Cytologic – malignant population of epithelial cells, often with signet ring cells, microvacuolation, and cellular pleomorphism.
  - Histopathologic – neoplastic epithelial cells arranged in haphazard nests and cords. May see signet ring cells as well (Figure 41.4).
    - World Health Organization classification system based on growth pattern: papillary, tubular, mucinous, signet ring, undifferentiated.
    - Also classified into interstitial and diffuse types.
    - Clinical and prognostic significance of subtypes is unknown.
- Leiomyosarcoma/GIST.
  - Gross – firm, submucosal masses with normal overlying mucosa.
  - Cytologic – mesenchymal tumors tend to exfoliate poorly.
  - Histopathologic – spindle to epithelioid cells arranged in streams and interlacing bundles, primarily involving the smooth muscle of the tunica muscularis. Leiomyosarcoma and GIST can only be differentiated by immunohistochemistry (IHC).
    - Leiomyosarcoma: IHC positive for smooth muscle actin, +/– desmin.
    - GIST: IHC positive for KIT (c-kit or CD117), +/– CD34.

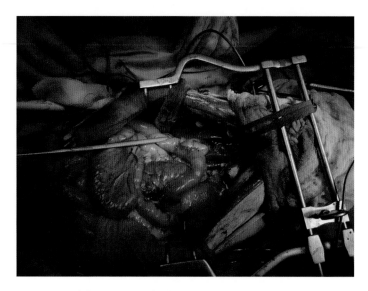

■ **Fig. 41.3.** Postoperative view following gastroduodenostomy, partial pancreatectomy, and cholecystoduodenostomy to excise the gastric mass in Figure 41.2. This image shows the incision line at the gastroduodenostomy (*lower*) and cholecystoduodenostomy (*upper*) sites. The Doyen forceps are placed aborad to the surgery sites, and the gallbladder is visible in the upper right of the image. Source: Courtesy of Dr Joel Takacs.

(a)   (b)

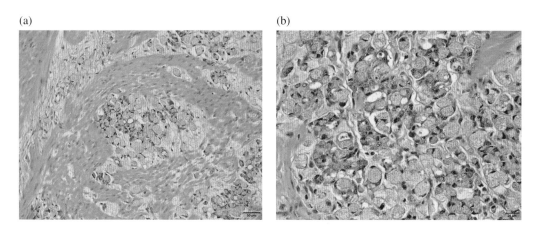

■ **Fig. 41.4.** (a) Histopathology specimen (20× magnification) from the gastric adenocarcinoma (*above*), showing invasion into the muscularis layer by the neoplastic epithelial cells. (b) 40× magnification showing the polygonal to round neoplastic cells arranged in haphazard nests and cords. Numerous signet ring cells are present (peripheralized nucleus with a single, granular cytoplasmic vacuole). Source: Courtesy of Dr Amy Durham, University of Pennsylvania School of Veterinary Medicine.

 THERAPEUTICS

Drug(s) of Choice

■ Chemotherapy.
- Adenocarcinomas – reports limited to case studies and series, with no known survival benefit over surgery alone. Protocols have included carboplatin, doxorubicin, cisplatin, 5-fluorouracil, and cyclophosphamide.
- GISTs – may respond to tyrosine kinase inhibitors (such as toceranib phosphate) given expression of KIT, although no specific studies to date.

Nursing Care

- Consider small, frequent meals during surgical recovery.
- Consider feeding tube placement if necessary.
- Antiemetics, antacids, analgesics for supportive care.
- Blood glucose monitoring in hypoglycemic patients, along with appropriate treatment (dextrose or glucose supplementation).

Surgical Considerations

- Surgical resection is the treatment of choice; however, gastric masses are often nonresectable due to the difficult locations (especially the pyloric antrum), extent of lesions, and debilitated status of patients.
- Carefully evaluate for metastasis before extensive surgery with staging (e.g., mesenteric lymph nodes, liver, and lungs).
- Perform a full abdominal exploratory surgery with biopsies of any other abnormal lesions.
- Surgical options.
  - Billroth I, if possible: wide partial gastrectomy/antrectomy, followed by gastro-duodenostomy.
  - Increased morbidity with Billroth II: gastrectomy/gastrojejunostomy.
  - Some lesions require biliary bypass or complete gastrectomy, associated with increased morbidity.
- Leiomyosarcomas and GISTs are more discrete and solitary, and may be removed with a gastrotomy and removal of the submucosa.

 COMMENTS

Patient Monitoring

- Regular physical exams.
- Regular postoperative abdominal ultrasound +/– thoracic radiographs.
- For patients with incomplete tumor excision – regular rechecks to provide palliative care and symptomatic support for clinical signs.

Possible Complications

Gastric perforation and sepsis, secondary to tumor growth or dehiscence of surgical site.

Expected Course and Prognosis

- Adenocarcinoma.
  - Most are nonresectable, and morbidity is high following radical surgical procedures.
  - Metastatic rate 50–90%, usually to regional lymph nodes, and later to distant sites including the liver, other abdominal sites, and/or lungs.
  - Reported median survival times range from one to 7.5 months.
- Leiomyosarcomas/GIST.
  - May metastasize to liver, regional lymph nodes, and other abdominal sites.
  - Hypoglycemia usually resolves after surgery, often within hours.
  - Median survival times approximately one year with surgery.
  - Behavior of GISTs can vary from benign to malignant.
  - Several studies have described reclassification of previously diagnosed smooth muscle tumors (leiomyosarcomas or leiomyomas) to GISTs based on immunohistochemistry.
    - No significant difference in survival reported among leiomyosarcoma, GIST, and leiomyoma; however, most studies include predominantly intestinal tumors with few gastric tumors.

- ○ One study reported median survival times of 7.8 months for gastrointestinal leiomyosarcomas and 11.6 months for GISTs (37.4 months for those that survived the perioperative period; overall no significant difference).
- ○ Tumor diameter prognostic in one study.
- ○ Even if high mitotic index or other malignant factors on histopathology, long-term prognosis can be good with complete surgical excision.

Abbreviations

- ■ FNA = fine-needle aspirate
- ■ GIST = gastrointestinal stromal tumor
- ■ IHC = immunohistochemistry

See Also

- ■ Gastric Neoplasia, Benign
- ■ Gastrointestinal Lymphoma, Canine
- ■ Gastrointestinal Lymphoma, Feline

Suggested Reading

Gillespie V, Baer K, Farrelly J, et al. Canine gastrointestinal stromal tumors: immunohistochemical expression of CD34 and examination of prognostic indicators including proliferation markers Ki67 and AgNOR. Vet Pathol 2011;48:283–291.

Hugen S, Thomas RE, German AJ, et al. Gastric carcinoma in canines and humans: a review. Vet Comp Oncol 2017;15:692–705.

Russell KN, Mehler SJ, Skorupski KA, et al. Clinical and immunohistochemical differentiation of gastrointestinal stromal tumors from leiomyosarcomas in dogs: 42 cases (1990–2003). J Am Vet Med Assoc 2007;230(9):1329–1333.

Swann HM, Holt DE. Canine gastric adenocarcinoma and leiomyosarcoma: a retrospective study of 21 cases (1986–1999) and literature review. J Am Anim Hosp Assoc 2002;38:157–164.

Willard MD. Alimentary neoplasia in geriatric dogs and cats. Vet Clin North Am Small Anim Pract 2012;42:693–706.

Acknowledgment: The author and editors acknowledge the prior contribution of Dr Laura D. Garrett.

Author: Jennifer A. Mahoney DVM, DACVIM (Oncology)

Chapter 42

Gastric Parasites

DEFINITION/OVERVIEW

- *Physaloptera* spp. occur in dogs and cats; adults attach to the gastric mucosa and there is no larval migration outside the gastrointestinal tract.
- Infective larvae of *Physaloptera* are acquired when the host ingests an intermediate arthropod host (beetle, cockroach, cricket) or in paratenic hosts (birds, mammals, reptiles).
- *Ollulanus* occurs in cats; adults are found attached to the gastric mucosa and eggs may hatch and mature without leaving the stomach.
- Infections can cause vomiting, gastritis, or no clinical signs.

ETIOLOGY/PATHOPHYSIOLOGY

- Animals become infected with gastric nematodes by ingesting L3 larvae.
- *Physaloptera* larvae are found within arthropod intermediate hosts.
- *Ollulanus* are ovoviviparous; larvae hatch and mature in the stomach. Therefore, the life cycle can be completed within a single host. It is thought that transmission occurs by ingesting vomit of an infected host.
- Adult worms adhere to the mucosa leading to gastritis and vomiting. *Ollulanus* infection leads to mucosal inflammation and fibrosis.

Systems Affected

Gastrointestinal.

SIGNALMENT/HISTORY

Dogs and cats, any breed, age, or sex. Infected animals may undergo extensive work-ups for suspected inflammatory bowel disease/ulcers, only to discover the nematodes at the time of endoscopy.

Risk Factors

- For *Physaloptera*, dogs and cats that roam outdoors and ingest arthropods and vertebrates are more at risk. Access to habitat frequented by wild reservoir hosts (raccoon, fox, coyote, and others).
- *Ollulanus* occurs more frequently in situations where there are many cats living together such as cat colonies or catteries. Large captive felines are also susceptible.

Blackwell's Five-Minute Veterinary Consult Clinical Companion: Small Animal Gastrointestinal Diseases,
First Edition. Edited by Jocelyn Mott and Jo Ann Morrison.
© 2019 John Wiley & Sons, Inc. Published 2019 by John Wiley & Sons, Inc.
Companion website: www.fiveminutevet.com/gastrointestinal

Historical Findings

- There may be no clinical signs.
- Chronic vomiting, weight loss.
- Signs can occur without finding parasite eggs in feces. Single sex or single worm infections are common for *Physaloptera*.
- Melena can occur.

 # CLINICAL FEATURES

Physical examination may be unremarkable.

 # DIFFERENTIAL DIAGNOSIS

- Other infectious causes of vomiting (parasites, viruses, bacteria).
- Other noninfectious causes of vomiting including dietary indiscretion, foreign objects in the stomach, noxious substances accidentally ingested, gastrointestinal neoplasia, metabolic diseases.
- In dogs, *Spirocerca* produces a larvated egg that is similar to but smaller than *Physaloptera*.

 # DIAGNOSTICS

Complete Blood Count/Biochemistry/Urinalysis

May be unremarkable or mild anemia and/or eosinophilia may be present.

Other Laboratory Tests

- For *Physaloptera* – direct smear, wet mount, or fecal flotation to detect eggs in vomitus or feces; eggs are dense and can be difficult to detect by fecal flotation using low specific gravity solutions; use flotation solution with specific gravity >1.25.
  - Eggs are larvated and colorless (42–58 × 29–42 μm). Intermittent egg shedding and/or single sex infections are common.
- For *Ollulanus* – larvae or eggs are seldom found in feces; it is thought they are digested in the intestine. Vomitus may be examined by Baermann sedimentation for larvae.

Imaging

- Abdominal radiography to eliminate other causes of vomiting.
- Abdominal ultrasound – may show gastric thickening with *Ollulanus*; rarely *see* Parasites.

Other Diagnostic Tests

- *Physaloptera* infections are often revealed by endoscopy (gastroscopy). A thorough search of the mucosa is needed as there are often few worms and they may be obscured by ingesta and rugae. Adults are 2–5 cm in length with an anterior cuticular collar. *P. praeputialis* has a posterior prepuce-like cuticular sheath.
- For *Ollulanus* – adults are very small and are unlikely to be discovered by endoscopy. Biopsy of the mucosa may reveal adults.
- Gastric lavage for *Ollulanus* – using saline collection followed by centrifugation to precipitate L3 larvae, or use Baermann technique.

THERAPEUTICS

- *Physaloptera* – endoscopic removal or anthelmintics.
- Outpatient treatment – anthelmintic with or without endoscopic removal of worms.
- Anthelmintic use is extra-label and anecdotal.

Drug(s) of Choice

- No labeled product available; doses are typically higher than for other internal nematodes. Pyrantel (20 mg/kg PO), every two weeks for at least three treatments is recommended. Fenbendazole 50 mg/kg PO q 24 h for 3–5 days may also be effective. Macrocyclic lactones have variable efficacy.
- Ivermectin (cats), 0.2 mg/kg PO or SQ once.
- Medication to reduce gastritis – histamine H2-antagonists (e.g., famotidine 0.5 mg/kg PO q 24 h); sucralfate 0.25–1 g PO q 8–12 h in the dog; 0.25 g PO q 8–12 h in the cat.
- *Ollulanus* – no labeled product available. Benzimidazoles and pyrantel are recommended but there is little data available for efficacy of these treatments.
- Tetramisole (2.5% formulation, 5 mg/kg PO) was reported to be effective; unavailable in the United States.

Appropriate Health Care

Patients with severe vomiting may require hospitalization with intravenous fluids and antiemetics.

 # COMMENTS

- Animals that ingest arthropods and/or paratenic hosts can become reinfected with *Physaloptera*.
- *Ollulanus* infection has been identified in a cat with concurrent gastric adenocarcinoma.

Patient Monitoring

- For *Physaloptera* – recheck 1–2 weeks post treatment and retreat with anthelmintic if eggs still present on fecal exam and/or if vomiting persists.
- For *Ollulanus* – warn owner to watch for further vomiting; treat with another round of tetramisole if it occurs.

Prevention/Avoidance

- Prompt removal and disposal of feces to prevent infection of arthropod intermediate hosts.
- Keep pets from roaming freely outdoors; prevent hunting and scavenging.

Expected Course and Prognosis

For *Physaloptera* – clinical signs and/or shedding of eggs in feces should resolve within two weeks of treatment.

See Also

- Parasites, Gastrointestinal
- Vomiting, Chronic

Suggested Reading

Barr SC, Bowman DD. *Ollulanus* infection. In: Canine and Feline Infectious Diseases and Parasitology. Ames: Blackwell, 2006, pp. 385–387.

Bowman DD. Georgis' Parasitology for Veterinarians, 9th ed. St Louis: Saunders Elsevier Science, 2009, pp. 89–91.

Bowman DD, Hendrix CM, Lindsay DS, et al. *Ollulanus tricuspis*. In: Feline Clinical Parasitology. Ames: Iowa State University Press, 2002, pp. 262–265.

Campbell KL, Graham JC. Physaloptera infection in dogs and cats. Compend Contin Educ Pract Vet 1999;21:299–314.

Authors: Jeba Jesudoss Chelladurai BVSc & AH, MS, DACVM, Matt T. Brewer DVM, PhD, DACVM

Chapter 43

Gastritis, Acute

DEFINITION/OVERVIEW

Acute gastritis is defined as an acute-onset syndrome of vomiting presumed to be associated with an acute insult or inflammation of the gastric mucosa.

ETIOLOGY/PATHOPHYSIOLOGY

- Mechanisms that protect the gastric mucosa from low pH (gastric acid), mechanical irritation (ingesta/food), and enzymatic digestion (pepsin, gastric lipase) include the tight layer of gastric epithelial cells, secretion of bicarbonate (diffusion over the epithelium) and mucus (produced by gastric epithelial cells), hydrophobic residues (phospholipids) of the epithelial cell surface, and maintenance of an abundant gastric mucosal blood flow supplying the tissue with nutrients and oxygen.
- A number of factors (see Risk Factors below) can break down this protective gastric mucosal barrier and can cause acute irritation followed by inflammation, which can range anywhere from mild self-limiting disease to severe gastritis with erosions or ulceration causing signs of systemic illness.

Systems Affected

- Gastrointestinal – esophagitis can develop as a result of vomiting. Chronic gastritis can result if the initial insult or inflammation persists.
- Respiratory – patients with vomiting are generally at risk for development of aspiration pneumonia.
- Cardiovascular – severe vomiting may cause hypovolemia, electrolyte changes (e.g., hypokalemia), and/or acid–base imbalances (e.g., hypochloremic metabolic alkalosis).

SIGNALMENT/HISTORY

- Acute gastritis is common in dogs and cats.
- There is no known breed, sex, or age predilection.
- No genetic basis.

Risk Factors

- Causes of acute gastritis include dietary indiscretion, nonimmunological food intolerance, immunological adverse food reaction (food allergy), ingestion of irritating substances (e.g., plants, cleaners) or foreign bodies (e.g. toys, rocks, bones, hairballs), medications

---

Blackwell's Five-Minute Veterinary Consult Clinical Companion: Small Animal Gastrointestinal Diseases, First Edition. Edited by Jocelyn Mott and Jo Ann Morrison.
© 2019 John Wiley & Sons, Inc. Published 2019 by John Wiley & Sons, Inc.
Companion website: www.fiveminutevet.com/gastrointestinal

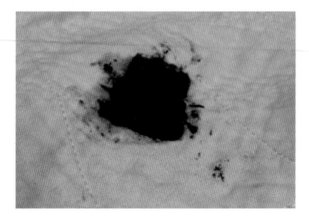

■ **Fig. 43.1.** Melena (tarry stool) in a dog with proximal gastrointestinal (gastric) bleeding.

(e.g., corticosteroids, nonsteroidal antiinflammatory drugs, certain antibiotics), toxins (e.g., dietary contaminants, organophosphates, herbicides, heavy metals), infections (e.g., endoparasites such as *Physaloptera* spp. or *Ollulanus* spp., parvoviral enteritis, bacterial toxins), or systemic diseases (e.g., uremia, hepatopathy, hypoadrenocorticism).

■ The role of *Helicobacter* sp. in naturally occurring canine and feline gastritis is currently not clear.

Historical Findings

■ Severity of clinical signs depends upon the underlying cause. Patients can also be asymptomatic.
■ Patients typically present with acute onset of vomiting and hyporexia or anorexia. Vomiting must be differentiated from regurgitation.
■ Hematemesis, melena (Figure 43.1), and/or concurrent diarrhea may be noted in some patients.
■ Signs of systemic involvement (e.g., lethargy) may be seen in severely affected patients.

 ## CLINICAL FEATURES

■ Physical examination is usually unremarkable.
■ Signs of dehydration may be evident in patients with severe vomiting.

 ## DIFFERENTIAL DIAGNOSIS

■ Several gastrointestinal and nongastrointestinal diseases can be associated with acute vomiting.
■ Endoparasites, including *Giardia* sp., can be a cause of vomiting and need to be ruled out. Gastrointestinal obstruction or intussusception, foreign bodies, primary (idiopathic) inflammation, or neoplasia (e.g., lymphoma) are also important differentials.
■ Infectious (e.g., parvovirus enteritis), metabolic (e.g., renal failure, pancreatitis, hepatobiliary disease), or endocrine diseases (e.g., hyperthyroidism, diabetes mellitus, hypoadrenocorticism) also need to be excluded as a cause of vomiting.

DIAGNOSTICS

Diagnostics should be performed if an underlying etiology or more complicated disease course is suspected.

Complete Blood Count/Biochemistry/Urinalysis

Results of the minimum database are usually unremarkable or nonspecific with mild and uncomplicated acute gastritis, but are important to rule out other etiologies (e.g., metabolic causes) or consequences (e.g., fluid and electrolyte disturbances) of vomiting. Hypokalemia or hypochloremic metabolic alkalosis may be seen with severe vomiting.

Other Laboratory Tests

- Serum specific canine pancreatic lipase (Spec cPL) concentration, together with abdominal ultrasound findings, can aid in diagnosing patients with pancreatitis.
- Fecal direct examination and flotation should be performed to detect endoparasites. *Giardia* sp. can be detected with an antigen enzyme-linked immunosorbent assay (ELISA).
- A baseline serum cortisol concentration or, if indicated, an adrenocorticotropic hormone (ACTH) stimulation test can help diagnose or exclude hypoadrenocorticism.

Imaging

Thoracic radiographs and abdominal ultrasound are usually unremarkable but should be performed to rule out other differentials or etiologies (e.g., gastric foreign bodies, gastrointestinal obstruction) and complications of vomiting (aspiration pneumonia).

Other Diagnostic Procedures

- Gastrointestinal endoscopy – mucosal erosions and edema can be detected during endoscopy (Figure 43.2). Gastroscopy may be indicated to remove a gastric foreign body.
- *Physaloptera* spp. infection can sometimes only be diagnosed endoscopically (Figure 43.3).

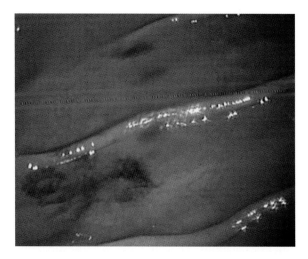

■ **Fig. 43.2.** Gastroscopic image showing multiple superficial mucosal hemorrhages due to erosions in a dog with acute gastritis.

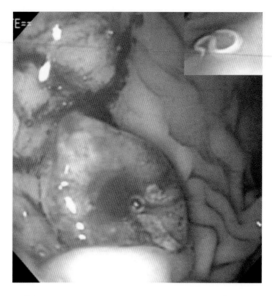

■ **Fig. 43.3.** Endoscopic view of the gastric mucosa revealing nodular lesions in a dog with parasitic gastritis (inset: *Physaloptera* spp. infection).

Pathologic Findings

Diagnosis of acute gastritis is usually based on clinical signs and response to symptomatic treatment, and is rarely confirmed by histopathology.

 THERAPEUTICS

Drug(s) of Choice

- Antiemetics are the most important part of symptomatic treatment for acute gastritis. Options include maropitant, ondansetron, dolasetron, metoclopramide (Table 43.1), or a combination.
- In addition, intravenous fluid therapy is recommended in moderately to severely dehydrated patients (Table 43.2). Balanced electrolyte solution (e.g., lactated Ringer's solution, supplemented with potassium if indicated; Table 43.3) are appropriate. Alternatively, an oral rehydration solution can be given to patients with mild dehydration provided that the animal is not vomiting.
- Antisecretory drugs including famotidine, ranitidine, omeprazole, esomeprazole, and pantoprazole (see Table 43.1) may be beneficial. Ranitidine also has mild gastric prokinetic effects.
- Gastric mucosal protectants, such as sucralfate or antacids (see Table 43.1), should be considered in patients with hematemesis or melena.

Precautions/Interactions

- Metoclopramide may cause nervousness, anxiety, or depression, and is contraindicated in animals with epilepsy.
- Proton pump inhibitors can interfere with cytochrome p450-dependent drug metabolism (e.g., cyclosporine, benzodiazepines).
- Sucralfate should be given on an empty stomach and at least two hours before or after administration of other medications. Antacids can cause constipation.
- Gastric prokinetic agents should not be administered in patients with gastrointestinal obstruction.

TABLE 43.1. Medications recommended for use in dogs and cats with acute gastritis.

Drug class	Drug	Dose
Antiemetics		
NK$_1$-receptor antagonist	Maropitant	1 mg/kg SQ q24h or 2 mg/kg PO q24h
5-HT$_3$-receptor antagonists	Ondansetron	0.1–0.3 mg/kg IV q12h or 0.2–0.5 mg/kg PO q12h
	Dolasetron	0.3–0.6 mg/kg IV, SQ, or PO q12h
D$_2$-receptor antagonist	Metoclopramide	0.2–0.4 mg/kg PO, SQ, or IV q8–12h or 5–20 µg/kg/h IV as a CRI
Antisecretory drugs		
H$_2$-receptor antagonists (H$_2$RA)	Famotidine	0.5–1 mg/kg q12h PO or IV
	Ranitidine	1–2 mg/kg q8–12h PO or IV
Proton pump inhibitors (PPI)	Omeprazole	0.7–1 mg/kg q12–24h PO
	Esomeprazole	0.5–1 mg/kg q24h PO or IV
	Pantoprazole	0.7–1 mg/kg q24h IV (give over ≥15 min)
Drugs for mucosal protection		
Direct cytoprotectant	Sucralfate	20–40 mg/kg q6–8h PO or 0.5–1.0 g q6–8h PO
Antacids	Aluminium hydroxide	100–200 mg q4–6h PO (dog) or 50–100 mg q4–6h PO (cat)
	Magnesium hydroxide	5–15 ml q12–24h PO

TABLE 43.2. Components and calculation of fluid therapy in patients with acute gastritis.

Component	Calculation
Replacement of fluid deficit	ml of fluid to be given (over 4–12 hours) = dehydration (%) × body weight (kg) × 10
Maintenance fluid requirement	ml of fluid to be given (over 24 hours) = (30 × body weight [kg]) + 70 or = 70 × (body weight [kg])$^{0.75}$ or = 40–60 × body weight (kg)
Replacement of ongoing losses	ml of fluid to be given (over 24 hours) = estimated ongoing losses due to vomiting/diarrhea

TABLE 43.3. Recommendation for potassium supplementation in patients with acute gastritis.

Plasma potassium level	KCl supplementation	Maximum fluid rate
3.6–5.5 mmol/L	20 mmol/L	24 mL/kg/h
3.1–3.5 mmol/L	30 mmol/L	16 mL/kg/h
2.6–3.0 mmol/L	40 mmol/L	12 mL/kg/h
2.0–2.5 mmol/L	60 mmol/L	8 mL/kg/h
<2.0 mmol/L	80 mmol/L	6 mL/kg/h

Appropriate Health Care

- Treatment of acute gastritis is mostly symptomatic and supportive, and most patients can be managed on an outpatient basis.
- Specific treatment is to be considered if an underlying etiology has been identified (e.g., endoscopic removal of a gastric foreign body).

Nursing Care

Additional supportive treatment options are recommended in patients with dehydration (intravenous fluids) and/or aspiration pneumonia (oxygen therapy, nebulization, coupage, appropriate antibiotics).

Diet

- Dietary restriction is usually recommended for a short (12–24 h) time, and provided that there is no contraindication.
- After vomiting has ceased, patients with acute gastritis should be given a highly digestible, fat-restricted diet in multiple small portions throughout the day for 3–5 days. Either a commercially available gastrointestinal diet or a bland home-prepared diet (consisting of boiled lean chicken or white fish with rice and low-fat cottage cheese) can be used.
- The patient is then slowly transitioned to its original diet over a period of 3–5 days.

Activity

Patients with acute gastritis can resume their normal level of activity.

Surgical Considerations

Acute gastritis is a nonsurgical disorder. Surgery may be needed if a gastric foreign body cannot be retrieved endoscopically.

 COMMENTS

Client Education

- Educate the client that further diagnostic evaluation will be needed if the patient does not respond to supportive treatment or if clinical signs recur after discontinuation of symptomatic treatment.
- Educate the client that careful monitoring for signs of possible aspiration pneumonia is needed.

Patient Monitoring

- Clinical signs of possible aspiration pneumonia include dyspnea, tachypnea, coughing, fever, and lethargy.
- Hydration status of the patient also needs to be carefully monitored.

Possible Complications

- Vomiting is a general risk for development of aspiration pneumonia.
- Esophagitis can also develop as a result of vomiting, with the potential for ensuing esophageal dysmotility or stricture formation.
- Chronic gastritis and gastric ulcers can develop if the initial insult or inflammation persists. Transient delayed gastric emptying due to gastritis usually subsides with successful treatment.

Expected Course and Prognosis

- Prognosis for acute gastritis is generally favorable to good, depending upon the underlying etiology, severity of clinical signs, and presence or development of complications.
- Most patients respond well to one of the above treatments (or a combination of these treatment options).
- In rare cases, acute gastritis can perpetuate and lead to chronic gastritis.
- Failure to respond to treatment suggests another underlying or causative factor.

Abbreviations

- ACTH = adrenocorticotropic hormone
- ELISA = enzyme-linked immunosorbent assay
- Spec cPL = specific canine pancreatic lipase

See Also

- Esophagitis
- Gastric Neoplasia, Malignant
- Gastritis, Chronic
- Gastroenteritis, Eosinophilic
- Gastroenteritis, Lymphocytic-Plasmacytic

Suggested Reading

Boothe DM. Small Animal Clinical Pharmacology and Therapeutics, 2nd ed. St Louis: Elsevier Saunders, 2006.

Elwood DC, Deveauchelle P, Elliot J, et al. Emesis in dogs: a review. J Small Anim Pract 2010;51(1):4–22.

Steiner JM. Small Animal Gastroenterology. Hannover: Schlütersche, 2008.

Washabau RJ, Day MJ. Canine and Feline Gastroenterology. St Louis: Elsevier, 2013.

Webb C, Twedt DC. Canine gastritis. Vet Clin North Am Small Anim Pract 2003;33(5):969–985.

Yalcin E, Kesar GO. Comparative efficacy of metoclopramide, ondansetron and maropitant in preventing parvoviral enteritis-induced emesis in dogs. J Vet Pharmacol Ther 2017;40:599–603.

Author: Romy M. Heilmann med.vet., Dr.med.vet., DACVIM (SAIM), DECVIM-CA, PhD

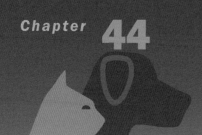

Gastritis, Atrophic

DEFINITION/OVERVIEW

A type of chronic gastritis characterized histologically by a focal or diffuse reduction in size and depth of gastric glands with associated inflammatory cells.

ETIOLOGY/PATHOPHYSIOLOGY

- Chronic vomiting, most often intermittent, with food, or bile stained.
- Anorexia, lethargy, weight loss, edema or ascites.

Systems Affected

Gastrointestinal (stomach).

SIGNALMENT/HISTORY

- Variable, uncommon in young patients.
- A high prevalence in the Norwegian lundehund (age range 4–13 years old); males are overrepresented.

Risk Factors

- A potential risk factor is preexisting idiopathic inflammatory gastroenteritis or other stomach infections/diseases.
- Suspect genetic predisposition in the Norwegian lundehund.

Historical Findings

- Patients have chronic vomiting, most often intermittent; vomitus can be food or have bile staining.
- Anorexia, lethargy, weight loss, edema or ascites can also be present.

CLINICAL FEATURES

- Thin body condition.
- Ascites.
- Norwegian lundehund.

Blackwell's Five-Minute Veterinary Consult Clinical Companion: Small Animal Gastrointestinal Diseases, First Edition. Edited by Jocelyn Mott and Jo Ann Morrison.
© 2019 John Wiley & Sons, Inc. Published 2019 by John Wiley & Sons, Inc.
Companion website: www.fiveminutevet.com/gastrointestinal

DIFFERENTIAL DIAGNOSIS

Other forms of chronic gastritis and chronic enteritis.

DIAGNOSTICS

Complete Blood Count/Biochemistry/Urinalysis

- Complete blood cell count – anemia with thrombocytopenia or thrombocytosis may be present if gastric ulceration is present.
- Biochemistry.
  - Panhypoproteinemia with an absence of proteinuria can be present with primary disease and in animals with concurrent protein-losing enteropathy.
  - Achlorhydria (absence of hydrochloric acid in gastric secretions) has been reported in dogs; may lead to intestinal dysbiosis.
- Urinalysis – most often normal; use to rule out protein-losing nephropathy if ascites present.

Other Laboratory Tests

- Cobalamin/folate – used to investigate further intestinal disease in cases of chronic vomiting; results are variable. Cobalamin can be low due to chronic malabsorption and affected patients should receive cobalamin supplementation.
- Hepatic function testing (bile acids) – used to rule out extragastrointestinal causes of chronic vomiting (hepatic dysfunction).
- Pancreatic lipase immunoreactivity – used to rule out extragastrointestinal causes of chronic vomiting (pancreatitis).

Imaging

- Survey radiographs of the thorax and abdomen are typically unremarkable. Stomach may contain ingesta despite adequate fasting, suggesting delayed gastric emptying. Can be used to identify abdominal masses or rule out extragastrointestinal causes of chronic vomiting.
- Ultrasonography of the abdomen may reveal a thickened or normal gastric wall, gastric masses, the presence or absence of mesenteric lymphadenopathy, thickened or normal intestinal walls, presence or absence of abdominal effusion. Lymphadenopathy and masses may be present with gastric neoplasia.

Other Diagnostic Tests

- Endoscopic biopsies of the stomach and the small intestines should be performed to evaluate for infiltrative disease.
- Definitive diagnosis – gastroscopy with biopsy and histopathologic evaluation.

Pathologic Findings

- Histopathologic examination of gastric biopsy specimens reveals glandular atrophy and inflammatory infiltrates (neutrophils or mononuclear cells). Majority of lesions are located in the fundic region. In non-lundehunds, lymphocytic plasmacytic gastritis may be found with gastric atrophy. Fibrosis may be present.
- Mucin staining in lundehunds reveals abnormal mucus neck cells and pseudopyloric metaplasia. Neoplastic transformation may be associated with linear hyperplasia of neuroendocrine cells (requires special staining, request in suspected cases: chromagrin A, synaptophysin, Sevier–Munger method).

- The role of *Helicobacter* infection is controversial. Cats developing atrophic gastritis have been found to have *H. pylori* infections, but active *Helicobacter* infections have not been documented in canine cases. Urease activity to diagnose *Helicobacter* infection in gastric biopsies is not diagnostic and poorly correlated with actual infection. Clinical infection is supported by histological documentation of characteristic spiral bacteria deep in gastric mucosa and pits with associated inflammation.

 THERAPEUTICS

Optimal therapy is unknown. Tylosin can be administered if the disorder has an antibiotic-responsive component. Treat any underlying etiology (e.g., inflammatory bowel disease) that is identified.

Drug(s) of Choice

- Tylosin 10–20 mg/kg PO q 12 h for bacterial overgrowth.
- Histamine type-2 receptor antagonists (e.g., famotidine 0.5–1 mg/kg PO q 12 h) or proton pump inhibitors (e.g., omeprazole 0.7–1.5 mg/kg PO q 12–24 h) to inhibit gastric acid secretion and prevent esophagitis. Long-term use of omeprazole should be avoided if possible in light of potential adverse effects (hypocalcemia, osteoporosis, intestinal dysbiosis, hypocobalaminemia, increased risk of diarrhea); if patient does well on proton pump inhibitor therapy then monitor for these changes q 3–6 months.
- If vomiting persists, antiemetics such as maropitant (1–2 mg/kg PO or SQ q 24 h, for five days in dogs, 15 days in cats) or ondansetron (0.5 mg/kg PO or SQ q 24 h for 5–7 days) or prokinetics such as metoclopramide (0.2–0.5 mg/kg PO q 8 h) or cisapride (0.3–0.5 mg/kg PO q 8–12 h) may be indicated.
- If infection with *Helicobacter* spp. is confirmed based upon histopathologic lesions in the stomach consistent with *Helicobacter* infection, consider triple therapy: amoxicillin 11–22 mg/kg PO q 12 h, metronidazole 10–15 mg/kg PO q 12 h and famotidine 0.5–1.0 mg/kg PO q 12 h or omeprazole 0.7–1.5 mg/kg PO q 24 h for two weeks. This infection may recur.

Precautions/Interactions

Be cautious with medications known to exacerbate gastritis, such as corticosteroids and non-steroidal antiinflammatory drugs.

Alternative Drugs

Metronidazole (10–15 mg/kg PO q 12 h) can be used if tylosin is not tolerated by patient.

Appropriate Health Care

Weight loss is a concern; appetite stimulants such as Entyce® (3 mg/kg PO q 24 h) could be tried but evidence for efficacy is lacking.

Nursing Care

- Treat dehydration or complications as they arise.
- Enteral feeding tube may be indicated in cachexic patients.

Diet

- Trial therapy for food-responsive gastropathy with an elimination diet can be tried. Novel protein and hydrolyzed diets are acceptable.
- If gastric emptying is delayed, low-residue, fat-restricted diets may aid in emptying.

Activity

No changes to activity needed.

 COMMENTS

- Correlation with progression to gastric cancer (adenocarcinoma or neuroendocrine carcinoma) is suspected but not proven. However, this has been documented in the Norwegian lundehund breed. If signs persist or recur, monitor for developing gastric tumors (thoracic radiographs, abdominal ultrasound).
- Hypergastrinemia and gastric hypoacidity are suspected but not proven in veterinary patients.

Client Education

Life-long disease with no cure; quality of life concerns can cause euthanasia decision.

Patient Monitoring

- Weight, muscle mass, body condition score q 30–60 days.
- Reassess any abnormal labwork (see diagnostics section) for improvement q 30–60 days.

Prevention/Avoidance

Identify chronic and stomach diseases early to start therapy.

Possible Complications

- Food intolerances, recurrence of gastrointestinal signs with gastric indiscretion.
- If *Helicobacter* is present, infection can recur even with successful treatment.

Expected Course and Prognosis

- Better prognosis if an underlying concurrent disease is found and treated.
- Progressive disease, poor prognosis.

Synonyms

Type A or Type B gastritis in humans

See Also

- Cobalamin Deficiency
- Gastritis, Chronic
- Gastric Neoplasia, Malignant
- *Helicobacter*-Associated Gastritis
- Inflammatory Bowel Disease
- Intestinal Dysbiosis
- Nutritional Approach to Chronic Enteropathies
- Protein-Losing Enteropathy
- Vomiting, Chronic

Suggested Reading

Berghoff N, Ruaux CG, Steiner JM, et al. Gastroenteropathy in Norwegian Lundehunds. Compend Contin Educ Pract Vet 2007;29(8):456–465, 468–470.

Qvigstad G, Kolbjornsen O, Skancke E, et al. Gastric neuroendocrine carcinoma associated with atrophic gastritis in the Norwegian Lundehund. J Comp Pathol 2008;139:194–201.

Simpson KW. Diseases of the stomach. In: Ettinger SJ, Feldman EC, eds. Textbook of Veterinary Internal Medicine, 6th ed. St Louis: Elsevier, 2005, pp. 1321–1326.

Author: Jessica M. Clemans DVM, DACVIM

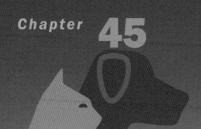

Chapter 45

Gastritis, Chronic

DEFINITION/OVERVIEW

- Intermittent vomiting of >1–2 weeks in duration, secondary to gastric inflammation.
- Presence of gastric erosions or ulcers dependent on the inciting cause and duration.

ETIOLOGY/PATHOPHYSIOLOGY

- Chronic irritation of the gastric mucosa by chemical irritants, drugs, foreign bodies, infectious agents, or hyperacidity syndromes resulting in an inflammatory response directed at the mucosal surface that may extend to involve submucosal layers.
- Chronic allergen exposure or immune-mediated disease may also produce chronic inflammation.
- Relatively common occurrence.

Systems Affected

- Gastrointestinal – esophagitis may result from chronic vomiting and/or gastroesophageal reflux.
- Respiratory – aspiration pneumonia is infrequently seen secondary to chronic vomiting; it is more likely if concurrent esophageal disease exists or if the patient is debilitated.

SIGNALMENT/HISTORY

- Dog and cat.
- Old, small-breed dogs (i.e., Lhasa apso, shih tzu, miniature poodle) are more commonly affected with antral mucosal hyperplasia and hypertrophy.
- Norwegian lundehunds are predisposed to chronic atrophic gastritis.
- Basenjis and the Drentse patrijshond (aka Dutch partridge dog or Drent) breed can develop chronic hypertrophic gastritis.
- Mean age and range varies with underlying cause.
- Predominant sex varies with underlying cause.

Risk Factors

- Medications – nonsteroidal antiinflammatory drugs (NSAIDs), glucocorticoids.
- Environmental – unsupervised/free-roaming pets are more likely to ingest inappropriate foods or materials. Young dogs are more likely to ingest foreign bodies.
- Ingestion of a dietary antigen to which an allergy or intolerance has been acquired.

Blackwell's Five-Minute Veterinary Consult Clinical Companion: Small Animal Gastrointestinal Diseases,
First Edition. Edited by Jocelyn Mott and Jo Ann Morrison.
© 2019 John Wiley & Sons, Inc. Published 2019 by John Wiley & Sons, Inc.
Companion website: www.fiveminutevet.com/gastrointestinal

Historical Findings

- Vomitus is frequently bile-stained and may contain undigested food, flecks of blood, or digested blood ("coffee grounds").
- Frequency varies from daily to every few weeks and increases as gastritis progresses.
- Vomiting may be stimulated by eating or drinking.
- Early morning vomiting before eating may indicate bilious vomiting syndrome.
- May see weight loss with chronic anorexia.
- May see melena with ulceration (not common).
- Increased water intake.
- Diarrhea, if concurrent intestinal disease.

CLINICAL FEATURES

- Physical exam generally within normal limits.
- May be thin with persistent anorexia.
- May have pale mucous membranes with anemia from chronic blood loss.
- May find cranial abdominal pain (rarely noted).

DIFFERENTIAL DIAGNOSIS

- Drugs – NSAIDs, glucocorticoids.
- Dietary indiscretion – plant material, foreign objects, chemical irritants.
- Idiopathic gastritis – diagnosis of exclusion; often characterized by a predominantly lymphoplasmacytic infiltrate (superficial or diffuse).
  - Can also be characterized by other types of infiltrates. Eosinophilic gastritis, hypertrophic gastritis, granulomatous/histiocytic gastritis, and atrophic gastritis are less common; often overlap of histologic changes exists in the types of inflammatory infiltrates.
  - Atrophic gastritis appears differently on endoscopic examination – visualization of the submucosal vessels secondary to thinning of the gastric mucosa.
  - Hypertrophic gastritis – prominent mucosal folds that do not flatten with gastric insufflation.
- Infectious – *Helicobacter* spp., pythiosis, viral (distemper in dogs, feline leukemia virus in cats).
- Inflammatory – immune mediated, dietary allergy or intolerance, idiopathic.
- Metabolic/endocrine disease – azotemia, chronic liver disease, hypoadrenocorticism, pancreatitis.
- Neoplastic.
  - Common causes – gastrointestinal lymphoma, gastric adenocarcinoma, small cell lymphoma (especially cats, recent increase in dogs).
  - Infrequent causes – gastric polyps, gastrinoma, leiomyosarcoma, plasma cell tumor, mast cell tumor.
- Parasitism – *Physaloptera* spp. (dogs, cats); *Ollulanus tricuspis* and *Gnathostoma* spp. (cats).
- Toxins – fertilizers, herbicides, cleaning agents, heavy metals.
- Miscellaneous – duodenogastric reflux (bilious vomiting syndrome), stress, achlorhydria.

Although the causes listed above are included in the differential diagnosis of chronic gastritis, an identifiable cause is often not found for the gastric inflammation. It is important to differentiate chronic vomiting from chronic regurgitation (active vs passive vomiting). This can be challenging and requires a very good history. A video of an event can be very helpful, especially when the client struggles to describe what they are seeing and hearing.

DIAGNOSTICS

Complete Blood Count/Biochemistry/Urinalysis

- Hemogram usually unremarkable unless systemic disease present.
  - Hemoconcentration if severe dehydration.
  - Nonregenerative (anemia of chronic disease) or regenerative anemia (blood loss).
  - Microcytic, hypochromic anemia associated with iron deficiency if prolonged, severe blood loss, such as might be seen with ulceration (uncommon; when seen, more likely associated with neoplastic infiltrates such as gastric adenocarcinoma).
  - Eosinophilia with eosinophilic gastroenteritis.
- Azotemia with low urine specific gravity in uremic gastritis.
- Increased serum hepatic enzyme activities, total bilirubin, or hypoalbuminemia with chronic hepatic disease.
- Hyperkalemia and hyponatremia suggests hypoadrenocorticism (Addison's disease).
- Hyponatremia, hypokalemia, hypochloremia, and an elevated bicarbonate level with an acidotic urine suggest a gastric outflow obstruction (hypochloremic metabolic alkalosis).

Other Laboratory Testing

- Elevated serum gastrin level without azotemia suggests a gastrinoma.
- Fecal flotation may reveal intestinal parasites. Trial treatment with a broad-spectrum dewormer such as fenbendazole is recommended, especially in areas where parasitism is more prevalent.

Imaging

- Survey abdominal radiographs – usually normal, but may reveal radiodense foreign objects, a thickened gastric wall or gastric outflow obstruction with persistent gastric distension. May reveal free gas within the abdominal cavity if perforation has occurred.
- Contrast radiography – may detect foreign objects, gastric outflow obstruction, delayed gastric emptying, or gastric wall defects or thickening.
- Ultrasonography – may detect gastric wall thickening, ulceration, and gastric foreign objects. If available, ultrasound is usually more useful than contrast radiography.

Other Diagnostic Procedures

- Gastroscopy – usually adequate for visualization of the gastric mucosa and for biopsy but in most cases one should also evaluate and biopsy the duodenum.
- Foreign objects can be identified and retrieved via endoscopy.
- Gastric biopsy and histopathology are required for diagnosis, even if gastric mucosa appears normal. Duodenoscopy with biopsy is also recommended at the same time.
- Exploratory celiotomy is indicated if a perforated ulcer or submucosal lesion of the gastric wall is suspected and partial gastrectomy or full-thickness biopsy is required.

Pathologic Findings

- Idiopathic gastritis (most common) – any combination of lymphocytes, plasma cells, neutrophils, eosinophils, and/or histiocytes.
- Mucosal changes can be degenerative, hyperplastic, or atrophic.

- May see varying degrees of edema and fibrous tissue; may see *Helicobacter* spp. Organisms must be noted within gastric glands to be significant and should be accompanied by a lymphofollicular gastritis; special stains can be requested for fungal hyphae and *Helicobacter*.
- May see lymphoplasmacytic inflammation along with *Helicobacter* spp. Treatment for *Helicobacter* may result in resolution of clinical signs without immunosuppressive therapy.
- If hyperplastic changes are noted, a gastrin level should be obtained before institution or after discontinuation of antacids, H2-blockers or proton pump inhibitors.

 # THERAPEUTICS

The objectives of treatment are to control vomiting by removing the cause (foreign body, gastric mass, polyp, infection) or reducing the inflammation found within the gastric and/or duodenal wall.

Drug(s) of Choice

- Treat any gastric erosions and ulcers (see Chapter 46).
- Give glucocorticoids (prednisone 2–4 mg/kg PO q 24 h, rarely requires high end of dose, additional medications should be added if refractory to low end prednisone dose; taper by 25% every 2–3 weeks over 2–3 months) for chronic gastritis secondary to suspected immune-mediated mechanisms if no clinical response to dietary management. Never exceed a total dose of 50 mg of prednisone/day no matter how heavy the dog is.
- Treatment for *Helicobacter* gastritis – amoxicillin (22 mg/kg PO q 12 h), peptobismol® (15 mg/kg PO q 6–8 h) and metronidazole (10 mg/kg PO q 12 h) for three weeks.
- Antiemetics (maropitant 1–2 mg/kg PO/SQ q 24 h) for fluid and electrolyte disorders caused by frequent or profuse vomiting.
- Metoclopramide (0.2–0.4 mg/kg PO q 6–8 h), cisapride (0.5–1 mg/kg PO q8–12 h), or low-dose erythromycin (0.5–1 mg/kg PO q 8 h) to increase gastric emptying and normalize intestinal motility if gastric emptying is delayed or gastroduodenal reflux is present. Metoclopramide is most effective as a constant rate infusion (CRI) administered at 1–2 mg/kg q 24 h for hospitalized patients.

Precautions/Interactions

- Steroids are immunosuppressive, making close monitoring for secondary infections important.
- Steroids may also inhibit the normal gastric mucosal barrier, leading to ulceration.
- Do not use prokinetics, metoclopramide, or cisapride if gastric outflow obstruction is present.
- Antacids are not indicated with atrophic gastritis and achlorhydria.
- Prednisone has been used safely in pregnant women; corticosteroids have been associated with increased incidence of congenital defects, abortion, and fetal death.
- Azathioprine has been used safely in pregnant women and may be a good substitute for corticosteroids in pregnant animals.
- Do not administer misoprostol to pregnant animals.

Alternative Drugs

- Synthetic prostaglandin E1 (misoprostol 1–3 μg/kg PO q 6–8 h) to prevent gastric mucosal ulcers with NSAID toxicity.
- For additional immunosuppression when in need of an immediate response, add chlorambucil (0.1–0.2 mg/kg q 24 h for seven days then q 48 h). Often used in place of azathioprine

but can be used in addition. A recent study suggests that this addition may be superior to adding azathioprine.

- Immunosuppressive drugs such as azathioprine (2.2 mg/kg PO q 24 h, tapering to q 48 h after 2–3 weeks in dogs) if an immune-mediated mechanism is suspected and response to dietary management and glucocorticoid administration is inadequate. Expect response to occur in 2–3 weeks. Avoid use of azathioprine in cats because the drug is markedly myelosuppressive.

Appropriate Health Care

- Most patients are stable at presentation unless vomiting is severe enough to cause dehydration.
- Can typically manage as outpatient, pending diagnostic testing or undergoing clinical trials of special diets or medications.
- If patient is dehydrated or if vomiting becomes severe, hospitalize and institute appropriate intravenous crystalloid fluid therapy.

Diet

- Soft, low-fat food ideally from a single carbohydrate and protein source.
- Nonfat cottage cheese, boiled skinless white meat chicken, boiled hamburger/turkey or tofu as a protein source, and rice, pasta, or potato as a carbohydrate source, in a ratio of 1:3.
- Frequent, small meals (q 4–6 h or more frequently).
- Can use novel protein source or hydrolyzed protein diet if dietary allergy is suspected.
- Feed diets for a minimum of 2–3 weeks to assess adequacy of response.
- Feed a late-night meal to help prevent bilious vomiting syndrome in the early morning hours.

Activity

Generally not limited. Control environment for patients prone to ingest foreign bodies.

Surgical Considerations

- Surgical management if a granulomatous mass or hypertrophy is causing a gastric outflow obstruction.
- Gastrotomy for removal of foreign objects if endoscopic retrieval is unsuccessful or is not available.

 COMMENTS

Client Education

- Gastritis has numerous causes.
- Diagnostic work-up – may be extensive; usually requires a biopsy for a definitive diagnosis.

Patient Monitoring

- Resolution of clinical signs indicates a positive response.
- Recheck electrolytes and acid–base status if initially abnormal.
- Complete blood counts should be obtained weekly and then reduced to q 6–8 weeks for patients on myelosuppressive drugs (i.e., azathioprine, chlorambucil). Additional chemistry monitoring q 2–3 months as well. Can cause bone marrow suppression which can be cumulative or immediate.

- Repeat diagnostic work-up and consider possible rebiopsy if signs decrease but do not resolve.
- Repeat diagnostic work-up and consider re-biopsy if signs resolve and then recur several months to years later, especially in cats. Inflammatory bowel disease (IBD) can progress to small cell lymphoma in the cat.

Prevention/Avoidance

- Avoid medications (e.g., corticosteroids, NSAIDs) and foods that cause gastric irritation or allergic response in the patient.
- Prevent free roaming and potential for dietary indiscretion.

Possible Complications

- Progression of gastritis from superficial to atrophic gastritis.
- Gastric erosions and ulcers with progressive mucosal damage.
- Aspiration pneumonia.
- Electrolyte or acid–base imbalances.

Expected Course and Prognosis

- Varies with underlying cause.
- Immediate resolution can be expected with foreign body removal or parasitic treatment (in cases with a parasitic etiology).
- Most animals will respond to antiinflammatory therapy quickly but may relapse as the medications are being tapered. A percentage of animals will require long-term (possibly lifelong) therapy to control their signs.

Abbreviations

- CRI = constant rate infusion
- IBD = inflammatory bowel disease
- NSAID = nonsteroidal antiinflammatory drug

See Also

- Bilious Vomiting Syndrome
- Gastritis, Atrophic
- Gastroduodenal Ulceration/Erosion
- Gastroenteritis, Eosinophilic
- Gastroenteritis, Lymphocytic-Plasmacytic
- *Helicobacter*-Associated Gastritis
- Hematemesis
- Hypertrophic Pyloric Gastropathy, Chronic
- Nutritional Approach to Chronic Enteropathies
- Vomiting, Acute

Suggested Reading

Dandrieux JR, Noble PJ, Scase TJ, Cripps PJ, German AJ. Comparison of a chlorambucil-prednisolone combination with an azathioprine-prednisolone combination for treatment of chronic enteropathy with concurrent protein-losing enteropathy in dogs: 27 cases (2007–2010). J Am Vet Med Assoc 2013;242(12):1705–1714.

Neiger R. Diseases of the stomach: chronic gastritis. In: Steiner JM, ed. Small Animal Gastroenterology. Hannover: Schlutersche, 2008, pp. 161–165.

Simpson KW. Diseases of the stomach. In: Ettinger SJ, Feldman EC, eds. Textbook of Veterinary Internal Medicine, 7th ed. St Louis: Elsevier, 2010, pp. 1515–1521.

Author: Michelle Pressel DVM, MS, DACVIM

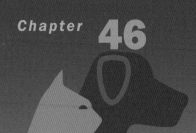

Chapter 46

Gastroduodenal Ulceration/Erosion

DEFINITION/OVERVIEW

Ulcers are defects that extend completely through the mucosa; erosions only extend part way through the mucosa.

ETIOLOGY/PATHOPHYSIOLOGY

- Gastroduodenal ulcers/erosions (GUE) result from various factors which damage or overwhelm normal gastric mucosal defense and repair mechanisms.
- Acid is a major factor in ulcer formation.
- Factors protecting the stomach from GUE include the mucous bicarbonate layer, gastric epithelial cell turnover, gastric mucosal blood flow, and locally produced prostaglandins.
- Forty percent to 60% of exercising Alaskan sled dogs have GUE, as have many military working dogs.
- Relatively common in dogs receiving nonsteroidal antiinflammatory drugs (NSAIDs) or dexamethasone.

Systems Affected

- Gastrointestinal (GI) – ulcers and/or erosions are most common in the stomach and then the proximal duodenum; however, neoplasia and some drugs (e.g., flunixin meglumine) can cause ulceration almost anywhere in GI tract.
- Cardiovascular – hemorrhage may cause anemia, tachycardia, systolic heart murmur, and/or hypotension.
- Peritoneal cavity – perforation may cause peritonitis/sepsis/systemic inflammatory response syndrome (SIRS).

Causes

Drugs

- NSAIDs – cyclooxygenase (COX-2) selective NSAIDs are usually safer than nonselective NSAIDs, although GUE and perforation can occur with all COX-2 selective NSAIDs. Coadministration of glucocorticoids (either systemic or local) enhances ulcerogenic potential of NSAIDs. Some NSAIDs are renowned for being extremely ulcerogenic (e.g., flunixin meglumine, naproxen, indomethacin).
- Glucocorticoid – dexamethasone is probably the most ulcerogenic. Prednisolone is less likely to cause GUE unless a high dose is administered and/or there are additional stress factors (e.g., hypoxemia, hypoperfusion) affecting the GI mucosa.

Blackwell's Five-Minute Veterinary Consult Clinical Companion: Small Animal Gastrointestinal Diseases,
First Edition. Edited by Jocelyn Mott and Jo Ann Morrison.
© 2019 John Wiley & Sons, Inc. Published 2019 by John Wiley & Sons, Inc.
Companion website: www.fiveminutevet.com/gastrointestinal

Gastrointestinal Diseases

- Gastrointestinal neoplasia – carcinomas are the most common cause of neoplastic ulceration, but leiomyomas/leiomyosarcomas are renowned for causing severe hemorrhage.
- Pythiosis can cause severe GUE. It is a regionally important disease and is becoming increasingly widespread in North America.
- Foreign bodies can be associated with GUE, but they are usually not an important cause in the stomach. Intestinal foreign bodies (especially linear foreign bodies) commonly cause intestinal ulceration/perforation.
- Gastric hyperacidity (e.g., gastrinomas, mast cell tumors).

Infectious Diseases

Pythiosis.

Metabolic Diseases

- Hepatic disease.
- Hypoadrenocorticism.
- Pancreatitis is typically mentioned as a cause, but it is of doubtful significance.

Toxicity

Heavy metal poisoning (arsenic, zinc, thallium, iron, or lead are very rare causes).

Neoplasia

- GI neoplasia (carcinoma, lymphoma, leiomyoma, GI stromal tumor (GIST)).
- Paraneoplastic hyperacidity (mastocytosis, gastrinoma).

Stress/Major Medical Illness

- Shock/severe hypotension (e.g., secondary to trauma or surgery).
- SIRS (heat stroke, sepsis).
- Burns.
- Sustained strenuous exercise (especially in extreme environments, either cold or hot).

SIGNALMENT/HISTORY

- Primarily dogs; cats uncommonly affected.
- Chow chows, rough-coated collies, Staffordshire bull terriers, and Belgian shepherds have increased incidence of gastric carcinoma.
- All ages. Neoplasia is more common in older animals.
- Male dogs are predisposed to gastric carcinoma.

Risk Factors

- Ulcerogenic drugs (NSAIDs, dexamethasone).
- Hypovolemic shock/SIRS.
- Extreme exercise.

Historical Findings

- Patients can be asymptomatic, hyporexic, vomiting, and/or have GI bleeding. Severity of clinical signs is not necessarily proportional to size and/or number of GUE.
- Some animals with GUE are asymptomatic (e.g., many patients taking NSAIDs or dexamethasone, dogs working in extreme environments).
- Hyporexia is probably the most common clinical sign.
- Vomiting, hematemesis, and/or melena may be seen (in decreasing order of frequency).
- Cranial abdominal pain ("praying position") is rarely seen.
- Weakness, pallor, lethargy, and/or collapse if severe anemia or SIRS develops.

CLINICAL FEATURES

- Physical examination often normal.
- Melena is rare.
- Pale mucous membranes and weakness if severely anemic (infrequent).
- Tachycardia, hypotension, and prolonged capillary refill time if hypovolemic shock or perforation/SIRS occur.

 ## DIFFERENTIAL DIAGNOSIS

- Esophageal disease (neoplasia, esophagitis, foreign body): diagnose with radiography and/or esophagoscopy.
- Coagulopathies (thrombocytopenia, anticoagulant poisoning): diagnose with platelet count, coagulation testing.
- Bronchopulmonary disease causing hemoptysis: diagnose with radiography and/or bronchoscopy.
- Regurgitation or vomiting of blood (hematemesis) swallowed from respiratory tract or swallowed with food.
- Pepto-Bismol or activated charcoal cause stool to resemble melena.

 ## DIAGNOSTICS

Complete Blood Count/Biochemistry/Urinalysis

- Acute blood loss (i.e., 3–5 days) – nonregenerative anemia/hypoalbuminemia.
- Blood loss >7 days – regenerative anemia/hypoalbuminemia.
- Chronic blood loss – iron deficiency anemia (i.e., microcytic, hypochromic, variable reticulocytosis) and hypoalbuminemia.
- BUN:creatinine ratio may be elevated with acute, severe GI hemorrhage, but this is hard to assess accurately without recent prebleed laboratory values.

Other Laboratory Tests

- Fecal flotation (parasitism).
- Serum bile acids (hepatic insufficiency).
- Resting serum cortisol (screen for hypoadrenocorticism).
- Serum gastrin concentrations (gastrinoma is rare).

Imaging

- Abdominal radiography (GI foreign body, abdominal mass, pancreatitis, pneumoperitoneum, effusion, hepatic disease).
- Barium contrast radiography is very insensitive for GUE.
- Ultrasonography has high specificity but poor sensitivity for GI ulcers and it cannot detect erosions.

Other Diagnostic Tests

- Endoscopy is most sensitive test for GUE (Figure 46.1), but gastric contents (especially excessive blood and large clots; Figure 46.2) can prevent detection. Endoscopy also allows biopsy of lesions. Very difficult and of questionable value to focus on biopsy of the margin of the ulcer. Typically biopsy of ulcerated base of ulcer and surrounding normal tissue is

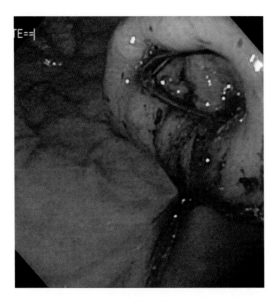

■ **Fig. 46.1.** Ulcerated tumor. Ulcerated leiomyoma visible at the lower esophageal sphincter.

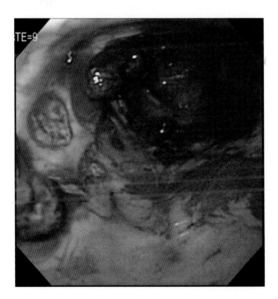

■ **Fig. 46.2.** Gastric blood clots. Endoscopic image at the incisura angularis looking towards the pylorus, showing gastric ulceration with large blood clots.

easier and just as informative. Be careful when biopsying center of ulcers as this rarely causes perforation. Generally, if endoscopic biopsy causes perforation of ulcer, it was going to perforate on its own sooner rather than later.

■ Fine needle aspirates or biopsies of infiltrative lesions in GI tract. Capsule endoscopy can be used if endoscopy is not an option. Capsule endoscopy can evaluate the entire GI tract for lesions.

■ Abdominocentesis may reveal septic peritonitis if ulcer perforates.

■ Exploratory surgery can be done to look for GUE, but it can be hard to see GUE or other mucosal lesions from serosal surface. It is easy to look into stomach through gastrostomy incision and miss erosions and ulcers, even large ulcers.

Pathologic Findings

- GUE are grossly visible.
- GUE can occur anywhere in stomach.
- Gastric body and antrum are most common sites of GUE (from NSAIDs, physiologic stress and glucocorticoids, especially dexamethasone).
- Scirrhous gastric carcinomas classically most common on incisura angularis.
- Proximal duodenal ulceration is classic but not diagnostic for excessive gastric acid secretion (mast cell tumor, gastrinoma).
- Microscopically can see inflammation, neoplasia, or fungal organisms.

 THERAPEUTICS

VERY IMPORTANT: Remove underlying cause if possible, especially drugs, toxins, and/or poor perfusion. Many GUE resolve spontaneously if cause is removed.

Drug(s) of Choice

- Proton pump inhibitors (PPIs) are currently the most potent inhibitors of gastric acid secretion. They irreversibly block the parietal cell proton pump. They require 3–5 days to achieve maximum efficacy, but their immediate effects are still superior to that of H2-receptor antagonists. They can be used as first-line therapy for any GUE, but they are especially indicated for gastrinomas. Omeprazole (1–2 mg/kg PO q 12 h, dog), is the most commonly used PPI. Esomeprazole or lansoprazole (1 mg/kg PO q 24 h, dog) can be administered orally whereas pantoprazole (1 mg/kg IV q 24 h, dog) can be administered parenterally. Twice-daily oral omeprazole is more effective than once-daily IV pantoprazole. Coadministration of PPIs and H2-receptor antagonists probably decreases the effectiveness of the PPI; therefore, dual therapy is not recommended
- Histamine receptor antagonists competitively inhibit gastric acid secretion and are clearly inferior to the proton pump inhibitors. Ranitidine (1–2 mg/kg SQ, PO, IV q 8–12 h, dog and cat); famotidine (0.5–1 mg/kg PO, IV q 12–24 h, dog and cat); nizatidine (5 mg/kg PO q 24 h, dog). Famotidine is most potent H2-receptor antagonist. Cimetidine should be avoided because of its short half-life and relative ineffectiveness. Lafutidine is a new H2-receptor antagonist that is supposed to be as effective as a PPI, but there is currently no experience with its use in veterinary medicine.
- Sucralfate (0.5–1 g PO q 6–8 h) protects ulcerated tissue by binding to ulcer sites and stimulating prostaglandin synthesis. The suspension is more effective than the tablets.
- Antiemetics if vomiting is frequent or nausea is severe. Maropitant (1 mg/kg SQ q 24 h, dog; 2 mg/kg PO q 24 h dog); ondansetron (0.5 mg/kg IV q 12 h, dog; 0.2 mg/kg IV q 12 h, cat).
- Oral antacids (e.g., calcium carbonate) are poorly effective and not recommended.

Precautions/Interactions

- Sucralfate may slow absorption of other drugs.
- Antacids may slow absorption of other drugs.

Alternative Drugs

Misoprostol, a synthetic prostaglandin E1 analog (2–5 µg/kg PO q 8–12 h), is used prophylactically to prevent NSAID-induced ulcers. Can be used to treat any existing ulcer or recent NSAID overdose. Do not use in pregnant patients (causes abortion).

Appropriate Health Care

- IV fluids if needed to maintain hydration and gastric mucosal perfusion, and/or treat shock.
- Transfusions if patient has severe GI hemorrhage.

Nursing Care

Do not ignore caloric requirements and adequate nutrition. Some patients may show extreme inappetence or complete anorexia.

Diet

- Discontinue oral intake if vomiting.
- When feeding is resumed, feed small amounts of low-fat/low-fiber diet.

Activity

Based upon patient's condition.

Surgical Considerations

- If GI blood loss is potentially life-threatening, perform gastroduodenoscopy to identify sites of hemorrhage and then either surgically resect lesions or cauterize sites endoscopically (either electrically or chemically).
- Surgical excision of ulcers is often reasonable if medical treatment shows no evidence of effect after 5–7 days.
- Rarely need to do intraoperative endoscopy to locate lesions which cannot be found at surgery.
- Rarely may need to have surgeon telescope intestines over the tip of the endoscope to allow thorough examination of most of the jejunal mucosa.

 COMMENTS

Client Education

- Dogs are especially prone to NSAID-induced GUE because these drugs usually have a longer half-life in dogs than in humans.
- Never administer an NSAID (especially if sold for human use) unless specifically told to use it by a veterinarian.
- Hyporexia is often the first sign of GUE and may be the only evidence of a gastric lesion (even a severe one).
- Adverse effects of NSAIDs reduced by giving drug with food.
- Proton pump inhibitors are probably as effective as misoprostol in preventing NSAID-induced GUE.
- At the time of this writing, no drug has been shown to be effective in preventing dexamethasone-induced GUE.

Patient Monitoring

If medications are going to be effective, the patient should show some definite evidence of clinical improvement within 5–7 days.

Prevention/Avoidance

- Administer NSAIDs with food.
- Concurrent use of PPI when chronically administering NSAIDs helps prevent GUE. If PPIs are inadequate, misoprostol is sometimes more effective.
- COX-2 selective or dual LOX/COX inhibitors are less likely to cause GUE than nonselective NSAIDs, but they can still cause GUE and perforation/peritonitis.

Possible Complications

Hemorrhage, ulcer perforation, and/or septic peritonitis.

Expected Course and Prognosis

- Varies with underlying causes.
- GUE not due to local malignancy can usually (not always) be treated successfully medically (especially if one can remove the cause). However, if perforation has occurred, surgery is necessary.

Abbreviations

- ACTH = adrenocorticotropic hormone
- COX = cyclooxygenase
- DIC = disseminated intravascular coagulation
- GI = gastrointestinal
- GIST = GI stromal tumor
- GUE = gastric ulceration/erosion
- IV = intravenous
- LOX = lipoxygenase
- NSAID = nonsteroidal antiinflammatory drug
- PPI = proton pump inhibitor
- SIRS = systemic inflammatory response syndrome

See Also

- Hematemesis
- Melena

Suggested Reading

Davignon DK, Lee ACY, Johnston AN, et al. Evaluation of capsule endoscopy to detect mucosal lesions associated with gastrointestinal bleeding in dogs. J Small Anim Pract 2016;57:148–158.

Mansfield CS, Abraham LA. Ulcer. In: Washabau RJ, Day MJ, eds. Canine and Feline Gastroenterology. St Louis, MO: Elsevier Saunders, 2013, pp. 637–642.

Neiger R. Gastric ulceration. In: Bonagura JD, Twedt DC, eds. Kirk's Current Veterinary Therapy XIV. St Louis: Elsevier Saunders, 2009, pp. 497–501.

Simpson KW. Diseases of stomach. In: Ettinger SJ, Feldman EC, eds. Textbook of Veterinary Internal Medicine, 7th ed. St Louis: Elsevier, 2010, pp. 1504–1526.

 Client Education Handout available online

Author: Michael D. Willard DVM, MS, DACVIM

Chapter 47

Gastroesophageal Reflux

DEFINITION/OVERVIEW

- Reflux of gastric and/or intestinal fluid into the esophageal lumen. The incidence is unknown but likely more common than clinically recognized.
- Transient relaxation of the gastroesophageal (GE) sphincter or vomiting may permit reflux of gastrointestinal juices into the esophageal lumen. A small amount of gastroesophageal reflux is normal and is rapidly cleared in healthy dogs and cats.

ETIOLOGY/PATHOPHYSIOLOGY

- Gastric acid, pepsin, trypsin, bicarbonate, and bile salts are all injurious to the esophageal mucosa with prolonged or repetitive contact.
- Esophagitis resulting from reflux may vary from mild inflammation of the superficial mucosa to severe ulceration involving the submucosa and muscularis.

Systems Affected

- Gastrointestinal.
- Respiratory – if aspiration pneumonia.

SIGNALMENT/HISTORY

- More common in dogs than cats.
- No breed predilections reported.
- May be associated with congenital hiatal hernia seen in Chinese shar-pei dogs and other brachycephalic breeds.
- Occurs at any age; younger animals may be at increased risk because of developmental immaturity of the gastroesophageal sphincter. Young animals with congenital hiatal hernia may also be at increased risk.
- Reflux is common in dogs with sliding hiatal hernias.

Risk Factors

- Anesthesia with relaxation of lower esophageal sphincter tone.
- Retained gastric contents.
- Foreign body ingestion with esophagitis.
- Pill ingestion in cats, especially associated with tetracyclines.
- Acquired or congenital hiatal hernia.
- Chronic vomiting with secondary esophagitis.

Blackwell's Five-Minute Veterinary Consult Clinical Companion: Small Animal Gastrointestinal Diseases,
First Edition. Edited by Jocelyn Mott and Jo Ann Morrison.
© 2019 John Wiley & Sons, Inc. Published 2019 by John Wiley & Sons, Inc.
Companion website: www.fiveminutevet.com/gastrointestinal

Historical Findings

- Regurgitation of food +/– blood with mucosal breach.
- Hypersalivation.
- Painful swallowing (odynophagia).
- Anorexia.

 # CLINICAL FEATURES

- Often unremarkable.
- Changes consistent with brachycephalic syndrome that can increase the likelihood of reflux and hiatal herniation.
- Hypersalivation – with severe ulcerative esophagitis; possible pain on palpation of cervical esophagus.

 # DIFFERENTIAL DIAGNOSIS

- Oral or pharyngeal disease.
- Ingestion of caustic agent.
- Esophageal foreign body.
- Esophageal tumor.
- Megaesophagus – idiopathic; focal myasthenia gravis; vascular ring anomaly.
- Hiatal hernia.
- Gastroesophageal intussusception.

 # DIAGNOSTICS

Complete Blood Count/Biochemistry/Urinalysis

Usually normal.

Imaging

- Survey thoracic radiography – usually unremarkable; may be air in the distal esophagus (nonspecific finding).
- Barium contrast radiography – *may* reveal irregular mucosal margins in some, but not all, animals. Aspiration pneumonia may be evident in the dependent portions of the lung fields.

Diagnostic Procedures

- Esophagoscopy – the best means of confirming reflux esophagitis; irregular mucosal surface with hyperemia or active bleeding (erosions) in the distal esophagus. Refluxed secretions may pool in the distal esophagus near the lower esophageal sphincter (LES) which may or may not be open.
- Radiography is of little value in confirming mucosal lesions of GE reflux.

 # THERAPEUTICS

Generally, managed as outpatient.

Drug(s) of Choice

- If there is significant mucosal injury, treatment is recommended.
- Sucralfate slurry (0.5–1 g/dog PO q 8 h) for mucosal cytoprotection and healing.
- Proton pump inhibitor (omeprazole or pantoprazole at 1 mg/kg q 12 h) for robust suppression of gastric secretions which may contribute to reflux esophagitis.
- Metoclopramide (0.2–0.5 mg/kg IV, SQ, PO q 8 h) or cisapride (0.5 mg/kg q 8–12 h PO for dogs; 2.5 mg/cat) is administered to stimulate gastric motility and emptying.
- Gastrostomy tube placement for enteral nutrition in animals with severe mucosal trauma.
- Viscous lidocaine gel administered with water and given 2–3 times daily can be used to help reduce esophageal pain if warranted.

Precautions/Interactions

Sucralfate suspension may interfere with the absorption of other drugs administered concurrently.

Diet

- Moderate-to-severe cases – may withhold food for 24 h to promote esophageal rest and to minimize further reflux; thereafter, give low-fat, high-protein meals in small, frequent feedings.
- Dietary fat decreases gastroesophageal sphincter pressure and delays gastric emptying.
- High protein meals stimulates gastric acid secretion and may precipitate gastroesophageal reflux (GER).

Activity

Not necessary to restrict activity.

 COMMENTS

Client Education

- Clients should avoid feeding high-fat foods; they promote gastric retention and might exacerbate reflux.
- Administer water ("wet" swallow = 5 mL) or soft food/meatball via syringe following pill administration in cats and dogs.

Patient Monitoring

- Patients rarely require follow-up endoscopy.
- It may be appropriate in many patients to simply monitor clinical signs.
- Consider endoscopy for patients that do not respond to empirical medical therapies. Severe mucosal damage (esophagitis) may progress to stricture.

Possible Complications

The most important complications are esophagitis and stricture formation.

Expected Course and Prognosis

- Many cases may be clinically silent.
- Mild-to-moderate cases typically respond favorably to medical management.
- Severe cases, up to and including esophageal stricture, may warrant a more guarded prognosis.

Synonyms

- GERD
- Gastroesophageal reflux disease

Abbreviations

- GE = gastroesophageal
- GER = gastroesophageal reflux
- LES = lower esophageal sphincter

See Also

- Esophageal Stricture
- Nutritional Approach to Gastroesophageal
  Reflux Disease and Megaesophagus

Suggested Reading

Kook PH, Kempf J, Ruetten M, Reusch CE. Wireless ambulatory esophageal pH monitoring in dogs with clinical signs interpreted as gastroesophageal reflux. J Vet Intern Med 2014;28(6):1716–1723.

Zacuto AC, Marks SL, Osborn J, et al. The influence of esomeprazole and cisapride on gastroesophageal reflux during anesthesia in dogs. J Vet Intern Med 2012;26(3):518–525.

Author: Albert E. Jergens DVM, PhD, DACVIM

Chapter 48

Helicobacter-Associated Gastritis

DEFINITION/OVERVIEW

- *Helicobacter* spp. are microaerophilic, gram-negative, urease-positive bacteria that range from coccoid to curved to spiral.
- *Helicobacter* spp. are frequently found in dogs and cats and are considered part of the normal microbiota (Figure 48.1), but have been associated with gastritis in a subset of animals.

ETIOLOGY/PATHOPHYSIOLOGY

- The discovery of an association of *H. pylori* with gastritis, peptic ulceration, and gastric neoplasia has fundamentally changed the understanding of gastric disease in humans.
- Putative mechanisms by which *H. pylori* alters gastric physiology in humans include disruption of the gastric mucosal barrier (due to secretion of phospholipases and vacuolating cytotoxins) and alteration of the gastric secretory activity (e.g., decreased somatostatin secretion leading to hypergastrinemia and hyperchlorhydria).
- *H. pylori* infection in humans has also been associated with increased secretion of proinflammatory cytokines, tumor necrosis factor-alpha (TNF-alpha), and nitric oxide.
- Several *Helicobacter* spp. other than *H. pylori* have been isolated from the stomach of dogs and cats. Typically, multiple species of *Helicobacter* are present.
- To date, *H. pylori*, the most important species affecting humans, has only been identified in a single colony of laboratory cats.
- A possible cause–effect relationship of *Helicobacter* spp. and gastric inflammation in cats and dogs remains unresolved; inflammation or glandular degeneration accompanies *Helicobacter* spp. in some but not all dogs and cats. There is no clear association between the presence of *Helicobacter* spp. and gastritis.
- Experiments to determine the pathogenicity of *H. pylori* in specific pathogen-free (SPF) cats and *H. pylori* and *H. felis* in gnotobiotic dogs demonstrated gastritis, lymphoid follicle proliferation, and humoral immune responses after infection.
- The role of *Helicobacter* spp. in intestinal and hepatic disease in dogs and cats is unclear.
- Several *Helicobacter*-like organisms (HLOs) have been identified in the large intestine and feces from normal and diarrheic dogs and cats.
- *H. canis* has also been isolated from the liver of a dog with active, multifocal hepatitis.
- Enterohepatic *Helicobacter* spp. were found to be more frequent in cats with mucinous adenocarcinomas in the large intestine in a recent report, but more studies are needed to conclude whether there is a significant association between the presence of organisms and intestinal neoplasia.

Blackwell's Five-Minute Veterinary Consult Clinical Companion: Small Animal Gastrointestinal Diseases,
First Edition. Edited by Jocelyn Mott and Jo Ann Morrison.
© 2019 John Wiley & Sons, Inc. Published 2019 by John Wiley & Sons, Inc.
Companion website: www.fiveminutevet.com/gastrointestinal

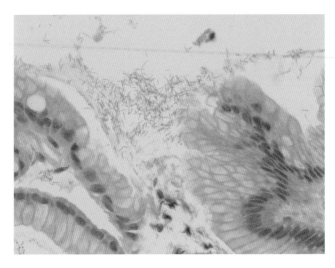

■ **Fig. 48.1.** Presence of *Helicobacter* spp. in the gastric mucosa of a healthy dog (H&E stain, 40×).

- Gastric *Helicobacter* spp. – *H. felis, H. heilmannii,* and *H. baculiformis* have been identified in cats. *Helicobacter felis, H. bizzozeronii, H. salomonis, H. heilmannii, H. bilis, Flexispira rappini,* and *H. cynogastricus* have been identified in dogs.
- Enterohepatic *Helicobacter* spp. – *H. bilis, H. canis, H. cinaedi,* and *Flexispira rappini* have been identified in feces from normal and diarrheic dogs. *H. cinaedi* has been identified in one cat but its significance is unknown. *H. canis* has been reported in one dog with acute hepatitis.
- Gastric HLOs are highly prevalent in dogs and cats – evidence for HLOs has been shown in 86% of random-source cats, 90% of clinically healthy pet cats, 67–86% of clinically healthy pet dogs.
- HLOs have been demonstrated in gastric biopsy specimens in 57–76% of cats and 61–82% of dogs presented for investigation of recurrent vomiting.
- To date, *H. pylori* has been reported only in laboratory cats. *H. pylori* appears not to be adapted to canine gastric mucosa, as *in vitro* studies have shown that canine gastric mucosa has a glycosylation profile that is different from the human gastric mucosa, preventing strong adhesion of *H. pylori* to the canine stomach.
- Enterohepatic *Helicobacter* spp. – *H. canis* has been isolated in 4% of 1000 dogs evaluated. However, only a single case of *H. canis*-associated hepatitis has been reported. The prevalence of *H. fennelliae* and *H. cinaedi* remains undetermined.
- *H. pylori* infection in human beings has a higher prevalence in less developed countries, and is higher in people living in poor environmental conditions.
- No information is available on the prevalence of infection in dogs and cats. *Helicobacter* spp. have been reported worldwide.

Systems Affected

- Stomach – *Helicobacter* spp. may lead to gastritis in a small subset of dogs and cats.
- Intestines – diarrhea can be observed in some dogs with *H. canis.*
- Hepatobiliary – acute hepatitis has been associated with *H. canis.*

SIGNALMENT/HISTORY

- Genetics – no genetic basis for susceptibility to *Helicobacter* spp. infection has been established.
- Species – dogs and cats.
- Mean age and range – infection with *Helicobacter* spp. appears to be acquired at a young age.

Risk Factors

Poor sanitary conditions and overcrowding may facilitate the spread of infection.

Historical Findings

- Asymptomatic presence of *Helicobacter* spp. is common.
- Vomiting, anorexia, abdominal pain, weight loss, and/or borborygmus have all been reported in dogs and cats with gastric *Helicobacter* spp.
- *H. canis* in dogs may be associated with diarrhea.
- Vomiting, weakness, and sudden death was reported in a dog with hepatic *H. canis*.

 # CLINICAL FEATURES

- Physical examination findings usually unremarkable.
- May have signs of dehydration from fluid and electrolyte loss due to vomiting and/or diarrhea.

 # DIFFERENTIAL DIAGNOSIS

- There is a high prevalence of *Helicobacter* spp. in both dogs and cats. Therefore, exclusion of other causes of gastric disease and a positive identification of *Helicobacter* spp. are crucial before a diagnosis of gastrointestinal disease due to *Helicobacter* spp. can be suspected.
- Gastric helicobacteriosis – must be distinguished from other causes of vomiting (both primary and secondary gastrointestinal diseases that can cause vomiting).
- Intestinal helicobacteriosis – must be distinguished from other causes of diarrhea (both primary and secondary gastrointestinal diseases).
- Hepatic helicobacteriosis – must be distinguished from other causes of hepatobiliary disease.

 # DIAGNOSTICS

Complete Blood Count/Biochemistry/Urinalysis

- May reflect fluid and electrolyte abnormalities secondary to vomiting and/or diarrhea.
- May reflect changes consistent with hepatic disease in patients with *H. canis*-associated hepatitis.

Additional Laboratory Tests

- Examination of impression smears of gastric mucosa or gastric washings using May-Grünwald-Giemsa, gram, or Diff-Quik stain is sensitive for *Helicobacter* spp. and can easily be performed, but this test cannot distinguish between different HLOs.

- Rapid urease test – requires gastric biopsy specimen, but is easy to perform in patients that undergo gastroduodenoscopy.
- ^{13}C-urea breath or blood test has been shown to be reliable in identifying infected dogs, but is currently not commercially available.
- Bacterial culture requires special techniques and media and is impractical.
- Polymerase chain reaction (PCR) of DNA extracted from biopsy specimens or from gastric juice.
- Serologic tests (enzyme-linked immunosorbent assay – ELISA) measure circulating IgG in serum, but this test cannot distinguish between different HLOs.
- Histopathology enables the definitive diagnosis of gastric *Helicobacter* spp. infection, but cannot distinguish between different HLOs.
- Evaluation of fecal samples for *Helicobacter* spp. by PCR or antigen testing has low sensitivity and is not recommended. Furthermore, fecal testing does not establish whether the organism is associated with gastric inflammation.

Imaging

Abdominal radiography and ultrasonography are usually normal in patients with *Helicobacter* spp. infection alone.

Diagnostic Procedures

- In cases of *Helicobacter*-associated gastritis, endoscopy may reveal superficial nodules that suggest hyperplasia of lymphoid follicles, diffuse gastric rugal thickening, punctate hemorrhages, and erosions.
- Hepatic helicobacteriosis – hepatic biopsy/histopathology (Warthin–Starry staining) and culture.

Pathologic Findings

- Identification of HLOs requires special staining of tissue samples with Warthin–Starry or modified Steiner stain. Routine H&E staining (see Figure 48.1) may reveal larger HLOs, but smaller organisms are often missed.
- In cases of *Helicobacter*-associated gastric disease – lymphocytic-plasmacytic gastritis and lymphoid follicle hyperplasia; rarely neutrophilic infiltrations. Gastric ulcers have not been reported in dogs and cats.
- In cases of *H. canis*-associated hepatitis – hepatocellular necrosis; infiltration of the hepatic parenchyma with mononuclear cells, and spiral-shaped to curved bacteria predominantly in biliary canaliculi.
- Role of *Helicobacter* spp. in the etiology of gastric carcinoma is questionable in dogs and cats.

 THERAPEUTICS

- The pathogenicity of *Helicobacter* spp. in dogs and cats is still unclear. Therefore, there are no generally accepted guidelines for the treatment of *Helicobacter* spp. infections in dogs and cats.
- Currently, there is no indication for treating asymptomatic animals with a *Helicobacter* spp. infection.
- Eradication of gastric *Helicobacter* spp. should only be considered in infected dogs and cats that have compatible clinical signs that cannot be attributed to another disease process.

Drug(s) of Choice

- A triple therapy (combination of two antibiotics and one antisecretory drug) is effective in humans with *H. pylori* infection, with cure rates of approximately 90%.
- Combination therapy may eliminate *Helicobacter* spp. infections in dogs and cats less effectively than in humans.
- Treat for 2–3 weeks.
- Antibiotics (two antibiotics with one antisecretory agent).
  - Clarithromycin (dogs 5 mg/kg PO q 12 h; cats 62.5 mg/cat PO q 12 h).
  - Metronidazole (dogs 11–15 mg/kg PO q 12 h; cats 12.5 mg/kg PO q 12 h).
  - Amoxicillin (22 mg/kg PO q 12 h; dogs and cats).
  - Azithromycin (5 mg/kg PO q 24 h; dogs and cats).
  - Tetracycline (20 mg/kg PO q 8 h; dogs and cats).
  - Bismuth subsalicylate has mucosal protectant, antiendotoxemic, and weak antibacterial properties; it remains unclear which property is responsible for its beneficial effects in HLO infections (0.22 mL/kg of 130 mg/15 mL solution of Pepto-Bismol® PO q 4–6 h; dogs and cats).
- Antisecretory agents (one with two antibiotics).
  - Omeprazole (0.7–1 mg/kg PO q 12 h; dogs and cats).
  - Famotidine (0.5 mg/kg PO q 12–24 h; dogs and cats).
  - Ranitidine (1–2 mg/kg PO q 12 h; dogs).
- Intestinal and hepatic *Helicobacter* spp. in dogs – a combination of amoxicillin and metronidazole at above dosages may be effective.

Precautions/Interactions

Hypersensitivity to one of the antibiotics.

Alternative Drugs

Patients with HLO infections and gastritis that do not respond to antibiotic therapy usually are given immunosuppressive therapy (prednisolone or others) for inflammatory bowel disease with gastric involvement.

Nursing Care

Fluid therapy in dehydrated patients.

Diet

Easily digestible diets in patients with gastrointestinal signs.

 COMMENTS

Client Education

- Explain the difficulty of establishing a definitive diagnosis, the high prevalence of various *Helicobacter* spp. in clinically normal dogs and cats, and the potential for recurrence.
- The zoonotic potential of canine and feline strains of *Helicobacter* spp. is low.
  - The high prevalence of *Helicobacter* spp. in dogs and cats raises the possibility that household pets may serve as a reservoir for the transmission of *Helicobacter* spp. to human beings.
  - *H. pylori*, *H. heilmannii*, and *H. felis* have been isolated from humans with gastritis.

- *H. fennelliae* and *H. cinaedi* have been isolated from immunocompromised humans with proctitis and colitis.
- *H. cinaedi* and *H. canis* have been associated with septicemia in humans.
- *H. pylori* has not been identified in pet dogs or pet cats.

Patient Monitoring

- Serologic tests are not useful to confirm eradication of gastric HLOs – serum IgG titers may not decrease for up to six months after a cleared infection.
- ^{13}C-urea breath and blood tests have been evaluated to monitor the eradication of HLOs in dogs and cats, but these tests are currently not commercially available.
- If vomiting persists or recurs after cessation of combination therapy, a repeat endoscopic biopsy to determine whether the infection has been successfully eradicated may be necessary.

Prevention/Avoidance

Avoid overcrowding and poor sanitation.

Possible Complications

- Other gastric diseases.
- Avoid metronidazole and tetracycline in pregnant animals.

Expected Course and Prognosis

- The efficacy of therapeutic regimens currently employed in dogs and cats for eradicating *Helicobacter* spp. infections is questionable.
- Metronidazole (20 mg/kg PO q 12 h), amoxicillin (20 mg/kg PO q 12 h), and famotidine (0.5 mg/kg PO q 12 h) for 14 days effectively eradicated *Helicobacter* spp. in 6/8 dogs when evaluated three days post treatment, but all dogs were recolonized by day 28 after completion of treatment.
- Clarithromycin (30 mg/cat PO q 12 h), metronidazole (30 mg/cat PO q 12 h), ranitidine (20 mg/cat PO q 12 h), and bismuth subsalicylate (40 mg PO q 12 h) for four days was effective in eradicating *H. heilmannii* in 11 of 11 cats by 10 days, but two cats were reinfected 42 days post treatment.
- Amoxicillin (20 mg/kg PO q 8 h), metronidazole (20 mg/kg PO q 8 h), and omeprazole (0.7 mg/kg PO q 24 h) for 21 days transiently eradicated *H. pylori* in six cats, but all were reinfected six weeks post treatment. (*Note:* this dose of metronidazole has the potential for toxicity.)

Synonyms

- Gastric spiral bacterial
- Gastrospirillum

Abbreviations

- ELISA = enzyme-linked immunosorbent assay
- HLO = *Helicobacter*-like organism
- PCR = polymerase chain reaction
- SPF = specific pathogen free
- TNF-alpha = tumor necrosis factor-alpha

See Also

- Gastritis, Chronic
- Vomiting, Chronic

Suggested Reading

Kubota-Aizawa S, Ohno K, Kanemoto H, et al. Epidemiological study on feline gastric *Helicobacter* spp. in Japan. J Vet Med Sci 2017;79 (5):876–880.

Leib MS, Duncan RB, Ward DL. Triple antimicrobial therapy and acid suppression in dogs with chronic vomiting and gastric *Helicobacter* spp. J Vet Intern Med 2007;21:1185–1192.

Simpson KW, Neiger R, DeNovo R, Sherding R. The relationship of *Helicobacter* spp. infection to gastric disease in dogs and cats. J Vet Intern Med 2000;14:223–227.

Swennes AG, Parry NM, Feng Y, et al. Enterohepatic Helicobacter spp. in cats with non-haematopoietic intestinal carcinoma: a survey of 55 cases. J Med Microbiol 2016;65(8):814–820.

Author: Jan S. Suchodolski Dr.med.vet., PhD, DACVM

Chapter 49

Hypertrophic Pyloric Gastropathy, Chronic

DEFINITION/OVERVIEW

Chronic hypertrophic pyloric gastropathy (CHPG) or acquired pyloric stenosis is an uncommon obstructive narrowing of the pyloric canal resulting from varying degrees of muscular hypertrophy or mucosal hyperplasia. The term chronic antral mucosal hypertrophy has been used to describe the condition when mucosal hyperplasia in implicated.

ETIOLOGY/PATHOPHYSIOLOGY

- Can result from a congenital lesion composed primarily of hypertrophy of the smooth muscle or be one of three types of acquired form – primarily circular muscle hypertrophy (type 1), a combination of muscular hypertrophy and mucosal hyperplasia (type 2), or primarily mucosal hyperplasia (type 3).
- The cause is unknown; proposed factors include increased gastrin concentrations (which have a trophic effect on the muscle and mucosa) or changes in the myenteric plexus that lead to chronic antral distension and its associated effects.

Systems Affected

- Gastrointestinal – chronic intermittent vomiting, regurgitation has also been reported.
- Musculoskeletal – weight loss.
- Respiratory – secondary to aspiration pneumonia.

SIGNALMENT/HISTORY

- Genetics – inheritance unknown.
- More common in dogs.
- Rare in cats.
- Congenital – brachycephalic breeds (boxer, Boston terrier, bulldog); Siamese cats.
- Acquired – Lhasa apso, shih tzu, Pekingese, poodle.
- Congenital – shortly after weaning (introduction of solid food) and up to one year of age.
- Acquired – 9.8 years of age.
- Twice as many males as females.

Risk Factors

Chronic stress, inflammatory disorders, chronic gastritis, gastric ulcers, and genetic predispositions influence the disease process in humans and may play a role in small animals.

Blackwell's Five-Minute Veterinary Consult Clinical Companion: Small Animal Gastrointestinal Diseases, First Edition. Edited by Jocelyn Mott and Jo Ann Morrison.
© 2019 John Wiley & Sons, Inc. Published 2019 by John Wiley & Sons, Inc.
Companion website: www.fiveminutevet.com/gastrointestinal

Historical Findings

- Chronic intermittent vomiting of undigested or partially digested food (rarely containing bile), often several hours after eating.
- Congenital lesions begin to produce clinical signs shortly after weaning.
- Frequency of vomiting increases with time.
- Lack of response to antiemetic agents or motility-modifying agents.
- Occasional anorexia with weight loss.
- Regurgitation.

 # CLINICAL FEATURES

- Clinical signs are related to the degree of pyloric narrowing.
- Projectile vomiting is generally not a presenting complaint. Animals are generally in good body condition.

 # DIFFERENTIAL DIAGNOSIS

- Gastric neoplasia.
- Gastric foreign body.
- Granulomatous fungal disease (e.g., pythiosis).
- Eosinophilic granuloma.
- Motility disorders.
- Cranial abdominal mass – pancreatic or duodenal.

 # DIAGNOSTICS

Complete Blood Count/Biochemistry/Urinalysis

- Findings vary, depending on the degree and chronicity of obstruction.
- Hypochloremic metabolic alkalosis (characteristic of pyloric outflow obstruction) or metabolic acidosis (or mixed acid–base imbalance).
- Hypokalemia.
- Anemia – if concurrent gastrointestinal (GI) ulceration.
- Prerenal azotemia – if dehydration present.

Additional Laboratory Tests

Venous blood gas analysis may indicate acid–base abnormalities.

Imaging

Abdominal Radiographs

- Normal to markedly distended stomach.

Upper GI Barium Contrast Study

- May display a "beak" sign created by pyloric narrowing, allowing minimal barium to pass into the pyloric antrum.
- Retention of most of the barium in the stomach after six hours indicates delayed gastric emptying.
- Intraluminal filling defects or pyloric wall thickening.

Fluoroscopy

- Normal gastric contractility.
- Delayed passage of barium through the pylorus.

Abdominal Ultrasound

- Measurable thickening of the wall of the pylorus and antrum.

Other Diagnostic Procedures

Endoscopy – allows evaluation of the mucosa for ulceration, hyperplasia, and mass lesions; specimens can be obtained for histopathologic evaluation.

Pathologic Findings

- Include focal to multifocal mucosal polyps, diffuse mucosal thickening, and pyloric wall thickening, with variable degree of pyloric narrowing.
- Changes range from hypertrophy of the circular smooth muscle to hyperplasia of the mucosa and associated glandular structures; a wide spectrum of inflammatory cell infiltration exists.

 # THERAPEUTICS

- Treatment should be aimed at resolving clinical signs. However, in some patients complete resolution may not be possible although the majority of patients do have a significant improvement in clinical signs and quality of life and are able to be ultimately weaned off medications or tapered to an infrequent dosing interval.
- Treatment is typically provided on an outpatient basis unless the patient is debilitated from dehydration, hypoproteinemia, or cachexia.

Drug(s) of Choice

- Antiemetics and motility modifiers are generally ineffective.
- H2 antagonists and proton pump inhibitors may provide symptomatic relief.

Appropriate Health Care

- Depends on severity of clinical signs.
- Patients should be evaluated and surgery scheduled at the earliest convenience.

Nursing Care

- Appropriate parenteral fluids to correct any electrolyte imbalances and metabolic alkalosis or acidosis.
- Isotonic saline (with potassium supplementation) is the fluid of choice for hypochloremic metabolic alkalosis.
- Consideration of postoperative nutritional support is important.
- In severe cases treated with gastroduodenostomy or gastrojejunostomy, surgical placement of a jejunostomy tube for enteral nutrition may be advantageous.

Diet

Highly digestible, low-fat diet until surgical intervention is feasible.

Activity

No restrictions.

Surgical Considerations

- Surgical intervention is the treatment of choice.
- Goals involve establishing a diagnosis with histopathologic samples, excising abnormal tissue, and restoring GI function with the least invasive procedure.
- Surgical procedures depend on the extent of obstruction – pyloromyotomy (Fredet–Ramstedt), pyloroplasty (Heineke–Mikulicz or antral advancement flap), gastroduodenostomy (Billroth 1), gastrojejunostomy (Billroth 2).

 ## COMMENTS

Client Education

- Surgical treatment is highly successful.
- If clinical signs recur postoperatively, more aggressive surgical procedures may be indicated.

Patient Monitoring

Postoperatively for recurrence of clinical signs because of poor choice of surgical procedure.

Possible Complications

Postoperative surgical complications include recurrence of clinical signs, gastric ulceration, pancreatitis, bile duct obstruction, and incisional dehiscence with peritonitis.

Expected Course and Prognosis

- 85% of dogs show good-to-excellent results with resolution of clinical signs upon proper surgical intervention.
- Poor prognosis if gastric neoplasia (especially adenocarcinoma) is an underlying cause.

Synonyms

- Chronic hypertrophic antral gastropathy
- Hypertrophic gastritis
- Acquired antral pyloric hypertrophy
- Acquired pyloric stenosis

Abbreviations

- CHPG – chronic hypertrophic pyloric gastropathy
- GI – gastrointestinal

See Also

- Regurgitation
- Vomiting, Chronic

Suggested Reading

Bellenger CR, Maddison JE, Macpherson GC, Ilkiw JE. Chronic hypertrophic pyloric gastropathy in 14 dogs. Aust Vet J 1990;67:317–320.

Fossum TW. Surgery of the digestive system. In: Fossum TW, ed. Small Animal Sugery. St Louis: Mosby, 2007, pp. 433–436.

Leib MS, Saunders GK, Moon ML, et al. Endoscopic diagnosis of chronic hypertrophic pyloric gastropathy in dogs. J Vet Intern Med 1993;7(6):335–341.

Author: Steven L. Marks BVSc, MS, MRCVS, DACVIM (SAIM)

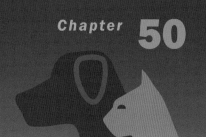

Chapter 50

Bilious Vomiting Syndrome

DEFINITION/OVERVIEW

Bilious vomiting syndrome (BVS) is a clinical condition that is associated with chronic intermittent or early morning vomiting of bile that is thought to be the result of reflux of duodenal contents (bile) into the stomach. Idiopathic bilious vomiting is considered a diagnosis of exclusion.

ETIOLOGY/PATHOPHYSIOLOGY

- The normal aborad gastric and intestinal motility along with a functional gastric pylorus normally prevent duodenogastric reflux of bile and other duodenal contents back into the stomach. When bile is refluxed into the stomach, it is normally rapidly removed by subsequent aborad peristaltic contractions of the stomach wall.
- Bile remaining in the gastric lumen along with the presence of gastric acid and pepsin (activated pepsinogen) can subsequently cause gastric mucosal irritation, loss of barrier function, damage, and inflammation which can further compromise gastric motility.
- Bilious vomiting syndrome is suspected to be secondary to alterations in normal gastrointestinal motility, especially the giant migrating motor complexes (MMC) during the interdigestive phase, rendering the stomach unable to maintain an intragastrical pressure that is greater than the duodenal pressure. Clinical signs usually occur early in the morning or with an empty stomach, suggesting that prolonged fasting or gastric inactivity may modify normal motility patterns, resulting in duodenogastric reflux of bile.

Systems Affected

- Gastrointestinal – chronic esophagitis can develop due to chronic vomiting of bile, with the risk of esophageal stricture development. Chronic gastritis often results from the duodenogastric reflux of bile and gastric erosions or ulcers can also develop.
- Respiratory – patients with chronic vomiting are generally at risk for development of aspiration pneumonia.

SIGNALMENT/HISTORY

- Commonly observed in dogs, rarely in cats.
- Most animals are middle-aged or older.
- No breed or sex predilection.
- No genetic basis.

Blackwell's Five-Minute Veterinary Consult Clinical Companion: Small Animal Gastrointestinal Diseases,
First Edition. Edited by Jocelyn Mott and Jo Ann Morrison.
© 2019 John Wiley & Sons, Inc. Published 2019 by John Wiley & Sons, Inc.
Companion website: www.fiveminutevet.com/gastrointestinal

Risk Factors

- The syndrome of idiopathic BVS is not entirely understood and the exact etiology is unknown at this point. Primary gastric hypomotility or abnormal (orad) intestinal peristaltic motility are suspected as the probable underlying causes.
- Disorders causing gastritis, proximal enteritis or intestinal obstructive disease may be responsible for altered proximal gastrointestinal motility and can cause bile reflux into the stomach. Patients should be investigated for *Giardia* sp. and *Physaloptera* sp. infection, food-responsive enteropathy or food intolerance, idiopathic inflammatory bowel disease, intestinal neoplasia, or obstructions as possible etiologies. Previous pyloric opening or resection surgery will also increase the risk of duodenogastric reflux.

Historical Findings

- Chronic intermittent vomiting of bile associated with an empty stomach. Signs generally occur late at night or early in the morning. Signs may also occur during the day but are usually more intermittent.
- Between bilious vomiting episodes, the animal appears normal in all other respects, and most dogs appear healthy immediately after vomiting episodes.

CLINICAL FEATURES

Results of the physical examination are usually unremarkable.

DIFFERENTIAL DIAGNOSIS

- A number of gastrointestinal and nongastrointestinal diseases can cause chronic vomiting. *Giardia* sp. should be excluded because the signs of this disease can mimic those of idiopathic bilious vomiting. Parasitic gastritis (e.g., *Physaloptera* sp.) can also be a cause of chronic vomiting and needs to be ruled out.
- Idiopathic inflammatory bowel disease and gastric neoplasia (e.g., adenocarcinoma, lymphoma) can result in duodenogastric bile reflux. Both need to be excluded as a cause of chronic vomiting.
- Intestinal obstruction or partial obstructions, which are also associated with chronic vomiting, should be ruled out using diagnostic imaging studies.
- Chronic pancreatitis can also cause vomiting. Serum specific pancreatic lipase and abdominal ultrasound can aid in diagnosing pancreatitis.
- Atypical hypoadrenocorticism is commonly associated with chronic gastrointestinal signs and should be ruled out.

DIAGNOSTICS

Complete Blood Count/Biochemistry/Urinalysis

Results are usually unremarkable but are important to rule out other etiologies (e.g., metabolic causes) of chronic vomiting.

Other Laboratory Tests

- A baseline cortisol and, if indicated, an adrenocorticotropic hormone (ACTH) stimulation test should be performed to rule out atypical hypoadrenocorticism.

- Serum specific canine pancreatic lipase (Spec cPL) should be measured and interpreted in light of the diagnostic imaging findings to evaluate the patient for possible pancreatitis.
- Fecal direct examination and flotation should be performed to detect endoparasites. *Giardia* sp. can be detected with an antigen enzyme-linked immunosorbent assay (ELISA).

Imaging

- Abdominal ultrasound and thoracic radiographs are usually unremarkable but are important to rule out other differential diagnoses or complications of chronic vomiting such as aspiration pneumonia.
- A barium contrast study may reveal delayed gastric emptying (normal gastric emptying: 6–8 h in dogs, 4–6 h in cats), although this must be interpreted with caution in the hospital setting. For a contrast study, barium can be given with meals or as radiopaque markers (barium-impregnated polyethylene spheres, BIPS).
- Gastric emptying ultrasonography (serial evaluation of the cross-sectional area or estimated volume of the pyloric antrum) or using a special noninvasive wireless motility capsule system (Smartpill™, which can detect pH, temperature, and pressure/contractions) (Figure 50.1) may also document delayed gastric motility.
- Alternative but less practical methods include ^{99m}Tc-radioscintigraphy and ^{13}C-sodium acetate breath testing.

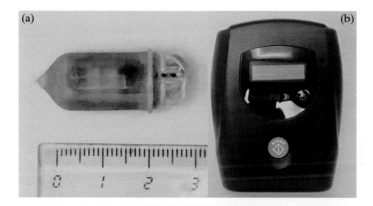

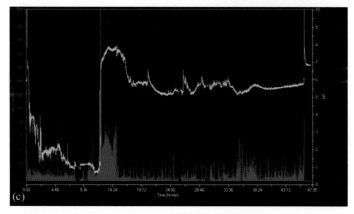

■ **Fig. 50.1.** Evaluation of gastric emptying in a dog using the SmartPill™ system. (a) Wireless capsule. (b) Monitoring device. (c) pH (*green line*), temperature (*blue line*), and pressure (*red spikes*) trace in a dog with normal gastric emptying. Note that the capsule is forced out of the stomach by the giant migrating motor complexes (MMC) during the interdigestive phase. Source: Image courtesy of Dr Jonathan Lidbury.

Other Diagnostic Procedures

Gastrointestinal endoscopy is usually unremarkable but is useful to rule out structural, primary inflammatory, or neoplastic diseases of the stomach or duodenum. *Physaloptera* sp. infection can sometimes only be diagnosed endoscopically.

Pathologic Findings

With idiopathic BVS, there may be evidence of bile in the stomach or gastritis noted in the antral region of the stomach.

THERAPEUTICS

Drug(s) of Choice

- If dietary modification fails, medical treatment options should be considered.
- Choices of drugs (Table 50.1) include agents for gastric mucosal protection against the refluxed bile or the use of gastric prokinetic agents to improve gastric motility. Often only a single evening dose of a medication may be required to prevent clinical signs if the signs occur at night or in the early morning. Alternatively, the prokinetic agent can be administered 30 min prior to feeding.
- Specific gastric prokinetic agents include metoclopramide and cisapride (see Table 50.1). Cisapride is only available through compounding pharmacies. Erythromycin given at

TABLE 50.1. Medications recommended for use in patients with bilious vomiting.

Drug class	Drug	Dose
Gastric prokinetic agents		
D_2-receptor antagonist	Metoclopramide	0.2–0.4 mg/kg PO q6–8h or 0.01–0.02 mg/kg/h IV as a CRI
5-HT_4-receptor agonist	Cisapride	0.2–0.5 mg/kg q8–12h PO
Motilin-receptor agonist	Erythromycin	0.5–1 mg/kg q8–12h IV
H_2-receptor antagonist	Ranitidine	1–2 mg/kg q8–12h PO or IV
Antisecretory drugs		
H_2-receptor antagonists (H_2RA)	Famotidine	0.5–1 mg/kg q12h PO or IV
	Ranitidine	1–2 mg/kg q8–12h PO or IV
Proton pump inhibitors (PPI)	Omeprazole	0.7–1 mg/kg q12–24h PO
	Esomeprazole	0.5–1 mg/kg q24h PO or IV
	Pantoprazole	0.7–1 mg/kg q24h IV (give over ≥15 min)
Drugs for mucosal protection		
Direct cytoprotectant	Sucralfate	20–40 mg/kg q6–8h PO or 0.5–1.0 g q6–8h PO
Antacids	Aluminium hydroxide	100–200 mg q4–6h PO (dog) or 50–100 mg q4–6h PO (cat)
	Magnesium hydroxide	5–15 ml q12–24h PO

physiologic doses stimulates gastric motility by activation of motilin receptors and may also resolve clinical signs.

- Drugs that reduce gastric acid production, including famotidine, ranitidine, omeprazole, esomeprazole, and pantoprazole, may be beneficial. Ranitidine also has mild gastric prokinetic effects *in vitro* and may be beneficial.
- Drugs for gastric mucosal protection include sucralfate or various antacids.
- Empirical deworming (fenbendazole 50 mg/kg PO q 24 h for 3–5 days) is also recommended.

Precautions/Interactions

- Gastric prokinetic agents should not be administered in patients with gastrointestinal obstruction. Metoclopramide can cause nervousness, anxiety, or depression, and is contraindicated in animals with epilepsy. Cisapride at higher doses can cause vomiting, diarrhea, or abdominal cramping. Erythromycin can cause vomiting.
- Famotidine and also ranitidine effects can wean with long-term administration due to drug tolerance. Proton pump inhibitors can interfere with cytochrome p450-dependent drug metabolism (e.g., cyclosporine, benzodiazepines). Antisecretory medications should be slowly tapered after long-term administration to prevent gastric acid rebound hypersecretion.
- Sucralfate should be given on an empty stomach and at least 2 h before or after administration after other medications. Antacids can cause constipation.

Appropriate Health Care

- Patients with idiopathic bilious vomiting are generally treated symptomatically on an outpatient basis and treatment response supports the suspected diagnosis.
- Objectives of treatment are the reduction of the frequency of vomiting or complete resolution of vomiting.

Diet

- Feeding the animal multiple small meals throughout the day, including a late evening meal or snack, often ameliorates or resolves the clinical signs. Food possibly can act as a buffer to the refluxed bile or may enhance gastrointestinal motility.
- A dietary trial using either a novel protein or hydrolyzed protein diet is also recommended.

Activity

Patients with idiopathic BVS can resume their normal level of activity.

Surgical Considerations

Idiopathic BVS is considered a nonsurgical disorder.

 COMMENTS

Possible Complications

- Esophagitis can develop as a result of chronic vomiting, which bears the risk of esophageal dysmotility or stricture development.
- Chronic gastritis and gastric ulcers can develop as a result of chronic duodenogastric reflux of bile.
- Vomiting patients are generally at risk for development of aspiration pneumonia.

Expected Course and Prognosis

- Idiopathic bilious vomiting is generally not a serious debilitating disorder if major underlying causes such as gastritis, idiopathic inflammatory bowel disease, or gastrointestinal neoplasia have been ruled out.
- Most patients respond to one of the above treatments (or a combination of these treatment options) and a clinical response supports the diagnosis. Failure to respond to treatment suggests another underlying or causative factor.

Abbreviations

- ACTH = adrenocorticotropic hormone
- BVS = bilious vomiting syndrome
- ELISA = enzyme-linked immunosorbent assay
- MMC = migrating motor complexes
- Spec cPL = specific canine pancreatic lipase

See Also

- Gastric and Intestinal Motility Disorders
- Gastritis, Acute
- Gastritis, Chronic
- Gastroesophageal Reflux
- Vomiting, Acute
- Vomiting, Chronic

Suggested Reading

Boillat CS, Gaschen FP, Gaschen L, et al. Variability associated with repeated measurements of gastrointestinal tract motility in dogs obtained by use of a wireless motility capsule system and scintigraphy. Am J Vet Res 2010;71(8):903–908.

Ferguson L, Wennogle S, Webb CB. Bilious vomiting syndrome in dogs: retrospective study of 20 cases (2002–2012). J Am Anim Hosp Assoc 2016;52(3):157–161.

McLellan J, Wyse CA, Dickie A, et al. Comparison of the carbon 13-labeled octanoic acid breath test and ultrasonography for assessment of gastric emptying of a semisolid meal in dogs. Am J Vet Res 2004;65(11):1557–1562.

Steiner JM. Small Animal Gastroenterology. Hannover: Schlütersche, 2008.

Tsukamoto A, Ohno K, Tsukagoshi T, et al. Real-time ultrasonographic evaluation of canine gastric motility in the postprandial state. J Vet Med Sci 2011;73(9):1133–1138.

Washabau RJ, Day MJ. Canine and Feline Gastroenterology. St Louis: Elsevier, 2013.

Webb C, Twedt DC. Canine gastritis. Vet Clin North Am (Small Anim Pract) 2003;33(5):969–985.

Authors: Romy M. Heilmann med.vet., Dr.med.vet., DACVIM (SAIM), DECVIM-CA, PhD, David C. Twedt DVM, DACVIM (SAIM)

Canine Parvovirus Infection

DEFINITION/OVERVIEW

- Canine parvovirus (CPV)-2 infection is an acute systemic illness of predominantly juvenile dogs characterized by vomiting and hemorrhagic enteritis.
- The disease may be fatal and dogs may present collapsed in a "shock-like" state and die suddenly without enteric signs, after only a brief period of illness.
- The myocardial form was observed in pups during the early outbreaks in the late 1970s when the dog population was fully susceptible, and is now rare.
- Monoclonal antibodies have revealed antigenic changes in CPV-2 since its emergence in 1978 and CPV-2a, b, and c strains have been identified.
- The original virus is now virtually extinct in the domestic dog population.
- CPV-2c viruses are more virulent than the original isolates, and case mortality rates appear to be higher than in the earliest outbreaks.
- The diagnosis is commonly made using a commercial fecal enzyme-linked immunosorbent assay (ELISA) with compatible clinical signs, but a negative result does not exclude canine parvoviral enteritis.
- Treatment is mainly supportive using intravenous fluid therapy, antiemetics, analgesics, nutritional support, and antibiotics and therefore may be intensive and costly.
- Survival rates are variable but may be improved with early and aggressive therapy.
- Vaccination for CPV is widely practiced but maternal antibodies may interfere with vaccination response and infection is possible even with an up-to-date vaccination history.
- The available commercial vaccines appear to confer adequate immunity against all known subtypes of CPV.
- In rare cases, CPV can cause clinical infections in cats which are indistinguishable from feline panleukopenia virus (FPV).

ETIOLOGY/PATHOPHYSIOLOGY

- CPV-2 is a small, nonenveloped, single-stranded DNA virus that is closely related to FPV and can persist in the environment for 5–7 months.
- Canine parvoviral enteritis has a world-wide distribution.
- Incidence and prevalence rates vary but are increased in breeding kennels, animal shelters, pet stores, or wherever pups are reared.
- Survival rates can be as low as 9% without treatment but can reach 95% with early and appropriate therapy.
- The main route of infection is oronasally through contact with fomites or the feces of infected dogs.

Blackwell's Five-Minute Veterinary Consult Clinical Companion: Small Animal Gastrointestinal Diseases, First Edition. Edited by Jocelyn Mott and Jo Ann Morrison.
© 2019 John Wiley & Sons, Inc. Published 2019 by John Wiley & Sons, Inc.
Companion website: www.fiveminutevet.com/gastrointestinal

- Parvoviruses, including CPV-2, require actively dividing cells for growth such as germinal epithelium of the intestinal crypts, bone marrow, lymphoid organs, and neonatal myocardiocytes.
- Clinical signs manifest after an incubation period of 3–7 days.
- After ingestion of virus, there is a 2–4-day period of viremia, with concomitant growth in oropharynx and local lymphoid tissue.
- Early lymphatic infection is accompanied by lymphopenia and precedes intestinal infection and clinical signs.
- By the third postinfection (PI) day, the rapidly dividing crypt cells of the small intestine are infected, with resultant collapse of the intestinal epithelium and loss of absorptive capacity.
- Intestinal epithelium infection is characterized by the development of hemorrhagic diarrhea 4–5 days after oral exposure and coincides with viral shedding in the feces.
- Virus ceases to be shed in detectable amounts by PI days 8–12.
- Antibodies start appearing within five days PI and increase to peak levels 7–10 days PI.
- Myocardiocyte proliferation is completed within two weeks of birth and myocarditis only occurs in neonates that are not covered by maternally derived antibodies during this period.
- Absorption of bacterial endotoxins from the damaged intestinal mucosa is believed to play a role in CPV-2 disease.
- Intensity of illness appears to be related to the viral dose and the antigenic type.
- Recovery from CPV infection confers long-lived immunity.

Systems Affected

- Cardiovascular – myocarditis with sudden death (now rare).
- Gastrointestinal – small intestinal crypt cells and adjacent mucosal epithelium; severe hemorrhagic diarrhea, vomiting, dehydration; hypovolemic and septic/endotoxic shock.
- Hemic/lymphatic/immune – thymus, lymph nodes, spleen, Peyer's patches.

 # SIGNALMENT/HISTORY

- Dogs and rarely cats.
- Certain breeds have been shown to be at increased risk for severe CPV enteritis, including American pit bull terriers, Doberman pinschers, English springer spaniels, German shepherd dogs, Labrador retrievers, rottweilers, and Yorkshire terriers. Mixed-breed dogs have been described as less susceptible compared to pure-breed dogs but several studies have failed to identify breed as a risk factor. Recent publications do not support breed-specific vaccine protocols but rather an evaluation of the environment. Dogs that reside in a high-risk environment may benefit from an extended vaccine protocol
- Illness may occur at any age. Infection is less likely in dogs older than one year but can still occur, especially if the dogs lack protective immunity.
- Most severe illness occurs in juvenile dogs 6–24 weeks of age.
- There is no apparent sex predilection in juvenile dogs but in dogs over six months of age, intact males are twice as likely as intact females to develop CPV infection.
- Parvovirus *per se* is not zoonotic, but these puppies may harbor coinfections with *Giardia* parasites which can be zoonotic.
- Pregnant animals are likely to abort due to the septicemia.

Risk Factors

- Unvaccinated or incompletely vaccinated young dogs.
- Unsanitary housing environments.

- Recent weaning – pups <4 months of age are at higher risk of severe infection.
- Comorbidity with other enteropathogens, such as parasites, viruses, and certain bacterial species (e.g., *Campylobacter* spp., *Clostridium* spp.), is hypothesized to exacerbate illness and dogs receiving anthelminthic prophylaxis were shown to be less likely to be CPV positive.
- Severe, often fatal, parvoviral infections have been demonstrated in pups exposed simultaneously to CPV-2 and canine coronavirus.
- Season, body weight, and sex are inconsistently associated with a positive CPV status.

Historical Findings

- Clinical signs of canine parvoviral enteritis are nonspecific and can vary. Suspect CPV-2 infection whenever pups have an enteric illness, especially with sudden-onset lethargy, vomiting, and/or diarrhea. Unvaccinated adult animals can be infected subclinically with resultant seroconversion.
- Sudden onset of bloody diarrhea, anorexia, and repeated episodes of vomiting.
- Rapid weight loss.
- Some pups may collapse in a shock-like state and die without enteric signs.
- In breeding kennels, several littermate pups may become ill simultaneously or within a short period of time.
- Occasionally, one or two pups in a litter have minimal or no signs, followed by the death of littermates that presumably encounter greater amounts of virus.

 ## CLINICAL FEATURES

- Most clinical signs are secondary to fluid losses following vomiting and small intestinal diarrhea, which is often hemorrhagic.
- Dehydration, weight loss, and abdominal discomfort or pain are consistent features.
- Some patients present in hypovolemic shock with characteristic findings of a prolonged capillary refill time, tachycardia, decreased mentation, poor pulse quality, hypotension, and cool extremities.
- Fluid-filled intestinal loops may be palpated.
- Occasionally enlarged mesenteric lymph nodes are palpable.
- May have fever or hypothermia.
- Some cases demonstrate evidence of sepsis including icterus, neurologic derangements, acute respiratory distress syndrome, presumably following intestinal bacterial translocation.
- Vomiting, anorexia, lethargy, and pyrexia often precede diarrhea and a diagnosis of CPV infection should not be excluded if diarrhea is absent.
- Protracted vomiting may precipitate esophagitis with hematemesis.

 ## DIFFERENTIAL DIAGNOSIS

- Canine coronavirus infection.
- Salmonellosis; colibacillosis; other enteric bacterial infections.
- Gastrointestinal foreign bodies.
- Gastrointestinal parasites.
- Hemorrhagic gastroenteritis.
- Intussusception.
- Toxin ingestion.

DIAGNOSTICS

Complete Blood Count/Biochemistry/Urinalysis

- Lymphopenia is the most consistent finding, characteristic of CPV-2 infection and commonly occurs between PI days 4 and 6 as a result of direct lymphocytolysis.
- Severely affected dogs often exhibit severe neutropenia concurrently with the onset of intestinal damage due to intestinal sequestration and the destruction of precursor cells in the bone marrow.
- Panleukopenia is seen in severe cases secondary to lymphoid necrosis and destruction of mitotically active bone marrow cells.
- Hemograms are an important part of the diagnostic regimen.
- Leukocytosis is common during recovery.
- Monocyte counts may aid in the evaluation of myelopoiesis due to a shorter duration of production compared to other leukocytes.
- Serum biochemistry profiles help assess electrolyte disturbances (especially hypokalemia), the presence of prerenal azotemia associated with dehydration, panhypoproteinemia, and hypoglycemia secondary to severe malnutrition or sepsis.

Other Laboratory Tests

- Canine serum pancreas specific lipase concentration may commonly be elevated but does not influence outcome.
- Hypercoagulability in the absence of disseminated intravascular coagulopathy has been reported, likely due to a reduction in antithrombin activity and hyperfibrinogenemia.
- In severe cases, thrombocytopenia, prolonged activated clotting time, prothrombin time, activated partial thromboplastin time, and elevated D-dimer levels may support a diagnosis of disseminated intravascular coagulopathy.

Imaging

- Diagnostic imaging is of value to investigate differential diagnoses with a similar clinical presentation or complications such as intussusceptions or diskospondylitis.
- Abdominal radiographs often reveal nonspecific changes such as generalized small intestinal ileus; exercise caution to prevent misdiagnosis of an intestinal obstruction or foreign body.
- Typical ultrasonographic changes include fluid-filled, atonic small and large intestines; duodenal and jejunal mucosal layer thinning with or without indistinct wall layers and irregular luminal-mucosal surfaces; extensive duodenal and/or jejunal hyperechoic mucosal speckling; and duodenal and/or jejunal corrugations.
- Intussusceptions can also occur.

Diagnostic Procedures

- Detection of virus antigen in stool or intestinal contents using a commercial immunochromatographic ELISA assays is the most commonly utilized diagnostic test which has high specificity but poor sensitivity due to a narrow detection window of a few days during infection.
- Repeating an ELISA a day following a negative result in a case with a high index of suspicion for CPV infection increases sensitivity in recent infections.
- Viral shedding can be detected post vaccination using a variety of molecular methods but this does not appear to cause false-positive results using commercial antigen ELISA assays.
- Real-time polymerase chain reaction assays have been developed with higher sensitivities and specificities than conventional assays and may identify and quantitate CPV-2 DNA.

- Electron microscopy is another method of detecting fecal virus during the early stages of infection.
- Samples for virus isolation should be submitted during the acute phase of infection; ship specimens refrigerated, not frozen.
- Serologic assays are widely available but not of much diagnostic use due to the seroprevalence of antibodies in vaccinated and recovered dogs.

Pathologic Findings

- Gross changes include subserosal congestion and hemorrhage or frank hemorrhage into the small intestinal lumen.
- Some dogs exhibit intestines that are empty or contain yellow or blood-tinged fluid.
- Mesenteric lymph nodes are often enlarged and edematous, with hemorrhages in the cortex.
- Thymic atrophy is common in young dogs.
- Pulmonary edema and hydropericardium may be the only gross change in pups with myocarditis and acute heart failure.
- Histopathology reveals intestinal inflammation, necrosis of the intestinal crypt germinal epithelium, severe villous atrophy or collapse, and disruption of the lamina propria.

 # THERAPEUTICS

Mild cases may be treated on an outpatient basis but most cases may benefit from admission for intensive monitoring, intravenous fluid therapy, intravenous medications, and nutritional support, at least until the gastrointestinal signs have subsided.

Drug(s) of Choice

- Supportive therapy is the cornerstone of treatment in cases with canine parvoviral enteritis.
- Intravenous fluid therapy, using a balanced electrolyte solution such as lactated Ringer's solution, to correct fluid and electrolyte imbalances is of the utmost importance.
- Immediate attention must be paid to correcting a hypovolemic state using appropriate crystalloids and colloids if necessary.
- Serial plasma lactate values and repeated blood pressure measurements may aid in goal-directed fluid resuscitation of animals presenting in a hypovolemic state.
- Fluid rates must be calculated and regularly adapted to correct dehydration and provide for maintenance requirements and continued fluid losses.
- Serial daily measurement of urinary specific gravity may aid in assessing the success of fluid therapy and tailoring fluid therapy to provide for ongoing losses which are difficult to estimate.
- Fluid supplementation with potassium chloride and dextrose must be guided by laboratory and clinical findings.
- Antiemetic therapy in the form of maropitant, ondansetron, and metoclopramide is commonly utilized.

Precautions/Interactions

- The use of subcutaneous fluids for dogs treated on an outpatient basis may fail to correct fluid imbalances in hypovolemic animals.
- In dogs with protracted vomiting, outpatient treatment may be a poor choice due to the dependence on oral medications.
- Particular attention must be paid to catheter sterility to prevent contamination with body fluids and potential resultant bacteremia in an immunocompromised patient.

- Biosecurity is important to prevent interpatient spread of comorbid enteropathogens as well as spread of CPV in the hospital environment.
- Aminoglycoside antibiotics such as gentamicin or amikacin can cause renal toxicity and the hydration status and urinary sediment of these patients should be monitored during use of these drugs.
- Maropitant is labeled for use in patients over eight weeks of age and the benefit of use in younger patients with severe vomiting should be compared against the risk of bone marrow hypoplasia in these patients.

Alternative Drugs

- Colloidal support using synthetic colloids such as hetastarch or dextran is indicated if the serum albumin is decreased below 2 g/dL or there is clinical evidence of third space losses.
- Blood transfusions may be necessary in cases presenting with anemia from intestinal blood loss.
- The use of plasma to improve perfusion or correct hypoalbuminemia is controversial due to the amount of plasma needed to cause clinically significant increases in albumin (22.5 mL/kg plasma will increase plasma albumin by 0.5 g/dL) and risk of immune reactions. Synthetic colloids have relatively fewer side effects, are more efficient at improving oncotic pressure, and are often less expensive than natural blood products.
- Analgesics are indicated in patients showing abdominal pain or discomfort and drugs such as buprenorphine, fentanyl, and lidocaine may be considered.
- The use of nonsteroidal antiinflammatory drugs in dogs with canine parvoviral enteritis is limited due to their gastrointestinal side effects and nephrotoxicity.
- Antibiotic therapy may not be indicated in mild cases with normal leukocyte counts.
- Short-duration, broad-spectrum, bactericidal antibiotics with anaerobic and gram-negative coverage are indicated in patients with evidence of septicemia and/or severe neutropenia to allow coverage against translocation until the mucosal barrier integrity has recovered.
- Feline interferon has been licensed for the treatment of canine parvoviral enteritis in some countries and has been shown to decrease the mortality rate.
- No clear advantages to the use of oseltamivir, the paraimmunity inducer PIND-ORF, single-dose immune plasma, antiendotoxin, granulocyte colony-stimulating factor or passive immunotherapy have been shown in the treatment of canine parvoviral enteritis.

Appropriate Health Care

- Symptomatic and supportive care. Therapies include intravenous fluids, antiemetics, analgesics, and antibiotics.
- Intensity depends on the severity of signs on examination.
- Goals are to provide intestinal nutrients, restore and maintain fluid and electrolyte balance, and resolve shock, sepsis, and endotoxemia.
- Prompt, intensive inpatient care leads to treatment success.
- Proper, strict isolation procedures are essential.
- Exercise care to prevent the spread of CPV-2, a very stable virus.

Nursing Care

- Hospitalize patients and monitor for dehydration and electrolyte imbalance.
- Fluids are usually supplemented with potassium chloride, 5% dextrose, and possibly sodium bicarbonate (if severe metabolic acidosis).

Diet

- Puppies that received early enteral nutrition via a nasoesophageal tube, compared to puppies that received nil PO until vomiting ceased, showed earlier clinical improvement, significant

weight gain, as well as improved gut barrier function, which could limit bacterial or endotoxin translocation.
■ A nasogastric tube may provide the additional advantage of allowing the measurement of residual gastric volume and has not been shown to have higher complication rates than a nasoesophageal tube.

Activity

Restrict until symptoms abate.

 # COMMENTS

■ Exercise caution to prevent misdiagnosis of an intestinal obstruction, especially if vomiting is the only clinical sign.
■ Although uncommon, intussusceptions can occur.
■ The use of a modified outpatient treatment protocol with maropitant (1 mg/kg SQ q 24 h), cefovecin (8 mg/kg SQ once) and subcutaneous fluid administrations (30 mL/kg SQ q 6 h) following intravenous fluid resuscitation yielded a similar outcome to conventional in-hospital treatment.

Client Education

■ Inform about the need for thorough disinfection, especially if other dogs are on the premises. Strict sanitation is essential.
■ A 1:30 dilution of bleach (5% sodium hypochlorite) destroys CPV-2 in a few minutes.
■ If possible, isolate pups until they reach three months of age and vaccinate repeatedly; typical protocols involve vaccination at six, nine, and 12 weeks of age.
■ Pups can be infected with virulent virus before any vaccine will engender immunity.
■ CPV-2 is shed for less than two weeks after infection; no carrier state has been substantiated.

Patient Monitoring

■ There seems to be an increased incidence of diskospondylitis in pups that had parvovirus infection.
■ Puppies with an incomplete vaccination history should present for follow-up vaccinations to induce immunoreactivity against other diseases covered in commonly used combination vaccines.

Prevention/Avoidance

■ Inactivated and live vaccines are available for prophylaxis and vaccines differ in their capacity to immunize pups with maternal antibodies.
■ Results of a recent study indicated that vaccination with a modified live vaccine at four weeks of age in pups with high maternally derived antibody concentrations resulted in seroconversion rates of up to 80% that may lead to a reduction in the window of susceptibility with respect to CPV infection and might be used as an adjunct control method in contaminated environments.
■ It is recommended that dogs are vaccinated from six weeks to 16 weeks of age and possibly 24 weeks in high-risk environments to minimize interference from maternally derived antibodies with vaccine response.
■ Control of CPV-2 infection requires efficacious vaccines, isolation of puppies, and stringent hygiene.
■ Owners must be warned that the virus is exceptionally resistant and may persist in the environment for up to six months for future acquisitions of new dogs.

Possible Complications

- Septicemia/endotoxemia.
- Secondary bacterial pneumonia.
- Intussusception.
- Diskospondylitis.
- Esophageal strictures following esophagitis.

Expected Course and Prognosis

- Prognosis is guarded in severely affected puppies.
- Prognosis is good for dogs that receive prompt initial treatment and survive the initial crisis of illness – approximately 80% survival rate.
- A patient is likely to have a poor prognosis if it is purebred, has a low body weight, and, after 24 h of intensive therapy the following biomarker levels are present: severe persistent leuko- and lymphopenia, a persistently elevated or rising serum cortisol concentration (>8.1 μg/dL), severe hypothyroxinemia (<0.2 μg/dL), hypocholesterolemia (<100 mg/dL), and persistently elevated serum CRP (>97.3 mg/L) and/or TNF concentrations.
- Conversely, the literature would suggest that puppies with a good prognosis are those that are of mixed breed, >6 months old, and show the following biomarker values: total leukocyte count >4.5 × 10^3/μL, lymphocyte count >1 × 10^3/μL, and mature neutrophil count >3 × 10^3/μL, all associated with a 100% survival when measured at 24 h post admission. Moreover, a serum cortisol <8.1 μg/dL is associated with a 96% survival when measured at 48 h after admission and a serum thyroxine concentration >0.2 μg/dL associated with 100% survival when measured at 24 h after admission. Lastly, a HDL cholesterol of >50.2 mg/dL is associated with a 100% survival when measured at admission.
- Coinfection with intestinal helminths and *Giardia* is indicative of unhygienic housing conditions and can worsen the clinical picture and contribute to morbidity if not treated.

Abbreviations

- CPV = canine parvovirus
- DNA = deoxyribonucleic acid
- ELISA = enzyme-linked immunosorbent assay
- FPV = feline panleukopenia virus
- PI = post infection

See Also

- Diarrhea, Acute
- Gastroenteritis, Hemorrhagic
- Intussusception
- Parasites, Gastrointestinal
- Vomiting, Acute

Suggested Reading

Goddard A, Leisewitz AL. Canine parvovirus. Vet Clin North Am Small Anim Pract 2010;40:1041–1053.

Mohr AJ, Leisewitz AL, Jacobson LS, Steiner JM, Ruaux CG, Williams DA. Effect of early enteral nutrition on intestinal permeability, intestinal protein loss, and outcome in dogs with severe parvoviral enteritis. J Vet Intern Med 2003;17:791–798.

Prittie J. Canine parvoviral enteritis: a review of diagnosis, management, and prevention. J Vet Emerg Crit Care 2004;14:167–176.

Schoeman JP, Goddard A, Herrtage ME. Serum cortisol and thyroxine concentrations as predictors of death in critically ill puppies with parvoviral diarrhea. J Am Vet Med Assoc 2007;231:1534–1539.

Venn EC, Preisner K, Boscan PL, Twedt DC, Sullivan LA. Evaluation of an outpatient protocol in the treatment of canine parvoviral enteritis. J Vet Emerg Crit Care 2017;27:52–65.

Authors: Willem J. Botha BSc, BVSc (Hons), Johan P. Schoeman BVSc, MMedVet (Med), PhD, DECVIM

Chapter 52

Cobalamin Deficiency

DEFINITION/OVERVIEW

- Cobalamin (vitamin B12) is a group of compounds that serve as essential cofactors for several important enzyme systems.
  - Transfer of propionyl-CoA to succinyl-CoA (essential for beta-oxidation of fatty acids).
  - Transformation of sulfur-containing amino acids.
  - Synthesis of tetrahydrofolate (essential for RNA and DNA synthesis).
  - Thus, cobalamin is needed in virtually all cells of the mammalian body.
- Cobalamin can only be synthesized by bacteria, but vertebrates have large body stores of cobalamin, mainly in the liver but also in other tissues.
- Animal-derived protein serves as the only natural source of cobalamin in dogs and cats. Thus, dogs and cats that are fed an exclusively vegan diet must receive cobalamin supplementation to avoid cobalamin deficiency.
- Cobalamin absorption is a complex process that involves multiple cobalamin carrier proteins.
  - Cobalamin bound to animal-based protein is ingested.
  - The animal-based protein is digested in the monogastric stomach by pepsin and HCl.
  - Cobalamin is released.
  - Free cobalamin is bound by R-protein (synthesized and secreted by the gastric mucosa).
  - The R-protein is digested by digestive proteases in the small intestine.
  - Cobalamin is released.
  - Free cobalamin is bound by intrinsic factor (in dogs and cats almost exclusively synthesized by the exocrine pancreas).
  - Intrinsic factor/cobalamin complexes are absorbed by specific receptors in the ileum.
  - In intestinal epithelial cells cobalamin is released.
  - Cobalamin is released into the vascular system and bound by transcobalamin.

ETIOLOGY/PATHOPHYSIOLOGY

- The main causes of cobalamin deficiency in dogs and cats include chronic gastrointestinal disease involving the ileum (e.g., inflammatory bowel disease, small intestinal dysbiosis, intestinal lymphoma), exocrine pancreatic insufficiency (EPI), short bowel syndrome, and, in rare cases, inherited cobalamin malabsorption or dietary deficiencies.

Blackwell's Five-Minute Veterinary Consult Clinical Companion: Small Animal Gastrointestinal Diseases,
First Edition. Edited by Jocelyn Mott and Jo Ann Morrison.
© 2019 John Wiley & Sons, Inc. Published 2019 by John Wiley & Sons, Inc.
Companion website: www.fiveminutevet.com/gastrointestinal

Cobalamin Deficiency Due to Chronic Gastrointestinal Disease

- If gastrointestinal disease involves the ileum, severe disease leads to cobalamin malabsorption due to destruction of cobalamin/intrinsic factor receptors in the ileum, leading to cobalamin malabsorption.
- To maintain cellular functions, cobalamin from body stores is being utilized.
- When body stores are used up, cobalamin deficiency ensues.

Exocrine Pancreatic Insufficiency

- Intrinsic factor, which is essential for cobalamin absorption is almost exclusively secreted by the exocrine pancreas in both dogs and cats.
- R-protein needs to be digested by pancreatic proteases in order to release cobalamin and make it accessible for absorption.
- Most patients with EPI have secondary small intestinal dysbiosis.

Short Bowel Syndrome

- In dogs and cats with short bowel syndrome, cobalamin can no longer be absorbed because the ileum, the main site of cobalamin absorption in dogs and cats, is no longer present.

Hereditary (Chinese Shar-Peis, Giant Schnauzers)

- Cobalamin deficiency is very common and believed to be inherited in the Chinese shar-pei in the US.
- The mutation has been localized to chromosome 13, but the actual mutation has not yet been identified.
- Isolated families of other breeds (e.g., Giant Schnauzers, Border Collie, and others) with familial cobalamin deficiency have been described.

Dietary

- Being fed an exclusively vegan or vegetarian diet without concurrent supplementation will lead to cobalamin deficiency long term.
- Cobalamin deficiency occurs in patients with cobalamin malabsorption when all body stores of cobalamin have been used up and cobalamin is deficient on a cellular level.
- Cobalamin deficiency is associated with gastrointestinal signs but also systemic complications, such as immunodeficiencies, central neuropathies, and peripheral neuropathies.

Clinical Signs

- Gastrointestinal signs – dogs and cats with cobalamin deficiency often have gastrointestinal signs, but it usually remains unclear whether the gastrointestinal disease leads to cobalamin deficiency or the deficiency leads to gastrointestinal signs.
- Immunodeficiencies – dogs and cats with cobalamin deficiency can present for recurrent septic episodes that may be associated with neutrophilia or neutropenia.
- Central neuropathies – in people with cobalamin deficiency, memory loss is a common clinical sign but in patients with more severe disease, seizures and clinical signs suggesting hepatoencephalopathy can be observed; seizure activity and hepatoencephalopathy have also been described in dogs and cats with cobalamin deficiency.
- Peripheral neuropathies – in people with cobalamin deficiency, tingling in toes or fingertips is common, but even quadriplegia has been observed; severe peripheral neuropathy was observed in cats with experimentally induced cobalamin deficiency.

Systems Affected

- Gastrointestinal.
- Nervous.
- Hemic/lymphatic/immune.

SIGNALMENT/HISTORY

- In the US, Chinese shar-peis have a high prevalence of cobalamin deficiency. Isolated families of other breeds, such as the giant schnauzer, beagle, border collie, and Australian shepherd dog, have also been described as having familial cobalamin deficiency.
- Also, exocrine pancreatic insufficiency, the second most common cause of cobalamin deficiency, is particularly common in German shepherd dogs. These patients are usually young adults at the time of presentation.
- Dogs and cats of any breed, sex, sexual status, and age can be affected by cobalamin deficiency.

Historical Findings

- Clinical signs reported by the owner can be due to the underlying disease process (e.g., diarrhea and weight loss in patients with chronic enteropathies or EPI) or due to cobalamin deficiency (e.g., clinical signs due to immunodeficiency, central, or peripheral neuropathy).
- Clinical signs attributable to the underlying disease process.
  - Chronic enteropathy – diarrhea, weight loss, vomiting, poor appetite, or others.
  - EPI – weight loss, failure to thrive, loose stools, steatorrhea, polyphagia or even pica, borborygmus, flatulence.
- Clinical signs attributable to cobalamin deficiency.
  - Weight loss, failure to thrive, poor hair coat, lethargy, anorexia.
  - Less commonly, clinical signs of central or peripheral neuropathies (e.g., encephalopathy, seizure activity); clinical signs of immunodeficiency (e.g., recurrent septic episodes).

CLINICAL FEATURES

- Poor hair coat.
- Poor body condition.
- Plantigrade stance and other clinical signs of a peripheral neuropathy.

DIFFERENTIAL DIAGNOSIS

- Other diseases causing chronic gastrointestinal disease, immunosuppression, central neuropathies, or peripheral neuropathies.
- Differential diagnoses for gastrointestinal signs – idiopathic inflammatory bowel disease, food-responsive enteropathy, antibiotic-responsive enteropathy, intestinal lymphoma, other.
- Differential diagnoses for central neurologic signs – hepatoencephalopathy, hypoglycemia, idiopathic epilepsy, other central neurologic disease.
- Differential diagnoses for peripheral neurologic signs – diabetic neuropathy, other central neuropathies.
- Differential diagnoses for immunosuppression – iatrogenic immunosuppression, feline immunodeficiency virus in cats.

DIAGNOSTICS

Complete Blood Count/Biochemistry Profile/Urinalysis

- May be within normal limits.
- May show changes associated with an underlying disease process (e.g., hypoalbuminemia in patients with severe inflammatory bowel disease).

- May show anemia, neutrophilia with left shift, or neutropenia. Rubricytes have been documented in cobalamin-deficient dogs and have been interpreted as evidence of ineffective erythropoiesis. Hypersegmented neutrophils can also be observed.

Serum Cobalamin Concentration

- Serum cobalamin is an indirect measure of cobalamin deficiency. As cobalamin is needed within cells, the amount of cobalamin in cells would be a better test for cobalamin deficiency. However, there is no direct way to measure cobalamin concentrations on a cellular level. In contrast, measurement of cobalamin concentration in serum is simple and widely available.
- It should be noted that all assays for the measurement of serum cobalamin concentrations were developed for use in humans. Since cobalamin is frequently bound to carrier proteins, not all assays developed for use in humans will accurately measure serum cobalamin concentrations in dogs and cats. Thus, all cobalamin assays must be validated for use in dogs and cats.
- Also, laboratory-specific reference intervals should be established. Decreased or low normal serum cobalamin concentrations are considered indicative of cobalamin deficiency. Studies measuring methylmalonic acid in serum (see below) in dogs and cats have shown that patients with low normal serum cobalamin concentrations may be cobalamin deficient on a cellular level.
- Serum and urine methylmalonic acid concentrations are increased in patients with cobalamin deficiency. However, analysis (by gas chromatography-mass spectrometry) is time-consuming and expensive and is not available for routine clinical use.

Imaging

Not useful.

Diagnostic Procedures

None for the diagnosis of cobalamin deficiency. However, intestinal biopsies may be useful to confirm and characterize chronic enteropathies.

 THERAPEUTICS

- Treatment of the underlying disease process if identified (e.g., inflammatory bowel disease, EPI, lymphoma, small intestinal dysbiosis).
- Cobalamin supplementation is the treatment of choice in patients with cobalamin deficiency.

Drug(s) of Choice

- Cobalamin supplements.
  - Cyanocobalamin (1000 μg/mL for parenteral use or 250 μg or 1 mg tablets for oral use).
  - Hydroxocobalamin (usually at 1000 μg/mL for parenteral use).
  - Methylcobalamin (usually 1 mg capsules for oral use).
- Traditionally, cobalamin supplementation in deficient patients has been administered parenterally (usually subcutaneously) using most commonly cyanocobalamin or rarely hydroxocobalamin.
- However, recent studies suggest that oral cobalamin supplementation is as efficacious as parenteral cobalamin supplementation, regardless of the underlying cause.
  - Parenteral supplementation protocol – cats receive 250 μg/injection; dogs receive between 250 μg (small dog) and 1500 μg (giant dog) per injection; others receive doses in between. In either species, six weekly injections are followed by a single injection a month later, and reevaluation of serum cobalamin concentration a month after the last dose.

- Oral supplementation protocol – cats receive 250 μg/day; dogs receive between 250 μg (small dog) and 1500 μg (giant dog) once a day; others receive doses in between. In either species, daily doses are given for 120 days followed by reevaluation of serum cobalamin concentration two weeks after the last dose.
- Continue parenteral therapy weekly or biweekly (daily for oral therapy) if serum cobalamin is still low; continue parenteral treatment monthly or bimonthly (or every other day for oral therapy) if cobalamin is in the mid-normal range; discontinue if serum cobalamin is supranormal or is in the high end of the normal range.

 ## COMMENTS

Client Education

- Cats are obligate carnivores and require a meat-based diet to supply them with cobalamin. Dogs and cats fed a vegetarian or vegan diet should be supplemented with cobalamin to avoid cobalamin deficiency.
- Cobalamin is not only an important diagnostic test that can help localize intestinal disease, but also is crucially important therapeutically. Dogs and cats with chronic intestinal disease or EPI that also have cobalamin deficiency have a worse prognosis than those that do not. Thus, supplementation with cobalamin is very important in these patients.
- While cyanocobalamin does contain a small amount of cyanide, there is no toxic risk when using cyanocobalamin for cobalamin supplementation.
- While methylcobalamin is one of the naturally occurring cobalamin forms within the cells of the body, it is not the only one and use of methylcobalamin for cobalamin supplementation does not carry any advantages over the use of cyanocobalamin, which is the cobalamin formulation most commonly used for supplementation.

Patient Monitoring

- Depending on the severity of the underlying disease process, the complications from cobalamin deficiency, and treatment response.
- Reevaluation of serum cobalamin concentration one month after the last cobalamin injection or two weeks after the last oral dose of cobalamin.
- Additional monitoring as required for the underlying disease process.

Abbreviations

- EPI = exocrine pancreatic insufficiency

Suggested Reading

Batchelor DJ, Noble P-JM, Taylor RH, et al. Prognostic factors in canine exocrine pancreatic insufficiency: prolonged survival is likely if clinical remission is achieved. J Vet Intern Med 2007;21:54–60.

Berghoff N, Parnell NK, Hill SL, et al. Serum cobalamin and methylmalonic acid concentrations in dogs with chronic gastrointestinal disease. Am J Vet Res 2013;74:84–89.

Bishop MA, Xenoulis PG, Berghoff N, et al. Partial characterization of cobalamin deficiency in Chinese Shar Peis. Vet J 2012;191:41–45.

Maunder CL, Day MJ, Hibbert A, et al. Serum cobalamin concentrations in cats with gastrointestinal signs: correlation with histopathological findings and duration of clinical signs. J Feline Med Surg 2012;14:686–693.

Ruaux CG, Steiner JM, Williams DA. Early biochemical and clinical responses to cobalamin supplementation in cats with signs of gastrointestinal disease and severe hypocobalaminemia. J Vet Intern Med 2005;19:155–160.

Toresson L, Steiner JM, Suchodolski JS, et al. Oral cobalamin supplementation in dogs with chronic enteropathies and hypocobalaminemia. J Vet Intern Med 2016;30:101–107.

Author: Jörg M. Steiner med.vet., Dr.med.vet., PhD, DACVIM, DECVIM-CA, AGAF

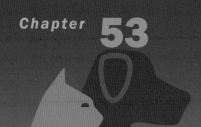

Cryptosporidiosis

DEFINITION/OVERVIEW

- *Cryptosporidium* is an apicomplexan protozoan parasite affecting the gastrointestinal tract.
- *Cryptosporidium canis* and *C. felis* parasitize the small intestine of the dog and cat, respectively. Occasionally *C. parvum* occurs in these hosts.
- Lesions includes villous blunting, villous fusion, and inflammation.
- Oocysts released in the feces are immediately infectious.
- Can cause bouts of acute small bowel diarrhea.

ETIOLOGY/PATHOPHYSIOLOGY

- Infection occurs when sporulated oocysts are ingested by consuming contaminated food or water, coprophagia, or grooming. Sporozoites are released and subsequently invade and replicate in enterocytes.
- Autoinfection is possible.
- Infection results in destruction of the brush border, shortening of the villi, and crypt hyperplasia.
- Clinical signs are associated with parasite multiplication in the small intestine.

Systems Affected

Gastrointestinal (GI).

SIGNALMENT/HISTORY

- Dogs and cats.
- There is no sex or breed predilection.
- Clinical signs are seen in young and newborn animals (dogs and cats) <6 months of age, immunosuppressed animals, those coinfected with *Giardia* or *Tritrichomonas foetus* and those with preexisting intestinal conditions such as intestinal lymphoma, inflammatory bowel disease, canine distemper virus (dogs), canine parvovirus (dogs), or feline leukemia virus (cats).
- Older dogs can excrete oocysts without clinical signs.

Risk Factors

- Stress associated with weaning increases susceptibility.
- Most clinical cases reported in immunocompromised cats.
- Contaminated environments increase the chances of reinfection.

Blackwell's Five-Minute Veterinary Consult Clinical Companion: Small Animal Gastrointestinal Diseases, First Edition. Edited by Jocelyn Mott and Jo Ann Morrison.
© 2019 John Wiley & Sons, Inc. Published 2019 by John Wiley & Sons, Inc.
Companion website: www.fiveminutevet.com/gastrointestinal

Historical Findings

- Signs are small bowel diarrhea mainly, but large bowel diarrhea may occur.
- Immunocompetent – usually asymptomatic intestinal infection with fecal oocyst shedding for two weeks.
- Immunocompromised – enteritis and possibly respiratory, liver, biliary, and pancreatic infections.

CLINICAL FEATURES

- Physical examination may be unremarkable.
- Other physical examination abnormalities may be present with concurrent immunocompromising diseases.

DIFFERENTIAL DIAGNOSIS

Other infectious and noninfectious causes of small bowel diarrhea, maldigestion, and malabsorption syndromes, especially exocrine pancreatic insufficiency, inflammatory bowel disease, intestinal lymphoma, other gastrointestinal parasites.

DIAGNOSTICS

Complete Blood Count/Biochemistry/Urinalysis

Complete blood cell count and serum chemistry are usually normal, unless an underlying immunosuppressive disease is present.

Other Laboratory Tests

- Detection of oocysts in the feces by fecal floatation using sugar or zinc sulfate flotation solutions. This concentrates fecal oocysts (oocysts are 5 µm and appear pale pink in color).
- Oocysts best visualized after staining of fecal smears with modified Ziehl–Neelsen (acid-fast) stain.
- Oocysts may be difficult to visualize; commercial antigen detection, immunofluorescence, and polymerase chain reaction (PCR) assays are available. PCR is approximately 10–100 times more sensitive for the diagnosis of cryptosporidiosis in cats than other techniques.
- Submitting feces to a laboratory – mix 1 part 100% formalin with 9 parts feces to inactivate oocysts and decrease health risk to laboratory personnel.

Pathologic Findings

- Gross lesions – enlarged mesenteric lymph nodes; hyperemic intestinal (particular ileum) mucosa; fix necropsy specimens in Bouin's or formalin solution within hours of death because autolysis causes rapid loss of the intestinal surface containing the organisms.
- Microscopic lesions – villous atrophy; reactive lymphoid tissue; inflammatory infiltrates in the lamina propria; parasites may be found throughout the intestines but most numerous in the distal small intestine.

THERAPEUTICS

Drug(s) of Choice

- All drug treatments are off label.

- Azithromycin 10 mg/kg PO q 24 h until clinical signs resolve for a minimum of 10 days; may cause mild gastrointestinal irritation.
- Paromomycin (Humatin) 125–165 mg/kg PO q 12 h for five days
- Tylosin 11 mg/kg PO q 12 h for 28 days; effective in treating an affected cat that also had lymphocytic duodenitis. Tylosin can cause irritation of the gastrointestinal tract.

Precautions/Interactions

Paromomycin may cause nephropathy in young animals with a damaged gastrointestinal barrier. Toxicity responds to diuresis; monitor renal toxicity by monitoring urine for casts.

Alternative Drugs

Nitazoxanide (Alinia) 25 mg/kg PO q 24 h for 7–28 days; stops oocyst shedding in cats; dosing usually associated with vomiting, which can be ameliorated by antiemetics (e.g., chlorpromazine). Has only been used in a limited number of cats with cryptosporidiosis and needs further evaluation.

Appropriate Health Care

In immunocompetent animals, diarrhea is usually mild and self-limiting. Withhold food for 24–48 h to control diarrhea; oral glucose-electrolyte solution in mild diarrhea; fluid therapy in severe diarrhea.

 COMMENTS

Client Education

- Genetic sequencing has revealed that dog and cat isolates of the parasite are host specific and transmission of *Cryptosporidium* from dogs and cats to people is extremely rare, although immunocompromised people may be at risk. Warn clients of potential zoonotic transmission.
- Oocysts are resistant to commercial bleach (5.25% sodium hypochlorite) and chlorination of drinking water.

Patient Monitoring

- Monitor clinical improvement for treatment efficacy.
- Monitor oocyst shedding in the feces two weeks after completion of treatment or if signs persist.

Prevention/Avoidance

- Solutions consisting of 10% formaldehyde, 5% ammonia, or 6% hydrogen peroxide will inactivate oocysts but may require long contact times (>18 h). Note that these solutions are potentially hazardous for humans and animals.
- Higher concentrations of ammonia (50%) will kill oocysts in 30 min; moist heat (steam or pasteurization, >55 °C), freezing and thawing, or thorough drying are effective.

Expected Course and Prognosis

Prognosis excellent if cause of immunosuppression can be overcome.

Abbreviations

- PCR = polymerase chain reaction

See Also

■ Diarrhea, Acute

Suggested Reading

Scorza V, Tangtrongsup S. Update on the diagnosis and management of *Cryptosporidium* spp infections in dogs and cats. Top Compan Anim Med 2010;25(3):163–169.

Thompson RC, Palmer CS, O'Handley R. The public health and clinical significance of *Giardia* and *Cryptosporidium* in domestic animals. Vet J 2008;177(1):18–25.

Authors: Jeba Jesudoss Chelladurai BVSc & AH, MS, DACVM, Matt T. Brewer DVM, PhD, DACVM

Chapter 54

Diarrhea, Antibiotic Responsive

DEFINITION/OVERVIEW

- Defined as antibiotic-responsive diarrhea without an identifiable underlying etiology.
- Antibiotic-responsive diarrhea (ARD) was previously termed idiopathic (primary) small intestinal bacterial overgrowth (SIBO). This term is no longer used as it was based on quantitative culture of bacteria in the upper gastrointestinal (GI) tract which could not be confirmed by newer polymerase chain reaction (PCR)-based methods. Secondary SIBO is a result of concurrent gastrointestinal diseases (e.g., exocrine pancreatic insufficiency – EPI).
- ARD is a subtype of disease within the broad diagnosis of chronic enteropathies (CE) in dogs. CE can further be subdivided retrospectively by response to treatment into the following groups.
  - Food-responsive enteropathy – FRE.
  - Antibiotic-responsive enteropathy – ARE.
  - Immunosuppressant-responsive enteropathy – IRE (dogs responding to steroids, usually reported as steroid-responsive diarrhea (SRD), are included in this group).
  - Nonresponsive chronic enteropathy – NRE. This implies that a sequential treatment approach is followed, with an elimination diet/hydrolyzed diet for at least two weeks, followed by an antibiotic trial for four weeks if there was no response to food, followed by immunosuppressive agents if the antibiotic trial failed to control clinical signs.

ETIOLOGY/PATHOPHYSIOLOGY

Current theories regarding pathogenesis center on the possibility of immune dysregulation, possibly associated with abnormal CD4+ T cells, IgA plasma cells, cytokine expression, and, in German shepherd dogs, mutations in pattern recognition receptors.

Systems Affected

- Gastrointestinal – typically chronic small intestinal and large intestinal diarrhea.
- Musculoskeletal – generalized muscle wasting and weakness can occur in severe disease.

SIGNALMENT/HISTORY

- May be increased incidence in German shepherds, boxers, and Chinese shar-peis.
- Recent studies show that the condition is more common in young dogs, with a median age of two years. In Finland, a tylosin-responsive from of ARD has been described in large-breed dogs of middle age.

Blackwell's Five-Minute Veterinary Consult Clinical Companion: Small Animal Gastrointestinal Diseases, First Edition. Edited by Jocelyn Mott and Jo Ann Morrison.
© 2019 John Wiley & Sons, Inc. Published 2019 by John Wiley & Sons, Inc.
Companion website: www.fiveminutevet.com/gastrointestinal

Risk Factors

- Genetic risk factors of mutations in pattern recognition genes (*TLR4*, *TLR5*, *NOD2*, and *MHCII*) have been associated with the disease. This is reminiscent of inflammatory bowel disease (IBD) in people, where mutations in innate immunity receptors and MHCII have been associated with the disease. The current thought is that the mutations in pattern recognition receptors lead to a misrepresentation of commensal bacteria as pathogens to the adaptive immune system in the mucosa. This subsequently leads to an increased proinflammatory response involving tumor necrosis factor (TNF) and interleukin (IL)-1beta. Treatment with antibiotics is thought to alter the microbiome in these dogs and reset the inflammation in the mucosa while the dog is on treatment. There is overlap in genetic mutations between dogs with food-responsive diarrhea, antibiotic-responsive diarrhea, and steroid-responsive diarrhea.
- Granulomatous colitis (GC) in boxers and French bulldogs is classified as an antibiotic-responsive diarrhea by some authors. Genetic risk factors have been identified for this, which render macrophages unable to effectively phagocytize bacteria. This leads to accumulation of macrophages in the cytoplasm and ulceration of the mucosa, which are the typical histological findings in GC.
- Adherent and invasive *Escherichia coli* of the pathotype AIEC have been associated with GC in boxers and French bulldogs, and rarely some other breeds. It is recommended to take biopsies to culture *E.coli* from the mucosa if GC is suspected and to tailor antibiotic treatment to the antibiotic sensitivity profile. Many GC cases have been shown to relapse after the first course of antibiotics is discontinued, with antibiotic-resistant *E.coli* strains being cultured more frequently.
- There is some debate whether frequent antibiotic treatment and/or severe mucosal infections such as parvoviral enteritis in young dogs can predispose them to the later development of a chronic enteropathy.

Historical Findings

- Small bowel signs – inappetence or anorexia, vomiting, weight loss, large-volume diarrhea.
- Large bowel signs – tenesmus, hematochezia, increased frequency of defecation.

 # CLINICAL FEATURES

- Physical examination findings – weight loss, poor body condition, borborygmus, and flatulence may be detected; hematochezia may be present if there is large bowel involvement.
- Clinical activity indices (canine IBD activity index (CIBDAI) and canine chronic enteropathy clinical activity index (CCECAI)) for chronic diarrhea are high in ARD, and are even more severe when the patients relapse after discontinuation of treatment. Most dogs will eventually need immunosuppressive treatment in order to keep them in remission.

 # DIFFERENTIAL DIAGNOSIS

- As in chronic enteropathy, it is crucial to achieve a clinical exclusion diagnosis for chronic diarrhea.
- EPI can be diagnosed by low serum trypsin-like immunoreactivity (TLI) levels, and can be difficult to differentiate from ARD as EPI may temporarily respond to antibiotic treatment due to the development of secondary bacterial dysbiosis.
- Once all other differential diagnoses for chronic diarrhea have been considered, CE (including food-responsive, antibiotic-responsive, and steroid-responsive diarrhea) can be

considered and are diagnosed by sequential treatment with an elimination diet/hydrolyzed diet for at least two weeks, followed by antibiotic trial therapy for 4–6 weeks.

- Immunosuppressive drugs should not be given before endoscopic biopsies have been taken in order to rule out the possibility of lymphoma or other GI tumors.
- Neoplasia (lymphoma, adenocarcinoma, gastrointestinal stromal tumors).

DIAGNOSTICS

Complete Blood Count/Biochemistry/Urinalysis

- Typically normal.
- Hypoalbuminemia is an uncommon finding in ARD.

Additional Laboratory Tests

- Tests that should be considered for work-up include fecal examination for parasitic diseases, hematology, biochemistry, and urinalysis to rule out metabolic diseases, possibly adrenocorticotropic hormone (ACTH) stimulation test if there is any suspicion for Addison's disease, canine pancreatic lipase (cPLI) to rule out chronic pancreatitis, TLI to rule out EPI, and abdominal ultrasound to rule out chronic partial obstructions, focal lesions, and masses.
- Fecal examination for bacterial pathogens is not often indicated in chronic diarrhea cases, as most positive culture or quantitative PCR (qPCR) results will reveal low levels of infection that are not the primary cause of disease. They should also not be done to guide antibiotic treatment in ARD, which is diagnosed by an empirical treatment trial.
- Serum cobalamin levels may be low and folate levels may be increased or decreased. Folate and cobalamin levels have been shown to be both insensitive and unspecific for the diagnosis of ARD. Most gastroenterologists will measure cobalamin and supplement if indicated, as a low serum cobalamin level has been shown to be associated with poor survival.
- Serum TLI levels (measured to rule out EPI) are normal in ARD. It is advised to repeat TLI measurement every 6–12 months, especially in younger animals and high-risk breeds, as it has been shown that some dogs will have decreased serum TLI levels over time. These dogs will benefit from supplementation with pancreatic enzymes.

Imaging

Routine abdominal imaging (radiographs and ultrasound) should be performed to rule out other causes for chronic diarrhea. Results of these tests are unremarkable in cases of ARD.

Diagnostic Procedures

- There is no definitive test for the diagnosis of ARD other than resolution of gastrointestinal signs following antibiotic administration.
- Diagnosis depends upon ruling out all other causes for chronic diarrhea (especially food-responsive diarrhea) and a clinical response to an appropriate course of antibiotic therapy, after FRD has been ruled out.

Pathologic Findings

- If endoscopy is performed and intestinal biopsies obtained, they will most commonly show mild-to-moderate lymphoplasmacytic inflammation on histopathological examination. Mild eosinophilic infiltration can also be seen.
- On endoscopy, there could be mild-to-moderate inflammatory changes seen in the duodenum, ileum, and colon. This is similar in food-responsive diarrhea and steroid-responsive diarrhea

cases and does not help to differentiate these subcategories of CE. Most gastroenterologists therefore recommend sequentially treating CE cases with diet and antibiotics, before taking biopsies.

 # THERAPEUTICS

- Hospitalization is generally not indicated and dogs may be managed on an outpatient basis.
- Restriction of physical activity is not indicated.
- The role of diet in ARD is unknown. Current recommendations are to feed a low-fat, highly digestible food or an elimination or hydrolyzed diet concurrently with the antibiotic treatment.

Drug(s) of Choice

- Tylosin (5–10 mg/kg PO q 24 h) for 4–6 weeks. Long-term maintenance regimens have been described with efficacy at 2–5 mg/kg PO q 24 h.
- Metronidazole (10–20 mg/kg PO q 12 h) for 4–6 weeks. Slow tapering to doses as low as 2 mg/kg PO q 24 h has been shown to be effective in selected cases.
- Oxytetracycline (10–20 mg/kg PO q 8 h) for 4–6 weeks.
- Enrofloxacin (5 mg/kg PO q 24 h) for 4–6 weeks. In some cases, combination therapy may be necessary.
- If serum cobalamin levels are decreased, cobalamin supplementation should be pursued. Dogs <15 kg body weight, 500 µg parenteral cobalamin; dogs >15 kg body weight, up to 1500 µg parenteral cobalamin. Doses are given as subcutaneous injections once weekly for six weeks, then once every other week for six weeks.
- Serum cobalamin levels should be reassessed at the end of therapy. Limited information is available regarding the effectiveness of oral cobalamin supplementation.
- Clinical resolution of diarrhea is the most important criterion.
- Relapses usually occur when the antibiotics are discontinued. Some dogs can be maintained on very low doses of antibiotics long term.
- Long-term outcome has been reported to be worst for ARD amongst all CE cases, possibly due to the frequent relapses that warrant veterinary treatment.

Precautions/Interactions

- Oxytetracycline may cause staining of tooth enamel. Doses should be decreased in animals with hepatic or renal insufficiency. Oxytetracycline has been associated with a high incidence of bacterial transfer of resistance genes.
- Metronidazole undergoes extensive hepatic metabolism; dosages should be reduced in animals with hepatic insufficiency.
- There is a concern among gastroenterologists that long-term antibiotic use should be avoided due to rising antibiotic resistance, particularly with the use of metronidazole.

Alternative Drugs

- Amoxicillin with or without clavulanic acid has been used by some to induce remission in ARD cases.
- Long-term management of ARD cases with amoxicillin or enrofloxacin is discouraged due to the high risk for development of antibiotic resistance.

Appropriate Health Care

Maintenance of adequate enteral nutrition and hydration is important during treatment.

Nursing Care

- If dehydration from prolonged diarrhea is present, rehydration with balanced electrolyte solutions will be necessary.
- This may be especially important at the time of discontinuation of the antibiotic treatment, as severe relapses with bouts of diarrhea are common.

Diet

- Maintenance of an adequate nutritional status is essential in all cases of chronic diarrhea.
- Many cases of ARD profit from being kept on an elimination hydrolyzed diet indefinitely.

Activity

No restrictions.

Surgical Considerations

Surgery is not indicated in cases of ARD. If biopsies of the intestinal mucosa are obtained, endoscopic biopsies of the duodenum, ileum, and/or colon will suffice to make a diagnosis. Bear in mind that histopathology is not pathognomonic for ARD and will be similar in FRD, ARD, and SRD.

 COMMENTS

Client Education

- Clients need to be informed about the fact that many dogs with ARD will have frequent severe relapses if they are not kept on antibiotic treatment.
- Long-term antibiotic treatment should be avoided due to the risk of antibiotic resistance; this needs to be communicated to the owners.
- Most ARD dogs will also be kept on long-term elimination or hydrolyzed diets which adds to cost and possible compliance issues with owners.

Patient Monitoring

- Check patients within first week after starting empirical antibiotic trial treatment. If there is no rapid response, the treatment should be discontinued and endoscopic biopsies considered.
- At the time of discontinuation, check patients as they frequently have severe relapses at that time.

Possible Complications

- Weight loss and debilitation in refractory cases.
- Antibiotic resistance – possible infections with multidrug-resistant (MDR) strains.
- Some antibiotics have been associated with long-term microbial dysbiosis in the gastrointestinal tract, which by itself can lead to chronic diarrhea.

Expected Course and Prognosis

- Patients should typically respond within 2–4 days of starting treatment.
- If patients respond within 2–4 days after starting antibiotic treatment, keep them on the treatment for 4–6 weeks before discontinuation.
- Long-term outcome has been reported to be the worst among the four causes for CE, with the most frequent and most severe clinical signs during phases of relapse (i.e., whenever antibiotics are discontinued).

- Most cases will eventually need immunosuppression to stay in remission.
- Due to this fact and the risk of antibiotic resistance development, ARD is difficult to control in the long term.

Synonyms

- Small intestinal bacterial overgrowth (SIBO)
- Intestinal dysbiosis

Abbreviations

- ACTH = adrenocorticotropic hormone
- ARD = antibiotic-responsive diarrhea
- ARE = antibiotic-responsive enteropathy
- CBC = complete blood count
- CCECAI = canine chronic enteropathy clinical activity index
- CE = chronic enteropathy
- CIBDAI = canine IBD activity index
- cPLI = canine pancreatic lipase
- EPI = exocrine pancreatic insufficiency
- FRE = food-responsive enteropathy
- GI = gastrointestinal.
- IBD = inflammatory bowel disease
- IL = interleukin

- IRE = immunosuppressant-responsive enteropathy
- MDR = multidrug resistant
- NAPDH = nicotinamide adenine dinucleotide phosphate
- NRE = nonresponsive chronic enteropathy
- PCR = polymerase chain reaction
- qPCR = quantitative PCR
- SIBO = small intestinal bacterial overgrowth
- SRD = steroid-responsive diarrhea
- TLI = trypsin-like immunoreactivity
- TNF = tumor necrosis factor

See Also

- Gastroenteritis, Lymphocytic-Plasmacytic
- Colitis, Granulomatous
- Fiber-Responsive Large Bowel Diarrhea
- Intestinal Dysbiosis

Suggested Reading

Allenspach K, Culverwell C, Chan D. Long-term outcome in dogs with chronic enteropathies: 203 cases. Vet Rec 2016;178(15):368.

German AJ, Day MJ, Ruaux CG, et al. Comparison of direct and indirect tests for small intestinal bacterial overgrowth and antibiotic-responsive diarrhea in dogs. J Vet Intern Med 2003;17:33–43.

Hostutler RA, Luria BJ, Johnson SE, et al. Antibiotic responsive histiocytic ulcerative colitis in 9 dogs. J Vet Intern Med 2004;18:499–504.

Westermarck E, Skrzypczak T, Harmoinen J, et al. Tylosin-responsive chronic diarrhea in dogs. J Vet Intern Med 2005;19:177–186.

Author: Karin Allenspach Dr.med.vet., DECVIM, PhD

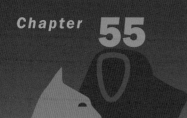

Chapter 55

Enteritis, Bacterial

DEFINITION/OVERVIEW

- Bacterial enteritis refers to infections caused by specific enteropathogens known to cause clinical signs in dogs and cats.
- Pathogens include *Salmonella*, *Campylobacter*, and *E. coli*.
- Clinical signs include diarrhea, weight loss, vomiting, lethargy, and abdominal pain.
- Transmission is fecal–oral.

ETIOLOGY/PATHOPHYSIOLOGY

Salmonella

- *Salmonella* is a ubiquitous, gram-negative facultative bacillus belonging to the family Enterobacteriaceae.
- The prevalence of *Salmonella* in healthy dogs (0–3.6%) and in dogs with diarrhea (0–3.5%) is similar.
- Many infections are subclinical.
- Prevalence in shelter or stay dogs and cats ranges from 0% to 51.4%.
- Virulence of *Salmonella* involves several factors related to both the bacteria and the host.
- Not all strains of *Salmonella* are equally able to cause disease.
- Many infected animals show no clinical signs.
- The majority of dogs are chronically and subclinically infected.
- When disease occurs, it begins 3–5 days after infection.
- The bacteria colonize the small intestine and invade enterocytes, eventually entering and multiplying in the lamina propria and mesenteric lymph nodes.
- Toxins (cytotoxin and enterotoxin) are produced, leading to inflammation and subsequent prostaglandin production, which results in mucosal sloughing and secretory diarrhea.
- In uncomplicated gastroenteritis, organisms are stopped at the mesenteric lymph nodes and the patient develops only diarrhea, vomiting, and dehydration. This is followed by persistent shedding for up to several weeks, after which animals can become latently infected.
- Bacteremia and septicemia can develop after gastroenteritis, resulting in extraintestinal infections (joint disease, abortion) or endotoxemia leading to organ infarction, generalized thrombosis, disseminated intravascular coagulation (DIC), and death.

Systems Affected

- Gastrointestinal – inflammation, mucosal sloughing, secretory diarrhea, watery mucoid diarrhea, anorexia, vomiting, abdominal pain, weight loss.

Blackwell's Five-Minute Veterinary Consult Clinical Companion: Small Animal Gastrointestinal Diseases,
First Edition. Edited by Jocelyn Mott and Jo Ann Morrison.
© 2019 John Wiley & Sons, Inc. Published 2019 by John Wiley & Sons, Inc.
Companion website: www.fiveminutevet.com/gastrointestinal

- All other body systems can be involved in systemic disease if complicated infection occurs, resulting in multiorgan infarction, abscess, osteomyelitis, arthritis, meningitis, abortion, endocarditis, pneumonia, pancreatitis, and death.

Campylobacter

- *Campylobacter* is a curved to spiral gram-negative bacterium belonging to the family Campylobacteraceae.
- It is found commonly in the gastrointestinal (GI) tracts of animals.
- It can survive for extended periods of time in water.
- It is commonly isolated from both healthy animals and those with diarrhea.
- 15–87% of healthy dogs shed *Campylobacter*.
- Up to 58% of cats with and without diarrhea shed *Campylobacter* (via polymerase chain reaction (PCR) testing).
- In dogs <1 year old, *C. jejuni* and *C. upsaliensis* have a prevalence rate two times greater in dogs with diarrhea versus those without; this was not observed in animals greater than one year old.
- *Campylobacter jejuni* is commonly implicated as a cause of diarrhea.
- The prevalence of *Campylobacter* carriage is particularly high in young dogs and cats housed in a group setting (kennels and shelters).
- The organism colonizes the lower intestinal tract (jejunum to colon).
- It possesses few virulence factors; host factors are important in determining the severity of disease.

Systems Affected

- Gastrointestinal – diarrhea (may be watery, bloody, or mucoid), abdominal pain, anorexia.
- Hepatobiliary – cholecystitis has rarely been reported.
- Reproductive – abortion has rarely been reported.

Escherichia coli

- *E. coli* is a gram-negative, non-spore forming rod belonging to the family Enterobacteriaceae.
- It can survive for long periods in dust, feces, and water.
- It is part of normal GI flora; however, enterocolitis can occur with impaired local or systemic immunity or in the presence of bacterial virulence factors.
- *E. coli* strains that cause GI disease are divided into seven distinct pathovars: enteropathogenic *E. coli* (EPEC), enterotoxigenic *E. coli* (ETEC), enterohemorrhagic *E. coli* (EHEC), necrotoxigenic *E. coli* (NTEC), enteroinvasive *E. coli* (EIEC), enteroaggregative *E. coli* (EAEC), and adherent-invasive *E. coli* (AIEC). Each pathovar is defined by a set of virulence factors acting in concert to determine the pathologic, clinical, and epidemiologic features of the disease they cause. Many strains have been isolated in both animals with diarrhea and those without.
- An association with EPEC and EHEC infection and diarrhea in dogs has been detected.
- AIEC is associated with granulomatous colitis of boxer dogs.
- ETEC pathovars have been associated with up to 31% of cases of canine diarrhea. Young dogs are overrepresented.
- EHEC pathovars produce Shiga-like toxins which cause diarrhea, hemorrhagic colitis, and hemolytic-uremic syndrome (HUS).
- It has been postulated that the cutaneous and renal vasculopathy of greyhounds ("Alabama rot") may result from infection with EHEC strains, as it bears a resemblance to HUS in humans and greyhounds are fed a mainly raw meat diet.
- NTEC has been associated with diarrhea in dogs.

Systems Affected
- Gastrointestinal – effacement of microvilli (EPEC), loss of tight junction integrity (EPEC), osmotic diarrhea (ETEC), hemorrhagic diarrhea, abdominal pain, vomiting, dehydration, thickened and irregular rectal wall on rectal palpation.
- Skin – cutaneous erythema and multifocal cutaneous ulcers on the limb that are well circumscribed (in HUS); peripheral edema.
- Renal/urologic – hematuria and renal failure can occur with HUS in greyhounds.

 # SIGNALMENT/HISTORY

Salmonella
- Cats and dogs can be infected; more commonly seen in young or pregnant dogs.
- It is typically an acute disease.
- Racing greyhounds and sled dogs are at increased risk as they are more commonly fed raw food diets.

Risk Factors
- Infections in dogs and cats have been associated with the feeding of a raw meat diet.
- Commercial dry and raw dog food, as well as pig ear treats, have become contaminated with *Salmonella*.
- Infections in cats have been associated with seasonal bird migration ("songbird fever") due to *S. ser. typhimurium*.
- Group-housed dogs, especially those eating a raw food diet, have the highest infection rates (racing sled dogs and greyhound breeding facilities).

Historical Findings
- Subclinical infection is common.
- Lethargy.
- Anorexia.
- Abdominal pain.
- Vomiting.
- Diarrhea, often mucoid, watery, and hemorrhagic, which may take weeks to resolve. Chronic intermittent diarrhea lasting up to eight weeks can be seen.
- Severely affected animals can develop septic shock.

Campylobacter
More common in young animals; has been occasionally reported in adults.

Risk Factors
- Puppies and kittens less than six months of age are most likely to have diarrhea associated with *Campylobacter*.
- Stress, crowding, and other intestinal infections (bacterial or parasitic) may also contribute to the severity of disease.

Historical Findings
- Dogs can be healthy carriers of *Campylobacter*.
- Mild diarrhea.
- Loose stool.
- Watery, blood, or mucoid diarrhea. Diarrhea is typically self-limiting within a 1–2-week timespan.
- Tenesmus.

- Lethargy.
- Decreased appetite.
- Vomiting (less common).

E. coli

- Puppies and kittens in the first week of life, young animals.
- Boxer dogs (in the case of granulomatous colitis), greyhounds eating raw meat (EHEC).

Risk Factors

- Young animals are overrepresented.
- The feeding of raw meat is a risk factor.
- Granulomatous colitis (associated with AIEC) occurs in the boxer dog (usually young adult boxers).

Historical Findings

- Lethargy.
- Diarrhea.
- Decreased appetite.
- Vomiting.
- Skin lesions as described can occur with possible HUS in greyhounds.

 ## CLINICAL FEATURES

Salmonella

- Infections are commonly subclinical.
- Fever up to 106 °F.
- Lethargy.
- Abdominal pain.
- Dehydration.
- Weight loss.
- Severe, extraintestinal infections.
  - Septic shock.
  - Neurologic signs.
  - Arthritis.

Campylobacter

- Lethargy.
- Dehydration.
- Fever.
- Abdominal pain.
- Diarrhea with blood or mucus can be found on rectal exam in dogs.

E. coli

- Fever.
- Dehydration.
- Abdominal pain.
- Weight loss.
- Thickened rectal wall on palpation.
- Acute infection in kittens and puppies in the first week of life characterized by septicemia and multiorgan involvement.

DIFFERENTIAL DIAGNOSIS

Differentials are similar for all three diseases covered (the three pathogens covered here are similar in disease presentation).

- *Salmonella, Campylobacter, E. coli.*
- Parvovirus.
- Distemper virus.
- *Giardia.*
- Various intestinal parasite infections (whipworms, roundworms).
- Dietary indiscretion.
- GI foreign body.
- Clostridial diarrhea.
- Inflammatory bowel disease.
- Pancreatitis.
- Hypoadrenocorticism.
- Pythiosis.
- Histoplasmosis.

DIAGNOSTICS

Salmonella

- The mere isolation of *Salmonella* alone is not sufficient to make a diagnosis of *Salmonella*-induced enteritis.

Complete Blood Count/Biochemistry/Urinalysis

- Complete blood cell count – may be normal or may show neutrophilia with a left shift, toxic neutrophils, anemia, thrombocytopenia.
- Chemistry panel – in severely affected animals: elevated liver enzymes, hyperbilirubinemia, azotemia, hypoalbuminemia, hypoglycemia, hypocholesterolemia, electrolyte changes.
- Urinalysis can have changes in cases of infection localized to the kidneys including isosthenuria, pyuria, proteinuria, casts, and bacteriuria.

Other Laboratory Tests

Coagulation profiles can show prolonged clotting times in animals with DIC.

Imaging

- Abdominal radiographs may show fluid-filled intestines, enlarged liver, or decreased serosal detail.
- Chest radiographs may show evidence of pneumonia or pleural effusion.
- Abdominal ultrasound may be unremarkable or may show enlarged mesenteric lymph nodes, thickened intestinal walls, fluid-filled intestines, enlarged spleen and liver, and ascites.

Other Diagnostic Tests

- Bacterial isolation – a salmonellosis diagnosis can be made when *Salmonella* is cultured from a normally sterile site (blood, synovial fluids, bronchoalveolar specimen, sterilely collected urine sample).
- Isolation of *Salmonella* from feces does not confirm it as the cause of disease, but it should raise suspicion.
- False negatives can occur after antibiotic administration.
- Bacterial isolation allows susceptibility testing.

- PCR – similar samples can be submitted as for bacterial isolation. Positive results from feces do not mean *Salmonella* is the cause of the disease. Does not allow for susceptibility testing. PCR should be performed after overnight enrichment in a nonselective broth, followed by culture of positive samples.

Pathologic Findings

- Grossly, animals with severe disease can have widespread petechial hemorrhage, hemorrhagic enteritis, abscesses, enlarged mesenteric lymph nodes, fibrinohemorrhagic ascites, pulmonary consolidation, and pleural effusion.
- Histopathologic lesions are variable and can include suppurative pneumonia, necrotizing hepatitis, fibrinohemorrhagic enterocolitis, typhlitis, and cholecystitis.

Campylobacter
Complete Blood Count/Biochemistry/Urinalysis

- Complete blood cell count – unremarkable or leukocytosis, neutrophilia, neutropenia, band neutrophils.
- Chemistry panel – unremarkable or elevated liver enzymes and total bilirubin

Other Laboratory Tests

- Microscopic examination – direct fecal smear cytology may show large numbers of S- or gull-shaped organisms. Detection in this manner suggests *Campylobacter* infection and should not be used as the sole method to diagnose campylobacteriosis.
- Bacterial isolation – *Campylobacter* cannot be isolated on routine media; selective media are needed.
- Molecular testing – PCR testing is available and can detect organisms that do not grow well in culture. Positive results do not imply that *Campylobacter* is the cause of the clinical signs.

Imaging

- Abdominal radiographs may be unremarkable or show fluid-filled intestinal loops.
- A thickened gallbladder wall may be seen on abdominal ultrasound.

Pathologic Findings

- Gross findings in infected puppies include fluid-filled intestines with mucosal edema and congestion, and enlarged mesenteric lymph nodes.
- Villous blunting, epithelial hyperplasia, congestion, and lymphoplasmacytic inflammation of the lamina propria.
- Silver stains and immunohistochemical stains can be used to identify *Campylobacter* in intestinal crypts.

E. coli

Diagnosis of intestinal *E. coli* infection is a challenge as both diarrheic and nondiarrheic animals shed *E. coli*. It is a combination of bacterial virulence factors and host immune competence that causes disease.

Complete Blood Count/Biochemistry/Urinalysis

- Complete blood count – leukocytosis, thrombocytopenia (with EHEC), microangiopathic hemolysis (EHEC), microcytic anemia (can be seen in granulomatous colitis).
- Chemistry panel – prerenal azotemia due to dehydration and electrolyte abnormalities. Dogs with EHEC can have hypoalbuminemia, increased alanine aminotransferase (ALT).
- Urinalysis – hematuria, proteinuria, and isosthenuria can be seen with HUS in greyhounds.

Other Laboratory Tests

Bacterial isolation – *E. coli* is commonly isolated on routine media from feces of dogs both with diarrhea and without diarrhea. In general, bacterial isolation is only performed to identify a cause of diarrhea for research purposes or when there is an outbreak.

Imaging

- Abdominal radiographs can be unremarkable or show fluid-filled intestinal loops.
- Abdominal ultrasound can show enlarged mesenteric or sublumbar lymph nodes and a thickened colon wall in granulomatous colitis.

Other Diagnostic Tests

- Colonoscopy/proctoscopy in boxer dogs with granulomatous colitis shows erythema, ulceration, and an irregularity of the rectal wall.
- *E. coli* can be isolated from endoscopic biopsies of the colon wall in dogs with granulomatous colitis. This allows susceptibility testing to direct treatment.

Pathologic Findings

- Dogs with suspected HUS – greyhounds with cutaneous lesions have fibrinoid vascular necrosis, dermal thrombosis, and leukocytoclastic vasculitis. Renal pathology shows hyaline fibrinous thrombi in glomerular capillaries and afferent arterioles, glomerular and multifocal tubular necrosis, and leukocytoclastic vasculitis with fibrinoid necrosis.
- Severe chronic histiocytic colitis is seen in boxer dogs with granulomatous colitis (AIEC). The disease is characterized by periodic acid–Schiff (PAS)-positive macrophages.

THERAPEUTICS

Salmonella

- Detection of *Salmonella* in feces of animals with uncomplicated diarrhea does not require antimicrobial therapy.
- Supportive care is recommended.
- Disease in this case is usually self-limiting.
- Antimicrobial therapy can prolong the carrier state and contribute to antibiotic resistance.
- If the owner is immune compromised, treatment of uncomplicated diarrhea with antibiotics is recommended.
- Animals with systemic salmonellosis require aggressive intravenous fluid therapy with crystalloids and potentially colloids to correct dehydration and hypovolemia.
- Parenteral antimicrobial therapy is warranted.

Drug(s) of Choice

- Antibiotic therapy ideally should be based on susceptibility testing.
- Empiric therapy with ampicillin (30 mg/kg IV q 8 h) and a fluoroquinolone (enrofloxacin 5–10 mg/kg IV q 24 h) is recommended with systemic disease while waiting for susceptibility testing.

Precautions/Interactions

Fluoroquinolones ideally should not be used in young animals due to adverse effects on cartilage.

Alternative Drugs

Alternatives should be based on antimicrobial susceptibility testing.

Nursing Care

- Care may be needed to prevent skin scald from diarrhea.
- Good intravenous catheter care is essential.

Diet

Oral intake should be instituted as soon as possible after vomiting is controlled.

Campylobacter

- Uncomplicated diarrhea is typically self-limiting; supportive care may be needed.
- Treatment in these cases can further disrupt intestinal flora.
- Antimicrobial treatment could be considered in seriously ill dogs.

Drug(s) of Choice

Macrolides (azithromycin 5–10 mg/kg PO q 24 h; this is the preferred drug in humans) and fluoroquinolones (enrofloxacin 5 mg/kg PO q 24 h for 5–7 days).

Precautions/Interactions

Fluoroquinolones ideally should not be used in young animals due to adverse effects on cartilage.

Nursing Care

- Care may be needed to prevent skin scald from diarrhea.
- Good intravenous catheter care is essential.

Diet

Oral intake should be instituted as soon as vomiting is controlled.

E. coli

Animals with severe diarrhea may need intravenous fluid therapy to correct dehydration and hypovolemia.

Drug(s) of Choice

- Dogs with granulomatous colitis are treated with enrofloxacin (10 mg/kg PO q 24 h) for a minimum of eight weeks. Typically, administration of enrofloxacin in these cases is associated with rapid improvement of clinical signs.
- Enrofloxacin resistance has been documented; isolation of *E. coli* from colonic biopsies is recommended to guide antimicrobial treatment.
- Antibiotics that penetrate intracellularly are recommended, based on susceptibility testing (fluoroquinolones, rifampin, chloramphenicol, trimethoprim-sulfonamides).

Precautions/Interactions

Fluoroquinolones ideally should not be used in young animals due to adverse effects on cartilage.

Alternative Drugs

Alternatives should be based on susceptibility testing in the case of granulomatous colitis as resistance to fluoroquinolones has been reported.

Nursing Care

- Care may be needed to prevent skin scald from diarrhea.
- Good intravenous catheter care is essential.

Diet

Oral intake should be instituted as soon as possible after vomiting is controlled.

COMMENTS

- Antimicrobial isolation for all diseases discussed should be interpreted in light of clinical signs and likelihood of the particular infection causing the disease.
- Diagnosis is made more difficult in all three infections by the fact that all three organisms have been isolated from both diarrheic and nondiarrheic animals.

Salmonella

Client Education

- There is the potential for zoonotic infection of *Salmonella*.
- Children, the elderly, and immune-compromised individuals are at greatest risk.
- People exposed to animals fed raw meat diets are at increased risk of exposure.
- Proper hand-washing can prevent zoonotic transmission, and appropriate techniques to prevent cross-contamination in the kitchen (separating raw meat from vegetables) should be implemented.
- Therapy dogs on a raw food diet should be excluded from animal-assisted intervention programs.

Patient Monitoring

Successive fecal cultures two weeks apart should be performed.

Prevention/Avoidance

- Prevention strategies include feeding cooked foods, hand-washing before and after handling pets and pet foods, and prevention of coprophagia.
- Food should be stored properly to prevent contamination by rodents and insects.
- In the hospital, instruments (thermometers, endoscopes) should be properly disinfected between uses.
- Cages should be properly disinfected between patients.
- Patients should be isolated until there is confirmation that shedding of organisms has ceased.
- Repeat fecal cultures should be performed every two weeks; three successive negative fecal cultures indicate shedding has stopped.

Expected Course and Prognosis

Uncomplicated diarrhea requires only supportive care and carries a good prognosis.

Campylobacter

Client Education

- Contact with infected animals can be a source of human infection.
- A direct link between pets and *C. jejuni* diarrhea in people has been shown.
- Immune-compromised people and children are especially at risk for more severe disease.

Prevention/Avoidance

Avoiding risk factors such as overcrowding and concurrent intestinal infection in puppies and kittens may lessen severity of diarrhea.

Expected Course and Prognosis

- Uncomplicated *Campylobacter* infection is typically self-limiting and resolves with only supportive care.
- Treated dogs will have a 50–73% response to treatment and 50% of cats will respond.
- Treatment failure may reflect antimicrobial resistance or incorrect diagnosis.

E. coli

Client Education

- The possibility of multidrug-resistant *E. coli* shed by dogs and cats passing to humans is an emerging concern.
- Possible risk of zoonotic transmission of enteropathogens should be discussed with owners.

Prevention/Avoidance

Proper disinfecting of hospital equipment (endoscopes, thermometers) is important to lessen spread of pathogens.

Expected Course and Prognosis

Dogs with granulomatous colitis can show dramatic responses to fluoroquinolone therapy.

Abbreviations

- AIEC = adherent-invasive *E. coli*
- ALT = alanine aminotransferase
- DIC = disseminated intravascular coagulation
- EAEC = enteroaggregative *E. coli*
- EHEC = enterohemorrhagic *E. coli*
- EIEC = enteroinvasive *E. coli*
- EPEC = enteropathogenic *E. coli*
- ETEC = enterotoxigenic *E. coli*
- GI = gastrointestinal
- HUS = hemolytic-uremic syndrome
- NTEC = necrotoxigenic *E. coli*
- PCR = polymerase chain reaction

See Also

- Canine Parvovirus Infection
- Clostridial Enterotoxicosis
- Colitis, Histiocytic Ulcerative
- Diarrhea, Acute
- Fungal Enteritides
- Gastroenteritis, Hemorrhagic
- Gastrointestinal Obstruction
- Giardiasis
- Hematochezia
- Inflammatory Bowel Disease
- Nutritional Approach to Acute Vomiting and Diarrhea
- Parasitism, Gastrointestinal
- Vomiting, Acute

Suggested Reading

Craven M, Dogan B, Schukken A, et al. Antimicrobial resistance impacts clinical outcome of granulomatous colitis in boxer dogs. J Vet Intern Med 2010;24:819–824.

Greene CE. Infectious Diseases of the Dog and Cat, 4th ed. St Louis: Elsevier, 2011.

Marks SL, Rankin SC, Byrne BA, Weese JS. Enteropathogenic bacteria in dogs and cats: diagnosis, epidemiology, treatment, and control. J Vet Intern Med 2011;25:1195–1208.

Sykes JE. Canine and Feline Infectious Disease. St Louis: Elsevier, 2014.

Acknowledgments: The author and editors acknowledge the prior contribution of Dr Patrick McDonough.

Author: Krysta Deitz DVM, MS, DACVIM

Chapter 56

Enterocolitis, Granulomatous

DEFINITION/OVERVIEW

- The term *granulomatous enteritis* describes an inflammation in the intestinal tract that is dominated by macrophages and/or multinucleated giant cells (fused macrophages). The inflammation may be diffuse and/or form organized granulomas. Other cell types such as neutrophils (pyogranulomatous enteritis), eosinophils, and/or plasma cells may be present.
- Granulomatous inflammation/granulomas typically develop due to foreign material (e.g., migrating foreign bodies, suture material, etc.) or due to invasive pathogens (e.g., bacteria, fungi) that are perceived as foreign but cannot be eliminated. The immune system attempts to wall off such pathogens by building a granuloma.
- In some cases (e.g., regional granulomatous enteritis), no cause can be found and the disease is suspected to be immune mediated.
- Dependent on the underlying disease, the patient might just show gastrointestinal (GI) signs or signs of systemic/disseminated disease.

ETIOLOGY/PATHOPHYSIOLOGY

- Infectious.
  - Bacteria: e.g., *E. coli*, *Mycobacteria* spp.
  - Fungi: e.g., *Histoplasma* spp.
  - Algae: e.g., *Prototheca zofii*, *Prototheca wickerhamii*.
  - Oomycetes: e.g., *Pythium insidiosum*.
  - Viruses: feline infectious peritonitis (FIP).
- Foreign body/material (e.g., migrating foreign body, suture material, etc.).
- Idiopathic/miscellaneous.
  - Regional granulomatous enteritis (very rare form of inflammatory bowel disease – IBD).
  - Diffuse granulomatous enterocolitis (very rare form of IBD).
  - Lipogranulomas associated with protein-losing enteropathy (PLE).
  - Focal intestinal lipogranulomatous lymphangitis.

Systems Affected
- Endocrine/metabolic.
- Gastrointestinal.
- Hemic/lymphatic/immune.

Blackwell's Five-Minute Veterinary Consult Clinical Companion: Small Animal Gastrointestinal Diseases, First Edition. Edited by Jocelyn Mott and Jo Ann Morrison.
© 2019 John Wiley & Sons, Inc. Published 2019 by John Wiley & Sons, Inc.
Companion website: www.fiveminutevet.com/gastrointestinal

SIGNALMENT/HISTORY

- Infectious and foreign-body related granulomatous enterocolitis: may occur in any dog or cat, including those living indoors.
- Histiocytic ulcerative colitis (HUC). Boxers and French bulldogs show a predisposition, very rarely described in other breeds.
- Pythiosis ("swamp cancer").
  - Occurs mostly in the south-eastern US and other tropical and subtropical areas in dogs with access to open water.
  - Cats are rarely affected.
  - GI pythiosis is characterized by severe segmental thickening of the intestinal wall (Figures 56.1 and 56.2).
  - The pyloric area, duodenum, and ileocolic junction are most commonly affected.
  - Severe mesenteric lymphadenopathy is common.
  - Other lesions such as cutaneous wounds or masses are commonly present.
- FIP.
  - Young male cats are predisposed.
  - Purebred cats (e.g., Abyssinians, Bengals, Birmans, Himalayans, Ragdolls and Rexes) may have an increased risk.
  - May cause granulomatous lesions in the GI tract and subsequently GI signs.
  - Other clinical signs and lesions such as lethargy, inappetence, pyrexia, effusions, icterus, dyspnea or neurologic signs usually dominate the clinical picture.
- Regional granulomatous enteritis.
  - Only reported in small-breed dogs.
  - Often regional and transmural.
  - Commonly associated with signs consistent with small bowel diarrhea and weight loss.
- PLE: Yorkshire terriers are predisposed.

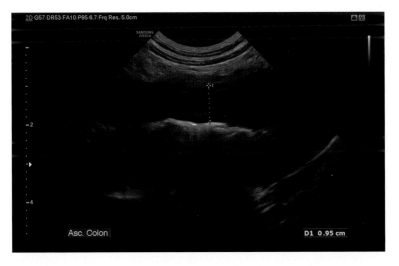

■ **Fig. 56.1.** Longitudinal plane sonographic image of the ascending colon in a five-year-old castrated male boxer dog with chronic, large bowel diarrhea. The intestinal wall is severely, diffusely thickened (between calipers; 0.95 cm) with loss of normal wall layering. The ileocolic junction, cecum, and transverse colon (not shown) were equally affected and the distal descending colon (not shown) was less severely affected. Differentials for the sonographic appearance of the colon in this patient include infectious and noninfectious inflammatory colitis and infiltrative neoplasia. Pythiosis was confirmed via positive serology. Source: Courtesy of Dr Lindsey Gilmour.

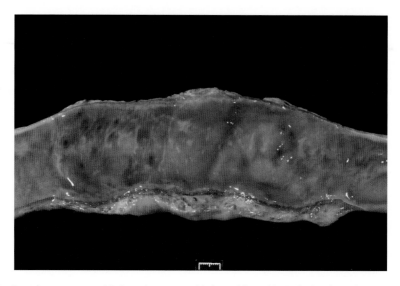

■ **Fig. 56.2.** Granulomatous enteritis in a three-year-old dog with pythiosis (*P. insidiosum*). The colon is locally affected by severe granulomatous inflammation and fibrosis, causing a thick, firm, and segmental lesion in the colonic wall. Marker = 1 cm. Source: Courtesy of Dr John Edwards.

Risk Factors

Immunocompromised dogs (e.g., on immunosuppressive medication) may be at higher risk of acquiring infections with facultative pathogens such as fungal infections causing granulomatous enterocolitis.

Historical Findings

- Dependent on the underlying disease and duration, clinical signs frequently observed are:
  - Diarrhea.
  - Weight loss.
  - Anorexia.
  - Tenesmus.
  - Hematochezia.
  - Lethargy.
  - Abdominal pain (e.g., prayer posture).
  - Vomiting.
  - Hematemesis.
  - Fever.
- In bacterial or fungal infections, lesions in other organs such as the skin or lungs may be found and may dominate the clinical picture.

 CLINICAL FEATURES

- Patients may be febrile, weak, or of poor body condition. Abdominal palpation may reveal pain, masses (e.g., lymphadenopathy, granulomas, etc.) or diffusely thickened bowel loops ("ropy loops").
- On rectal exam, thickened mucosa, masses or hematochezia may be found. Small dogs with regional granulomatous enteritis are commonly reported to have a palpable, firm, tubular soft mass in the cranial abdomen.

DIFFERENTIAL DIAGNOSIS

- Extraintestinal or systemic diseases causing clinical signs of GI disease.
- Intestinal disease.
    - Infectious – intestinal parasites and infectious agents such as hookworms, whipworms, *Giardia* spp., *Campylobacter* spp., *Cryptosporidium* spp., *Salmonella* spp.
    - Rectoanal polyp.
    - Neoplasia (gastrointestinal, rectoanal, anal glands, etc.).
    - Perineal hernia.
    - Chronic intussusception.
    - Rectal stricture.

DIAGNOSTICS

Complete Blood Count/Biochemistry/Urinalysis

Complete Blood Count

- Stress leukogram (mild leukocytosis with mature neutrophilia, lymphopenia, monocytosis and eosinopenia) can occur in any disease process.
- Systemic inflammation (moderate to severe leukocytosis, band neutrophils, etc.), e.g., in systemic fungal disease, HUC, foreign bodies, etc.

Biochemistry

- Hypoalbuminemia (GI loss or negative acute phase reaction).
- Panhypoproteinemia (GI loss).
- Hyperproteinemia or hyperglobulinemia (FIP, neoplasia, chronic inflammation).
- Hypocholesterolemia (GI loss).
- Low creatinine (weight/muscle mass loss).
- Other unspecific changes.

Urinalysis

Usually normal unless kidneys are affected (e.g., fungal disease, prototer cosis etc.).

Imaging

- Abdominal radiographs may reveal mass lesions, foreign bodies, signs of obstruction or abdominal effusion. Generally low yield in diagnosis of chronic gastrointestinal diseases.
- Abdominal ultrasound may show thickening of the intestinal wall, mass lesions, lymphadenopathy, foreign bodies, signs of obstruction or abdominal effusion (see Figure 56.1). Abdominal ultrasound is most helpful in assisting in the decision on the next diagnostic step, i.e., abdominocentesis, endoscopy, exploratory laparotomy, fine needle aspiration (FNA), Tru-cut biopsies, etc.
- Computed tomography (CT) scans might be helpful for identification of foreign bodies, bone lesions, and thoracic lesions (e.g., fungal disease, foreign body, etc.).

Specific Testing

- Infectious causes.
    - *E. coli* – colonoscopy and mucosal biopsies.
        - Histopathology including hemotoxylin and eosin (H&E) and periodic acid–Schiff (PAS) staining.
        - Fluorescence *in situ* hybridization – FISH (can be performed on formalin-fixed paraffin-embedded colonic mucosal biopsies).
        - Culture of colonic mucosa biopsies and susceptibility testing (enteroinvasive *E. coli* are increasingly resistant to enrofloxacin).

- *Mycobacteria* spp.
  - ○ Ziehl–Neelsen staining may reveal acid-fast bacteria in biopsies or fine needle aspirates.
  - ○ Culture.
  - ○ Polymerase chain reaction (PCR).
- *Histoplasma* spp.
  - ○ Organisms might be found upon microscopic examination of rectal scrapings which can be performed on a conscious or sedated patient.
  - ○ *Histoplasma* spp. antigen testing can be performed on serum or urine samples.
  - ○ Histopathologic examination of intestinal biopsies including H&E, Grocott's methenamine silver (GMS), and PAS staining.
- *Prototheca* spp.
  - ○ Culture from aspirates or biopsies.
  - ○ Capsules of the organisms might be found upon microscopic examination of urine samples, rectal scrapings, FNAs or tissue sections.
  - ○ Histopathologic examination of intestinal biopsies including H&E, GMS, and PAS staining.
- *Pythium insidiosum.*
  - ○ Serology (enzyme-linked immunosorbent assay (ELISA) or immunoblot) for anti-*P. insidiosum* antibodies.
  - ○ Isolating the organism by PCR or culture from affected tissue.
  - ○ Histopathologic examination of intestinal biopsies including H&E, GMS, and PAS staining.
- FIP.
  - ○ Reverse transcriptase polymerase chain reaction (RT-PCR) for mutated coronavirus in serum, effusion, etc.
  - ○ Immunofluorescence staining of effusion or FNA for feline coronavirus antigen in macrophages.
  - ○ Histopathology of affected organs.
- Foreign body/material (e.g., migrating foreign body, suture material, etc.) – imaging (radiographs, ultrasound, CT), exploratory laparotomy.
- Idiopathic/miscellaneous – histopathologic examination of intestinal biopsies (endoscopic or surgical).

Pathologic Findings

- See discussion under specific diseases.
- Dependent on the underlying disease, granulomatous lesions may be found focally or disseminated within the GI tract as well as in other organs (see Figures 56.1 and 56.2).
- Figures 56.3 and 56.4 show histopathologic lesions in a dog with granulomatous colitis. The epithelium on the surface is flattened. The lamina propria is expanded by an inflammatory infiltrate, dominated by epithelioid macrophages and fibrosis.

 # THERAPEUTICS

Drug(s) of Choice

- HUC – enrofloxacin 5 mg/kg q 12 h for eight weeks. If the disease is unresponsive, mucosal biopsies should be submitted for culture and sensitivity testing.
- Histoplasmosis – itraconazole 10 mg/kg q 12–24 h in dogs and 5 mg/kg q 12 h in cats. Continue treatment for about two months after resolution of clinical signs and a minimum of 4–6 months.

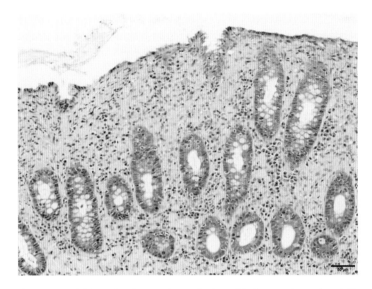

■ **Fig. 56.3.** Granulomatous colitis in a dog (H&E stain, 10×). The epithelium on the surface is flattened. The lamina propria is expanded by an inflammatory infiltrate, dominated by epithelioid macrophages and fibrosis. Source: Courtesy of Dr Paula Giaretta.

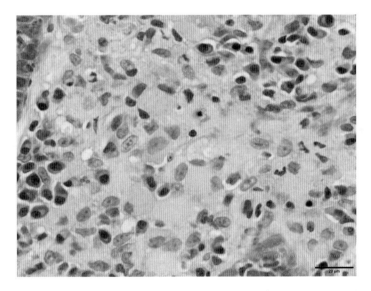

■ **Fig. 56.4.** Granulomatous colitis in a dog (H&E stain, 40×). Infiltration of the lamina propria by epithelioid macrophages and plasma cells indicating predominantly granulomatous inflammation. Source: Courtesy of Dr Paula Giaretta.

- Protothecosis – no effective treatment for disseminated protothecosis has been reported. Palliative therapy with amphotericin B and itraconazole might slow disease progression.
- Pythiosis – palliative therapy using itraconazole and terbinafine may be attempted.
- FIP – no effective treatment available. Palliative treatment to reduce inflammation using corticosteroids, pentoxifylline, etc. may be considered.

- Regional granulomatous enteritis – in cases with signs of obstruction, enterectomy followed by medical management with corticosteroids, sulfasalazine, cytotoxic drugs, and antibiotics have been reported to be successful. In cases without signs of obstruction, medical management similar to that in IBD may be attempted.
- Diffuse granulomatous enterocolitis – medical management as for IBD.
- Lipogranulomas associated with PLE: medical management as for PLE.
- Focal intestinal lipogranulomatous lymphangitis – enterectomy followed by medical management similar to that for PLE has been reported to be effective in some dogs.

Precautions/Interactions

See discussion under specific diseases.

Alternative Drugs

See discussion under specific diseases.

Appropriate Health Care

See discussion under specific diseases.

Nursing Care

See discussion under specific diseases.

Diet

- Limiting dietary antigens by feeding a novel protein or hydrolyzed diet might be beneficial for cases of idiopathic granulomatous enteritis.
- Patients with PLE or lipogranulomatous lymphangitis should be fed a low-fat diet.

Activity

See discussion under specific diseases.

Surgical Considerations

Surgical resection of affected areas in the GI tract may be considered for cases with pythiosis, regional granulomatous enteritis, and focal intestinal lipogranulomatous lymphangitis.

    COMMENTS

Client Education

See discussion under specific diseases.

Patient Monitoring

See discussion under specific diseases.

Prevention/Avoidance

See discussion under specific diseases.

Possible Complications

- Cases with pythiosis or regional granulomatous enteritis may develop GI obstruction at any point in time.
- Histoplasmosis, pythiosis, and prototothecosis are likely to be disseminated.

Expected Course and Prognosis

- The prognosis is dependent on the specific underlying disease.
- The prognosis for idiopathic forms of granulomatous enterocolitis (regional and diffuse forms, lipogranulomas, and focal intestinal lipogranulomatous lymphangitis) is generally considered to be guarded.

Abbreviations

- CT = computed tomography
- ELISA = enzyme-linked immunosorbent assay
- FIP = feline infectious peritonitis
- FISH = fluorescence *in situ* hybridization
- FNA = fine needle aspirate/aspiration
- GMS = Grocott's methenamine silver
- GI = gastrointestinal

- H&E = hemotoxylin and eosin (histologic staining)
- HUC = histiocytic ulcerative colitis
- IBD = inflammatory bowel disease
- PAS = periodic acid–Schiff (histologic staining)
- PLE = protein-losing enteropathy
- RT-PCR = reverse transcriptase polymerase chain reaction

See Also

- Colitis, Histiocytic Ulcerative
- Fungal Enteritides
- Inflammatory Bowel Disease

- Nutritional Approach to Chronic Enteropathies
- Protein-Losing Enteropathy
- Pythiosis

Suggested Reading

Hall EJ. Granulomatous enteritis: small intestine. In: Washabau RJ, Day MJ, eds. Canine and Feline Gastroenterology. St Louis: Saunders Elsevier, 2013, p. 672.

Lecoindre P, Gouni V, Chevallier M, et al. Regional granulomatous enteritis in 14 dogs. J Vet Intern Med 2012;26(3):773–774 (abstract).

Watson VE, Hobday MM, Durham AC. Focal intestinal lipogranulomatous lymphangitis in 6 dogs (2008–2011). J Vet Intern Med 2014;28(1):48–51.

Author: Sina Marsilio Dr.med.vet., DVM, DACVIM (SAIM), DECVIM-CA

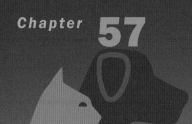
Feline Viral Enterides

DEFINITION/OVERVIEW

- Feline viral enterides encompass several important viral pathogens infecting the feline gastrointestinal tract, including feline panleukopenia virus (FPV), feline coronavirus (FCoV), feline leukemia virus (FeLV), and feline immunodeficiency virus (FIV).
- Additionally, other pathogenic viral pathogens have been recognized which include astrovirus, rotavirus, norovirus, reovirus, torovirus-like agent, and canine parvovirus infection in cats.

ETIOLOGY/PATHOPHYSIOLOGY

- The majority of feline viral enterides are transmitted by the fecal–oral or intranasal routes, or are spread by contact with infected body fluids including blood, saliva, feces, and fomites. Some of these viruses can be life threatening (FPV, FCoV, FIV, FeLV), and some of them have been found in clinically healthy cats.
- Cats infected with FPV typically have acute, severe clinical signs accompanied by high mortality, especially in unvaccinated and juvenile populations. It is worth noting that canine parvovirus infection in cats is distinct from FPV. Canine parvovirus (CPV) 2a and 2b replicate and can induce disease in cats with exposure to infected dog feces.
- Retrovirus (FIV, FeLV)-infected cats may experience a prolonged period of clinical latency. Cats with FIV have low viral loads and typically become infected via bite wounds. Cats with FeLV typically have abundant levels of circulating core viral antigen (p27) and become infected via vertical or horizontal transmission. FeLV is more pathogenic and, interestingly, can lead to several outcomes including a progressive infection, regressive infection, abortive exposure, or focal infection.
- FCoV-infected cats may stay healthy or show mild enteritis. Within one week of infection, cats can shed FCoV for weeks, months, or become lifelong carriers. Only a portion of cats develop feline infectious peritonitis (FIP) which has two forms: the effusive (wet) and the noneffusive (dry) forms. FIP occurs in part as a result of mutations arising during bursts of replications in monocytes and macrophages. Multiple factors dictate whether a cat will develop FIP, including viral load and the individual cat's immune response.
- Other enteric viruses have been described that are less pathogenic, including astroviruses (very uncommon) and noroviruses which have recently been detected in some kittens in New York. Experimental inoculation of norovirus can induce enteric signs, but further epidemiological studies need to be performed to elucidate the true pathogenic nature of this virus.
- Rotaviruses have worldwide distribution and are classified into serogroups A–G. Infection in cats is common but clinical disease is rare.

Blackwell's Five-Minute Veterinary Consult Clinical Companion: Small Animal Gastrointestinal Diseases,
First Edition. Edited by Jocelyn Mott and Jo Ann Morrison.
© 2019 John Wiley & Sons, Inc. Published 2019 by John Wiley & Sons, Inc.
Companion website: www.fiveminutevet.com/gastrointestinal

- Three types of reoviruses have been isolated from cats. The significance of torovirus-like infection in cats is unknown as many cats have antibodies to this virus, but most lack clinical disease.

Systems Affected

- Gastrointestinal –anorexia, diarrhea, vomiting, stomatitis.
- Hemic/lymphatic/immune – fever, anemia, leukopenia, thrombocytopenia, vasculitis, hematopoietic tumors such as lymphoma or leukemia, ascites or effusion (Figures 57.1, 57.2).
- Neurologic – cerebellar ataxia, nystagmus, seizures, behavioral changes, hydrocephalus (most commonly with FPV).

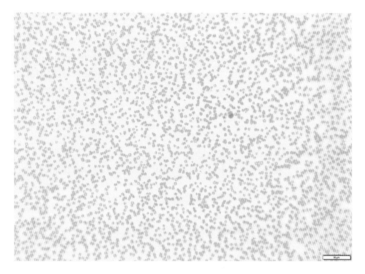

■ **Fig. 57.1.** Magnification at 10× of a blood smear from a cat with FIV. Note pale red blood cell color and lack of platelets or white blood cells. Source: Image courtesy of Dr Ilaria Cerchiaro.

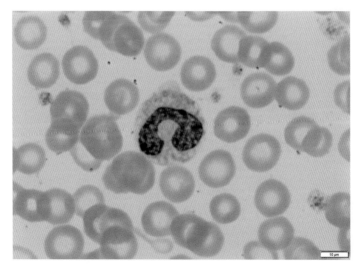

■ **Fig. 57.2.** Magnification at 100× of a blood smear from a parvovirus-positive patient. Note the toxic changes in the neutrophil: cytoplasmic basophilia and vacuolation, Döhle bodies, and toxic granulation. Source: Image courtesy of Dr. Ilaria Cerchiaro.

- Ophthalmic – protrusion of nictitating membranes, uveitis.
- Reproductive – *in utero* infection can lead to fetal death, resorption, abortion, or mummified fetus.

 # SIGNALMENT/HISTORY

- Kittens and juveniles (<6 months to one year of age) are most commonly clinically affected.
- Infections occur most commonly in cats residing in crowded, high-stress environments including shelters, catteries, and multi-cat households.
- However, older cats with diarrhea have also been found to harbor many of these viruses.

Risk Factors

- Young, unvaccinated (FPV, FeLV) cats.
- Outdoor exposure may increase the risk of some viruses (retroviruses); crowded, contaminated, stressful living conditions may exacerbate some infections. Additionally, secondary or coinfections (especially respiratory) may exacerbate viral enterides infections.

Historical Findings

- Weight loss, lethargy, and decreased appetite.
- Signs can be slow and insidious or acute.
- Outdoor lifestyle, multi-cat household or recently obtained from a shelter or cattery.
- Incomplete or no vaccination history.

 # CLINICAL FEATURES

- Infected cats may be asymptomatic or have transient illness of several days' duration.
- A fever refractive to antibiotics may or may not be present on physical examination.
- Dehydration and poor body condition may also be present, depending on the chronicity.
- Additional clinical signs can be variable but may include diarrhea, anorexia, vomiting, ascites (especially common in the "wet" form of FIP), or ataxia.
- Other disease conditions that may also be present include immune-mediated diseases, secondary infections, and neoplasia (depending on the virus responsible).
- Death can occur from septicemia and/or disseminated intravascular coagulation.

 # DIFFERENTIAL DIAGNOSIS

- Differentials are dependent on the presenting clinical signs.
- Gastrointestinal signs may be consistent with parasitism, chronic enteropathies, or lymphoma.
- Many of these diseases (FPV, FIV, FeLV, FIP) can be mistaken for one another.
- Appropriate diagnostic testing and evaluation must be performed.

 # DIAGNOSTICS

Complete Blood Count/Biochemistry/Urinalysis

- Anemia, leukopenia, leukocytosis, panleukopenia, thrombocytopenia, and/or lymphocytosis.
- Hyperglobulinemia and hyperbilirubinemia may or may not be present.

Other Laboratory Tests

- Point-of-care testing from stool or blood is important for diagnosing FPV (utilizing canine tests to detect CPV-2a or -2a-derived strains and/or FPV antigen).
- FIV/FeLV (snap tests, antibody testing for FIV, and antigen testing for FeLV).
- Polymerase chain reaction (PCR) may also be performed on feces, blood or infected tissue.
- It is important to note that a serologic diagnosis of FCoV is not indicative of FIP. Obtaining an antemortem diagnosis of FIP is difficult at best. Fecal RT-PCR can be used to identify asymptomatic FCoV shedding (multiple positive samples over an eight-month period). Additionally, PCR can be used to detect FCoV in abdominal fluid, blood, or tissues (spleen, liver, or kidney) in suspect cases of FIP. Additionally, the Rivalta test and the albumin to globulin ratio (A:G <0.6) have been used to rule out FIP in suspect patients.

THERAPEUTICS

May or may not be needed, depending on the severity of the condition in the cat. Some of these viral enterides have transient or self-limiting effects. Others require intensive care. In many advanced cases of FIP, FIV, FeLV, FPV, no cure exists.

Drug(s) of Choice

- Specifically, in cases of FIP, medications are given to control the immune response. Therefore, prednisolone has been given at antiinflammatory doses to reduce inflammation and improve the cat's quality of life.
- Immune modulators such as proprenyl immunostimulant or acemannan have been used in treatment of FIP with no documented efficacy.
- Tylosin, the macrolide antibiotic which also has "immunomodulatory" effects, has also been utilized in clinical FIP cases.
- Most antiviral compounds act by inhibiting the retroviral enzyme reverse transcriptase (RT). This is done by three different classes of RT. Additionally, there are drugs that inhibit other viral enzymes which interfere with virus genome replication.
- Antiviral therapy including feline recombinant interferon-omega administered subcutaneously (available in Japan, Australia, and Europe), oral and/or parenteral human recombinant IFN-alpha (HR alpha-interferon (Roferon A) diluted in saline at 30 units/day PO for seven days every other week; may increase survival rates and improve clinical status; high-dose recombinant feline interferon-omega (Virbagen Omega) at 1 million units/kg/day SQ daily for five days at three intervals (d0–4, d14–18, d60–64) or lower-dose oral protocols may be effective), and zidovudine (AZT) (5–15 mg/kg PO q 12 h) has been administered to cats with various viral infections, but efficacy has not been consistently and convincingly proven.
- Recent investigations iton the use of antiviral medications (specifically, protease and nucleoside inhibitors) for FIP have demonstrated promising early results. Commercially available products have not yet been developed.

Appropriate Health Care

Symptomatic treatment for these conditions may include hospitalization with intravenous fluids, antibiotic use in cases of neutropenia/bacteremia, antiemetics, nasoesophageal/nasogastric nutritional support, and colloid assistance for hypovolemia.

Nursing Care

- Primary consideration – manage secondary and opportunistic infections.
- Supportive therapy – parenteral fluids and nutritional supplements, as required.

COMMENTS

Client Education

FPV

- Inform client that all current and future cats in the household must be vaccinated against FPV before exposure.
- Inform client that the virus will remain infectious on the premises for years unless the environment can be adequately disinfected with household bleach.

FIV

- Inform client that the infection is only slowly progressive and healthy antibody-positive cats may remain healthy for years.
- Advise client that cats with clinical signs will have recurrent or chronic health problems that require medical attention.
- Discuss the importance of keeping cats indoors to protect them from exposure to secondary pathogens and to prevent spread of FIV.

FeCoV

- Discuss the various aspects of disease, including the grave prognosis; once clinical FIP is confirmed, nearly 100% of cats will eventually die of the disease.
- Inform client of the high prevalence of FCoV infection but low incidence of actual clinical disease; <10% of FCoV antibody-positive cats <2 years of age eventually develop clinical disease.

FeLV

- Discuss importance of keeping cats indoors and separated from FeLV-negative cats to protect them from exposure to secondary pathogens and to prevent spread of FeLV.
- Discuss good nutrition and routine husbandry for control of secondary bacterial, viral, and parasitic infections.

Patient Monitoring

- Monitor hydration and electrolyte balance closely.
- Monitor complete blood cell count daily or at least every two days until recovery with FPV.
- Recovered cats are immune against FPV infection for life and do not require further vaccination.

Prevention/Avoidance

- Housing cats indoors in low-stress environments.
- Retroviral screen for new cats prior to introduction into a household.
- Strict hygiene practices including separating feeding and waste spaces, providing multiple litter pans, and frequently cleaning them will help to minimize viral fecal–oral transmission.
- Adhering to proper vaccine protocols to prevent FPV.
- Vaccinate at-risk (outdoor) cats for FeLV.
- In order to prevent FIP, one must prevent infection of FCoV in cats.

Expected Course and Prognosis

- FPV-infected cats that survive the first five days usually recover.
- FIV-infected cats have mean survival of 4.9–6 years post diagnosis.
- FeLV-infected cats have a median survival of 2.4 years.

- FIP-infected cats have a generally poor prognosis, with median survival times ranging from seven to 477 days. Typically, FIP cats with low platelet and lymphocyte counts and elevated bilirubin and effusions have a poorer prognosis.

Abbreviations

- CPV = canine parvovirus
- FCoV = feline coronavirus
- FeLV = feline leukemia virus
- FIP = feline infectious peritonitis
- FIV = feline immunodeficiency virus

- FPV = feline panleukopenia virus
- PCR = polymerase chain reaction
- RT = enzyme reverse transcriptase
- RT-PCR = reverse transcriptase polymerase chain reaction

See Also

- Diarrhea, Acute

- Vomiting, Acute

Suggested Reading

Addie D, Belak S, Boucraut-Baralon C, et al. Feline infectious peritonitis: ABCD guidelines on prevention & management. J Feline Med Surg 2009;11:594–604.

Di Marino B, di Profio F, Melegari I, et al. A novel feline norovirus in diarrheic cats. Inf Gen Evol 2016;38:132–137.

Green CE. Infectious Diseases of the Dog and Cat, 4th ed. St Louis: Elsevier, 2012, p. 9.

Levy J, Harmann K, Hofann-Lehmann R, et al. 2008 American Association of Feline Practitioners' Feline Retrovirus Management Guidelines. J Feline Med Surg 2008;10:300–316.

Pedersen NC, Kim Y, Liu H, et al. Efficacy of a 3C-like protease inhibitor in treating various forms of acquired feline infectious peritonitis. J Feline Med Surg 2018;20:378–392.

Stuetzer B, Harmann K. Feline parvovirus infection and associated diseases. Vet J 2014;201:150–155.

Sykes JE. Canine and Feline Infectious Diseases. St Louis: Elsevier, 2014, p. 19.

Acknowledgments: The authors and editors acknowledge the prior contribution of Dr Margaret Barr and Dr Fred Scott.

Author: Jennifer E. Slovak DVM, MS, DACVIM

Chapter 58

Food Reactions (Gastrointestinal), Adverse

DEFINITION/OVERVIEW

- The term *adverse food reaction* encompasses disorders with an immunologic etiology (food allergies), a nonimmunologic etiology (food intolerances), and toxic reactions (food intoxication).
- Adverse food reactions are often associated with gastrointestinal signs (vomiting, diarrhea) in dogs and cats. Practically speaking, it can be difficult to distinguish between food allergies manifesting with gastrointestinal signs and food intolerances.
- Diet-responsive chronic enteropathy describes gastrointestinal signs that resolve with dietary management. Since some enteropathies with underlying etiologies unrelated to food allergy or intolerance may respond to diet due to other dietary properties (high digestibility, etc.), this is technically not a gastrointestinal adverse food reaction but is treated similarly. A diet-responsive chronic enteropathy may not consistently relapse after provocation with the original diet, unlike food allergy or food intolerance.

ETIOLOGY/PATHOPHYSIOLOGY

- Food allergy occurs due to a disruption of the complex gastrointestinal immune system which likely involves a combination of a breakdown in the anatomic and physiologic gastrointestinal barrier function (tight junctions, mucus layer, normal peristalsis, pH, and bile acids), loss of oral tolerance, and dysregulated immune responses.
- Food allergy is most commonly a type I hypersensitivity reaction in humans. In dogs and cats, type I, III, and IV hypersensitivity reactions have been thought to occur and may occur in combination. Food allergy requires previous exposure to an antigen (sensitization) to occur prior to development of the allergy.
- Food intolerance may be due to idiosyncratic reactions to various food ingredients or additives, pharmacologic reactions to compounds in the diet, or defects or deficiencies in enzymes or pathways needed to digest or utilize certain ingredients (e.g. lactose intolerance). Unlike food allergy, food intolerance requires no previous exposure to the food product.
- Toxicity reactions occur when food contains toxins (e.g. aflatoxin, a hepatotoxin produced by *Aspergillus* spp.) or has spoiled or been contaminated by bacterial growth.

Systems Affected

- Gastrointestinal – small intestine, colon, and/or stomach can be affected by adverse food reactions.
- Skin/exocrine – food allergy can manifest with concurrent dermatologic signs or exclusive dermatologic signs.

Blackwell's Five-Minute Veterinary Consult Clinical Companion: Small Animal Gastrointestinal Diseases, First Edition. Edited by Jocelyn Mott and Jo Ann Morrison.
© 2019 John Wiley & Sons, Inc. Published 2019 by John Wiley & Sons, Inc.
Companion website: www.fiveminutevet.com/gastrointestinal

SIGNALMENT/HISTORY

- Soft-coated wheaten terriers affected with the syndrome of protein-losing enteropathy (PLE) and/or protein-losing nephropathy (PLN) have been shown to be affected by food allergies, which may play a role in the development of PLE/PLN.
- Gluten-sensitive enteropathy is an autosomal recessive trait seen in some Irish setters.
- Dogs affected with diet-responsive chronic enteropathy tend to be young (median age 3.4 years in one study).
- Cats of all ages have been reported to be affected by gastrointestinal adverse food reactions (median age five years).

Risk Factors

- Young Irish setters susceptible to gluten-sensitive enteropathy may be at greater risk to develop the disease if exposed to gluten at an early age.
- Host genetic susceptibility is suspected in wheaten terriers and German shepherd dogs.

Historical Findings

- Mild to moderate vomiting, usually no more frequent than once daily.
- Diarrhea – large bowel, small bowel, or mixed. Some studies have shown a predominance of large bowel diarrhea.
- Flatulence, borborygmus, abdominal pain.
- Anorexia.
- Weight loss – can uncommonly be the sole presenting complaint.

 # CLINICAL FEATURES

- The physical exam is often normal, but this depends on the severity and chronicity of the problem.
- Weight loss or muscle wasting may be noted.
- Dehydration can be present if there has been recent severe vomiting or diarrhea.
- Concurrent pruritic dermatologic lesions may be seen in food allergy.

 # DIFFERENTIAL DIAGNOSES

- Infectious diseases – intestinal nematodes, *Giardia*, histoplasmosis, salmonellosis, toxoplasmosis (cats), feline infectious peritonitis.
- Infiltrative gastrointestinal diseases – inflammatory bowel disease, histiocytic ulcerative colitis (boxers, French bulldogs).
- Endocrine diseases – hypoadrenocorticism, hyperthyroidism (cats).
- Exocrine pancreatic insufficiency.
- Lymphangiectasia.
- Gastrointestinal motility disorders.
- Pancreatitis.
- Metabolic diseases (renal disease, liver disease).

 # DIAGNOSTICS

Exclusion of relevant differential diagnoses is recommended prior to diagnosing an adverse food reaction; however, there are no laboratory tests that reliably diagnose adverse food reaction and an elimination diet trial is the test of choice.

Complete Blood Count/Biochemistry/Urinalysis

- Often normal but should be performed to screen for complicating factors or differential diagnoses (hypoalbuminemia, evidence of hypoadrenocorticism, etc.).
- Eosinophilia can sometimes be seen in patients with food allergies.

Other Laboratory Tests

- Fecal flotation and fecal smear. Perform 2–3 tests over several days to increase sensitivity. Empiric deworming with a broad-spectrum anthelminthic may be considered to address possible undetected parasitism.
- Few diagnostic tests are specific to adverse food reactions but the following are helpful to rule out differential diagnoses and to identify complicating factors.
    - Serum cobalamin and folate – can help determine involvement of proximal and distal small intestine as well as identify possible need for cobalamin supplementation.
    - Trypsin-like immunoreactivity (TLI) – gold standard test for exocrine pancreatic insufficiency.
    - Baseline cortisol or adrenocorticotropic hormone (ACTH) stimulation test – to rule out hypoadrenocorticism, if clinically suspected.
    - Total T4 (cats) – to evaluate for hyperthyroidism, if clinically suspected.
    - Fecal alpha-1 proteinase inhibitor – this test can be performed if there is a suspicion of protein-losing enteropathy but other lab results are equivocal or there is complicating proteinuria.
    - Perinuclear antineutrophilic cytoplasmic autoantibodies (pANCA) – this test is currently limited to use in a research setting, but has shown promise in early detection of PLE and PLN, believed to be due to underlying food allergy, in soft-coated wheaten terriers. Additionally, it may help to differentiate between dogs with diet-responsive enteropathies and enteropathies requiring treatment with glucocorticoids.

Imaging

- Abdominal radiographs or ultrasound may be useful in eliminating some differential diagnoses but are generally unhelpful in determining the underlying cause of diarrhea unless there is high suspicion of neoplasia.
- Doppler evaluation (ultrasound) may detect changes in blood flow through the celiac and cranial mesenteric arteries in dogs shortly after a dietary challenge, prior to the development of clinical signs. This has little practical application in a clinical setting.

Other Diagnostic Tests

- Elimination diet trial.
    - Resolution of clinical signs on an elimination diet followed by recurrence of clinical signs after provocation with the patient's original diet or ingredients from the original diet is the gold standard test for the diagnosis of adverse food reactions in dogs and cats.
    - Prior to performing an elimination diet, obtaining a thorough dietary history is critical to choosing an appropriate food for the trial.
    - A trial with exclusive feeding of a novel protein diet or a hydrolyzed protein diet is then performed. The trial diet should be administered for a minimum of two weeks when gastrointestinal (GI) signs predominate, although clinical improvement may be seen in days, particularly in cats. It may take up to 8–12 weeks to see improvement in dermatologic signs.
    - A dietary provocation test should be performed once clinical signs have resolved on the elimination diet. During this time, the original diet is reintroduced. Ideally, if GI signs return within a few days of feeding the original diet, an adverse food reaction is confirmed.

- • Alternatively, individual ingredients can be introduced in a dietary provocation test. It is important to introduce each ingredient one at a time and wait several days before confirming no reaction.
- • Practically, many owners are relieved to see resolution of clinical signs and are reluctant to perform a dietary provocation and elect to continue feeding the trial diet.
- ▪ GI histopathology – endoscopic or surgical gastrointestinal biopsies may be taken to help rule out other differential diagnoses. Histologic lesions have not been shown to help differentiate between dogs with diet-responsive enteropathies, adverse food reactions, and enteropathies requiring glucocorticoids. No indication for biopsy unless they fail diet trial.
- ▪ Serology and gastroscopic food sensitivity testing are unreliable and are not recommended.

Pathologic Findings

- ▪ Villous atrophy and mild lymphoplasmacytic inflammation, eosinophilic inflammation, or mixed inflammation may be seen with food allergy.
- ▪ Gastric and intestinal morphology can also be normal.

 # THERAPEUTICS

Drug(s) of Choice

Generally, no medications are used or are necessary if effective dietary management is implemented.

Nursing Care

- ▪ These patients are typically treated on an outpatient basis.
- ▪ If an adverse food reaction is severe, intravenous fluid therapy, administration of antiemetics, and nutritional support via enteral-assisted feeding may be temporarily required.

Diet

- ▪ Lifelong dietary management is essential for animals with food intolerance and food allergy.
- ▪ Diets that can be chosen for an elimination diet trial include veterinary prescription hydrolyzed protein diets, commercial novel protein diets (available as veterinary prescription diets or over-the-counter products), or a home-cooked novel protein diet.
- ▪ Novel protein diets are foods containing only protein sources to which the animal has not been previously exposed and are selected based on a careful dietary history.
- ▪ Over-the-counter novel protein diets have been found to contain proteins other than those listed on the label, which may be due to contamination during processing; veterinary prescription products are prepared specifically for animals with food allergy and should be chosen when possible.
- ▪ Home-prepared novel protein diets can uncommonly result in a beneficial response in animals who did not respond to a commercial diet containing the same protein. Considerations for home-prepared novel protein diets are that many are not suitable for long-term feeding (unless the diet is complete and balanced with the help of a veterinary nutritionist) and the owner inconvenience of home preparation of meals.
- ▪ Hydrolyzed protein diets are created by enzymatic hydrolysis of the intact protein into peptides small enough to reduce the potential of the protein to induce an allergic response.
- ▪ Hydrolyzed diets are ideal when an animal has been exposed to many different protein sources or when a reliable dietary history cannot be obtained.
- ▪ Hydrolyzed protein diets can retain some antigenicity and, if possible, the parent protein of the hydrolyzed diet should be a protein to which the animal does not have a known sensitivity.
- ▪ Hydrolyzed protein diets may also benefit animals without true food allergy due to the improved digestibility of the diet.

Activity

No restrictions.

COMMENTS

Client Education

- Owners should be aware of possible sources of food antigen during an elimination trial that may make the animal's response difficult to interpret, including table scraps, flavored medications and toothpastes, and coprophagy.
- Counsel clients on the necessity of lifelong avoidance of ingredients to which their animal is sensitive.

Patient Monitoring

- Assess efficacy of elimination diet trial by observing improvement in gastrointestinal signs.
- Failure to improve in 2–3 weeks may warrant a subsequent trial with another diet if adverse food reaction is strongly suspected or continued work-up for other causes of gastrointestinal signs, including endoscopy with biopsies.

Expected Course and Prognosis

The prognosis is excellent as long as the offending dietary components are successfully identified and avoided.

Abbreviations

- ACTH = adrenocorticotropic hormone
- GI = gastrointestinal
- pANCA = perinuclear antineutrophilic cytoplasmic autoantibodies
- PLE = protein-losing enteropathy
- PLN = protein-losing nephropathy
- TLI = trypsin-like immunoreactivity

See Also

- Diarrhea, Chronic – Canine
- Diarrhea, Chronic – Feline
- Flatulence
- Inflammatory Bowel Disease
- Gastroenteritis, Eosinophilic
- Gastroenteritis, Lymphocytic-Plasmacytic
- Gluten-Sensitive Enteropathy in Irish Setters
- Vomiting, Chronic

Suggested Reading

Gaschen FP, Merchant SR. Adverse food reactions in dogs and cats. Vet Clin North Am 2011;41:361–379.

Guilford WG, Jones BR, Markwell PJ, Arthur DG, Collett MG, Harte JG. Food sensitivity in cats with chronic idiopathic gastrointestinal problems. J Vet Intern Med 2001;15:7–13.

Luckschander N, Allenspach K, Hall J. Perinuclear antineutrophilic cytoplasmic antibody and response to treatment in diarrheic dogs with food responsive disease or inflammatory bowel disease. J Vet Intern Med 2006;20:221–227.

Mandigers PJJ, Biourge V, van den Ingh TSGAM, Ankringa N, German AJ. A randomized, open-label, positively-controlled field trial of a hydrolyzed protein diet in dogs with chronic small bowel enteropathy. J Vet Intern Med 2010;24:1350–1357.

Vaden SL, Hammerberg B, Davenport DJ, et al. Food hypersensitivity reactions in Soft Coated Wheaten Terriers with protein losing enteropathy or protein-losing nephropathy or both: gastroscopic food sensitivity testing, dietary provocation, and fecal immunoglobulin E. J Vet Intern Med 2000;14:60–67.

Authors: Laura Van Vertloo DVM, MS, DACVIM, Albert E. Jergens DVM, PhD, DACVIM

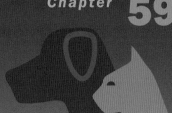

Chapter 59

Fungal Enteritides

DEFINITION/OVERVIEW

Infection of the gastrointestinal tract by pathogenic fungal organisms, most commonly *Histoplasma capsulatum* and *Pythium insidiosum*.

ETIOLOGY/PATHOPHYSIOLOGY

- Although almost all pathogenic fungal organisms have the capacity to infect the gastrointestinal (GI) tract, fungal enteritis is generally a rare occurrence except in *Histoplasma capsulatum* and *Pythium insidiosum* infections.
- *Pythium insidiosum* is a pathogenic oomycete that exists in aquatic environments as a biflagellate zoospore. Infection typically occurs when the biflagellate encysts in damaged skin or GI mucosa.
- *Histoplasma capsulatum* is a dimorphic fungus present in the soil and is especially prevalent in bat and bird excrement. Infection occurs through the inhalation of microconidia that are released during the mycelial stage of the organism's growth. Once in the host, the microconidia transform to a yeast form, which are phagocytized by the pulmonary macrophages. Yeast organisms are capable of surviving indefinitely within these immune cells. Infection can then remain limited to the pulmonary tree or can disseminate to other organs (skin, lymph nodes, bone, heart, central nervous system (CNS) and GI tract). The existence of *Histoplasma* cases with only GI involvement and no respiratory signs suggests that direct infection of the GI tract by ingestion of the organisms is also possible.

Systems Affected

- Gastrointestinal.
  - Pythiosis – infection and inflammation cause marked segmental transmural thickening of various areas of the GI tract. The gastric outflow tract, duodenum, and ileocolic junction are most commonly affected. Occasionally, infection of the esophagus can occur. Disease can extend into the mesenteric vessels causing intestinal ischemia, perforation, and peritonitis.
  - Histoplasmosis – infection of the intestinal tract causes focal to diffuse thickening, erosion, and ulceration of the GI mucosa.
- Hemic/lymphatic/immune.
  - Pythiosis – draining lymph nodes (mesenteric) are often enlarged secondary to reactive inflammation, not infection by the organism. GI blood loss can result in significant anemia.
  - Histoplasmosis – disseminated disease often involves the abdominal lymph nodes.

Blackwell's Five-Minute Veterinary Consult Clinical Companion: Small Animal Gastrointestinal Diseases, First Edition. Edited by Jocelyn Mott and Jo Ann Morrison.
© 2019 John Wiley & Sons, Inc. Published 2019 by John Wiley & Sons, Inc.
Companion website: www.fiveminutevet.com/gastrointestinal

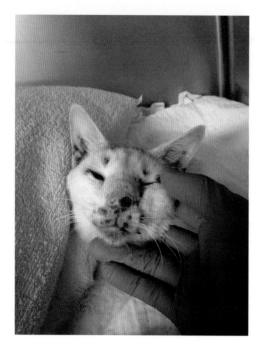

■ **Fig. 59.1.** Cat with ulcerative cutaneous lesions secondary to disseminated histoplasmosis.

■ Skin/exocrine.
  • Pythiosis – alhough a cutaneous form of pythiosis exists, concurrent dermatologic and gastrointestinal pathology is extremely rare.
  • Histoplasmosis – disseminated histoplasmosis can localize to the skin, causing ulcerative lesions (Figure 59.1).

 ## SIGNALMENT/HISTORY

■ Pythiosis – infection typically occurs in young active large-breed male dogs. Although few feline cases have been reported, young cats (<12 months) appear to be overrepresented. Pythiosis occurs mostly in tropical or subtropical areas. Most cases reported in the USA occur in the states surrounding the Gulf of Mexico but cases have been reported in the Midwest as well as in California.
■ Histoplasmosis – most commonly reported in young and active sporting breed dogs. While most reports have been from the American Midwest (specifically the areas drained by the Mississippi, Missouri, and Ohio Rivers), cases have been reported in all continents with temperate to subtropical climates.

Risk Factors

■ Fungal enteritides are more commonly reported in dogs than in cats.
■ Immunosuppressed animals might be at increased risk of infection.
■ Access to warm freshwater areas (pythiosis) or freshly disturbed soil that is rich in bird or bat excrement (histoplasmosis) has been associated with increased risk of infection.

Historical Findings

■ Pythiosis – weight loss, anorexia, vomiting, diarrhea, hematochezia.
■ Histoplasmosis – large bowel diarrhea, hematochezia, melena.

CLINICAL FEATURES

- Dogs with fungal enteritides will commonly display signs of chronic weight loss. Abdominal palpation might reveal the presence of an abdominal mass caused by either a fungal granuloma or mesenteric lymphadenopathy.
- Patients with significant GI bleeding can have pale mucous membranes and be clinically dehydrated. Frank blood and a thickened rectal mucosa are often present on rectal examination.

DIFFERENTIAL DIAGNOSIS

- Infectious disease (intestinal parasites, parvovirus, *Campylobacter*, *Salmonella*, *Clostridium*) – presence of ova or protozoal organisms on fecal floatation test; positive *Giardia* enzyme-linked immunosorbent assay (ELISA); positive fecal parvovirus ELISA antigen test; positive bacterial fecal culture or polymerase chain reaction (PCR).
- Inflammatory disease (inflammatory bowel disease, pancreatitis) – hypoechoic pancreas on ultrasonographic examination, positive pancreatic lipase immunoreactivity (SNAP cPL or SPEC cPL); gastrointestinal biopsies are necessary to distinguish inflammatory masses from fungal disease.
- Neoplasia (lymphoma, carcinoma, gastrointestinal stromal tumor (GIST)) – presence of cells displaying criteria of malignancy on fine needle aspirates or biopsies of mass or lymph nodes.

DIAGNOSTICS

Complete Blood Count/Biochemistry/Urinalysis

- Complete blood cell count – mild to moderate nonregenerative anemia, eosinophilia.
- Chemistry – intestinal protein loss will manifest with hypoalbuminemia. Serum globulins can be low due to GI loss but chronic inflammation can occasionally cause a hyperglobulinemia. Hypercalcemia has been reported in cats with histoplasmosis.
- Urinalysis – mild proteinuria.

Imaging

- Thoracic radiographs.
  - Pythiosis – cases with esophageal involvement can show a mediastinal mass with possible tracheal deviation.
  - Histoplasmosis – cases with pulmonary involvement commonly have a diffuse miliary to nodular pulmonary pattern.
- Abdominal radiographs – poor serosal detail due to severe weight loss or abdominal effusion. GI perforation can occur. An abdominal mass with possible signs of GI obstruction can occur with cases of pythiosis.
- Abdominal ultrasound – moderate to severe segmental thickening of the GI tract with possible mesenteric lymphadenopathy. While pythiosis lesions are focal, histoplasmosis lesions can be focal to diffuse.
- Computed tomography – allows a more global assessment of the abdomen and can also determine the extent of vascular invasion, if present.

Other Diagnostic Tests

■ Endoscopy – with fungal enteritides, the mucosa of the small intestines and/or colon will often appear thickened and granular with multifocal erosions and ulcerations (Figure 59.2).

■ Cytology – samples from abdominal lymph nodes, mass lesions, or rectal scrapings will reveal granulomatous or pyogranulomatous inflammation. *Pythium insidiosum* organisms will appear as broad, poorly septate hyphae. When stained with Wright or Giemsa stain, *Histoplasma* organisms will often be intraphagocytic and will appear round, measuring 2–4 μm in diameter with a basophilic center (Figure 59.3).

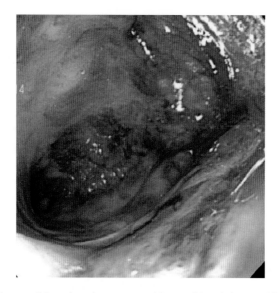

■ **Fig. 59.2.** Endoscopic image of the colon of a one-year-old spayed female boxer with intestinal pythiosis.

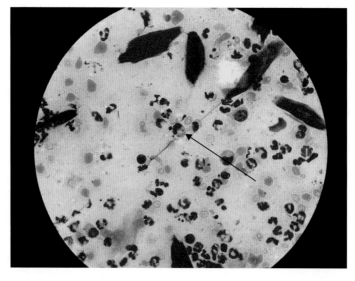

■ **Fig. 59.3.** Cytological sample showing intracellular *Histoplasma capsulatum* organisms.

- Culture.
  - Pythiosis – the organism is readily cultured from fresh tissue samples. However, since distinctive sexual reproductive structures rarely develop in culture, PCR is necessary for positive identification.
  - Histoplasmosis – due to its tendency to revert to the hyphal (infectious) form when cultured, fungal culture of *Histoplasma* is not recommended.
- Serology.
  - Pythiosis – immunoblot and ELISA assays show very high sensitivity and specificity. Moreover, antibody titers measured using the ELISA assay have been shown to correlate with success of treatment.
  - Histoplasmosis – serologic testing for anti-*Histoplasma* antibodies is not recommended due to the high rates of false-negative and false-positive results.
- Antigen testing – a highly sensitive commercial ELISA assay is available for detection of *Histoplasma* antigen. Although either serum or urine can be used for the assay, urine is recommended due to the greater sensitivity when compared to serum. Since cross-reactivity can occur with other systemic mycoses, a positive result should always be confirmed with additional testing (cytology, histopathology). This assay can also be used to gauge response to treatment
- PCR.
  - Pythiosis – a highly specific PCR is available.
  - Histoplasmosis – although PCR has been used for diagnosis in humans, this test is not widely available in veterinary medicine.

Pathologic Findings

- A common finding in tissues from fungal enteritides is the presence of granulomatous to pyogranulomatous inflammation. An eosinophilic component is also often present, especially in cases of pythiosis.
- Intralesional organisms are often identified.
- In the case of histoplasmosis, small, often intracellular organisms can be seen. Infections with pseudofungal organisms such as pythiosis will be characterized by the presence of broad and sparsely septate hyphae.
- Since hyphae may not stain with routine hematoxylin-eosin stains, use of Gomori's methenamine silver stain is recommended as it allows easy visualization.

 # THERAPEUTICS

- Surgical excision is recommended for treatment of pythiosis. Wide margins (3 cm) should be taken.
- While regional lymphadenopathy is usually not caused by extension of disease, biopsies are recommended to aid in prognostication.

Drug(s) of Choice

- Medical therapy for pythiosis is most effective when combined with surgical excision of the mass(es). Combination therapy of itraconazole (10 mg/kg once daily PO) with terbinafine (10 mg/kg once daily PO) should be continued for at least 2–3 months following surgery. If serology results at that time show significant decrease of the titers (>50% from baseline), medical therapy can be discontinued. Otherwise, therapy should be continued until titers decrease to baseline.
- The current drug of choice for treatment of histoplasmosis is itraconazole (5–10 mg/kg once daily). However, newer azoles (voriconazole and posaconazole) have been shown to be very

effective in treated histoplasmosis in disseminated disease models. In severe cases of histo-plasmosis, combination of itraconazole with amphotericin B (0.5 mg/kg every other day IV) might improve outcome.

■ Therapy should be continued until 2 months after a negative result is obtained on urine anti-gen testing. Long-term therapy (4–6 months) is often necessary for resolution of disease.

Precautions/Interactions

■ Many antifungal medications carry risks of toxicity. In patients receiving systemic azole medi-cations, liver values should be regularly assessed to monitor for possible hepatotoxicity.

■ Ulcerative dermatitis has been reported in dogs receiving higher doses of itraconazole (10 mg/kg or above).

■ Likewise, patients receiving amphotericin should be monitored closely for acute kidney injury through regular review of urine sediment and serum creatinine measurements.

Alternative Drugs

■ Although medical therapy alone is rarely successful for treatment of pythiosis, cures have been reported using combination therapy. Also, the addition of the agricultural fungicide mefenoxam was successful in treating a dog with GI pythiosis in one case report.

■ Although fluconazole (5 mg/kg twice daily PO) can be used in patients with reactions to itraconazole, its efficacy in treating histoplasmosis might be inferior to other antifungals.

■ Immunotherapy, surgical resection, and antifungal medications have been used to treat pythiosis in some cases.

Diet

■ Patients should be provided with high-quality, easily digestible food.

■ If voluntary intake is not sufficient due to systemic disease, placement of an esophageal or gastric feeding tube should be considered in order to provide adequate caloric intake.

Surgical Considerations

As opposed to histoplasmosis, where systemic presence of the organism is often suspected, pythiosis is usually limited to one area of the intestinal tract. Therefore, aggressive surgical excision of the lesion is the most important component of successful therapy.

 COMMENTS

Client Education

■ Since *Histoplasma* infection occurs through the production of microconidia by the hyphal form of the organism, transmission from host to host is not possible and has not been reported. However, since humans and their pets will often reside in the same environment, concurrent infection is possible.

■ Owners should be informed to avoid areas where soil is heavily contaminated with bird or bat excrement.

Patient Monitoring

■ Pythiosis – serologic testing using ELISA has been shown to correlate with fungal burden. A marked decrease in antibody levels should be seen with 2–3 months of successful surgical resection.

- Histoplasmosis – urine antigen testing should be monitored every 1–2 months during therapy to assess response. Although no consensus exists on length of treatment, the author recommends therapy be continued two months after negative urine antigen levels are obtained. Antigen levels should be monitored every 3–6 months for the first year of remission.

Prevention/Avoidance

Owner should be informed to limit exposure to recently disturbed soil or areas rich in bird or bat excrement.

Possible Complications

- Pythiosis – recurrence of disease is relatively common at the site of surgical excision.
- Histoplasmosis – involvement of other organ systems (CNS, bone, skin, lungs, eyes, liver) is common with this disease. Relapse can occur following cessation of treatment.

Expected Course and Prognosis

- Long-term medical therapy (4–6 months) is generally necessary for resolution of disease.
- Pythiosis – prognosis is fair to good in cases where complete surgical excision is possible. However, prognosis is more guarded in cases treated with medical therapy alone.
- Histoplasmosis – prognosis for intestinal histoplasmosis is fair to good depending on the severity of disease and involvement of other body systems.
- Patients with compromised immune systems (medical immunosuppression, diabetes, hyperadrenocorticism) will likely have a poorer prognosis.

Abbreviations

- CNS = central nervous system
- ELISA = enzyme-linked immunosorbent assay
- GI = gastrointestinal
- GIST = gastrointestinal stromal tumor
- PCR = polymerase chain reaction
- PLI = pancreatic lipase immunoreactivity

See Also

- Enterocolitis, Granulomatous
- Protein-Losing Enteropathy

Suggested Reading

Grooters AM. Pythiosis, lagenidiosis, and zygomycosis. In: Sykes JE, ed. Canine and Feline Infectious Diseases. St Louis: Saunders Elsevier, 2014, pp. 668–678.

Hanzlicek AS, Meinkoth JH, Renschler JS, Goad C, Wheat LJ. Antigen concentrations as an indicator of clinical remission and disease relapse in cats with histoplasmosis. J Vet Intern Med 2016;30:1065–1073.

Hensel P, Greene CE, Medleau L, Latimer KS, Mendoza L. Immunotherapy for treatment of multicentric cutaneous pythiosis in a dog. J Am Vet Med Assoc 2003;223(2):215–218.

Hummel J, Grooters A, Davidson G, Jennings S, Nicklas J, Birkenheuer A. Successful management of gastrointestinal pythiosis in a dog using itraconazole, terbinafine, and mefenoxam. Med Mycol 2011;49:539–542.

Lin Blache J, Ryan K, Arceneaux K. Histoplasmosis. Compend Contin Educ Vet 2011;33:E1–10.

Schmiedt CW, Stratton-Phelps M, Torres BT, et al. Treatment of intestinal pythiosis in a dog with a combination of marginal excision, chemotherapy, and immunotherapy. J Am Vet Med Assoc 2012;241(3):358–363.

Acknowledgments: The author and editors acknowledge the prior contribution of Dr Amy Grooters and Dr Daniel Foy.

Author: Jean-Sébastien Palerme DVM, MSc, DACVIM

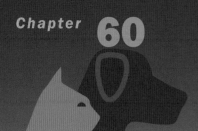

Chapter 60

Gastroenteritis, Eosinophilic

DEFINITION/OVERVIEW

An inflammatory disease of the stomach and intestine, characterized by an infiltration of eosinophils, usually into the lamina propria, but occasionally involving the submucosa and muscularis.

ETIOLOGY/PATHOPHYSIOLOGY

- Antigens bind to IgE on the surface of mast cells, resulting in mast cell degranulation.
- Some of the products released are potent eosinophil chemotactants.
- Eosinophils contain granules with substances that directly damage the surrounding tissues.
- Eosinophils also can activate mast cells directly, setting up a vicious cycle of degranulation and tissue destruction.

Systems Affected

- Gastrointestinal – generally affects the stomach and small intestine; however, large intestine may be affected.
- Hypereosinophilic syndrome in the cat can involve the gastrointestinal (GI) tract, liver, spleen, kidney, adrenal glands, and heart. There are also rare reports in the dog, particularly rottweilers. This disease is very severe and is often fatal as it does not always respond to therapy well.

SIGNALMENT/HISTORY

- Dog and cat. Eosinophilic gastroenteritis is reportedly more common in dogs than in cats.
- German shepherds, rottweilers, soft-coated wheaten terriers, and shar-peis may be predisposed.
- Dogs – most common in animals <5 years of age, although any age may be affected.
- Cats – median age eight years; range, 1.5–11 years reported.
- No predominant sex reported.

Historical Findings

- Intermittent, usually chronic, vomiting, small bowel diarrhea, anorexia/hyporexia, and/or weight loss are the most common findings, similar to other causes of gastroenteritis. Any combination of these signs is possible, including just one alone. For example, a patient

---

Blackwell's Five-Minute Veterinary Consult Clinical Companion: Small Animal Gastrointestinal Diseases,
First Edition. Edited by Jocelyn Mott and Jo Ann Morrison.
© 2019 John Wiley & Sons, Inc. Published 2019 by John Wiley & Sons, Inc.
Companion website: www.fiveminutevet.com/gastrointestinal

could be eating normally, not vomiting or having diarrhea but continue to lose weight. Or another patient might be vomiting but is eating normally, has normal stools, and is maintaining its weight. This latter scenario appears to be fairly common in the cat and therapy may not be needed if the owner is not bothered by the vomiting. One must always weigh the pros and cons of therapy against the severity of the signs. These cats also often respond to diet change alone.

- One report states that 50% of cats with eosinophilic gastritis/enteritis had hematochezia or melena.
- Less common than lymphocytic-plasmacytic gastroenteritis. This latter form is the most common form of chronic gastroenteritis, often referred to as inflammatory bowel disease (IBD).
- A mixed cellular infiltrate of eosinophils, lymphocytes, and plasma cells may be present on occasion.

 # CLINICAL FEATURES

- Cats – thickened bowel loops may be palpated, often more so in caudal abdomen.
- Evidence of weight loss is often present and can occasionally be the only sign seen.
- If hypereosinophilic syndrome is the cause of the GI disease, enlarged peripheral lymph nodes, mesenteric lymphadenopathy, hepatomegaly, and splenomegaly may also be noted.

 # DIFFERENTIAL DIAGNOSIS

- Idiopathic eosinophilic gastroenteritis.
- Parasitic.
- Immune mediated – food allergy; adverse drug reaction; associated with other forms of inflammatory bowel disease.
- Systemic mastocytosis.
- Hypereosinophilic syndrome.
- Eosinophilic leukemia.
- Eosinophilic granuloma.

All the causes listed above are included in the differential diagnosis of eosinophilic infiltrates in the stomach and small intestine. Idiopathic eosinophilic gastroenteritis is a diagnosis of exclusion.

 # DIAGNOSTICS

Complete Blood Count/Biochemistry/Urinalysis

- Hemogram may reveal a peripheral eosinophilia – more common in cats than dogs, especially common and pronounced in hypereosinophilic syndrome.
- Panhypoproteinemia or hypoalbuminemia may be present if a protein-losing enteropathy is also present. Keep in mind that low normal albumin levels are common in cases of IBD and should be looked at critically. Most dogs/cats do not have low normal levels of albumin when they are clinically healthy. Dogs tend to have midrange albumins and cats have upper end of normal albumin levels when healthy.
- Liver enzyme elevations and/or azotemia may be seen with hypereosinophilic syndrome due to the infiltration of eosinophils into these respective organs.
- Urinalysis is usually normal.

Other Laboratory Tests

- Serum cobalamin levels may be low, suggesting ileal disease; folate levels may be increased, suggesting small intestinal bacterial overgrowth.
- Buffy coat smear can be used to help rule out systemic mastocytosis, when suspected. This test is rarely necessary.
- Multiple fecal flotations and direct smears are imperative to rule in or rule out intestinal parasitism. Fecal polymerase chain reaction (PCR) testing could also be useful. Routine deworming with a broad-spectrum product such as fenbendazole is commonly indicated, even when all fecal examinations are negative.

Imaging

- Plain abdominal radiographs provide little information but are useful to rule out other diseases that may present with similar clinical signs.
- Barium contrast radiography may demonstrate thick intestinal walls and mucosal irregularities but does not provide any information about etiology or the nature of the thickening. This is rarely needed as ultrasound, when available, offers more conclusive information on bowel wall thickness.
- Ultrasonography – used to measure stomach and intestinal wall thickness and to rule out other diseases; used to examine the liver, spleen, and mesenteric lymph nodes in animals with hypereosinophilic syndrome. When the latter is seen, aspirates of these organs are often indicated. Ultrasound can also be unremarkable and does not necessarily rule out disease.

Diagnostic Procedures

- Definitive diagnosis often requires histopathology of biopsy samples obtained via endoscopy or laparotomy.
- Bone marrow aspirates are recommended if systemic mastocytosis or significant peripheral eosinophilia is apparent. This is especially true if hypereosinophilic syndrome is suspected.
- Exploratory laparotomy may be indicated if distal small intestine is involved or abdominal organomegaly is present.
- Intestinal biopsy differentiates the other causes of IBD from eosinophilic gastroenteritis.
- Dietary trials can be used to rule in or rule out food allergy or hypersensitivity but diet alone may not always be enough to improve the clinical status of the patient. The addition of immune suppression may be needed in the short term to gain control over the clinical signs. Then diet can be used to keep the disease in check long term. Some dermatologists believe that food allergies are not always lifelong but rather can resolve with time.

Pathologic Findings

- Thickened rugal folds, erosions, ulcers, and increased mucosal friability may be present in the stomach, although grossly it can appear normal.
- Ulcerations and erosions may be seen in the intestine.
- Eosinophilic infiltrates can be patchy in the intestine; multiple biopsies may be necessary to obtain a diagnosis.
- Histopathology reveals a diffuse infiltrate of eosinophils into the lamina propria; the submucosa and muscularis can also be involved (more common in cats).

 # THERAPEUTICS

The goal of therapy is to resolve the associated clinical signs with a combination of drug therapy and diet.

Drug(s) of Choice

- Glucocorticoids – prednisone 2–4 mg/kg PO q 24 h. Most dogs/cats can be treated success-fully starting at 2 mg/kg. It is rarely necessary to go to the high end of the dose range. At this point, additional medications should be added. Never exceed a total dose of 50 mg/day in a dog, no matter how heavy. Prednisolone is often preferred for cats due to the inability to metabolize prednisone into prednisolone in some individuals.
- Gradually taper corticosteroids approximately 25% every 2–3 weeks until at 25% of original dose, then extend to 4–8-week intervals before discontinuing; relapses are more common in patients that are taken off corticosteroids too quickly.
- Occasionally other immunosuppressive drugs can be used to allow a reduction in corticosteroid dose and avoid some of the adverse effects of steroid therapy. These medications can also be added in refractory cases.
  - Chlorambucil – when in need of rapid immunosuppression or with refractory cases, add chlorambucil (0.1–0.2 mg/kg q 24 h for seven days then q 48 h). Often used in place of azathioprine but can be used in addition. A recent study suggests that this addition may be superior to adding azathioprine. Avoid the simultaneous implementa-tion of three different immunosuppressive drugs at one time.
  - Azathioprine – azathioprine (2.2 mg/kg PO q 24 h, tapering to q 48 h after 2–3 weeks) can be added if an immune-mediated mechanism is suspected and response to dietary management and glucocorticoid administration is inadequate. Expect response to occur in 2–3 weeks.
  - Budesonide – an orally administered glucocorticoid with a high first-pass effect; has been used successfully in some cases to treat cats and dogs with IBD; it appears to have more of a topical effect on the intestinal tract. Reports have shown that some absorp-tion and secondary effects on the adrenal pituitary axis still occur and one study showed no difference in the reported side effects when compared to prednisone. The literature also shows some difference in outcome when this drug has been studied. Current dose recommendations are:
    - 3–7 kg: 1 mg PO q 24 h
    - 7.1–15 kg: 2 mg PO q 24 h
    - 15.1–30 kg: 3 mg PO q 24 h
    - >30 kg: 5 mg PO q 24 h.
    Dosing often requires compounding for smaller dogs and cats. The dose is then gradually tapered over the course of 8–10 weeks. One study would suggest that pure powder-based forms are superior to the controlled-release formulation which is more commonly used in humans.

Precautions/Interactions

- Prednisone and budesonide (less commonly) can cause GI ulceration. Once evidence has been seen, the addition of gastric protectants is indicated. Use of gastric protectants has not been shown to prevent damage but is effective as a treatment.
- Azathioprine and chlorambucil can cause bone marrow suppression in dogs; avoid the use of azathioprine in cats due to its myelosuppressive effects. All patients receiving azathio-prine or chlorambucil should have a complete blood count 10–14 days after the start of treatment, with rechecks monthly and then bimonthly thereafter for the entire treatment period; bone marrow suppression can be seen at any time during treatment but is usually cumulative. It is generally reversible with drug discontinuation if caught early. A chemistry panel should also be regularly evaluated.

Appropriate Health Care

- Most treated on an outpatient basis.
- Patients with systemic mastocytosis, protein-losing enteropathies, or other concurrent illnesses may require hospitalization until they are stabilized.

Nursing Care

- If the patient is dehydrated or must be NPO because of vomiting, any balanced crystalloid solution such as lactated Ringer's solution is adequate; otherwise, select fluids on the basis of secondary diseases.
- If severe hypoalbuminemia from protein-losing enteropathy, consider colloids such as hetastarch. Small dogs under 15 pounds (7 kg) may benefit from a plasma transfusion resulting in transient increase in albumin. This may lead to improved stability during anesthesia, allowing for further diagnostics and biopsies.

Diet

- Dietary manipulation is usually a critical component of therapy and may take several forms.
- Highly digestible diets with limited macronutrient sources (elimination or hydrolyzed diets) – are extremely useful for eliciting remission; can be used as maintenance diets once the patient is stabilized. Most cases are managed successfully long term in this way.
- Dogs – examples include Hill's Prescription Diet d/d and Hill's z/d; Purina HA; Royal Canin Hypoallergenic diets; Royal Canin Ultamino; balanced home-made diets (recommend consultation with a veterinary nutritionist to ensure complete nutrition).
- Cats – examples include Hill's Prescription Diet z/d and d/d; Purina HA; Royal Canin Hypoallergenic diets.
- Monomeric diets (e.g., elemental diet) – have nonallergenic components; can be used in patients that are not vomiting but have moderate-to-severe GI inflammation; useful if a food allergy is suspected. However, treatment with monomeric diets is rarely necessary.
- In patients with severe intestinal involvement and significant protein-losing enteropathy, total parenteral nutrition may be indicated until remission is obtained. Total parenteral nutrition is almost never necessary.
- Once the patient is stabilized, an elimination diet trial may be instituted if food allergy or intolerance is the suspected cause to determine the offending nutrient. This is generally not done as prescription diets are readily available.

Activity

No need to restrict unless severely debilitated.

 COMMENTS

Client Education

Explain the waxing and waning nature of the disease, the necessity for lifelong vigilance regarding inciting factors, and the potential need for long-term therapy.

Patient Monitoring

- Initially frequent for severely affected patients; monitoring peripheral eosinophil counts may be helpful; the corticosteroid dosage is usually adjusted during these visits.
- Patients with less severe disease may be checked 2–5 weeks after the initial evaluation; monthly to bimonthly thereafter until corticosteroid therapy is completed.

- Patients receiving azathioprine or chlorambucil – monitor as mentioned above.
- Patients usually do not require long-term follow-up unless the problem recurs.

Prevention/Avoidance

If a food intolerance or allergy is suspected or documented, avoid that particular nutrient and adhere strictly to dietary restrictions.

Possible Complications

- Weight loss, debilitation in refractory cases.
- Adverse effects of corticosteroid therapy.
- Bone marrow suppression, pancreatitis, hepatitis, or anorexia caused by azathioprine and/or chlorambucil.

Expected Course and Prognosis

- The vast majority of dogs with eosinophilic gastroenteritis respond to a combination of dietary manipulation and steroid therapy.
- Cats often have a more severe form of the disease, with a poorer prognosis than dogs.
- Cats often require higher doses of corticosteroids for longer periods of time to elicit remission.

Abbreviations

- GI = gastrointestinal
- IBD = inflammatory bowel disease
- PCR = polymerase chain reaction

See Also

- Diarrhea, Chronic
- Gastroenteritis, Lymphocytic-Plasmacytic
- Hematemesis
- Inflammatory Bowel Disease
- Melena
- Nutritional Approach to Chronic Enteropathies
- Vomiting, Chronic

Suggested Reading

Dandrieux JR, Noble PJ, Scale TJ, et al. Comparison of a chlorambucil-prednisolone combination with an azathioprine-prednisolone combination for treatment of chronic enteropathy with concurrent protein-losing enteropathy in dogs: 27 cases (2007–2010). J Am Vet Med Assoc 2013;242(12):1705–1714.

Dye TL, Diehl KJ, Wheeler SL, Westfall DS. Randomized, controlled trial of budesonide and prednisone for the treatment of idiopathic inflammatory bowel disease in dogs. J Vet Intern Med. 2013;27(6):1385–1391.

Hall EJ, German AJ. Diseases that affect more than one organ of the gastrointestinal tract: Inflammatory bowel disease In: Steiner JM, ed. Small Animal Gastroenterology. Hannover: Schlutersche, 2008, pp. 311–327.

Rychlik A, Kołodziejska-Sawerska A, Nowicki M, Szweda M. Clinical, endoscopic and histopathological evaluation of the efficacy of budesonide in the treatment of inflammatory bowel disease in dogs. Pol J Vet Sci 2016;19(1):159–164.

Sattasathuchana P. Steiner J. Canine eosinophilic gastrointestinal disorders. Anim Health Res Rev 2014;15(1):76–86.

Simpson KW. Diseases of the stomach. In: Ettinger SJ, Feldman EC, eds. Textbook of Veterinary Internal Medicine, 7th ed. St Louis: Elsevier, 2010, pp. 1515–1521.

Tumulty J, Broussard J, Steiner JM, Peterson ME, Williams DA. Clinical effects of short-term oral budesonide on the hypothalamic-pituitary-adrenal axis in dogs with inflammatory bowel disease. J Am Anim Hosp Assoc 2004;40:120–123.

Author: Michelle Pressel DVM, MS, DACVIM

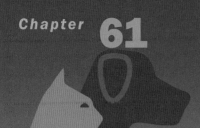

Chapter 61

Gastroenteritis, Hemorrhagic

DEFINITION/OVERVIEW

- In dogs, hemorrhagic gastroenteritis is characterized by peracute severe hemorrhagic diarrhea. The diarrhea is frequently explosive and is typically associated with a dramatic loss of water and electrolytes into the intestinal lumen.
- The shift of water and electrolytes results in marked hypovolemia, hemoconcentration, and hypovolemic shock.
- Initially, there is often associated vomiting which may progress to hematemesis; however, the source of the blood is not usually from the stomach lining. Histologically, damage to the gastric mucosa is not usually evident, and mucosal damage is typically confined to the small and large intestines.
- It is suspected that when hematemesis occurs, the source of blood is secondary to duodenal erosion. Thus, a more appropriate name for the disorder may be acute hemorrhagic diarrhea syndrome (AHDS).

ETIOLOGY/PATHOPHYSIOLOGY

- Hemorrhagic diarrhea can be a feature of a number of disorders in the dog; however, AHDS has specific clinical features which are unique and distinguish it from other conditions.
- The definitive etiology of this disease remains unknown but allergic reaction, hereditary factors, autoimmune disease, and infectious agents have been proposed as potential contributors.
- The most significant clinical features of AHDS develop as a result of acute mucosal hemorrhagic necrosis and severe neutrophilic inflammation of both small and large intestines, resulting in an increase in intestinal permeability. The loss of the normal intestinal barrier allows extravasation of water, plasma protein, and red blood cells into the lumen. Subsequently, hypovolemic shock develops quickly, followed by dehydration. Traditional concepts of bacterial translocation suggest that the loss of mucosal integrity leads to movement of bacteria and toxins out of the gastrointestinal (GI) tract into the circulation, increasing the potential for septicemia and endotoxemia.
- The organism *Clostridium perfringens* has been linked to AHDS, but it is unclear whether the association represents cause or effect. The dysbiosis associated with GI disease in general, and with diarrhea in particular, can dramatically alter the conditions within the intestinal tract, leading to promotion or inhibition of specific organism growth. While clostridial overgrowth is commonly encountered in gastrointestinal disease, a novel pore-forming enterotoxin has been identified from a specific strain of *C. perfringens* type A and may play a significant role in the etiology of AHDS.

Blackwell's Five-Minute Veterinary Consult Clinical Companion: Small Animal Gastrointestinal Diseases,
First Edition. Edited by Jocelyn Mott and Jo Ann Morrison.
© 2019 John Wiley & Sons, Inc. Published 2019 by John Wiley & Sons, Inc.
Companion website: www.fiveminutevet.com/gastrointestinal

- Because the progression of AHDS is rapid, patients are often presented with severe dehydration and tachycardia along with varying degrees of shock, vomiting, and large-volume hemorrhagic diarrhea progressing to a "raspberry jam" consistency.

Systems Affected

- Gastrointestinal – mucosal necrosis of the large and small intestines results in large-volume fluid loss into the GI tract and a subsequent hemorrhagic diarrhea. Vomiting is noted in most patients and hematemesis may develop in some dogs.
- Cardiovascular – rapid and significant fluid loss into the intestinal tract leads to the development of hypovolemic shock. Tachycardia and hypotension are found in patients as fluid loss progresses. Dehydration develops if hypovolemic shock is not treated. Cardiac dysrhythmias may be noted in the later stages of the disease.
- Hemic – in AHDS, hemoconcentration is associated with loss of intravascular fluid. However, plasma protein is not increased, because a larger proportion of plasma protein is lost into the GI tract relative to the red blood cells.
- Overall – left untreated, AHDS may progress and involve all body systems. Severe loss of circulating volume can lead to inadequate organ perfusion and oxygen delivery and development of systemic inflammation. In addition, loss of intestinal mucosal integrity may lead to sepsis and/or endotoxemia. Multiple organ dysfunction is possible without appropriate intervention.

 SIGNALMENT/HISTORY

- AHDS can affect any breed, but has a higher incidence in the small and toy breeds.
  - Although a genetic predisposition has not been confirmed, an association has been suggested between the higher incidence in small-breed dogs and the documented adverse effects of breed-related excitability and potential nervous dispositions on resultant gut motility and permeability.
  - The miniature schnauzer, dachshund, Yorkshire terrier, miniature poodle, and Maltese are more frequently affected.
- Although there is no gender predilection, young to middle-aged dogs appear to be most frequently affected (average age is five years old).
- Although the clinical findings, progression, and severity of AHDS are highly variable among patients, it is always characterized by peracute signs which rapidly progress to hypovolemic shock.
- Stress and diet change may contribute to initiation of AHDS but no clear association has been established. Most patients are previously healthy and have had no history of changes in environment.

Risk Factors

- AHDS is a common clinical condition but definitive risk factors contributing to the incidence of this disease have not been elucidated.
- Hyperactivity, excitability, and stress experienced by small-breed dogs are considered by many to be factors contributing to development of AHDS. This association is consistent with research linking body weight inversely to these variables. The subsequent stress-related alteration of intestinal motility and bacterial overgrowth may contribute to disease progression.
- Concurrent disease is unlikely.
- Findings from one study suggest that AHDS was observed more frequently during the winter season.
- There are no recognized geographic boundaries for AHDS.

Historical Findings

- Initial signs begin with an acute onset of vomiting in up to 80% of dogs, associated with anorexia, lethargy, and abdominal pain. Vomiting may progress to hematemesis, and also in this time period, diarrhea develops. At first, diarrhea may be watery but rapidly progresses to hemorrhagic (median time approximately 10 h after the onset of symptoms).
- Disease severity progresses rapidly over 8–12 h as hypovolemic shock worsens secondary to loss of fluid, blood, and protein from the circulatory system into the intestinal lumen.

 CLINICAL FEATURES

- At initial presentation, dogs are weak and lethargic with depressed mentation.
- Early in the course of the disease, pulse rate and quality, mucous membrane color, capillary refill time (CRT), and hydration status may appear normal to hyperdynamic. As shock progresses, tachycardia, weak pulses, pale mucous membranes, and prolonged CRT are observed.
- Dehydration as assessed by skin turgor may not be apparent, because the disease is peracute and time is required for fluid compartment shifts.
- Normally, abdominal palpation causes mild to moderate discomfort and reveals fluid-filled bowel loops and, less frequently, a distended or "doughy" colon.
- Rectal exam reveals fresh dark blood. Later in the course of disease, the feces appear like "raspberry jam."
- In some cases, rectal temperature is elevated; however, normal or subnormal body temperature is more frequently observed.

 DIFFERENTIAL DIAGNOSIS

- Viral – parvovirus.
- Bacterial – *Salmonella*, *Campylobacter*.
- Acute GI ulceration.
- Dietary indiscretion.
- Intestinal obstruction, intussusception or volvulus.
- Toxicity.
- Hypoadrenocorticism.
- Heat stroke.
- Pancreatitis.
- Coagulopathy.
- Other causes of hypovolemic or endotoxic shock.
- The typical presentation involves large-volume hemorrhagic diarrhea in a young to middle-aged small-breed dog. Onset is rapid without prior illness; hypovolemic shock is evident, as is hemoconcentration without an associated elevation of plasma protein.

 DIAGNOSTICS

Packed Cell Volume/Total Protein (PCV/TP)

- AHDS cannot be ruled out on the basis of a normal PCV. Previously, hemoconcentration with a PCV >60% was considered a hallmark feature but in a recent study of 108 dogs with AHDS, 52% had a PCV within the reference range and only 31% had a PCV greater than 60%.

- Plasma protein is normal to decreased secondary to loss into the GI tract. If PCV is increased and the plasma protein is not similarly increased, then protein loss is a more likely cause for the plasma protein levels than severe dehydration. Determination of albumin and globulin fractions may be helpful. Albumin levels are more commonly affected by hydration status. Albumin and globulins tend to be lost at a similar rate into the GI tract.

Complete Blood Count/Biochemistry/Urinalysis

- Complete blood count shows a stress leukogram, but neutrophilia with a left shift or degenerative left shift may be present. Platelet count may be decreased, primarily due to loss in the GI tract.
- Biochemistry profile may reveal an increase in blood urea nitrogen and alanine aminotransferase secondary to organ hypoperfusion. Hypokalemia may be present, as well as mildly decreased albumin and total protein levels.
- Urinalysis is typically unremarkable.

Additional Laboratory Tests

- Frequently, lactate will be elevated with hypovolemia, and degree of elevation can be loosely correlated to severity of volume depletion. This test can be useful to evaluate serially for assessment of the efficacy of volume replacement.
- Fecal smear and microscopic examination would be negative for parasites in most cases, and show increased red blood cells and occasional white blood cells.
- Clostridial spores (observed as "safety pins") may be present.
- Negative parvovirus enzyme-linked immunosorbent assay (ELISA) antigen test, although false positives may be uncommonly noted.
- Culture, ELISA, and polymerase chain reaction (PCR) for the detection of clostridium and associated toxins are not useful for diagnosis as there is no clear association between the presence of the organism and the incidence or severity of disease.
- Coagulation profile is usually normal early in the disease but may become abnormal later if the clinical course deteriorates and disseminated intravascular coagulation (DIC) develops.

Imaging

- Abdominal radiographs and/or ultrasound show signs of ileus and fluid- and gas-filled small and large intestines.
- Imaging is also helpful to rule out other differential diagnoses (e.g., GI foreign body, obstruction, volvulus, etc.).

Diagnostic Procedures

- Cardiac dysrhythmias, such as ventricular premature contractions or ventricular tachycardia secondary to hypovolemia or toxemia, may be observed with an electrocardiogram.
- Endoscopy is not indicated in most cases.
- The stomach will typically not have lesions, but the large and small intestine will have diffuse mucosal hemorrhage, ulceration, and hyperemia.

Pathologic Findings

- The most important histological changes noted in the intestine are acute mucosal necrosis and neutrophilic infiltration. Notably, in many of the small intestine lesions, a dense layer of large rod-shaped bacteria were adhered to the necrotic mucosal surfaces.
- Grossly, the stomach will typically not have lesions, but the large and small intestine will have diffuse mucosal hemorrhage, ulceration, and hyperemia.

THERAPEUTICS

- Suspicion of AHDS requires hospitalization with rapid and aggressive replacement and maintenance of intravascular volume, and supportive care.
- Without treatment, clinical deterioration can occur quickly and may be fatal.

Drug(s) of Choice

- Parenteral antibiotics have frequently been recommended and used, but their use in an aseptic patient has been questioned. Although we recognize the intestinal barrier in AHDS dogs is compromised and translocation is probably occurring, research looking at bacteremia and septicemia in AHDS dogs indicates that the incidence is very low, if these patients are treated appropriately relative to hypovolemia. When present, bacteremia had no influence on the clinical course of disease or survival. Treatment of the aseptic AHDS patient with amoxicillin/clavulanic acid did not change survival outcome or time to recovery. It is recognized that antibiotics will disrupt protective intestinal flora and may stimulate toxin production.
- Antibiotics are clearly indicated if there is a suspicion of sepsis in the AHDS patient, and should be used as directed in the guidelines for treatment of septic patients.
- Antiemetics and prokinetics are generally not needed in these patients, but if vomiting is persistent, maropitant (1 mg/kg q 24 h) can be used to control nausea.
- Antacids are also not usually needed, but if there is an indication for their use, pantoprazole (1 mg/kg q 12 h) can be administered intravenously.

Precautions/Interactions

Septic and hypovolemic shock can develop rapidly and patients should be closely monitored for the development of this complication in a hospital setting.

Alternative Drugs

- Oral antibiotics are not typically administered in the aseptic patient, as previously discussed. Gastrointestinal protectants have not been shown to be beneficial and thus are not administered.
- Antidiarrheal drugs are contraindicated.

Appropriate Health Care

The most critical aspect of treatment for the AHDS patient is appropriate fluid therapy for volume resuscitation and replacement of losses into the GI tract. This will enable correction of hypovolemic shock and stop progression.

Nursing Care

- Treat pain as soon as possible; a mu agonist opioid is appropriate in most cases.
- In the absence of recognized comorbidities, large-volume resuscitation with a balanced isotonic crystalloid (20–30 mL/kg over 15–30 min) is indicated when hypovolemic shock is present. Assess the patient for normal endpoints (normalization of heart rate, blood pressure, mucous membrane color, capillary refill time, pulse quality, PCV, and lactate). Repeat resuscitation therapy as needed up to 80–90 mL/kg.
- Colloid therapy is generally not required for these patients, but with significant blood loss, red blood cell replacement may be needed (uncommon). Despite the loss of protein in these patients, synthetic colloid (e.g., Vetstarch®) use is controversial. There is some evidence that morbidity and mortality may be increased with these products, particularly when coagulation abnormalities or acute kidney injury are present. Historically, they have been used in

many cases without incident as a 5–10 mL/kg bolus to supplement and enhance the fluid resuscitation when normal endpoints are difficult to achieve with crystalloid therapy alone. In rare instances of severe protein loss, plasma or plasma products can be considered.

- Maintenance fluid therapy should be initiated to maintain fluid balance and circulatory function and correct electrolyte abnormalities when satisfactory endpoints are reached. Ongoing GI fluid loss should be estimated and added to the fluid requirements.

Diet

- Nothing by mouth (NPO) during the acute disease (vomiting, 12–48 h). Parenteral and enteral (via tube) feeding has not been demonstrated to improve outcome to date in the normal course of this disease, but early enteral nutrition is recognized as beneficial for most GI disease. Placement of a nasogastric tube may be helpful to manage persistent vomiting and reduce the risk of aspiration pneumonia, and would then serve as a route for nutrition when vomiting is under control.
- Small amounts of a bland, low-fat, low-fiber food are offered once vomiting is resolved and should be continued for several days.
- Increased dietary fiber is normally recommended to decrease recurrent diarrhea. There is no definitive evidence to support this supplement for AHDS.

Activity

Restricted.

Surgical Considerations

None unless GI ulceration results in bowel perforation.

 ## COMMENTS

- In general, a suspicion of AHDS is based on historical information, classic physical exam findings, and preliminary blood testing of PCV and TP.
- While the recommended diagnostic testing is valuable to rule out other differentials, rapid recognition of hypovolemic shock should trigger the initiation of appropriate fluid therapy which is the primary treatment to reverse this disorder.
- Clients should be advised of the need for hospital-based care for immediate and aggressive medical management.
- With appropriate medical care, mortality rate is low.

Client Education

- After resolution of clinical signs, home care includes restricted activity for 5–7 days, with an appropriate GI diet provided in small frequent feedings for 2–3 days, gradually transitioned to a normal diet over 2–3 days.
- Owners should contact a veterinarian if lethargy, anorexia or recurrent symptoms are observed.

Patient Monitoring

- Monitor heart rate, blood pressure, pulse quality, mucous membranes, CRT, temperature, and ongoing fluid loss every 2–4 h. Adjust fluid therapy as needed to normal endpoints.
- Monitor PCV and total solids every 2–4 h, and lactate every 2 h until normal.
- Failure to improve within 24–48 h may indicate that other causes for the hemorrhagic diarrhea are probable.

Prevention/Avoidance

- The recurrence rate of AHDS is typically 10–15%.
- Owners should be advised to try and minimize stress in the home environment as much as possible, and to follow the dietary recommendations above.

Possible Complications

- DIC may develop but is uncommon. Neurologic signs secondary to the hemoconcentration and poor brain perfusion may occur.
- Cardiac dysrhythmias may be noted secondary to poor perfusion, potential reperfusion injury, toxemia, electrolyte imbalance or elevated cytokine levels.
- Hemolytic-uremic syndrome may occur in rare cases.
- Most dogs will improve with appropriate treatment, but mortality can be high in untreated dogs. Fewer than 10% of treated dogs die, and this may be due to a proposed variant form of AHDS that is particularly severe.

Expected Course and Prognosis

- The course of the disease is usually short, 24–72 h.
- The prognosis is good with appropriate therapy, and most dogs recover without complications.
- Sudden death is uncommon.

Synonyms

- HGE

Abbreviations

- AHDS = acute hemorrhagic diarrhea syndrome
- CRT = capillary refill time
- DIC = disseminated intravascular coagulation
- ELISA = enzyme-linked immunosorbent assay
- GI = gastrointestinal
- HGE = hemorrhagic gastroenteritis
- NPO = nothing by mouth (*nil per os*)
- PCR = polymerase chain reaction
- PCV = packed cell volume
- RBC = red blood cell
- TP = total protein
- WBC = white blood cell

See Also

- Hematemesis
- Melena

Suggested Reading

Mortier F, Strohmeyer K, Hartmann K, Unterer S. Acute haemorrhagic diarrhoea syndrome in dogs: 108 cases. Vet Rec 2015;176(24):627.

Spielman BL, Garvey MS. Hemorrhagic diarrhea in dogs. J Am Anim Hosp Assoc 1993;29:341–344.

Trotman TK. Gastroenteritis. In: Silverstein DC, Hopper K, eds. Small Animal Critical Care Medicine, 2nd ed. St Louis: Elsevier, 2015, pp. 622–626.

Unterer S, Busch K, Leipig M, et al. Endoscopically visualized lesions, histological findings, and bacterial invasion in the gastrointestinal mucosa of dogs with acute hemorrhagic diarrhea syndrome. J Vet Intern Med 2014;28:52–58.

Unterer S, Lechner E, Mueller RS, et al. Prospective study of bacteraemia in acute hemorrhagic diarrhea syndrome in dogs. Vet Rec 2015;176(12):309.

Acknowledgments: The author and editors acknowledge the prior contribution of Dr David Twedt.

Author: Michael Curtis DVM, PhD, DACVA

Chapter 62

Gastroenteritis, Lymphocytic-Plasmacytic

DEFINITION/OVERVIEW

- The most common form of inflammatory bowel disease characterized by lymphocyte and plasma cell infiltration into the lamina propria of the stomach and intestine; usually accompanied by other criteria of mucosal inflammation.
- Less commonly, the infiltrates may extend into the submucosa and muscularis.

ETIOLOGY/PATHOPHYSIOLOGY

- An aberrant immune response to environmental stimuli likely resulting in loss of mucosal homeostasis; alterations in intestinal microbiota (i.e., dysbiosis) may be a trigger.
- Continued antigen exposure, coupled with dysregulated inflammation, results in disease, although the exact mechanisms and patient factors remain unknown.
- Pathogenesis is likely multifactorial.

Systems Affected

- Gastrointestinal – typically the small intestine and occasionally stomach; the colon can be independently or simultaneously affected.
- Hematologic – rarely mild thrombocytopenia may be observed although this is not well characterized.
- Cardiovascular – hypovolemia or electrolyte and acid–base imbalances may occur due to severe vomiting and/or diarrhea.
- Respiratory – hypoproteinemia may develop in cases that develop protein-losing enteropathy leading to pleural or abdominal effusion; in severe cases pleural effusion may result in tachypnea and/or respiratory compromise.
- Musculoskeletal – generalized muscle wasting/cachexia may occur during severe cases of prolonged disease.
- Renal – dehydration may result in prerenal azotemia.

SIGNALMENT/HISTORY

- Genetics – basenjis, lundehunds, and soft-coated wheaten terriers have familial forms of inflammatory bowel disease.
- Gluten-sensitive enteropathy affects Irish setters.

Blackwell's Five-Minute Veterinary Consult Clinical Companion: Small Animal Gastrointestinal Diseases,
First Edition. Edited by Jocelyn Mott and Jo Ann Morrison.
© 2019 John Wiley & Sons, Inc. Published 2019 by John Wiley & Sons, Inc.
Companion website: www.fiveminutevet.com/gastrointestinal

- Protein-losing enteropathy affects soft-coated wheaten terriers and Yorkshire terriers; concurrent protein-losing nephropathy may occur in soft-coated wheaten terriers.
- German shepherds and Chinese shar-peis are predisposed to lymphocytic-plasmacytic gastroenteritis.
- Pure-breed cats (Asian breeds) may have a higher incidence.
- Most common in middle-aged and older animals.
- Dogs as young as eight months and cats as young as five months of age have been reported.

Risk Factors

- Infectious organisms such as *Giardia*, *Salmonella*, and *Campylobacter*, and alterations in numbers of normal gastrointestinal microbiota have been implicated. Increased mucosally associated bacteria have been observed in dogs and cats with inflammatory bowel disease (IBD) compared to healthy animals.
- Dietary agents – meat proteins, food additives, artificial coloring, preservatives, milk proteins, and gluten (wheat) may contribute to the pathogenesis of chronic mucosal inflammation.
- Certain forms of IBD are more common in some breeds of dogs (see above).
- Certain major histocompatibility genes may render an individual susceptible to development of IBD.

Historical Findings

- Signs associated with lymphocytic-plasmacytic gastritis with or without enteritis can vary in type, severity, and frequency, depending on which areas of the gastrointestinal tract are affected. Disease affecting the stomach and duodenum may result in vomiting and anorexia. Disease affecting the duodenum, jejunum, and ileum may result in small intestinal diarrhea. Disease affecting the colon may result in large bowel diarrhea. Concurrent involvement of multiple areas of the gastrointestinal tract may result in a combination of these signs, e.g., mixed bowel diarrhea and/or concurrent vomiting and anorexia.
- Generally have an intermittent or cyclical, chronic course over time. Flares are characterized by spontaneous exacerbations and remissions.
- Cats – intermittent, chronic vomiting is the most common; chronic small bowel diarrhea is second.
- Dogs – chronic small bowel diarrhea is the most common; if only the stomach is involved, vomiting is the most common.
- Dogs and cats – anorexia and chronic weight loss are common; hematochezia, hematemesis, and melena are occasionally noted.

 ## CLINICAL FEATURES

- Physical examination may vary significantly depending on severity of disease. Examination may be normal in mild or early stage of disease. In severe or chronic conditions, lethargy, dehydration, and muscle wasting/cachexia may be noted.
- Diarrhea, hematochezia, or melena may be noted on rectal examination.

 ## DIFFERENTIAL DIAGNOSIS

- Other infiltrative gastrointestinal conditions (e.g., eosinophilic/granulomatous gastroenteritis).
- Mechanical gastrointestinal obstruction if severe/persistent vomiting and anorexia.

- Food hypersensitivity.
- Metabolic disorders.
- Endocrine disorders such as hypoadrenocorticism (canine), hyperthyroidism (feline).
- Neoplasia.
- Parasitic infections (e.g. *Physaloptera, Toxocara, Ancylostoma, Trichuris*).
- Infectious diseases (e.g., histoplasmosis, toxoplasmosis, giardiasis, salmonellosis, *Campylobacter* enteritis, and bacterial overgrowth).
- Pancreatic disorders – pancreatitis, exocrine pancreatic insufficiency.
- Biliary disease – biliary mucocele, cholangitis/cholangiohepatitis.
- Miscellaneous gastrointestinal diseases (e.g., lymphangiectasia, gastrointestinal motility disorders).
- In the cat, consider systemic viral infection (e.g., FeLV, FIV, FIP).

DIAGNOSTICS

Complete Blood Count/Biochemistry/Urinalysis

- Often normal.
- Mild nonregenerative anemia and mild leukocytosis with or without a mild left shift.
- Hypoproteinemia (hypoalbuminemia typically in conjunction with panhypoproteinemia) is more common in dogs than cats with IBD.

Additional Laboratory Tests

- Baseline cortisol testing if clinical signs and CBC/chemistry findings are consistent with this differential. If baseline cortisol is greater than 2 µg/dL, hypoadrenocorticism is ruled out. If less than 2 µg/dL, then adrenocorticotropic hormone (ACTH) stimulation testing is warranted.
- Alterations in serum cobalamin and folate may serve to localize enteric regions of small intestinal disease.
- Serum pancreatic specific lipase to screen for pancreatic inflammation.
- Fecal alpha-1-proteinase inhibitor to evaluate for protein-losing enteropathy.
- Trypsin-like immunoreactivity to evaluate for exocrine pancreatic insufficiency.
- Cats – T4 and FeLV/FIV/toxoplasmosis serology are recommended to screen for infectious causes for gastrointestinal signs.
- Always perform direct and indirect fecal examinations for parasites. Empirical deworming should also be considered (pyrantel pamoate for *Physaloptera*, fenbendazole for other parasitic infections).

Imaging

- Survey abdominal radiographs are usually normal.
- Barium contrast studies occasionally reveal mucosal abnormalities and thickened bowel loops but are typically not helpful in establishing a definitive diagnosis.
- Abdominal ultrasound may aid in ruling out foreign bodies/obstructive lesions or nongastrointestinal differentials such as pancreatitis, biliary disease, and masses. Ultrasound may also show if there is overt diffuse or segmental disease, which may guide the route of biopsy (endoscopy versus surgery).

Diagnostic Procedures

- Initiate a hypoallergenic dietary trial to rule out adverse food reactions; if signs resolve then additional diagnostics are not necessary.

- Definitive diagnosis requires mucosal biopsy and histopathology, usually obtained via endoscopy (Figure 62.1). Gross endoscopic abnormalities are typically present supporting the presence of microscopic disease. Endoscopic lesions vary in severity and type but may include granularity (Figure 62.2), erosions (Figure 62.3), and friability. Lacteal dilation may be seen in cases of protein-losing enteropathy (Figure 62.4).
- Exploratory laparotomy or laparoscopy may be indicated when portions of the GI tract, unapproachable by endoscopy, are involved or if abdominal organomegaly, lymphadeno-megaly, or masses are present necessitating biopsy of additional structures.
- Clinical assessment of disease severity using the canine IBD activity index (CIBDAI) is a useful tool for baseline and subsequent therapeutic monitoring.

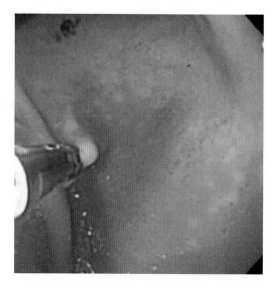

■ **Fig. 62.1.** Endoscopic gastric biopsy in a dog with lymphocytic-plasmacytic gastroenteritis.

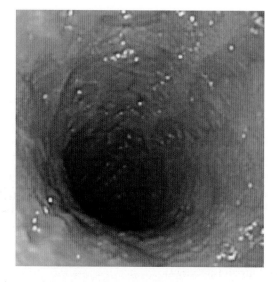

■ **Fig. 62.2.** Severe granularity in the duodenum of a dog with lymphocytic-plasmacytic gastroenteritis.

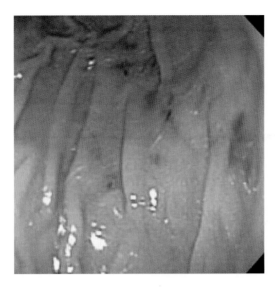

■ **Fig. 62.3.** Gastric erosions identified in a dog with lymphocytic-plasmacytic gastroenteritis.

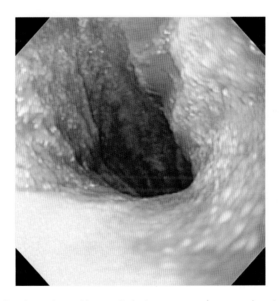

■ **Fig. 62.4.** Lacteal dilation in a dog with protein-losing enteropathy secondary to lymphocytic-plasmacytic gastroenteritis.

Pathologic Findings

- Grossly, stomach and intestinal appearance can range from normal to edematous, thickened, and ulcerated.
- The hallmark histopathologic finding is an infiltrate of lymphocytes and plasma cells in the lamina propria (Figure 62.5); architectural changes including villus atrophy, fusion, fibrosis, crypt abscessation, and lymphangiectasia may be present to varying degrees.
- The distribution may be patchy so multiple biopsy specimens are necessary to make the diagnosis.
- Lymphocytic and plasmacytic infiltrates typically are found in the areas of the gastrointestinal tract that correspond with the most severe clinical signs (e.g., stomach or proximal small

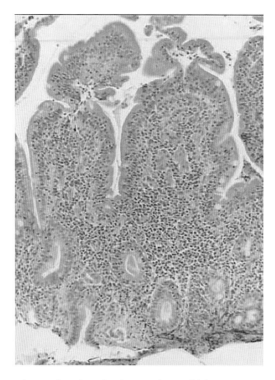

■ **Fig. 62.5.** Histopathology of severe lymphocytic-plasmacytic enteritis in a cat.

intestine in vomiting patients, duodenum/jejunum/ileum in small intestinal diarrhea, colon in large intestinal diarrhea). While biopsies of the duodenum may provide a diagnosis in small intestinal diarrhea, concurrent ileal biopsies should be considered if feasible as this may aid in diagnosis, especially in felines.

 # THERAPEUTICS

- Treatment should be aimed at resolving clinical signs. In some patients a complete resolution may not be possible. The majority of patients do have a significant improvement in clinical signs and quality of life and are able to be ultimately weaned off medications or tapered to an infrequent dosing interval.
- Treatment is typically provided on an outpatient basis unless the patient is debilitated from dehydration, hypoproteinemia, or cachexia.
- Monitor therapeutic responses using CIBDAI scores.

Drug(s) of Choice

- Corticosteroids – the mainstay of treatment for idiopathic lymphocytic-plasmacytic enteritis; prednisone or prednisolone is used most frequently (1 mg/kg PO q 12h) in dogs and cats; cats may require a higher dose to control their disease. Gradually taper the corticosteroid dose after 2–4 weeks of induction therapy when clinical signs are resolved; relapses are common if patients are tapered too quickly. Maintenance dosages q 48–72h may be necessary in some patients. Cats may respond better to prednisolone than prednisone. Budesonide, a locally active steroid, may be used in patients that cannot tolerate the systemic side effects of prednisone. Parenteral steroids may be needed in severe cases in which oral absorption may be limited.

- Azathioprine (2 mg/kg q 24–48 h PO in dogs; not recommended in cats) – an immunosuppressive drug that can be used to allow a reduction in corticosteroid dose; delayed onset of activity (up to three weeks) limits effectiveness in acute cases.
- Chlorambucil (2 mg q 48–72 h PO in cats) is an effective alternative to azathioprine.
- Metronidazole – has antibacterial and antiprotozoal properties; some evidence that it also has immune-modulating effects in rodents; the dosage for IBD in dogs and cats is 10–12 mg/kg PO q 12 h.

Alternative Drugs

- Cyclosporine – may be useful in the therapy of refractory cases of lymphocytic-plasmacytic gastroenteritis; using Atopica®, 5 mg/kg PO q 12 h, dosage is very individualized so monitoring trough levels is recommended. Monitoring of T cell function may provide a more adequate estimate of efficacy of immunosuppression provided and guide dosage adjustments if needed.
- Sulfasalazine – a sulfa analog that is broken down by luminal bacteria into sulfapyridine and mesalamine, the latter of which provides antiinflammatory effects in the colon; dosage for dogs with colonic IBD is 10–30 mg/kg PO q 8–12 h. Use cautiously in cats and at reduced dosage due to the potential for salicylate toxicity.
- Mycophenolate – 10–15 mg/kg PO q 12 h in dogs may be tried for some refractory cases.

Precautions/Interactions

- Azathioprine – causes bone marrow suppression, especially in cats; routine CBCs are recommended at two weeks, one month, and then bimonthly; bone marrow suppression is typically reversible if the drug is discontinued as soon as suppression is noted.
- Metronidazole – can cause reversible neurotoxicity at high dosages; discontinuation of the drug usually reverses the neurologic signs.
- Cyclosporine – can cause vomiting, gingival hyperplasia, and papillomatosis; associated with the development of lymphoma in humans.
- Mycophenolate – can cause diarrhea that may be dose dependent. If the primary clinical problem is diarrhea then differentiation of disease-based versus pharmacologic side effects may be difficult.
- Cyclosporine can interfere with the metabolism of phenobarbital and phenytoin.
- Ketoconazole, erythromycin, and cimetidine can decrease hepatic metabolism of cyclosporine.
- Any drugs that are potentially nephrotoxic should be used with caution in conjunction with cyclosporine.

Appropriate Health Care

Maintenance of adequate enteral nutrition and hydration is essential during treatment.

Nursing Care

- If the patient is dehydrated or must be NPO because of severe vomiting, a balanced crystalloid (e.g., lactated Ringer's solution) is adequate; additional electrolyte supplementation may be necessary if alterations are present (e.g., potassium chloride).
- Colloids (dextrans or hetastarch) should be given if severe hypoalbuminemia from protein-losing enteropathy is present.

Diet

- Dietary therapy with an elimination or hydrolyzed diet is an essential component of patient management. Trying several commercial brands/formulations of diets may be needed based on patient palatability and clinical responsiveness.

- Patients with severe intestinal involvement and protein-losing enteropathy may require total parenteral nutrition until stable.
- Highly digestible diets decrease the intestinal antigenic load, thus helping to reduce mucosal inflammation; appropriate diet therapy can contribute to clinical remission and can be used as a maintenance diet.
- Modification of the n3:n6 fatty acid ratio may also help to modulate the inflammatory response.
- Parenteral cobalamin supplementation is essential if serum levels are subnormal. Deficiencies in cobalamin can contribute to clinical signs and limit the effectiveness of dietary and medical therapy.
- Numerous commercial elimination diets that meet the above criteria are available for dogs and cats; home-cooked diets are also an excellent option but are more time-consuming for owners and should be formulated by a board-certified veterinary nutritionist to ensure complete and balanced nutritional profile.
- Use fiber supplementation in dogs and cats with colitis.

Activity

No restrictions.

Surgical Considerations

- If severe hypoproteinemia is present then surgical gastrointestinal biopsies should be avoided if possible or performed with owner understanding that the chance of dehiscence is significantly increased.
- Pleural effusion secondary to hypoproteinemia may compromise respiratory function. Colloidal therapy for 1–2 days prior to anesthesia and/or thoracocentesis may improve patient stability for anesthesia.

 COMMENTS

Client Education

- Patience is required during the various food and medication trials that are often necessary.
- IBD is more likely to be controlled rather than cured, as relapses are common.
- The majority of animals do have a significant reduction in clinical signs. Some patients may need to be maintained on low-dosage maintenance therapy (e.g., every other or every third day prednisone) to keep clinical signs in remission.

Patient Monitoring

- Severely affected patients on bone marrow-suppressive medications require frequent monitoring (see above); adjust medications during these visits based on bloodwork and clinical signs.
- Check patients with less severe disease 2–3 weeks after their initial evaluation and then monthly to bimonthly until medications are tapered and clinical signs are resolved.

Prevention/Avoidance

When a food intolerance or allergy is suspected or documented, avoid that particular item and adhere strictly to dietary restriction.

Possible Complications

- Weight loss and debilitation in refractory cases.
- Iatrogenic hyperadrenocorticism and steroid side effects.

- Bone marrow suppression, pancreatitis, hepatopathy, or anorexia can be caused by azathioprine.
- Vomiting, diarrhea, and anorexia with cyclosporine; decreasing the dosage temporarily typically will result in resolution of gastrointestinal signs.
- Diarrhea with mycophenolate; discontinuation and decrease in dosage typically will result in resolution of gastrointestinal signs.
- Keratoconjunctivitis sicca with sulfasalazine.

Expected Course and Prognosis

- Dogs and cats with mild-to-moderate inflammation have a good-to-excellent prognosis for full recovery.
- Patients with severe infiltrates, particularly if other portions of the GI tract are involved, have a more guarded prognosis.
- Other prognostic indices associated with negative long-term outcome include severe mucosal lesions on endoscopy, hypocobalaminemia, and especially hypoalbuminemia.
- Often the initial response to therapy sets the tone for a given individual's ability to recover.

Synonyms

Frequently referred to as inflammatory bowel disease. However, inflammatory bowel disease may also encompass other variations in gastrointestinal inflammatory disease.

Abbreviations

- CIBDAI = canine IBD activity index
- FeLV = feline leukemia virus
- FIP = feline infectious peritonitis
- FIV = feline immunodeficiency virus
- GI = gastrointestinal
- IBD = inflammatory bowel disease

See Also

- Gastroenteritis, Eosinophilic
- Inflammatory Bowel Disease
- Nutritional Approach to Chronic Enteropathies

Suggested Reading

Day MJ, Bilzer T, Mansell J, et al. Histopathological standards for the diagnosis of gastrointestinal inflammation in endoscopic biopsy samples from the dog and cat: a report from the World Small Animal Veterinary Association Gastrointestinal Standardization Group. J Comp Pathol 2008;138 Suppl 1:S1–43.

Hall EJ. Diseases of the large intestine. In: Ettinger SJ, Feldman EC, Cote E, eds. Textbook of Veterinary Internal Medicine, 8th ed. St Louis: Elsevier, 2017, pp. 1565–1592.

Hall EJ, Day M. Diseases of the small intestine. In: Ettinger SJ, Feldman EC, Cote E, eds. Textbook of Veterinary Internal Medicine, 8th ed. St Louis: Elsevier, 2017, pp. 1516–1564.

Jergens AE, Schreiner CA, Frank DE, et al. A scoring index for disease activity in canine inflammatory bowel disease. J Vet Intern Med 2003;17:291–297.

Jergens AE, Willard MD, Allenspach K. Maximizing the diagnostic utility of endoscopic biopsy in dogs and cats with gastrointestinal disease. Vet J 2016;214:50–60.

Author: John M. Crandell DVM, DACVIM

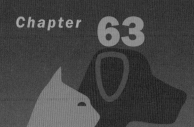

Chapter 63

Gastrointestinal Obstruction

DEFINITION/OVERVIEW

- Gastrointestinal (GI) obstructions are a common cause of presentation of companion animals to veterinary clinics.
- Causes of GI obstruction are classically divided into either functional (also known as ileus) or mechanical causes.
- Ileus is usually transient and secondary to systemic causes such as inflammatory diseases, neurologic and metabolic diseases or the use of certain drugs (opioids and anticholinergics).
- Common mechanical causes of GI obstruction (the focus of this chapter) include foreign bodies, intestinal neoplasia, gastric dilation-volvulus (GDV), and intussusceptions.

ETIOLOGY/PATHOPHYSIOLOGY

- Mechanical obstruction most commonly results from indiscriminate ingestion of foreign material, the presence of a gastrointestinal mass or intussusception.
- The accumulation of ingesta and gastrointestinal secretions orad to the obstruction causes local vascular compromise resulting in intestinal wall edema, necrosis, and possible sepsis.
- Decreased oral intake, vomiting, and sequestration of GI secretions results in acid–base and electrolyte imbalances.

Systems Affected

- Cardiovascular – hypovolemic or septic shock can result from fluid loss or gastrointestinal translocation of bacteria.
- Gastrointestinal – GI obstructions cause pathology by distension and compression of the GI tract orad to the obstruction. This results in decreased blood flow to the area with resulting edema, ulceration, and necrosis of the mucosa. In addition, direct physical damage to the GI mucosa by foreign bodies (especially linear foreign bodies) can result in ulceration and possible perforation of the intestinal wall.
- Hemic/lymphatic/immune – sepsis secondary to necrosis of the intestinal tract.

SIGNALMENT/HISTORY

Risk Factors

- GDV is more commonly reported in large-breed dogs (Great Dane, German shepherd).
- No breed predilections have been identified for gastrointestinal foreign bodies. However, foreign bodies are more commonly found in young dogs and cats (mean age of 2–4 years)

Blackwell's Five-Minute Veterinary Consult Clinical Companion: Small Animal Gastrointestinal Diseases, First Edition. Edited by Jocelyn Mott and Jo Ann Morrison.
© 2019 John Wiley & Sons, Inc. Published 2019 by John Wiley & Sons, Inc.
Companion website: www.fiveminutevet.com/gastrointestinal

due to their indiscriminate oral behavior. Linear foreign bodies are found more commonly in cats.

- Gastrointestinal tumors are more common in older cats and dogs.

Historical Findings

- Severity of clinical signs is strongly influenced by location and completeness of obstruction.
- Patients with gastric outflow tract obstruction (GOTO) tend to have a more acute onset and severity of vomiting. Some patients can present as an acute abdomen (acute and severe abdominal pain, vomiting). Partial obstructions can have more chronic and intermittent clinical signs.
- Duration of clinical signs can be variable but is usually 2–3 days.
- Patients may have a history of eating foreign material or even of previous episodes of GI foreign bodies.

 # CLINICAL FEATURES

- Patients will commonly have a moderate to severe degree of dehydration.
- Careful oral examination is recommended as linear foreign bodies can often be tangeled around the base of the tongue.
- Abdominal palpation may elicit a painful response; sometimes patients will vomit in response to palpation.
- With various causes of GI obstruction, an abdominal mass can be palpated.
- Cranial abdominal distension and tympany are often seen with GDV.

 # DIFFERENTIAL DIAGNOSIS

- Benign pyloric outflow tract obstruction.
- Foreign body.
- Gastroenteritis (infectious, granulomatous).
- GDV.
- GI neoplasia.
- Intussusception.
- Mesenteric torsion/volvulus.
- Pancreatitis.
- Peritonitis.
- Pyloric stenosis.
- Stricture.

 # DIAGNOSTICS

Complete Blood Count/ Biochemistry/Urinalysis

- Complete blood cell count – bloodwork will often reflect systemic consequences of the obstruction. Variable degrees of neutrophilia with left shift and possible toxic changes are seen with cases of sepsis.
- Chemistry – often reveals changes secondary to dehydration (increased BUN and creatinine) as well as electrolyte and acid–base disturbances. Animals with GOTOs classically have a hypokalemic and hypochloremic metabolic acidosis.
- Urinalysis – urine specific gravity will be increased secondary to dehydration.
- Lactate – hypoperfusion can often result in hyperlactatemia (>2.5 mmol/L).

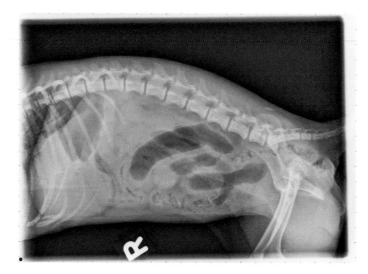

■ **Fig. 63.1.** Right lateral radiograph showing excessive gas dilation of bowel loops with foreign material in a dog with an intestinal foreign body.

Imaging

■ Survey abdominal radiographs – radiopaque foreign material can occasionally be seen in the GI lumen. The presence of soft tissue opacity in the stomach in a patient with a recent history of vomiting and anorexia is highly suspicious for a GOTO. Indirect signs of GI obstruction can include gastric or intestinal distension with fluid or gas (Figure 63.1). Linear foreign bodies characteristically cause grouping of the intestinal loops on the right of the midline with small luminal gas bubbles (apostrophe shaped). The presence of free gas in the abdomen is consistent with GI perforation and septic peritonitis.

■ Contrast abdominal radiographs – positive contrast agents (liquid barium) can be used to identify intraluminal radiolucent material in the GI tract. Retained contrast material in the stomach 4–6 h after administration is consistent with a GOTO. Use of barium contrast agents is contraindicated if GI perforation is suspected. In these instances, use of noniodinated contrast agents (e.g., iohexol) is recommended if imaging is performed.

■ Abdominal ultrasound – ultrasound can be very effective at identifying GI foreign bodies and intraluminal masses as well as assessing for integrity of the GI tract and the presence of abdominal fluid/air. Luminal foreign bodies will cause distal acoustic shadowing while linear foreign bodies often appear as hyperechoic linear objects within the intestinal lumen (Figure 63.2).

■ Advanced diagnostics – in cases where intestinal neoplasia is suspected, advanced imaging techniques such as computed tomography (CT) and GI endoscopy with biopsies, if indicated, can provide additional information such as the nature of the mass and its degree of invasion.

 ## THERAPEUTICS

■ Cases of GI obstruction are surgical emergencies.
■ Therapeutic goals should include (1) stabilization and correction of electrolyte and acid–base abnormalities, (2) surgical or endoscopic removal of the foreign body/mass or correction of volvulus, and (3) identification and excision of any nonviable tissue or gastrointestinal perforation.

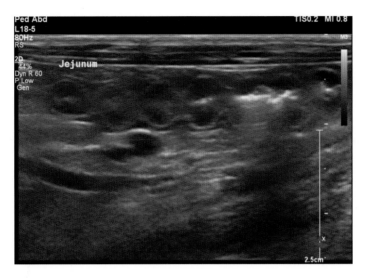

■ **Fig. 63.2.** Ultrasonographic image showing plication of the small intestines in a dog with a linear foreign body.

Drug(s) of Choice

■ Parenteral broad-spectrum intravenous antibiotic therapy (ampicillin-sulbactam 30 mg/kg IV three times daily with enrofloxacin 10 mg/kg IV once daily) should be initiated prophylactically as soon as possible in patients with suspected GI obstruction.
■ In cases where GI ulceration is suspected or confirmed, use of a proton pump inhibitor is recommended (omeprazole or pantoprazole 1 mg/kg twice daily orally or intravenously, respectively).
■ Appropriate analgesia should be provided before, during, and after surgery. Mu-agonist opioids (fentanyl 2–5 μg/kg/h IV as a constant rate infusion, hydromorphone 0.1 mg/kg IV q 4–6 h) are recommended given their strong analgesic effect.

Precautions/Interactions

■ Use of antiemetic medications is contraindicated in patients with suspected GI obstructions.
■ Nonsteroidal antiinflammatory drugs should not be used in patients with GI obstructions due to their adverse effects on the GI mucosa and renal function in patients that are not hemodynamically stable.

Appropriate Health Care

■ Prior to definitive treatment of the obstruction, stabilization of the patient and correction of dehydration as well as electrolyte and acid–base abnormalities are imperative.
■ Dogs with GDV should have gastric decompression first using orogastric intubation or percutaneous gastrocentesis in order to relieve gastric pressure.

Nursing Care

■ Aggressive intravenous administration of isotonic crystalloids is recommended to correct dehydration and hypovolemia, if present. Recommendation is to administer ¼ shock bolus of 20 mL/kg (dogs) or 10 mL/kg (cat) over 15 min and reevaluate the patient's status (heart rate, blood pressure, blood lactate). Repeat 1–2 times if vital parameters fail to normalize. If crystalloid therapy is not successful in stabilizing patient, colloid solutions such as Voluven®

or hetastarch can be administered at 5 mL/kg (dogs) and 2.5 mL/kg (cats) to a maximum of 20 mL/kg (dogs) and 10 mL/kg (cats).

- Colloids should be used with caution, especially in cases where sepsis is suspected, due to their association with acute kidney injury.

Diet

- Food should be withheld from patients as long as vomiting is not controlled. Feeding of small portions of a bland diet can be initiated once emesis has subsided.
- If necessary, use of tube feeding or parenteral feeding should be considered following relief of the obstruction.

Activity

Activity should be restricted for the first 10–14 days after surgery.

Surgical Considerations

- Surgical exploration of the abdomen allows for removal of the foreign body as well as resection of any nonviable tissue. If the obstruction is neoplastic, infectious or inflammatory in nature, surgical intervention can be therapeutic as well as diagnostic as long as excised tissue is submitted for histopathology and culture.
- When GI obstruction is caused by a gastric foreign body, endoscopic removal can be attempted. If unsuccessful, foreign material can be removed from the stomach by gastrotomy.
- GOTOs – GDV should be corrected and future volvulus prevented with a gastropexy.
- Intestinal obstruction – the full length of the intestinal tract should be examined and palpated. Enterotomy should be performed to remove any luminal foreign material. If nonviable or perforated sections are present, resection and anastomosis should be performed.
- Although intussusceptions can be percutaneously reduced, recurrence is very common. Surgical reduction and/or resection with or without enteropexy is recommended (Figure 63.3).

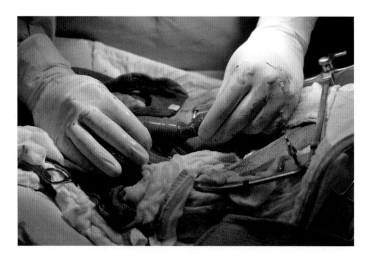

■ **Fig. 63.3.** Intraoperative picture of an intussusception in a dog.

COMMENTS

Client Education

Animals with a history of GI foreign bodies have a tendency to repeat this behavior. Owners should be counseled on ways to minimize ingestion of these objects.

Patient Monitoring

- Dehiscence of gastrotomy and enterotomy sites can occur 3–5 days postoperatively. Patients should be watched closely during this period for signs of lethargy, recurrence of vomiting, and fever.
- Ventricular arrhythmias are documented in approximately 40% of GDV patients. In these cases, electrolyte and acid–base disturbances should be identified and treated, if present. Antiarrhythmic therapy (lidocaine 2 mg/kg IV bolus to effect followed by a constant rate infusion at 50–75 µg/kg/min thereafter) has traditionally been recommended only in:
  - cases with clinical signs (syncope, weakness) or
  - cases fulfilling certain cardiac criteria (heart rate over 160 beats per minute, R on T phenomenon, multiform ventricular premature contractions (VPCs), torsades de pointes).
- However, some evidence suggests that preemptive treatment of all GDV patients with lidocaine is associated with a better outcome.

Possible Complications

- Aspiration pneumonia.
- Septic peritonitis.
- Functional ileus.

Expected Course and Prognosis

- With rapid surgical intervention of uncomplicated cases of GI foreign bodies, the prognosis is good (>95%). However, the prognosis associated with septic peritonitis is significantly lower (50%). Negative prognostic factors that have been identified include a longer duration of clinical signs, presence of a linear foreign body, and multiple surgical procedures.
- With intestinal neoplasia, the prognosis remains guarded to poor with the exception of small cell lymphoma in cats. With gastric carcinoma, complete surgical excision is rarely attainable and intestinal carcinoma has a high rate of metastasis at the time of diagnosis. Large cell GI lymphoma has a relatively poor response rate to commonly used chemotherapy protocols and median survival times in cats and dogs are 4–6 months and 110 days, respectively.

Abbreviations

- CT = computed tomography
- GDV = gastric dilation-volvulus
- GI = gastrointestinal disease
- GOTO = gastric outflow tract obstruction
- VPC = ventricular premature beats

See Also

- Acute Abdomen
- Esophageal Foreign Bodies
- Esophageal Neoplasia
- Esophageal Stricture.
- Gastric Dilation-Volvulus
- Gastric Neoplasia, Benign
- Gastric Neoplasia, Malignant
- Gastrointestinal Lymphoma, Canine
- Gastrointestinal Lymphoma, Feline
- Hiatal Hernia
- Hypertrophic Pyloric Gastropathy, Chronic
- Intestinal Neoplasia, Benign

- Intestinal Neoplasia, Malignant
- Intussusception
- Megaesophagus

- Regurgitation
- Vomiting, Acute

Suggested Reading

Boag AK, Coe RJ, Martinez T, Hughes D. Acid-base and electrolyte abnormalities in dogs with gastrointestinal foreign bodies. J Vet Intern Med 2005;19:816–821.

Fossum TW. Small Animal Surgery, 3rd ed. St Louis: Mosby, 2007.

Hayes G. Gastrointestinal foreign bodies in dogs and cats: a retrospective study of 208 cases. J Small Anim Pract 2009;50:576–583.

Hobday MM, Pachtinger GE, Drobatz KJ, Syring RS. Linea versus non-linear gastrointestinal foreign bodies in 499 dogs: clinical presentation, management and short-term outcome. J Small Anim Pract 2014;55:560–565.

Authors: Jean-Sébastien Palerme DVM, MSc, DACVIM, Albert E. Jergens DVM, PhD, DACVIM

Chapter 64

Gastrointestinal Lymphoma, Canine

DEFINITION/OVERVIEW

- Clonal proliferation of B, T, or non-B-/non-T type (null cell) lymphoblasts found primarily in enlarged peripheral lymph nodes (LN).
- Cells can spread systemically to invade bone marrow, peripheral blood, central nervous system (CNS), and visceral organs.

ETIOLOGY/PATHOPHYSIOLOGY

- ~85% of cases are multicentric (involving more than one lymph node).
- ~75% are B cell in origin and ~25% are T cell in origin.
- T cell lymphoma (LSA) is usually associated with hypercalcemia. Multicentric T cell LSA includes aggressive (peripheral T cell lymphoma not otherwise specified (PTCL-NOS) and indolent (T-zone lymphoma (TZL), follicular LSA (FL)) subtypes.
- Multicentric B cell lymphoma is an aggressive disease.
- Aggressive lymphomas respond to treatment quickly, but have a shorter overall survival.
- 20–107 LSA cases per 100 000 dogs.
- LSA comprises up to 24% of all canine neoplasms and 83% of all canine hematopoietic malignancies.

Systems Affected

- Lymphatic (~85%) – generalized peripheral lymphadenopathy with or without splenic, hepatic, peripheral blood, and/or bone marrow involvement.
- Gastrointestinal (~5–7%) – focal or diffuse infiltration of intestines, and associated lymph nodes.
- Mediastinal (~5%) – proliferation of neoplastic lymphocytes in mediastinal lymph nodes, thymus, or both.
- Skin – divided into cutaneous nonepitheliotropic B and T cell LSA and mycosis fungoides (epitheliotropic T cell LSA).
- Hepatosplenic gamma-delta T cell LSA (rare) – liver/spleen sinusoidal infiltration of T cells with eventual bone marrow infiltration.
- Intravascular LSA (rare) – typically T or null cell proliferation in lumen or wall of blood vessel.

Blackwell's Five-Minute Veterinary Consult Clinical Companion: Small Animal Gastrointestinal Diseases, First Edition. Edited by Jocelyn Mott and Jo Ann Morrison.
© 2019 John Wiley & Sons, Inc. Published 2019 by John Wiley & Sons, Inc.
Companion website: www.fiveminutevet.com/gastrointestinal

Comparative Cytogenetics and Gene Expression Profiling

- Some chromosome copy number aberrations are shared between human and canine lymphomas.
- Gene expression profiling can be used to separate distinct subtypes of human and canine lymphoma.
- Canine diffuse large B cell lymphoma and marginal zone lymphoma may be a continuum of the same disease.

 # SIGNALMENT/HISTORY

- Boxer, basset hound, golden retriever, St Bernard, Scottish terrier, Airedale terrier, and bulldog – reported high-risk breeds.
- Dachshund and Pomeranian – reported low-risk breeds.
- Breed determines relative risk for B cell or T cell disease: ~85% of boxer LSAs are T cell in origin, while golden retrievers develop both B and T cell LSA in a ~50:50 ratio.
- Historically, 6–9 years of age.

Risk Factors

Suggested causes include heritable breed risks, chromosomal aberrations, increased telomerase activity, germline and somatic genetic mutations, epigenetic changes, retroviral infection, Epstein–Barr virus infection, and environmental factors.

Historical Findings

- Multicentric – from no clinical signs to anorexia, lethargy, vomiting, diarrhea, weight loss, fever, polydipsia, and polyuria secondary to hypercalcemia.
- Gastrointestinal (GI) – vomiting, diarrhea, anorexia, weight loss, malabsorption.
- Mediastinal – respiratory distress, pleural effusion, coughing, difficulty swallowing, caval syndrome.
- Skin.
  - Cutaneous LSA – lesions usually generalized or multifocal: nodules, plaques, ulcers, focal alopecia, and hypopigmentation.
  - Mycosis fungoides – initial scaling, alopecia, pruritus progressing to thickened, ulcerated, exudative lesions. Later stages include proliferative plaques and nodules with progressive ulceration. Oral mucosa many times involved.
- Extranodal – varies with the anatomic site: ocular: photophobia and conjunctivitis; central nervous system: neurologic deficits, paresis, paralysis, seizures; hepatosplenic: lethargy, inappetence, weakness, icterus.

 # CLINICAL FEATURES

- Multicentric – generalized, painless, enlarged peripheral lymph node(s) with or without hepatosplenomegaly.
- Gastrointestinal – unremarkable to palpable thickened gut loops and/or abdominal mass, rectal mucosal irregularities, ascites.
- Mediastinal – dyspnea; tachypnea; muffled heart sounds secondary to pleural effusion, pitting edema of head, neck, forelimbs.
- Skin – raised plaques that may coalesce, patch lesions, and erythematous, exudative lesions.
- Extranodal – ocular: anterior uveitis, retinal hemorrhages, and hyphema; CNS: dementia, seizures, and paralysis.

DIFFERENTIAL DIAGNOSIS

- Multicentric – disseminated infections, metastatic disease, immune-mediated disorders, other hematopoietic tumors.
- Gastrointestinal – other GI tumors, foreign body, enteritis, GI ulceration, systemic mycosis.
- Mediastinal – other tumors (thymoma, chemodectoma, ectopic thyroid), infectious disease.
- Skin – infectious dermatitis, pyoderma, immune-mediated dermatitis, histiocytic or mast cell disease.
- Extranodal – depends on affected site.

DIAGNOSTICS

Complete Blood Count/Biochemistry/Urinalysis

- Anemia of chronic disease, thrombocytopenia, lymphocytosis, lymphopenia, neutrophilia, monocytosis, circulating blasts, hypoproteinemia (with gastrointestinal involvement).
- Hypercalcemia, increased liver enzymes with hepatic involvement, increased blood urea nitrogen (BUN) or creatinine with renal involvement.
- Urinalysis usually normal.

Other Laboratory Tests

- Immunohistochemistry (LN biopsy/resection) – to determine immunophenotype.
- Flow cytometry or polymerase chain reaction (PCR) for antigen receptor rearrangements (PARR) (LN or affected organ fine needle aspirates) – to determine immunophenotype.

Imaging

- Thoracic radiography – sternal or tracheobronchial lymphadenopathy, widened mediastinum, pulmonary densities, and pleural effusion.
- Abdominal ultrasonography – abdominal lymphadenopathy, hepatosplenic involvement, thickened bowel loops, other visceral organ involvement, ascites.

Other Diagnostic Tests

- Fine needle aspirate cytology of enlarged lymph nodes or other affected organs for cytopathologic confirmation.
- Lymph node biopsy or resection for accurate histopathologic classification.
- Bone marrow cytology for accurate prognosis.
- Cerebral spinal fluid analysis if patient has neurologic signs.
- Electrocardiogram to identify arrhythmias before doxorubicin administration.

Pathologic Findings

- Multicentric – effacement of LN parenchyma with large, neoplastic CD3+ T cells (PTCL-NOS) or small, CD3+ cell proliferation between fading follicles (TZL). Effacement of LN parenchyma with large, neoplastic CD79a+B cells (high-grade diffuse, large B cell lymphoma (DLBCL)) or perifollicular proliferation of CD79a+ cells (marginal zone lymphoma (MZL)) or CD79a+ cell proliferation that maintains follicle architecture (FL).
- Gastrointestinal – infiltration of neoplastic lymphocytes throughout mucosa and submucosa, with occasional transmural infiltration.

- Skin – CD79a+B cells infiltrating mucosa and submucosa, but sparing the epidermis (non-epitheliotropic) LSA or CD3+ T cells invading the epidermis –Pautrier's microabcesses (mycosis fungoides).
- Hepatosplenic – sinusoidal infiltration of erythrophagocytic CD3+ T cells.

Staging

- I – one enlarged LN.
- II – regionally enlarged LNs.
- III – generalized LN involvement.
- IV – visceral organ involvement.
- V – blood or bone marrow involvement.
- Substage a – not sick.
- Substage b – sick.

 THERAPEUTICS

- High-grade LSAs are exquisitely sensitive to both chemotherapy and radiation.
- Systemic multiagent chemotherapy is the therapy of choice.
- Radiation therapy for refractory lymphadenopathy, large mediastinal masses, and solitary cutaneous areas.
- Surgery – rarely used unless an acutely obstructive gastrointestinal mass is identified or to remove a refractory lymphadenopathy.
- Autologous and allogeneic bone marrow transplantation can be considered.

Drug(s) of Choice

- Always consult a veterinary oncologist to discuss various treatment options, precautions, chemotherapy dosing schedules, and potential side effects.
- Consider combination chemotherapy protocols to treat intermediate and high-grade diseases and single-agent protocols to treat indolent diseases.
- Most multiagent protocols have superior remission and survival times when compared to single-agent protocols.
- Corticosteroids alone can induce significant multidrug resistance.

Intermediate and High-Grade Lymphomas

- L-CHOP – L-asparaginase 10000 IU/m², vincristine (Oncovin) 0.7 mg/m² IV, cyclophosphamide (Cytoxan) 250 mg/m² IV or PO, doxorubicin (Adriamycin) 30 mg/m² IV, prednisone 30, 20, 10 mg/m² PO q 24 h tapering for three weeks. Consult a veterinary oncologist concerning the treatment schedule.
- COP – vincristine 0.7 mg/m² IV, cyclophosphamide (Cytoxan) 250 mg/m² IV or PO, prednisone 30, 20, 10 mg/m² PO q 24 h tapering for three weeks. Each drug given weekly.

Single Agent

- Any drug of L-CHOP can be used as a single agent, but expect shorter overall survival than multiagent.
- Doxorubicin (Adriamycin) 30 mg/m² IV every three weeks (1 mg/kg for dog <15 kg) 5–6 treatments.
- CCNU (lomustine) 70 mg/m² PO every three weeks, prednisone 2 mg/kg PO daily.

Low-Grade Lymphomas

- Chlorambucil (Leukeran) 6 mg/m² PO daily for 7–14 days, prednisone 2 mg/kg PO daily. Consider reducing chlorambucil dose to 3 mg/m² for maintenance.
- CCNU (lomustine) as above.

Precautions/Interactions

- Doxorubicin – use dexrazoxane (Zinecard) in conjunction with doxorubicin or substitute epirubicin for dogs with cardiac issues.
- Always use a freshly placed catheter when administering intravenous doxorubicin.
- L-asparaginase and doxorubicin – pretreat with diphenhydramine (1–2 mg/kg SQ) 15 min before administration.
- Most chemotherapy drugs have overlapping gastrointestinal and bone marrow toxicities. Consider antidiarrheal drugs (metronidazole, loperamide) and antiemetics (metoclopramide, maropitant, ondansetron) to abrogate these effects.

Alternative (Rescue) Protocols

- Many published rescue protocols have been reported; therefore always consult with a medical oncologist.
- MOPP – methchlorethamine (Mustargen), vincristine, procarbazine, and prednisone.
- DMAC – dexamethasone, melphalan, actinomycin-D, and cytosine arabinoside.
- CCNU ± L-asparaginase, prednisone, or DTIC (dacarabazine).
- Mitoxantrone alone or Adriamycin/DTIC.

Appropriate Health Care

Fluid therapy – for advanced disease to treat clinically ill, azotemic, and/or dehydrated patients. Also to prevent tumor lysis syndrome and/or reduce calcium levels.

Surgical Considerations

Surgery is rarely used unless an acutely obstructive GI mass is identified or to remove a refractory lymphadenopathy.

 COMMENTS

Client Education

- Canine LSA is a treatable but rarely curable disease.
- Side effects of chemotherapy drugs include reversible GI tract and bone marrow toxicities.
- The vast majority of dogs receiving chemotherapy enjoy an excellent quality of life.

Patient Monitoring

- Weekly physical examination to assess response and complete blood cell counts to gauge bone marrow toxicities.
- If neutropenia (neutrophils <1500 cells/mm³) is noted, reduce dosage (20–25%) of drug when given again.

Possible Complications

- Reversible neutropenia 4–7 days after chemotherapy.
- Temporary vomiting, diarrhea, and anorexia 2–5 days after chemotherapy.
- Alopecia in certain dog breeds (poodle, shih tzu, etc.).
- Febrile neutropenia (treated with broad-spectrum antibiotics).

Expected Course and Prognosis

- More than 80% of dogs will go into clinical remission during the first month of induction chemotherapy.
- Stage, substage, and immunophenotype are important prognostic indicators.
- Expect median survivals of ~12–14 months and ~6–9 months in dogs with high-grade multicentric B and T cell LSA, respectively, when treated with a multiagent protocol. Dogs with indolent disease can live years. Gastrointestinal, mediastinal (T cell ± hypercalcemia), and mycosis fungoides are associated with poorer response to treatment and an overall shorter survival time.

Synonyms

- Lymphosarcoma
- Malignant lymphoma

Abbreviations

- CNS = central nervous system
- DLBCL = diffuse, large B cell lymphoma
- FL = follicular LSA
- GI = gastrointestinal
- LN = lymph node
- LSA = lymphoma
- MZL = marginal zone lymphoma

- PARR = polymerase chain reaction for antigen receptor rearrangements
- PCR = polymerase chain reaction
- PTCL-NOS − peripheral T cell lymphoma not otherwise specified
- TZL = T-zone lymphoma

See Also

- Gastrointestinal Lymphoma, Feline

Suggested Reading

Bienzle D, Vernau W. The diagnostic assessment of canine lymphoma: implications for treatment. Clin Lab Med 2011;31(1):21–39.

Flood-Knapik KE, Durham AC, Gregor TP, et al. Clinical, histopathological, and immunohistochemical characterization of canine indolent lymphoma. Vet Comp Oncol 2013;11(4):272–286.

Garrett LD, Thamm DH, Chun R, et al. Evaluation of a 6-month chemotherapy protocol with no maintenance therapy for dogs with lymphoma. J Vet Intern Med 2002;16(6):704–709.

Rassnick KM, McEntee MC, Erb HN, et al. Comparison of 3 protocols for treatment after induction of remission in dogs with lymphoma. J Vet Intern Med 2007;21(6):1364–1373.

Acknowledgments: The author and editors acknowledge the prior contribution of Wallace B. Morrison.

Client Education Handout available online

Author: Steven E. Suter VMD, MS, PhD, DACVIM (Oncology)

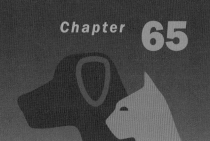

Chapter 65

Gastrointestinal Lymphoma, Feline

DEFINITION/OVERVIEW

Malignant transformation of lymphocytes (large lymphoblasts or small lymphocytes) in the gastrointestinal (GI) tract.

ETIOLOGY/PATHOPHYSIOLOGY

- Viral oncogenesis (feline leukemia virus – FeLV) is rare, although feline immunodeficiency virus (FIV) infection may predispose to alimentary B cell lymphoma.
- Chemical (tobacco smoke) exposure increases risk of developing lymphoma.
- Chronic inflammation (inflammatory bowel disease – IBD) may be associated with development of lymphoma. Up to 41% of cats with gastrointestinal lymphoma have concurrent lymphoplasmacytic enteritis (IBD), and progression of IBD to lymphoma has been reported.
- Incidence – most common gastrointestinal tumor in cats.
- Small cell lymphoma accounts for approximately 30–40% of gastrointestinal lymphoma cases.
- Large granular lymphoma (LGL) accounts for approximately 6–7% of gastrointestinal lymphoma cases.

Systems Affected

- Mainly gastrointestinal.
- Disease may also be multicentric, affecting:
  - Hemic/lymphatic/immune.
  - Hepatobiliary.
  - Renal/urologic (associated with high rate of relapse in central nervous system).
  - Respiratory.

SIGNALMENT/HISTORY

- Breed predilection: Siamese/Oriental breeds overrepresented.
- Median age and range.
  - Small cell (low-grade) lymphoma: 13 years.
  - Large/intermediate cell (high-grade) lymphoma: 10 years.
  - Large granular lymphoma (LGL): 9–10 years.

Historical Findings

- Small cell lymphoma – weight loss, vomiting and/or diarrhea, anorexia; clinical signs are usually present for a median of six months prior to presentation.

Blackwell's Five-Minute Veterinary Consult Clinical Companion: Small Animal Gastrointestinal Diseases,
First Edition. Edited by Jocelyn Mott and Jo Ann Morrison.
© 2019 John Wiley & Sons, Inc. Published 2019 by John Wiley & Sons, Inc.
Companion website: www.fiveminutevet.com/gastrointestinal

- Large cell lymphoma – as above, but progression over days to weeks; melena; hematochezia, and/or tenesmus if colon is involved. Rarely may present with signs of acute abdomen if intestinal obstruction or GI perforation and concurrent peritonitis.
- Large granular lymphoma – anorexia, weight loss, lethargy, vomiting; usually acute presentation as with large cell lymphoma.

 CLINICAL FEATURES

- Presentation and progression of clinical signs vary between large and small cell GI lymphoma, and will be separated accordingly below.
  - Small cell lymphoma – thickened intestines (50%); palpable abdominal mass is uncommon.
  - Large cell lymphoma – more likely to present with palpable abdominal mass (GI tract or mesenteric nodes); more likely to present with icterus or involvement with other organs (e.g., renal, etc.).
  - Large granular lymphoma – palpable mass in approximately 50% of cases.
  - All forms – cachexia will be noted in some patients.

 DIFFERENTIAL DIAGNOSIS

Foreign body ingestion; intestinal ulceration; inflammatory bowel disease (IBD); intussusception; other gastrointestinal tumor (adenocarcinoma, mast cell tumor); lymphangiectasia; intestinal fungal infection.

 DIAGNOSTICS

Complete Blood Count/Biochemistry/Urinalysis

- Anemia, leukocytosis (neutrophils, lymphocytes, or lymphoblasts).
- Hypoproteinemia (hypoalbuminemia), hypoglycemia, high hepatic enzyme activity (if hepatic infiltration, concurrent pancreatitis, etc.), azotemia (if renal involvement), hypercalcemia (rare), and monoclonal gammopathy (rare).

Additional Laboratory Tests

- FeLV testing – usually negative in older cats with gastrointestinal lymphoma, but may be positive in younger cats and those with multicentric lymphoma.
- FIV testing – may be associated with alimentary B cell lymphoma.
- Serum cobalamin – 78% of cats with small cell lymphoma had decreased serum cobalamin concentrations.
- ± Bone marrow aspirate depending on CBC findings (leukemia, cytopenias).

Imaging

- Thoracic radiography – may be useful if clinical suspicion of respiratory disease, but uncommon to see abnormal pulmonary parenchymal pattern, perihilar or retrosternal lymphadenomegaly, mediastinal mass, or pleural effusion associated with alimentary lymphoma.
- Abdominal ultrasonography.
  - Small cell lymphoma – diffuse small intestinal wall thickening, predominantly the muscularis and submucosa; mesenteric lymphadenopathy. Focal mural masses, abnormalities in other organs (liver, spleen) and peritoneal effusion are less common findings.
    - Despite thickening of intestines, layering may be preserved.
    - Thickened muscularis layer and lymph node enlargement are suggestive of small cell lymphoma over IBD.

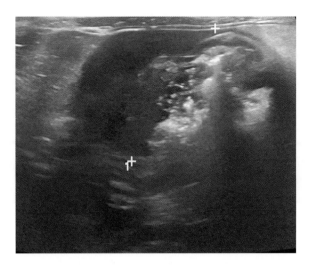

■ **Fig. 65.1.** Ultrasonographic image of a large gastric mass in a cat. The mass is diffusely hypoechoic with loss of wall layering, and extends circumferentially around the body of the stomach. Fine needle aspirate confirmed a diagnosis of large cell lymphoma. Source: Courtesy of Dr Wilfried Mai, University of Pennsylvania School of Veterinary Medicine.

- Large cell lymphoma – focal transmural mass in the stomach or intestines (Figure 65.1); mesenteric lymphadenopathy; abnormalities in the liver and/or spleen; renomegaly; peritoneal effusion.
- LGL lymphoma most commonly affects the intestine and mesenteric lymph nodes.

Other Diagnostic Procedures

- Aspiration or biopsy of a mass or lymph node.
- Aspirate often sufficient to diagnose large cell lymphoma; biopsy or molecular diagnostics often required for small cell lymphoma in order to differentiate from IBD.
- Intestinal biopsies may be collected by endoscopy or laparotomy for full-thickness biopsies.
- Immunohistochemistry can be performed on histopathology specimens for confirmation of diagnosis and to determine immunophenotype.
- PARR (polymerase chain reaction (PCR) for antigen receptor rearrangement) testing can be done on cytology slides to determine if lymphocyte population is monoclonal (consistent with lymphoma) vs polyclonal; sensitivity in cats is approximately 80%.
- Staging as described above.

Pathologic Findings

- Gross – usually white to gray in color with areas of hemorrhage and necrosis (Figure 65.2).
- Cytologic – monomorphic population of lymphoid cells (small lymphocytes or lymphoblasts), sometimes with prominent, multiple nucleoli and coarse nuclear chromatin (Figure 65.3).
    - Large granular lymphoma – characteristic magenta or azurophilic granules.
- Histopathologic – vary; several morphologic classification schemes in use.
    - B cell most common in stomach (100%) and large intestine (88%), T cell most common in small intestine (52%, most common location in the gastrointestinal tract).
    - Most B cell tumors are transmural, while most T cell variants are mucosal.
    - Epitheliotropism present in about 40% of T cell lymphomas, but rare in B cell.
    - Differentiating small cell lymphoma vs IBD on histology.
        - Lymphoid infiltration of the intestinal wall beyond the mucosa.
        - Pattern of epitheliotropism.
        - Nuclear size of lymphocytes.
        - Infiltration into mesenteric lymph nodes.

(a) (b)

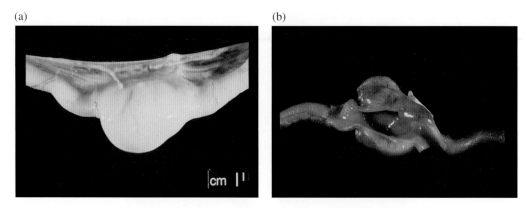

■ **Fig. 65.2.** (a) Gross specimen of a pale gray, mural intestinal mass in a cat. Histopathology confirmed a diagnosis of lymphoblastic lymphoma. (b) Gross specimen of an intestinal mass in a cat, cut to show diffuse transmural infiltrate of lymphoblastic lymphoma. Source: Courtesy of Dr Amy Durham, University of Pennsylvania School of Veterinary Medicine.

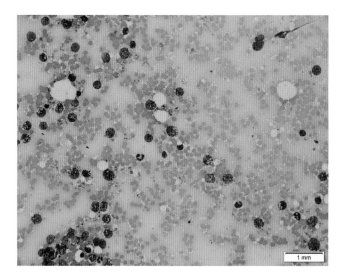

■ **Fig. 65.3.** Cytology from an intestinal mass in a cat, showing vacuolated lymphocytes with an eccentrically located round to ovoid nucleus, granular chromatin, and a medium to large lavender nucleolus. This was diagnostic for lymphoblastic lymphoma. Vacuolated lymphoma is anecdotally seen in feline intestinal, renal, and nasal lymphoma. Source: Courtesy of Dr Koranda Walsh, University of Pennsylvania School of Veterinary Medicine.

 THERAPEUTICS

- Chemotherapy is the mainstay of treatment for both small and large cell lymphoma.
- For intermediate/large cell lymphoma, there are many variations of combination protocols, all with similar efficacy.

Drug(s) of Choice

- Small cell lymphoma – oral chlorambucil, an alkylating agent, in combination with prednisolone. Chlorambucil is given either at continuous low doses (daily or every other day) or at higher pulse doses (once every two weeks; usually reserved for cats resistant to oral medications).

- Intermediate/large cell lymphoma.
    - Responds to CHOP-based protocols (cyclophosphamide, doxorubicin, vincristine, prednisone/prednisolone) such as the University of Wisconsin-Madison protocol (alternating drugs in repeated sequence) or COP-based protocols (cyclophosphamide, vincristine, prednisone/prednisolone).
    - Vinblastine has similar efficacy but less GI toxicity compared to vincristine, and can be substituted for cats who experience significant GI side effects to vincristine.
    - CCNU (lomustine) also has reported activity, primarily partial responses.
    - L-asparaginase has a lower response rate in cats compared to dogs.
- Consult a veterinary oncologist for doses, schedules, and to help assess best option(s) for treatment.
- Prednisone/prednisolone alone can result in short-lived responses.
- Cyanocobalamin can be supplemented in patients who are deficient.

Precautions/Interactions

- Avoid doxorubicin in cats with preexisting renal failure as the drug can potentially be nephrotoxic. Renal function should be monitored closely throughout therapy.
- Dose reductions of vincristine/vinblastine may be required in patients with hyperbilirubinemia.
- Myelosuppression secondary to chemotherapy – may be more severe in FeLV- or FIV-positive cats.
- Seek advice before initiating treatment if you are unfamiliar with cytotoxic drugs. Some drugs such as vincristine and doxorubicin are vesicants and can cause tissue sloughing if leaked outside the vein during administration.
- Prednisone/prednisolone side effects – risk of diabetes, worsening underlying heart disease.
- Do not use chemotherapy in pregnant animals.

Appropriate Health Care

Outpatient whenever possible, supportive care as needed.

Nursing Care

Fluid therapy, antiemetics, appetite stimulants, antidiarrheal agents, etc. when indicated.

Diet

- No change; can add n-3 fatty acids to diet (fish oil origin).
- Feeding tubes may be placed for nutritional support in patients with prolonged anorexia.

Surgical Considerations

- To relieve intestinal obstructions or perforations and remove solitary masses.
- To obtain specimens for histopathologic examination, via endoscopy/colonoscopy or exploratory laparotomy.

Radiation Therapy (RT)

Two preliminary studies have evaluated RT as a possible option for cats that have progressive disease following chemotherapy, or as additional treatment in conjunction with chemotherapy.

 COMMENTS

Client Education

- Emphasize that chemotherapy side effects are treatable and should be addressed promptly.
- Inform client that the goal is to induce remission and achieve a good quality of life for as long as possible.

- Discuss the risk of gastric or intestinal perforation in patients with intermediate/large cell transmural lymphoma, as a result of treatment or tumor progression.
- Discuss risks of chemotherapy exposure to the client, from handling oral capsules or handling eliminations (litterbox, etc.).

Patient Monitoring

- Physical examination and complete blood cell count – before each chemotherapy treatment and one week after each new drug is administered, or if there are concerns about low cell counts.
- Serum biochemistry as indicated, i.e., if any hepatic enzyme elevation or azotemia is noted at the start of treatment. Periodically monitor blood glucose in patients on long-term prednisone/prednisolone (to screen for potential development of diabetes mellitus).
- Diagnostic imaging – recheck ultrasound and/or thoracic radiographs (depending on organ involvement at diagnosis) as necessary to assess response to therapy.

Prevention/Avoidance

Avoid exposure to or breeding of FeLV-positive or FIV-positive cats.

Possible Complications

- Leukopenia/neutropenia.
- Sepsis.
- Anorexia, vomiting, weight loss; may need imaging tests to distinguish between chemotherapy side effects and lymphoma progression.
- Gastrointestinal perforation, mostly a concern for high-grade, transmural masses. May occur as a result of disease progression, or as a result of chemotherapy if there is a rapid, full-thickness die-off of lymphoma cells.

Expected Course and Prognosis

- Depends on tumor grade, initial response to chemotherapy, and tumor burden.
- Small cell lymphoma of gastrointestinal tract, with or without additional visceral involvement – greater than 90% overall response rate to chlorambucil and prednisone/prednisolone for median survival time of 1–2 years. Longer survival times (>2 years) reported for cats with complete response to therapy.
- Large cell lymphoma.
  - Overall response rate of 50–80% to CHOP/COP-based protocols, with complete response rates approximately 30–40%.
  - Median survival times reported range from two to 10 months, with durable responses rare.
  - Prednisone/prednisolone alone – median survival time 1.5–2 months.
  - Doxorubicin-based and lomustine rescue therapy reported for refractory LSA.
  - Large granular lymphoma – approximately 30% response for median survival of approximately two months.
  - Weight loss during first month of treatment of large cell lymphoma associated with shorter survival times.
  - Clinical response to chemotherapy associated with longer survival times.
  - Immunophenotype has not been shown to be associated with prognosis.
  - Surgery – one recent study of cats with discrete gastrointestinal intermediate/large cell lymphoma masses that underwent surgery prior to chemotherapy reported a median survival time of 13.9 months, longer than other reports of treatment with chemotherapy alone.

- Abdominal radiation therapy.
  - ○ Two preliminary studies showed survival times of 8–44 months in five respond-ers treated with radiation and combination CHOP-based chemotherapy, and a median survival time of approximately one year when radiation was used as a rescue therapy in cats that progressed after chemotherapy.

Synonyms

- Lymphosarcoma
- Malignant lymphoma

Abbreviations

- FeLV = feline leukemia virus
- FIV = feline immunodeficiency virus
- GI = gastrointestinal
- IBD = inflammatory bowel disease
- IHC = immunohistochemistry

- LGL = large granular lymphoma
- LSA = lymphoma
- PARR = PCR (polymerase chain reaction) for antigen receptor rearrangement
- RT = radiation therapy

See Also

- Cobalamin Deficiency
- Gastrointestinal Neoplasia, Malignant

- Inflammatory Bowel Disease

Suggested Reading

Barrs V, Beatty J. Feline alimentary lymphoma: clinical review. J Fel Med Surg 2012;14:182–201.

Gouldin ED, Mullin C, Morges M, et al. Feline discrete high-grade gastrointestinal lymphoma treated with surgical resection and adjuvant CHOP-based chemotherapy: retrospective study of 20 cases. Vet Comp Oncol 2017;15 (2):328–335.

Kiselow MA, Rassnick KM, McDonough SP, et al. Outcome of cats with low-grade lymphocytic lymphoma: 41 cases (1995-2005). J Am Vet Med Assoc 2008;232(3):405–410.

Krick EL, Little L, Patel R, et al. Description of clinical and pathological findings, treatment and outcome of feline large granular lymphocyte lymphoma (1996–2004). Vet Comp Oncol 2008; 6(2):102–110.

Rissetto K, Villamil JA, Selting KA, et al. Recent trends in feline intestinal neoplasia: an epidemiological study of 1,129 cases in the veterinary medical database from 1964–2004. J Am Anim Hosp Assoc 2011;47(1):28–36.

Acknowledgment: The author and editors acknowledge the prior contributions of Dr Kim A. Selting and Dr Erika L. Krick.

Author: Jennifer A. Mahoney DVM, DACVIM (Oncology)

Giardiasis

DEFINITION/OVERVIEW

- *Giardia* is a flagellated protozoan and obligate parasite of the gastrointestinal tract.
- In dogs and cats, *Giardia* is a parasite of the small intestine.
- Motile trophozoites adhere to and damage the intestinal mucosa.
- Cysts are shed in feces and are immediately infectious.
- Can cause small bowel diarrhea but is also frequently asymptomatic.

ETIOLOGY/PATHOPHYSIOLOGY

- Infection occurs when animal ingests cysts from feces present in food, water, fur, or elsewhere in the environment.
- Trophozoites emerge from cysts in the gastrointestinal tract and attach to intestinal epithelial cells with an adhesive disk.
- Infection results in increased rates of enterocyte apoptosis and disrupts intestinal function.
- Impaired mucosal function leads to malabsorptive maldigestive diarrhea.

Systems Affected

Gastrointestinal.

SIGNALMENT/HISTORY

- Clinical signs are often more common in young or immunocompromised hosts. Older dogs and cats are usually asymptomatic.
- Dogs –up to 50% for puppies, up to 100% in some kennels.
- Cats – up to 11%.

Risk Factors

- Ongoing problems occur more frequently in kennels, catteries, shelters, and research facilities.
- Transmitted by ingestion of cysts from feces in/on food, water, environment, or fur.
- Indirect water-borne transmission most common; cool, moist conditions favor cyst survival.
- Higher risk of infection in puppies and kittens, in high-density populations (kennels, catteries, animals shelters), and in dogs/cats with compromised immunity.

Historical Findings

- Signs can be acute, transient, intermittent, or chronic.
- Malabsorption syndrome with soft, frothy, greasy, voluminous feces (diarrhea), often with rancid odor.

Blackwell's Five-Minute Veterinary Consult Clinical Companion: Small Animal Gastrointestinal Diseases, First Edition. Edited by Jocelyn Mott and Jo Ann Morrison.
© 2019 John Wiley & Sons, Inc. Published 2019 by John Wiley & Sons, Inc.
Companion website: www.fiveminutevet.com/gastrointestinal

CLINICAL FEATURES

- Physical examination may be unremarkable.
- Occasional weight loss.

DIFFERENTIAL DIAGNOSIS

- Other infectious and noninfectious causes of small bowel diarrhea, maldigestion, and malabsorption syndromes, especially pancreatic exocrine insufficiency, inflammatory bowel disease, and other parasitic diseases.
- In cats, differentiate from infection with *Tritrichomonas foetus*, a cause of large bowel diarrhea.

DIAGNOSTICS

Complete Blood Count/Biochemistry/Urinalysis
Usually normal.

Other Laboratory Tests
- Detection of *Giardia* cysts, trophozoites, or antigen in feces.
- Cysts (~12 μm long), oval with 2–4 nuclei are shed intermittently; centrifugal flotation of fresh feces in zinc sulfate (s.g. 1.18) is the preferred method. Examination of three samples collected at 2–3-day intervals detects >70% of infections. In sugar flotations, cysts become distorted and resemble ping-pong balls with kinked-in sides. Iodine improves cyst visualization.
- Commercial antigen detection enzyme-linked immunosorbent assay (ELISA) kits are available. These kits often have very high sensitivity and should be used as a confirmatory test rather than a screening tool as many asymptomatic animals are potentially antigen positive.
- Trophozoites (15×8 μm) are more rarely detected and more likely to be found in fresh diarrhea or duodenal aspirates obtained by endoscopy. Diff-Quik or Lugol's iodine helps to highlight the teardrop-shaped cells with two nuclei. In wet mounts, trophozoites have a "falling leaf" motility.
- Flotation solutions lyze trophozoites.

THERAPEUTICS

Drug(s) of Choice
- All drug treatment is extra label. Fenbendazole and/or metronidazole are recommended.
- For dogs – oral fenbendazole (50 mg/kg q 24 h) for five days. This treatment can be combined with oral metronidazole (25 mg/kg q 12 h) for five days. Combination treatment may achieve better outcomes, but treatment efficacy can be as low as 50–60%. Treatment can be extended for an additional 10 days if signs do not resolve.
- Commercial antiparasitic preparations containing febantel may also be effective.
- For cats – metronidazole benzoate (25 mg/kg q 12 h) for five days.

Precautions/Interactions
- Metronidazole only 67% effective in dogs; bitter taste; can cause anorexia; vomiting, central nervous system signs. Note that metronidazole may induce salivation and inappetence in cats.

- Albendazole (25 mg/kg PO q 12 h for two days in dogs or five days in cats) is effective but not recommended because it can be teratogenic and/or cause anorexia, depression, vomiting, ataxia, diarrhea, abortion, or myelosuppression.

Appropriate Health Care

- The objective of therapy for giardiasis is to resolve diarrhea and associated clinical signs.
- Treat as outpatient unless debilitated or dehydrated; fluid therapy may be warranted in some cases.

COMMENTS

Client Education

- *Giardia* is a common parasite in humans. Molecular data indicate that dog and cat isolates are host-specific and there is little evidence of transmission of the parasite from cats or dogs to humans. There is likely a greater zoonotic threat for a human who is immunocompromised.
- Most human *Giardia* infections are anthroponotic (may be transferred to other animals) or originate from livestock.

Patient Monitoring

- Repeat fecal examinations to confirm efficacy of treatment and to detect reinfection.
- Chronic infection can lead to debilitation.

Prevention/Avoidance

- Drug therapy should be combined with environmental cleaning and disinfection plus bathing of the patient. It is thought that ingestion of material contained on the hair coat is adequate to cause reinfection and/or cause animals to be antigen ELISA positive.
- In asymptomatic animals, a single course of therapy is recommended. It is common for asymptomatic animals to be antigen ELISA positive, so the antigen test should not be used as a screening test.
- *Giardia* vaccines are commercially available. Efficacy is poor and the vaccine is not widely used.

Abbreviations

- ELISA = enzyme-linked immunosorbent assay

See Also

- Diarrhea, Acute
- Diarrhea, Chronic
- Nutritional Approach to Chronic Enteropathies
- Trichomoniasis

Suggested Reading

Bowman DD. Georgis' Parasitology for Veterinarians, 9th ed. St Louis: Saunders Elsevier, 2009, pp. 89–91.
Tysnes KR, Skancke E, Robertson LJ. Subclinical *Giardia* in dogs: a veterinary conundrum relevant to human infection. Trends Parasitol 2014;30:520–527.

Authors: Jeba Jesudoss Chelladurai BVSc & AH, MS, DACVM, Matt T. Brewer DVM, PhD, DACVM

Chapter 67

Gluten-Sensitive Enteropathy in Irish Setters

DEFINITION/OVERVIEW

- Gluten-sensitive enteropathy (GSE) is a rare, naturally occurring enteropathy in Irish setters that resembles celiac disease in humans. It is a genetic disease.
- Clinical signs are induced by the presence of gluten, which is found in wheat and other grains, in the diet of susceptible individuals.

ETIOLOGY/PATHOPHYSIOLOGY

- Gluten-sensitive enteropathy is a genetic disease of Irish setters with an autosomal recessive mode of inheritance.
- Prevalence of gluten hypersensitivity in dogs as a whole has not been reported.
- Clinical signs develop in young to middle-aged, gluten-sensitive Irish setters when gluten, the storage component of wheat, is consumed.
- Clinical signs resolve once gluten is removed from the diet and return when gluten is reintroduced.

Systems Affected

- Gastrointestinal.
  - Brush border enzyme expression is reduced and villi become atrophied.
  - There is increased intestinal permeability.
  - Inflammation is characterized by increased numbers of lymphocytes in the lamina propria and epithelium of the small intestine histopathologically.

SIGNALMENT/HISTORY

- Gluten-sensitive enteropathy has mainly been described in the Irish setter. However, recently a presumptive case of gluten sensitivity was described in a border terrier with neurologic signs and atopy.
- Affected Irish setters are typically young to middle-aged.
- There is no sex predilection.
- Genetic transmission is under the control of a single autosomal recessive locus.
- Clinical signs include small intestinal diarrhea (which can be intermittent), weight loss or failure to gain weight, decreased appetite, and vomiting (although this is not always present).

Risk Factors

The main risk factor is genetic predisposition in combination with consumption of a diet containing wheat gluten.

Blackwell's Five-Minute Veterinary Consult Clinical Companion: Small Animal Gastrointestinal Diseases, First Edition. Edited by Jocelyn Mott and Jo Ann Morrison.
© 2019 John Wiley & Sons, Inc. Published 2019 by John Wiley & Sons, Inc.
Companion website: www.fiveminutevet.com/gastrointestinal

Historical Findings

Owners report small bowel diarrhea, decreased appetite, weight loss or failure to gain weight, poor body condition, and occasionally vomiting.

 CLINICAL FEATURES

Weight loss or failure to gain weight and poor body condition can be found on physical exam.

 DIFFERENTIAL DIAGNOSIS

- Inflammatory bowel disease.
- Parasitism (*Giardia*, hookworms, roundworms) – fecal flotation and routine deworming should be performed to eliminate this as a differential.
- Lymphangiectasia.
- Other food allergy/intolerance.
- Metabolic abnormalities – routine blood work and resting cortisol should be performed to eliminate metabolic disease, including hypoadrenocorticism, as a differential.
- Exocrine pancreatic insufficiency (EPI) – a gastrointestinal (GI) malabsorption panel should be performed to eliminate EPI as a differential.

 DIAGNOSTICS

Complete Blood Count/Biochemistry/Urinalysis

- A chemistry panel may reveal panhypoproteinemia in some patients.
- Complete blood count is typically normal but may reveal eosinophilia.

Other Laboratory Tests

- Serum folate concentrations are subnormal in some patients due to chronic malabsorption.
- Fecal flotation and routine deworming should be performed to eliminate parasitism.
- A food trial using a gluten-free diet resolves the clinical signs in affected Irish setters.

Pathologic Findings

Histopathology of small intestinal mucosa shows villus stunting and increased numbers of lymphocytes in the lamina propria and epithelium.

 THERAPEUTICS

- The goal of therapy is to eliminate clinical signs (diarrhea, poor body condition) and decrease intestinal inflammation.
- Clinical signs and intestinal biopsy specimens improve following gluten withdrawal.

Drug(s) of Choice

Patients with decreased folate levels may benefit from folate supplementation (0.5–2 mg PO q 24 h for 2–4 weeks).

Diet

Therapy is lifelong elimination of gluten from the diet.

Activity

Activity restriction is not necessary.

COMMENTS

Client Education

- Clients should be counseled about the importance of a lifelong gluten-free diet.
- Affected dogs should not be bred.

Patient Monitoring

- In dogs with panhypoproteinemia, proteins should be monitored once a gluten-free diet is initiated.
- Weight and body condition should be monitored once a gluten-free diet is initiated.

Prevention/Avoidance

Avoiding gluten in the diet will prevent recurrence.

Possible Complications

Complications occur when gluten is not avoided and include diarrhea, weight loss, decreased appetite, and vomiting.

Expected Course and Prognosis

Prognosis is good with dietary management.

Synonyms

- Gluten enteropathy

Abbreviations

- EPI = exocrine pancreatic insufficiency
- GI = gastrointestinal
- GSE = gluten-sensitive enteropathy

See Also

- Nutritional Approach to Chronic Enteropathies

Suggested Reading

Garden OA, Manners HK, Sorensen SH, et al. Intestinal permeability of Irish Setter puppies challenged with a controlled oral dose of gluten. Res Vet Sci 1998;65:23–28.

Garden OA, Pidduck H, Lakhani KH, et al. Inheritance of gluten-sensitive enteropathy in Irish Setters. Am J Vet Res 2000;61:462–468.

Manners HK, Hart CA, Getty B, et al. Characterization of intestinal morphologic, biochemical, and ultrastructural features in gluten sensitive Irish Setters during controlled oral gluten challenge exposure after weaning. Am J Vet Res 1998;59:1435–1440.

Author: Krysta Deitz DVM, MS, DACVIM

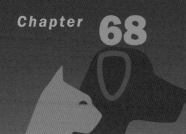

Immunoproliferative Enteropathy of Basenjis

DEFINITION/OVERVIEW

An immunologically mediated small intestinal infiltrative disease characterized by progressive, chronic intermittent diarrhea, anorexia, and weight loss.

ETIOLOGY/PATHOPHYSIOLOGY

- Intense lymphoplasmacytic, infiltrative gastroenteritis or enteritis and concurrent evidence of protein-losing enteropathy, malabsorption, and maldigestion.
- Hypergammaglobulinemia is present due to increased concentrations of serum immunoglobulin A (IgA).

Systems Affected

- Gastrointestinal – diarrhea with possible vomiting.
- Immune – appears to be an immune-mediated response.
- Skin – can be accompanied by alopecia.
- Renal – glomerulonephritis.
- Endocrine – thyroid parafollicular cell atrophy.
- Hepatobiliary – elevated liver enzymes.

SIGNALMENT/HISTORY

- Young to middle-aged basenji, usually <3 years of age.
- Related dogs often affected.
- No known sex predisposition.
- Chronic intermittent diarrhea.
- Severe progressive weight loss.
- Anorexia often preceding diarrhea.
- Bilaterally symmetric alopecia.
- Decreased body condition score.
- Attitude – usually bright and alert.
- Vomiting is variable in severity but common.

Risk Factors

- Pathogenesis is unclear but an interaction between abnormal immune responses, genotype and possibly a contribution by environmental factors is hypothesized.

Blackwell's Five-Minute Veterinary Consult Clinical Companion: Small Animal Gastrointestinal Diseases, First Edition. Edited by Jocelyn Mott and Jo Ann Morrison.
© 2019 John Wiley & Sons, Inc. Published 2019 by John Wiley & Sons, Inc.
Companion website: www.fiveminutevet.com/gastrointestinal

- Mode of inheritance is not known.
- Episodic worsening of symptoms has been associated with stressful events – boarding, estrus, transport, vaccination, etc.

Historical Findings

Owners most often notice gastrointestinal signs (vomiting/diarrhea) first.

 # CLINICAL FEATURES

Thin body condition with diarrhea often noted on rectal examination; alopecia can sometimes be noted.

 # DIFFERENTIAL DIAGNOSIS

Lymphangiectasia, lymphoplasmacytic enteritis, eosinophilic enteritis, histoplasmosis, exocrine pancreatic insufficiency, intestinal lymphoma, intestinal microbial dysbiosis, giardiasis, metabolic disorders, intestinal parasitism.

 # DIAGNOSTICS

Complete Blood Count/Biochemistry/Urinalysis

- Hypoproteinemia.
- Severe hypoalbuminemia.
- Hyperglobulinemia.
- Mature neutrophilia often present.
- Poorly regenerative anemia associated with chronic inflammatory disease.
- Moderately increased hepatic enzymes – seen with advanced disease.

Other Laboratory Tests

- Electrophoresis may yield hypergammaglobulinemia due to increased serum IgA.
- Depression of xylose absorption curve correlates with severity of clinical disease.
- May have hypergastrinemia and hyperchlorhydria, if specifically measured.
- No single test or histologic finding is definitive or pathognomonic.

Imaging

Abdominal ultrasound may demonstrate diffuse small bowel thickening (4–6 mm) or normal gastrointestinal wall layering, and lack of other visceral abnormalities.

Other Diagnostic Procedures

- Endoscopic appearance of the small bowel usually appears abnormal but may be normal. Biopsies (stomach and duodenum, but ileal biopsies are also beneficial) are always required for an accurate diagnosis.
- Genetic testing (DNA) is not available at this time.

Pathologic Findings

- Consistent pathologic lesions include uniform thickening of the small bowel, generalized infiltration of the intestinal lamina propria with lymphocytes and plasma cells, and blunting and fusion of villous tips.

- May be gastric rugal fold hypertrophy, lymphocytic gastritis and/or gastric mucosal atrophy, blunting and widening of intestinal villi, and mild dilation of lacteals.
- Presence and severity of gastric lesions do not correlate with severity of intestinal lesions.
- Other associated lesions include thyroid parafollicular cell atrophy, ulceration of the pinna, gastric acinar atrophy, and glomerulonephritis.
- Immunohistochemical (IHC) staining or polymerase chain reaction (PCR) for antigen receptor rearrangement (PARR) may help differentiate from lymphoma (discriminating may be difficult; in human literature, immunoproliferative enteropathy is often considered an early type of lymphoma).

 THERAPEUTICS

- Outpatient medical management possible unless dehydration or other severe complications exist.
- The disease is expected to be progressive over months to years, but clinical signs can be controlled (at first).

Drug(s) of Choice

Immunosuppressive/Antiinflammatory Drugs
- Variable success reported but considered the mainstay of treatment.
- Prednisone (2 mg/kg/day PO for 2–4 weeks, then slowly taper over 3–4 months to achieve 0.5–1 mg/kg PO q 48 h).
- Chlorambucil (0.25 mg/kg PO q 72 h with monitoring for adverse effects) or other immunosuppressive medications can be tried.

Antibiotics
- Trials of antibiotics are variably helpful for affected individuals that may have intestinal microbial dysbiosis.
- Metronidazole (10–15 mg/kg PO q 12–24 h).
- Tylosin (5–10 mg/kg PO q 24 h).
- *Helicobacter*, *Campylobacter*, and other infectious causes have been associated with immunoproliferative disease in humans, and these patients are occasionally responsive to various antibiotics (including *Helicobacter* eradication protocols, tetracycline, and others).

Chemotherapy
- CHOP (chemotherapy protocol often involving cyclophosphamide, doxorubicin, vincristine and prednisone), or other protocol, may be utilized if disease has progressed to, or is identified as, lymphoma.

Nutritional Supplements/Adjunctive Treatment
- Use of omega-3 fatty acid-rich diets or supplements is thought to potentially favor improved membrane stability and decreased inflammatory responses in the affected gut but there is little specific information available to support this hypothesis.
- Use of probiotics is commonly advised and may favor reduced risk of dysbiosis and a lowered state of inflammatory responses by the gut-associated lymphoid tissues but no specific data are available to support this hypothesis.

Precautions/Interactions
Anticholinergics contraindicated.

Alternative Drugs

See Drug(s) of Choice above.

Nursing Care

No specific nursing care other than that associated with chronic diarrhea.

Diet

Use dietary trials, often with reduced long chain triglycerides, to determine what diet is best tolerated.

Activity

Minimize stressful episodes.

Surgical Considerations

Hypoalbuminemia should be considered with regard to healing if surgical biopsies are elected.

 # COMMENTS

Client Education

This is a chronic condition and recurrence of signs is common.

Patient Monitoring

Monitor weight, gastrointestinal signs, and minimum database.

Prevention/Avoidance

Avoid breeding affected dogs or their littermates.

Possible Complications

Continued weight loss and eventual death are possible.

Expected Course and Prognosis

Clinical signs will initially improve but will often worsen/reoccur in the future; long-term prognosis is poor.

Abbreviations

- CHOP = chemotherapy protocol often involving cyclophosphamide, doxorubicin, vincristine, and prednisone
- IgA = immunoglobulin A
- IHC = immunohistochemistry
- PARR = polymerase chain reaction (PCR) for antigen receptor rearrangement

See Also

- Diarrhea, Chronic – Canine
- Gastroenteritis, Lymphocytic-Plasmacytic
- Gastrointestinal Lymphoma, Canine
- Inflammatory Bowel Disease
- Intestinal Dysbiosis
- Nutritional Approach to Chronic Enteropathies

Suggested Reading

Breitschwerdt EB. Immuno-proliferative enteropathy of Basenjis. Semin Vet Med Surg Small Anim 1992;7:153–161.

Coeuret S, de la Blanchardiere A, Saguet-Rysanek V, et al. Campylobacter coli cultured from the stools of a patient with immunoproliferative small intestinal disease. Clin Microbiol Infect 2014;20(9):908–911.

Dutta U, Udawat H, Noor MT, et al. Regression of immunoproliferative small intestinal disease after eradication of Helicobacter pylori. J Gastrointest Cancer 2010;41(3):212–215.

MacLachlan NJ, Breitschwerdt EB, Chambers JM, et al. Gastroenteritis of Basenji dogs. Vet Pathol 1988;25(1):36–41.

Spohr A, Koch J, Jensen AL. Ultrasonographic findings in a Basenji with immunoproliferative enteropathy. J Small Anim Pract 1995;36:79–82.

Acknowledgments: The author and editors acknowledge the prior contribution of Dr Mark E. Hitt and Dr Stanley L. Marks.

Author: Gavin Olsen DVM, DACVIM (SAIM)

Chapter 69

Inflammatory Bowel Disease

DEFINITION/OVERVIEW

- A group of idiopathic, chronic enteropathies characterized by persistent/intermittent gastrointestinal (GI) signs with histopathologic evidence of intestinal inflammation.
- Inflammatory bowel disease (IBD) is a diagnosis of exclusion to be primarily differentiated from food-responsive enteropathy (FRE), antibiotic-responsive enteropathy (ARE), and intestinal cancer.
- IBD is generally characterized by the predominant mucosal cellular infiltrate, such as lymphocytic-plasmacytic, eosinophilic, or granulomatous enterocolitis.

ETIOLOGY/PATHOPHYSIOLOGY

- Poorly understood but likely due to interactions between mucosal immunity and environmental factors (i.e., dietary constituents and bacterial antigens) in genetically susceptible hosts. Dysregulated host responses are likely triggered by and directed against members of the intestinal microbiota resulting in chronic inflammation to the gut mucosa.
- Damage results from the elaboration of proinflammatory cytokines, release of proteolytic and lysosomal enzymes, complement activation secondary to immune complex deposition, and generation of oxygen free radicals which damage the intestinal epithelial barrier.
- Host genetic susceptibility involving defects in innate immunity has been confirmed in dogs, and is suspected in cats.

Systems Affected

- Gastrointestinal.
- Hepatobiliary – most common in cats.
- Pancreas – pancreatitis seen in cats.
- Hemic/lymphatic/immune – rarely.
- Skin/exocrine – rarely.

SIGNALMENT/HISTORY

- Increased susceptibility has been identified in the German shepherd dog, boxer, and soft-coated wheaten terrier; possible increased prevalence in Asian-breed cats.
- Predominantly occurs in middle-aged animals but any age affected.

Blackwell's Five-Minute Veterinary Consult Clinical Companion: Small Animal Gastrointestinal Diseases, First Edition. Edited by Jocelyn Mott and Jo Ann Morrison.
© 2019 John Wiley & Sons, Inc. Published 2019 by John Wiley & Sons, Inc.
Companion website: www.fiveminutevet.com/gastrointestinal

Risk Factors

- Defects in innate immunity (mutations in toll-like receptors) are seen in German shepherd dogs and may increase susceptibility to IBD.
- Boxers with granulomatous colitis (GC) have mutations in the NCF2 gene which impairs bacterial clearance and contributes to mucosal association of adherent invasive *Escherichia coli* (AIEC) bacteria.

Historical Findings

- Intermittent chronic GI signs (>3 weeks' duration) that wax and wane are often reported.
- Clinical signs are related to GI organs of involvement and may include vomiting, small/large bowel diarrhea, decreased appetite, and/or weight loss.
- Severe inflammation may cause protein-losing enteropathy (PLE) in dogs.

 CLINICAL FEATURES

- Varies from an apparently healthy animal to a thin, lethargic animal.
- Poor hair coat is noted with chronic disease and nutritional deficiencies.
- Abdominal palpation may reveal pain, thickened bowel loops, and mesenteric lymphadenopathy (especially in cats).
- Abdominal pain may be present in cats with concurrent pancreatic involvement.
- Ascites may occur in dogs with PLE.
- Hematochezia, fecal mucus, and tenesmus seen with colonic involvement.

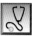 **DIFFERENTIAL DIAGNOSIS**

- Cats – hyperthyroidism, intestinal neoplasia (especially small cell lymphoma), adverse food reactions, granulomatous feline infectious peritonitis (FIP) and other viral infections (e.g., feline leukemia virus (FeLV) and feline immunodeficiency virus (FIV)), renal and hepatic insufficiency, exocrine pancreatic insufficiency, intestinal parasitism, and antibiotic responsive diarrhea (ARD) are primary differentials.
- Dogs – intestinal neoplasia, motility disorders, adverse food reactions, lymphangiectasia, exocrine pancreatic insufficiency, intestinal parasitism, GI histoplasmosis, and ARD are primary differentials.

 DIAGNOSTICS

Complete Blood Count/Biochemistry/Urinalysis

- Results may be unremarkable; these tests more often serve to eliminate other differential diagnoses.
- Mild, nonregenerative anemia of chronic disease. Mild leukocytosis ± a left shift is sometimes seen with mucosal disruption. Mild peripheral eosinophilia may be seen with eosinophilic enteritis.
- Cats with IBD may show alterations in serum total protein (i.e., hyperproteinemia) with increased liver enzyme (e.g., ALT and/or ALP) activities.
- Hypoproteinemia (hypoglobulinemia + hypoalbuminemia) is common in dogs with PLE.

Other Laboratory Tests

- Useful to eliminate other differential diagnoses.
- Cobalamin deficiency is often observed with involvement of the ileum.

- Dogs – tests include evaluation of exocrine pancreatic function (trypsin-like immunoreactivity (cTLI)), serology for pancreatitis (canine pancreatic lipase activity (Spec PLI)), serum cobalamin and folate assays to localize small intestinal disease, and urine antigen testing for *Histoplasma* spp. infection.
- Cats – T4 and FeLV/FIV serology are recommended; fasting serum TLI (if exocrine pancreatic insufficiency is suspected); serology for pancreatitis (Spec fPLI), and serum cobalamin and folate assays to localize small intestinal disease.

Imaging

- Abdominal radiographs – usually unremarkable. Diagnostic imaging is most useful in documenting abnormalities outside the GI tract.
- Barium contrast studies – may reveal mucosal abnormalities and thickened bowel loops. Normal findings do not eliminate the possibility of IBD.
- Ultrasonography – may indicate increased intestinal wall thickness (particularly the muscularis propria/submucosal layers), ± mesenteric lymphadenopathy. However, these abnormalities, even if present, are not specific for IBD.

Diagnostic Procedures

- Perform an elimination dietary trial to rule out adverse food reactions. If GI signs resolve within two weeks, then a diagnosis of adverse food reaction is made and no further diagnostic work-up is required.
- Always perform fecal testing for nematode and protozoal parasites.
- Definitive diagnosis of IBD requires intestinal biopsy and histopathology, usually obtained via GI endoscopy. WSAVA guidelines should be used to define the severity of mucosal inflammation.
- Laparotomy is indicated if GI endoscopy is unavailable or to collect full-thickness mucosal specimens.
- Use scoring indices (canine inflammatory bowel disease activity index (CIBDAI)) to define clinical disease severity and assess response to therapy.

 # THERAPEUTICS

- IBD is a controllable disease but is not curable – expect disease flares. Most animals are well managed as outpatients.
- Cornerstones of therapy include feeding an elimination diet and administration of drugs to reduce intestinal inflammation.
- Since no optimal treatment has been designed, sequential therapy using diet → antibiotics → immunosuppressive drugs is often utilized.
- Treat nutritional deficiencies if present.

Drug(s) of Choice

- Empirical deworming with fenbendazole (50 mg/kg PO q 24 h for three days).
- Evidence-based data indicate that glucocorticoids are effective drugs for inducing remission in the majority of dogs and cats. Use prednisone or prednisolone in dogs dosed at 1–2 mg/kg PO daily for 21 days to induce remission. If clinical remission occurs, taper steroid dose by 25% every two weeks.
- Note that large dogs, weighing greater than 30 kg, will require a lower steroid dosage to provide comparable clinical efficacy. This will also reduce adverse effects of the glucocorticoid.

- Treat IBD cats with oral prednisolone at a dosage of 1–2 mg/kg for 14–21 days; then taper as above. Avoid glucocorticoids in cats with diabetes mellitus and those with a history of adverse effects.
- Budesonide may be used to minimize adverse steroid effects and to maintain remission in some dogs and cats. Dosage ranges for dogs are 1–3 mg/m² daily; for cats, 1 mg/day.
- Antibiotics (metronidazole, tylosin) are generally *not* indicated for treatment of IBD. These drugs may cause significant disruption to the gut microbiota even after administration is discontinued.
- Enrofloxacin (5 mg/kg PO q 24 h for 14–21 days alone or with metronidazole and amoxicillin) is recommended for treatment of granulomatous colitis (GC) in boxers. Antimicrobial therapy should be guided by mucosal culture with antimicrobial sensitivity testing.
- There is some evidence that oral cyclosporine is of value in dogs with steroid-refractory disease and PLE. This drug is dosed at 5 mg/kg PO daily for 4–6 weeks or as needed to induce remission.
- Empirical use of other immunosuppressive drugs, including azathioprine, chlorambucil, leflunomide, and mycophenolate, for treatment of IBD has been reported.

Diet

- Feed an intact protein or hydrolyzed elimination diet to help reduce intestinal inflammation.
- Correct hypocobalaminemia by means of weekly parenteral cobalamin injections for the first six weeks and thereafter every 2–3 weeks or as needed based on repeat testing of cobalamin concentrations.
- Fiber supplementation (e.g., fermentable fiber such as pumpkin, Metamucil™) is recommended in dogs and cats with colitis.
- Probiotics may be of benefit in some animals but are clinically unproven at this time. These supplements must be given continuously over several weeks for potential benefit to be realized.

 COMMENTS

Client Education

- Emphasize to the client that IBD is not curable but is controllable in most instances.
- Relapses are common; clients should be patient during the various food and medication trials that are often necessary to get the disease under control.

Patient Monitoring

- Periodic (q 2–4 weeks) physical and laboratory evaluations may be necessary until the patient's condition stabilizes. Serum albumin provides important prognostic information in dogs; serum cobalamin deficiency will delay complete clinical recovery in both dogs and cats.
- Monitor serum cobalamin concentrations in hypocobalaminemic dogs and cats.
- No other follow-up may be required except yearly physical examinations and assessment during relapse.

Expected Course and Prognosis

- Generally a good-to-excellent short-term prognosis.
- Poor long-term prognosis in dogs with IBD has been associated with severe clinical disease, marked endoscopic (duodenal) abnormalities, ascites, and hypoalbuminemia.

Abbreviations

- AIEC = adherent invasive *E. coli*
- ALP = alkaline phosphatase
- ALT = alanine aminotransferase
- ARD = antibiotic-responsive diarrhea
- ARE = antibiotic-responsive enteropathy
- CIBDAI = canine IBD activity index
- FeLV = feline leukemia virus
- FIP = feline infectious peritonitis
- FIV = feline immunodeficiency virus
- FRE = food-responsive enteropathy
- GC = granulomatous colitis
- GI = gastrointestinal
- IBD = inflammatory bowel disease
- PLE = protein losing enteropathy
- Spec cPL or fPL = canine or feline pancreatic lipase activity
- T4 = thyroxine
- TLI = trypsin-like immunoreactivity
- WSAVA = World Small Animal Veterinary Association

See Also

- Diarrhea, Antibiotic Responsive
- Food Reactions (Gastrointestinal), Adverse
- Gastroenteritis, Eosinophilic
- Gastroenteritis, Lymphocytic-Plasmacytic
- Nutritional Approach to Chronic Enteropathies
- Protein-Losing Enteropathy

Suggested Reading

Allenspach K, Wieland B, Grone A. et al. Chronic enteropathies in dogs: evaluation of risk factors for negative outcome. J Vet Intern Med 2007;21:700–708.

Simpson KW, Jergens AE. Pitfalls and progress in the diagnosis and management of canine inflammatory bowel disease. Vet Clin North Am Small Anim Pract 2011;41(2):381–398.

Slovak JE, Wang C, Sun Y, et al. Development and validation of an endoscopic activity score for canine inflammatory bowel disease. Vet J 2015;203(3):290–295.

Washabau RJ, Day MJ, Willard MD, et al. Endoscopic, biopsy, and histopathologic guidelines for the evaluation of gastrointestinal inflammation in companion animals. J Vet Intern Med 2010;24(1):10–26.

Author: Albert E. Jergens DVM, PhD, DACVIM

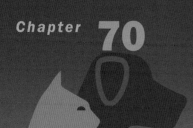

Chapter 70

Intestinal Dysbiosis

DEFINITION/OVERVIEW

- Small intestinal dysbiosis (SID) is a clinical syndrome caused by an alteration of the small intestinal microbiota.
- Previously, a variety of different terms have been used to describe small intestinal dysbiosis.
  - Small intestinal bacterial overgrowth (SIBO) has been defined as $>10^4$ anaerobic and/or $>10^5$ total bacterial colony-forming units (cfu)/mL in duodenal juice from dogs. However, these criteria are now controversial. In cats, the culture-based quantitative assessment of the gut microbiota was too variable to define normal.
  - The term antibiotic-responsive diarrhea (ARD) has been used by several authors to describe patients that have diarrhea that responds to antibiotic therapy. Neither the type of bacteria nor the type of antibiotic that is effective has been defined for ARD.
  - Tylosin-responsive diarrhea (TRD) has been described by a group in Finland. The term was coined based on the fact that several dogs with chronic diarrhea failed to respond to a variety of antibiotics or corticosteroids, but did respond to treatment with tylosin.
- Recent molecular studies have shown that the qualitative make-up of the small intestinal microbiota is highly individualized for each dog and cat.
- It should be emphasized that SID differs from colonization of the alimentary tract by known enteropathogens (e.g., *Salmonella* spp., *Campylobacter jejuni*, enterotoxigenic *Clostridium perfringens*, enterotoxic *Escherichia coli*, or others).
- Intestinal dysbiosis can be primary or secondary to other conditions associated with chronic enteropathy, such as food-responsive diarrhea or idiopathic inflammatory bowel disease (IBD).

ETIOLOGY/PATHOPHYSIOLOGY

- The normal intestinal tract of dogs and cats harbors a highly complex microbiota (i.e., bacteria, fungi, protozoa, and viruses). Bacteria make up the vast majority of the microbiota. In the colon, the number of cultivable bacteria is much higher compared to the small intestine. The small intestine harbors a mixture of aerobic and facultative anaerobic bacteria, while the large intestine is home to mostly anaerobic bacteria.
- A normal balanced microbial ecosystem is important to host health, as the microbiota provides proper stimuli for the immune system, helps defend against enteropathogens, and provides nutrients to the host.

Blackwell's Five-Minute Veterinary Consult Clinical Companion: Small Animal Gastrointestinal Diseases,
First Edition. Edited by Jocelyn Mott and Jo Ann Morrison.
© 2019 John Wiley & Sons, Inc. Published 2019 by John Wiley & Sons, Inc.
Companion website: www.fiveminutevet.com/gastrointestinal

- Host-protective mechanisms prevent overgrowth of pathogenic or potentially pathogenic bacteria through gastric acid secretion, intestinal motility (peristalsis), secretion of antimicrobial substances in bile and pancreatic juice, and local enteric IgA production.
- The ileocolic valve is a physiologic barrier between the large bowel, which is populated by large numbers of bacteria, and the less populated small bowel.
- When these natural defense mechanisms fail and excessive numbers of certain bacterial species persist in the upper small intestine, they may cause pathology, even though they are not considered enteropathogens.
- Primary SID is probably uncommon, but a definitive cause of secondary SID often remains undiagnosed and thus many dogs are diagnosed with idiopathic SID.
- Secondary SID (more common).
  - Altered small intestinal anatomy – inherited or acquired (e.g., partial obstructions, neoplasia, foreign body, intussusception, stricture, adhesion, or diverticulum).
  - Altered intestinal motility (e.g., hypothyroidism, autonomic neuropathies).
  - Exocrine pancreatic insufficiency (EPI) – approximately 70% of dogs with EPI have concurrent SID.
  - Hypochlorhydria or achlorhydria – spontaneous or iatrogenic (e.g., proton pump inhibitor treatment).
  - Altered immune system – immunodeficiency, decreased mucosal defense, and preexisting intestinal disease.
  - Antibiotic induced – in most animals, the microbiota recovers within a few weeks after cessation of antibiotic administration, but some animals may have prolonged dysbiosis, potentially causing signs of intestinal disease.

Systems Affected

- Gastrointestinal – normal absorptive function is disrupted, resulting in loose stool and weight loss.
- Hepatobiliary – the portal vein carries bacterial toxins and other substances to the liver, which may lead to hepatic changes.

 # SIGNALMENT/HISTORY

- Genetics – no genetic basis for SID has yet been identified. However, recent studies would suggest that histiocytic ulcerative colitis should be considered a type of dysbiosis of the large intestine. Since the majority of cases have been described in the boxer, genetic factors that predispose dogs of this breed to this type of dysbiosis are likely.
- Certain canine breeds (e.g., German shepherd, Chinese shar-pei, and beagles) appear to be at an increased risk for SID.
- The exact incidence/prevalence is unknown.
- Intestinal dysbiosis is observed in dogs and cats.
- The mean age and age range are unknown, and dysbiosis can be seen in dogs and cats of any age and, depending on the underlying disease, even in very young animals.
- Alterations of the small intestinal microbiota can cause clinical signs of small intestinal disease, such as loose stool or diarrhea, weight loss, and/or others.

Risk Factors

- Intestinal diseases that affect local defense mechanisms (e.g., IBD, adverse food reactions, parasite infestation, others).

- SID has been suspected as a cause of IBD in some patients.
- Consider the possibility of concurrent EPI.

Historical Findings

- Chronic loose stools or diarrhea (small bowel or large bowel type diarrhea) – common.
- Weight loss, despite a reasonable appetite – common.
- Borborygmus and flatulence – common.
- Vomiting – occasional/variable.
- Clinical signs of the underlying disease process may be seen in cases of secondary SID.
- Clinical signs may wax and wane or be continuous.

CLINICAL FEATURES

Unremarkable or evidence of weight loss and decreased body condition.

DIFFERENTIAL DIAGNOSIS

- Secondary gastrointestinal disease (e.g., hepatic failure, renal failure, EPI, chronic pancreatitis, hypothyroidism, hypoadrenocorticism).
- Primary gastrointestinal disease (i.e., infectious, inflammatory, neoplastic, mechanical, toxic, or other).

DIAGNOSTICS

Complete Blood Count/Biochemistry/Urinalysis

- Usually unremarkable.
- Hypoalbuminemia – uncommon finding; when present, it suggests particularly severe intestinal disease and warrants an aggressive diagnostic and therapeutic approach.

Additional Laboratory Tests

- Serum cobalamin and folate concentrations.
  - Serum folate concentration may be increased as many bacterial species synthesize folate and an increased abundance of folate-producing bacterial species will lead to an overabundance of folic acid in the small intestine.
  - Serum cobalamin concentration may be decreased – many bacterial species compete with the host for dietary cobalamin.
  - The finding of an increased serum folate concentration and a decreased serum cobalamin concentration is suggestive, but not specific for SID in dogs. In addition, not all patients with SID show this pattern.
- Dysbiosis index (DI).
  - Fecal dysbiosis occurs commonly in dogs with chronic enteropathies (i.e., dogs with food- and antibiotic-responsive diarrhea, and dogs with IBD).
  - The intestinal tract harbors many anaerobic bacterial species; routine bacterial culture of feces does not provide an accurate assessment of the fecal microbiota.
  - The fecal DI is a polymerase chain reaction (PCR)-based assay that quantifies the abundances of eight bacterial groups in fecal samples of dogs and summarizes them in one single number. A DI below 0 indicates a normal fecal microbiota; a DI above 0 indicates dysbiosis. Approximately 15% of clinically healthy dogs have an increased DI, with most of them falling into the equivocal range between 0 and 2.

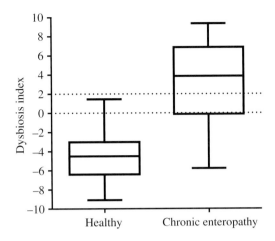

■ **Fig. 70.1.** Fecal dysbiosis index (DI) for assessment of fecal dysbiosis in dogs. A DI below 0 indicates normal fecal microbiota, while a DI above 0 indicates fecal dysbiosis. A DI between 0 and 2 is equivocal.

- Many dogs with chronic enteropathy or EPI have an abnormal fecal DI (Figure 70.1). Also, a small subset of dogs with acute diarrhea and acute hemorrhagic diarrhea syndrome may have a DI between 0 and 2, but the microbiota normalizes within 7–14 days (DI below 0).
- Due to anatomical and physiological differences along the intestine, evaluation of the fecal DI may not accurately reflect microbiota changes in the small intestine. Concurrent evaluation of serum concentration of cobalamin/folate with assessment of the fecal dysbiosis index may help in the diagnosis of small intestinal dysbiosis.

Imaging

Not useful for the diagnosis of primary SID. However, may reveal findings indicative of an underlying cause of secondary SID.

Diagnostic Procedures

- A therapeutic trial can be performed by treating patients with suspected SID with an antibiotic, a diet containing a prebiotic, or a probiotic, or a combination thereof.
- Interpreting the results of a therapeutic trial may be difficult as more than one disease (e.g., IBD plus SID, dietary intolerance plus SID) may be present, and lack of a clinical response might lead to the incorrect conclusion that SID is absent; incorrect selection of the treatment that is trialed might also cause failure of a clinical response.

Pathologic Findings

- No macroscopic findings upon exploratory laparotomy or endoscopy.
- Histopathology of small intestinal mucosal biopsies is typically unremarkable.

 # THERAPEUTICS

Drug(s) of Choice

- Broad-spectrum, orally administered antibiotics effective against both aerobic and anaerobic bacteria are preferred.
- Tylosin (10–25 mg/kg PO q 12 h for six weeks) is the primary choice. Tylosin is usually used in a powder formulation that is marketed for use in poultry and pigs. It is administered in

food because of its bitter taste. It can be used long term. For small dogs and cats, the drug should be reformulated into capsules. For larger dogs, the dose can be approximated by using a teaspoon and administering the drug in food.

- Metronidazole (10–15 mg/kg PO q 12h for six weeks) is used commonly because of its activity against anaerobic bacteria. Metronidazole may also have immunomodulatory effects. However, metronidazole can have significant side effects.
- Dogs with SID may be cobalamin deficient, and oral or parenteral supplementation of vitamin B12 is indicated: 250 µg cats; 250–1500 µg dogs, weekly for six weeks with one more dose a month later when administered SQ and daily for 120 days if administered PO; dose depends on body size; serum cobalamin concentrations should be reevaluated a week (oral dosing regimen) or month (parenteral dosing regimen) after the last dose to determine the need for continued supplementation.

Alternative Drugs

In dogs with EPI and SID, concurrent therapy for SID is only indicated if enzyme replacement alone does not resolve the diarrhea and/or lead to weight gain.

Precautions/Interactions

- Metronidazole can be associated with gastrointestinal side effects and in rare cases with neurologic side effects.
- Avoid metronidazole during early pregnancy.

Appropriate Health Care

- Outpatient medical management.
- SID can be managed with antibiotics, prebiotics (can be administered through the diet or as a nutritional supplement), probiotics, or a combination thereof. Also, fecal transplantation has been used on a limited basis for patients that fail any of the other treatments.
- Antibiotics – see as for medications.
- Prebiotics – see as for diet.
- Probiotics – there has been a lot of interest in probiotic use for dogs and cats with chronic diarrhea, although little is known about their efficacy. Currently, because of quality issues with many products, only probiotics from major manufacturers can be recommended.
- Improvement may take a few days to several weeks.

Nursing Care

- Usually none.
- Supportive care for emaciated or hypoalbuminemic patients.

Diet

- Highly digestible diet.
- A diet containing fructooligosaccharides has been shown to be beneficial in dogs with small intestinal dysbiosis.

Activity

Unrestricted.

Surgical Considerations

Only indicated for some underlying causes of SID (i.e., partial obstruction, diverticulum, or intestinal mass).

COMMENTS

Client Education

- Some patients show clinical improvement within days, but treatment must be continued long term (6–8 weeks minimum).
- Some patients require weeks of therapy before demonstrating improvement; treat for 2–3 weeks before concluding that therapy is ineffective.
- Any concurrent or predisposing diseases (e.g., IBD, EPI, dietary intolerance/allergy, alimentary tract neoplasia, partial obstruction) must also be treated.
- Continuous or repeated treatment is often required.

Patient Monitoring

- Body weight and, in hypoproteinemic patients, serum albumin concentrations are the most important parameters; improvement suggests effective therapy.
- Diarrhea should also resolve.
- If diarrhea persists despite improved body weight and/or increased serum albumin concentration, investigation for concurrent intestinal disease is indicated.

Expected Course and Prognosis

Primary SID without complicating factors (e.g., IBD, lymphoma) – prognosis with appropriate therapy is usually good, although relapses can be seen following cessation of antibiotic therapy.

Synonyms

- Antibiotic-responsive diarrhea
- Tylosin-responsive diarrhea
- Small intestinal bacterial overgrowth

Abbreviations

- ARD = antibiotic-responsive diarrhea
- cfu = colony-forming units
- DI = dysbiosis index
- EPI = exocrine pancreatic insufficiency
- IBD = inflammatory bowel disease
- PCR = polymerase chain reaction
- SIBO = small intestinal bacterial overgrowth
- SID = small intestinal dysbiosis
- TRD = tylosin-responsive diarrhea

See Also

- Diarrhea, Chronic – Feline
- Diarrhea, Chronic – Canine
- Exocrine Pancreatic Insufficiency
- Inflammatory Bowel Disease
- Gastrointestinal Lymphoma, Feline
- Gastrointestinal Lymphoma, Canine

Suggested Reading

German AJ, Day MJ, Ruaux CG, Steiner JM, Williams DA. Comparison of direct and indirect tests for small intestinal bacterial overgrowth and antibiotic-responsive diarrhea in dogs. J Vet Intern Med 2003;17(1):33–43.

Kilpinen S, Spillmann T, Westermarck E. Efficacy of two low-dose oral tylosin regimens in controlling the relapse of diarrhea in dogs with tylosin-responsive diarrhea: a prospective, single-blinded, two-arm parallel, clinical field trial. Acta Vet Scand 2014;56:43.

Suchodolski JS. Microbes in intestinal health of dogs and cats. J Anim Sci 2011;89:1520–1530.

Suchodolski JS. Diagnosis and interpretation of intestinal dysbiosis in dogs and cats. Vet J 2016;215:30–37.

Authors: Jan S. Suchodolski Dr.med.vet., PhD, DACVM, Jörg M. Steiner med.vet., Dr.med.vet., PhD, DACVIM, DECVIM-CA, AGAF

Chapter 71

Intestinal Neoplasia, Benign

DEFINITION/OVERVIEW

- Tumors that are located in the small intestine that lack the ability to invade neighboring tissues or metastasize.
- Although the tumors are benign, in some locations the masses can cause life-threatening clinical symptoms.
- Common tumor types are adenomatous polyps, lipoma, hamartoma, and ganglioneuromatosis.
- Adenomatous polyps are pedunculated, sessile or diffuse (Figure 71.1).
- Lipoma – most common subcutaneous tumor in dogs, can cause more severe signs when located within the abdominal cavity.
- Hamartoma.
  - Rare intestinal tumor that results from a benign, focal malformation of normal tissue. The tissue is histologically normal but proliferates in a disorganized fashion.
  - In humans, associated with long-term increase in neoplasia development. No long-term follow-up in canine cases.
- Ganglioneuromatosis.
  - Diffuse proliferation of ganglia cells in the mucosa and submucosa of the small intestines. Cells originate in the autonomic nervous system of the intestinal tract and are histologically normal tissue.

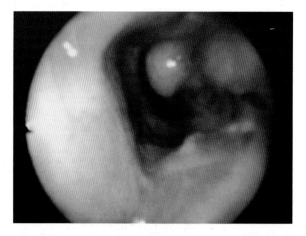

■ **Fig. 71.1.** Endoscopic appearance of benign adenomatous polyps in the duodenum of a dog.

Blackwell's Five-Minute Veterinary Consult Clinical Companion: Small Animal Gastrointestinal Diseases,
First Edition. Edited by Jocelyn Mott and Jo Ann Morrison.
© 2019 John Wiley & Sons, Inc. Published 2019 by John Wiley & Sons, Inc.
Companion website: www.fiveminutevet.com/gastrointestinal

- Two distinct syndromes described in humans: transmural disease associated with a specific genetic mutation (RET protooncogene) in young children; mucosal disease described in older patients and not associated with genetic abnormalities.
- Unknown if disease in veterinary patients correlates with human disease syndrome.

ETIOLOGY/PATHOPHYSIOLOGY

- Unknown; some breeds may be predisposed to adenomatous polyps.
- Chronic inflammation may be a risk factor with progression from metaplasia to dysplasia seen in some patients.

Systems Affected

Gastrointestinal.

SIGNALMENT/HISTORY

- Will affect any age – range from <1 year to 12 years.
- Very rare in cats but Asian breeds are overrepresented.
- Affects a variety of breeds of dogs.
- Hamartoma – rare reports in dogs, never reported in cats.
- Ganglioneuromatosis – case reports in both young and older dogs.

Historical Findings

- Most commonly present with hematemesis and chronic vomiting, occasionally hematochezia.
- Adenomatous polyps.
  - Pedunculated masses more likely to cause signs related to obstruction or intussusception. Ingested food passing by the mass may cause traction on the intestine, resulting in invagination of the wall and an increased risk for intussusception. Larger polyps may act like a valve and intermittently obstruct the intestinal lumen.
  - Pedunculated masses may cause more acute signs of intestinal intussusception or strangulation, including acute abdominal pain with dehydration, severe vomiting, and possibly shock.
- Lipoma.
  - Signs will relate to organs that are entrapped or compressed. Large intraabdominal lipomas will cause abdominal distension and possibly vomiting if the stomach and small intestines are significantly compressed.
  - Pedunculated mesenteric lipomas can cause acute life-threatening intestinal strangulation. More common in older horses; rare reports in the canine species.

CLINICAL FEATURES

Abdominal distension can occur when large abdominal lipoma is present.

DIFFERENTIAL DIAGNOSIS

- Foreign body.
- Viral enteritis.
- Inflammatory bowel disease.

- Pancreatitis.
- Intestinal parasites.

DIAGNOSTICS

Complete Blood Count/Biochemistry/Urinalysis

Minimum database of a complete blood cell count, chemistry, and urinalysis is recommended.

Imaging

- Plain film abdominal radiographs are of limited utility; most masses are intraluminal and cannot be visualized.
- Contrast radiography – may reveal benign mass but will also delay the ability to perform surgery.
- Abdominal ultrasonography is consistently superior to contrast radiography. With the advent of portable, high-quality ultrasound units, this test is available to most veterinarians through mobile services. Operator experience and skill are paramount.
- Abdominal ultrasound also allows for imaging mass and determining location.

Other Diagnostic Tests

- Ultrasound-guided mass aspiration generally unrewarding for benign lesions but can be useful in ruling out lymphoma.
- Endoscopy and mucosal biopsy – results must be interpreted with caution; frequently nondiagnostic for tumors that are deep to the mucosal surface. Complete removal of a polyp via endoscopy is preferred to ensure that there are no focal areas of dysplasia or neoplasia present within the mass on histopathology.

THERAPEUTICS

Drug(s) of Choice

- Adenomatous polyps of the colon will overexpress cyclooxygenase-2 (COX-2).
- Nonsteroidal antiinflammatories such as deracoxib, firocoxib, meloxicam, and piroxicam may play a role in treatment; uncertain if the same is true for small intestinal polyps as the disease is much less common.

Surgical Considerations

- Adenomatous polyps.
  - Preferred treatment is surgical resection and anastomoses when an obstruction or intussusception is present.
  - Endoscopy with snare polypectomy may be possible for tumors that can be reached. Risk for recurrence when polyps are not completely excised. Small risk for intestinal perforation when endocautery is used. Best performed at a referral practice with an individual who is experienced in the procedure.
  - Sessile lesions may be too large for endoscopy, may require surgical intervention with resection and anastomosis.
  - Diffuse lesions respond best to treatment with resection and anastomosis.
- Hamartoma – treatment with surgical resection and anastomosis of affected areas of the small intestine causes complete resolution of clinical signs in reported cases.
- Ganglioneuromatosis – treat with surgical excision; relieves clinical syndromes but limited long-term follow-up for this very rare disease.

COMMENTS

Expected Course and Prognosis

- Complete excision of masses either through surgery or endoscopy curative for most patients.
- Masses will recur locally if incompletely excised.
- Recurrence may increase the risk for malignant transformation.

Abbreviations

- COX 2 = cyclooxygenase 2

See Also

- Hematemesis
- Hematochezia
- Intestinal Neoplasia, Malignant
- Vomiting, Chronic

Suggested Reading

Brown, PJ, Adam S, Wotton P, et al. Hamartomatous polyps in the intestine of two dogs. J Comp Pathol 1994;110(1):97–102.

Foy D. Endoscopic polypectomy using endocautery in three dogs and one cat. J Am Anim Hosp Assoc 2010;46:168–173.

McLaughlin R, Kuzma,AB. Intestinal strangulation caused by intra-abdominal lipomas in a dog. J Am Vet Med Assoc 1991;199(11):1610–1611.

Osborn SD, Ludwig L, Johnson S, et al. What is your diagnosis? Cranial displacement of the small intestine and substanial abdominal distention caused by a large intra-abdominal lipoma. J Am Vet Med Assoc 1996;208(8):1235–1236.

Paris JK, McCandlish I, Schwarz T, et al. Small intestinal ganglioneuromatosis in a dog. J Comp Pathol 2013;148(4):323–328.

Schwandt CS. Low-grade or benign intestinal tumours contribute to intussusception: a report on one feline and two canine cases. J Small Anim Pract 2008;49(12):651–654.

Author: Carrie A. Wood DVM, DACVIM (Oncology)

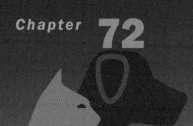
Intestinal Neoplasia, Malignant

DEFINITION/OVERVIEW

- Tumors that are located in the small intestine that are not lymphoma.
- Adenocarcinoma, leiomyoma/leiomyosarcoma, gastrointestinal stromal tumors (GIST), carcinoids, and mast cell tumor (MCT).

ETIOLOGY/PATHOPHYSIOLOGY

- Adenocarcinoma is the most common intestinal tumor in both dogs and cats.
- Polypoid growths may be premalignant and can represent a risk factor.
- Intestinal adenocarcinoma.
  - Typically jejunal in location.
  - High rate (approximately 45%) of metastatic disease to regional lymph nodes, liver, and mesentery.
- Leiomyosarcoma.
  - Second most common tumor in dogs; rare in cats.
  - Actual incidence may have been overstated in the past; likely to decrease with more accurate diagnosis through the use of immunohistochemistry.
  - Arises from the smooth muscle lining of the gastrointestinal tract; tumors are positive for smooth muscle actin (SMA).
  - Low to moderate rate of metastases (30–50%); typically to liver and regional lymph nodes.
  - Hypoglycemia may be present.
  - Must be differentiated from a gastrointestinal stromal tumor via immunohistochemistry.
- Gastrointestinal stromal tumor.
  - Arises from the smooth muscle of the gastrointestinal tract, specifically the interstitial cells of Cajal which are the pacemaker cells of the small intestinal tract.
  - Tumors are positive for KIT protein (CD 117) and vimentin on immunohistochemistry.
  - Dogs more commonly affected, rare reports in cats.
  - Variable clinical course, still not well understood with lack of long-term follow-up in literature.
  - Larger tumors and tumors with a heterogeneous appearance and irregular margins on ultrasound are more likely to be metastatic.
  - Metastasize to liver most frequently and regional lymph nodes.
- Non-GIST non-smooth muscle sarcoma.
  - Likely peripheral nerve sheath tissue in origin.
  - Low rate of metastases for well-differentiated tumors.

Blackwell's Five-Minute Veterinary Consult Clinical Companion: Small Animal Gastrointestinal Diseases,
First Edition. Edited by Jocelyn Mott and Jo Ann Morrison.
© 2019 John Wiley & Sons, Inc. Published 2019 by John Wiley & Sons, Inc.
Companion website: www.fiveminutevet.com/gastrointestinal

- Carcinoid.
    - May also be classified as a goblet cell carcinoid.
    - Neuroendocrine tumor occurring in the intestinal tract of both dogs and cats, can release serotonin, 5-hydroxytryptophan, histamine, bradykinins, tachykinins, and prostaglandins. May present with a unique paraneoplastic syndrome of cutaneous flushing, secretory diarrhea, and/or bronchospasm.
    - Overt metastases to regional nodes with lymphatic invasion often found at surgery; generally carries a poor prognosis.
- Mast cell tumor.
    - Rare in dogs, 5% of all intestinal tumor in cats.
    - Commonly metastasizes to mesenteric lymph nodes.
    - Sclerosing subtype is more aggressive in cats.

Systems Affected

- Gastrointestinal.
- Hepatic/lymphatic/others with metastatic disease.

 # SIGNALMENT/HISTORY

- Middle-aged to older patients (>6 years).
- Siamese cats, collies, and German shepherd dogs have increased rates of intestinal adenocarcinoma.

Historical Findings

- Most commonly present with melena, diarrhea, and weight loss.
- Vomiting occurs with tumors located in the duodenum or jejunum.
- Diarrhea and weight loss seen more often with jejunal and ileal tumors.
- Almost two-thirdsof cats will have vomiting as a symptom.
- Anorexia and weight loss are common and may be severe, resulting in cachexia (Figure 72.1).

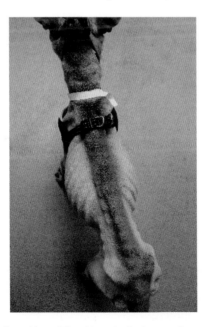

■ **Fig. 72.1.** Severe cachexia in a dog with multifocal intestinal adenocarcinoma.

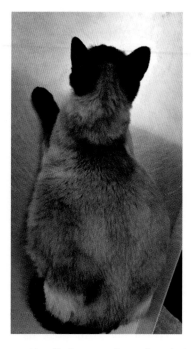

■ **Fig. 72.2.** Abdominal distension caused by effusion secondary to intestinal carcinoma in a cat.

CLINICAL FEATURES

- Abdominal distension can occur when a malignant effusion develops (Figure 72.2).
- Midabdominal mass may be palpable.
- Obstruction may occur, causing an acute exacerbation of vomiting.
- Septic peritonitis may develop and will present with collapse, fever, and abdominal pain.

DIFFERENTIAL DIAGNOSIS

- Foreign body.
- Lymphoma.
- Inflammatory bowel disease.
- Pancreatitis.
- Intestinal parasites.

DIAGNOSTICS

Complete Blood Count/Biochemistry/Urinalysis

- Minimum database of a complete blood cell count, chemistry, and urinalysis is recommended.
- Anemia and leukocytosis are common findings; microcytic, hypochromic anemia can occur when chronic blood loss is present.
- Paraneoplastic hypoglycemia can be seen with mesenchymal tumors in dogs.

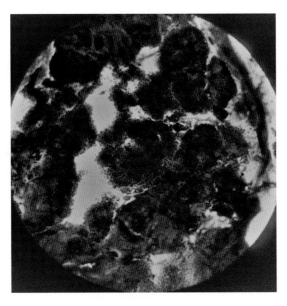

■ **Fig. 72.3.** Aspiration cytology of metastatic intestinal adenocarcinoma showing nests of malignant epithelial cells.

Imaging

■ Thoracic radiographs may reveal metastatic lesions; finding is rare but carries grave consequences when metastasis is found.
■ Plain film abdominal radiographs are of limited utility, most commonly not revealing the mass and instead showing gas-filled intestinal loops. In cases of intestinal perforation, pneuomoperitoneum may be identified.
■ Contrast radiography – filling defect associated with mass.
■ Abdominal ultrasonography is consistently superior to contrast radiography. With the advent of portable, high-quality ultrasound units, this test is available to most veterinarians through mobile services. Operator experience and skill are paramount.
■ Abdominal ultrasound also allows for imaging of regional lymph nodes, liver, and spleen to screen for metastatic disease. Loss of gastrointestinal wall layering correlated significantly with presence of neoplasia.

Other Diagnostic Tests

■ Ultrasound-guided mass aspiration can assist in diagnosis. Carcinomas may exfoliate, typically nondiagnostic for mesenchymal tumors but can be essential for ruling out lymphoma (Figure 72.3).
■ Endoscopy and mucosal biopsy – most helpful for adenocarcinomas; frequently nondiagnostic for tumors that are deep to the mucosal surface (Figure 72.4).

 THERAPEUTICS

Drug(s) of Choice

■ Intestinal adenocarcinoma.
  • Many carcinomas will overexpress cyclooxygenase (COX) 2; NSAIDs such as deracoxib, firocoxib, meloxicam, and piroxicam may play a role in treatment.

(a)   (b)

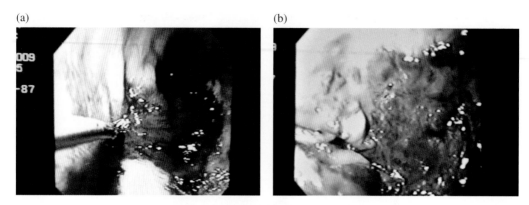

■ **Fig. 72.4.** (a,b) Intestinal bleeding and hematochezia seen via endoscopy in a patient with intestinal carcinoma.

- Chemotherapy with doxorubicin, carboplatin, and toceranib reported anecdotally. No compelling evidence for use in patients with solitary lesions that are completely excised.
- Gastrointestinal stromal tumor – may respond positively to targeted therapy with imatinib or toceranib if metastases are present or mass is not resectable; ideal case selection for adjunctive therapy is unknown.
- Mast cell tumor.
  - Treatment with surgery, prednisolone, lomustine, chlorambucil, and toceranib have been attempted with variable results; additional studies are needed.
  - Feline mast cell tumors can respond to prednisolone.

Appropriate Health Care

Supportive nutritional care vital for postsurgical recovery in debilitated, cachectic patients.

Surgical Considerations

- Intestinal adenocarcinoma – preferred treatment is surgical resection and anastomoses with removal of 5 cm of normal bowel on either side of the affected area.
- Leiomyosarcoma – surgical resection is the treatment of choice; survival variably reported as one (80%) to two years (67%).
- Non-GIST non-smooth muscle sarcomas – treat with wide surgical excision.
- Mast cell tumors – treatment with surgery, prednisolone, lomustine, chlorambucil, and toceranib has been attempted with variable results; additional studies are needed.

 COMMENTS

Expected Course and Prognosis

- Canine intestinal adenocarcinoma – annular tumors are associated with the shortest survival time with surgery (two months), multifocal nodular or "cobblestone" lesions (12 months), and solitary lesions (32 months).
- Feline intestinal mast cell tumors – prognosis for feline MCT thought to be poor due to inability to resect with wide margins and metastases at the time of diagnosis. More recent studies show variability in outcomes with survival times in cats ranging from two to 39 months with treatment. Dogs generally have a very poor prognosis (<2-month survival).

- GIST – two-year survival not uncommon for fully resected tumors; larger or metastatic tumors may benefit from tyrosine kinase inhibitors.
- Leiomyosarcoma – true extent of disease and outcomes not well understood as many tumors in the past were misdiagnosed due to lack of immunohistochemistry.

Abbreviations

- COX = cyclooxygenase
- GIST = gastrointestinal stromal tumor
- MCT = mast cell tumor
- NSAID = nonsteroidal antiinflammatory drug
- SMA = smooth muscle actin

See Also

- Diarrhea, Acute
- Hematemesis
- Hematochezia
- Intestinal Neoplasia, Benign
- Melena
- Vomiting, Acute

Suggested Reading

Barrett LE, Skorupski K, Brown DC, et al. Outcome following treatment of feline gastrointestinal mast cell tumours. Vet Comp Oncol 2018;16:188–193.

Church EM, Mehlhaff CJ, Patnaik AK. Colorectal adenocarcinoma in dogs: 78 cases (1973–1984). J Am Vet Med Assoc 1987;191(6):727–730.

Crawshaw J, Berg J, Sardinas J, et al. Prognosis for dogs with nonlymphomatous, small intestinal tumors treated by surgical excision. J Am Anim Hosp Assoc 1998;34(6):451–456.

Frost D, Lasota J, Miettinen M. Gastrointestinal stromal tumors and leiomyomas in the dog: a histopathologic, immunohistochemical, and molecular genetic study of 50 cases. Vet Pathol 2003;40(1):42–54.

Halsey CHC, Powers BE, Kamstock DA. Feline intestinal sclerosing mast cell tumour: 50 cases (1997–2008). Vet Comp Oncol 2010;8:72–79.

Hanazono K, Fukumoto S, Hirayama K, et al. Predicting metastatic potential of gastrointestinal stromal tumors in dog by ultrasonography. J Vet Med Sci 2012;74(11):1477–1482.

Hayes S, Yuzbasiyan-Gurkan V, Gregory-Bryson E, Kiupel M. Classification of canine nonangiogenic, nonlymphogenic, gastrointestinal sarcomas based on microscopic, immunohistochemical, and molecular characteristics. Vet Pathol 2013;50(5):779–788.

Irie M, Takeuchi Y, Ohtake Y, et al. Imatinib mesylate treatment in a dog with gastrointestinal stromal tumors with a c-kit mutation. J Vet Med Sci 2015;77(11):1535–1539.

Maas C, ter Haar G, van der Gaag I, Kirpensteijn J. Reclassification of small intestinal and cecal smooth muscle tumors in 72 dogs: clinical, histologic, and immunohistochemical evaluation. Vet Surg 2007;36(4):302–313.

McEntee MF, Cates J, Neilsen N. Cyclooxygenase-2 expression in spontaneous intestinal neoplasia of domestic dogs. Vet Pathol 2002;39(4):428–436.

Author: Carrie A. Wood DVM, DACVIM (Oncology)

Chapter 73

Intussusception

DEFINITION/OVERVIEW

- Telescoping or invagination of one intestinal segment into the lumen of an adjoining segment.
- Intussusceptions are classified based on localization of the affected segment within the gastrointestinal (GI) tract.
- Ileocolic and jejunojejunal intussusceptions are most commonly described. Other types include gastroesophageal, pylorogastric, duodenojejunal, cecocolic, and colocolic intussusceptions.
- The intussusceptum is more commonly the proximal intestinal segment. It is the segment entrapped within another portion of intestine.
- The intussuscipien is often the more distal intestinal segment. It is the segment that engulfs the adjacent bowel segment.

ETIOLOGY/PATHOPHYSIOLOGY

- The exact mechanism is not known, but it is often associated with enteritis (from parasitism, viral or bacterial infections, dietary indiscretion, foreign body, and masses).
- Intestinal irritation results in hypermotility of one intestinal segment, allowing it to invaginate into another. The direction of intussusception can be from proximal to distal or vice versa.
- Intussusceptions can occur at one or multiple sites.
- Initial invagination causes partial intestinal obstruction which can progress to complete obstruction.
- Vascular compromise commonly occurs in the intussusceptum due to increased intraluminal pressure or vessel avulsion, resulting in marked edema, intramural hemorrhage, and blood extravasation into the intestinal lumen.
- Eventual intestinal devitalization occurs from decreased oxygen delivery to the mucosal layer. This leads to a lack of effective mucosal barrier to bacteria, resulting in endotoxin transfer into the bloodstream, along with intestinal contents into the abdominal cavity.

Systems Affected

- Gastrointestinal – mechanical obstruction, ileus, peritonitis.
- Cardiovascular – fluid loss (vomiting, diarrhea), hypovolemia.

Blackwell's Five-Minute Veterinary Consult Clinical Companion: Small Animal Gastrointestinal Diseases,
First Edition. Edited by Jocelyn Mott and Jo Ann Morrison.
© 2019 John Wiley & Sons, Inc. Published 2019 by John Wiley & Sons, Inc.
Companion website: www.fiveminutevet.com/gastrointestinal

SIGNALMENT/HISTORY

- More commonly reported in dogs than cats.
- German shepherds, Siamese, and Burmese cats more commonly reported with intestinal intussusception than other breeds. German shepherds are also more predisposed to gastroesophageal intussusception.
- Most intussusceptions occur in immature animals <1 year old.
- Adult dogs should be screened for diseases such as intestinal neoplasia or other mural disease.
- Cats can have a bimodal occurrence: young cats (<1 year) have idiopathic lesions, and those >6 years tend to have concurrent inflammatory bowel disease or alimentary lymphoma.
- There is no documented sex predilection for intestinal intussusception in small animals.

Risk Factors

- Intestinal parasitism, dietary indiscretion, linear foreign bodies, intestinal masses, bacterial/viral induced enteritis (especially postparvoviral enteritis), environmental change, or prior abdominal surgery are reported risk factors.
- Association of intussusception with previous surgery may be due to ileus, adhesion or anastomotic malfunction.

Historical Findings

- Most patients have a history of illness, environmental change, or recent surgery.
- Vomiting.
- Abdominal pain.
- Scant, bloody diarrhea.
- Abdominal distension.
- Anorexia.
- Weight loss.
- If chronic, often show intractable, intermittent diarrhea, depression, emaciation.

CLINICAL FEATURES

- Clinical signs can span several weeks, with progression from partial to complete obstruction.
- Gastroesophageal intussusceptions typically cause more severe clinical signs of regurgitation than intussusceptions located in a more aboral location.
- May have overt abdominal pain or discomfort.
- An elongated, thickened (sausage-shaped) intestinal loop may be palpable within the abdomen (53% have palpable abdominal mass).
- Signs of dehydration can exist: tacky mucous membrane, prolonged capillary refill time, increased skin tent.
- Depression, lethargy, anorexia, emaciation, and poor body condition can be observed.
- Pyrexia or hypothermia (cats) can be present.
- Ileocolic intussusception may protrude from the rectum. This can be differentiated from a rectal prolapse via probing along the side of the protruding tissue. The presence of a blind-ending fornix indicates the existence of a rectal prolapse rather than an intussusception.
- Any disease that alters gastrointestinal motility may lead to an intussusception.

DIFFERENTIAL DIAGNOSIS

- Enteritis (e.g., bacterial – clostridial, viral – parvovirus, distemper virus, inflammatory).
- Intestinal obstruction: foreign body, neoplasia, granuloma, previous adhesion from surgery, intestinal volvulus or torsion, incarceration, strictures, abscesses, granulomas.
- Physiologic ileus secondary to inflammation, e.g., parvovirus or peritonitis.

DIAGNOSTICS

Complete Blood Count/Biochemistry/Urinalysis

- Leukogram – can range from normal to leukopenia (especially with sepsis or parvoviral infection) to leukocytosis (either stress response or sepsis).
- Hematocrit can be elevated (dehydration or underlying hemorrhagic gastroenteritis) or decreased (cases of intraluminal hemorrhage).
- Biochemistry – can show electrolyte abnormalities due to loss through vomiting or diarrhea, including hyponatremia, hypochloremia, and hypokalemia. May be azotemic (prerenal) if significantly dehydrated. May also be hypoalbuminemic due to effusive loss into intestinal lumen or from chronic intussusception (protein loss from congested mucosa).
- Urinalysis – may reveal elevated specific gravity in response to dehydration.

Other Laboratory Tests

- Lactate: may be elevated due to sepsis, septic abdomen, or vascular compromise from loss of intestinal integrity.
- Blood gas: may show metabolic acidosis secondary to vomiting, dehydration, hypovolemia, hypoperfusion. A hypochloremic, hypokalemic, metabolic alkalosis can result if primarily gastric vomiting (e.g., pyloric obstruction).
- Fecal examination: may reveal parasite infestation.

Imaging

- Survey radiographs may reveal area of obstruction, such as a tubular soft tissue mass, or gas highlighting area of intussusception. An obstructive intestinal pattern is more commonly identified with jejunojejunal intussusception than ileocolic intussusception (Figure 73.1).
- A barium contrast study may assist in localization of intussusception, a filling defect may be present when barium within the lumen surrounds the intussusceptum, or contrast accumulation between the intussusceptum and intussuscipien walls.
- Gastroesophageal intussusceptions often show a soft tissue mass within the lumen of the thoracic esophagus near the esophageal hiatus at the diaphragm.
- Ultrasound is most helpful in the diagnosis of intussusceptions. In the transverse plane, a target-like lesion with multilayers of concentric rings is pathognomonic. Longitudinal sections can demonstrate multiple parallel lines (Figures 73.2, 73.3). Other concurrent abnormalities that may be detected include lymphadenopathy, infiltrative intestinal lesions, and masses.
- Coloscopy may identify invaginated intestine in the colon with ileocolic or cecocolic intussusception. Gentle and careful application of the scope is required.

Pathologic Findings

- Gross examination of affected segment reveals a telescoping segment of bowel into an adjacent segment.
- Histopathologic examination reveals variable severity of venous congestion, edema, vascular compromise, intestinal ischemia or necrosis and peritonitis.

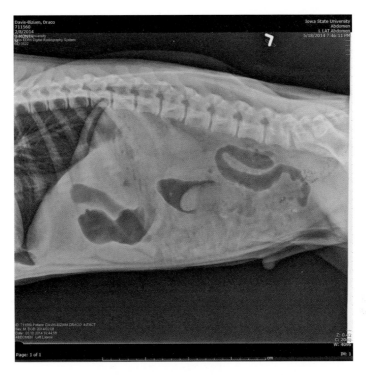

■ **Fig. 73.1.** Left lateral abdominal radiograph of a juvenile canine. In the midabdomen, there is a single loop of intestine that contains a tubular soft tissue opacity projecting into the bowel lumen, consistent with an intussusception. This tubular structure is surrounded cranially by a cap of intraluminal gas, and the intestinal loop is moderately dilated. The two populations of small intestine are consistent with a mechanical obstruction. Source: Courtesy of Iowa State University.

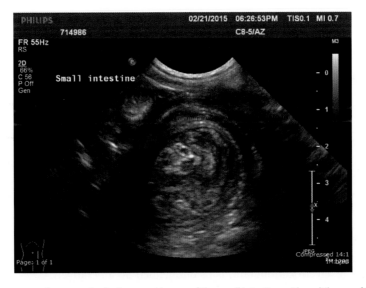

■ **Fig. 73.2.** A transverse (cross-section) ultrasound image of the small intestine with multilayers of intestine, similar to a tube within a tube. This is consistent with an intussusception. Source: Courtesy of Iowa State University.

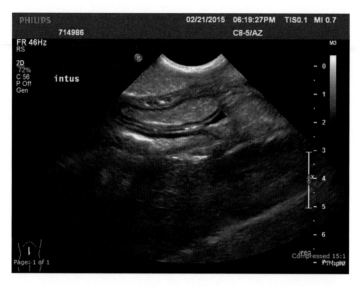

■ **Fig. 73.3.** A longitudinal ultrasound image of the small intestine. A loop of small intestine has telescoped into another, resulting in a thickened structure with too many intestinal layers, consistent with an intestinal intussusception. Source: Courtesy of Iowa State University.

 # THERAPEUTICS

Drug(s) of Choice

■ Medical therapy should be aimed at correcting fluid, electrolyte, and acid–base imbalance.
■ Antibiotics are not recommended except in cases where septic peritonitis is present.
■ Empiric deworming (praziquantel/pyrantel pamoate/febantel) is recommended, especially in puppies.

Precautions/Interactions

■ Pediatric patients should not be fasted for longer than 4–8 hours to prevent hypoglycemia.
■ The use of promotility agents, e.g., metoclopramide, is contraindicated by some surgeons due to potential for recurrence of intussusception.

Alternative Drugs

Other antiemetics such as maropitant, dolasetron or ondansetron can be used instead of metoclopramide if nausea or vomiting becomes persistent.

Appropriate Health Care

■ Patient stabilization is paramount if there are signs of septic peritonitis or systemic illness.
■ If septic peritonitis exists, appropriate antibiotics should be initiated as soon as feasible, along with adjusting fluid administration and electrolyte/blood gas management.
■ Appropriate analgesics should be provided.

Nursing Care

■ Appropriate patient management with fluid therapy, acid–base balance, and vital monitoring (blood pressure, electrocardiogram) is recommended perioperatively.
■ Keep the perineum clean, especially if diarrhea is present.
■ Appropriate maintenance and utilization of any feeding tubes is required.

Diet

- Most patients should be fed within 24 hours of surgical correction. If vomiting intractably, appropriate therapy should be instituted with antiemetics or careful use of prokinetics.
- Management with a temporary feeding tube may be necessary, e.g., via enterostomy tube, if the patient is debilitated, hypoalbuminemic, vomiting or anorectic. Other forms of nutritional support may be necessary (esophagostomy or gastrostomy tube, parenteral nutrition) if sepsis is present.

Activity

Restricted, controlled activity for 10–14 days postoperatively.

Surgical Considerations

- Surgery is the treatment of choice. Intussusceptions are considered a surgical emergency and surgery should be performed as soon as the patient is stable enough to withstand anesthesia and surgery (Figure 73.4).
- A thorough abdominal exploratory procedure should be performed, in addition to identification of the affected segment.
- Surgical treatments include simple reduction, manual reduction with plication, intestinal resection/anastomosis, and intestinal resection/anastomosis with plication. There was no statistically significant difference in recurrence rate of intussusceptions when various surgical techniques were compared.
- Occasionally, percutaneous manual reduction of the intussusception can be achieved (under general anesthesia); however, most cases require surgical reduction and ancillary procedures to prevent recurrence. Reduction may occur simply with general anesthesia leading to negative exploratory laparotomy findings.
- Intraoperative reduction of the intussusception can be performed manually by applying gentle traction and milking the intussusceptum out of the intussuscipien.
- If manual reduction is not possible, or if the bowel has questionable viability, an intestinal resection and anastomosis may be necessary. Submission of the resected segment for histopathology is strongly recommended.

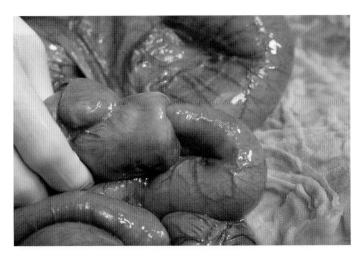

■ **Fig. 73.4.** An intraoperative image of a jejunocolic intussusception. The orad end of the jejunum (intussusceptum) has telescoped into the lumen of the ileum and colon (intussuscipien) held by the hand. Source: Courtesy of Iowa State University.

- Careful evaluation for viability, perforation, and serosal damage of the affected and adjacent segments of bowel will dictate whether simple reduction or a resection and anastomosis should be performed.
- Biopsy of the intestine at the time of surgical correction may help identify the cause of intussusception.
- Enteroplication or enteroenteropexy has been previously reported to help prevent recurrence. However, recent articles contraindicate this, as it does not show any benefit. It is also important to exercise care when performing this procedure. The loops created in the bowel should be gently handled; any sharp turns of the bowel loops are to be avoided. The submucosal layer of the adjacent loops of bowel should be included in the sutures, but the lumen should not be entered.
- Use of absorbable monofilament sutures and gentle handling of the intestinal loops is required.
- If intestinal perforation or signs of septic peritonitis exist, appropriate lavage and source control are necessary.
- Placement of a temporary feeding tube (esophagostomy, gastrostomy or jejunostomy) should be considered during surgery as the case indicates.
- Surgical reduction of gastroesophageal intussusception is recommended with left- and right-sided gastropexy performed along with hiatal reduction.

COMMENTS

Client Education

- Surgical management is strongly recommended as this is a surgical emergency.
- Identification and correcting underlying disease is ideal, but many cases have an unknown etiology (idiopathic).
- Spontaneous reduction of intussusception is possible but uncommon.

Patient Monitoring

- Postoperative management would include fluid therapy, appropriate analgesia, and correction of nausea, acid–base abnormalities, and nutritional support.
- Intestinal dehiscence typically occurs 3–5 days postoperatively.

Prevention/Avoidance

Prevention of underlying causes can be variable, such as vaccinations against parvovirus, intestinal parasite control, limiting opportunities for dietary indiscretion or foreign body ingestion.

Possible Complications

- Recurrence usually occurs proximal to anastomotic site or plicated section of bowel (up to 27% reported).
- Recurrence of an intussusception was not related to either the bowel segment involved or whether a simple reduction, bowel resection, or intestinal plication was performed at the initial surgery.
- Most recurrences happen within the first few days of surgery, but recurrences have been reported up to three weeks after surgery.
- Septic peritonitis – may result from postoperative intestinal dehiscence, intraoperative contamination, or preexisting septic peritonitis.
- Short bowel syndrome is possible if large sections of small intestine are resected.
- Megaesophagus may persist in patients with gastroesophageal intussusception.

Expected Course and Prognosis

Generally good prognosis for intestinal intussusception with early recognition of intussusception, aggressive fluid therapy, and prompt surgical correction. However, recurrence rates are approximately 11–25%.

Synonyms

- Intestinal invagination
- Intestinal telescoping

Abbreviations

- GI = gastrointestinal

See Also

- Acute Abdomen
- Canine Parvovirus Infection
- Gastrointestinal Obstruction
- Hiatal Hernia
- Parasites, Gastrointestinal
- Rectal and Anal Prolapse
- Short Bowel Syndrome

Suggested Reading

Burkitt JM, Drobatz KJ, Saunders HM, Washabau RJ. Signalment, history, and outcome of cats with gastrointestinal tract intussusception: 20 cases (1986-2000). J Am Vet Med Assoc 2009;234(6):771–776.

Levitt L, Bauer MS. Intussusception in dogs and cats: a review of 36 cases. Can Vet J 1992;33(10):660–664.

Radlinsky MG. Surgery of the digestive system. In: Fossum TW, ed. Small Animal Surgery, 4th edn. St Louis: Elsevier, 2013, pp. 524–528.

Acknowledgments: The authors and editors acknowledge the prior contribution of Dr S. Brent Reimer.

Authors: Louisa Ho-Eckart BVSc Hons, MS, DACVS-SA, Eric Zellner DVM, DACVS-SA

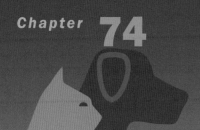

Chapter 74

Irritable Bowel Syndrome

DEFINITION/OVERVIEW

- Chronic idiopathic large bowel diarrhea (CILBD), previously known as irritable bowel syndrome (IBS), is a diagnosis of exclusion. Patients with CILBD experience intermittent chronic large bowel gastrointestinal (GI) signs (diarrhea, constipation, tenesmus, hematochezia) in the absence of significant structural intestinal pathology or other identifiable disease.
- The prevalence of CILBD in dogs as a primary disorder ranges in the literature from 5% to 26%.
- CILBD prevalence may be underrepresented as empiric fiber response and diet trials may resolve clinical signs in many patients that would otherwise be diagnosed with CILBD.

ETIOLOGY/PATHOPHYSIOLOGY

- The pathophysiology of CILBD is incompletely understood. Studies in affected dogs are lacking.
- Underlying etiology is likely multifactorial and includes altered motility, visceral hypersensitivity, and a psychosomatic relationship relating to stress and behavioral disorders.

Systems Affected

Gastrointestinal.

SIGNALMENT/HISTORY

- Dog (uncommon); cat (rare).
- Any breed; suspected to be more common in active working dogs or individual dogs with anxious temperaments.

Risk Factors

- Stress (e.g., changes in the household, change of diet, separation anxiety) may or may not be associated with episodes in some patients.
- Behavioral disorders – anxiety, aggression, etc. may be associated with CILBD.

Historical Findings

- Chronic, intermittent, large bowel signs (tenesmus, frequent small volumes of diarrhea, hematochezia, dyschezia, etc.).
- Large bowel signs may be mixed with periods of diarrhea, normal stool, and constipation.
- Abdominal pain, ileus, vomiting, anal pruritus, and anorexia are variably present.

Blackwell's Five-Minute Veterinary Consult Clinical Companion: Small Animal Gastrointestinal Diseases,
First Edition. Edited by Jocelyn Mott and Jo Ann Morrison.
© 2019 John Wiley & Sons, Inc. Published 2019 by John Wiley & Sons, Inc.
Companion website: www.fiveminutevet.com/gastrointestinal

CLINICAL FEATURES

- Physical exam findings are typically unremarkable but helpful in ruling out other causes of signs, i.e., anal sac and prostatic disease.
- Rectal palpation may reveal signs consistent with large bowel diarrhea.

 DIFFERENTIAL DIAGNOSIS

Causes of Large Bowel Disease

- Whipworms.
- Inflammatory bowel disease (IBD).
- *Clostridium perfringens* or *C. difficile*-associated diarrhea.
- Invasive adherent *Escherichia coli*-associated granulomatous colitis.
- Diet-responsive enteropathy.
- Dietary indiscretion (foreign body-induced coloproctitis) or intolerance.
- Pancreatitis can cause inflammation of the transverse colon with signs of colitis.
- Histoplasmosis.
- Pythiosis.
- Colorectal neoplasia.
- Cecal inversion.
- Gluten enteropathy.
- Anal sacculitis.
- Megacolon (colorectal pseudoobstruction).

Diseases with Similar Signs

- Dysuria/stranguria – exclude with observation, urinalysis, and imaging.
- Prostatic disease – exclude with rectal examination and imaging.
- Peritoneal adhesions.
- Perineal hernia – exclude with imaging and physical examination.
- Disorders or injury affecting innervation of the GI tract via intestinal intrinsic nervous system, vagal nerve, and pelvic nerve plexuses.

 DIAGNOSTICS

- Based on the exclusion of all other potential causes of large bowel signs.
- Criteria – history of recurrent large bowel signs, negative fecal exam, unremarkable complete blood count (CBC), serum chemistry and absence of significant abnormalities on abdominal imaging, colonoscopy and histopathology and a failure to respond with empiric deworming (particularly for whipworm) or a hypoallergenic diet. (Figure 74.1).

Complete Blood Count/Biochemistry/Urinalysis

- Typically unremarkable – used to rule out other diseases.
- Evidence of dehydration (hypernatremia, hyperalbuminemia, etc.) – uncommon.

Other Laboratory Tests

Fecal flotation and rectal scraping cytology typically unremarkable but should be performed to rule out other etiologies, prior to invasive procedures.

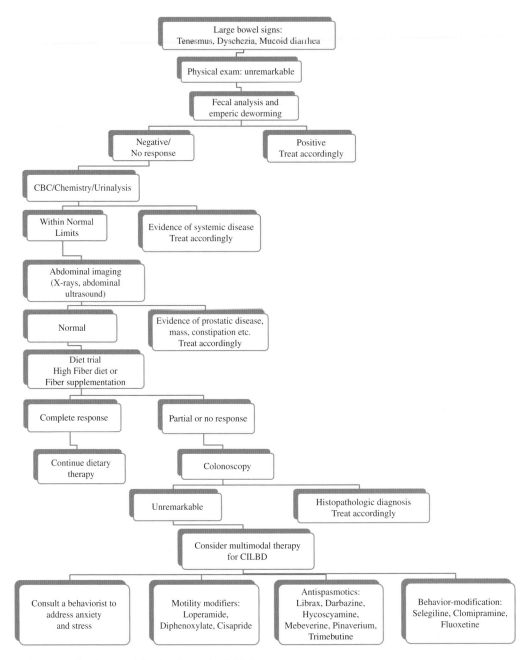

■ Fig. 74.1. Flowchart to aid in the diagnosis of CILBD.

Imaging

- Survey and contrast radiographic studies of the abdomen – unremarkable or may show segmental luminal gas distension.
- Abdominal ultrasonography – unremarkable.

Other Diagnostic Procedures

- Endoscopy/colonoscopy – minimal changes (increased friability, granularity, hyperemia) have been reported (Figure 74.2).
- Exploratory surgery with biopsy generally unremarkable.

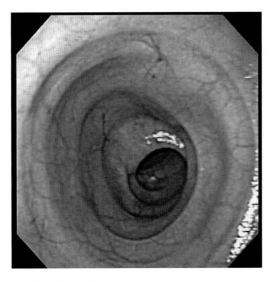

■ **Fig. 74.2.** Normal colonoscopy in a dog with CILBD.

Pathologic Findings

- Histopathology – usually unremarkable; minimal changes (increased/decreased lymphoid follicles, decreased visualization of vascularity, local colonic spasm, etc.) have been reported.
- Concurrent chronic intestinal disease (e.g., IBD) may be present and needs to be successfully managed prior to consideration of a diagnosis and treatment for CILBD.

 # THERAPEUTICS

- Many dogs with CILBD respond to fiber supplementation as a sole treatment. The lack of response to fiber justifies the use of pharmaceutical behavior therapy.
- The use of motility modifiers and antispasmodics may be attempted in acute, severe flare-ups with variable success.

Drug(s) of Choice

- Drug therapy may range from short term (days) to life-long.
- Most cases of CILBD can involve both gastrointestinal hypermotility (spasmodic) and potential sensory changes thought to result in forms of dysmotility via interference with GI intrinsic nervous system activity. Librax™ (an antispasmodic with anxiolytic) or gabapentin (5–10 mg/kg q 12 h) for possible neuropathic pain (if pelvic plexus stimulation is suspected) may be prescribed.
- Start at lower end of dosage range.

Motility Modifiers

Antidiarrheals

Opiates improve signs by increasing rhythmic segmentation.
- Loperamide: 0.1–0.2 mg/kg PO q 8–12 h.
- Diphenoxylate: 0.05–0.2 mg/kg PO q 8–12 h.

Prokinetics

May help in cases of constipation (once GI obstruction has been ruled out).
- Cisapride: (prokinetic) 0.5 mg/kg to maximum of 10 mg PO q 8–12 h.
- Gabapentin: 1–10 mg/kg PO q 12 h for possible neuropathic pain.

Antispasmodics (Neurotropics)/Tranquilizers/Anxiolytics

Used to relieve anxiety, abdominal cramping, bloating, and distress.

- Librax (chlordiazepoxide (anxiolytic), and clidinium bromide (anticholinergic)): 0.1–0.25 mg of clidinium/kg PO q 8–24 h. Given at time of stressful event or anticipated clinical signs. Give for a few days only.
- Darbazine™ (isopropamide (anticholinergic) and prochlorperazine (tranquilizer)): 0.14–0.22 mg/kg SQ q 12 h. Use during acute paroxysms.
- Hycoscyamine: 0.003–0.006 mg/kg PO q 8–12 h. Use during acute paroxysms only.

Antispasmodics (Musculotropic)

- Mebeverine: 2.5–5 mg/kg PO q 12 h.
- Pinaverium: 1 mg/kg PO q 12 h.
- Trimebutine: 0.33 mg/kg PO q 8 h.

Parenteral Antiemetics

Can be used parenterally if nausea and vomiting preclude the use of oral medication.

- Maropitant: 1 mg/kg SQ dogs q 24 h in dogs.
- Prochlorperazine: 0.1–0.5 mg/kg q 6–24 h SQ or IM.

Behavior-Modifying Agents

- Selegiline (dopamine agonist): 0.5 mg/kg PO q 24 h; titrate up to 2 mg/kg q 24 h if no response within two months.
- Clomipramine (tricyclic antidepressant): 1 mg/kg PO q 12 h; titrate up to 3 mg/kg PO q 12 h if no response within 14 days.
- Fluoxetine (selective serotonin reuptake inhibitor (SSRI)): 1–2 mg/kg PO q 24 h.

Precautions/Interactions

- Opiates – respiratory dysfunction, hepatic encephalopathy, constipation and/or severe debilitation. Be aware of potential risk for diversion/human abuse with veterinary prescriptions.
- Anticholinergics – cardiac disease, renal disease, hypertension, constipation, and/or hyperthyroidism.

Appropriate Health Care

Patients must retain the ability to successfully pass fecal material, with appropriate analgesic intervention as necessary.

Nursing Care

- The perineal area may become soiled and the presence of matted hair/stool may preclude fecal passage. Keep the perineum clean; hair may need to be clipped.
- Gently clean skin and use topical medications if clinically indicated.
- Prevent self-trauma.

Diet

- A high-fiber diet is recommended with or without a known behavior disorder. Many dogs with CILBD respond to diet alone. A diet with a blend of soluble and insoluble fiber can be fed. Many veterinary prescription and commercially available diets are supplemented with fiber. Alternatively, psyllium can be added to the diet. If not helpful, the addition of insoluble (methylcellulose) fiber can be attempted with variable success.
- Psyllium – approximately 1.3 mg/kg. Daily dose:
  - toy-breed dogs – 0.5 tablespoons (T).
  - small-breed dogs – 1 T.
  - medium-breed dogs – 2 T.
  - large-breed dogs – 3 T.

Activity

- Regular controlled exercise may help with GI motility.
- For high-energy dogs prone to anxious behaviors, regular exercise/training/activity is encouraged.

 COMMENTS

Client Education

- Reduce environmental stress as able.
- If possible, identify stressful triggers and remove from the environment.
- Monitor elimination habits closely and pursue veterinary consultation if concerns exist.

Prevention/Avoidance

- Maintain dietary consistency.
- Environmental manipulations as described above.

Expected Course and Prognosis

- Improvement in signs (improved stool, decreased mucus, tenesmus, dyschezia, etc.) should be noted within a few days of starting therapy.
- Prognosis is excellent if patients respond to fiber manipulation of the diet; however, dogs may require lifelong fiber supplementation.
- Most dogs will respond to medical management (diet/fiber, medication, etc.); however, a small subset may have no long-term resolution of signs.

Synonyms

- Chronic idiopathic large bowel diarrhea
- IBS
- IBD
- Large bowel diarrhea
- Stress colitis

Abbreviations

- CBC = complete blood count
- CILBD = chronic idiopathic large bowel diarrhea
- GI = gastrointestinal
- IBD = inflammatory bowel disease
- IBS = irritable bowel syndrome
- SSRI = selective serotonin reuptake inhibitor
- T = tablespoon

See Also

- Colitis and Proctitis
- Diarrhea, Chronic – Canine
- Diarrhea, Chronic – Feline
- Dyschezia and Tenesmus
- Fiber-responsive Large Bowel Diarrhea
- Hematochezia
- Inflammatory Bowel Disease
- Nutritional Approach to Chronic Enteropathies

Suggested Reading

Lecoindre P, Gaschen FP. Chronic idiopathic large bowel diarrhea in the dog. Vet Clin North Am Small Anim Pract 2001;41(2):447–456.

Acknowledgments: The author and editors acknowledge the previous contribution of Dr Mark E. Hitt.

Author: Alana Redfern DVM, MSc, DACVIM

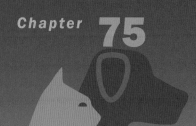
Lymphangiectasia

DEFINITION/OVERVIEW

An idiopathic, obstructive disorder of the gastrointestinal (GI) lymphatic system causing lymphatic hypertension and protein-losing enteropathy (PLE).

ETIOLOGY/PATHOPHYSIOLOGY

- Lymphatic obstruction produces dilation and rupture of intestinal lacteals with subsequent loss of lymph (i.e., plasma proteins, chylomicrons, and lymphocytes) into the intestinal lumen.
- Although some of the proteins may be digested and reabsorbed, excessive enteric loss of plasma proteins ultimately causes hypoalbuminemia with or without hypoglobulinemia.
- Hypoalbuminemia decreases plasma oncotic pressure, which, if severe, may lead to edema, ascites, and/or pleural effusion.

Causes

Primary Lymphangiectasia
Intestinal lymphatic dilation, often with intestinal crypt abscesses and/or intestinal lipogranu-lomas; intestinal inflammatory infiltrates range from essentially absent to moderately severe.

Secondary Lymphangiectasia
- Infiltrative intestinal disorders.
- Neoplasia (lymphosarcoma).
- Right-sided congestive heart failure – a rare cause of PLE in dogs.

Systems Affected
- Gastrointestinal – diarrhea.
- Respiratory – pleural effusion.
- Skin – subcutaneous edema; uncommon.
- Systemic – ascites.
- Vascular – thromboembolic disease; uncommon.

SIGNALMENT/HISTORY

- Occurs in dogs
- Increased prevalence in soft-coated wheaten terrier, Norwegian lundehund, and Yorkshire terrier. Soft-coated wheaten terriers may have concurrent protein-losing nephropathy.

Blackwell's Five-Minute Veterinary Consult Clinical Companion: Small Animal Gastrointestinal Diseases, First Edition. Edited by Jocelyn Mott and Jo Ann Morrison.
© 2019 John Wiley & Sons, Inc. Published 2019 by John Wiley & Sons, Inc.
Companion website: www.fiveminutevet.com/gastrointestinal

- Dogs of any age can be affected. Most common in young adult to middle-aged dogs.
- An increased prevalence has been reported in female soft-coated wheaten terriers; no sex predilection has been reported for other breeds.

Risk Factors

A familial tendency for lymphangiectasia has been reported for soft-coated wheaten terriers, Yorkshire terriers, and Norwegian Lundehunds, but the genetic basis has not been defined.

Historical Findings

- Clinical signs are variable.
- Diarrhea– chronic, intermittent, or continuous, watery to semi-solid consistency (typically small bowel type diarrhea); however, some animals do not have diarrhea.
- Normal to decreased appetite.
- Weight loss.
- Vomiting – uncommon.

CLINICAL FEATURES

- Physical examination findings are variable.
- Weight loss
- Diarrhea (varies in severity; may be absent).
- Ascites.
- Subcutaneous edema – uncommon.
- Dyspnea from pleural effusion.

DIFFERENTIAL DIAGNOSIS

- Lymphangiectasia must be differentiated from other causes of PLE (e.g., lymphoma, fungal infections).
- PLE must be differentiated from other causes of hypoalbuminemia.

DIAGNOSTICS

Complete Blood Count/Biochemistry/Urinalysis

- Hypoalbuminemia with or without hypoglobulinemia.
- Hypocholesterolemia.
- Hypocalcemia.
- Hypomagnesemia.
- Lymphopenia – inconsistent.

Other Laboratory Tests

Tests to Differentiate PLE from Other Causes of Hypoalbuminemia

- Serum chemistry profile and pre- and postprandial serum bile acids concentrations to rule out hepatic insufficiency.
- Urine protein:creatinine ratio to rule out protein-losing nephropathy.
- Fecal alpha-1-protease inhibitor concentration to help confirm intestinal protein loss, although this test is almost never necessary.

Tests to Differentiate Other Causes of Excessive Protein Loss into the GI Tract

- Fecal smear and flotation to rule out intestinal parasites.
- Serum trypsin-like immunoreactivity – exocrine pancreatic insufficiency is rarely associated with severe hypoalbuminemia.
- Fluid analysis of body cavity effusions – the effusion associated with lymphangiectasia is a low-protein transudate, but chyloabdomen and chylothorax may rarely be seen.

Imaging

- Abdominal ultrasound to help rule out infiltrative intestinal disease and other causes of PLE.
- Abdominal ultrasound sometimes shows hyperechoic mucosal striations, which are very suggestive of lymphangiectasia; corn oil administered orally 60–90 minutes before abdominal ultrasonography improves sensitivity.
- Survey thoracic radiographs or cardiac ultrasound to rule out cardiac disease and neoplasia.

Other Diagnostic Tests

- Endoscopy allows mucosal biopsy and sometimes allows visualization of dilated lacteals engorged with white chyle (Figure 75.1). Ileal biopsies should always be obtained because some patients have lymphangiectasia localized to the ileum.
- Laparotomy sometimes reveals "white spots" on the intestine which are lipogranulomas which are very suggestive of lymphangiectasia. Very rarely, one may see dilated intestinal lymphatics on the intestines. Laparotomy allows biopsies of intestines (full thickness) and lymph nodes, but may be risky in patients with severe hypoproteinemia.
- Capsule endoscopy after a fatty meal may be diagnostic.

Pathologic Findings

- Gross findings at necropsy rarely include dilated lymphatics visible as a web-like network throughout the mesentery and serosal surface.
- May see lipogranulomas (i.e., yellow-white nodules on the intestinal serosa or in the intestinal wall).
- Classic histopathology findings include ballooning distortion of villi caused by markedly dilated lacteals. Lipogranulomas in the mucosa or wall of the intestine are often seen. Intestinal crypt lesions are often seen in severely affected patients.

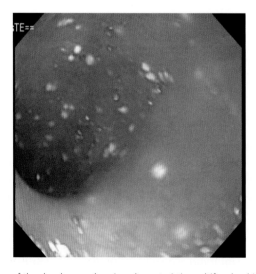

■ **Fig. 75.1.** Endoscopic view of the duodenum showing characteristic multifocal, white, grossly dilated lacteals.

- Villi can be edematous; some have a blunted appearance.
- Occasionally see mucosal edema or diffuse or multifocal accumulations of lymphocytes and plasma cells in the lamina propria.

 # THERAPEUTICS

Objectives of treatment are to control intestinal protein and lymphatic loss and facilitate intestinal nutrient absorption, stabilizing plasma oncotic pressure.

Drug(s) of Choice

- First, wait to see if dietary therapy alone is effective (i.e., the serum albumin clearly and obviously increases within 10 days). If dietary therapy is effective, then administer antiinflammatory therapy for 6–12 weeks and then stop.
- If dietary therapy by itself is not effective, then the antiinflammatory drugs are administered for 2–4 months and then gradually tapered off while monitoring the serum albumin concentration. If the serum albumin concentration clearly begins to decrease as the drugs are tapered off, then the tapering is stopped.
- Glucocorticoids (e.g., prednisolone 2 mg/kg PO daily) or cyclosporine (3-6 mg/kg PO q 12 h) are commonly used.
- Sometimes either azathioprine (2.2 mg/kg PO q 48 h) or chlorambucil (4–6 mg/m² PO q 24 h) – do not use both; may be combined with prednisolone if cyclosporine is too expensive. In large-breed dogs, the starting dose of cyclosporine, chlorambucil, and azathioprine should be more conservative than in small-breed dogs.
- Diuretics such as furosemide (1 mg/kg q 12 h) or spironolactone (1 mg/kg q 12 h) are reasonable in animals that are not responding to dietary/medical therapy but with severe ascites causing excessive pressure on the diaphragm, resulting in respiratory compromise (abdominocentesis is typically the first step in such cases).

Precautions/Interactions

Severe protein loss and resultant hypoproteinemia may affect distribution of highly protein-bound drugs.

Appropriate Health Care

- Monitoring and maintenance of lean body mass as much as possible.
- Cobalamin may be administered if the patient is hypocobalaminemic.
- May need hospitalization if complications due to hypoalbuminemia develop.

Nursing Care

Monitor for respiratory difficulty secondary to severe ascites causing excessive pressure on diaphragm or severe pleural effusion.

Diet

- Ultra low-fat diet with high-quality protein. Avoid diets that are excessively high in fiber. If dietary therapy alone is effective, will see serum albumin clearly and obviously increase within 7–10 days.
- Dogs with concurrent lymphangiectasia and inflammatory bowel disease (a relatively uncommon situation) may benefit from a commercial hypoallergenic hydrolyzed protein diet that is severely restricted in dietary fat.

- Long-chain triglycerides stimulate intestinal lymph flow and may lead to increased intestinal protein loss. Supplementation of medium chain triglycerides (MCT) oil is not recommended.

Activity

Normal.

Surgical Considerations

- When intestinal lymphangiectasia is secondary to an identifiable lymphatic obstruction, consider surgery to relieve the obstruction. Patients that benefit from surgical intervention are very rare.
- Pericardiectomy may be indicated in cases of constrictive pericarditis – this is very rare in dogs.
- Anesthesia may be challenging due to low plasma oncotic pressure and the presence of body cavity effusions impinging on the diaphragm.

 COMMENTS

Client Education

- Discuss unpredictable disease progression and response to therapy.
- Explain that this is a disease that is often controlled but almost never cured once and for all.

Patient Monitoring

- Patients need to be reevaluated periodically since this disease has a propensity for recurrence or relapse.
- Body weight, serum albumin concentrations, and evidence of recurrent clinical signs (pleural effusion, ascites, and/or edema).
- It is imperative to use the same laboratory when repeating measurement of serum albumin and lipemic, hemolyzed or icteric serum must be avoided.

Possible Complications

- Respiratory difficulty from pleural effusion.
- Severe protein-calorie depletion.
- Intractable diarrhea.

Expected Course and Prognosis

- Prognosis is uncertain. Early diagnosis seems to be associated with better prognosis.
- Some animals fail to respond to treatment.
- Remissions of several months to more than two years can be achieved in many patients if they are diagnosed early.

Abbreviations

- GI = gastrointestinal
- MCT = medium chain triglyceride
- PLE = protein-losing enteropathy

See Also

- Cobalamin Deficiency
- Diarrhea, Chronic – Canine
- Nutritional Approach to Chronic Enteropathies
- Protein-Losing Enteropathy

Suggested Reading

Bota D, Lecoindre A, Poujade A, et al. Protein-losing enteropathy in Yorkshire terriers – retrospective study in 31 dogs. Rev Med Vet 2016;167:2–9.

Larson RN, Ginn JA, Bell CM, et al. Duodenal endoscopic findings and histopathologic confirmation of intestinal lymphangiectasia in dogs. J Vet Intern Med 2012;26:1087–1092.

Okanishi H, Yoshioka R, Kagawa Y, et al. The clinical efficacy of dietary fat restriction in treatment of dogs with intestinal lymphangiectasia. J Vet Intern Med 2014;28:809–817.

Pollard RE, Johnson EG, Pesavento PA, et al. Effects of corn oil administered orally on conspicuity of ultrasonographic small intestinal lesions in dogs with lymphangiectasia. Vet Radiol Ultrasound 2013;54:390–397.

Rudinsky AJ, Howard JP, Bishop MA, et al. Dietary management of presumptive protein-losing etneropathy in Yorkshire terriers. J Small Anim Pract 2017;58:103–108.

Author: Michael D. Willard DVM, MS, DACVIM

Chapter 76

Nutritional Approach to Chronic Enteropathies

The gastrointestinal (GI) tract represents the body's largest organ of communication with the external environment, surpassing even the surface area of the skin. As such, healthy GI function is essential for overall health and well-being, while dysfunction risks exposing the body to external pathogens and toxins. Enterocytes lining the GI tract are responsible for the uptake of all dietary nutrients, while immune cells, making up the GI tract's own specialized mucosa-associated and gut-associated lymphoid tissues, are the first line of defense against potential invading pathogens. Chronic conditions of the GI tract not only impair nutrient uptake, resulting in malnutrition, but compromised immune defenses also allow disease to establish within the body.

A critical consideration for nutritional therapy of patients with chronic GI compromise is the amenability of many of these disorders to either mostly or entirely with dietary management. Food types can have direct effects on the structure and function of the GI tract by influencing enterocyte health, luminal pH, gut microflora, motility, and secretion. Optimal nutritional support, therefore, is crucial to maintain normal gut function and assist recovery in patients with chronic GI disorders. The underlying cause must be addressed, where possible, by following key nutritional factors, while additional nutritional considerations can promote healing and return of normal gut function.

Common chronic enteropathies encountered in companion animal practice may be divided into the following categories: dietary, inflammatory, and functional. The causes and types of chronic enteropathies in dogs and cats are quite similar, although prevalence may be different between the two species. Although there are numerous pathogeneses of chronic enteropathies, most animals present with similar, nonspecific signs: diarrhea and/or vomiting, malaise, inappetence, dyschezia, tenesmus, and weight loss. General recommendations for nutritional approaches to chronic enteropathies focus on maintaining sufficient caloric intake, avoiding foods which irritate the gut or exacerbate the animal's condition, and supporting maintenance of lean tissue. These general recommendations, as outlined below (and provided in Table 76.1), are sufficient for most patients, although specific nutritional recommendations for the most commonly encountered enteropathies are covered as well.

OVERALL NUTRITIONAL CONSIDERATIONS

Energy

Adequate energy intake is a critical factor for all patients with enteropathies. Sufficient provision of nonprotein calories, i.e., fat and carbohydrates, ensures that dietary and body stores of protein are spared from catabolism for energy production and that dietary protein is instead utilized to regenerate damaged enterocytes (Harris et al. 2017). It is important that sufficient

---

Blackwell's Five-Minute Veterinary Consult Clinical Companion: Small Animal Gastrointestinal Diseases,
First Edition. Edited by Jocelyn Mott and Jo Ann Morrison.
© 2019 John Wiley & Sons, Inc. Published 2019 by John Wiley & Sons, Inc.
Companion website: www.fiveminutevet.com/gastrointestinal

TABLE 76.1. **Recommended components for nutritional support in chronic enteropathies.**

Key nutritional factor	Requirement	Cats (DM basis)	Dogs (DM basis)
Energy density	High	>4200 kcal/kg	>4000 kcal/kg
Protein	>87% digestible*	30–40%**	20–30%**
Carbohydrates	>90% digestible	<40%	<60%
Fiber	Low	<5%	<5%
	Moderate†	7–15%	7–15%
Fat	Moderate††	15–22%	12–15%

*Hydrolyzed proteins are highly digestible and are particularly indicated in cases of hypersensitivity.
**May be increased if the animal is underweight or has evidence of muscle wasting and/or low serum albumin and total protein concentrations.
†Fiber-enhanced diets may not meet >4000 kcal/kg recommendation due to decreased energy density.
††Low (<10%) in cases with lymphangiectasia.
DM, dry matter.

nonprotein calories from highly digestible sources are provided to maintain, or achieve, an optimal body condition. Highly digestible, energy-dense diets also reduce the load on the gut and allow energy requirements to be met with smaller meals, an important consideration in animals with decreased appetite.

Protein

A high intake of dietary protein is often indicated, in order to provide enough amino acids for recovery and regeneration of affected tissues and to prevent protein-calorie malnutrition. Also, in animals with protein-losing enteropathies (PLE), provision of adequate protein is essential to replace luminal losses. Protein quality and digestibility must also be high, as undigested amino acids reaching the colon can feed pathogenic bacterial populations and exacerbate disease. Hydrolyzed protein sources are particularly highly digestible and also beneficial in cases with dietary hypersensitivity.

Carbohydrates and Fiber

Provision of ample nonprotein calories is essential to reduce amino acid catabolism for energy; thus adequate levels of carbohydrates, particularly highly digestible starch sources, are indicated. Addition of fiber, a group of indigestible carbohydrates, can also play a key role in managing stool quality and promoting colonocyte health, although fiber decreases digestibility and energy density and should thus be added in moderate quantities. Soluble fibers act to slow GI transit time, bind toxins and irritating bile acids, and are fermented by bacteria in the colon to short-chain fatty acids (SCFA). These SCFAs are beneficial to the distal small intestine and colon where they nourish enterocytes and colonocytes, modulate gut motility, blood flow, and intestinal electrolyte and fluid balance. Due to their physical gelling/binding properties, soluble fibers are indicated for improving fecal consistency in cases with diarrhea of small or large bowel origin (Guilford and Matz 2003; Leib 2000). Furthermore, they may promote beneficial bacterial populations while inhibiting growth of pathogenic bacteria. Insoluble fibers act to normalize GI transit time, trap irritating and toxic compounds within fecal material, increase fecal bulk and often are particularly useful in cases with large bowel diarrhea (Guilford and Matz 2003).

Pectins, gums, psyllium, and indigestible oligosaccharides are common sources of soluble, fermentable fiber included in pet diets or easily available as supplements (Simpson 1998). Brans, soy fiber, pea fiber, and beet pulp are mixed fiber sources, meaning they contain both soluble and insoluble fibers, whereas cellulose provides only insoluble fiber (de Godoy et al. 2013). Although useful for some conditions, fiber-enhanced diets may not meet the recommended energy density and may not be appropriate for animals with decreased appetites or increased energy requirements.

Fats

Modest reduction of dietary fat is often beneficial for any animal with GI disease, although fat is a valuable source of nonprotein energy, increases the energy density and palatability of diets, is the only source of essential fatty acids, and is a vehicle for fat-soluble vitamins. Thus, dietary fat levels should not be unduly restricted unless specifically indicated. For instance, for some disease processes, such as lymphangiectasia, severe fat restriction is absolutely required (see below). For many other chronic enteropathies, reduction in the functional surface area of the intestinal mucosa, particularly secondary to inflammation, may result in malabsorption of dietary fats even in cases where fat is not a primary consideration. Undigested fats reaching the large intestine can feed pathogenic bacterial populations, resulting in production of hydroxy fatty acids, bacterial overgrowth, and exacerbation of deconjugation of irritating bile salts, all of which contribute to secretory diarrhea (Melgarejo et al. 2000). Fat also delays gastric emptying and increases GI transit time, so high levels of fat are contraindicated in cases of vomiting and diarrhea. Thus, conservative or modest fat content is indicated in diets to be fed to patients with chronic enteropathy.

Additional Nutritional Considerations

Chronic diarrhea can result in losses of body water, electrolytes, and water-soluble nutrients, so dietary supplementation of potassium and B-complex vitamins up to double their recommended inclusion rate may be warranted (Guilford and Matz 2003). In animals with muscle wasting and decreased body condition score, increase in dietary intake or parenteral supplementation of fat-soluble vitamins A, D, E, and K is also indicated.

General Feeding Recommendations

All patients with chronic enteropathies will benefit from multiple small meals spaced throughout the day. If voluntary intake is insufficient, assisted enteral nutritional support may be indicated. Placement of a nasoesophageal tube may be required if the patient is unfit for anesthesia or only very short-term (3–5 days) support is anticipated. Nasoesophageal tubes are well tolerated in the short term by many patients, but only liquid diets may be provided due to the small luminal diameter of the tube. Longer term support may be provided through use of an esophagostomy or gastrostomy (surgically or percutaneously placed) tube, which are typically well tolerated both in hospital and after discharge, and allow administration of homogenized canned diets (Yam and Cave 2003).

Key Points

- Small frequent meals.
- High energy density.
- Highly digestible, high-quality protein source.
- Moderate fat for most cases of chronic enteropathy.
- Soluble fiber for small bowel diarrhea, mixed fiber for large bowel diarrhea.

DIETARY: ADVERSE REACTIONS TO FOOD

Adverse reactions to food include intolerances, which are nonimmunological in pathogenesis, and true hypersensitivity or allergic reactions. Differentiation between intolerance and hypersensitivity may seem straightforward as dietary allergens are typically proteins and require sensitization prior to exhibition of clinical signs, while an animal may be intolerant of any dietary component and may show signs upon their first exposure and thus present with more acute signs (Guilford et al. 2001). However, clinical appearance may be very similar as a food intolerance often mimics true allergies.

Food Intolerances

There are few common dietary ingredients to which intolerances are recognized in dogs and cats. Lactose intolerance is the most common, and arises from a lack of lactase production in the enterocyte brush border (Davenport and Remillard 2010). Puppies and kittens produce small but sufficient amounts of lactase to digest the lactose within their mother's milk but after weaning, lactase production decreases by around 90% as milk is not typically consumed by adults of any species. When unabsorbed lactose reaches the colon, rapid bacterial fermentation results in flatulence, pain, and osmotic diarrhea (Vesa et al. 2000). Irish setter dogs are currently the only companion animals for which an inheritable sensitivity to gluten, or more specifically to gliadin, a glycoprotein component of gluten found in grains such as wheat, rye, and barley, has been described. If affected, Irish setter puppies typically show chronic, intermittent small bowel diarrhea and weight loss (Garden et al. 2000). Intolerance to other dietary compounds is seen more sporadically and not recognized as having any genetic association. This includes intolerance to food additives such as coloring agents, binding agents, food toxins and biologically active compounds, preservatives, and pharmacologically active products (Guilford et al. 2001).

Specific Nutritional Considerations

If the offending dietary component is avoided, these animals may be fed any complete and balanced diet appropriate for their life-stage.

Additional Nutritional Considerations

Avoidance of scromboid fish (tuna, mackerel, skipjack, bonito), liver, processed meats, cheese, tomato, and avocado will reduce exposure to dietary vasoactive or biogenic amines which may exacerbate adverse reactions.

Feeding Recommendations

No specific feeding recommendations exist as long as the offending dietary agent is avoided.

Key Points

- Healthy adult dogs and cats may have decreased tolerance for lactose.
- An inheritable gluten-sensitive enteropathy is known to exist among Irish setter dogs.

Dietary Hypersensitivity

Dietary hypersensitivities or allergies are true immunological responses mounted against a dietary component and thus require sensitization prior to exhibition of clinical signs. Hypersensitivity may arise as a primary allergic condition or as a sequel to GI inflammation and may be a complication of IBD (Guilford and Matz 2003). Animals with dietary hypersensitivities often present with either gastrointestinal signs or dermatological signs, or a combination of both.

Specific Nutritional Considerations

Dietary allergens typically consist of glycoproteins; thus, protein is the main nutrient of concern in management of dietary hypersensitivity. Common dietary allergens for both dogs and cats include beef, dairy, and chicken, while cats are commonly also allergic to fish (Mueller et al. 2016). Incompletely digested dietary proteins and polypeptides large enough to bridge IgE receptors on mucosal mast cells (>10 kDa) may be absorbed and instigate an inflammatory response within the lamina propria and submucosa (Cave 2006; Guilford and Matz 2003). Protein sources in pet foods are primarily from animal products (meats, meals, and digests) and legumes (beans or peas), though grains and even some vegetables also contain protein (corn, wheat, potato). Furthermore, carbohydrates and even lipids have also been implicated as potential allergens and warrant consideration in selection/formulation of a suitable diet (Cave 2006). It is unclear whether the carbohydrates or lipids themselves are the causative agent or whether the source of the carbohydrates or lipids contains protein to which the animal is sensitive.

Management of dietary hypersensitivity involves feeding of an elimination diet with a novel or hydrolyzed protein source and a novel carbohydrate and fat source, which may function in both diagnosis and therapy. The term *novel* refers to an ingredient to which the animal has not had previous exposure and thus should not be sensitized to, whereas hydrolyzation cleaves intact dietary proteins into polypeptides prior to consumption and further digestion. The hydrolyzation process reduces the number of protein molecules large enough to stimulate an immune response within the mucosa, and is effective enough that most animals sensitive to the intact protein source may consume the hydrolyzed protein source without any clinical signs (Cave 2006). That being said, hydrolyzed protein diets are not effective in 100% of cases, and other potential allergens may yet remain within the diets (other intact proteins, carbohydrates or lipids), and some animals may react even to the hydrolyzed peptides.

While both novel ingredient diets and hydrolyzed protein diets act by avoiding stimulation of the immune system, one may be more suitable than the other for feeding while the animal is symptomatic. Inflamed GI mucosa has altered permeability which may allow leakage of more and larger nutrients from the lumen (Cave 2006; Guilford and Matz 2003). By nature, hydrolyzed proteins are less able to initiate mast cell degranulation than intact proteins, thus rendering them relatively inert even in animals with poor mucosal integrity. Comparatively, while novel proteins will not elicit a response initially, exposure can result in sensitization and thus development of a new hypersensitivity to that protein. It is thus suggested that hydrolyzed diets may be preferable while the animal is showing clinical signs, which can be gradually replaced with a novel protein diet once the animal is stable and mucosal inflammation has resolved (Table 76.2).

Additional Nutritional Considerations

Addition of eicosapentaenoic acid (EPA) and docosahexaenoic acid (DHA), omega-3 fatty acids with antiinflammatory properties, may help ameliorate clinical signs associated with the inflammation (Ontsouka et al. 2012). Both DHA and EPA can be supplemented with marine oils

TABLE 76.2. Recommended components for nutritional support in dietary hypersensitivity.

Key nutritional factor	Requirement	Cats (DM basis)	Dogs (DM basis)
Protein	Novel or hydrolyzed	30–40%*	20–30%*
Carbohydrates	Novel	<40%	<60%
Fat	Ideally vegetable source	15–22%	12–15%

*Increased (>30% for dogs, >40% for cats) if patient is underweight, has muscle wasting or low plasma protein levels.
DM, dry matter.

TABLE 76.3. Recommended omega 3 fatty acid supplementation.

Key nutritional factor	Requirement	Cats (DM basis)	Dogs (DM basis)
DHA and EPA	Increased	0.35–1.8%	0.35–1.8%

DHA, docosahexaenoic acid; DM, dry matter; EPA, eicosahexaenoic acid.

(Kumari et al. 2010). Fish oils are most commonly utilized, though oils derived from algae or seaweed are also suitable and remove any concerns about potential animal protein contamination (Table 76.3).

Feeding Recommendations

A trial utilizing an elimination diet should be implemented to facilitate diagnosis by response to treatment (Gaschen et al. 2008; Guilford and Matz 2003). Elimination diets are particular to individual cases and must be devoid of ingredients, particularly protein and carbohydrate sources, to which the animal has been previously exposed. A thorough dietary history is required to determine all ingredients, including treats, medication, and supplements, which the animal has consumed in the past. Commercial diets marketed as being hypoallergenic may not in fact be hypoallergenic to that particular patient if they have had previous exposure to the ingredients (Guilford and Matz 2003).

Typical elimination diets contain minimal ingredients to reduce possible antigen exposure and thus often consist of only one novel or hydrolyzed protein, one novel carbohydrate, fat, vitamins and minerals. Veterinary therapeutic diets or home-made diets may be used, although homemade diets must be nutritionally complete and balanced if they are to be continued for longer than a 12-week elimination trial. All other foods, including treats, pill pockets, snacks, supplements, flavored medications, human foods and scavenged foods (including coprophagia), must be eliminated during the course of the trial. Commercial diets other than veterinary therapeutic elimination diets are not recommended, even if the protein sources appear novel, as the risk of cross-contamination is high and may negatively impact the trial.

Improvement in GI signs is expected within the first 2–4 weeks, although an elimination trial may take up to six weeks if solely GI signs or even 12 weeks, especially if dermatological signs are also present.

After clinical signs resolve during the dietary elimination trial, the gold standard protocol is to challenge the animal with the original diet, or to add single ingredients to the elimination diet, to provoke clinical signs and definitively diagnose an adverse reaction to that food/ingredient (Guilford et al. 2001; Verlinden et al. 2006). Challenge with individual ingredients can identify which is the culprit, whereas challenge with the original diet will confirm only that one or more of the ingredients in that diet are responsible. Pet owners are often not willing to go back to the original diet once clinical signs have resolved, but they may be open to add individual protein or carbohydrate sources to the elimination diet and observe for recurrence of clinical signs for 1–2 weeks. While this process allows the identification of each offensive food component and development of an appropriate long-term management plan for the animal, it can be a lengthy process and some owners may not be willing to perform such a thorough investigation. Alternatively, the original elimination diet may be fed to the animal long term if it is, or can be, formulated to be nutritionally complete and balanced.

Key Points

- An elimination diet can be diagnostic as well as therapeutic.
- Strict dietary elimination trials should be six weeks in duration if solely GI signs and up to 12 weeks if concurrent dermatological signs. This includes elimination of treats, snacks, pill pockets, scavenging, coprophagia.

- Novel or hydrolyzed protein is the cornerstone of therapy.
- Carbohydrate and fat sources may also need to be considered as potential dietary allergens.

INFLAMMATORY: INFLAMMATORY BOWEL DISEASE

Inflammatory bowel diseases (IBD) are the most commonly recognized chronic enteropathies in companion animals (Simpson 1998). The etiology is not always known and likely differs between cases, with endoparasitism, genetic susceptibility, stress, dietary factors, and reduced immune tolerance likely playing roles (Inness et al. 2007). Idiopathic IBD is a diagnosis of exclusion, supported by histopathological changes characteristic of IBD with no identifiable underlying factors (Sturgess 2005).

The diseases are characterized by the predominant inflammatory cellular infiltrate (Gaschen et al. 2008; German et al. 2003a). In dogs, lymphoplasmacytic enterocolitis is most common, and some dog breeds are predisposed to unique forms of IBD, such as histiocytic ulcerative colitis in boxers and immunoproliferative small intestinal disease in basenjis and lundehunds. In cats, lymphoplasmacytic and eosinophilic enteritis are both commonly diagnosed. The underlying mechanism is thought to be immunological in origin, differentiating IBD from primary gastrointestinal food intolerances. What is currently accepted is that an inflammatory response in the GI mucosa can lead to persistent inflammation and further mucosal sensitization, resulting in the clinical presentation of IBD (Guilford and Matz 2003). Animals with IBD may present with small intestinal diarrhea, large intestinal diarrhea, or a combination of both. Severe cases may be complicated by protein loss (Dossin and Lavoué 2011); see section on PLE under Lymphangiectasia.

Regardless of the underlying cause, the characteristic inflamed mucosa is a primary source of clinical signs in and of itself, and also allows infiltration by dietary antigens, perpetuating inflammation and predisposing the animal to development of new dietary hypersensitivities (Cave 2006; Foster et al. 2003; Guilford and Matz 2003). Thus, differentiation of IBD from dietary allergies can be challenging, and many animals may suffer from both conditions concurrently. Despite uncertainty regarding the exact immunological mechanisms underlying the inflammation, nutritional considerations for IBD are very similar to those for dietary hypersensitivity.

Specific Nutritional Considerations

The primary consideration for animals with IBD is replacement of potential dietary antigens to avoid exacerbation of inflammatory responses. This is particularly true of proteins, which are the most common source of allergens in dogs and cats (Cave 2006). Due to the increased permeability of inflamed mucosa, animals with IBD are at risk of developing new dietary hypersensitivities during periods of inflammation (Simpson 1998). For this reason, it is suggested that *diets with hydrolyzed protein are utilized when animals are showing clinical signs of IBD, reserving novel proteins for long-term management once the inflammation is resolved.* Use of novel proteins during periods of inflammation risks "sacrificing" that protein source when the animal develops hypersensitivity to it, necessitating a switch to a new novel protein source (Cave 2006; Sturgess 2005).

Single, novel carbohydrate sources are also recommended, as it is possible that dogs and cats may develop hypersensitivity to dietary components of these ingredients (Mueller et al. 2016; Verlinden et al. 2006). Manipulation of dietary fibers may also be indicated to physically improve clinical signs of diarrhea, nourish the colonocytes, and provide substrate for beneficial intestinal microbes by acting as prebiotics (Segarra et al. 2016). For large bowel diarrhea, addition of both soluble and insoluble fibers can be beneficial, while for small bowel diarrhea soluble fibers are preferred. High inclusion levels of fiber, however, decreases overall diet digestibility which may

TABLE 76.4. Recommended components for nutritional support in inflammatory bowel disease.

Key nutritional factor	Requirement	Cats (DM basis)	Dogs (DM basis)
Protein	Hydrolyzed > novel*	30–40%**	20–30%**
Fat	Vegetable oil	15–22%	12–15%
Carbohydrates	Single, novel	<40%	<60%
Fiber	If large bowel diarrhea[†]	7–15%	7–15%

*Hydrolyzed protein, at least until clinical signs have been resolved for ≥6 weeks, to avoid development of new hypersensitivities, then a transition to novel proteins may be made if desired.
**Increased (>30% for dogs, >40% for cats) if patient is underweight, has muscle wasting or decreased plasma protein levels.
[†]Fiber may not ameliorate clinical signs in all cases and may worsen signs in some, so fiber should be decreased (<5%) if clinical signs worsen at a moderate inclusion level, or if increased energy density is indicated.
DM, dry matter.

result in increased nutritional content of digesta reaching the large intestine, which risks exacerbation of inflammation if dietary antigens are still present (Guildford and Matz 2003). If clinical signs are worsened by fiber, the animal should be switched to another appropriate hydrolyzed (or novel) protein diet with lower fiber content, or supplementary fiber should be discontinued. Dietary fats may also be a source of antigens and may require consideration in some patients (Cave 2006). For this reason, vegetable oil is a preferred fat source (Table 76.4).

Additional Nutritional Considerations

Antiinflammatory support is highly indicated, with some cases even requiring medical therapy including antiinflammatory corticosteroids or sulfasalazine, or immunosuppressive medications such as cyclosporine. Dietary antiinflammatory support for the GI tract includes supplementation with fiber, as discussed, as well as the omega-3 fatty acids DHA and EPA (see Table 76.3) (Ontsouka et al. 2012).

Although probiotics, live cultures of perceived beneficial bacteria, are commonly recommended by veterinarians in practice, only a few studies have been performed on their use as an adjunctive therapy for IBD in dogs. Research regarding the use of probiotics in IBD cases have been plagued by complications and most failed to yield convincing results (Sauter et al. 2006; Schmitz et al. 2015). So far, the most convincing evidence of efficacy was demonstrated utilizing a commercial probiotic supplement containing *Lactobacillus casei, L. plantarus, L. acidophilus, L. delbrueckii, Bifidobacterium longum, B. breve, B. infantis,* and *Streptococcus sulivarius* subsp. *thermophiles* (Rossi et al. 2014). Findings suggested that treatment with probiotics was equally efficacious as treatment with metronidazole and prednisone in reducing GI mucosal inflammation based on histology, though slower to resolve clinical signs according to the owners' descriptions. While their use may appear promising, or at least safe, rigorous scientific evidence supporting the use of probiotics in canine and feline IBD patients is lacking at this time.

Feeding Recommendations

As with dietary hypersensitivity, a trial utilizing an elimination diet should be implemented to reduce potential for mucosal sensitization.

Key Points

- Antiinflammatory support.
- Hydrolyzed protein to avoid mucosal sensitization and development of dietary hypersensitivities.
- May transition to a novel protein diet for long-term maintenance once clinical signs abate.

FUNCTIONAL

Lymphangiectasia

Intestinal lymphangiectasia describes the dilation of the lymphatics of the small intestine resulting in leakage of protein- and lipid-rich lymph fluid into the lumen of the intestine (Dossin and Lavoué 2011; Okanishi et al. 2014). Lymphangiectasia may occur due to a primary lymphatic defect or it may occur secondarily to any condition resulting in lymphatic hypertension. Animals presenting with lymphangiectasia typically have a long-standing history of waxing and waning, signs of diarrhea or vomiting and paradoxical weight loss despite polyphagia. In cases with hypoalbuminemia due to protein loss, signs of ascites, edema, and pleural or thoracic effusion may be evident (Box 76.1).

BOX 76.1. Protein-losing Enteropathy

The term *protein-losing enteropathy* (PLE) is used to describe any condition causing a net loss of protein from the intestinal lumen, resulting in hypoalbuminemia. This condition is more common in dogs than cats, and is a consequence of either lymphatic defect or severe manifestations of infiltrative disease such as IBD and intestinal lymphoma (Dossin and Lavoué 2011; Okanishi et al. 2014). Clearly, a key nutritional consideration for these patients is protein, as patients with PLE may be cachectic and metabolizing body protein stores to compensate for their intestinal losses. Thus, these patients benefit from a diet rich in highly digestible protein (>30% DM for dogs, >40% DM for cats) with a relatively high energy density (>3.5 kcal/g). In cases where the PLE is secondary to lymphangiectasia, energy density of the diet may be decreased by reduced fat levels but in general, the appropriate diet with the highest energy density should be selected. Protein hydrolyzates are highly digestible and are particularly suitable for patients with PLE secondary to severe IBD. However, most veterinary therapeutic diets formulated with hydrolyzed proteins do not contain the required protein levels to compensate for ongoing losses from PLE, so supplementary hydrolyzed protein powders, oligomeric or elemental diets may be required. For dogs, supplementation with hydrolyzed cat food, being generally higher in protein than dog food, may also be an option. Restriction of dietary fiber (<5% DM) is prudent to maintain high digestibility and energy density of the diet, particularly in cases with severe IBD to decrease the potential antigen load.

Specific Nutritional Considerations

Animals with lymphangiectasia suffer from severe lipid malabsorption, with dietary intake directly affecting their condition. Digestion of most dietary fats leads to absorption of long-chain triglycerides (LCT) into the intestinal lymphatic system. In animals with lymphangiectasia, absorption of fats into distended lacteals is impaired, and lymphatic hypertension can be exacerbated by dietary fats. Rupture of overdistended lymph vessels results in loss of plasma proteins, lymphocytes, and lipids into the intestinal lumen (Kull et al. 2001). These patients can often present in a state of marked negative energy and protein balance (Dossin and Lavoué 2011). An energy-dense, high-protein and low-fat diet is thus indicated for these patients (Table 76.5). Fat should not be decreased below AAFCO minimum recommendation (5.5% on a dry matter basis for dogs, 9% for cats) due to risk of essential fatty acid and fat-soluble vitamin deficiencies, as well as decreased palatability and energy density. It has been suggested that medium-chain triglycerides (MCT) may be of use to increase dietary energy density without increasing lymphatic LCT load. Medium chain triglycerides may be better tolerated by patients with lymphangiectasia as they are thought to be more water soluble and mostly absorbed directly into the portal venous circulation, thus being incorporated less into chylomicrons absorbed into the lymphatic system (Beynen et al. 2002; Trevizan et al. 2010). Given that MCT do not exclusively bypass lymphatic uptake (Jensen et al. 1994), this practice may be unreliable. If included, MCT content should be

TABLE 76.5. Recommended components for nutritional support in lymphangiectasia.

Key nutritional factor	Requirement	Cats (DM basis)	Dogs (DM basis)
Energy density	High**	>3500 kcal/kg	>3500 kcal/kg
Protein	Highly digestible	>40%	>30%
Fiber	Restricted	<5%	<5%
Fat	Restricted*	<15%	<10%

*Supplementation with MCT may be appropriate.
**As energy dense as possible with restricted fat.
DM, dry matter.

conservative, maximum 5% on a dry matter basis, as there may still be some stimulation of lymphatic flow and many dogs find them to be poorly palatable (Dossin and Lavoué 2011). Dietary supplementation with oligomeric or elemental diets may be required in severe cases to provide readily available small peptides and free amino acids to maintain plasma protein levels.

Additional Nutritional Considerations

Animals with restricted dietary fat intake, lipid malabsorption, steatorrhea, or a low body condition score may require parenteral supplementation with fat-soluble vitamins A, D, E, and K. Intramuscular injection of 1 mL of a proprietary ADE combination provides 100 000 IU vitamin A, 10 000 IU vitamin D and 300 IU vitamin E, sufficient to most dogs for three months (small dogs may require only 0.5 mL). Vitamin K can be given separately at 0.5–1 mg/kg body weight if coagulopathy is suspected.

Feeding Recommendations

Multiple small meals are required to minimize stimulation of intestinal lymph flow.

Key Points
- Fat restriction.
- High protein (hydrolyzed if concurrent IBD).
- Low fiber.

Idiopathic Bowel Syndrome

Idiopathic bowel syndrome (IBS), also known as irritable bowel syndrome, is a cause of large bowel dyschezia/diarrhea in dogs with no detectable underlying cause. This condition is not recognized in cats. Clinical signs are suggested to arise from colonic dysmotility and/or visceral sensation, resulting from abnormalities in enteral neurotransmission (Lecoindre and Gaschen 2011). The syndrome may be precipitated by stressful situations and is characterized by bloating, dyschezia and/or large bowel diarrhea, often with abdominal pain. Large-breed working and showing dogs are at highest risk of developing IBS, although small, nervous breeds are also overrepresented (Lecoindre and Gaschen 2011; Leib 2000).

Specific Considerations

Removal of the stressor is the most effective management approach, although there are also nutritional strategies which are recognized to improve clinical signs. Dietary fiber is likely the most important factor (Table 76.6), reinforced by clinical findings to support its use (Lecoindre and Gaschen 2011; Leib 2000). Efficacy of fiber type may vary between cases, with some responding to soluble fiber (pectins, gums, and psyllium), some to insoluble fiber (cellulose, peanut hulls), and some to mixed fiber (rice bran, oat bran, wheat bran, soy fiber, pea fiber, beet pulp). Fiber can be added to a highly digestible veterinary therapeutic diet, as opposed

TABLE 76.6. Recommended components for nutritional support in idiopathic bowel syndrome.

Key nutritional factor	Requirement	DM basis
Soluble fiber *or*	Increased	1–5%
Mixed fiber *or*	Increased	5–10%
Insoluble fiber *or*	Increased	10–15%
Crude fiber*	Increased	>10%
Fat	Moderate	12–15%

*Crude fiber is the only fiber measurement obligatory on pet food labels, but only represents insoluble fiber. Total dietary fiber including both soluble and insoluble fiber may be available in product guides from veterinary therapeutic diet companies. DM, dry matter.

to simply feeding a commercial diet high in fiber, to minimize production of gas. Some fiber-supplemented highly digestible veterinary therapeutic diets are also available. Modest reduction of dietary fat may also help by minimizing irritating bile acids reaching the colon (Guilford and Matz 2003).

Additional Nutritional Considerations

Some patients may benefit from an elimination diet, as described for dietary hypersensitivity.

Feeding Recommendations

Follow general feeding recommendations for chronic enteropathies, as described above.

Key Points

- Choose a high-fiber diet or supplement with fiber.
- If one type of fiber (soluble, insoluble, mixed) is not effective, try another.
- Avoid high-fat diets.
- Hydrolyzed or novel protein elimination diet may be required.

Constipation

The term *constipation* refers to infrequent and/or challenging passage of feces. Frequently, constipation arises secondary to dehydration, resulting in dry, hard feces, and electrolyte imbalance which can alter colonic muscular activity (Washbau 2003). Animals commonly present with tenesmus, dyschezia, anorexia and, paradoxically, diarrhea. Small amounts of mucoid feces may pass impacted feces, giving the impression of diarrhea when the primary issue is in fact constipation. Long-standing, severe, or uncorrected constipation can result in obstipation, or complete inability to pass feces, at which point physical intervention is indicated to remove the impacted fecal material. A potential sequel of severe chronic constipation and obstipation is megacolon (Box 76.2).

BOX 76.2. Megacolon

Megacolon refers to the pathologic dilation of the colon, which occurs most commonly in cats although dogs may be afflicted as well. Megacolon can occur secondarily to chronic constipation and obstipation, or can occur primarily. Primary megacolon is also termed *idiopathic megacolon* and results from a disorder of colonic motility, thought to be caused by neurogenic and neuromuscular disorders (Byers et al. 2006; Prokić et al. 2010; Washbau 2003). Regardless of etiology, the disorder manifests as obstipation with severe colonic dilation and fecal impaction and the animal typically presents with anorexia, vomiting, dyschezia, and cachexia. Some cases may respond to dietary therapy and medical management, though severe megacolon may require surgical correction by subtotal colectomy. Nutritional considerations for patients with early and less severe megacolon are the same as for patients with constipation: manipulation of dietary fiber to increase fecal moisture and support colonic motility. In severe cases, however, fiber supplementation is strongly contraindicated, as increasing fecal bulk will only exacerbate colonic impaction. Instead, increased energy density and a highly digestible diet are indicated for these cases.

Specific Considerations

Rehydration and correction of electrolyte imbalances, particularly of calcium and potassium, are key to initial management of constipation. Nutritional management of chronic or recurring cases of constipation requires maintaining hydration and fecal water content (Table 76.7). Dietary water content should be greater than 75%, and additional water intake should be encouraged, such as by feeding moistened foods, adding warm water to food, adding flavor enhancers to water, and always ensuring access to clean, fresh water. For constipation, fiber-enriched diets can have a laxative effect from increasing fecal water content, moderating intestinal transit, and stimulating colonic motility (Frieche et al. 2011; Rondeau et al. 2003). Supplementation with fermentable soluble fiber is also an option, which may be achieved by adding psyllium husk, fruit pectin, or guar gum (1 tsp per 5–10 kg body weight) to an otherwise highly digestible therapeutic diet. Bulk-forming insoluble fiber such as cellulose and peanut hulls, or mixed fiber such as bran and pea fiber are only beneficial in constipation and should be avoided in cases where the colonic motility is completely abolished, i.e., megacolon, as colonic stretching can only stimulate contraction when the musculature is actually capable of doing so, otherwise increased bulk will only add to the already impacted feces (Byers et al. 2006).

Additional Nutritional Considerations

Additional supplementation with lactulose, a synthetic fermentable fiber with hyperosmotic laxative properties, at 0.25–0.5 mg/kg per day may also be beneficial in patients with a normal hydration status. Lactulose has quite a sweet flavor and is palatable to most dogs simply top-dressed on their food, but cats may resent the taste. Bones and raw food are particularly contraindicated as aside from the risks of microbial contamination, these are also associated with constipation and obstipation in dogs (Freeman and Michel 2001).

Feeding Recommendations

Frequent small meals may be beneficial to promote colonic motility and reduce the load in the large bowel at a given time. Gentle exercise, such as a short quiet walk, immediately after eating is encouraged.

TABLE 76.7. Recommended components for nutritional support in constipation.

Key nutritional factor	Requirement	DM basis
Soluble fiber	Increased	1–5%
Crude fiber	Increased*	7%
Moisture	Increased	>75%
Energy density	Increased**	>4000 kcal/kg

*Except in cases of severe megacolon or obstipation, in which case crude fiber should be <5%.
**Particularly for cases of severe megacolon or obstipation.
DM, dry matter.

Key Points

- Moist/wet food and stimulation of water intake.
- Various fiber sources (soluble, mixed, insoluble) increase fecal water content and promote colonic motility.
- Patients with megacolon benefit more from low-fiber diets as especially insoluble fiber may add to the already impacted feces if colonic motility is abolished.

Altered GI Microbiome

The healthy GI tract contains an estimated 10^{12}–10^{14} microbial cells representing around 80–100 different bacterial genera and 15–30 fungal genera in dogs and cats. (Handl et al. 2011; Suchodolski 2016). Alterations in the GI microbiome can result in enteropathy, typically associated with diarrhea, and are frequently termed antibiotic-responsive diarrhea (ARD). These alterations can be a change in number, known as small intestinal bacterial overgrowth (SIBO), or a change in the types of microbes present, known as dysbiosis. Controversy persists, however, regarding the nomenclature of these conditions, as not all dogs with ARD have quantitative differences in small intestinal bacteria when compared with clinically normal animals, nor do all dogs with SIBO respond to antibiotic therapy (German et al. 2003b). Dysbiosis is thought to arise from disruption of the healthy microbial community allowing a relative proliferation of pathogenic species, even when the overall number of microbes present is within recognized normal limits (Minamoto et al. 2014).

Changes in the number or type of bacteria in the small intestine may occur secondary to surgical resection of the ileocolic valve, antibiotic therapy, or in cases with malabsorptive conditions such as exocrine pancreatic insufficiency or IBD (German et al. 2003b; Suchodolski 2016; Suchodolski et al. 2012). Animals with reduced or altered immune function may also exhibit changes in their microflora (Littler et al. 2006). Furthermore, while these changes in the host's GI tract may cause changes in the microbiome secondarily, it is also thought that change in the microbiome can itself be a cause of or exacerbate enteropathy (Minamoto et al. 2014; Suchodolski 2016).

Specific Considerations

Feeding a diet with highly digestible macronutrients will result in greater absorption of nutrients in the proximal GI tract and reduce the amount of substrate for bacterial growth. Similarly, lower amounts of dietary residues will decrease the osmolarity of intestinal contents, thus ameliorating osmotic diarrhea (Table 76.8). Fat is calorically dense; therefore reducing the amount of food required to meet daily caloric intake, thus dietary restriction of fat, is not indicated. However, high levels of fat may exacerbate osmotic diarrhea, so a moderate fat content is recommended, with the potential to increase fat and feed more energy-dense foods as tolerated.

Additional Nutritional Considerations

Changes in gut flora can allow proliferation of bacteria which utilize cobalamin, thus decreasing the availability of the vitamin for absorption by the animal (German et al. 2003b). For cases with decreased cobalamin status, subcutaneous administration of injectable vitamin B12 can be dosed

TABLE 76.8. Recommended components for nutritional support in dysbiosis.

Key nutritional factor	Requirement	Cats (DM basis)	Dogs (DM basis)
Protein	Highly digestible	26–40%	18–30%
Fiber	Soluble	<5%	<5%
Fat	Moderate	15–25%	12–15%

DM, dry matter.

at 30–55 μg/kg as required. Administration of antibiotics, a common therapy when ARD is suspected, may hinder vitamin K synthesis by destroying beneficial gut flora. Thus, dietary supplementation of vitamin K may also be beneficial. Addition of prebiotics – soluble fibers which are included in the diet to promote healthy gut flora – may support or reinstate beneficial intestinal bacteria such as *Lactobacillus* and *Bifidobacterium* species (Barry et al. 2010). Care must be taken, however, not to overly reduce the digestibility of the diet with oversupplementation of fiber.

Probiotics, live microorganisms, have been suggested as a means of inoculating the intestine with beneficial bacteria. Provision of perceived beneficial bacteria, particularly *Lactobacillus* and *Bifidobacterium* species, has been reported to modify intestinal pH, enhance local immune system, and inhibit growth of pathogenic bacteria in dogs with chronic enteropathies (Jugan et al. 2017; Pascher et al. 2008; Rossi et al. 2014). That said, there are currently only a few studies suggesting clinical efficacy; sample sizes have been small and the results mediocre. More thorough scientific evidence is needed before strong recommendations for or against use of probiotics can be made.

References

Barry KA, Wojcicki BJ, Middelbos IS, Vester BM, Swanson KS, Fahey GC. Dietary cellulose, fructooligo-saccharides, and pectin modify fecal protein catabolites and microbial populations in adult cats. J Anim Sci 2010;88:2978–2987.

Beynen AC, Kappert HJ, Lemmens AG, van Dongen AM. Plasma lipid concentrations, macronutrient digestibility and mineral absorption in dogs fed a dry food containing medium-chain triglycerides. J Anim Physiol Anim Nutr 2002;86:306–312.

Byers C, Leasure C, Sanders N. Feline idiopathic megacolon. Compend Contin Educ Vet 2006;28(9):658–664.

Cave NJ. Hydrolyzed protein diets for dogs and cats. Vet Clin Small Anim Pract 2006;36:1251–1268.

Davenport DJ, Remillard RL. Introduction to small intestinal diseases. In: Hand MS, Thatcher CD, Remillard RL, Roudebush P, Novotny BJ, eds. Small Animal Clinical Nutrition, 5th edn. Topeka: Mark Morris Institute, 2010.

De Godoy MRC, Kerr KR, Fahey GC Jr. Alternative dietary fiber sources in companion animal nutrition. Nutrients 2013;5:3099–3117.

Dossin O, Lavoué R. Protein-losing enteropathies in dogs. Vet Clin North Am Small Anim Pract 2011;41:399–418.

Foster AP, Knowles TG, Moore AH, Cousins PDG, Day MJ, Hall EJ. Serum IgE and IgG responses to food antigens in normal and atopic dogs, and dogs with gastrointestinal disease. Vet Immunol Immunopathol 2003;92:113–124.

Freeman LM, Michel KE. Evaluation of raw food diets for dogs. J Am Vet Med Assoc 2001;218(5): 705–709.

Frieche V, Houston D, Weese H, et al. Uncontrolled study assessing the impact of a psyllium-enriched extruded dry diet on faecal consistency in cats with constipation. J Feline Med Surg 2011;13:903–911.

Garden OA, Pidduck H, Lakhani KH, Walker D, Wood JLN, Batt RM. Inheritance of gluten-sensitive enteropathy in Irish Setters. Am J Vet Res 2000;61(4):462–468.

Gaschen L, Kircher P, Stüssi A, et al. Comparison of ultrasonographic findings with clinical activity index (CIBDAI) ad diagnosis in dogs with chronic enteropathies. Vet Radiol Ultrasound 2008;49(1):56–64.

German AJ, Hall EJ, Day MJ. Chronic intestinal inflammation and intestinal disease in dogs. J Vet Intern Med 2003a;17:8–20.

German AJ, Day MJ, Ruaux CG, Steiner JM, Williams DA, Hall EJ. Comparison of direct and indirect tests for small intestinal bacterial overgrowth and antibiotic-responsive diarrhea in dogs. J Vet Intern Med 2003b;17:33–43.

Guilford WG, Matz ME. The nutritional management of gastrointestinal tract disorders in companion animals. NZ Vet J 2003;51(6):284–291.

Guilford WG, Jones BR, Markwell PJ, Aruther DG, Collett MG, Harte JG. Food sensitivity in cats with chronic idiopathic gastrointestinal problems. J Vet Intern Med 2001;15:7–13.

Handl S, Dowd SE, Garcia-Mazcorro JF, Steiner JM, Suchodolski JS. Massive parallel 16s rRNA gene pyrosequencing reveals highly diverse fecal bacterial and fungal communities in healthy dogs and cats FEMS Microbiol Ecol 2011;76:301–310.

Harris JP, Parnell NK, Griffith EH, Saker KE. Retrospective evaluation of the impact of early enteral nutrition on clinical outcomes in dogs with pancreatitis: 34 cases (2010-2013). J Vet Emerg Crit Care 2017;27(4):425–433.

Inness VL, McCartney AL, Khoo C, Gross KL, Gibson GR. Molecular characterisation of the gut microflora of healthy and inflammatory bowel disease cats using fluorescence in situ hybridisation with special reference to Desulfovibrio spp. J Anim Physiol Anim Nutr 2007;91:48–53.

Jensen GL, McGarvey N, Taraszewski R, et al. Lymphatic absorption of enterally fed structured triacylglycerol vs physical mix in a canine model. Am J Clin Nutr 1994;60:518–524.

Jugan MC, Rudinsky AJ, Parker VJ, Gilor C. Use of probiotics in small animal veterinary medicine. J Am Vet Med Assoc 2017;250(5):519–528.

Kull PA, Hess RS, Craig LE, Saunders HM, Washabau RJ. Clinical, clinicopathologic, radiographic, and ultrasonographic characteristics of intestinal lymphangiectasia in dogs: 17 cases (1996-1998). J Am Vet Med Assoc 2001;219(2):197–202.

Kumari P, Kumar M, Gupta V, Reddy CRK, Jha B. Tropical marine macroalgae as potential sources of nutritionally important PUFAs. Food Chem 2010;120:749–757.

Lecoindre P, Gaschen FP. Chronic idiopathic large bowel diarrhea in the dog. Vet Clin North Am Small Anim Pract 2011;41(2):447–456.

Leib MS. Treatment of chronic idiopathic large-bowel diarrhea in dogs with a highly digestible diet and soluble fiber: a retrospective review of 37 cases. J Vet Intern Med 2000;14(1):27–32.

Littler RM, Batt RM, Lloyd DH. Total and relative deficiency of gut mucosal IgA in German shepherd dogs demonstrated by faecal analysis. Vet Rec 2006;158(10):334–341.

Melgarejo T, Williams DA, O'Connell NC, Setchell KDR. Serum unconjugated bile acids as a test for intestinal bacterial overgrowth in dogs. Dig Dis Sci 2000;45(2):407–414.

Minamoto Y, Dhanani N, Markel ME, Steiner JM, Suchodolski JS. Prevalence of Clostridium perfringens, Clostridium perfringens enterotoxin and dysbiosis in fecal samples of dogs with diarrhea. Vet Microbiol 2014;174:463–473.

Mueller RS, Olivry T, Prélaud P. Critically appraised topic on adverse food reactions of companion animals (2): common food allergen sources in dogs and cats. BMC Vet Res 2016;14:24.

Okanishi H, Yoshioka R, Kagawa Y, Watari T. The clinical efficacy of dietary fat restriction in treatment of dogs with intestinal lymphangiectasia. J Vet Intern Med 2014;28:809–817.

Ontsouka EC, Curgener IA, Luckschandler-Zeller N, Blum JW, Albrecht C. Fish-meal diet enriched with omega-3 PUFA and treatment of canine chronic enteropathies. Eur J Lipid Sci Technol 2012;114:412–422.

Pascher M, Hellweg P, Khol-Parisini A, Zentek J. Effects of a probiotic Lactobacillus acidophilus strain on feed tolerance in dogs with non-specific dietary sensitivity. Arch Anim Nutr 2008;62(2):107–116.

Prokić B, Todorović V, Mitrović O, Vignjević S, Savić VS. Ethiopathogenesis, diagnosis and therapy of acquired megacolon in dogs. Acta Vet 2010;60(2-3):273–284.

Rondeau MP, Meltzer K, Michel KE, McManus CM, Washbau RJ. Short chain fatty acids stimulate feline colonic smooth muscle contraction. J Feline Med Surg 2003;5:167–173.

Rossi G, Pengo G, Caldin M, et al. Comparison of microbiological, histological, and immunomodulatory parameters in response to treatment with either combination therapy with prednisone and metronidazole or probiotic VSL#3 strains in dogs with idiopathic inflammatory bowel disease. PLoS One 2014;9(4):e94699.

Sauter SN, Benyacoub J, Allenspach K, et al. Effects of probiotic bacteria in dogs with food responsive diarrhea treated with an elimination diet. J Anim Physiol Anim Nutr (Berl) 2006;90(7-8):269–277.

Schmitz S, Werling D, Allenspach K. Effects of ex-vivo and in-vivo treatment with probiotics on the inflammasome in dogs with chronic enteropathy. PLoS One 2015;10:0120779.

Segarra S, Martínez-Subiela S, Cerdà-Cuéllar M, et al. Oral chondroitin sulfate and prebiotics for the treatment of canine inflammatory bowel disease: a randomized, controlled clinical trial. BMC Vet Res 2016;12:49.

Simpson JW. Diet and large intestinal disease in dogs and cats. J Nutr 1998;128:2717S–2722S.

Sturgess K. Diagnosis and management of idiopathic inflammatory bowel disease in dogs and cats. In Practice 2005;27:293–301.

Suchodolski JS. Diagnosis and interpretation of intestinal dysbiosis in dogs and cats. Vet J 2016;215:30–37.

Suchodolski JS, Markel ME, Garcia-Mazcorro JF, et al. The fecal microbiome in dogs with acute diarrhea and idiopathic inflammatory bowel disease. PLoS One 2012;7(12):e51907.

Trevizan L, de Mello Kessler A, Bigley KE, Anderson WH, Waldron MK, Bauer JE. Effects of dietary medium-chain triglycerides on plasma lipids and lipoprotein distribution and food aversion in cats. Am J Vet Res 2010;71(4):435–440.

Verlinden A, Hesta M, Millet S, Janssens GPJ. Food allergy in dogs and cats: a review. Crit Rev Food Sci Nutr 2006;46:259–273.

Vesa TH, Marteau P, Korpela R. Lactose intolerance. J Am Coll Nutr 2000;19(2):165S–175S.

Washbau RJ. Gastrointestinal motility disorders and gastrointestinal prokinetic therapy. Vet Clin North Am Small Anim Pract 2003;33(5):1007–1028.

Yam P, Cave C. Enteral nutrition: options and feeding protocols. In Practice 2003;25(3):118–159.

Suggested Reading

AAFCO. 2017 Official Publication. Champaign: Association of American Feed Control Officials, 2017.

Ali T, Shakir F, Morton J. Curcumin and inflammatory bowel disease: biological mechanisms and clinical implication. Digestion 2012;85:249–255.

Bauer JE. Responses of dogs to dietary omega-3 fatty acids. J Am Vet Med Assoc 2007;231(11):1657–1661.

Evans SE, Bonczynski JJ, Broussard JD, Han E, Baer KE. Comparison of endoscopic and full-thickness biopsy specimens for diagnosis of inflammatory bowel disease and alimentary tract lymphoma in cats. J Am Vet Med Assoc 2006;229(9):1447–1450.

Hand M, Thatcher CD, Remillard RL, Roudebush P, Novotny BJ. Small Animal Clinical Nutrition, 5th edn. Topeka: Mark Morris Institute, 2010.

Jergens AE, Schreiner CA, Frank DE, et al. A scoring index for disease activity in canine inflammatory bowel disease. J Vet Intern Med 2003;17:291–297.

Morris JG. Idiosyncratic nutrient requirements of cats appear to be diet-induced evolutionary adaptations. Nutr Rev Rev 2002;15:153–168.

Schmitz S, Suchodolski J. Understanding the canine intestinal microbiota and its modification by pro-, pre- and synbiotics – what is the evidence? Vet Med Sci 2016;2(2):71–94.

Authors: Sarah Dodd DVM, BSc, Caitlin Grant DVM, BSc, Adronie Verbrugghe DVM, PhD, Dip ECVCN

Chapter 77

Parasites, Gastrointestinal

DEFINITION/OVERVIEW

- Intestinal helminthiasis can be caused by *Ancylostoma caninum* (dogs) and *A. tubaeforme* (cats), *Uncinaria stenocephala* (dogs and cats), *Toxocara canis* (dogs), *T. cati* (cats), *Toxascaris leonina* (dogs and cats), *Trichuris vulpis* (dogs) and *Trichuris felis* (cats). *Baylisascaris procyonis* of raccoons can also infect dogs.
- Hookworms (*Ancylostoma* spp., *Uncinaria* spp.) attach to the intestinal mucosa, suck blood, and cause anemia and enteritis; *Ancylostoma* can be transmitted via colostrum/milk to pups and can cause cutaneous larval migrans (CLM) in humans. Respiratory disease may result from larval migration in lungs.
- Heavy infections with ascarids cause distended intestines, colic, and intestinal rupture; *Toxocara canis* can be transplacentally transmitted from bitch's tissues to pups; causes visceral larval migrans (VLM) in humans.
- The whipworm, *Trichuris*, occurs in the cecum of dogs (*T. vulpis*) and cats (*T. felis*). Feline trichuriasis is rare in the United States. Infection can be asymptomatic or cause bloody diarrhea and large bowel inflammation.
- Dog-specific: *Cystoisospora canis*, *C. ohioensis*, *C. burrowsi*, *C. neorivolta* and cat- specific: *Cystoisospora felis* and *C. rivolta* can cause coccidiosis in dogs and cats, respectively; infection is generally subclinical and shedding of oocysts is associated with stress.

ETIOLOGY/PATHOPHYSIOLOGY

Hookworms

- Infection with hookworm occurs by ingestion of infective third-stage larvae from the environment; transmammary through the milk while nursing through the reactivation and migration of somatic larvae to the mammary glands in nursing bitches (*Ancylostoma caninum*); or through larval invasion of the skin resulting in CLM (*Ancylostoma* spp,).
- Adults and fourth-stage larvae of *A. caninum* and *A. tubaeforme* are blood feeders, causing hypochromic, microcytic anemia, enteritis, and even death in puppies and kittens. Former bite sites continue to hemorrhage. Mature dogs may harbor adult worms and be asymptomatic.

Roundworms

- Ascariasis is acquired by ingestion of larvated infectious eggs from the environment; transplacental transmission of *T. canis* larvae from bitch's tissues to pups, causing prenatal infection; transmammary transmission of *T.canis* and *T. cati* larvae; or predation on vertebrate transport hosts. No transplacental or transmammary transmission occurs with *Toxascaris*.

Blackwell's Five-Minute Veterinary Consult Clinical Companion: Small Animal Gastrointestinal Diseases,
First Edition. Edited by Jocelyn Mott and Jo Ann Morrison.
© 2019 John Wiley & Sons, Inc. Published 2019 by John Wiley & Sons, Inc.
Companion website: www.fiveminutevet.com/gastrointestinal

- Adult ascarids reside in the lumen of the small intestine, and can distend the intestine, interfere with gut motility and nutrient utilization, and cause intestinal rupture.
- Larval stages of *Toxocara* spp. migrate in liver, lungs, and other organs, causing granulomatous inflammation (VLM), and persist as somatic larvae in adult animals.

Whipworms

- *Trichuris* infections are acquired by ingestion of larvated infectious eggs that can persist in the environment for years.
- Adults are found attached to the mucosa of the cecum, terminal small intestine, or colon, and consume blood, epithelia, and tissue fluids.
- Clinical signs can occur before patency, i.e., before eggs are shed in feces.

Coccidia

- *Cystoisospora* infections are acquired by ingestion of sporulated oocysts from the environment or from transport hosts that carry extraintestinal stages. Oocysts release zoites that invade enterocytes and undergo asexual and sexual multiplication, causing destruction of host cells.
- *Cystoisospora* can also invade extraintestinal tissue and persist as a latent stage without causing clinical disease.

Systems Affected

Gastrointestinal (GI).

 # SIGNALMENT/HISTORY

- For ancylostomiasis, neonatal animals are at highest risk for clinical disease, while infected bitches or queens are asymptomatic reservoirs. Transmission of *A. caninum* larvae from bitch to offspring in colostrum/milk results in a high rate of infection in pups. Peracute to acute disease is seen in young animals; asymptomatic or chronic disease is seen in mature dogs and cats. Clinical severity greater in dogs than cats.
- Toxocariasis is important clinically in pups and kittens due to transmission *in utero* and/or in colostrum/milk.
- Trichuriasis is not common in very young animals because of long prepatent periods (74–90 days). Many infections are asymptomatic or subclinical. Transmission does not occur from paratenic hosts, transmammary or transplacental routes. Trichuriasis is rare in cats in North America.
- For cystoisosporiasis/coccidiosis, young animals are at higher risk of becoming clinically infected, while adult animals can be asymptomatic.

Risk Factors

- For ancylostomiasis, concurrent enteric infections and compromising conditions (e.g., pregnancy, malnutrition) may exacerbate disease. Environment contaminated with feces of hookworm-infected dog/cat.
- For ascariasis, infection of bitch with dormant larvae in tissues; infection of queen during late pregnancy or early lactation; access to predation of infected transport hosts; and concurrent enteric infections are risk factors.
- For trichuriasis, ingestion of infective (larvated) eggs from environment contaminated with feces of infected dog. Eggs accumulate in environment and remain infective for months to years, especially in soil and dirt runs in moist, shady areas. Return of dog to an environment contaminated with infective eggs after anthelmintic treatment will result in reinfection.

- For cystoisosporiasis/coccidiosis, contaminated environments, concurrent infections, immunosuppression, environmental/travel stress, and predation are risk factors.

Historical Findings

- For ancylostomiasis, melena, diarrhea, loss of condition, poor appetite, dry cough, and sudden death.
- For ascarids, abdominal distension ("pot belly"), weakness, loss of condition, cachexia, poor nursing or appetite, scant feces, coughing; condition affecting entire litters.
- For trichuriasis, diarrhea with mucus and fresh blood indicative of large bowel diarrhea are historical findings of importance.
- For cystoisosporiasis, diarrhea with weight loss, and dehydration are typical findings.

 CLINICAL FEATURES

Hookworms

- Pale mucous membranes, poor body condition, ill thrift, poor hair coat are seen in ancyclostomiasis.
- Erythematous, prurutic lesions, papules on feet, especially between toes are caused by hookworm larvae.

Roundworms

- Abdominal distension ("pot belly"), often with palpable intestinal distension, loss of condition, cachexia, poor nursing or appetite, scant feces, coughing due to larval lung migration are clinical signs associated with toxocariasis in young animals.
- Expulsion of adult *Toxocara* worms in vomitus and/or feces also occurs in severe infections.

Whipworms

- Clinical signs range from asymptomatic to severe with trichuriasis. Intermittent large bowel diarrhea often containing mucus and fresh blood (hematochezia), and in severe cases diarrhea with dehydration, anemia, and weight loss is seen.
- Signs of trichuriasis can occur before eggs are detectable in feces.

Coccidia

- Diarrhea, weight loss, and, rarely, hemorrhage are seen in cystoisosporiasis/coccidiosis.
- Severe infections may manifest with anorexia, vomiting, depression, and even death.

 DIFFERENTIAL DIAGNOSIS

- Anemia and melena are seen with hookworm infections, other causes of erythrocyte destruction or blood loss, physalopterosis, gastrointestinal ulcers.
- GI signs without anemia can be ascribed to dietary indiscretion, ascariasis (large roundworm infection), coccidiosis, strongyloidosis, giardiasis, other bacterial and viral causes. Examine feces to identify eggs, larvae, or cysts. *Physaloptera* can also be seen in vomitus.
- Large bowel diarrhea – bacterial infections of cecum, trichuriasis.
- Inflammatory bowel disease.
- Capillarid infections (*Pearsonema*, *Eucoleus*) – eggs similar in appearance to *Trichuris* but smaller with roughened surface; infect urinary or respiratory tracts, respectively, rather than GI tract; usually asymptomatic.

- Secondary pseudohypoadrenocorticism in severe trichuriasis with metabolic acidosis, hyponatremia, hyperkalemia, and dehydration; normal adrenocorticotropic hormone (ACTH) stimulation response in trichuriasis.
- *Eimeria* pseudoparasites may be seen in fecal floats of dogs and are indicative of coprophagy.

DIAGNOSTICS

Complete Blood Count/Biochemistry/Urinalysis

- For ancylostomiasis, eosinophilia; anemia usually acute normochromic, normocytic, and regenerative; can become microcytic, hypochromic due to chronic iron deficiency.
- For ascarids, usually unremarkable.
- For trichuriasis, usually normal; hyponatremia, hyperkalemia, and metabolic acidosis can occur in very severe cases.

Other Laboratory Tests

- Note that disease/death due to ancylostomiasis may occur prior to egg shedding by adult worms.
- Fecal flotation in hookworm infections reveals typical morulated strongylid eggs with minor size differences among species. Eggs of *Uncinaria* slightly longer than *Ancylostoma* spp.
- Toxocariasis can be diagnosed by fecal flotation to detect eggs; *Toxocara* eggs have a spherical pitted outer shell membrane, single dark cell filling interior, 80–85 μm (*T. canis*), ~75 μm (*T. cati*). *Baylisascaris* eggs appear similar to *T. canis* eggs but smaller (~76 × 60 μm), more finely pitted shell. *Toxascaris* eggs are ovoid, with a smooth exterior shell membrane, 1–2 cells with light-colored cytoplasm; cells do not fill interior of egg; 80 × 70 μm in diameter.
- Ascarids in feces, vomitus, or small intestine can be identified by large size, presence of three lips, and cervical alae.
- Centrifugal flotation of feces in sugar solution (s.g. >1.2) is preferred for the detection of *Trichuris* eggs. *Trichuris* eggs (brown, ovoid or lemon shaped with prominent bipolar plugs, smooth shell, single cell within egg, ~90 × 45 μm) can be differentiated from similar capillarid eggs (smaller, roughened shell surface).
- Centrifugal flotation can be used to visualize unsporulated *Cystoisospora* oocysts in fresh feces. Sporulation in a moist environment can help differentiate *Cystoisospora* oocysts (with two sporocysts) from *Eimeria* oocysts (with four sporocysts).
- Commercial fecal antigen tests are available to specifically detect and differentiate between the intestinal helminths.
- ACTH stimulation test in severe cases with electrolyte disturbances to differentiate trichuriasis from hypoadrenocorticism.

Other Diagnostic Tests

Necropsy of littermates that died of similar signs can be helpful.

Pathologic Findings

- For ancylostomiasis, hookworms attached to small intestinal mucosa may be observed, along with multifocal hemorrhagic ulcerations ("bite sites") on mucosa and blood in the intestinal lumen. Microscopically, eosinophilic enteritis is observed.
- In toxocariasis, enteritis and presence of adult worms are seen.
- Typhlitis, with observation of whipworms attached to large intestinal mucosa, is indicative of trichuriasis.

THERAPEUTICS

Drug(s) of Choice

Hookworms

- *Ancylostoma* adulticide/larvicide therapy can be instituted using one of the following: fenbendazole 50 mg/kg PO q 24 h for three consecutive days in dogs; milbemycin oxime 0.5 mg/kg (dogs) or 2 mg/kg (cats) PO q 30 days; emodepside (3 mg/kg)/praziquantel (12 mg/kg) topically once in cats; moxidectin 0.17 mg/kg SQ q 6 months in dogs; moxidectin 2.5 mg/kg (dogs) or 1.0 mg/kg (cats)/imidoclopramide 10 mg/kg, topically q 30 days; ivermectin 24 µg/kg PO q 30 days in cats.
- Adulticide-only drugs that act against *Ancylostoma* include pyrantel pamoate, label dose in dogs; 10–20 mg/kg PO in cats (extra-label); praziquantel/pyrantel pamoate/febantel, label dose for dogs; praziquantel/pyrantel pamoate, label dose for cats; ivermectin/pyrantel pamoate or ivermectin/pyrantel pamoate/praziquantel, label dose for dogs; selamectin 6 mg/kg topically q 30 days in cats.

Roundworms

- *Toxocara*: milbemycin or other anthelmintic effective against *T. canis* suggested for treatment (extra-label) of *Baylisascaris* in dog. Treat bitch or queen with adulticide/larvicide anthelmintic to remove intestinal stages and to limit transmission to subsequent litters.
- *Toxocara*: adulticide/larvicide therapy can be instituted with fenbendazole 50 mg/kg PO q 24 h for three days; milbemycin oxime 0.5 mg/kg (dogs) or 2 mg/kg (cats) PO q 30 days; emodepside (3 mg/kg) or praziquantel (12 mg/kg) topically once for cats ≥8 weeks old, repeat in 30 days if cat is reinfected.
- Anthelminthics that act against *Toxocara* adult worms but not larvae include pyrantel 5 mg/kg (dogs) or 10–20 mg/kg (cats, extra-label) PO; pyrantel/praziquantel, label dose for cats; febantel/praziquantel/pyrantel, label dose for dogs; ivermectin/pyrantel, label dose for dogs; pyrantel pamoate 5 mg/kg (dogs) or 10–20 mg/kg (cats, extra-label); selamectin 6 mg/kg topically once (*T. cati*, cats), extra-label in dogs; milbemycin oxime, label dosages for dogs and cats; moxidectin, label dosages topically for dogs and cats.

Whipworms

- *Trichuris*: fenbendazole 50 mg/kg PO q 24 h for three days, repeat monthly three times; extra-label use in cats; febantel/praziquantel/pyrantel pamoate, label dose PO in dogs; milbemycin oxime 0.5 mg/kg PO q 30 days in dogs; moxidectin/imidacloprid, label dose in dogs.

Coccidia

- *Cystoisospora*: sulfamethoxine 50–60 mg/kg daily for 5–20 days in dogs and cats is the only label approved drug. Other drugs with some efficacy include sulfaguanidine 150–200 mg/kg daily for six days in dogs and cats; furazolidone 8–20 mg/kg q 24 h or q 12 h for five days for dogs and cats; trimethoprim/sulfonamide, 30–60 mg/kg trimethoprim q 24 h for six days in animals ≥4 kg or 15–30 mg/kg trimethoprim for six days in animals ≤4 kg; sulfadimethoxine/ ormetoprim, 55 mg/kg of sulfadimethoxine and 11 mg/kg of ormetaprim for 7–23 days for dogs; quinacrine 10 mg/kg daily for five days for cats; amprolium 300–400 mg (total) for five days for dogs, 110–200 mg (total) daily for 7–12 days for dogs, 60–100 mg/kg (total) daily for seven days for cats, 1.5 tbsp (23 cc)/gal (sole water source) not to exceed 10 days for dogs; amprolium/sulfadimethoxine, 150 mg/kg of amprolium and 25 mg/kg of sulfadimethoxine for 14 days for dogs; toltrazuril 10–30 mg/kg daily for 1–3 days for dogs; diclazuril 25 mg/kg daily for one day for cats; ponazuril 20 mg/kg daily for 1–3 days for dogs and cats.

Appropriate Health Care

- *Ancylostoma*: peracute and severe acute cases need treatment as inpatients; anthelmintic plus fluid therapy, blood transfusion, supplemental oxygen as indicated by severity of anemia and clinical signs. Sudden death can occur in spite of treatment. In chronic compensatory cases, treat with anthelmintic; if noncompensatory, provide nutritional support (along with iron supplementation).
- *Toxocara*: anthelmintic treatment as outpatient. Acute severe cases treated as inpatients; supplement with intravenous fluids.
- *Trichuris*: outpatient treatment with anthelmintic for most cases. Severe cases with dehydration and electrolyte disturbances require inpatient fluid therapy plus anthelmintic.

 COMMENTS

Client Education

- All hookworms, especially *A. braziliense*, cause CLM when infective larvae penetrate human skin. *A. caninum* larvae can cause CLM or migrate to GI tract, causing abdominal pain and eosinophilia without becoming patent.
- Visceral larva migrans, ocular larva migrans, neural larva migrans, chronic abdominal or cutaneous problems may follow ingestion of infective *Toxocara* spp. or *Baylisascaris* eggs by humans. Most likely cause of neural larva migrans is *Baylisascaris*. Virtually all raccoons become infected with *Baylisascaris* and therefore extreme caution should be exercised with clients having raccoons as "pets."
- *Trichuris* is thought to be host adapted and is less likely to cause zoonotic infections.
- *Cystoisospora* infecting dogs and cats do not commonly infect humans.

Patient Monitoring

- For *Ancylostoma*, monitor fecal egg counts after treatment and hematocrit in anemic patients.
- For ascarids, repeat posttreatment fecal exams on pups/kittens and/or repeat anthelmintic treatment every 2–3 weeks until old enough for monthly anthelmintic product because migrating larvae acquired from bitch or dam will continue to mature.
- For *Trichuris*, repeat fecal examination for trichurid eggs and/or retreat with anthelmintic at three weeks and three months following initial treatment or once a month for three months to detect and eliminate recently matured adults.

Prevention/Avoidance

- Promptly remove and dispose of feces to prevent contamination of environment with larvae of hookworms, eggs of roundworms and whipworms, and oocysts of coccidia.
- Prevent hunting and scavenging to prevent ingestion of potential transport hosts.
- Extra-label treatment of bitch or queen with adulticide/larvicide anthelmintic to remove intestinal stages and decrease vertical transmission to offspring. Treat queen with adulticide/larvicide anthelmintic prior to breeding and after parturition.
- To eliminate intestinal stages and activated dormant larvae of *Ancylostoma* in breeding bitch: fenbendazole at 50 mg/kg/day from day 40 of gestation to day 14 of lactation or ivermectin at 0.5 mg/kg 4–9 days prior to whelping and again 10 days later.
- Begin biweekly anthelmintic treatment of pups at two weeks of age; continue until weaned, especially pups at high risk of infection from bitch or environment; treat monthly after weaned. Begin treatment of kittens at 3–4 weeks of age; treat monthly thereafter.

Possible Complications

- For ascarids, transplacental transmission of large numbers of larvae can result in fetal death or birth of weak, nonviable pups.
- Infection with large numbers of ascarids can cause blockage, possible rupture of small intestine.

Expected Course and Prognosis

- Good prognosis following treatment and implementation of preventive measures.
- Guarded with severe prenatal *T. canis* infection.
- Puppies with peracute or acute *A. caninum* infection may die in spite of treatment. Expect full recovery in cases with anthelmintic treatment and nutritional support. Anthelmintic treatment of adult dogs with dormant larvae in their tissues can result in larval activation and repopulation of small intestine.

Abbreviations

- ACTH = adrenocorticotropic hormone
- CLM = cutaneous larval migrans
- GI = gastrointestinal
- VLM = visceral larval migrans

See Also

- Diarrhea, Acute
- Hematemesis
- Hematochezia

Suggested Reading

Bowman DD. Georgis' Parasitology for Veterinarians, 9th edn. St Louis: Saunders Elsevier, 2009.

Lee AC, Shantz P, Kazacos K, et al. Epidemiologic and zoonotic aspects of ascarid infections in dogs and cats. Trends Parasitol 2010;26:155–161.

Authors: Jeba Jesudoss Chelladurai BVSc & AH, MS, DACVM, Matt T. Brewer DVM, PhD, DACVM

Chapter 78

Protein-Losing Enteropathy

DEFINITION/OVERVIEW

- Any disease process that is characterized by excessive loss of protein into the gastrointestinal lumen.
- Diseases associated with protein-losing enteropathy (PLE) include primary gastrointestinal diseases such as inflammatory bowel disease, intestinal lymphoma, or intestinal lymphangiectasia. In addition, there are other, less common, gastrointestinal diseases that can be associated with excessive gastrointestinal (GI) protein loss, such as fungal disease, other intestinal cancers, intussusceptions, or others. Also, occasionally, systemic disorders such as congestive heart failure may lead to excessive intestinal protein loss, but of course these conditions are not associated with a primary enteropathy.

ETIOLOGY/PATHOPHYSIOLOGY

- The gastrointestinal mucosa serves as an efficient barrier against loss of plasma proteins into the gastrointestinal lumen.
- However, even under physiologic conditions small amounts of plasma proteins are being lost into the gastrointestinal lumen.
- While there are also other sites of protein loss, under physiologic conditions, two-thirds of normal protein loss in dogs occurs through the small intestine.
- Plasma proteins that leak into the gastrointestinal lumen are rapidly digested into oligopeptides and also constituent amino acids. Amino acids can be reabsorbed and used for the synthesis of new proteins.
- This normal loss of plasma proteins can be accelerated by gastrointestinal mucosal disease or by increased leakage of lymph into the gastrointestinal lumen.
- Gastrointestinal protein loss is associated with loss of both albumin and globulin.
- In response to increased gastrointestinal protein loss, the liver increases albumin synthesis. However, the liver cannot increase albumin synthesis to more than twice the normal rate.
- When protein loss exceeds protein synthesis, hypoproteinemia ensues.
- Severe hypoproteinemia causes decreased plasma oncotic pressure, which may be associated with hemodynamic changes and may lead to effusion into body cavities or, less commonly, peripheral edema.
- However, dogs and cats with PLE are not always panhypoproteinemic, and can have a low-normal serum globulin concentration with hypoalbuminemia. This is due to the fact that while globulin is being lost at an increased rate, globulin production may also be equally increased due to the underlying disease process.

Blackwell's Five-Minute Veterinary Consult Clinical Companion: Small Animal Gastrointestinal Diseases, First Edition. Edited by Jocelyn Mott and Jo Ann Morrison.
© 2019 John Wiley & Sons, Inc. Published 2019 by John Wiley & Sons, Inc.
Companion website: www.fiveminutevet.com/gastrointestinal

Systems Affected

- Coagulation – patients with PLE lose antithrombin and may become hypercoagulable.
- Gastrointestinal – as mentioned, PLE may be due to a primary gastrointestinal disease that may be associated with diarrhea, vomiting, or other clinical signs of GI disease.
- Hemodynamic – ascites or pleural effusion due to decreased oncotic pressure leading to abdominal discomfort or even dyspnea.
- Lymphatic – lymphangiectasia.
- Respiratory – dyspnea due to pleural effusion.
- Skin – subcutaneous edema.

 # SIGNALMENT/HISTORY

- In general, PLE is considered to be far more common in dogs than in cats. However, more recent data would suggest that PLE also frequently occurs in cats with severe chronic enteropathy, but in contrast to dogs, the disease is usually not as severe in cats.
- Several breeds appear to have a breed predilection: soft-coated Wheaten Terrier, Basenji, Yorkshire Terrier, and Norwegian Lundehund. However, a dog or cat of any breed or sex can be affected. Also, there is no age predilection.

Risk Factors

Any of the possible underlying conditions should be considered risk factors for PLE.

Historical Findings

- Diarrhea (chronic, continuous or intermittent, watery to semi-solid), weight loss, and lethargy are most frequently reported. However, a significant number of dogs with PLE have normal stools.
- Vomiting is uncommon.
- Dogs can be presented for apparent weight gain or abdominal distension as the only clinical sign.
- Cats with PLE generally are presented for chronic diarrhea, vomiting, and/or weight loss.

 # CLINICAL FEATURES

- There are no specific clinical features of PLE itself. However, many dogs and cats with PLE show a poor body condition and/or a poor hair coat.
- Physical examination may reveal features of chronic enteropathy, such as thickened bowel loops. However, many dogs with intestinal lymphangiectasia do not have thickened bowel loops.
- Also, physical examination may reveal clinical signs of complications of PLE, such as ascites, while dependent edema and dyspnea from pleural effusion may be detected with marked hypoproteinemia.

 # DIFFERENTIAL DIAGNOSES

Hypoalbuminemia due to PLE must be differentiated from other causes of hypoalbuminemia.
- Hypoalbuminemia due to liver failure.
  - Hypoalbuminemia due to hepatic failure is most often associated with a normal or even increased serum globulin concentration.
  - Hepatic enzyme activities may be increased, although in late-stage hepatic failure serum liver enzyme activities may not be increased.

- Serum concentrations of synthetic markers, such as blood urea nitrogen (BUN), cholesterol, or glucose, may also be decreased, although less residual hepatic function is needed to maintain BUN, cholesterol, and especially glucose homeostasis than albumin homeostasis.
  - Serum pre- and postprandial bile acids concentrations may be increased.
  - Serum bilirubin concentration may be increased.
  - Liver failure can usually easily be ruled out by a simple serum chemistry profile. In some patients, further diagnostics, such as serum bile acids concentrations or abdominal ultrasound, are needed to confirm hepatic failure.
- Hypoalbuminemia due to protein-losing nephropathy (PLN).
  - Mild urinary protein loss may occur in patients with fever or hyperadrenocorticism. However, this is rarely severe enough to cause hypoalbuminemia.
  - Moderate to severe urinary protein loss can occur in patients with glomerulonephritis or amyloidosis. Hypoalbuminemia in these patients is commonly associated with a normal or even increased serum globulin concentration.
  - PLN can be ruled out by a normal urine protein:creatinine ratio.
- Hypoalbuminemia due to severe blood loss.
  - Hypoalbuminemia of blood loss is usually associated with hypoglobulinemia.
  - Blood loss can be excluded by assessment of the erythrogram on the complete blood count (CBC) and a thorough physical examination; in some cases a test for fecal occult blood may be necessary (tests based on o-toluidine are considered more reliable than guaiac-based tests as they are less affected by the patient's diet).
- Inadequate protein intake (i.e., starvation) is a rare cause of hypoalbuminemia.
- Hypoalbuminemia due to PLE is often associated with hypoglobulinemia. PLE can be confirmed by measurement of an increased fecal alpha-1-protease inhibitor concentration (must be assessed in naturally passed and freshly frozen fecal samples from three consecutive days).

 # DIAGNOSTICS

- Serum chemistry profile: essential for the diagnosis of hypoalbuminemia.
- CBC, serum chemistry profile, serum bile acids concentrations, and urine protein/creatinine ratio for a basic differentiation of the cause of hypoalbuminemia.
- Fecal occult blood to rule out blood loss into the gastrointestinal tract. In general, there are two different types of occult blood tests for use in dogs and cats. One is based on guaiac, the other on o-toluidine. Guaiac tests appear to be more likely to be affected by a meat-based diet and thus o-toluidine-based tests are preferred.
- A definitive diagnosis of gastrointestinal protein loss is only possible by chromium-labeled albumin (^{51}Cr-albumin) in both dogs and cats or measurement of fecal concentrations of alpha-1-protease inhibitor.
  - A ^{51}Cr-albumin test can be performed by administering a known amount of ^{51}Cr intravenously and then collecting all urine and fecal matter for a period of several days. The ^{51}Cr binds to albumin in the circulation and is only slowly released as ^{51}Cr-albumin is being metabolized. Thus, in healthy dogs and cats, almost no radioactivity should be recovered in either urine or feces. In patients with PLE fecal radioactivity will be increased. This test exposes both patient and personnel to unacceptable amounts of radioactivity and is thus no longer being routinely performed.
  - The measurement of fecal alpha-1-protease inhibitor concentration can be used to document excessive gastrointestinal protein loss. Alpha-1-protease inhibitor is a plasma protein with a similar molecular weight to albumin and is thus lost at a similar rate to

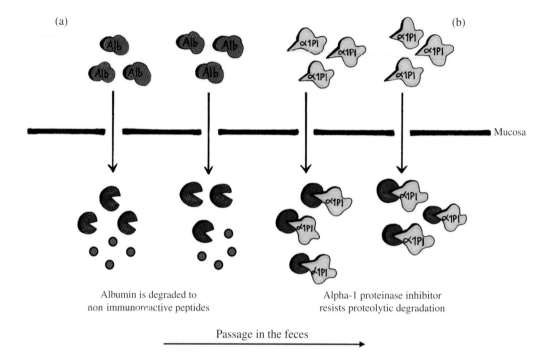

(a)

(b)

Mucosa

Albumin is degraded to
non immunoreactive peptides

Alpha-1 proteinase inhibitor
resists proteolytic degradation

Passage in the feces

■ **Fig. 78.1.** (a) After being lost into the intestinal lumen, albumin and other plasma proteins are readily degraded by digestive and bacterial proteinases. The resulting degradation products are not immunoreactive and, thus cannot be measured by immunoassays. (b) Alpha-1-PI has a similar molecular size to albumin and is thus lost into the gastrointestinal tract at a similar rate to albumin. Unlike albumin, alpha-1-PI resists degradation by proteinases present in the intestinal lumen and can thus be detected in feces by immunoassays. Source: ©GI Lab, Texas A&M University; reproduced with permission.

albumin. Assays for the measurement of alpha-1-protease inhibitor are species specific for dogs and cats and at the moment, only an assay for dogs is available for routine clinical use. This assay is only available through the Gastrointestinal Laboratory at Texas A&M University. Samples from three consecutive defecations need to be collected in special preweighed fecal tubes that can be sourced from the GI Lab (Figure 78.1).

■ For a more general work-up of gastrointestinal signs.
  • Fecal smear, fecal flotation, and broad-spectrum antihelmintic agent to evaluate and treat for potential parasitism with a variety of gastrointestinal endoparasites.
  • Measurement of serum folate and cobalamin concentrations to localize the gastrointestinal disease and diagnose complicating cobalamin deficiency.
  • Feeding trial using an elimination diet containing a novel or hydrolyzed protein source to rule out adverse reactions to food.
  • Antibiotic therapy with tylosin to rule out an antibiotic-responsive diarrhea.
  • Rectal mucosal scraping to help rule out histoplasmosis in geographic regions where histoplasmosis is endemic.
  • Abdominal ultrasound may reveal intestinal "striations", which represent dilated lacteals. This finding is not pathognomonic for a particular etiology.
  • Gastroduodenoscopy and colonoscopy to visualize the gastrointestinal mucosa and to collect endoscopic biopsies for histopathologic evaluation. Visualizing white "plaques" (e.g., chylomicron distended lacteals) along the mucosa suggests lymphangiectasia (Figure 78.2). Endoscopic biopsies should contain full-thickness mucosa to maximize the diagnostic yield of tissue specimens.

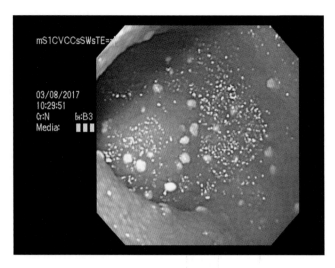

■ **Fig. 78.2.** Visualizing white "plaques" (e.g., chylomicron distended lacteals) along the mucosa during endoscopy suggests lymphangiectasia.

- Abdominal exploratory laparotomy may show dilated intestinal lymphatics and allows for full-thickness biopsies of intestines and lymph nodes. However, full-thickness biopsies are not recommended in patients with severe hypoalbuminemia.
- Other diagnostics as necessary.

Pathologic Findings

- PLE is not associated with any specific gross or histopathologic lesions. Lesions identified are those of the specific cause of PLE.
  - Inflammatory bowel disease.
  - Intestinal lymphoma.
  - Lymphangiectasia.
  - Histoplasmosis.
  - Other.

 # THERAPEUTICS

There is no specific treatment for PLE. Instead, the underlying disease process needs to be managed appropriately. This, of course, requires definitive diagnosis, which in turn requires collecting intestinal biopsies, by either endoscopy or exploratory laparotomy. This can be especially challenging as many patients with severe PLE are hypoalbuminemic and are thus poor anesthetic risks and also show poor healing of the intestinal biopsy site. Because of this, the author prefers endoscopy to collect biopsy samples as this will help to mitigate any issues of biopsy site dehiscence. If the primary diagnosis is idiopathic inflammatory bowel disease, a hypoallergenic diet and immunosuppressive agents should be chosen. Intestinal lymphoma should be therapeutically addressed with chemotherapy, and lymphangiectasia can be addressed by an ultra-low-fat diet. However, even after histopathologic evaluation of intestinal biopsies, the diagnosis is often unclear and many times lymphangiectasia coexists with IBD.

Drug(s) of Choice

- There is no pharmacologic therapy for PLE itself. Instead, the underlying cause of PLE must be addressed.

- However, patients with PLE lose antithrombin and can be hypercoagulable. Thus, patients should be treated with a platelet aggregation inhibitor.
  - In dogs or cats: clopidogrel bisulfate 3–5 mg/kg q 24 h PO in dogs; 18.75 mg/cat q 24 h PO, which equals one-fourth of a 75 mg tablet.
  - In dogs: low-dose aspirin 0.5 mg/kg q 12 h PO; use an 81 mg tablet of aspirin and put into the barrel of a 10 mL syringe, add 8.1 mL of water and shake until completely dissolved to make a 10 mg/mL solution; discard unused portion immediately.

Precautions/Interactions

- Aspirin and clopidogrel should not be used concurrently.
- Clopidogrel should also not be used with other nonsteroidal antiinflammatory drugs (NSAIDs), phenytoin, torsemide, or warfarin.

Alternative Drugs

- Octreotide, a long-acting somatostatin inhibitor, has been successfully used in some patients with PLE; the mechanism of action for improving intestinal protein loss is not clear and no specific dosage for this indication has been published.
- Diuretics such as furosemide have been used by some clinicians to control edema and pleural effusion. However, they do not work well in patients with PLE because of decreased plasma oncotic pressure and may be associated with side effects.

Appropriate Health Care

The most important consideration in dogs with PLE is identifying and treating the underlying disease process. This is followed by preventing complications from hypoalbuminemia and preserving plasma oncotic pressure.

Nursing Care

- In cases of severe hypoalbuminemia that are associated with clinical signs due to edema or effusion, plasma transfusions or colloids (such as hetastarch or dextran) should be considered to increase plasma oncotic pressure.
- Abdominocentesis to remove ascites or pleurocentesis to remove pleural effusion in cases with compromise from severe effusion.

Diet

- The choice of an appropriate diet should depend on the underlying disease process that has been identified.
  - Idiopathic inflammatory bowel disease: a limited antigen or hypoallergenic diet should be chosen. Limited antigen diets contain a single protein source to which the patient should not have been previously exposed to. The diet should also only contain a single carbohydrate source because each carbohydrate source contains a small amount of proteins that could have negative effects. Hypoallergenic diets usually contain a hydrolyzed protein. Various diets are available and may differ based on the protein source, level of hydrolyzation, and evenness of hydrolyzation.
  - Lymphangiectasia: traditionally, an ultra-low-fat diet is chosen in dogs with lymphangiectasia. However, data are very limited. Ultra-low-fat diets contain less than 20 g of fat per 1000 kcal, but are not energy restricted (i.e., they are not weight loss diets).

Activity

Normal, unless there are severe complications from hypoalbuminemia.

Surgical Considerations

- Hypoalbuminemia increases postoperative morbidity because of slow wound healing.
- Some rare causes of PLE (e.g., intussusception, chronic foreign body, and some intestinal neoplasias) may require surgical intervention.

 COMMENTS

- PLE is a complex condition as it describes a compilation of a group of diseases rather than one single disease entity.
- Patients with hypoalbuminemia need to be assessed for the various causes to definitively identify the GI tract as the site of protein loss.
- Excessive gastrointestinal protein loss should prompt the clinician to immediately undertake a systematic evaluation of the patient for chronic enteropathy (i.e., comprehensive history and physical examination; evaluation and treatment for gastrointestinal parasites; differentiation of primary and secondary causes of GI signs; evaluation of serum cobalamin and folate concentrations and cobalamin supplementation if indicated; definitive diagnosis of the underlying enteropathy by abdominal ultrasound, gastroduodenoscopy, rectal scrape, and others as needed).

Client Education

- PLE is a severe disease process that has a guarded to poor prognosis. Thus, work-up might be complex and management may involve multiple interventions that all may or may not have a beneficial effect.
- The clinical signs of complications from hypoalbuminemia should be discussed with the client.

Patient Monitoring

- The most important parameter to monitor is serum albumin concentration. Depending on the value at the time of diagnosis, serum albumin concentration should be reevaluated after a couple of days initially and with decreasing frequency as serum albumin concentrations normalize.
- Also, evaluation of body weight and clinical signs from the complications of hypoalbuminemia (i.e., pleural effusion, ascites, and/or edema) should be monitored in patients with severe hypoalbuminemia.

Prevention/Avoidance

Manage the patient long term, i.e., diet and antiinflammatory agents should be continued long term to avoid recurrence of the disease.

Possible Complications

- Respiratory difficulty from pleural effusion.
- Severe protein-calorie malnutrition.
- Intractable diarrhea.

Expected Course and Prognosis

- Prognosis is guarded. Smaller breed dogs carry a more favorable prognosis since nutritional support is easier to accomplish.
- The primary disease cannot be treated in many cases.

Abbreviations

- ^{51}Cr-albumin – chromium-labeled albumin
- BUN = blood urea nitrogen
- CBC = complete blood count
- GI = gastrointestinal
- IBD = idiopathic inflammatory bowel disease (some authors translate IBD as inflammatory bowel disease; however, this author finds it more useful to reserve the term IBD for cases that are idiopathic)
- NSAID = nonsteroidal antiinflammatory drug
- PCV = packed cell volume
- PLE = protein-losing enteropathy
- PLN = protein-losing nephropathy

See Also

- Inflammatory Bowel Disease
- Lymphangiectasia

Suggested Reading

Burke KF, Broussard JD, Ruaux CG, Suchodolski JS, Williams DA, Steiner JM. Evaluation of fecal alpha1-proteinase inhibitor concentrations in cats with idiopathic inflammatory bowel disease and cats with gastrointestinal neoplasia. Vet J 2013;196:189–196.

Dossin O, Lavoué R. Protein-losing enteropathies in dogs. Vet Clin North Am Small Anim Pract 2011;41:399–418.

Littman MP, Dambach DM, Vaden SL, et al. Familial protein-losing enteropathy and protein-losing nephropathy in soft coated Wheaten Terriers: 222 cases (1983–1997). J Vet Intern Med 2000;14:68–80.

Simmerson SM, Armstrong PJ, Wunschmann A, Jessen CR, Crews LJ, Washabau RJ. Clinical features, intestinal histopathology, and outcome in protein-losing enteropathy in Yorkshire Terrier dogs. J Vet Intern Med 2014;28:331–337.

Vaden SL. Protein-losing enteropathies. In: Steiner JM, ed. Small Animal Gastroenterology. Hannover: Schlütersche, 2008, pp. 207–210.

Author: Jörg M. Steiner med.vet., Dr.med.vet., PhD, DACVIM, DECVIM-CA, AGAF

Chapter 79

Salmon Poisoning Disease

DEFINITION/OVERVIEW

- Salmon poisoning disease (SPD) is caused by the rickettsial organism *Neorickettsia helminthoeca*.
- The gram-negative coccobacillary rickettsia organisms are approximately 0.3 μm in size and reside in the trematode (fluke) vector, *Nanophyetus salmincola*.
- Three hosts are required for the fluke life cycle: snails, fish, mammals or birds.
- Coinfections with other bacteria or strains of *N. helminthoeca* can occur (Elokomin fluke fever and *Stellanchasmus falcatus*).
- SPD occurs in dogs, foxes, and coyotes after consuming raw, undercooked, infected, salmonid fish. It should be noted that salmonid fish includes salmon, char, trout, and other freshwater fishes.

ETIOLOGY/PATHOPHYSIOLOGY

- The typical geographic distribution for SPD is the coastal Pacific Northwest, extending from northern California to southern British Columbia, but can also be inland along the Columbia River basin.
- The fluke initially infects the first intermediate host, an aquatic snail (*Oxytrema silicula*), prevalent in fresh or brackish coastal streams, to help complete its life cycle. These coastal streams and the rivers that coalesce in these areas reflect the distribution of the snail.
- The fluke then leaves the snail as a cercaria and penetrates the skin of or is ingested by the second intermediate host, the salmonid fish. The fish are infected in fresh water but maintain the trematode and rickettsial infection throughout their ocean migration.
- Ingestion of raw or undercooked infected salmonids by dogs, foxes, and coyotes leads to SPD.
- Domestic cats do not become infected with SPD.
- *Neorickettsia helminthoeca* is not zoonotic, and does not cause disease in humans.
- *N. salmincola* (fluke) can cause gastrointestinal signs and possibly an eosinophilia in humans.

Systems Affected

- Gastrointestinal – vomiting occurs in >80% of dogs and >70% have diarrhea.
- Hemic/lymphatic/immune – peripheral lymphadenopathy occurs in >70% of dogs.

Blackwell's Five-Minute Veterinary Consult Clinical Companion: Small Animal Gastrointestinal Diseases, First Edition. Edited by Jocelyn Mott and Jo Ann Morrison.
© 2019 John Wiley & Sons, Inc. Published 2019 by John Wiley & Sons, Inc.
Companion website: www.fiveminutevet.com/gastrointestinal

- Respiratory – a serous nasal discharge, mucopurulent conjunctivitis, or tachypnea may occur.
- Nervous – fewer than 20% of dogs exhibit mental changes, neck pain, or seizures.

 SIGNALMENT/HISTORY

- Most commonly occurs in domestic and wild canidae, but has been reported in captive bears.
- SPD does not occur in domestic cats.
- Intact male dogs and Labrador retrievers are overrepresented but this may be the result of lifestyle and recreation.
- The median age of infection was three years in one study.

Risk Factors

- Dogs engaged in swimming, water and outdoor activities in endemic areas.
- Any dog with a history of exposure to raw or undercooked salmon, trout or other salmonids.

Historical Findings

- Incubation of SPD can range from two to seven days post exposure, but can be as long as 33 days.
- Typically, an owner notes inappetence, lethargy, and other gastrointestinal signs (vomit and or diarrhea) for several days.
- All these findings may also be accompanied by a marked fever (104–107 °F).

 CLINICAL FEATURES

- A mild to marked fever is noted in many dogs infected with SPD.
- Additionally, peripheral lymphadenopathy is quite common.
- Other signs include clinical dehydration, weak pulses, abdominal discomfort, tachypnea, tachycardia, and splenomegaly.
- Most dogs are depressed and exhibit weight loss and inappetence.

 DIFFERENTIAL DIAGNOSIS

- Many diseases and conditions present similarly to SPD.
- Some notable rule-outs include pancreatitis, hypoadrenocorticism, parvovirus, acute hemorrhagic diarrhea syndrome, canine distemper, lymphoma, toxin ingestion, *Ehrlichia*, and other tick-borne illnesses.
- Careful consideration of the signalment and history of the patient may help in prioritizing the differential list.

 DIAGNOSTICS

Complete Blood Count/Biochemistry/Urinalysis

- Thrombocytopenia (present in 90% of dogs), neutropenia to neutrophilia, lymphopenia, and nonregenerative anemia.
- Hypoproteinemia, hypocholesterolemia, hypochloremia, hyponatremia, hyperkalemia.
- Proteinuria, bilirubinuria, cylindruria.

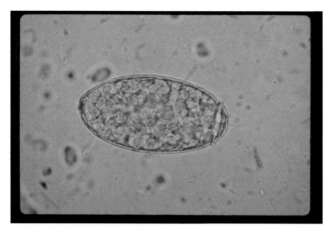

■ **Fig. 79.1.** Ova from *N. salmincola* in a fecal sample from a dog diagnosed with SPD. Source: Image courtesy of Dr William Foreyt.

Other Laboratory Tests

■ Coagulation panel: elevated prothrombin, activated partial thromboplastin time, decreased antithrombin activity, elevated d-dimers. SPD dogs are diagnosed with disseminated intravascular coagulation.

■ Fecal smear/centrifugation/sedimentation: *N. salmincola* ova detected in fecal specimens within 5–8 days post ingestion of infected fish. Multiple fecal methods may be needed to detect ova (Figure 79.1).

■ Polymerase chain reaction (PCR): DNA can be detected from clinical specimens (blood, lymph node aspirates, splenic aspirates, stool) if ova in the stool or the rickettsial organism cannot be detected in the blood or lymph node/organ aspirate cytology.

■ Specific testing including a quantitative canine pancreatic lipase immunoreactivity, SNAP parvo test, screening cortisol/adrenocorticotropic stimulation test, SNAP 4Dx Plus test, and tick serology may also be helpful to rule out other differentials or concurrent disease.

Imaging

■ Abdominal ultrasound may reveal splenomegaly with a mottled echotexture and abdominal lymphadenomegaly.

■ Fluid-distended intestinal loops with wall thickening, corrugation, hypermotility or hypomotility may also be seen using ultrasonographic examination.

Other Diagnostic Tests

■ Cytology findings: lymph node aspirates contain rickettsial organisms and associated histiocytic hyperplasia and lymphoid reactivity (Figure 79.2).

Pathologic Findings

■ Lymphoid tissue enlargement – tissues are often yellowish with prominent white foci.
■ Petechial hemorrhages.
■ Gastrointestinal tract thickening with white nodules.
■ Intestinal contents – frequently contain free blood. Flukes may not be visible grossly.
■ Histopathology reveals depletion of lymph node follicles and infiltration of lymphoid tissues and the intestinal submucosa by histiocytes, the cytoplasm of which contains numerous lymphoid follicles. Flukes may also be found embedded in the gastrointestinal mucosa.

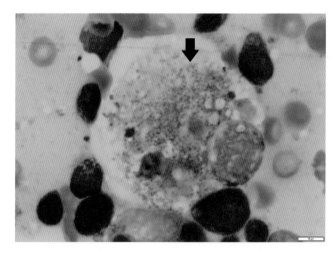

■ **Fig. 79.2.** Magnification 100×, lymph node aspirate cytology of a dog with SPD. Intracytoplasmic *N. helminthoeca* in the macrophage. Source: Image courtesy of Dr Ilaria Cerchiaro.

 THERAPEUTICS

- May be dependent on how acutely the animal presents in the course of the disease.
- It is worth noting that parenteral antibiotic therapy may be needed in vomiting and/or debilitated animals.

Drug(s) of Choice

- The overall treatment of choice for *Neorickettsia helminthoeca* is doxycycline (5 mg/kg PO q 12 h) or tetracycline (22 mg/kg q 8 h PO). This should be given for a minimum of 1–2 weeks. It is worth noting that parenteral antibiotic therapy may be needed in vomiting and/or debilitated animals.
- One dose of the anthelmintic praziquantel (10–30 mg/kg PO) is often given as treatment for the flukes (*Nanophyetus salmincola*), and may be repeated. Parenteral therapy may be needed in vomiting and/or debilitated animals.
- It is suggested that SPD-affected dogs should also be tested and treated for other parasitic infections.

Appropriate Health Care

An acutely ill patient that is febrile, dehydrated and anorexic/hyporexic may need hospitalization and supportive care consisting of intravenous fluid therapy, antiemetics, nutritional support (nasoesophageal or nasogastric feeding), whole blood, packed red blood cell transfusion, plasma transfusion, or other colloids if anemic or hypovolemic.

 COMMENTS

Patient Monitoring

Monitor hydration, electrolytes, acid–base balance, and body temperature.

Prevention/Avoidance

- *Neorickettsia helminthoeca* metacercariae are destroyed by proper cooking or freezing of fish.
- Dogs should be discouraged from eating raw fish. If dogs have access to raw fish in endemic areas, they should be closely monitored for signs of lethargy, hyporexia, or vomiting within two weeks of exposure.
- There are no vaccines for SPD in dogs.
- Recovered dogs may be reinfected with SPD if their antibodies fail to cross-react with an alternate strain of *N. helminthoeca*.

Possible Complications

Complications that can occur as a result of SPD are disseminated intravascular coagulation, septicemia, cardiac arrhythmias, adverse drug reactions, and intussusceptions.

Expected Course and Prognosis

If diagnosed early, SPD has an excellent prognosis for recovery. However, without treatment, the patient can succumb to the disease in 5–10 days.

Abbreviations

- DNA = deoxyribonucleic acid
- PCR = polymerase chain reaction
- SPD = salmon poisoning disease

See Also

- Canine Parvovirus Infection
- Diarrhea, Acute
- Gastroenteritis, Hemorrhagic
- Hematochezia
- Melena
- Vomiting, Acute

Suggested Reading

Green CE. Infectious Diseases of the Dog and Cat, 4th edn. St Louis: Elsevier, 2012, p.25.

Greiman SE, Kent ML, Betts J, et al. *Nanophyetus salmincola*, vector of the salmon poisoning agent *Neorickettsia helminthoeca*, harbors a second pathogenic *Neorickettsia* species. Vet Parasit 2016;229:107–109.

Sykes JE. Canine and Feline Infectious Diseases. St Louis: Elsevier, 2014, p. 31.

Sykes JE, Marks SL, Mapes RM, et al. Salmon poisoning disease in dogs: 29 cases. J Vet Intern Med 2010;24:504–513.

Acknowledgments: The author and editors acknowledge the prior contribution of Dr Jane Sykes.

Author: Jennifer E. Slovak DVM, MS, DACVIM

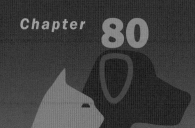

Chapter 80

Short Bowel Syndrome

DEFINITION/OVERVIEW

- Short bowel syndrome (SBS) refers to the clinical signs that develop after extensive resection of the small intestine (SI).
- SBS in animals frequently results when 75% or more of the SI is resected.
- The decreased absorptive surface area of the SI that results from extensive resection often causes inadequate digestion and malabsorption.
- Common causes for extensive bowel resection include intestinal foreign bodies, volvulus, intussusception, trauma, infarction, neoplasia, and fungal infection.

ETIOLOGY/PATHOPHYSIOLOGY

- Removal of a significant portion of the duodenum and jejunum results in decreased pancreaticobiliary and mucosal enzyme concentrations.
    - There is insufficient digestion and transport of fat, carbohydrates, and proteins.
    - Absorption of glucose, monosaccharides, amino acids, vitamins, and microelements is impaired.
    - A faster than normal transit time contributes to malabsorption where there is decreased contact time of nutrients with the intestinal mucosa.
    - A hypertonic environment is created by undigested or partially digested carbohydrates and fats, which causes the flow of water from the vascular space to the intestinal lumen.
    - Faster than normal intestinal transit time through the ileum means the colon cannot respond to increased loads of water, which contributes to diarrhea, dehydration, hyponatremia, hypokalemia, and hypovolemia.
- In cases of ileal resection, bile salt reabsorption and transport via the portal vein to the liver is impaired. This eventually leads to fat malabsorption and steatorrhea.
- Loss of significant portions of the jejunum and ileum interferes with absorption of trace elements (iron, zinc, copper) and vitamins (such as cobalamin).
- Loss of extensive portions of the jejunum can lead to vitamin D deficiency, contributing to impaired calcium, phosphorus, and magnesium homeostasis.
- Resection of the ileocolic valve can result in small intestinal bacterial overgrowth (SIBO), which may become serious if left untreated.
- Loss of intestinal hormones (gastrin, cholecystokinin, and secretin, among others) can occur. These enzymes are responsible for regulation of motility, intestinal secretion, and mucosal adaption.

Blackwell's Five-Minute Veterinary Consult Clinical Companion: Small Animal Gastrointestinal Diseases, First Edition. Edited by Jocelyn Mott and Jo Ann Morrison.
© 2019 John Wiley & Sons, Inc. Published 2019 by John Wiley & Sons, Inc.
Companion website: www.fiveminutevet.com/gastrointestinal

- The goal of intestinal adaptation is to increase absorption of nutrients in the remaining intestine and increase intestinal transit time.
  - The ability of the intestine to adapt when extensive resection has occurred is very important in the prognosis of patients with SBS. During adaption, the intestinal mucosa undergoes histologic and functional changes to maintain nutritional balance. Villi elongate, crypts deepen, and there are increased numbers of cells per villus column.
  - The ileum possesses the greatest adaptive ability. Clinical improvement of diarrhea in patients with SBS is a result of adaptation, which allows for improved absorptive ability and mucosal enzyme activity.

Systems Affected

- Gastrointestinal – loose, watery diarrhea, malabsorption, weight loss, dehydration, and electrolyte imbalances can occur postoperatively. Occasionally polyphagia can occur after postoperative shock subsides. Long term, malnutrition, hypergastrinemia, and steatorrhea can occur.
- Hemic/lymphatic/immune – normocytic, normochromic anemia can develop postoperatively as a result of chronic disease. Persistent malnutrition leading to hypoalbuminemia and hypoproteinemia can lead to a depressed immune system.

 # SIGNALMENT/HISTORY

Any animal can develop SBS after extensive resection of the SI.

Risk Factors

- The main risk factor is extensive resection of the SI.
- SBS frequently develops when 75% or more of the SI is resected.

Historical Findings

Clinical signs occur after extensive resection of the SI.
- Loose, watery diarrhea.
- Weight loss or failure to gain weight.
- Polyphagia can develop as postoperative shock subsides.
- Ascites and edema can develop in hypoalbuminemic patients.

 # CLINICAL FEATURES

- Animals may initially be in shock in the immediate postoperative period (depressed, hypovolemic).
- Physical exam reveals weight loss and dehydration.

 # DIAGNOSTICS

Diagnosis is based on the presence of clinical signs and history of extensive SI resection.

Complete Blood Count/Biochemistry/Urinalysis

- In the immediate postoperative period, a chemistry panel may show hyponatremia, hypokalemia, azotemia, metabolic acidosis, and hypoalbuminemia.
- A complete blood count may show nonregenerative anemia.

Other Laboratory Tests

A gastrointestinal malabsorption panel may show hypocobalaminemia with ileal resection.

Imaging

Abdominal radiographs and contrast studies may show dilated intestinal segments and a fast intestinal transit time.

 THERAPEUTICS

- Treatment is directed at maintaining adequate nutritional support, minimizing electrolyte abnormalities, and controlling diarrhea.
- Intravenous fluid therapy and electrolyte support are important during the initial period after resection to maintain hydration and minimize electrolyte abnormalities.

Drug(s) of Choice

- Gastric acid hypersecretion can occur, which can be an important contributor to diarrhea. H2-receptor antagonists such as famotidine at 0.5–1 mg/kg/day PO q 12–24 h in dogs and cats or proton pump inhibitors such as omeprazole at 1–2 mg/kg/day PO in dogs should be administered.
- Intestinal bacterial overgrowth is common and should be managed with antibiotics. Metronidazole (15 mg/kg PO twice daily in dogs and cats) and amoxicillin (6–20 mg/kg PO q 8 h in dogs and cats) or enrofloxacin (5–10 mg/kg PO once daily in dogs) should be used initially. Choices for long-term management include metronidazole or tylosin (7–15 mg/kg PO q 12–24 h in dogs and cats).
- Occasionally pancreatic enzyme replacement such as Pancrezyme™ (2 teaspoons of powder per 20 kg of body weight in dogs) is useful if extensive resection of the duodenum has disrupted the pancreatic duct.
- Persisent, loose, watery diarrhea can be treated with an antidiarrheal such as loperamide (0.1 mg/kg PO q 8–12 h in dogs and 0.08 mg/kg PO q 12 h in cats).
- Ursodeoxycholate (UDCA) improved fecal characteristics experimentally. The recommended dose is 10–15 mg/kg PO once daily.
- Hydrophilic laxatives may decrease fluidity of existing bowel contents and may increase fecal bulk. Psyllium (Metamucil™ 1 teaspoon/5–10 kg added to each meal for dogs and cats).
- Micronutrient supplementation (vitamins, calcium, zinc, magnesium) of food may be needed.
- Patients may be hypocobalaminemic if the ileum has been resected. Cobalamin supplementation is recommended (250–1500 μg/week in dogs depending on weight; 250 μg/week in cats; see http://vetmed.tamu.edu/gilab/research/cobalamin-information for dosing information).

Precautions/Interactions

Hydration status should be monitored in patients on long-term laxatives if used to improve fecal consistency (as described above).

Appropriate Health Care

The animal's nutritional status and food tolerance should be closely monitored long term to avoid starvation.

Diet

- During the initial postoperative period, ideal nutritional support may be provided via total parenteral nutrition (TPN).

- Partial parenteral nutrition (PPN) can also be used.
- Limited oral intake should be started as early as possible after surgery to help stimulate intestinal adaptation. Initially, elemental or polymeric diets (such as Clinicare™) can be fed. Polymeric diets can be fed via nasoesophageal or nasogastric tube. Some animals are polyphagic soon after surgery; care should be taken not to feed these animals large amounts as this can contribute to diarrhea.
- Low-fat, highly digestible diets fed as frequent, small meals should be used long term.

Activity

Once the patient is home, and hydration status is normal, activity level can return to normal.

Surgical Considerations

- Surgery may be considered when medical and dietary therapy fails to control clinical signs.
- The goal of surgical management is to increase intestinal absorptive capacity.
- Clinical data regarding use of surgery to improve clinical signs in SBS are lacking.
- Surgical options have only been described in case reports or in experimental animals and include reversed small intestinal segment, colonic interposition, and creation of intestinal valves.
- Close anesthetic monitoring of hypoalbuminemic patients is warranted and drugs that are highly protein bound should be avoided. Hypotension is the main complication and colloidal support with hetastarch is recommended.

 # COMMENTS

Early and aggressive management of SBS typically leads to a better outcome.

Client Education

- Clients should be informed that treatment may be long term and at considerable cost.
- It may take weeks or months of aggressive therapy for diarrhea or loose stool to improve to an acceptable level.
- It is important to allow time for intestinal adaptation to occur prior to making any decisions about euthanasia.

Patient Monitoring

- Weight and body condition scores should be monitored closely.
- Electrolytes should be monitored daily while patients are hospitalized.
- Protein levels should be monitored every 2–3 weeks initially after patients are discharged from the hospital, especially if the patient is initially hypoalbuminemic.

Possible Complications

Possible complications include malnutrition, failure to gain weight, chronic diarrhea, mild to moderate nonregenerative anemia, poor healing, ascites, and edema.

Expected Course and Prognosis

- Factors involved in determining the clinical course are status of the ileocolic valve (if resected, clinical signs are consistently worse), extent and site of bowel resection, functional capacity of remaining bowel and other digestive organs, degree of adaptation that occurs in the remaining intestine, and client determination to pursue management with significant cost.

- Experimental studies and clinical reports generally show that resection of less than 70% of the SI is usually well tolerated. Dogs with 30–40 cm of remaining SI and cats with approximately 20 cm have a great chance of surviving without intensive treatment.
- A decision to euthanize should not be made too hastily as time is needed for remaining intestines to adapt.
- Prognosis seems better in patients with early aggressive management.
- Persistent malabsorption and steatorrhea are associated with a poor prognosis if enough time has passed for adaptation of the intestines to occur. This is especially common in patients whose ileocolic valves have not been preserved.
- In one retrospective study, most animals had diarrhea or loose stools for a few weeks or months postoperatively and then developed normal fecal consistency or had only mild clinical signs that were deemed acceptable to the owner.

Abbreviations

- PPN = partial parenteral nutrition
- SBS = short bowel syndrome
- SI = small intestine
- SIBO = small intestinal bacterial overgrowth
- TPN = total parenteral nutrition
- UDCA = ursodeoxycholate

See Also

- Cobalamin Deficiency
- Intestinal Dysbiosis

Suggested Reading

Gorman SC, Freeman LM, Mitchell SL, Chan DL. Extensive small bowel resection in dogs and cats: 20 cases (1998–2004). J Am Vet Med Assoc 2006;228(3):403–407.

Imamura M, Yamauchi H. Effects of massive bowel resection on metabolism of bile acids and vitamin D_3 and gastrin release in dogs. Tohoku J Exper Med 1992;168:515–528.

Kouti VI, Papazoglou LG, Rallis T. Short bowel syndrome in dogs and cats. Compend Contin Educ Vet 2006;28(3):182–195.

Author: Krysta Deitz DVM, MS, DACVIM

Diseases of the Colon

Chapter 81

Atresia Ani

DEFINITION/OVERVIEW

Failure of the urogenital and rectal tracts to separate or retaining a membrane over the anus.

ETIOLOGY/PATHOPHYSIOLOGY

- Urorectal fold normally separates the urogenital and rectal tracts at seven weeks of development.
- Failure of this division leads to a shared cloaca.
- The anal membrane normally ruptures to form the anus.
- Retained anal membrane leads to the rectum terminating in a blind pouch.
- Atresia ani is rare in dogs, but it is the most frequent congenital anomaly of the anus.
- Four types are recognized.
  - Type I: Congenital anal stenosis with opening.
  - Type II: Imperforate membrane over anus.
  - Type III: Imperforate membrane with rectum terminating more cranially in a blind pouch.
  - Type IV: Lack of connection between cranial rectum and terminal rectum.

Systems Affected

- Gastrointestinal – constipation, vomiting, and tenesmus may result due to not being able to void the rectum.
- Renal/urologic – urinary tract infections may be more frequent if a rectovaginal fistula develops.
- Skin – fistulas may develop in the perineal region or vulva.

SIGNALMENT/HISTORY

- Puppies and kittens within the first few weeks of life.
- There is a female predisposition of 1.79:1 males.
- Miniature or toy poodles, Boston terriers, Finnish spitz, Maltese, chow chow, German short-haired pointer, and miniature schnauzer have an increased incidence.

Risk Factors

Atresia ani is a congenital anomaly that may be of an inherited origin.

Blackwell's Five-Minute Veterinary Consult Clinical Companion: Small Animal Gastrointestinal Diseases, First Edition. Edited by Jocelyn Mott and Jo Ann Morrison.
© 2019 John Wiley & Sons, Inc. Published 2019 by John Wiley & Sons, Inc.
Companion website: www.fiveminutevet.com/gastrointestinal

Historical Findings

- Constipation.
- Tenesmus.
- Hematochezia.
- Voiding feces through vulva.
- Vomiting.

 ## CLINICAL FEATURES

- Presence of feces in vulva.
- Abdominal distension and discomfort usually after weaning.
- Perineal bulging.
- Stenosis or absence of anus (Figure 81.1). There is often a thinner appearance of the skin over the predicted location of the anus (Figure 81.2).
- Perineal or anal reflex should be monitored.

 ## DIFFERENTIAL DIAGNOSIS

- Megacolon.
- Constipation.
- Rectal/anal stricture.

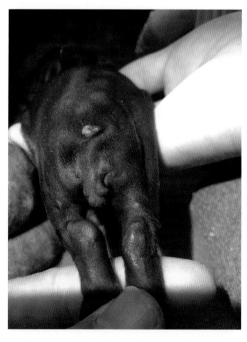

■ **Fig. 81.1.** Classic appearance of a puppy with atresia ani. There is no anus present between the base of the tail and vulva. Source: Courtesy of Dr Peter Tazawa. Reproduced with permission of Iowa State University.

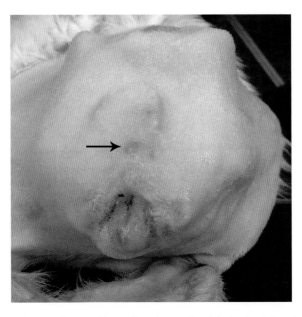

■ **Fig. 81.2.** A preoperative image of a cat with atresia ani. Note the pink circular defect above the vulva as an area of thinner skin is present where the anus is normally. Source: Courtesy of Dr Bryden Stanley. Reproduced with permission of Iowa State University.

 # DIAGNOSTICS

Complete Blood Count/Biochemistry/Urinalysis

Biochemistry may reveal electrolyte abnormalities from inappetence or vomiting, depending on severity of disease.

Imaging

- Plain radiographs can highlight the blind pouch of the rectum if gas is present (Figure 81.3).
- A contrast study (fistulogram) using iodinated contrast may be useful in determining course of fistula.
- Advanced imaging, such as CT scan, may help characterize the specific type of atresia ani and assist in surgical planning.

 # THERAPEUTICS

- Surgical reconstruction of the anus with resolution of fistulous tracts is the recommended treatment (Figure 81.4).
- Fistulous tracts may be rerouted to the correct position of the anus if large diameter and limited surgical options exist.
- Membrane over anus is excised and anal opening is reconstructed, attaching rectal mucosa to skin.
- Patient may become more malnourished or develop worsening electrolyte imbalances if surgery is not performed as soon as possible.

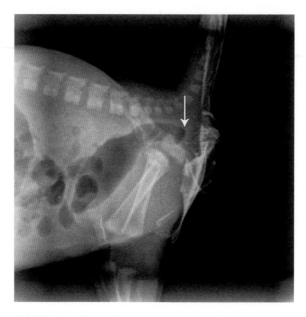

■ **Fig. 81.3.** A lateral radiograph of a kitten with atresia ani. Note the blunt end to the gas-filled rectum with no communication to the perineal skin. Source: Courtesy of Dr Hye-Yeon Jang. Reproduced with permission of Iowa State University.

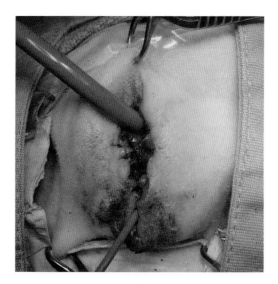

■ **Fig. 81.4.** A postoperative image of the cat in Figure 81.2 with a small red rubber catheter present in the urethra and a large red rubber catheter coursing through the recent anoplasty site. Source: Courtesy of Dr Bryden Stanley. Reproduced with permission of Iowa State University.

Precautions/Interactions

■ Lactulose or other stool softeners should be used with caution due to potential dehydration from loss of water content in a pediatric patient.
■ If imperforate anus is present, this can lead to further distension of large intestine.

Appropriate Health Care

- Cleaning of perineal soiling or soiling of the vulva may be required.
- Feeding a liquid diet until surgery is performed may reduce colonic distension.

Nursing Care

- Routine monitoring of the perineum and gentle cleaning when necessary to prevent secondary urogenital infections.
- Following anoplasty surgery, the surgical site should be disturbed as little as possible to reduce chance of stricture formation.

Diet

- A liquid diet may be administered prior to surgical correction to prevent obstipation.
- Following surgery, a diet with increased fiber should be used short term to promote colonic activity and decrease diarrhea.

Activity

- Patient should have short frequent walks to have ample opportunity to defecate if the anus is stenotic to help relieve obstipation.
- Post surgery, patients should be activity restricted for 10–14 days, and provided short frequent walks for defecation.

Surgical Considerations

- Anesthetic concerns due to young patient with possible electrolyte imbalances from malnutrition or obstipation, along with hypothermia and hypoglycemia as increased anesthetic risks.
- Reconstruction of the anus is complicated, and can involve disturbance of the external anal sphincter. Hence, owners should be aware of the potential for incontinence (temporary or permanent).
- Colotomy at the time of reconstructive surgery may be recommended to relieve obstipated feces and initial tenesmus on anoplasty site.

 COMMENTS

Client Education

Although genetic inheritance is unknown for atresia ani, it is recommended that affected animals be neutered at an appropriate age.

Patient Monitoring

- Patients should be observed for any continued signs of tenesmus or constipation post surgery.
- If dehiscence is present, signs of peritonitis may be present such as lethargy, depression, abdominal pain and distension, vomiting; other signs may include perineal abscessation or fistulas.
- Most patients have continued tenesmus for 2–5 weeks following surgery.

Prevention/Avoidance

Due to possibility of genetic inheritance, affected animals should not be bred.

Possible Complications

- Megacolon may result from persistent distension of the colon. This may or may not resolve as the patient develops.
- Stricture formation and fecal incontinence are possible complications following corrective surgery.

Expected Course and Prognosis

- Type 1 and type 2 atresia ani have a good prognosis, with many surviving past one year with 66% fecal continence postoperatively.
- Stricture of the anoplasty site may occur in up to 50% of cases and require surgical revision.
- Lack of an anal reflex may reduce the potential for fecal continence following surgery.
- Type 3 atresia ani cases have a guarded prognosis for long-term survival due to persistent complications and clinical signs.

Synonyms

- Rectal atresia
- Rectal agenesis

See Also

- Constipation and Obstipation
- Hematochezia
- Megacolon
- Rectal Stricture

Suggested Reading

Ellison GW, Papazoglou LG. Long-term results of surgery for atresia ani with and without anogenital malformations in puppies and a kitten: 12 cases (1983–2010). J Am Vet Med Assoc 2012;240:186–192.

Rahal SC, Vicente CS, Mortari AC, Mamprim MJ, Caporalli EH. Rectovaginal fistula with anal atresia in 5 dogs. Can Vet J 2007;48:827–830.

Vianna ML, Tobias KM. Atresia ani in the dog: a retrospective study. J Am Anim Hosp Assoc 2005;41: 317–322.

Authors: Eric Zellner DVM, DACVS-SA, Louisa Ho-Eckart BVSc Hons, MS, DACVS-SA

Chapter 82

Clostridial Enterotoxicosis

DEFINITION/OVERVIEW

- *Clostridium difficile* and *C. perfringens* are both spore-forming, gram-positive bacilli. They cause diarrhea by producing toxins.
- Clostridia species produce the most toxins among bacteria.
- *C. difficile* is common and well described in the human and equine literature, especially in cases of hospital- and antibiotic-associated diarrhea.
- *C. perfringens* has a widespread distribution as it is part of the normal microbiota of humans and animals.

ETIOLOGY/PATHOPHYSIOLOGY

- Hosts for Clostridia spp. includes humans, horses, dogs, cats, and many other animals. Infection can be the result of direct and indirect contact with contaminated environments and animals. Interestingly, in veterinary medicine, unlike human medicine, a history of antibiotic use has not been largely associated with colonization of Clostridia spp.
- *C. difficile* has been implicated in community-acquired infections in humans as it is the most common cause of hospital- and antimicrobial-associated diarrhea. Recently, in human medicine there have been reports of "hypervirulent" strains that have led to an increased incidence of relapse rates, and even mortality.
- In veterinary medicine, *C. difficile* has been associated with nosocomial diarrhea in dogs and cats. Currently, there is concern that animals are a potential source of *C. difficile* epidemic strains. *C. difficile* can produce up to five toxins, but toxins A and B are most often described, as they are most important in cases of diarrhea. Toxins A and B disrupt the cell cytoskeleton which leads to death of intestinal epithelial cells and leaky tight junctions. Additionally, the toxins release inflammatory cytokines from mast cells, macrophages, and epithelial cells. Clinical disease results from the growth of toxin-producing strains of *C. difficile* in the intestinal tract.
- *C. perfringens* is an important cause of food-borne illness in humans. It is found in the soil and dust. *C. perfringens* is the largest toxin producer within the Clostridia, is a normal inhabitant of the intestine, and is responsible for several enteric diseases in the dog and cat. *C. perfringens* consists of five biotypes (A–E). Biotype A occurs most commonly in dogs and cats, but biotype C has also been reported. Each biotype expresses a subset of other established toxins which may include *C. perfringens* enterotoxin (CPE). CPE, a virulent pore-forming protein, is released when vegetative clostridial cells lyze and release spores. CPE's role in diarrhea in dogs and cats is unclear as it can be found in nondiarrheic pets. Clinical disease may be the result

Blackwell's Five-Minute Veterinary Consult Clinical Companion: Small Animal Gastrointestinal Diseases,
First Edition. Edited by Jocelyn Mott and Jo Ann Morrison.
© 2019 John Wiley & Sons, Inc. Published 2019 by John Wiley & Sons, Inc.
Companion website: www.fiveminutevet.com/gastrointestinal

of food-borne or nonfood-borne illness or from triggered enterotoxigenic strains (from diet changes, antibiotic administration, or coinfection with another pathogen). There is suggestion that *C. perfringens* CPE may be involved in the pathogenesis of acute hemorrhagic diarrhea (AHD), formerly known as hemorrhagic gastroenteritis (HGE). This is based on characteristic histologic lesions, occurrence of *Clostridium* spp. identified by mass spectrometry, and necrosis of the superficial intestinal epithelium found in AHD patients and patients with *C. perfringens* infection. However, it is still possible that clostridial overgrowth in patients with AHD may not be the cause, but rather the sequela of the disease.

- It is worth noting that studies in cats have failed to show an association with diarrhea and CPE *C. perfringens* strains in stool samples.

Systems Affected

Gastrointestinal – small, large, or mixed bowel diarrhea can be noted although traditionally, clostridial diarrhea has been described as a large bowel type of diarrhea. Vomiting and or anorexia may also accompany lower gastrointestinal (GI) signs. Severity can range from mild and self-limiting to hemorrhagic, profound, and fatal.

 SIGNALMENT/HISTORY

- Variable age, breed, and sex.
- May have a history of diarrhea (possibly hemorrhagic) that clinically cannot be differentiated from enteritis from other pathogens.

Risk Factors

There may be a history of stress, diet change or antimicrobial use.

Historical Findings

- May have a history of small, large, or mixed bowel diarrhea (possibly hemorrhagic or mucoid), that clinically cannot be differentiated from enteritis from other pathogens.
- Other signs include vomiting, flatulence, hematochezia, abdominal discomfort, or a generalized unthriftiness in chronic cases.

 CLINICAL FEATURES

- There are no specific or pathognomonic clinical signs implicating a clostridial infection in cats and dogs.
- Gastrointestinal discomfort or distress may occur.
- Rectal exam may reveal fresh blood/mucus.
- An infection with Clostridia spp. may be subclinical, acute, or severe, and may lead to a fatal hemorrhagic diarrheal syndrome.

 DIFFERENTIAL DIAGNOSIS

- Cannot be grossly differentiated from any cause of enteritis, including small, large, or mixed bowel diarrhea.
- Examples include parvovirus, inflammatory bowel disease, food-responsive diarrhea, parasites, *Giardia*, etc.

DIAGNOSTICS

Challenging at best. There are no specific clinical predictors or values for Clostridia infections.

Complete Blood Count/Biochemistry/Urinalysis

- Complete blood count may show hemoconcentration or an inflammatory leukogram.
- The serum chemistry may have a low-normal total protein.

Other Laboratory Tests

- A fecal smear stained with Wright stain may show a high number of Clostridia endospores per high-power field. The endospores have a "tennis racquet" or "safety pin" appearance. There is no association between the number of endospores seen on a fecal smear and diarrhea, or pathogenicity. Therefore, although sporulation is associated with enterotoxin production, fecal endospore counts are discouraged as a means of diagnosing Clostridia enterotoxicosis as sporulation occurs in fecal specimens of diarrheic and nondiarrheic dogs.
- *C. difficile* can be cultured to procure strains for detection of toxin genes and typing. Several enzyme linked immunosorbent assay (ELISA) tests are used in veterinary reference laboratories to detect glutamate dehydrogenase (GDH), which is produced by toxigenic and nontoxigenic strains, as well as *C. difficile* A and B toxins.
- Molecular detection may also occur by performing polymerase chain reaction (PCR) on fecal specimens. For best results, fecal culture followed by PCR testing of *C. difficile* isolates for toxin genes improves specificity of the culture.
- *C. perfringens* may be cultured from a fecal sample; however, it is a normal commensal organism.
- Fecal enteroxin immunodetection of CPE, utilizing an ELISA procedure, is a common diagnostic tool in human medicine but has not been validated in dogs and cats (Figures 82.1, 82.2).
- Molecular techniques (PCR) have also routinely been employed to detect enterotoxigenic *C. perfringens* (Figure 82.3).

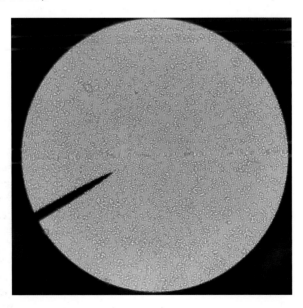

■ **Fig. 82.1.** Magnification at 60× of a fecal sample mixed with diluted antitoxin and incubated and transferred to a microtiter well to form a cellular monolayer. Demonstrates cytopathic effect due to the presence of *C. difficile* toxin, as cells are rounded and separating from each other. Source: Images courtesy of Dr Claire Miller.

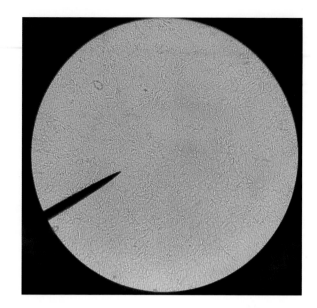

■ **Fig. 82.2.** Magnification at 60× of fecal sample prepared as in Figure 82.1 but which has no cytopathic effect; *C. difficile* toxin has not been detected. The cells are confluent and plump. Source: Images courtesy of Dr Claire Miller.

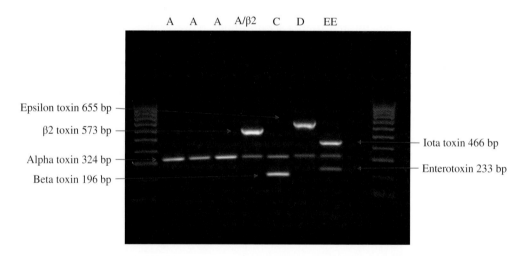

■ **Fig. 82.3.** *C. perfringens* toxin genotyping PCR gel. Lanes 1 and 10 contain molecular size markers. Lanes 2 and 3 are test samples and are of type A. Lanes 4–8 represent the positive controls for varying toxin types. Lane 4 represents type A (alpha toxin only). Lane 5 represents type A with beta-2 toxin. Lane 6 represents type C (alpha and beta toxin). Lane 7 represents type D (alpha and epsilon toxin). Lane 8 represents type E (alpha and iota toxin with enterotoxin). Lane 9 contains the negative control (NC). The enterotoxin gene can be present in any toxin type; in this case, the type E positive control carries the enterotoxin gene. Source: Images courtesy of Dr Claire Miller.

Imaging

Abdominal radiography may reveal fluid-filled intestinal loops.

Pathologic Findings

■ Patients with *C. perfringens* enterotoxicosis may have colonoscopic evidence of hyperemic or ulcerated mucosa.

- Histology may show catarrhal or suppurative colitis.
- Occasionally a mild lymphocytic and plasmacytic enteritis is present.

 THERAPEUTICS

- Systemically ill animals with clostridial enterocolitis (inflammatory/toxic leukogram, fever, hemorrhagic gastroenteritis) may benefit from antimicrobial therapy.
- Supportive care, including adequate intravenous hydration, with uncomplicated *Clostridium* enterotoxicosis may not require antimicrobial therapy and has recently been reported in the literature.

Drug(s) of Choice

- The most commonly recommended drug for the treatment of a clostridial infection is metronidazole given at 10 mg/kg q 12 h for 5–7 days; however, in human medicine, concerns exist about metronidazole-resistant clostridial strains.
- Additional antimicrobials used in the treatment of clostridial infections include intravenous ampicillin at 22 mg/kg q 8 h for 5–7 days, or oral amoxicillin at 22 mg/kg q 12 h for 5–7 days.
- Oral tylosin at 5–10 mg/kg q 24 h for 5–7 days has also been clinically popular and useful in some cases.
- Clinical improvement usually occurs within 24–36 hours. Some cases may be mild and self-limiting and may warrant conservative management, including a temporary diet modification. Probiotics have been utilized in some instances.

Precautions/Interactions

Macrolides and tetracyclines are not generally recommended for clostridial infections as resistance to these types of antimicrobials has been reported.

Appropriate Health Care

- Most treated as outpatients.
- When diarrhea or vomiting is severe, resulting in dehydration and electrolyte imbalance, hospitalization may be required.

Nursing Care

Fluid and electrolyte therapy may be required to replace losses occurring from diarrhea, particularly in dogs with AHD.

Activity

Restricted during acute disease.

Diet

- Dietary manipulation plays a role in the treatment and management of cases with chronic recurring disease.
- Diets high in fiber, either soluble (fermentable) or insoluble fiber, often result in clinical improvement by reducing enteric clostridial numbers. This may be due to acidification of the distal intestine, potentially limiting *C. perfringens* sporulation and enterotoxin production.
- Commercial high-fiber diets can be supplemented with psyllium (1/2–2 tsp/day) as a source of soluble fiber.
- Diets low in fiber should be supplemented with fiber (coarse bran 1–3 tbs/day) as a source of insoluble fiber or psyllium added as a source of soluble fiber.

COMMENTS

Client Education

- Acute disease is often self-limiting.
- There have been no documented reports of zoonotic transmission of *C. perfringens* from animals to humans.

Patient Monitoring

- The patient's response to antibiotic therapy does not confirm a diagnosis of *C. perfringens*-associated diarrhea.
- Monitoring for hydration status and electrolyte imbalances is warranted in dogs with moderate to severe disease.

Prevention/Avoidance

- There are no vaccines available for clostridial diarrhea prevention in dogs. Infections can be sporadic.
- Hand washing is imperative to try and reduce transmission and infection in a hospital setting. Hand hygiene (washing versus hand sanitizing) is important for prevention as endospores are alcohol resistant.
- Barrier precautions should be in place and direct and indirect contact between infected and uninfected animals should be prevented.
- Clostridia spp. are not typically considered zoonotic, although many species affect both humans and animals.
- Many human cases occur from contamination, especially through improperly handled or contaminated food sources.
- Notably, *C. difficile* spores are resistant to many disinfectants. Sodium hypochlorite (bleach) has very good sporicidal activity, and quaternary ammonium and phenol compounds are effective when *C. difficile* is in the vegetative state.
- Dogs may shed *C. difficile* strains similar to those that infect humans, but human disease usually is the result of hospital-acquired infection. *C. perfringens* infections are usually sporadic and are typically associated with food poisoning. Therefore, *C. perfringens* isolates from affected dogs and cats are not typically zoonotic, but may need further investigation.

Expected Course and Prognosis

- Many animals with clostridial enterotoxicosis have a good to favorable prognosis.
- However, infections may be deadly if there is acute, severe, hemorrhagic diarrhea that leads to severe intestinal mucosal inflammation, dehydration, and decompensation.

Abbreviations

- AHD = acute hemorrhagic diarrhea
- CPE = *C. perfringens* enterotoxin
- ELISA = enzyme linked immunosorbent assay
- GDH = glutamate dehydrogenase
- GI = gastrointestinal
- HE = hemorrhagic gastroenteritis
- PCR = polymerase chain reaction

See Also

- Colitis and Proctitis
- Gastroenteritis, Hemorrhagic
- Intestinal Dysbiosis

Suggested Reading

Green CE. Infectious Diseases of the Dog and Cat, 4th ed. St Louis: Elsevier, 2012, p. 37.

Orden C, Blanco JL, Alvarez-Perez S, et al. Isolation of *Clostridium difficile* from dogs with digestive disorders, including stable metronidazole-resistant strains. Anaerobe 2017;43:78–81.

Sykes JE. Canine and Feline Infectious Diseases. St Louis: Elsevier, 2014, p. 48.

Silva ROS, Lobato FCF. Clostridium perfringens: a review of enteric diseases in dogs, cats and wild animals. Anaerobe 2015;33:14–17.

Unterer S, Strohmeyer K, Kruse BD, et al. Treatment of aseptic dogs with hemorrhagic gastroenteritis with amoxicillin/clavulanic acid: a prospective blinded study. J Vet Intern Med 2011;25:973–979.

Acknowledgments: The author and editors acknowledge the prior contribution of Dr Stanley L. Marks.

Author: Jennifer E. Slovak DVM, MS, DACVIM

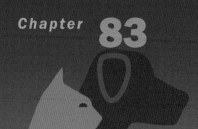

Colitis and Proctitis

DEFINITION/OVERVIEW

- Colitis – inflammation of the colon (large intestine).
- Proctitis – inflammation of the rectum.

ETIOLOGY/PATHOPHYSIOLOGY

- Multiple etiologies for colitis and proctitis exist, including parasitic, neoplastic, infectious, metabolic, immune mediated, and toxic agents. As such, the diagnostic work-up may be relatively standardized, especially if patients have chronic disease and complete diagnostic evaluations are pursued.
- The incidence of colitis/proctitis is relatively common although etiologies may differ by geography (e.g., fungal infections in endemic areas) and patient signalment (e.g., parasitic infections in younger patients).
- Dietary etiologies: food-responsive enteropathy, dietary indiscretion, food intolerance.
- Drug administration etiologies: antibiotics, nonsteroidal antiinflammatory drugs (NSAIDs), corticosteroids.
- Infectious etiologies: *Trichuris vulpis*, *Entamoeba histolytica*, *Balantidium coli*, *Tritrichomonas foetus*, *Clostridium perfringens* and *C. difficile*, *Campylobacter jejuni* and *C. coli*, *Yersinia enterocolitica*, *Prototheca*, *Histoplasma capsulatum*, and pythiosis/phycomycosis. More recent literature indicates that intestinal dysbiosis may be linked to the development of chronic enteropathies.
- Traumatic etiologies: foreign body, abrasive material.
- Inflammatory etiologies: secondary to pancreatitis (transverse colitis).
- Inflammatory/immune etiologies: inflammatory bowel disease (IBD), irritable bowel syndrome (IBS), colitis (of varying forms).
- The pathophysiology is consistent with what is seen in other sections of the intestinal tract. Inflammation may cause any or all of the following.
    - Accumulation of proinflammatory cytokines.
    - Generation of oxygen free radicals.
    - Disruption of tight junctions between epithelial cells.
    - Release of proteolytic and lysosomal enzymes.
    - Complement activation.
    - Stimulation of colonic goblet cell secretion.
    - Disruption of normal motility.
- As the colon is the main site of water resorption, along with conservation of electrolytes, inflammation may result in dehydration and electrolyte disturbances. When present, diarrhea commonly contains mucus and may contain frank blood.

Blackwell's Five-Minute Veterinary Consult Clinical Companion: Small Animal Gastrointestinal Diseases, First Edition. Edited by Jocelyn Mott and Jo Ann Morrison.
© 2019 John Wiley & Sons, Inc. Published 2019 by John Wiley & Sons, Inc.
Companion website: www.fiveminutevet.com/gastrointestinal

Systems Affected

- Cardiovascular – signs of dehydration/electrolyte disorders when severe.
- Gastrointestinal (GI) – signs of large bowel diarrhea.
- Hemic/lymphatic/immune – signs of dehydration/anemia with severe cases.

SIGNALMENT/HISTORY

- Any age or breed of dog and cat may develop signs of colitis/proctitis.
- Certain subsets of colitis do have breed dispositions. Histiocytic ulcerative colitis (HUC) is more commonly seen in younger dogs and predisposed breeds include boxers, French bulldogs, Doberman pinschers, mastiffs, and Alaskan malamutes. German shepherd dogs are predisposed to perianal fistulas that can be associated with colitis. Pure-bred cats may be predisposed to certain parasitic infections (e.g., *Tritrichomonas foetus*).
- Historical signs (in decreasing order of frequency) include:
  - Increase in defecation frequency.
  - Decrease in fecal volume.
  - Tenesmus.
  - Increased fecal mucus.
  - Hematochezia.
  - Dyschezia.
- Upper GI signs (vomiting, decreased appetite, weight loss) are less common and depend upon etiology.

Risk Factors

- Genetic predispositions for certain subsets of colitis.
- Environmental factors may predispose to certain parasitic (e.g., whipworms, *Tritrichomonas*) and infectious diseases (e.g., histoplasmosis, pythiosis). Immune-compromised hosts may be predisposed to parasitic and infectious etiologies. Older patients may be predisposed to neoplastic disorders.

Historical Findings

Along with the historical signs listed above, owners may report increase in needing to go outside or trips to the litterbox, increased urgency in defecation, increased "accidents" in the house, or unsuccessful defecation (note that straining to defecate may be confused with straining to urinate and owners may present pets for suspected urinary obstruction)

CLINICAL FEATURES

- May be unremarkable.
- Rectal palpation should be performed in all patients being presented with signs of colitis (when possible and accepted by the patient). Palpation may reveal irregular, thickened, rough mucosa with mucus and hematochezia. Patients may resent rectal palpation or may exhibit significant pain/discomfort so caution should be exercised.
- German shepherds may present with perianal fistulas.
- In cases of colonic neoplasia, enlarged sublumbar lymph nodes may be palpable.
- Patients with severe or systemic disease may show dehydration and weight loss.

DIFFERENTIAL DIAGNOSIS

- Neoplasia – colonic lymphoma, adenocarcinoma, sarcomas. It is more common for the colon to be the primary site of neoplasia, rather than a metastatic site.
- Irritable bowel syndrome.
- Lower urinary tract/prostatic disease.
- Hypoadrenocorticism.
- Gastrointestinal (GI) intussusception.
- Intestinal parasitism.

DIAGNOSTICS

- As a general rule, evaluation of a patient with signs of intestinal disease should proceed as follows: complete history and physical examination (including rectal palpation). Evaluation for disease/etiology outside the GI tract should be pursued next, then proceed with evaluation for disease arising from the GI tract.
- Testing for parasitic disease/empiric treatment for parasites should not be overlooked.

Complete Blood Count/Biochemistry/Urinalysis

- Results may be unremarkable; with severe inflammation, a neutrophilia with a left shift may be present; parasitic etiologies may induce an eosinophilia.
- Anemia may result from chronic inflammation, and intestinal blood loss may induce an iron deficiency anemia (microcytic, hypochromic).
- Hyperglobulinemia and hypercalcemia may be seen in some patients with infectious or neoplastic conditions.
- Urinalysis is typically unremarkable but should be evaluated to rule out lower urinary tract disease which may present with similar historical findings.

Other Laboratory Tests

- Parasitic etiologies must be ruled out. Depending on the signalment, this testing may include fecal centrifugation flotation, direct fecal smear, fecal culture and sensitivity, fecal bacterial toxin immunoassays (*C. perfringens* enterotoxin and *C. difficile* toxins A and B), polymerase chain reaction (PCR) for bacteria and other etiologies, enzyme linked immunosorbent assay (ELISA) testing for intestinal parasites, *Pythium*, and submission of feces for *Tritrichomonas* testing (InPouch™).
- Rectal scraping for cytology or urine antigen testing for *Histoplasma* may be performed.
- In rare cases where hypoadrenocorticism is suspected, baseline cortisol and adrenocorticotropic hormone (ACTH) stimulation testing is diagnostic.

Imaging

- Abdominal radiographs – will usually be unremarkable, but may show an underlying etiology (e.g., ileus, neoplasia).
- Abdominal ultrasonography – may be unremarkable but may also reveal masses, diffuse thickening or altered architecture of the colon, or enlarged associated lymph nodes.

Other Diagnostic Procedures

- Colonoscopy with biopsy – when the etiology of the clinical signs has been narrowed down to the mucosal/submucosal layers of the colon/rectum. Along with direct visualization of the mucosa, samples may be obtained for cytology, histopathology, and tissue culture and sensitivity. Mucosal lesions that may be visualized include loss of grossly visible submucosal blood vessels, granular or "cobblestone" mucosal appearance, hyperemia, mucus, erosions or ulcerations, hemorrhage (which may be linear in appearance), mass(es) or parasitic organisms.

- Any visible lesions should be sampled and it is important to obtain multiple samples from all portions of the colon/rectum, even if the mucosa appears grossly normal.
- Adequate preparation for colonoscopy is critical to the procurement of diagnostic samples. Fasting for a minimum of 12 hours is recommended (however, fresh water should always be available). Depending on the protocol followed, osmotic cathartics such as Golytely™ (dosed at 60 mL/kg PO) are administered starting the night before the procedure and continued the morning of the procedure. Warm water enemas (20 mL/kg) are also administered. Dogs should be frequently walked outside to encourage elimination. Cats may require manual evacuation of feces once under anesthesia.
- Oral administration of osmotic cathartics can be challenging. Some dogs may readily drink the solution but others will require orogastric intubation. A nasogastric tube may be utilized in cats.

Pathologic Findings

- Gross findings include the mucosal lesions described above. Regional lymphadenopathy may also be present.
- Histopathologic findings will depend upon the histologic type and etiology of colitis. The most common subtypes of colitis include lymphoplasmacytic, eosinophilic, and histiocytic ulcerative. Special stains and molecular techniques such as fluorescent *in situ* hybridization (FISH) may be utilized to investigate infectious etiologies.

  THERAPEUTICS

- Objectives of treatment are to eliminate, when possible, the underlying etiology of the disease, thereby removing the need for chronic management.
- When a "cure" is not possible, long-term control of clinical signs with minimal impact (e.g., medication side effects) to the patient is the goal.
- If a complete diagnostic evaluation is not possible, it has become common to pursue empiric deworming (e.g., fenbendazole) first, followed by a dietary trial (see below), an antibiotic trial (metronidazole or tylosin), and then consider immune suppressant therapy.

Drug(s) of Choice

Parasitic/Bacterial Etiologies

- *Trichuris* – fenbendazole (50 mg/kg PO q24h for five consecutive days, repeat in three months).
- *Tritrichomonas foetus* – ronidazole (30 mg/kg q24h for 14 days).
- *Clostridium perfringens* – metronidazole (10 mg/kg PO q12h for five days), tylosin (5–10 mg/kg PO q24h for five days).
- *Clostridium difficile* – metronidazole (10 mg/kg PO q12h for five days).
- *Campylobacter* spp. – erythromycin (10–15 mg/kg PO q8h) or azithromycin (5–10 mg/kg PO q24h) for 7–10 days.
- *Histoplasma* – itraconazole (dogs, 10 mg/kg PO q24h; cats, 5 mg/kg PO q12h; several months of therapy is necessary); amphotericin B (0.25–0.5 mg/kg slow IV q48h up to cumulative dose of 4–8 mg/kg) in advanced cases.

- Pythiosis – itraconazole (10 mg/kg PO q24h) and terbinafine (10 mg/kg PO q24h) are the drugs of choice following surgical debridement of affected portions of bowel, though prognosis is poor.
- Fluoroquinolones are the antibiotic of choice for HUC. Historically, enrofloxacin (10 mg/kg PO q 24 h for 4–6 weeks) was recommended but recent literature indicates that resistance to this antibiotic may be increasing. Ideally, therapy should be tailored based on the results of tissue culture and sensitivity.

Inflammatory/Immune-Mediated Colitis

- Sulfasalazine or other 5-ASA drugs – may be a reasonable consideration following assessment of response to dietary therapy. This is typically reserved for cases with mild signs of disease before considering more aggressive therapy. Dosing: dogs, 25–40 mg/kg PO q8h for 3–6 weeks with a progressive tapering of the dose throughout the course of drug therapy; cats, 20 mg/kg PO q12h for three weeks. See precautions below.
- Metronidazole – both antimicrobial and immune-modulating properties have been described and therapy is not associated with the degree of immune suppression that may be seen with other medications. Dosing: 10 mg/kg PO q12h for five days is typically a sufficient duration to determine clinical benefit.
- Corticosteroids – have the highest level of evidence for efficacy in immune-mediated disease. Therapy consists of prednisone for dogs and prednisolone for cats. Dosing: 1–2 mg/kg PO q12h until clinical remission, with gradual, progressive tapering of dose. Never use more than 50 mg total of prednisone per day for any animal, regardless of size.
- Azathioprine – for use in dogs only and may take several weeks for benefits to be realized. Dosing: 1–2 mg/kg PO q24h for 10–14 days followed by a taper to 1–2 mg/kg q48h for 4–6 weeks. See precautions below.
- Chlorambucil – an effective immunomodulator in both dogs and cats and is usually administered in conjunction with prednisone or prednisolone. Dosing: dogs, 0.1–0.2 mg/kg PO q24h for 8–12 weeks for immune disease, with gradual tapering of dose over the course of therapy; cats, 2 mg per cat q3–4 days for 2–3 months (or longer if managing lymphoma) or 15 mg/m^2 given for four consecutive days every three weeks for 2–3 months.
- Cyclosporine – also used as a potent immunomodulatory agent; chronic therapy has been associated with the development of lymphoreticular neoplasia in people. Dosing: 5 mg/kg PO q12–24 h for six weeks.

Precautions/Interactions

- Sulfasalazine – has been associated with keratoconjunctivitis sicca (KCS). Measure tear production (Schirmer tear test) at baseline and every two weeks throughout the course of therapy. Avoid use or use extreme caution in breeds predisposed to KCS (e.g., American cocker spaniel). Discontinue drug if tear production decreases. Hepatotoxicity to sulfa drugs has been reported in certain breeds (e.g., Doberman pinscher). Avoid use or use extreme caution with regular monitoring of hepatic enzymes in predisposed breeds.
- Azathioprine – monitor patients on azathioprine for bone marrow suppression via complete blood count (CBC) every 2–3 weeks; stop treatment or go to alternate day if white blood cell (WBC) count falls below 3000 cells/µL. Azathioprine can also increase the risk of pancreatitis, especially when combined with prednisone, and should be used extremely cautiously in any dog at increased risk for pancreatitis. Azathioprine can also cause a hepatopathy and liver enzymes should be measured at baseline and monitored over time.
- Chlorambucil – is generally well tolerated but can cause a progressive neutropenia; CBC should be repeated every 2–3 weeks in all patients receiving this drug.

- Cyclosporine – can cause hepatotoxicity and may cause profound emesis in some patients. A chemistry panel should be performed as baseline before starting the drug and repeated every 2–3 months.

Alternative Drugs

In lieu of empiric immune suppression, some patients will respond to a dietary trial, empiric deworming, and/or an antibiotic trial.

Appropriate Health Care

- Immune suppression should ideally only be considered when an immune-mediated etiology is proven.
- Opportunistic infections have been reported in patients on long-term immune suppression.

Nursing Care

- Rarely, animals will require hospitalization for fluid support and correction of electrolyte imbalances.
- German shepherds with perianal fistulas will require more intensive support and analgesic medications.
- Patients with profound diarrhea may benefit from routine, gentle cleaning of the perineal area and topical medications for inflammation.

Diet

- When medically appropriate, consider a dietary trial of an elimination or hypoallergenic diet for at least two weeks. The response to dietary therapy is typically seen within the first 5–7 days following dietary implementation. Obtain a comprehensive dietary history to optimize selection of a novel, single protein and carbohydrate source for the trial diet. Strict dietary compliance is pivotal during this trial period to optimize interpretation of the clinical response.
- If the patient responds well to the dietary trial, ingredients may be individually added to the diet in an attempt to identify the offending antigens. Alternatively, a veterinary nutritionist may be consulted to develop a complete and balanced nutritional plan based on the preferred ingredients.
- Fiber supplementation with an insoluble fiber (e.g., bran) is recommended to increase fecal bulk. This will also improve colonic contractility and motility, and bind fecal water to produce formed feces.
- Soluble fiber sources (e.g., psyllium or a diet containing beet pulp or fructooligosaccharides) may be beneficial. Short-chain fatty acids produced by fermentation may be beneficial for colonocyte function.

Activity

In general, activity restriction is typically not necessary.

Surgical Considerations

Unless an underlying neoplastic condition is diagnosed, most etiologies of colitis/proctitis are treated medically.

 COMMENTS

Client Education

Certain etiologies have zoonotic potential (e.g., parasitic infections).

Patient Monitoring

- Mild disease may be self-limiting.
- For chronic conditions, or for patients on immunosuppressant therapies, rechecks of clinical response and potential bloodwork as listed above are recommended.

Prevention/Avoidance

- Minimize exposure to infectious agents (e.g., other dogs, contaminated foods, moist environments) when possible.
- Avoid abrupt dietary changes and minimize dietary variety.
- Encourage veterinary consultation if clinical signs do not resolve.
- Follow Companion Animal Parasite Council (CAPC) recommendations for routine antiparasitic treatments.

Possible Complications

- Recurrence of signs without treatment, when treatment is tapered, and with progression of disease.
- Patients on immune suppressive therapy may be at risk for opportunistic infections.
- Some etiologies may have zoonotic potential.

Expected Course and Prognosis

- Course and prognosis depend primarily on etiologic agent and also individual animal response to therapy/complicating factors.
- Most primary bacterial and parasitic infectious causes have an excellent prognosis with a high likelihood of cure following appropriate therapy.
- *Histoplasma* spp. – with advanced or disseminated disease the prognosis is poor; mild-to-moderate cases generally respond to therapy with dedicated owners. Therapeutic drug monitoring is available to help tailor therapy.
- Pythiosis/phycomycosis – poor to grave long-term prognosis in most animals, despite surgical intervention and aggressive medical management.
- Inflammatory – fair to good with treatment in patients with lymphoplasmacytic, eosinophilic, and granulomatous colitis. Prognosis worsens with more diffuse GI tract involvement.

Synonyms

- Inflammatory bowel disease
- Irritable bowel syndrome
- Large bowel diarrhea

Abbreviations

- 5-ASA = 5-aminosalicylic acid
- ACTH = adrenocorticotropic hormone
- CAPC = Companion Animal Parasite Council
- CBC = complete blood count
- ELISA = enzyme linked immunosorbent assay
- FISH = fluorescent *in situ* hybridization
- GI = gastrointestinal
- HUC = histiocytic ulcerative colitis
- IBD = inflammatory bowel disease
- IBS = irritable bowel syndrome
- KCS = keratoconjunctivitis sicca
- NSAID = nonsteroidal antiinflammatory drug
- PCR = polymerase chain reaction
- WBC = white blood cell

See Also

- Colitis, Histiocytic Ulcerative
- Dyschezia and Tenesmus
- Fiber responsive Large Bowel Diarrhea
- Hematochezia
- Inflammatory Bowel Disease
- Irritable Bowel Disease
- Nutritional Approach to Chronic Enteropathies
- Individual chapters on infectious and parasitic agents

Suggested Reading

Cassman E, White R, Atherly T, et al. Alterations of the ileal and colonic mucosal microbiota in canine chronic enteropathies. PLoS One https://doi.org/10.1371/journal.pone.0147321

Hahn H, Freiche V, Baril A, et al. Ultrasonographical, endoscopic and histological appearance of the caecum in clinically healthy cats. J Feline Med Surg 2017;19(2):94–104.

Kathrani A, Fascetti AJ, Larsen JA, et al. Whole-blood taurine concentrations in cats with intestinal disease. J Vet Intern Med 2017;31:1067–1073.

Lechowski R, Cotard JP, Boulouis HJ, et al. Proper use of quinolones for canine colitis ambulatory treatment: literature review and REQUEST guidelines. Polish J Vet Sci 2013;16(1):193–197.

Acknowledgments: The author and editors acknowledge the previous contribution of Dr Stanley L. Marks.

Author: Jo Ann Morrison DVM, MS, DACVIM

Colitis, Histiocytic Ulcerative

DEFINITION/OVERVIEW

- Histiocytic ulcerative colitis (HUC) is described as a variant of granulomatous colitis, with an adherent-invasive *Escherichia coli* (AIEC) serving as the etiologic agent.
- A defined breed association has been described (see below).

ETIOLOGY/PATHOPHYSIOLOGY

- The primary pathophysiology appears to be a result of impaired macrophage phagocytic function (likely genetic in origin due to the breed predispositions identified).
- Intestinal macrophages are unable to kill and phagocytize AIEC, leading to clinical signs of large bowel diarrhea: tenesmus, hematochezia, increased frequency in defecation, and reduced volumes of defecation.
- Severely affected cases may show more diffuse gastrointestinal (GI) involvement, including weight loss and hypoalbuminemia.
- This somewhat common disease was initially thought to be immune mediated in origin. Further studies elucidated the primary bacterial etiology.

Systems Affected

- Gastrointestinal – expected signs of large bowel diarrhea, with more diffuse GI signs in severe cases. Severe cases may also present with a protein-losing enteropathy.
- Hemic/lymphatic/immune – macrophage phagocytic defects have been identified in affected dogs.
- Musculoskeletal – severely affected cases may show generalized cachexia and loss of lean body mass.

SIGNALMENT/HISTORY

- The initial descriptions of the condition were primarily from young boxer dogs (previously, the condition was also described as boxer colitis). Further investigations have shown French bulldogs may also have HUC.
- A similar granulomatous colitis syndrome, not specifically identified as HUC, has been described in:
  - Dobermans.
  - English bulldogs.
  - Mastiffs.
  - Alaskan malamutes.

Blackwell's Five-Minute Veterinary Consult Clinical Companion: Small Animal Gastrointestinal Diseases,
First Edition. Edited by Jocelyn Mott and Jo Ann Morrison.
© 2019 John Wiley & Sons, Inc. Published 2019 by John Wiley & Sons, Inc.
Companion website: www.fiveminutevet.com/gastrointestinal

- Younger dogs appear to be at risk, with most cases being diagnosed before two years of age. No sex predilection has been identified.

Risk Factors

- Predisposed breeds as described.
- The macrophage phagocytic defect is suspected to be genetic in origin, although a specific genetic defect/mutation has not been identified.

Historical Findings

- Hematochezia.
- Tenesmus.
- Increased frequency of defecation (house soiling).
- Fecal mucus.

 # CLINICAL FEATURES

- Rectal palpation may show hematochezia and mucus.
- Patients may be painful on rectal palpation.
- Irregular, firm, raised rectal mucosa may be palpable on rectal examination.
- Severely affected patients may exhibit weight loss, cachexia, and loss of lean body mass.

 # DIFFERENTIAL DIAGNOSIS

- Primary differentials are other etiologies for large bowel diarrhea.
  - Anatomic: intussusception, cecal inversion, etc.
  - Metabolic: hypoadrenocorticism, etc.
  - Neoplasia: lymphoma, adenocarcinoma, colorectal polyps, etc.
  - Infectious diseases: *Salmonella*, *Campylobacter*, *Pythium*, etc.
  - Immune-mediated diseases: lymphoplasmacytic colitis, eosinophilic colitis, food intolerance, food allergy, etc.
  - Parasitic infections: *Giardia*, whipworms, etc.
- The signalment, history, and physical examination findings are important differentiators of HUC from other differential diagnoses.

 # DIAGNOSTICS

Complete Blood Count/Biochemistry/Urinalysis

- Minimum database performed to investigate other differentials and determine overall health and stability for more invasive diagnostics.
- Minimum database may be unremarkable, depending on severity and duration of disease.
- If GI hemorrhage has been chronic, microcytic, hypochromic anemia may be seen.
- Biochemical analysis may show hypoalbuminemia and azotemia (prerenal), along with electrolyte abnormalities.
- Urinalysis may demonstrate hypersthenuria if dehydrated.

Imaging

- Radiographs may be unremarkable but may demonstrate loss of abdominal detail if peritoneal effusion is present in severe cases. Increased intestinal gas may be visualized.

- Abdominal ultrasound may be unremarkable. Reported changes include thickening of colonic wall and loss of normal layering architecture. Enlarged mesenteric and/or sublumbar lymph nodes may be identified.

Colonoscopy

- Colonoscopy should be utilized to visualize the mucosal surfaces of the large intestine and obtain representative samples for cytology and histopathology.
- Samples should be taken from all areas of the large intestine, even if mucosa appears grossly normal.
- Patients should undergo appropriate preparation prior to colonoscopy to ensure adequate visualization of tissues.
- Different protocols describe this technique. It is common to use a polyethylene glycol solution (e.g., GoLytely®) to help clear the intestines and aid visualization. Solid food is withheld prior to the procedure for roughly 24 hours. A dose of 60 mL/kg of the polyethylene glycol solution is administered by mouth or via orogastric tube the night before the procedure, and is repeated roughly 2–4 hours later. Warm water enemas are administered after each oral gavage and a third enema is administered again the morning of the procedure. Allow the patient ample time outdoors for elimination.
- Surgical (full-thickness) biopsies obtained during exploratory laparotomy are not typically pursued in cases of HUC due to concerns about wound dehiscence and contamination.

Pathologic Findings

- Gross pathology demonstrates lymphadenopathy and thickened, irregular intestinal walls. Hemorrhage may be noted on mucosal surfaces.
- Histopathology shows characteristic periodic acid–Schiff (PAS)-positive macrophages in the mucosal and submucosal intestinal tissues. Other findings consistent with HUC include neutrophilic inflammation, epithelial necrosis, and ulceration.
- Fluorescent *in situ* hybridization (FISH) testing highlights the presence of *E. coli* organisms within the tissues. These findings are considered pathognomonic for HUC.

 # THERAPEUTICS

- Antibiotic therapy is the mainstay of treatment for HUC and is associated with a good prognosis.
- Fluoroquinolones have historically been prescribed although there have been reports of antimicrobial resistance.

Drug(s) of Choice

- Enrofloxacin (10 mg/kg PO q 24 h × 6–8 weeks) has been recommended.
- More cases have been identified as having a population resistant to fluoroquinolones, and so current recommendations include performing culture and sensitivity on isolated *E. coli* specimens from biopsy samples.
- Antibiotic therapy can then be directed based on culture and sensitivity results.
- Chloramphenicol, trimethoprim sulfa, and amikacin may be options in cases that exhibit resistance to fluoroquinolones.

Precautions/Interactions

- As a general rule, antidiarrheal medications should not be used on patients with an infectious etiology for diarrhea.

- Patients undergoing concurrent therapy with theophylline and fluoroquinolones are at risk for drug toxicity. Consider reducing theophylline dosage by 30%.

Nursing Care

- Severely affected patients may require hospitalization for crystalloid fluid and electrolyte support.
- Nursing care for diarrhea may be indicated (gentle cleaning, topical medications) in cases of associated dermatitis.

Diet

- Long-term dietary therapy is not commonly indicated.
- Short-term dietary manipulation to increase digestibility and soluble fiber concentrations may be considered.

Activity

No restriction of activity is typically needed, beyond what the patient may self-impose.

 COMMENTS

- Previous empiric or inappropriate antibiotic therapy, especially with fluoroquinolones, may increase the risk of resistant AIEC populations.
- In general, antibiotic therapy should be prescribed in those cases with defined bacterial etiologies and, ideally, based on culture and sensitivity results.
- Resistant AIEC populations may be more difficult to treat.

Client Education

- Clinical signs should start to improve within days of starting appropriate antibiotic therapy. If clinical signs do not improve, or worsen, the patient should be reevaluated.
- The entire course of prescribed antibiotics should be administered, even in the face of clinical improvement.

Patient Monitoring

- Monitoring for resolution of clinical signs should show notable improvement in signs of large bowel diarrhea.
- More severely affected patients should demonstrate weight gain and improved body condition.
- Abnormal blood work results (e.g., hypoalbuminemia) should be rechecked to ensure resolution with clinical improvement.

Possible Complications

Very severely affected patients may show rectal stricture formation as a result of long-standing inflammation but this is considered a rare complication.

Expected Course and Prognosis

Prognosis is considered to be good, with appropriate diagnosis and targeted therapy.

Synonyms

- Boxer colitis

Abbreviations

- AIEC = adherent invasive *Escherichia coli*
- FISH = fluorescent *in situ* hybridization
- GC = granulomatous colitis
- GI = gastrointestinal
- HUC = histiocytic ulcerative colitis
- PAS = periodic acid–Schiff

See Also

- Diarrhea, Acute
- Diarrhea, Chronic – Canine
- Dyschezia and Tenesmus
- Hematochezia
- Irritable Bowel Syndrome
- Colitis and Proctitis
- Fiber-responsive Large Bowel Diarrhea

Suggested Reading

Cassman E, White R, Atherly T, et al. Alterations of the ileal and colonic mucosal microbiota in canine chronic enteropathies. PLoS One https://doi.org/10.1371/journal.pone.0147321

Craven M, Dogan B, Schukken A, et al. Antimicrobial resistance impacts clinical outcome of granulomatous colitis in boxer dogs. J Vet Intern Med 2010;24(4):819–824.

Manchester AC, Hill S, Sabatino B, et al. Association between granulomatous colitis in French Bulldogs and invasive Escherichia coli and response to fluoroquinolone antimicrobials. J Vet Intern Med 2013;27:56–61.

Simpson DW, Dogan B, Rishniw M, et al. Adherent and invasive Escherichia coli is associated with granulomatous colitis in boxer dogs. Infect Immun 2006;74:4778–4792.

Acknowledgments: The author and editors acknowledge the previous contribution of Dr Stanley Marks.

Author: Jo Ann Morrison DVM, MS, DACVIM

Chapter 85

Colonic Neoplasia, Benign

DEFINITION/OVERVIEW

- Tumors located in the large intestine that lack the ability to invade neighboring tissues or metastasize.
- Adenomatous polyps, inflammatory pseudopolyposis, and body cavity lipomas.
- Piroxicam and other cyclooxygenase-2 (COX-2) inhibiting nonsteroidal antiinflammatory drugss (NSAIDs) have been used as a palliative measure in the management of canine rectal tubulopapillary polyps.
- Surgical treatment usually involves excision through the anus and/or cryosurgery, although electrotherapy using snares has also been used to resect small, pedunculated polyps.

ETIOLOGY/PATHOPHYSIOLOGY

- May be related to chronic inflammation in the colon.
- Benign polyps left untreated can progress to neoplasia.

Adenomatous Polyps

- Typically colorectal in location.
- Three types – tubular, papillary or papillotubular.
  - Solitary – single polyp; 7% risk of malignant transformation.
  - Multiple – more than one polypoid mass; 25% risk of malignant transformation (Figure 85.1).
  - Diffuse – greater than 50% of the mucosal surface is involved; high risk (75–100%) of malignant transformation (Figure 85.2).
- Carcinoma *in situ* (CIS) – areas of dysplasia within a polyp indicating malignant transformation – not a benign disease. Uncertain how progression occurs; no specific risk factors or markers have been identified in the dog.

Lipoma

- Benign tumor in a location where space-occupying lesions will cause symptoms.
- When located within the pelvic canal (Figure 85.3) or as a pedunculated abdominal mass near the colon, may can cause obstruction, tenesmus, or compression of nearby viscera and structures.

Systems Affected

Gastrointestinal.

Blackwell's Five-Minute Veterinary Consult Clinical Companion: Small Animal Gastrointestinal Diseases,
First Edition. Edited by Jocelyn Mott and Jo Ann Morrison.
© 2019 John Wiley & Sons, Inc. Published 2019 by John Wiley & Sons, Inc.
Companion website: www.fiveminutevet.com/gastrointestinal

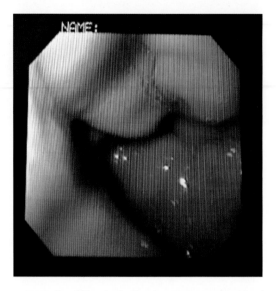

■ **Fig. 85.1.** Endoscopic appearance of multifocal colonic adenomatous polyps in a dog.

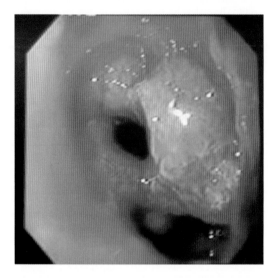

■ **Fig. 85.2.** Endoscopic appearance of diffuse adenomatous colonic polyps in a dog.

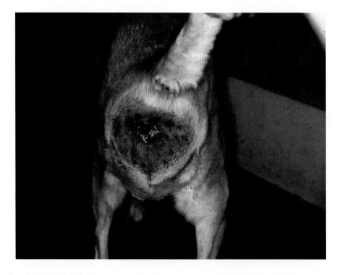

■ **Fig. 85.3.** Intrapelvic lipoma in a dog.

SIGNALMENT/HISTORY

- Primarily affects dogs; extremely rare in cats with only scattered case reports.
- Median age of onset of symptoms is eight years, more frequently in male dogs.
- West Highland white terriers, miniature dachshunds, collies, German shepherds and Labrador retrievers are overrepresented in dogs with colorectal adenomatous polyps.

Historical Findings

- Most commonly present with hematochezia, increased fecal mucus, and tenesmus.
- More severe cases may have constipation or obstipation with passing of thin-diameter stools.

CLINICAL FEATURES

- Weight loss is uncommon.
- Rectal examination may reveal polyps or masses.

DIFFERENTIAL DIAGNOSIS

- Foreign body.
- Viral enteritis.
- Inflammatory bowel disease.
- Intestinal parasites.
- Dietary indiscretion.
- Food allergy.

DIAGNOSTICS

Complete Blood Count/Biochemistry/Urinalysis

Minimum database of a complete blood count, chemistry, and urinalysis often unremarkable.

Imaging

- Plain film abdominal radiographs are of limited utility; most masses are intraluminal or within the pelvic colon and cannot be visualized.
- Contrast radiography – unlikely to highlight mass and delays the ability to perform endoscopy.
- Abdominal ultrasonography is less effective in colonic lesions unless the bowel has been prepared. Large amounts of stool and gas in the colon may interfere with imaging.

Other Diagnostic Tests

- Ultrasound-guided mass aspiration is generally unrewarding for benign lesions; lesions may not be imaged if deep within the pelvic canal.
- Colonoscopy and mucosal biopsy – results must be interpreted with caution; frequently nondiagnostic for tumors that are deep to the mucosal surface; focal areas of dysplasia or neoplasia can be present within the mass on histopathology.

THERAPEUTICS

Drug(s) of Choice

- NSAIDs will significantly decrease the risk of colorectal neoplasia and decrease the risk of malignant transformation or adenomatous polyps in humans.
- NSAIDs such as deracoxib, firocoxib, meloxicam, and piroxicam may play a role in treatment of veterinary patients.
- Piroxicam can be administered PO or as a suppository to treat nonresectable or diffuse polyps. Will relieve clinical symptoms in most patients for a prolonged period of time.
- NSAIDs have been investigated as an alternative to excision of masses. In dogs, piroxicam suppositories relieved clinical signs in a small group of patients with adenomatous polyps.

Precautions/Interactions

Use NSAIDS with caution in patients with preexisting renal or hepatic disease.

Surgical Considerations

Surgical treatment usually involves excision through the anus and/or cryosurgery, although electrotherapy using snares has also been used to resect small, pedunculated polyps.

Adenomatous Polyps

- Endoscopic mucosal resection (EMR) and snare electrocautery are considered the treatments of choice for solitary or multiple lesions. Risk for recurrence exists when polyps are not completely excised. Small risk for intestinal perforation when endocautery is used. Best performed at a referral practice by an individual who is experienced in the procedure.
- Diffuse lesions are best treated with surgical resection. Significant risk for postoperative complications such as colonic stricture, infection, dehiscence, and fecal incontinence exists.

Inflammatory Polyps

Surgical resection is treatment of choice; survival variably reported as one (80%) to two years (67%).

Lipoma

Complete surgical excision generally curative.

COMMENTS

Client Education

- Owners should be advised that some dogs are predisposed and may develop multiple polyps.
- Owners need to be well informed of risks associated with colorectal surgery.

Patient Monitoring

Follow up with recheck and rectal exam every three months after removal.

Prevention/Avoidance

Consider NSAIDs as a preventive for dogs with recurrent disease.

Expected Course and Prognosis

- All polyps should be removed due to risk for malignant transformation.
- The prognosis after radical surgery is poor.

- Even with benign tumors, the postoperative morbidity is high, with prolonged tenesmus and fecal incontinence a frequent complication.
- For inflammatory polyps, surgical resection treatment of choice; survival variably reported as one (80%) to two years (67%).

Abbreviations

- CIS = carcinoma *in situ*
- COX-2 = cyclooxygenase-2
- EMR = endoscopic mucosal resection
- NSAID = nonsteroidal antiinflammatory drug

See Also

- Colonic Neoplasia, Malignant
- Constipation and Obstipation
- Dyschezia and Tenesmus
- Hematochezia

Suggested Reading

Coleman KA, Berent A, Weisse C. Endoscopic mucosal resection and snare polypectomy for treatment of a colorectal polypoid adenoma in a dog. J Am Vet Med Assoc 2014;244(12):1435–1440.

Danova NA, Robles-Emanuelli J, Bjorling D. Surgical excision of primary canine rectal tumors by an anal approach in twenty-three dogs. Vet Surg 2006;35(4):337–340.

Holt PE. Evaluation of transanal endoscopic treatment of benign canine rectal neoplasia. J Small Anim Pract 2007;48(1):17–25.

Knottenbelt CM, Simpson J, Tasker S, et al. Preliminary clinical observations on the use of piroxicam in the management of rectal tubulopapillary polyps. J Small Anim Pract 2000;41(9):393–397.

Mayhew PD, Brockman DJ. Body cavity lipomas in six dogs. J Small Anim Pract 2002;43(4):177–181.

Ohmi,A, Tsukamoto A, Ohno K, et al. A retrospective study of inflammatory colorectal polyps in miniature dachshunds. J Vet Med Sci 2012;74(1):59–64.

Valerius KD, Powers B, McPherron M, et al. Adenomatous polyps and carcinoma in situ of the canine colon and rectum: 34 cases (1982-1994). J Am Anim Hosp Assoc 1997;33(2):156–160.

Author: Carrie A. Wood DVM, DACVIM (Oncology)

Chapter 86

Colonic Neoplasia, Malignant

DEFINITION/OVERVIEW

Nonhematopoietic neoplasia of the large bowel with the potential to metastasize to other sites.

ETIOLOGY/PATHOPHYSIOLOGY

- The cause of colon cancer in dogs and cats is unknown.
- Some animals may have multiple lesions, ranging from benign adenomas to invasive adenocarcinomas.
- The incidence is unknown, but colon cancer in dogs and cats is rare.

Systems Affected

- Gastrointestinal – obstruction.
- Lymphatic – metastasis.
- Hepatic – metastasis.

SIGNALMENT/HISTORY

Dogs

- Male preponderance.
- Mean age 8.5–10 years; median 11 years (range 2–24 years).
- Clinical signs: tenesmus, hematochezia, dyschezia, anorexia, diarrhea, vomiting.
- No reported breed predilections or genetic basis.

Cats

- Male preponderance.
- Siamese cats may have a higher incidence.
- Mean age 10.6–12.5 years; median 11–13 years (range 6–18 years).
- Clinical signs: vomiting, diarrhea, anorexia/hyporexia, weight loss, hematochezia, tenesmus/constipation.

Risk Factors

None known.

Blackwell's Five-Minute Veterinary Consult Clinical Companion: Small Animal Gastrointestinal Diseases, First Edition. Edited by Jocelyn Mott and Jo Ann Morrison.
© 2019 John Wiley & Sons, Inc. Published 2019 by John Wiley & Sons, Inc.
Companion website: www.fiveminutevet.com/gastrointestinal

Historical Findings

- Most signs present less than three months.
- Tenesmus.
- Hematochezia.
- Vomiting.
- Hyporexia/anorexia.

 # CLINICAL FEATURES

- Approximately half of all colorectal masses are palpable.
- Dogs are more likely to have rectal masses than colonic masses.
- Cats have colonic masses more frequently than rectal masses.
- Multiple masses are estimated to be present in <10% of dogs.

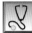 # DIFFERENTIAL DIAGNOSIS

- Adenomas (mass present) – biopsy required to differentiate.
- Carcinoma *in situ* (mass present) – biopsy required to differentiate.
- Inflammatory bowel disease (signs related to colorectal disease) – biopsy required to differentiate.
- Lymphoma – aspirate/biopsy required to differentiate.
- Megacolon in cats (straining) – distended colon on radiographs and feces-filled colon identified via abdominal palpation.
- Parasitic infection, e.g., *Giardia* (hematochezia) – positive fecal examination.
- Any systemic disease (weight loss) – other abnormalities on bloodwork, physical exam.

 # DIAGNOSTICS

Complete Blood Count/Biochemistry/Urinalysis

Often unremarkable.

Imaging

- Abdominal ultrasound is useful for identifying a mass and determining the mass to be of colonic origin.
- Abdominal ultrasound is helpful in identifying possible sites of metastasis.
- Thoracic radiographs may demonstrate pulmonary metastasis.

Other Diagnostic Tests

- Cytology of the mass or possible metastatic lesions can help with differentiation from hematopoietic intestinal tumors (e.g., lymphoma, mast cell tumor, plasmacytoma).
- Colonoscopy may be performed to visualize mass and obtain biopsies (Figure 86.1).
- Surgical biopsy is most accurate means of obtaining a definitive diagnosis.

Pathologic Findings

- Gross: masses may be covered by mucosa or ulcerated; pedunculated, sessile or annular; solitary or multiple.
- Microscopic: most malignant tumors are adenocarcinoma; neuroendocrine tumors also occur in this location.
- Plasmacytomas, lymphoma, adenomas or carcinoma *in situ* are also found in the colon or rectum.

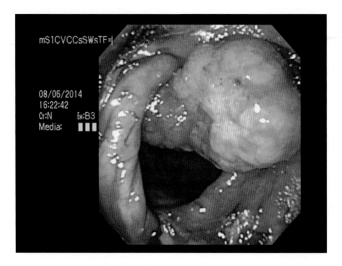

■ **Fig. 86.1.** Colonic adenocarcinoma visualized via endoscopy. Source: Courtesy of Dr Michael Willard.

THERAPEUTICS

- The primary goal of treatment is complete surgical removal of the primary tumor to slow progression and alleviate clinical signs.
- Complete resection appears to improve survival.
- Chemotherapy may improve survival in cats.

Drug(s) of Choice

- Doxorubicin appears to improve survival in cats (1 mg/kg IV every three weeks).
- Two dogs treated with surgery and multiple chemotherapy agents both lived >17 months.
- Stool softeners may be beneficial in patients not undergoing surgical excision (e.g., docusate sodium, 50 mg capsules, 1 capsule/cat or small dog, up to 4/day in a large dog).

Precautions/Interactions

Intestinal stimulants should not be used in any patients with a bowel obstruction as they could result in intestinal rupture.

Alternative Drugs

There are no known alternative drugs.

Appropriate Health Care

If surgical excision is not elected, and the animal becomes obstructed, euthanasia is necessary.

Nursing Care

The addition of canned pumpkin may help maintain a soft stool (1–4 tsp/day).

Diet

Soft, moist foods may help maintain a soft fecal consistency.

Surgical Considerations

- Complete surgical excision appears to improve survival for patients with this condition.
- Metastasis within the abdomen is common (approximately 50%), so the surgeon should be prepared to biopsy and/or remove suspicious tissues.

 # COMMENTS

Although historical reports of this condition suggest a poor prognosis, more recent reports employing oncologic surgical techniques suggest long-term survivals are common for most colorectal adenocarcinomas where complete excision can be obtained.

Client Education

Patients should be monitored for continued ability to defecate.

Patient Monitoring

Abdominal ultrasound and thoracic radiographs should be evaluated every three months for evidence of metastasis or disease progression.

Possible Complications

- Obstruction due to the primary tumor or metastasis is possible.
- Advanced metastatic disease may present as cachexia, decreased quality of life.

Expected Course and Prognosis

- At necropsy, 75% of cats had metastasis: 45% to abdominal lymph nodes, 50% to omentum/ peritoneum, 9% to lungs, 8% to liver/spleen.
- Mean survival of 11 dogs treated with *en bloc* excision of a single colorectal adenocarcinoma was 44.6 months, with no dogs developing additional documented metastatic disease (one dog had lymph node metastasis resected); two dogs had local recurrence.
- A median survival of 15 months was reported for dogs treated with stool softeners (no surgery).
- The appearance of the mass (annular/nodular/pedunculated) may affect survival, with annular masses having the shortest survival.
- The metastatic rate of colonic and rectal tumors is unknown (has been reported to range from 0% to 80% and many studies do not differentiate between small and large intestinal tumors).
- Adenocarcinoma *in situ* can progress to invasive disease.
- Dogs with colorectal plasmacytomas (8/9 treated surgically) had a median survival of 15 months.

See Also

- Colonic Neoplasia, Benign
- Dyschezia and Tenesmus
- Hematochezia

Suggested Reading

Church EM, Mehlhaff CJ, Patnaik AK. Colorectal adenocarcinoma in dogs: 78 cases (1973-1984). J Am Vet Med Assoc 1987;191(6):727–730.

Morello E, Martano M, Squassino C, et al. Transanal pull-through rectal amputation for treatment of colorectal carcinoma in 11 dogs. Vet Surg 2008;37(5):420–426.

Selting KA. Intestinal tumors. In: Withrow SJ, Vail DM, Page RL, eds. Small Animal Clinical Oncology, 5th ed. St Louis: Elsevier, 2013.

Slawienski MJ, Mauldin GE, Mauldin GN, Patnaik AK. Malignant colonic neoplasia in cats: 46 cases (1990–1996). J Am Vet Med Assoc 1997;211(7):878–881.

Author: Marlene L. Hauck DVM, PhD, DACVIM (Oncology)

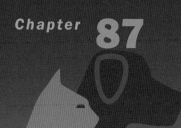

Chapter 87

Fiber-Responsive Large Bowel Diarrhea

DEFINITION/OVERVIEW

- A form of chronic idiopathic large bowel diarrhea that occurs in dogs that responds favorably to dietary fiber supplementation (usually with soluble fiber).
- At the author's institution, chronic idiopathic large bowel diarrhea is diagnosed in approximately 25% of dogs referred for evaluation of chronic large bowel diarrhea.
- Exclusion diagnosis that requires eliminating known causes of chronic large bowel diarrhea.
- No pathophysiologic studies have been performed.
- Only three reports of this condition in the veterinary literature, containing 83 dogs.
- May overlap with another chronic idiopathic large bowel diarrheal syndrome in dogs called irritable bowel syndrome, also referred to as nervous colitis, spastic colon, or mucus colitis. Irritable bowel syndrome is stress associated and is poorly defined in dogs. Some affected dogs respond to dietary fiber supplementation, while others require stress alleviation, antispasmodic medications, and/or antianxiety drugs.

ETIOLOGY/PATHOPHYSIOLOGY

- Unknown as pathophysiologic studies have not been performed. Stress or abnormal personality traits may play a role in some dogs.
- Clinical response to dietary soluble fiber supplementation suggests abnormal colonic motility and/or dysbiosis. Dysbiosis is defined as a microbial imbalance within the GI tract. Soluble dietary fiber is a prebiotic, fermented by colonic bacteria, resulting in altered composition or activity of bacteria. Prebiotics are not digested by mammalian digestive enzymes and "feed" the colonic bacteria, potentially correcting dysbiosis. Soluble fibers also absorb water, improving stool quality. Fermentation of soluble fiber by colonic bacteria produces volatile fatty acids, which are an energy source for colonic epithelial cells.
- Insoluble dietary fiber helps to distend the colonic lumen; distension is necessary for normal fecal storage and colonic motility.
- Psyllium is the fiber often fed to affected dogs. It comes from the seeds or husks of the plant ispaghula and consists of approximately 90% soluble fiber. Psyllium has been shown to be an effective treatment in some children with chronic nonspecific diarrhea and in people with several diarrheal disorders.

Systems Affected

Gastrointestinal.

Blackwell's Five-Minute Veterinary Consult Clinical Companion: Small Animal Gastrointestinal Diseases,
First Edition. Edited by Jocelyn Mott and Jo Ann Morrison.
© 2019 John Wiley & Sons, Inc. Published 2019 by John Wiley & Sons, Inc.
Companion website: www.fiveminutevet.com/gastrointestinal

SIGNALMENT/HISTORY

- Dogs of all ages (0.5–14 years); median six years.
- Many breeds, including mixed breeds; common breeds include German shepherd dog, miniature schnauzer, cocker spaniel, and miniature or toy poodle.

Risk Factors

- Stress factors or abnormal personality traits occur in approximately 35% of dogs.
- Diarrhea has been associated with visitation, travel, moving, construction, invisible fence installment, recent adoption or personality disorders such as being considered nervous, high-strung, aggressive, sensitive, or having noise phobia, anxiety or depressive disorders.

Historical Findings

- Chronic diarrhea (soft to liquid) with classic large bowel characteristics: tenesmus, excess fecal mucus, hematochezia, increased frequency (median 3.5 times/day), and urgency.
- Diarrhea is usually episodic, alternating with periods of normal stool; however, diarrhea may be continuous in approximately 25% of dogs.
- Less common signs include occasional vomiting, decreased appetite during episodes of diarrhea, abdominal pain, and anal pruritus.
- Weight loss is rare.

 # CLINICAL FEATURES

- Physical examination reveals no significant abnormalities.
- Digital rectal examination is usually normal. Feces may be normal due to episodic nature of the disease. Loose stool may be present and may contain hematochezia (red blood) or excess mucus.

 # DIFFERENTIAL DIAGNOSIS

- Dietary indiscretion.
- GI diet-responsive diarrhea.
- Hypoallergenic diet-responsive diarrhea.
- Whipworms.
- *Clostridium perfringens*-associated diarrhea.
- Lymphocytic plasmacytic colitis.
- Eosinophilic colitis
- Miscellaneous types of colitis.
- Irritable bowel syndrome.
- Colonic neoplasia (adenocarcinoma, lymphoma, and adenoma are most common).
- Cecal inversion.

 # DIAGNOSTICS

- CBC, biochemistry, and urinalysis are normal. Eosinophilia may occur in dogs with whipworms, eosinophilic colitis, and dietary hypersensitivity.
- Fecal flotations by zinc sulfate are negative for whipworms and other parasites. Due to intermittent shedding of whipworm ova, dogs not receiving monthly heartworm prophylaxis with milbemycin or moxidectin should have three fecal examinations performed.

■ Therapeutic deworming for whipworms (fenbendazole 50 mg/kg PO q24h for three days) should be performed in dogs not receiving milbemycin or moxidectin for heartworm prevention. No improvement will occur in dogs with fiber-responsive large bowel diarrhea.

■ *Clostridium perfringens* enterotoxin fecal ELISA will be negative.

■ "GI" diet trial for 2–4 weeks. No improvement in stool quality occurs in dogs with fiber-responsive large bowel diarrhea. Prescription diets such as Hills i/d®, Purina EN®, and Royal Canin Digestive Low Fat® are often used. During the food trial, the dog must not receive any other nutrients. These diets are highly digestible, low in fiber, and restricted in fat. If the dog's stool becomes normal during this diet trial, no further diagnostic tests are indicated. The "GI" diet can be fed for another 2–4 weeks and then the original diet can be slowly introduced. Some dogs develop diarrhea again; others can be maintained on their original diet.

■ Hypoallergenic diet trial for 2–3 weeks. No improvement in stool quality occurs in dogs with fiber-responsive large bowel diarrhea. During the food trial, the dog must not receive any other nutrients, including flavored heartworm preveatives, vitamins, or any other supplements. For this diet trial, the author recommends using a hydrolyzed diet, such as Hills z/d®, Purina HA®, or Royal Canin HP®. The hydrolyzed protein in these diets is hypoallergenic. If the dog's stool becomes normal during this diet trial, a diagnosis of dietary hypersensitivity or inflammatory bowel disease can be made. These hydrolyzed diets are also highly digestible, low in fiber, and restricted in fat. Some clinicians skip the "GI" diet trial and go directly to the hydrolyzed diet trial. Without performing a "GI" diet trial first, response to the hydrolyzed diet trial could also be due to the digestibility, fat, and fiber content and not due to dietary hypersensitivity.

■ Abdominal imaging is rarely performed in dogs with chronic large bowel diarrhea, absence of weight loss, and a normal physical examination and digital rectal examination. If performed, abdominal radiographs and abdominal ultrasound will be normal.

■ Colonoscopy is usually within normal limits (Figure 87.1), or only very mild nonspecific findings, such as slight increases in granularity or friability, occur.

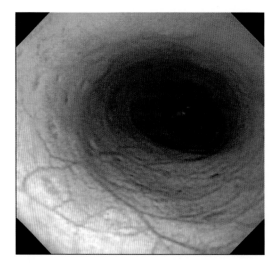

■ **Fig. 87.1.** Endoscopic appearance of a normal descending colon in a dog. The mucosa is pink, smooth, and glistening. Submucosal blood vessels are clearly visible. There are several dimples at 9:00 that are lymphoid follicles. There is a minute amount of scattered brown fecal material coating the mucosa, most obvious at the 10:00 to 1:00 position. A diagnosis of idiopathic large bowel diarrhea requires a grossly normal colon during colonoscopy.

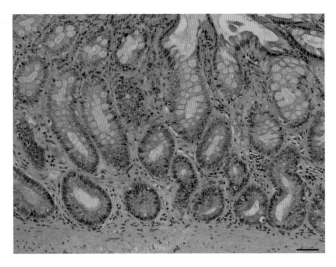

■ **Fig. 87.2.** Histological appearance of a normal colon in a dog. Multiple biopsy samples should be collected from the cecum to the descending colon and evaluated microscopically. A diagnosis of idiopathic large bowel diarrhea requires a microscopically normal colon. The image extends from the luminal surface (*top*) to the muscularis mucosa (*bottom*) and includes the lamina propria. The surface epithelial cells are not damaged, the crypts are uniform in diameter and length, there is no fibrosis between crypts, and there are a normal number of lymphocytes and plasma cells within the lamina propria. Bar = 50 μg. Source: Courtesy of Dr Tom Cecere.

Pathologic Findings

■ Histopathologic evaluation of multiple colonic biopsy samples is within normal limits (Figure 87.2). Histopathologic standards from the 2008 WSAVA report should be utilized.

■ Multiple biopsy specimens should be evaluated from throughout the colon, from the cecum to the rectum. Usually 5–6 locations are sampled.

 THERAPEUTICS

■ Health care can be provided on an outpatient basis and consists of dietary fiber supplementation of a GI diet.

■ If stresses have been identified in the history, they should be reduced or modified if possible. In addition, if abnormal personality factors are present, they should be addressed with behavioral therapy or medication.

■ A highly digestible "GI" diet should initially be supplemented with 1–3 tbsp daily (divided into 2–3 meals/day) of psyllium hydrophobic mucilloid (Metamucil® contains 10.2 g psyllium/tbsp).

■ Median dose is 2 tbsp/day, or 0.13 tbsp/kg/day, or 1.3 g psyllium/kg/day.

■ Initial response to less fiber supplementation or the use of other fiber types is not as successful.

■ After 2–3 months without diarrhea, the amount of fiber can be slowly reduced successfully in approximately 50% of dogs.

Diet

■ After resolution of diarrhea with psyllium supplementation, owners may switch to a commercial high-fiber diet (usually containing insoluble fiber) that may be more convenient to feed. Diarrhea will return in some dogs.

- After resolution of diarrhea with psyllium supplementation, owners may also be able to switch from the highly digestible "GI" diet to a high-quality maintenance dog food. Diarrhea will return in some dogs.
- Lack of response to fiber supplementation suggests that the chronic idiopathic large bowel diarrhea may be due to irritable bowel syndrome and pharmacologic management of that disorder should be instituted.

Activity

Activity level does not have to be modified.

 COMMENTS

Patient Monitoring

Patient monitoring requires periodic assessment of the stool quality, performed during recheck office examinations or via telephone interviews.

Expected Course and Prognosis

- Dietary soluble fiber supplementation can occasionally produce excessive flatulence, which can be managed by reduction in the fiber dosage.
- Prognosis is very favorable as approximately 85% of dogs have an excellent or very good long-term response to fiber supplementation.

Abbreviations

- GI – gastrointestinal

See Also

- Colitis and Proctitis
- Irritable Bowel Syndrome
- Nutritional Approach to Chronic Enteropathies

Suggested Reading

Day MJ, Bilzer T, Mansell J, et al. Histopathological standards for the diagnosis of gastrointestinal inflammation in endoscopic biopsy samples from the dog and cat: a report from the World Small Animal Veterinary Association Gastrointestinal Standardization Group. J Comp Pathol 2008:138 Suppl 1:S1–S43.

Dimski DS, Buffington CA. Dietary fiber in small animal therapeutics. J Am Vet Med Assoc 1991;199:1142–1146.

Lecoindre P, Gaschen FP. Chronic idiopathic large bowel diarrhea in the dog. Vet Clin North Am 2011;41:447–456.

Leib MS. Treatment of chronic idiopathic large bowel diarrhea in dogs with a highly digestible diet and soluble fiber: a retrospective review of 37 cases. J Vet Intern Med 2000;14:27–32.

Author: Michael S. Leib DVM, MS, DACVIM

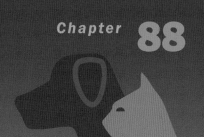

Megacolon

Chapter 88

DEFINITION/OVERVIEW

A persistent, irreversible dilation of the colon associated with permanent loss of function that is often the end-result of chronic constipation/obstipation.

ETIOLOGY/PATHOPHYSIOLOGY

- Megacolon is seen most commonly in cats. Idiopathic dilated megacolon is the most common diagnosis in this species and occurs due to generalized colonic smooth muscle dysfunction.
- The diagnosis of idiopathic dilated megacolon is often preceded by months to years of chronic, recurrent constipation so it is unclear whether a primary disorder of colonic smooth muscle occurs first or whether smooth muscle dysfunction results from prolonged colonic distension.
- Megacolon can also occur secondary to abnormal neurologic function of the colon.
- Reported neurogenic causes of megacolon include dysautonomia, spinal cord injury or deformities, pelvic nerve injury, and autonomic ganglioneuritis. Colonic aganglionosis/hypoganglionosis (Hirschsprung's disease in humans) is a congenital absence of ganglia in the colonic smooth muscle; affected segments are unable to relax and megacolon develops as a result.
- Hypertrophic megacolon can develop as a consequence of obstructive lesions and will progress to irreversible dilated megacolon if the obstruction is not corrected.

Systems Affected

- Gastrointestinal.
- Neuromuscular – megacolon can be seen as a consequence of neuromuscular disorders, and concurrent neurologic abnormalities may be seen along with megacolon, depending on the underlying disease process.
- Musculoskeletal – megacolon can occur secondary to pelvic fractures, causing obstruction to normal defecation.
- Endocrine/metabolic – megacolon can result in electrolyte derangements due to prolonged vomiting. Electrolyte and endocrine abnormalities (hypercalcemia, hypokalemia, hypothyroidism) can promote constipation and possibly lead to or exacerbate megacolon.
- Hepatobiliary – cats with megacolon may have a history of prolonged anorexia and as a result should be evaluated for hepatic lipidosis.

Blackwell's Five-Minute Veterinary Consult Clinical Companion: Small Animal Gastrointestinal Diseases,
First Edition. Edited by Jocelyn Mott and Jo Ann Morrison.
© 2019 John Wiley & Sons, Inc. Published 2019 by John Wiley & Sons, Inc.
Companion website: www.fiveminutevet.com/gastrointestinal

SIGNALMENT/HISTORY

- For feline idiopathic megacolon.
  - Domestic shorthair, domestic long hair, and Siamese cats have been most commonly reported.
  - Young adult cats affected most commonly (average age approximately six years) although cats of any age can be affected.
  - Males overrepresented.
- Dogs and cats of any age and breed can develop megacolon that occurs secondary to neurogenic or obstructive processes.

Risk Factors

- History of chronic constipation.
- Conditions leading to obstruction or difficulty defecating, including prior trauma and pelvic fractures and spinal cord injury or deformity.
- Possible association with low physical activity and obesity as well as the consumption of bone meal in dogs.

Historical Findings

- The most common historical finding is chronic and recurrent constipation.
- Dyschezia and tenesmus, characterized by frequent trips to the litterbox in cats. Owners may not witness failed attempts to defecate but may report their cat sitting in the litterbox for prolonged periods. Clients need to distinguish between dyschezia and dysuria.
- Small amounts of diarrhea and hematochezia may also be seen due to irritation of the colonic mucosa by impacted feces.
- Vomiting, anorexia, and weight loss are frequently seen with prolonged inability to defecate and may be the primary presenting complaint.

CLINICAL FEATURES

- The classic physical examination finding is a distended, feces-filled colon on abdominal palpation. The feces are often very firm.
- Rectal exam confirms fecal impaction and may reveal an underlying obstructive cause such as narrowing of the pelvic canal or an intraluminal mass.
- With chronic constipation/obstipation, dehydration and evidence of weight loss may be present.
- A complete neurologic exam and rectal exam should be performed in all patients with suspected megacolon. Sedation may be necessary in cats or if animals are resistant to rectal exam.

DIFFERENTIAL DIAGNOSES

- Mechanical obstruction: pelvic fractures, neoplasia, rectal foreign body, rectal stricture, atresia ani, prostatomegaly.
- Neurologic disease: dysautonomia, sacral spinal cord deformities (Manx cat), cauda equina syndrome, pelvic nerve injury or dysfunction.
- Endocrine/metabolic: hypercalcemia, hypokalemia, hypothyroidism, severe dehydration.
- Administration of drugs: opioids, anticholinergics, phenothiazines.

DIAGNOSTICS

Complete Blood Count/Biochemistry/Urinalysis

■ A minimum laboratory database is often normal and, while not required to reach a definitive diagnosis in affected patients, it is essential to evaluate for possible complicating factors, especially if there has been prolonged anorexia or vomiting.

■ Complete blood count may show evidence of dehydration (elevated packed cell volume, total protein) and stress leukogram.

■ Chemistry: electrolyte abnormalities may develop with chronic illness, and certain electrolyte abnormalities (hypokalemia, hypercalcemia) can contribute to or exacerbate constipation. Prerenal azotemia may occur with severe dehydration.

■ Urinalysis: important to confirm normal renal function in dehydrated animals and to investigate lower urinary tract disease as a differential diagnosis for tenesmus.

Total T4

■ Evaluation of thyroid status should be considered in feline patients if they have other clinical signs of hypothyroidism or a history of being treated for hyperthyroidism.

■ Congenital hypothyroidism in the cat is frequently associated with chronic constipation (rare).

Imaging

■ An enlarged, feces-filled colon is easily identified on survey abdominal radiographs (Figures 88.1 and 88.2).

■ In the cat, a maximal colonic diameter of L5 vertebral body length ratio of >1.48 is suggestive of megacolon. Bear in mind that radiographic information should be used in combination with a history of the animal being refractory to appropriate medical therapy before surgical intervention is selected.

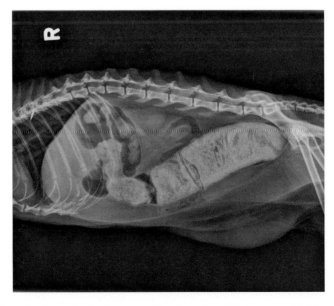

■ **Fig. 88.1.** Right lateral radiograph of a four-year-old male neutered Maine coon with idiopathic megacolon and concurrent hepatic lipidosis. Source: Courtesy of Dr Elizabeth Riedesel.

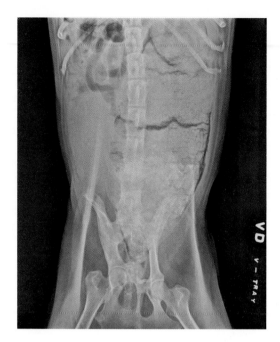

■ **Fig. 88.2.** Ventrodorsal radiograph of a 10-year-old male neutered mixed-breed dog with a history of chronic constipation following pelvic fracture after vehicular trauma years earlier. Source: Courtesy of Dr Elizabeth Riedesel.

Additional Diagnostics

■ Advanced abdominal imaging, such as abdominal ultrasound or computed tomography, may be needed to gain additional information about possible causes of extraluminal compression of the gastrointestinal (GI) tract.
■ Colonoscopy or proctoscopy, after manual evacuation of feces, may be needed to visualize intraluminal masses, strictures, or foreign bodies.
■ Advanced neurologic diagnostics, such as magnetic resonance imaging, cerebrospinal fluid analysis, and electrodiagnostics, may be useful if the animal has other signs of neurologic dysfunction.

Pathologic Findings

■ Gross pathologic features: a distended, feces-filled colon is observed at necropsy. Mesenteric lymphadenopathy can be seen with severe cases.
■ Histopathologic features.
  • Feline idiopathic megacolon has no defining histologic changes. Smooth muscle typically appears normal with evidence of normal innervation. Mucosal and submucosal ulceration, fibrosis, and inflammation can be variably present and are secondary to chronic fecal impaction.
  • Megacolon resulting from other etiologies may have other features such as abnormalities in or reduced numbers of ganglia (ganglioneuritis or hypogangliosis), or smooth muscle hypertrophy (believed to be a compensatory mechanism in obstructive megacolon).

THERAPEUTICS

- For animals with a distended, feces-impacted colon for which a clear, reversible obstructive or neurologic cause cannot be identified, inpatient medical management for severe constipation should be attempted.
- Megacolon is associated with a permanent loss of normal colonic function and is, by definition, refractory to medical therapy. Surgery (sub-total colectomy) will be indicated if medical therapy is unsuccessful.

Drug(s) of Choice

- Colonic prokinetic agents: cisapride is a 5-HT receptor agonist that has been shown to stimulate colonic smooth muscle motility in cats and dogs with constipation. The dose for dogs and cats is 0.1–0.5 mg/kg PO q 8–12 h. This dosage may be increased up to 1 mg/kg if well tolerated. Metoclopramide does not affect colonic motility and should not be used for constipation.
- Hyperosmotic laxatives: polyethylene glycol 3350 powder (Miralax®) 1/8–¼ tsp with food q 12 h; lactulose 0.5 mL/kg PO q 8–12 h to effect. Polyethylene glycol electrolyte solution (GoLytely®, Colyte®) can be given via nasogastric or nasoesophageal feeding tube as a trickle for 12–48 h in a 24-h care hospital setting to facilitate passage of feces in cats with severe constipation, either as an alternative to or in preparation for manual evacuation of feces. Administer at a rate of 6–10 mL/kg/h.
- Enemas: 5–10 mL/kg warm water or a 50–50 mixture of warm water and water-soluble lubricant administered slowly via a lubricated 10–12 Fr red rubber catheter gently passed into the rectum. Lactulose can also be administered as an enema at a dose of 5–10 mL/kg.

Precautions/Interactions

- Patients should be adequately hydrated prior to administration of hyperosmotic laxatives (orally or via enema) as these agents will draw water into the GI tract and may exacerbate dehydration.
- Sodium phosphate (Fleet) enemas should never be administered to cats as life-threatening electrolyte derangements can result.
- When administering polyethylene glycol electrolyte solution via feeding tube, patients should be monitored for aspiration. Confirm placement of the tube radiographically and discontinue administration if vomiting or increased respiratory rate develops.

Alternative Drugs

- Psyllium acts as a bulk-forming laxative and can be added to food at a dose of ¼–1 tsp twice a day. Fiber may be beneficial in early stages but may exacerbate clinical signs in cats with loss of colonic muscle function.
- Dioctyl sodium sulfosuccinate (Colace®) is an emollient laxative that can be given as an alternative to lactulose or polyethylene glycol.
- Ranitidine, a member of the H2-receptor antagonist drug class, may stimulate colonic motility and can be given if cisapride is unavailable. The dose is 3.5 mg/kg PO q 12 h for cats or 2.5 mg/kg IV q 12 h.

Appropriate Health Care

- If administration of laxatives or enemas fails to resolve fecal impaction, manual evacuation of feces will be necessary.
- For manual evacuation of feces, the patient should be placed under general anesthesia and intubated to prevent aspiration should manipulation of the colon trigger vomiting or regurgitation.

- Warm water enemas combined with a water-based lubricant can be administered before and during the procedure to help facilitate removal of feces. Feces are then removed manually while providing gentle assistance with abdominal palpation of the colon.
- Periprocedural administration of an intravenous antibiotic with a good anaerobic spectrum can be considered in case manipulation of the compromised colon results in bacterial translocation.
- This procedure may need to be repeated if the impaction is too severe to safely accomplish removal of all feces under one anesthetic event.
- Trickle administration of polyethylene glycol 3350 via nasogastric tube for 24–48 h prior to manual extraction will result in better fecal hydration and may facilitate stool removal.

Nursing Care

- Intravenous fluid therapy for rehydration and correction of any electrolyte abnormalities.
- Nutritional support should be initiated with placement of a feeding tube if anorexia has been prolonged (three or more days) or if ongoing anorexia is anticipated.
- Control nausea and vomiting with antiemetic medications.
- Analgesia should be considered.

Diet

- While fiber supplementation can increase colonic smooth muscle contraction and may be beneficial in patients with mild constipation, a diet with high insoluble fiber that increases fecal bulk may worsen clinical signs in patients with impaired colonic motility.
- Low-residue diets are preferred in patients with megacolon.

Activity

Because there is some association between low activity and obesity and the development of megacolon, increasing exercise is recommended when practical.

Surgical Considerations

- An underlying obstructive cause should be surgically corrected, if possible. Alternatively, subtotal colectomy has been described in the successful management of megacolon occurring secondary to pelvic fracture malunion (Figure 88.3).
- Patients with permanent loss of colonic function and structure do not respond favorably to medical treatment and subtotal colectomy is the treatment of choice for these patients.
- Subtotal colectomy may also be required with obstructive megacolon even if the obstruction is corrected if irreversible changes in colonic motility have already occurred.
- Avoid enema administration or attempts at colonic evacuation prior to surgery. These efforts are usually unsuccessful and may result in increased likelihood of fecal contamination of the abdomen during surgery.
- Subtotal colectomy can be performed with either an ileorectal or colorectal anastomosis. Preservation of the ileocolic junction has been recommended since cats that have subtotal colectomy with excision of the ileocolic junction have been reported to have looser stools long term than cats who have the ileocolic junction preserved.

 COMMENTS

Client Education

- It is difficult to differentiate between reversible severe constipation with significant colonic distension and the irreversible colonic dysfunction seen with megacolon.

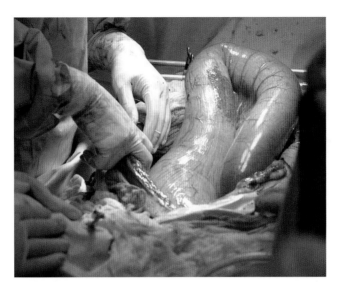

■ **Fig. 88.3.** Intraoperative picture of a dog with megacolon secondary to pelvic fracture. Source: Courtesy of Dr Louisa Ho-Eckart.

- Following treatment for constipation, medical therapy, including dietary management, laxatives, and/or colonic prokinetics, may be required long term and has the potential to fail.
- Subtotal colectomy is indicated in cases of medical treatment failure.

Patient Monitoring
- Owner monitoring of patient defecation at home.
- Concerns for recurrent clinical signs should be addressed promptly with physical exam and abdominal radiographs, if indicated.

Prevention/Avoidance
- Encourage physical activity and maintenance of a healthy lean body condition.
- Maintain hydration.
- Early correction of colonic obstruction may prevent progression to megacolon with permanent dysfunction.

Possible Complications
- Recurrent or persistent constipation is the most common complication following subtotal colectomy or medical management.
- Potential surgical complications include infection, persistent diarrhea, and stricture formation.
- Traumatic perforation of the colon is a potential complication of manual evacuation of feces.

Expected Course and Prognosis
- Medical management is typically unrewarding if there is true megacolon.
- Subtotal colectomy is well tolerated by cats and dogs and the prognosis is generally good. Recurrent constipation can occur years following surgery.
- Diarrhea is expected following subtotal colectomy but typically improves within about six weeks of surgery as the remaining bowel adapts by increasing reservoir capacity and water absorption.

Abbreviations

- GI – gastrointestinal

See Also

- Constipation and Obstipation.

Suggested Reading

Carr AP, Gaunt MC. Constipation resolution with administration of polyethylene-glycol solution in cats (abstract). J Vet Intern Med 2010;24:753.

Nemeth T, Solymosi N, Balka G. Long-term results of subtotal colectomy for acquired hypertrophic megacolon in eight dogs. J Small Anim Pract 2008;49:618–624.

Rosin E, Walshaw R, Mehlhaff C, Matthiesen, Orshner R, Kusba J. Subtotal colectomy for treatment of chronic constipation associated with idiopathic megacolon in cats: 38 cases (1979–1985). J Am Vet Med Assoc 1988;193:850–853.

Travail T, Gunn-Moore D, Carrera I, Courcier E, Sullivan M. Radiographic diameter of the colon in normal and constipated cats and in cats with megacolon. Vet Radiol Ultrasound 2011;52:516–520.

Washabau RJ, Holt D. Pathogenesis, diagnosis, and therapy of feline idiopathic megacolon. Vet Clin North Am 1999;29:589–603.

Authors: Laura Van Vertloo DVM, MS, DACVIM, Albert E. Jergens DVM, PhD, DACVIM

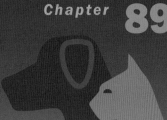

Chapter 89

Perianal Fistula

DEFINITION/OVERVIEW

- Chronic inflammatory condition characterized by multiple, painful, malodorous, progressive, ulcerating sinuses or, much less frequently, true fistulous tracts involving the perianal region.
- Secondary involvement of the anal sacs is common in advanced cases.

ETIOLOGY/PATHOPHYSIOLOGY

- Cause not clearly defined, but a multifactorial immune-mediated mechanism is strongly suspected based on the similarities to perianal Crohn's disease in humans and the response to immunosuppressive drugs.
- Immunohistochemical studies of affected tissues indicate the inflammatory process is characterized by infiltration of T lymphocytes, plasma cells, and eosinophils with local formation of ectopic lymphoid follicles.
- A genetic predisposition in German shepherds (Figure 89.1) is suspected based on the high incidence in this breed and genetic studies have shown an association with the major histocompatibility complex genes. The potential involvement of other gene loci is being explored.

Systems Affected

- Gastrointestinal.
- Skin/exocrine.

SIGNALMENT/HISTORY

- Middle-aged, large breed dogs with mean age of 5–7 years; range 7 months–14 years.
- German shepherd dogs primarily.
- Also reported in many other breeds including Irish setters, Labrador retrievers, Old English sheep dogs, collies, bouvier des Flandres, bulldogs, beagles, various spaniels, and mixed breeds.
- A convincing sex predilection has not been demonstrated because incidence varies between studies.

Blackwell's Five-Minute Veterinary Consult Clinical Companion: Small Animal Gastrointestinal Diseases, First Edition. Edited by Jocelyn Mott and Jo Ann Morrison.
© 2019 John Wiley & Sons, Inc. Published 2019 by John Wiley & Sons, Inc.
Companion website: www.fiveminutevet.com/gastrointestinal

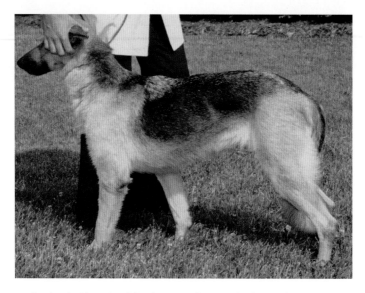

■ **Fig. 89.1.** German shepherd with perianal fistulas. Note the typical tail tucked stance.

Risk Factors

- Anatomic factors have been implicated, particularly in German shepherds. Low tail carriage with a broad tail base and dense fur create a moist contaminated environment (see Figure 89.1).
- High density of apocrine sweat glands in the cutaneous zone of the anal canal of German shepherd dogs potentially predisposing to inflammation and infection of the glands and hair follicles.
- An association with colitis has also been proposed, particularly in German shepherd dogs.

Historical Findings

- Usually presented because of anal discomfort, scooting, licking, odor, straining to defecate sometimes with thin ribbon-shaped stools, diarrhea or constipation, serosanguineous to mucopurulent discharge, fecal incontinence.
- Weight loss, decreased appetite.
- Behavioral changes, especially reluctance/aggression with attempts to manipulate the tail or examine the perineal area due to the severe pain.

 ## CLINICAL FEATURES

- Complete examination often requires heavy sedation or general anesthesia because of the severe pain.
- Anal sphincter tone should be assessed prior to sedation or anesthesia, since fecal incontinence may be present.
- The number of draining tracts varies from a few tracts to 360° involvement with extension a significant distance from the perianal region (Figures 89.2 and 89.3).
- Rectal examination is essential to evaluate for anal or rectal stenosis which may occur secondary to the inflammation, concomitant perineal hernia or weakening of the pelvic diaphragm, integrity of the anal sacs, and anal tone if not done previously.
- Express and flush the anal sacs. Flushing the anal sacs with saline may identify previously unobserved communications with the draining tracts.
- Gently probe the draining tracts to assess their depth and extent and also identify anocutaneous or rectocutaneous fistula (Figure 89.4).

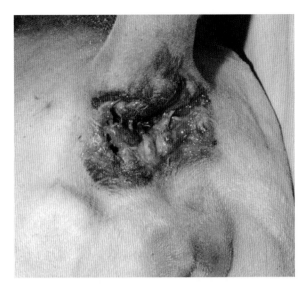

■ **Fig. 89.2.** Severe perianal fistulas with 360° involvement around the anus were found after clipping the hair and cleaning the perineum under general anesthesia.

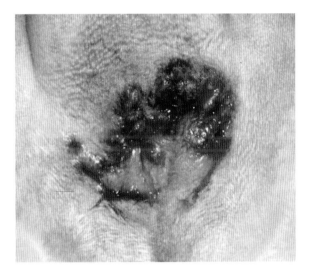

■ **Fig. 89.3.** Moderate case of perianal fistulas. The sinus tracts were superficial and confined to the perianal region.

 # DIFFERENTIAL DIAGNOSIS

- Other inflammatory processes.
- Chronic anal sac abscess.
- Perianal adenoma or adenocarcinoma with ulceration and drainage.
- Squamous cell carcinoma.
- Atypical bacterial infection.
- Oomycosis, e.g., pythiosis.
- Anocutaneous or rectocutaneous fistula.

(a)   (b)

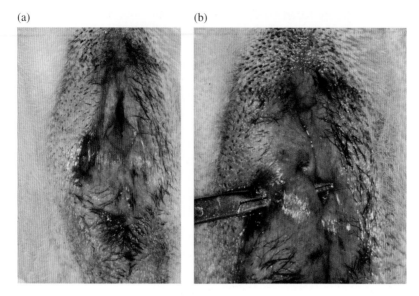

■ **Fig. 89.4.** (a) Perineal fistulas in the ventrolateral areas around the anus should raise suspicion of anal sac involvement. (b) A true rectocutaneous fistula (very uncommon) was identified by probing the fistula.

DIAGNOSTICS

Complete Blood Count/Biochemistry/Urinalysis

Often unremarkable.

Pathologic Findings

Immunohistochemical studies of affected tissues indicate the inflammatory process is characterized by infiltration of T lymphocytes, plasma cells, and eosinophils with local formation of ectopic lymphoid follicles.

THERAPEUTICS

Various immunosuppressive drug protocols and dosage regimens have been reported. Surgery is indicated when a complete response is not achieved.

Drug(s) of Choice

- Approximately 85–90% of cases will show significant improvement with immunosuppressive therapy. Multiple drugs and protocols have been reported but the following options appear to be very effective.
- Moderate to severe cases.
  - Combination of cyclosporine and ketoconazole has produced good results with reduced cost compared to cyclosporine alone.
  - Definitive dosage regimens have not been established because dogs on the same dose often have large differences in blood cyclosporine levels due to variations in absorption and metabolism.
  - Cyclosporine A (CsA) 0.5–1 mg/kg PO q12h depending on severity of lesions and ketoconazole 5.8–8.3 mg/kg PO q12h. Higher CsA doses (4–8 mg/kg q24h) typically necessary if CsA is used alone.

- Dosage is adjusted based on clinical response. Improvement is generally seen within 1–2 weeks with complete resolution in 3–10 weeks. Taper administration while monitoring for recurrence.
- Due to the variability in absorption and bioavailability, measure trough cyclosporine levels in those patients which fail to show improvement and when side effects are persistent or severe. Several techniques are used to measure cyclosporine levels. High-pressure liquid chromatography (HPLC) appears to be the most accurate but is expensive and not widely available. Radioimmune assay (RIA) is cheaper and faster to perform but may overestimate cyclosporine levels. A target range of 200 ng/mL appears to be adequate when HPLC is used while a target range of 400–600 ng/mL is recommended when RIA is utilized.
- If most lesions resolve but draining tracts persist ventral and lateral to the anus, previously unidentified involvement of the anal sacs should be suspected. Bilateral anal sacculectomy is necessary in these cases.

- Mild cases and maintenance therapy.
  - 0.1% tacrolimus ointment applied q12h topically with a gloved hand initially and then tapering to q24–72h as lesions resolve.
  - Continue for at least four weeks after complete resolution. Monitor regularly for recurrence if discontinued.
  - Tacrolimus therapy often instituted as CsA/ketoconazole dose is being tapered off.
  - The temperament of the patient must be considered before recommending this therapy.
- Antimicrobials.
  - Infection is common.
  - Broad-spectrum antibiotics such as amoxicillin-clavulanic acid (13.75 mg/kg PO q12h) effective against gram-negative and anaerobic bacteria.

Precautions/Interactions

- Cyclosporine and ketoconazole have a wide safety margin.
- Side effects are uncommon at these dosages and most are transient. Most reactions are related to the cyclosporine administration and may include inappetence, vomiting and diarrhea, hypertrichosis, gingival hyperplasia, and lameness.

Alternative Drugs

- Prednisone alone or combined with azathioprine or metronidazole.
- Azathioprine and metronidazole – typically reduce but do not completely resolve the lesions; can be used to reduce the severity of the lesions prior to surgery.

Nursing Care

- Clipping the hair and cleaning the perineum.
- Chemical restraint is usually necessary until the pain and inflammation are controlled.

Diet

Novel protein diets may be beneficial with concurrent colitis, particularly in German shepherds.

Surgical Considerations

- Surgery is considered in cases which fail to respond to immunotherapy, response is incomplete, and when true fistulas or anal sac involvement are identified.
- Bilateral anal sacculectomy should be performed when any other surgical procedure is performed because of the high incidence of secondary involvement of the anal sacs.

- Medical management is often effective in reducing the severity of the lesions, making a less aggressive surgery possible.
- Make an incision in healthy skin beyond the extent of draining tracts. Establish a dissection plane deep to the tracts and work toward the anus. All diseased tissue and fibrous tissue must be removed. The use of electrosurgery or a surgical laser is highly recommended to control bleeding, which may be brisk, and improve visualization as the dissection proceeds.
- Involvement of the anal sphincter is common. Attempt to preserve as much anal sphincter as possible while still removing the affected tissue.
- Thoroughly lavage the wound and suture the wound closed if enough skin is present. Otherwise, allow the wound to heal by second intention.
- Complete anoplasty, excision of the anocutaneous junction with modified rectal pull-through, is often necessary with 360° involvement.
- Fecal incontinence is a common complication of the more radical excision techniques and when multiple surgeries are performed but can often be manageable with dietary modification.

 COMMENTS

A recent open-label study using intralesional injections of human embryonic stem cell-derived mesenchymal stem cells in dogs with lesions refractory to cyclosporine as a model for humans with fistulizing Crohn's disease showed promising results and could lead to the development of novel treatments for dogs with perianal fistula.

Client Education

- Although significant improvement and occasionally complete remission can be achieved, recurrence is common.
- Owners should be committed to life-long therapy, if needed.
- Therapy can be expensive.

Patient Monitoring

- Regular monitoring for recurrence is essential if immunosuppression is discontinued.
- The incidence of recurrence has been estimated at 40–60%.

Possible Complications

- Vomiting, diarrhea, anorexia.
- Weight loss.
- Failure to heal.
- Dehiscence if surgical procedures are performed.
- Tenesmus.
- Anal stricture.
- Fecal incontinence.
- Flatulence.
- Reversible alopecia and gingival hyperplasia with CsA administration.
- Iatrogenic Cushing's disease from corticosteroids.

Expected Course and Prognosis

- Complete cure is uncommon. Most patients require multiple rounds of treatment or life-long maintenance therapy.
- Owner frustration is common due to inability to completely resolve the problem, expense, required home care, and perceived decrease in quality of life in some patients.

Synonyms

- Anal furunculosis
- Perianal sinus
- Perianal hidradenitis

Abbreviations

- CsA = cyclosporine A
- HPLC = high-pressure liquid chromatography
- RIA = radioimmune assay

See Also

- Colitis and Proctitis
- Colonic Neoplasia, Benign
- Colonic Neoplasia, Malignant
- Dyschezia and Tenesmus
- Fungal Enteritides
- Perineal Hernia
- Rectal Stricture

Suggested Reading

Aronson LR. Rectum, anus, perineum. In: Tobias KM, Johnston SA, eds. Veterinary Small Animal Surgery. St Louis: Elsevier Saunders, 2012, pp. 1564–1600.

Ellison GW. Excisional techniques for perianal fistulas. In: Bojrab MJ, Waldron D, Toombs JR, eds. Current Techniques in Small Animal Surgery, 5th ed. Jackson: Teton NewMedia, 2014, pp. 315–317.

Fallipowicz D. Nonsurgical management of perianal fistulae. In: Bojrab MJ, Waldron D, Toombs JR, eds. Current Techniques in Small Animal Surgery, 5th ed. Jackson: Teton NewMedia, 2014, 309–315.

Ferrer L, Kimbrel EA, Lam A, et al. Treatment of perianal fistulas with human embryonic stem cell-derived mesenchymal stem cells: a canine model of human fistulizing Crohn's disease. Regen.Med 2016;11(1):33–43.

Kennedy LJ, O'Neill T, House A, et al. Risk of anal furunculosis in German Shepherd dogs is associated with the major histocompatibility complex. Tissue Antigens 2008;71(1):51–56.

Stanley BJ, Hauptman JG. Long-term prospective evaluation of topically applied 0.1% tacrolimus ointment for treatment of perianal sinuses in dogs. J Am Vet Med Assoc 2009;235:397–404.

Author: Eric R. Pope DVM, MS, DACVS

Chapter 90

Perineal Hernia

DEFINITION/OVERVIEW

- Perineal hernia is a weakening or tearing of the pelvic diaphragm, causing loss of support and abnormal function during defecation. Herniation of pelvic and abdominal viscera can occur with severity and chronicity.
- Pelvic diaphragm weakening is postulated to be caused by hormonal influences in intact male dogs, but may also occur from any condition causing chronic or excessive straining to defecate, or neuropathic weakness in the muscles.
- The levator ani and coccygeus muscles separate from the anal sphincter and rectum to allow lateral bulging of the rectum when the animal strains, causing incoordination in defecation. Separation of the muscles also allows pelvic and abdominal viscera to migrate caudally and enter the pelvic cavity.
- Abdominal organs which most frequently herniate into the pelvic cavity are the prostate and bladder, which can cause ureteral or urethral obstruction, and intestines which can potentially become strangulated.

ETIOLOGY/PATHOPHYSIOLOGY

- Any underlying pathology related to the colon and pelvis may cause excessive straining and lead to perineal hernia.
- Straining leads to weakening of the muscles, which separate and allow the rectum to bulge. Bulging is usually lateral and ventrolateral to the anus.

Systems Affected

The gastrointestinal system is primarily affected.

SIGNALMENT/HISTORY

- Primarily affects older intact male dogs.
- Can occur in cats.
- Can occur in female dogs.

Risk Factors

- Intact status in older male dogs.
- Underlying pathology leading to excessive straining: prostatomegaly in male dogs. Megacolon and malunion of pelvic fractures can predispose to perineal laxity in cats.
- Caudal neuropathy, malformation or injury such as tail traction.

Blackwell's Five-Minute Veterinary Consult Clinical Companion: Small Animal Gastrointestinal Diseases,
First Edition. Edited by Jocelyn Mott and Jo Ann Morrison.
© 2019 John Wiley & Sons, Inc. Published 2019 by John Wiley & Sons, Inc.
Companion website: www.fiveminutevet.com/gastrointestinal

Historical Findings

- Chronic straining to defecate or urinate (can be acute).
- Constipation is the main feature, but diarrhea can be a presenting sign if liquid feces are leaking out past firm impacted stool.
- Visible unilateral or bilateral bulge in the perineal area which is impacted feces or displaced organs. This can be a main feature in cats.

 ## CLINICAL FEATURES

- Perineal palpation reveals bulges between the tailhead and anus. Anus is generally positioned more caudally than usual. Normal anal position is dorsal and slightly cranial to the caudal extent of the tuber ischii. When the perineal diaphragm breaks down, the anus migrates caudally.
- Thorough but gentle rectal examination should confirm fecal accumulation in the dilated rectum and perineal laxity once the feces are removed.
- Carefully evaluate both sides of the perineum since laxity is often present or developing on both sides even if complete hernia is present only on one side.

 ## DIFFERENTIAL DIAGNOSIS

- Prostatomegaly in older intact male dogs.
- Megacolon in cats.
- Malunion of pelvic fractures with pelvic narrowing.
- Caudal neuropathy, malformation, or tail traction injury.
- Perineal neoplasia such as adenoma or adenocarcinoma.
- Sublumbar lymphadenopathy secondary to malignancy (anal sac adenocarcinoma), rectal tumors, perineal or pelvic lipomas, paraprostatic cyst.
- Perineal abscesses (migrating foreign body or anal sac abscess).

 ## DIAGNOSTICS

Complete Blood Count/Biochemistry/Urinalysis

No specific complete blood count or chemistry abnormalities with the exception of postrenal azotemia if urinary obstruction is present.

Imaging

- Abdominal radiographs can confirm constipation/obstipation, prostatomegaly, sublumbar lymphadenopathy, megacolon in cats.
- Pelvic radiographs confirm pelvic fracture malunion, intrapelvic mass, feces bulging in the perineum.
- Abdominal ultrasonography to evaluate the size and consistency of the prostate.
- Perineal ultrasonography to evaluate herniated viscera or masses.

 ## THERAPEUTICS

- Medical therapy with low-residue food and stool softeners may ease but not resolve the condition.
- Lactulose (1 mL/4.5 kg PO q8h to effect) is preferred over high-fiber stool softeners.

- Bladder retroflexion is considered an emergency due to high potential for urinary obstruction or strangulation and devitalization.
  - Urethral catheterization is preferred.
  - Percutaneous perineal cystocentesis may be required to decrease bladder size and facilitate manual rectal repositioning of the bladder to allow urethral catheter placement.
- Intravenous treatment of azotemia (with crystalloid fluid therapy) prior to and during treatment of azotemia and hyperkalemia due to urinary obstruction, if present.
- Definitive therapy for perineal hernia is surgical reconstruction of the pelvic diaphragm.
- Castration of intact male dogs should be performed prior to or concurrently with perineal herniorrhaphy.

Diet

Low-bulk diet is fed to promote soft stool but not diarrhea.

Activity

Activity is restricted while the incisions are healing.

Surgical Considerations

- Under anesthesia, manual fecal evacuation is performed.
- Enemas are avoided due to increased risk of fecal contamination at surgery from liquid feces.
- Purse-string suture is placed in the anus and anal sacs should be expressed.
- Entire perineum is clipped, including tail base and laterally to the greater trochanters of the femur.
- Scrotum and prescrotal area should be prepared for either prescrotal or caudal castration. Surgeon preference determines approach for castration.
- Once in perineal position, perineal incision, either vertical or curvilinear, is made 1–2 cm lateral to the anus extending ventrally past the tuber ischium. Subcutaneous tissues are incised and the hernia sac is exposed. Incision of the sac often allows a small to large amount of clear to serosanguinous fluid to escape.
- Omentum is the most common organ in the hernia and there are frequently areas of saponified fat or organizing hematomas which can be resected as needed. Loose connective tissue is dissected to expose the coccygeal muscles dorsally and laterally, the anal sphincter medially and the internal obturator muscle ventrally on the ischial table.
- Identify and avoid the pudendal nerve and artery as it crosses the dorsal aspect of the internal obturator toward the anus.
- Internal obturator transposition is the most frequently selected technique to close the defect with the least tension (Figure 90.1).
- Internal obturator muscle is elevated and transposed into the defect and secured to the anal sphincter medially and the coccygeal muscles laterally. Interrupted sutures of either absorbable or nonabsorbable suture material can be utilized.
- Site is lavaged and routine closure of subcutaneous tissues and skin performed. Purse-string suture is removed.
- If bladder retroflexion is present, abdominal surgical approach can be made and cystopexy and/or colopexy to the body wall performed. Recurrence rates are not affected by this procedure, but herniorrhaphy may be more easily performed afterwards.
- Some patients have poor perineal muscle development and additional supporting materials may be utilized. Prosthetic mesh, porcine submucosal intestinal or dermal implant, superficial gluteal muscle flap, and semitendinosus muscle transposition can be used in severe cases. Autogenous fascia lata graft has been successfully used also.

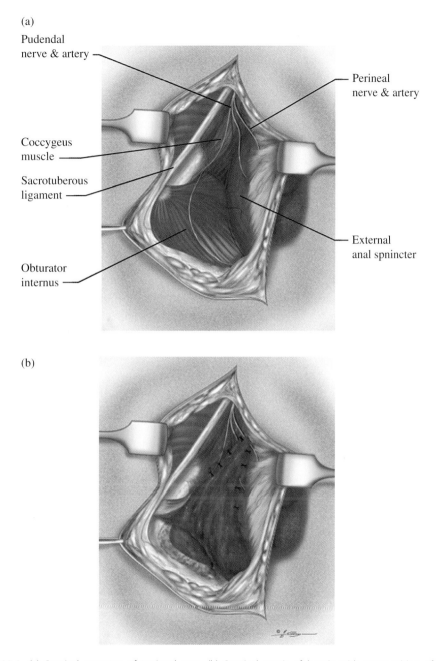

(a)

Pudendal nerve & artery

Perineal nerve & artery

Coccygeus muscle

Sacrotuberous ligament

External anal spnincter

Obturator internus

(b)

■ **Fig. 90.1.** (a) Surgical anatomy of perineal area. (b) Surgical repair of hernia with transposition of internal obturator muscle. Source: Monnet E. Small Animal Soft Tissue Surgery. Hoboken: Wiley-Blackwell, 2013.

- Bilateral perineal herniorrhaphy can be performed in a single anesthetic episode.
- Ice perineal incisions to reduce pain and swelling.
- Elizabethan collars are used postoperatively.
- Fecal softeners can be used if needed but care should be taken to avoid liquid fecal soiling of the incisions.
- Due to the complexity of the surgical technique and risks of iatrogenic damage, referral to a board-certified surgical specialist is recommended.

COMMENTS

- Greatest risk of perineal herniorrhaphy is recurrence of the hernia; the likelihood of this is decreased with internal obturator transposition technique and concurrent castration.
- Additional risk of temporary dysfunction of the anal sphincter due to stretching in cases of large bilateral repairs.
- Fecal/urinary incontinence can occur if excessive dissection is performed around the pudendal nerve or peritoneal reflection.

Patient Monitoring

- The patient should be evaluated thoroughly for the first 48 h following surgery, with particular attention paid to urination and defecation. A rectal examination should be performed at the time of suture removal if feasible.
- Efficacy of the procedure is evaluated by client monitoring of ease and duration of defecation and rectal examination during rechecks.

Prevention/Avoidance

The major factor known to reduce the risk of recurrence following surgery is castration.

Expected Course and Prognosis

- Recovery and function after surgery are good to excellent.
- There is a 10–50% risk of recurrence depending on resolution of underlying conditions and intact status of the dog.

See Also

- Colitis and Proctitis
- Constipation and Obstipation
- Dyschezia and Tenesmus
- Megacolon

Suggested Reading

Bellenger CR, Canfield RB. Perineal hernia. In: Slatter D, Textbook of Small Animal Surgery, 3rd ed. St Louis: Elsevier, 2003, pp. 487–498.

Bongartz A, Carofglio F, Balligand M, et al. Use of autogenous fascia lata graft for perineal herniorrhaphy in dogs. Vet Surg 2005;34(4):405–413.

Grand JG, Bureau S, Monnet E. Effects of urinary bladder retroflexion and surgical technique on postoperative complication rates and long-term outcome in dogs with perineal hernia: 41 cases. J Am Vet Med Assoc 2013;243(10):1442–1447.

Lee AJ, Chung WH, Kim DH, et al. Use of canine small intestinal submucosa allograft for treating perineal hernias in two dogs. J Vet Sci 2012;13(3):327–330.

Morello E, Martano M, Zabarino S, et al. Modified semitendinosus muscle transposition to repair ventral perineal hernia in 14 dogs. J Small Anim Pract 2015;56(6):370–376.

Shaughnessy M, Monnet E. Internal obturator muscle transposition for treatment of perineal hernia in dogs: 34 cases (1998–2012). J Am Vet Med Assoc 2015;246(3):321–326.

Souza C, Mann T. Perineal hernias. In: Monnet E, ed. Small Animal Soft Tissue Surgery. Hoboken: Wiley-Blackwell, 2013, pp. 286–296.

Acknowledgments: The author and editors acknowledge the prior contribution of Dr Geraldine Briony Hunt.

Author: Fiona M. Little VMD, DACVS

Chapter 91

Rectal Stricture

DEFINITION/OVERVIEW

- Diminution in the size of the rectal or anal lumen either from cicatricial contracture or scarring as a result of wound healing or chronic inflammation or from proliferative neoplastic disease.
- Anorectal stricture can also be a component of congenital malformations such as atresia ani.

ETIOLOGY/PATHOPHYSIOLOGY

Systems Affected

Gastrointestinal – interference with the normal passage of feces through the rectum may lead to colonic dilation or megacolon orad to the stricture.

SIGNALMENT/HISTORY

- Dog and cat.
- No age, breed, or gender predilection reported.

Risk Factors

- Inflammatory – rectoanal abscess, anal sacculitis, perianal fistulas, proctitis, foreign body, fungal infection (e.g., histoplasmosis, pythiosis).
- Traumatic – lacerations.
- Neoplastic – rectal adenocarcinoma, leiomyoma, rectal polyps.
- Iatrogenic – rectal anastomosis, rectal mass excision, rectal biopsy. Strictures following rectal resection and anastomosis usually become apparent within weeks after surgery.
- Congenital – atresia ani.

Historical Findings

The most common presenting complaints are tenesmus, hematochezia, diarrhea, and bleeding from the rectum.

CLINICAL FEATURES

- Vary with severity of the lesion.
- Tenesmus.
- Dyschezia.

Blackwell's Five-Minute Veterinary Consult Clinical Companion: Small Animal Gastrointestinal Diseases, First Edition. Edited by Jocelyn Mott and Jo Ann Morrison.
© 2019 John Wiley & Sons, Inc. Published 2019 by John Wiley & Sons, Inc.
Companion website: www.fiveminutevet.com/gastrointestinal

- Constipation.
- Hematochezia.
- Mucoid feces.
- Large bowel diarrhea.
- Secondary megacolon can develop.

DIFFERENTIAL DIAGNOSIS

Space-occupying processes that lead to diminished rectal capacity (extraluminal rectal compression, e.g., prostatic disease, pelvic fractures, intraluminal rectal obstruction, e.g., pseudocoprostasis, foreign body) and functional constriction (rectal muscle spasms).

DIAGNOSTICS

Digital rectal palpation – all strictures were palpable during rectal examination in one study.

Complete Blood Count/Biochemistry/Urinalysis

Often unremarkable.

Imaging

- Survey abdominal radiography may show colonic dilation/megacolon.
- Contrast studies (e.g., barium, air, or double-contrast enema and barium gastrointestinal series) may reveal consistent narrowing of the rectal luminal diameter. A combination of air and barium allows the best visualization of the colonic mucosa and aids in determining the extent of the lesion.
- Abdominal ultrasonography may reveal thickening and altered architecture if infiltrative rectocolonic disease is present (e.g., pythiosis, neoplasia). The sublumbar lymph nodes can also be evaluated for evidence of metastasis in cases with neoplasia.

Other Diagnostic Procedures

- Proctoscopy/colonoscopy may be useful to visualize a stricture, determine the extent of the lesion, and procure a biopsy specimen.
- Colonic scrapings may aid in cytologic diagnosis of fungal (histoplasmosis) and neoplastic diseases.
- Biopsy and evaluate the lesion histopathologically to classify the disease process and establish a prognosis.

Pathologic Findings

The pathologic findings vary with the underlying cause.

THERAPEUTICS

- Resolve the underlying cause before specifically treating the stricture when possible.
- Medical treatment directed at either palliation by use of stool softeners and enemas or the elimination of infective agents or inflammatory conditions.

Drug(s) of Choice

- Stool softeners – docusate sodium (dogs, 50–200 mg PO q8–12 h; cats, 50 mg PO q12–24 h) or docusate calcium (dogs, 50–100 mg PO q12–24 h; cats, 50 mg PO q12–24 h).
- Alternative stool softener – lactulose (1 mL/4.5 kg PO q8h to effect).

- Intralesional injection of corticosteroids such as triamcinolone in conjunction with balloon dilation of the stricture may improve outcome and reduce the likelihood of recurrence. Injection can be repeated one time if additional dilations are necessary.
- Corticosteroids – can use prednisolone to treat noninfectious inflammatory conditions (0.5–1 mg/kg PO q24h or divided q12h).
- Chemotherapy may be indicated for various neoplasms.
- Antifungal therapy if fungal infection present.
- Appropriate perioperative antimicrobial therapy with a broad spectrum of activity against anaerobes and coliforms (e.g., cefoxitin sodium 30 mg/kg IV) in conjunction with balloon dilation or surgical therapy.
- Antibiotics can be administered after dilation if mucosal tearing occurs (e.g., amoxicillin/clavulanic acid [13.75 mg/kg PO q12h] or metronidazole [10–15 mg/kg PO q12h]).

Precautions/Interactions

- Appropriate precautions must be followed when using chemotherapeutic drugs.
- Corticosteroids when infection is possible.
- Corticosteroids may adversely affect healing after surgical correction of the stricture.

Diet

- High-fiber bulk-forming diets or addition of fiber additives such as pumpkin pie filling (1–5 tsp daily) or commercial sources of psyllium (1–5 tsp daily) to the regular diet.
- Dietary therapy may be effective in cases with minor stenotic lesions.

Activity

Provide daily exercise and frequent opportunities to defecate.

Surgical Considerations

- Balloon dilation is very successful, especially in the management of strictures resulting from mechanical trauma such as foreign bodies, lacerations, and those following surgery.
- Balloon dilation of nonneoplastic and postoperative strictures – more than one procedure may be needed based on patient response.
- Balloon dilation is performed under general anesthesia by inflating progressively larger cylindrical balloons under direct endoscopic guidance and visualization.
- Guidelines for the amount of dilation typically needed are as follows.
  - Dogs <15 kg – dilate to 18–20 mm diameter.
  - Dogs 15–30 kg – dilate to 20 25 mm diameter.
  - Dogs >30 kg – dilate to 30–35 mm diameter.
- Repeat at 2–3-week intervals if clinical signs persist and a stricture is palpable.
- Triamcinolone (10 mg/mL) 0.5–1.0 mL injected submucosally divided between four equally spaced locations or oral prednisolone administered postoperatively may help prevent recurrence.
- Mitomycin C – topical mitomycin has been used with success following balloon dilation of esophageal strictures to inhibit recurrence.
  - Follow routine precautions for handling and use of chemotherapeutic drugs.
  - Reconstitute 5 mg of mitomycin in 10 mL of sterile water.
  - Soak a gauze sponge in the solution and then apply the sponge to the area of stricture.
  - Leave the sponge in place for five minutes and then remove.
  - Flush the area thoroughly with sterile water and suction/aspirate the fluid from the area.

Surgical Reconstruction

Focal (narrow) strictures (Figure 91.1), e.g., postoperative complication or those associated with foreign bodies or trauma, and may be amenable to reconstruction using plasty procedures similar to the Heineke–Mikulicz pyloroplasty for pyloric outflow obstruction. This technique can also be used for strictures involving just the anal ring.

- Expose the stricture either transanally (preferred and possible in most cases) or by dorsal approach to the rectum.
- Place atraumatic forceps (e.g., Babcock forceps) or stay sutures to expose the stricture (Figure 91.2).
- Beginning at the 6 o'clock location, place two stay sutures through the stricture, leaving just enough space to be able to incise between them.
- Incise through the stricture longitudinally (cranial to caudal) as deeply as needed to divide the stricture.
- Place lateral tension on the stay sutures to reorient the incision from longitudinal to transverse (Figure 91.3).
- Suture the incisions with 3/0–4/0 synthetic absorbable suture material (Figure 91.4).
- Reassess the stricture by digital palpation. If necessary, repeat the same procedure at 12 o'clock and then 3 and 9 o'clock until all narrowing is relieved.
- Consider applying topical mitomycin as described above to inhibit stricture reformation.
- More extensive strictures such as those associated with infiltrative and neoplastic diseases may require resection and anastomosis using either the rectal pull-through procedure (Figures 91.5 and 91.6) or dorsal approach to the rectum. Consult surgery textbooks for details on these procedures.
- Extensive resection may result in fecal incontinence and postoperative strictures may occur.
- Placement of a colorectal stent may be successful in relieving obstructions due to nonresectable neoplasms and potentially for nonneoplastic lesions but large studies evaluating effectiveness have not been reported.

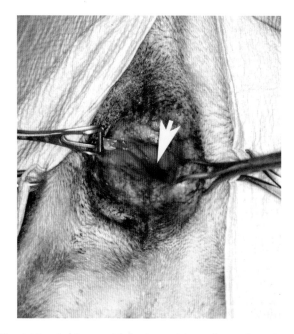

■ **Fig. 91.1.** Postoperative stricture (*white arrow*) following rectal resection and anastomosis.

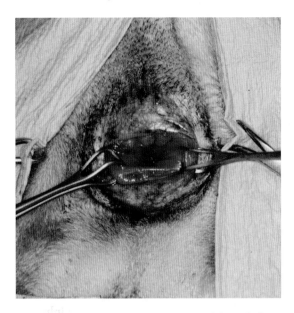

■ **Fig. 91.2.** The ventral portion of the rectal stricture has been everted through the anus with the aid of Babcock forceps.

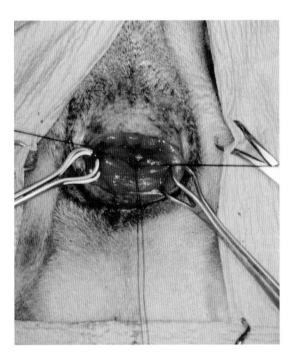

■ **Fig. 91.3.** After placing stay sutures at the midpoint of the stricture, the stricture was incised longitudinally until the lateral traction on the stay sutures confirmed complete transection of the restricting band.

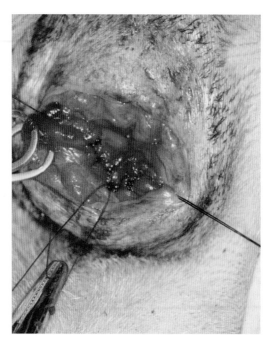

■ **Fig. 91.4.** The incision was closed transversely with interrupted sutures. The stay sutures were removed and rectal palpation was performed to evaluate the stricture. In this case, one additional incision dorsally closed similarly was sufficient to relieve the stricture.

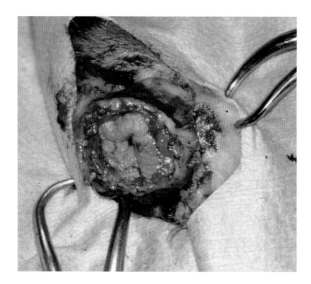

■ **Fig. 91.5.** Congenital anorectal stricture in a cat. Resection of the anal ring and distal rectum by rectal pull-through was necessary to relieve the stricture.

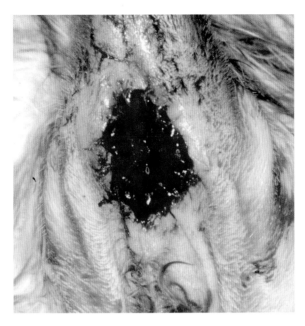

■ **Fig. 91.6.** Completed rectoanal anastomosis. Fecal incontinence is a common complication of these pull-through procedures.

  COMMENTS

The outcomes for strictures secondary to neoplasia and inflammatory/infiltrative disease depend on the ability to treat the underlying disease. The management of malignant neoplastic disease can be quite challenging due to incidence of recurrence and morbidities associated with extensive surgical procedures.

Client Education

- Outcomes are influenced by the underlying cause and ability to effectively manage it.
- Clinical signs may not completely resolve.
- More than one treatment may be needed.
- Long-term dietary modification may be needed.
- Recurrence may be seen.

Patient Monitoring

Reexamination after balloon dilation or surgical management to detect recurrence of the stenosis.

Possible Complications

- Medical treatment – can include inefficacy, diarrhea, and adverse effects of medications.
- Balloon dilation can result in deep rectal tears, hemorrhage, or possibly full-thickness perforation.
- Surgical treatment – fecal incontinence, secondary stricture formation, and wound dehiscence.

Expected Course and Prognosis

- Varies with the severity of the stricture.
- Patients with benign strictures that are readily managed medically or with balloon dilation may have a good long-term outcome.
- Surgical resection has a more guarded prognosis because of the frequency of complications.
- Most patients with recognizable clinical signs due to neoplasia have a guarded to poor prognosis for complete resolution.

See Also

- Colitis and Proctitis
- Constipation and Obstipation
- Dyschezia and Hematochezia
- Fungal Enteritides
- Perianal Fistula
- Pythiosis
- Rectoanal Polyps

Suggested Reading

Culp WT, Macphail CM, Perry JA, Jensen TD. Use of a nitinol stent to palliate a colorectal neoplastic obstruction in a dog. J Am Vet Med Assoc 2011;239:222–227.

Webb CB, McCord KW, Twedt DC. Rectal strictures in 19 dogs: 1197–2005. J Am Anim Hosp Assoc 2007;43:332–336.

Author: Eric R. Pope DVM, MS, DACVS

Rectoanal Polyps

DEFINITION/OVERVIEW

- Most rectoanal polyps are benign growths located in the distal rectum.
- Histopathologic evaluation typically reveals hyperplasia or adenomas, but lesions may undergo malignant transformation.

ETIOLOGY/PATHOPHYSIOLOGY

- The etiology is unknown. Clinical signs are primarily related to the presence of a mass or masses in the rectum/anal canal that result in tenesmus. The masses are often friable and result in bleeding from the rectum or the presence of bright red blood on the feces.
- Malignant transformation is possible.

Systems Affected

Gastrointestinal – rectoanal polyps are benign masses and effects are local.

SIGNALMENT/HISTORY

- Dog and rarely cat.
- A breed predilection has not been proven but German shepherds, collies, and West Highland white terriers are commonly affected breeds in some studies.
- No sex predilection.

Risk Factors

None known.

Historical Findings

- May be an incidental finding on wellness exam.
- Owners notice blood on the stool and/or straining to defecate and/or painful defecation.
- Occasionally the mass is seen everted through the anus after defecation.

CLINICAL FEATURES

- Hematochezia with relatively well-formed feces.
- Tenesmus.
- Dyschezia.

Blackwell's Five-Minute Veterinary Consult Clinical Companion: Small Animal Gastrointestinal Diseases,
First Edition. Edited by Jocelyn Mott and Jo Ann Morrison.
© 2019 John Wiley & Sons, Inc. Published 2019 by John Wiley & Sons, Inc.
Companion website: www.fiveminutevet.com/gastrointestinal

- Mucus-covered feces.
- Pencil-thin or ribbon-like feces.
- Soft, well-vascularized, friable, and often ulcerated mass(es) may be seen or palpated rectally.
- Usually single but multiple polyps can occur. A single mass was seen in 93% of dogs in one study.

DIFFERENTIAL DIAGNOSIS

- Carcinoma *in situ* and adenocarcinoma.
- Other neoplasias – leiomyoma, fibroma, lymphoma, papilloma.
- Inflammatory polyps.
    - Inflammatory polyps have primarily been reported in miniature dachshunds in Japan.
    - The lesions are typically small round white polyps diffusely spread throughout the rectum and descending colon.
    - Immunosuppressive therapy with prednisolone (1.6 mg/kg/day, range 0.6–3.8 mg/kg/day), and cyclosporine (4.7 mg/kg/day, range 2.3–8.4 mg/kg/day) was effective in 80% of cases. Prednisolone dose tapered at 2–4-week intervals to lowest maintaining response with or without cyclosporine. Refractory cases responded to leflunomide (5 mg/kg/day) but was associated with more adverse effects.
- Proctitis.
- Pythiosis.

DIAGNOSTICS

- Rectal palpation – over 50% of colorectal masses are diagnosed on palpation.
- Direct visualization through anus.

Complete Blood Count/Biochemistry/Urinalysis

Often unremarkable.

Other Diagnostic Procedures

- Proctoscopy – viable low-cost procedure that allows one to visualize the descending colon after cleansing the animal's colon. This method is suitable in most dogs and cats because the polyps are usually localized to the rectoanal or colorectal region and tend not to metastasize.
- Colonoscopy – often recommended to evaluate the entire rectum and colon for additional polyps but lesions orad to the rectum were not found in one study reviewing 82 dogs with rectal masses.
- Cytologic examination of polyp aspirate or scraping may help the initial diagnosis, although cytology should be interpreted with caution given the inherent challenges of differentiating benign adenomas from adenocarcinomas cytologically.
- Histopathologic examination of excised tissue is required for definitive diagnosis and to assess completeness of the excision.

Pathologic Findings

- May be pedunculated or broad-based sessile masses.
- Adenomatous polyps are typically friable and bleed easily.
- Annular and diffuse lesions (involving 50% of rectal circumference) are more likely to be invasive carcinomas rather than benign polyps.

- Histopathologic assessment of excised masses should be performed regardless of whether preoperative cytology or endoscopic biopsies were done because in one study endoscopic biopsies underestimated the severity of the lesion in 30% of cases. This is probably related to the fact that endoscopic biopsies are typically small and superficial.
- Histologically, adenomatous polyps appear as well-differentiated proliferative masses composed of branching glands and papillary projections that are confined to the mucosa.
- Carcinoma *in situ* is diagnosed when there are foci of dysplasia (i.e., greater cellular atypia indicative of malignancy) but the lesions are still confined to the mucosa.
- Lesions invading through the mucosal basement membrane into the submucosa are classified as invasive carcinoma.
- Malignant transformation of benign lesions is possible.

 ## THERAPEUTICS

Most polyps are readily exteriorized through the rectum and can be excised with minimal risk of complications.

Drug(s) of Choice

- Appropriate perioperative antibiotics are recommended (e.g., cefoxitin sodium 30 mg/kg IV).
- Stool softeners may help decrease tenesmus – docusate sodium (dogs, 50–200 mg PO q8–12h; cats, 50 mg PO q12–24h) or docusate calcium (dogs, 50–100 mg PO q12–24h; cats, 50 mg PO q12–24h).
- Alternative stool softener – lactulose (1 mL/4.5 kg PO q8h to effect).

Alternative Drugs

- One study in dogs showed significant improvement in clinical signs following administration of piroxicam (20 mg suppositories [adjust size of suppository to approximate oral dose of 0.3 mg/kg placed every 2–3 days] or dose should be 0.34 mg/kg q48h), but long-term follow-up is not available.
- There is evidence in humans that aspirin and NSAIDs inhibit the development of benign and malignant colorectal neoplasia, although the exact mechanism of action, dosage, and duration of administration have not been clearly defined.

Diet

High-fiber bulk-forming diets or fiber additives such as pumpkin pie filling (1–5 tsp daily) or commercial sources of psyllium (1–5 tsp daily).

Activity

Provide daily exercise and frequent opportunities to defecate.

Surgical Considerations

- Surgical excision is the treatment of choice.
- Pedunculated polyps.
  - Most pedunculated polyps can be exteriorized directly through the anus and removed with mucosal resection at the base (Figure 92.1).
  - There are numerous methods of removing the mass, including tonsil snares +/– electrosurgery, electrosurgery alone, simple ligation of the pedicle, sharp excision followed by suturing of the defect, and cryosurgery (Figure 92.2).

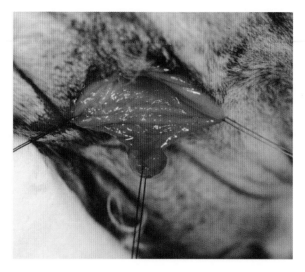

■ **Fig. 92.1.** Discrete polyp exteriorized through the anus with the aid of stay sutures.

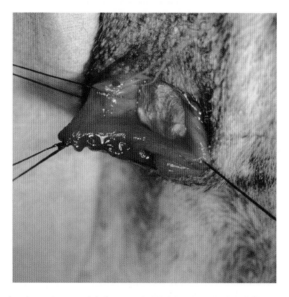

■ **Fig. 92.2.** Polyp excised at base. Mucosal defects such as this can be sutured with simple continuous or interrupted sutures.

■ Sessile polyps.
  • Sessile polyps that are mobile and where the cranial extent of the lesion can be reached by rectal palpation can usually be removed by everting the rectal mucosa though the anus by the use of stay sutures (Figure 92.3).
  • Epidural anesthesia relaxes the anal sphincter, facilitating eversion of the rectal mucosa through the anus.
  • Place stay sutures (e.g., 2/0–3/0 nylon) cranial to the lesion and then slowly evert the mucosa through the anus by placing caudal traction on the stay sutures.

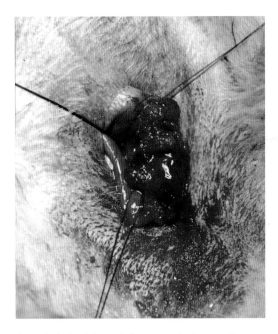

■ **Fig. 92.3.** Larger sessile polyp exteriorized through the anus prior to resection.

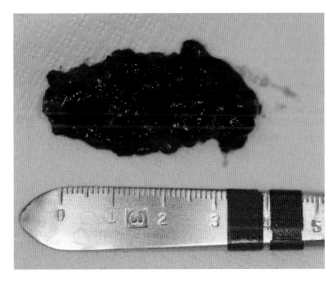

■ **Fig. 92.4.** Complete excision of the mass in Figure 92.3 was performed with 0.5 cm margins.

- Excise the mass(es) with scissors (e.g., Metzenbaum), electrosurgery, or surgical laser (Figure 92.4).
- Suture the mucosal defect with interrupted or simple continuous sutures using 3/0–4/0 synthetic absorbable suture material.

■ Lesions that cannot be exteriorized may be removable transanally by electrosurgery with endoscopic guidance or can be directly exposed through a dorsal rectal approach.

COMMENTS

Complete excision of pedunculated and focal masses is curative. Recurrence is common in dogs with multiple or diffuse masses and with malignant masses (Figure 92.5).

Client Education

- Clinical signs usually resolve within a few days.
- Patients with persistent clinical signs should be examined for complications.

Patient Monitoring

- Observe for excessive or persistent tenesmus postoperatively which could lead to rectal prolapse.
- Examine the excision site 14 days after surgery and again at three and six months to ensure absence of recurrence or stricture.
- Twice-yearly examination thereafter to assess for recurrence.

Possible Complications

- Recurrence.
- Rectal stricture (rare).
- Fecal incontinence with more extensive resections, e.g., rectal pull-through.

Expected Course and Prognosis

- Recovery following polypectomy is usually uneventful with resolution of clinical signs within a few days.
- Dogs with focal single adenomas have a good prognosis with a low rate of recurrence.
- Dogs with multiple and/or diffuse lesions (involvement of >50% of circumference of rectal wall) have much higher rates of recurrence.
- Malignant transformation of benign lesions can occur.

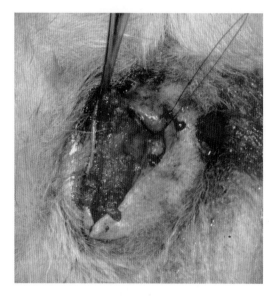

■ **Fig. 92.5.** Diffuse polyp(s) involving more than 50% of the circumference of the rectal wall are more frequently malignant. Invasive carcinoma was diagnosed in this case.

Synonyms

- Adenomatous polyp
- Adenomatous hyperplasia

Abbreviations

- NSAID = nonsteroidal antiinflammatory drug

See Also

- Colitis and Proctitis
- Colonic Neoplasia, Benign
- Colonic Neoplasia, Malignant
- Dyschezia and Hematochezia
- Fungal Enteritides
- Perineal Hernia
- Rectal and Anal Prolapse
- Rectal Stricture

Suggested Reading

Adamovich-Rippe KN, Mayhew PD, Marks SL, et al. Colonoscopic and histologic features of rectal masses in dogs: 82 cases (1995–2012). J Am Vet Med Assoc 2017;250:424–430.

Aronson LR. Rectum, anus, perineum. In: Tobias KM, Johnston SA, eds. Veterinary Small Animal Surgery. St Louis: Elsevier Saunders, 2012, pp. 1564–1600.

Ohmi A, Tsukamoto A, Ohno K, et al. A retrospective study of inflammatory colorectal polyps in miniature dachshunds. J Vet.Med Sci 2012;74(1):59–64.

Valerius KD, Powers BE, McPherron MA, et al. Adenomatous polyps and carcinoma in situ of the canine colon and rectum – 34 cases (1982–1994). J Am Anim Hosp Assoc 1997;33:156–160.

Author: Eric R. Pope DVM, MS, DACVS

DEFINITION/OVERVIEW

- *Tritrichomonas foetus* is a parasite of the bovine reproductive tract and the feline digestive tract.
- There is a proposal to rename the cat-adapted parasite as *T. blagburni*, but this is currently not accepted by many parasitologists.
- *Tritrichomonas* is a cause of large bowel diarrhea in cats.
- Nonpathogenic trichomonads inhabit the gastrointestinal tract of many vertebrates such as reptiles. *Pentatrichomonas* inhabits the intestines of cats, dogs, and other mammals, and is not thought to be pathogenic.

ETIOLOGY/PATHOPHYSIOLOGY

- *T. foetus* is transmitted by a fecal–oral route.
- There is no environmentally resistant cyst; pear-shaped trophozoites are the only life cycle stage.
- Contaminated food and water may play a role in transmission. The organism also apparently survives within slugs which could possibly facilitate transmission.
- Trophozoites bind receptors on epithelial cells of the large intestine.

Systems Affected

Gastrointestinal.

SIGNALMENT/HISTORY

- Clinical signs are thought to occur in young cats although cats of any age may be affected.
- Ongoing problems occur more frequently in shelters and particularly in catteries.
- Pure-bred cats appear to be at increased risk.
- Coinfection with other parasites (*Giardia, Cryptosporidium, Cystoisospora, Toxoplasma*) occurs.

Risk Factors

- *T. blagburni* – high prevalence in catteries and show cats, but very low in feral or indoor cats.
- Pathogenic factors leading to infected cats developing diarrhea – endogenous bacterial flora, adherence of parasite to host epithelium, and cytotoxin and enzyme elaboration.

Blackwell's Five-Minute Veterinary Consult Clinical Companion: Small Animal Gastrointestinal Diseases, First Edition. Edited by Jocelyn Mott and Jo Ann Morrison.
© 2019 John Wiley & Sons, Inc. Published 2019 by John Wiley & Sons, Inc.
Companion website: www.fiveminutevet.com/gastrointestinal

Historical Findings

- Intermittent large bowel diarrhea.
- Diarrhea occasionally contains blood and mucus.
- May be accompanied by pyrexia, flatulence, hematochezia, and vomiting.
- Stools are soft and malodorous; the feces are semi-formed.
- Diarrhea – improves with antibiotic treatment but reoccurs when treatment stops.
- Median length of time of diarrhea is about nine months, with resolution in most cats by two years.
- Persistence of infection after the resolution of diarrhea is common.

 # CLINICAL FEATURES

- Anus – may become edematous, erythematous, and painful in kittens.
- Rectal prolapse – if anal irritation becomes severe.

 # DIFFERENTIAL DIAGNOSIS

- Other infectious and noninfectious causes of small bowel diarrhea, maldigestion, and malabsorption syndromes, especially pancreatic exocrine insufficiency, inflammatory bowel disease.
- In cats, differentiate from infection with *Giardia*. Coinfections with both parasites are known to occur.

 # DIAGNOSTICS

Complete Blood Count/Biochemistry/Urinalysis

Usually normal – may reflect diarrhea.

Other Laboratory Tests

- Only trophozoite stages are present.
- Trophozoites may be found in saline wet mounts of feces but the sensitivity of this method is low.
    - Method – dilute fresh feces 50:50 in saline, cover slip, examine at 40× objective with condenser lowered to increase contrast.
    - Distinguish from *Giardia* (concave ventral disk, spiral forward motion) – *T. blagburni* has jerky forward motion, spindle-shaped, undulating membranes.
    - *T. blagburni* trophozoites – are not seen on fecal flotation.
    - *T. blagburni* trophozoites – will not survive refrigeration.
- Fecal protozoal culture – use commercial media in a 37 °C incubator (In Pouch™ TF, Biomed Diagnostics, San Jose, CA).
    - Method – inoculate with 0.05 g of fresh feces, examine for motile trophozoites daily for 12 days.
    - *Giardia* and *P. hominis* – do not grow after 24 hours in In Pouch culture system.
    - Feces can be used to inoculate commercial growth medium that can be subsequently assessed by microscopy or polymerase chain reaction (PCR). PCR more sensitive than fecal culture in cats.
    - Antigen detection tests for *Giardia* can be used to help differentiate the two parasites.
- Flotation solutions lyse trophozoites.

THERAPEUTICS

- Essential to rule out coexisting disease (cryptosporidiosis, giardiasis, bacterial), especially if diarrhea persists after specific treatment.
- Treatment may decrease the severity of diarrhea but may also prolong time to resolution of diarrhea.

Drug(s) of Choice

- Metronidazole (50 mg/kg for 5–10 days) has been used; this regimen does not always reliably clear the infection.
- Ronidazole (30 mg/kg q24h for 14 days) is recommended, but some cats experience neurotoxic (ataxia, tremors, hyperesthesia) signs associated with this treatment.

Precautions/Interactions

- Glucocorticoids may exacerbate clinical disease.
- High doses of metronidazole (usually >30 mg/kg) for extended periods may cause neurologic signs.

Diet

Alterations in diet may improve clinical signs.

COMMENTS

Client Education

- Relapses of diarrhea are common and often precipitated by dietary changes, stress of travel, and treatments of other conditions.
- Possible zoonotic transmission should be discussed with owner.
- Limit contact of infected cats with uninfected individuals.

Patient Monitoring

Most cats spontaneously resolve their diarrhea but this may take years (range: 4 months–2 years).

Abbreviations

- GI = gastrointestinal
- PCR = polymerase chain reaction

See Also

- Diarrhea, Chronic – Canine/Feline
- Giardiasis
- Hematochezia
- Parasites, Gastrointestinal
- Rectal and Anal Prolapse
- Nutritional Approach to Chronic Enteropathies

Suggested Reading

Bowman DD. Georgis' Parasitology for Veterinarians, 9th ed. St Louis: Saunders Elsevier Science, 2009, pp. 89–91.
Yao C, Koster LS. Tritrichomonas foetus infections, a cause of chronic diarrhea in the domestic cat. Vet Res 2015;46:35.

Authors: Jeba Jesudoss Chelladurai BVSc & AH, MS, DACVM, Matt T. Brewer DVM, PhD, DACVM

Diseases of the Pancreas

Chapter 94

Nutritional Approach to Exocrine Pancreas Disease

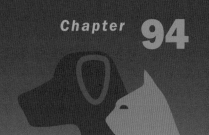

The pancreas is a vital organ that has both endocrine and exocrine functions. This chapter will focus on the nutritional management of disorders affecting the exocrine pancreas.

The exocrine pancreas is responsible for the production and secretion of enzymes that digest protein, fat, and carbohydrates and break them down into simpler, absorbable forms. The pancreas also secretes other substances important for digestion and gut health, including bicarbonate, intrinsic factor, and bacteriostatic substances. When a disease process affects the function of the pancreas, either inflammatory (pancreatitis) or atrophy of functional cells (exocrine pancreatic insufficiency, EPI), important dietary considerations must be taken into account in the management of these conditions. Animals with disorders of the exocrine pancreas often are malnourished and underweight and therefore need to be on a highly digestible, energy-dense diet in order to achieve ideal body condition.

EXOCRINE PANCREATIC INSUFFICIENCY

Exocrine pancreatic insufficiency is the most common cause of maldigestion in dogs and refers to either a partial or complete deficiency of pancreatic enzymes. This condition of the pancreas can be either primary or secondary, with the primary form being more common in dogs and the secondary more common in cats. Primary EPI is a disease process in which there is selective atrophy of the pancreatic acinar cells, which are responsible for the production and storage of digestive enzymes. Clinical signs do not typically develop until 85–90% of functional exocrine tissue is lost, therefore animals are usually 6–18 months old when diagnosed. There is a genetic basis to EPI in dogs and the majority of cases are diagnosed in German shepherd dogs and rough collies.

The secondary form of EPI arises as a result of severe inflammation and fibrosis of the pancreas as a consequence of end-stage chronic pancreatitis. As with the primary form, clinical signs of EPI will not develop until there is almost a 90% loss of functional exocrine pancreatic tissue. This condition can also occur as a consequence of pancreatic adenocarcinoma or cholecystoduodenostomy.

Severe nutrient malassimilation may occur in animals with this condition. Due to the deficiency in pancreatic enzymes, intraluminal digestion is impaired, leading to the inability to effectively use nutrients, weight loss, malnutrition, and failure to thrive. Animals with this condition produce voluminous, loose and foul-smelling stools. Diarrhea and steatorrhea are common. Animals often have a voracious appetite but excessive weight loss is seen which might lead to emaciation. The pancreas is also responsible for the production and release of secretory products including bicarbonate, gastrointestinal (GI) trophic factors, antimicrobial factors, and intrinsic factor. The deficiency of these products in animals with EPI contributes to impaired GI function and nutrient malassimilation. Small intestinal bacterial overgrowth (SIBO) is also commonly seen in dogs with EPI due to the lack of antimicrobial factors found in pancreatic secretions as well as impaired immunity secondary to malnutrition.

Blackwell's Five-Minute Veterinary Consult Clinical Companion: Small Animal Gastrointestinal Diseases, First Edition. Edited by Jocelyn Mott and Jo Ann Morrison.
© 2019 John Wiley & Sons, Inc. Published 2019 by John Wiley & Sons, Inc.
Companion website: www.fiveminutevet.com/gastrointestinal

TABLE 94.1. Recommended components for nutritional support in exocrine pancreatic insufficiency.

Key nutritional factor	Requirement	Cats (DM basis)	Dogs (DM basis)
Energy density	High	>4200 kcal/kg	>4000 kcal/kg
Protein*	Highly digestible	>87% digestibility	>87% digestibility
	Moderate	30–40%	15–30%
	to high	>40%	>30%
Carbohydrates	Highly digestible	<90% digestibility	<90% digestibility
Fat	Low to moderate	15–25%	10–15%
Crude fiber	Low	<5%	<5%

*Moderate protein is generally recommended, except for emaciated patients which require high protein.
DM, dry matter.

Main Considerations

The main nutritional goals for management of EPI are to provide sufficient energy for healthy body condition, provide nutrients to avoid deficiencies, and minimize steatorrhea (Table 94.1). Choosing a veterinary therapeutic diet that is highly digestible is of utmost importance. This should be coupled with addition of pancreatic enzyme preparations to the food and micronutrient supplementation as required. Veterinary products for enzyme supplementation come in powdered or uncoated tablet formulations and enzyme activity of the different products varies. Powdered enzyme preparations are the most common form of supplementation used and should be fed at a dose of 1 tsp per 10 kg body weight, with the minimum being 1 tsp per meal. The dose can be adjusted based on response of the animal. The enzyme powder must be mixed in with the food directly before feeding.

Although feeding raw pancreas has been done in the past, this is not the best choice. It poses the same risk as feeding other raw meat, including the possibility of bacterial contamination and the potential for spread of zoonotic disease. Other risks include lack of availability as well as storage and handling difficulties.

Protein

Animals with EPI have impaired protein digestion and absorption and therefore require a highly digestible protein source in their diet. The recommended protein digestibility is >87% and the protein source should contain all essential amino acids in their correct proportions. A moderate to high protein diet with protein level >30% for cats and 15–30% for dogs, and even higher if the animal is emaciated, is recommended for weight gain (including muscle) that is needed for these emaciated patients. Protein hydrolyzate-based diets may have some use in the management of EPI because they are highly digestible and contain protein that has been predigested.

Carbohydrates

A diet with a highly digestible (>90%) carbohydrate source is beneficial for animals with EPI due to their impaired ability to digest and assimilate nutrients.

Fat

Traditionally, restriction of dietary fat has been recommended in the management of EPI. In a more recent canine model, dogs with EPI were fed a high-fat diet. As these dogs absorbed protein, fat, and carbohydrates more efficiently than when fed a lower fat diet, this study failed to demonstrate a benefit to severe fat restriction (Biourge and Fontaine 2004). These dogs absorbed protein, fat, and carbohydrates more efficiently than when fed a lower fat diet. This could be due to newer pancreatic enzymes, especially lipase, having better preservation. Most animals when initially diagnosed with EPI have poor body condition. A higher fat diet, if tolerated by the animal, could also help the animal to achieve ideal body condition at a quicker rate. A higher fat content increases the energy density of the diet which is important for animals with EPI that have an increased caloric demand. When feeding a high-energy density (high-fat) diet, smaller volumes of food can be fed to achieve the same energy requirement. Other benefits of a higher fat diet include absorption of fat-soluble vitamins as well as increased palatability of the diet. Feeding highly digestible foods with the use of pancreatic enzyme supplementation is more effective than decreasing the fat content of the current diet.

Overall, significant individual variation has been observed when it comes to the tolerability of fat levels in the diet and a period of trial and error may be required to determine which diet is best for each individual. General guidelines are to start with a moderate dietary fat content for animals with EPI: 10–15% for dogs and 15–25% for cats.

Medium chain triglycerides (MCT) are more water soluble and are digested and absorbed by mechanisms independent of those used for long chain triglycerides. Therefore, the addition of MCT to the food can increase total fat assimilation. However, MCT supplements generally decrease palatability and therefore food intake, which becomes counterproductive. This is not the case with currently available veterinary GI diets that contain a source of MCT, such as coconut oil.

Fiber

Low-fiber diets should be selected for animals with EPI in order to maximize food digestibility and energy density. Crude fiber content should be 5% or less on a dry matter basis.

Additional Nutritional Considerations

Nutrients/Vitamins/Trace Elements

Animals with EPI have decreased absorption of the fat-soluble vitamins A, D, E, and K due to lack of the pancreatic enzyme lipase. Vitamins A and D can be supplemented via intramuscular injections (0.5–1 mL divided into two intramuscular sites every three months) to patients that have demonstrated low levels and in patients that are emaciated. If serum concentrations of vitamin E are low, or again if the patient is emaciated, then supplementation may be beneficial (400–500 IU PO q24h). Vitamin K1 supplementation (5–20 mg PO q12h) is recommended in animals with EPI if coagulopathies are detected.

Low serum concentrations of cobalamin (vitamin B12) are frequently documented due to deficiency of intrinsic factor which is responsible for binding cobalamin to allow for absorption in the ileum (Batchelor et al. 2007). Small intestinal bacterial overgrowth also plays a role in cobalamin deficiency because there is consumption of vitamin B12 by microflora in the GI tract. Parenteral administration of cyanocobalamin weekly for six weeks and then a final dose after 30 days is recommended for animals with low serum cobalamin. Serum level should be rechecked after 30 days and further supplementation is indicated if serum levels remain subnormal. Oral supplementation of cobalamin has also been used and is just as effective as the parenteral route. Oral dosing is once per day for three months and should be discontinued for a total of one week before rechecking serum levels (Table 94.2). Pancreatic enzyme supplementation does not improve cobalamin absorption. Serum folate can either be increased or decreased in animals with EPI. In most dogs, it is increased due to SIBO and bacterial elaboration of folate. If, however, serum folate is low, it should be supplemented parenterally (0.5–1 mg PO q24 h).

TABLE 94.2. Doses of cobalamin.

Dogs							
Weight	<10 lbs	10–20 lbs	20–40 lbs	40–60 lbs	60–80 lbs	80–100 lbs	>100 lbs
Parenteral – daily for 6 weeks+one final dose after 30 days							
Dose	250 µg	400 µg	600 µg	800 µg	1000 µg	1200 µg	1500 µg
Oral – daily for 3 months							
Dose	250 µg		500 µg	1000 µg			
Cats							
250 µg orally once daily for 3 months or parenterally weekly for 6 weeks plus one final dose after 30 days							

Feeding Recommendations

Assess the food the animal is currently being fed and compare digestibility and nutrient levels to the recommended levels as described above. If nutritional factors in the current food do not match the recommended levels, changing to a more appropriate food is indicated. Feeding a highly digestible, moderate-fat, low-fiber veterinary therapeutic diet can eventually allow a decrease in the amount of pancreatic enzyme supplementation required.

Animals with EPI are polyphagic when first diagnosed but are unable to absorb the nutrients they ingest, so despite eating large volumes of food they are underweight. They will require a higher daily energy intake to meet their requirements and initially, we support their increased appetite and give them as much as they need. To determine how much to offer initially, calculate current energy intake. If the animal is underweight, increase calories fed by 10%. Monitor the animal closely and if it is still losing weight at the time of follow-up, increase again by 10%. Continue to increase total caloric intake by 10% increments until body weight is stabilized. Animals with EPI benefit from having their total caloric intake split into multiple small meals per day (at least 2–3 times daily) along with pancreatic enzyme supplementation. Once pancreatic enzymes have been added and the right dose is found, digestion processes will improve and therefore energy needs will go down. Some animals, however, may require higher amounts of food even after ideal body condition is achieved due to persistent malabsorption even with the addition of pancreatic enzymes.

Key Points

- Lifelong enzyme replacement therapy.
- Feed a highly digestible diet.
- Moderate dietary fat levels.
- Assess individual needs for vitamin supplementation as needed.
- Variation seen with response to treatment – expect to make adjustments as needed based on individual response and clinical signs.

ACUTE AND CHRONIC PANCREATITIS

Pancreatitis is a condition affecting both dogs and cats and can be classified as acute, recurrent acute, or chronic. The pancreas is responsible for the synthesis and secretion of enzymes essential for the digestion of nutrients. In a normal healthy environment, mechanisms are in place to prevent activation of these enzymes until they reach the intestinal lumen. Pancreatitis occurs when there is premature activation of the enzymes within the acinar cells of the pancreas, resulting in autodigestion. In the acute situation, there is sudden inflammation of the pancreatic acinar tissue. This usually resolves with no lesions of necrosis or atrophy of the acinar cells; however, severe cases can lead to rapid tissue necrosis and death. The chronic form of pancreatitis is a constant low-grade inflammatory condition that leads to permanent damage of pancreatic tissue and therefore can result in decreased exocrine function of the pancreas.

Animals with pancreatitis usually present with vomiting, abdominal pain, diarrhea, anorexia, and lethargy. Risk factors for the development of pancreatitis include obesity, dietary indiscretion, and hyperlipidemia. Drugs such as corticosteroids and phenobarbital, as well as endocrinopathies such as diabetes mellitus, hyperadrenocorticism, and hypothyroidism have also been linked as potential factors contributing to pancreatitis.

Main Considerations

When managing a case of pancreatitis and considering nutritional management, the goal is to keep in mind is to provide the animal with adequate nutrient levels to facilitate recovery and repair of damaged tissue. The first step in nutritional management for an animal with pancreatitis is to return the animal to a hemodynamically stable condition. Once that has been achieved, food is introduced in small amounts or fed through a feeding tube if the patient is anorexic. Initially, energy-dense diets with high protein and moderate to high fat are selected. Once the animal is no longer showing clinical signs of pancreatitis and has returned to its appropriate daily caloric intake, the diet choice should be adjusted to a long-term GI diet especially considering fat content, as outlined in Table 94.3.

Water

The most important nutritional factor to consider when managing a case of pancreatitis is water. Animals can become quickly dehydrated due to losses from vomiting as well as decreased intake when animals are anorexic and unable to properly replace the fluid loss. Hydration status of the patient should be assessed and in moderate to severe cases, dehydration should be corrected with appropriate parenteral fluid therapy. Further nutritional support should be postponed until dehydration has been resolved and electrolyte and acid–base disturbances have been corrected.

Protein

Consideration of protein content in the diet for animals recovering from pancreatitis is important for two reasons. First, free amino acids in the duodenum of the small intestine can act as a strong stimulus for pancreatic secretion. Animals with pancreatitis, however, will also have impaired protein digestion and absorption. This can lead to protein malnutrition and therefore animals require higher dietary protein to allow for recovery and tissue repair. Initially, a high-protein, high-fat veterinary therapeutic recovery diet is recommended. Once the animal is back to its proper daily caloric intake, a GI diet with less protein and moderate fat can be used. The diet should have a high-quality, easily digestible protein source which contains all amino acids

TABLE 94.3. Recommended components for nutritional support in pancreatitis.			
Key nutritional factor	Requirement	Cats (DM basis)	Dogs (DM basis)
Protein	Moderate	30–40%	15–30%
Fat*	Moderate	15–25%	10–15%
	to low	<15%	<10%
Fiber	Low	<5%	<5%

*Moderate fat is generally recommended, except for obese/overweight or hyperlipidemic patients which require low fat.

in correct proportions. Recommended dry matter protein levels for animals with pancreatitis eating their full maintenance energy requirement (MER) are 15–30% for dogs and 30–40% for cats. Adverse reactions to food can also be seen in some dogs and cats with pancreatitis, so in some cases selection of a food with a single and novel protein source or a hydrolyzed protein diet may be warranted.

Fat

Fat digestion and assimilation are severely impaired in animals with pancreatitis. As with protein, however, it is recommended to initially feed a recovery diet with higher fat content if the animal is anorexic. It is acceptable to feed a higher fat diet to an anorexic animal with pancreatitis because they are eating less than their MER and are also being fed multiple small meals per day. Therefore, the absolute amount of fat consumed in each meal is actually less, even though the diet is high fat.

Once the animal is eating full MER, a diet with moderate or low fat can be selected depending on the animal. Diet history, hypertriglyceridemia, breed, body condition score, and other underlying conditions are factors to consider when selecting an appropriate fat level for the diet. If the inciting cause for the pancreatitis episode was dietary indiscretion, it may not be necessary to switch the animal to a fat-restricted diet. Obese animals and animals with hyperlipidemia are at risk for future episodes, and therefore may benefit from a lower fat diet. Also, high serum triglyceride levels are directly linked to dietary fat content and are indicative of diet-induced pancreatitis. It is recommended that obese animals or animals that have high triglyceride levels should be fed a lower fat diet (<10% for dogs and <15% for cats) than animals with ideal body conditions and normal triglyceride levels (<15% for dogs and <25% for cats).

Fiber

Animals with pancreatitis should be fed a highly digestible diet that is low in fiber. Crude fiber content should be 5% or less on a dry matter basis. In the long term after recovery, for patients that are obese/overweight and need to be on a weight loss plan, higher fiber weight loss diets can be used for gradual weight loss.

Additional Nutritional Considerations

Cobalamin

Some cats with pancreatitis may have low cobalamin levels, especially if their pancreatitis is complicated by inflammatory bowel disease or triaditis. If cobalamin levels are low, supplementation via weekly subcutaneous injections (250 µg/cat) for 4–6 weeks or until serum levels are in the normal range is needed.

Antiemetics

Use of antiemetics to control nausea and vomiting is recommended when clinically indicated.

Feeding Recommendations

Historically, when managing a case of acute pancreatitis, a strict period of fasting was recommended to allow for "pancreatic rest." The thought was that by eliminating any stimulation to the pancreas and GI tract, secretions would be reduced and tissue repair could occur more rapidly. New information indicates that a period of nothing *per os* is actually less ideal for recovery as it can lead to intestinal mucosal atrophy and breakdown of the intestinal barrier, likely resulting in increased intestinal permeability and sepsis. Instead, nutritional management has moved to accept early enteral nutrition (EEN) feeding. Experimental models have shown a benefit to intraluminal nutrition, including stimulation of intestinal mucosal regeneration, decreased bacterial translocation, and decreased severity of inflammation. Early enteral nutrition delivered proximal to the jejunum is well tolerated in dogs with severe pancreatitis

(Mansfield et al. 2011) and EEN may actually help to minimize ileus and vomiting, thus improving gut health. Therefore, it is now recommended to begin feeding as soon as the animal is hemodynamically stable and if the animal is anorexic, placement of an esophagostomy or gastrostomy tube to facilitate EEN is advised.

If the animal is anorexic, choose a high-fat, high-protein recovery diet initially. Begin by feeding one-third of resting energy requirement (RER) on day 1, dividing that amount into multiple small meals to be fed throughout the day. If there is no vomiting and the diet is well tolerated, increase total volume each day. For example, one-third RER day 1, two-thirds RER day 2, and full RER by day 3. The animal should be offered food to eat on its own as well and once the period of anorexia has passed and the animal is eating voluntarily, assisted feeding through the feeding tube can be stopped. The goal is to have the animal eating its full RER daily in hospital and once it is home, gradual increase to full MER according to the patient's body condition is recommended. Obese animals will need to be on a weight loss plan as obesity is a risk factor for pancreatitis, but it is not recommended to begin the weight loss plan until the animal is fully recovered from pancreatitis.

The type of diet to be fed at home will depend on the inciting cause of the episode of pancreatitis. For animals with recurrent episodes or hypertriglyceridemia, or breeds at risk (e.g., schnauzers), a highly digestible diet with low (10% dogs, 15% cats) fat is recommended. For other animals, a highly digestible diet with moderate fat (12–15% dogs, 20–25% cats) is usually acceptable. The current diet of the animal should be evaluated for nutrient levels and if this diet does not meet the proper criteria with recommended fat and protein levels, a more appropriate diet should be selected, especially if the animal has risk factors which make it more susceptible to a second pancreatic episode.

Key Points

- Assess hydration and initiate parenteral fluid therapy if indicated.
- Initiate oral feeding once animal is hemodynamically stable.
- Early enteral feeding via feeding tube if anorexia is prolonged.
- In the ICU setting initially select a high protein, high fat recovery diet.
- Feed very small meals frequently throughout the day and increase total caloric intake gradually each day.
- Once animal is eating full MER, the diet plan can be adjusted with consideration of the individual animal when selecting a highly digestible low or moderate fat diet.
- Address potential underlying causes i.e. obesity, hyperlipidemia and dietary indiscretion, to prevent future bouts of pancreatitis.

References

Batchelor DJ, Noble PJM, Taylor RH, et al. Prognostic factors in canine exocrine pancreatic insufficiency: prolonged survival is likely if clinical remission is achieved. J Vet Intern Med 2007;21:54–60.

Biourge VC, Fontaine J. Exocrine pancreatic insufficiency and adverse reaction to food in dogs: a positive response to a high-fat, soy isolate hydrolysate-based diet. J Nutr 2004;134:2166S–2168S.

Mansfield CS, James FE, Steiner JM, et al. A pilot study to assess tolerability of early enteral nutrition via esophagostomy tube feeding in dogs with severe acute pancreatitis. J Vet Intern Med 2011;25:419–425.

Suggested Reading

Batchelor DJ, Noble PJM, Cripps PJ, et al. Breed associations for canine exocrine pancreatic insufficiency. J Vet Intern Med 2007;21:207–214.

Chan DL, Freeman LM, Labato MA, et al. Retrospective evaluation of partial parenteral nutrition in dogs and cats. J Vet Intern Med 2002;16(4):440–445.

German AJ. Exocrine pancreatic insufficiency in the dog: breed associations, nutritional considerations, and long-term outcome. Topics Compan Anim Med 2012;27:104–108.

Hess RS, Kass PH, Shofer FS, et al. Evaluation of risk factors for fatal acute pancreatitis in dogs. J Am Vet Med Assoc 1999;214:46–51.

Kalfarentzos F, Kehagias J, Mead N, et al. Enteral nutrition is superior to parenteral nutrition in severe acute pancreatitis: results of a randomised prospective trial. Br J Surg 1997;84:1665–1669.

Lem KY, Fosgate GT, Norby B, Steiner JM. Associations between dietary factors and pancreatitis in dogs. J Am Vet Med Assoc 2008;233:1425–1431.

McClave SA, Greene LM, Snider HL, et al. Comparison of the safety of early enteral vs parenteral nutrition in mild acute pancreatitis. J Parenter Enteral Nutr 1997;21:14–20.

Moore LE, Morgan JA. A quick review of canine exocrine pancreatic insufficiency. Vet Med 2009;427–433.

Steiner JM. Cobalamin: Diagnostic use and therapeutic considerations. Gastrointestinal Laboratory, Texas A&M University, College Station, Texas. Available from: http://vetmed.tamu.edu/gilab/research/cobalamin-information.

Vu MK, van der Veek PP, Frolich M, et al. Does jejunal feeding activate exocrine pancreatic secretion? Eur J CLin Invest 1999;29:1053–1059.

Westermarck E, Wiberg M. Exocrine pancreatic insufficiency in dogs. Vet Clin Small Anim 2003;33:1165–1179.

Westermarck E, Wiberg M. Exocrine pancreatic insufficiency in the dog: historical background, diagnosis, and treatment. Topics Compan Anim Med 2012;27:96–103.

Authors: Caitlin Grant DVM, BSc, Sarah Dodd DVM, BSc, Adronie Verbrugghe DVM, PhD, Dip ECVCN

Chapter 95

Exocrine Pancreatic Insufficiency

DEFINITION/OVERVIEW

Syndrome that is caused by inadequate amounts of pancreatic digestive enzymes in the small intestinal lumen.

ETIOLOGY/PATHOPHYSIOLOGY

- Most commonly caused by insufficient synthesis and secretion of pancreatic enzymes by pancreatic acinar cells.
  - Due to chronic pancreatitis; most common cause in cats and dogs of breeds that are not commonly affected by pancreatic acinar atrophy (PAA).
  - Due to PAA; most common cause of exocrine pancreatic insufficiency in German shepherd dogs and Eurasians.
  - In rare cases, can be caused by an obstruction of the pancreatic duct or pancreatic hypoplasia.
- Deficient exocrine pancreatic secretion results in maldigestion. Additionally, there is nutrient malabsorption, probably due to lack of trophic factors from the exocrine pancreas that physiologically stimulate mucosal proliferation.
- Maldigestion and malabsorption lead to weight loss and loose stools with steatorrhea.
- Malassimilation of nutrients contributes to small intestinal dysbiosis.

Systems Affected

- Endocrine/metabolic – lack of important nutrients due to malassimilation. Diabetes mellitus may occur concurrently in patients with exocrine pancreatic insufficiency (EPI) that are due to chronic pancreatitis.
- Gastrointestinal – decreased mucosal proliferation due to lack of trophic factors.
- Immune – potential immunosuppression secondarily to cobalamin deficiency.
- Nervous/neuromuscular – peripheral and central neuropathies secondary to cobalamin deficiency.
- Dermatologic – changes in hair coat and quality, likely due to nutritional deficiency.
- Musculoskeletal – loss of lean muscle mass may be noticed with chronic malabsorption.

SIGNALMENT/HISTORY

- Pancreatic acinar atrophy, which is believed to be an immune-mediated disease, almost exclusively occurs in the German shepherd dog and also much less frequently in the rough-coated collie and the Eurasians. In the German shepherd dog, PAA used to be believed to be

Blackwell's Five-Minute Veterinary Consult Clinical Companion: Small Animal Gastrointestinal Diseases,
First Edition. Edited by Jocelyn Mott and Jo Ann Morrison.
© 2019 John Wiley & Sons, Inc. Published 2019 by John Wiley & Sons, Inc.
Companion website: www.fiveminutevet.com/gastrointestinal

inherited as an autosomal recessive trait. However, a more recent breeding trial has shown that the trait is not inherited as a simple autosomal recessive trait, but that inheritance is more likely complex and multifactorial.

- EPI due to chronic pancreatitis can occur at any age (even puppies and kittens less than six months of age can be affected), while EPI due to PAA is mostly first diagnosed in young adult dogs (often between one and three years of age).

Risk Factors

There are no specific risk factors for EPI due to chronic pancreatitis. However, there are some known risk factors for chronic pancreatitis in dogs and cats. In dogs, dietary indiscretion, hypertriglyceridemia, hypercalcemia, some medications (e.g., potassium bromide and pheno-barbital), and concurrent inflammatory conditions of other abdominal organs (e.g., idiopathic inflammatory bowel disease (IBD) or chronic hepatitis) are known risk factors for chronic pancreatitis, while in cats only hypercalcemia and concurrent inflammatory conditions of other abdominal organs (e.g., IBD or chronic cholangitis) are known risk factors.

Historical Findings

- Weight loss with a normal to increased appetite.
- Chronically loose stools or diarrhea.
- Diarrhea often resembles cow feces and may be continuous or intermittent (Figure 95.1).
- Fecal volumes are larger than normal and may be associated with steatorrhea.
- Flatulence and borborygmus are common, especially in dogs.
- May show coprophagia and/or pica.
- May be accompanied by polyuria/polydipsia with diabetes mellitus as a sequel to chronic pancreatitis.
- Signs of clinical complications from cobalamin deficiency (e.g., clinical signs of peripheral or central neuropathies).

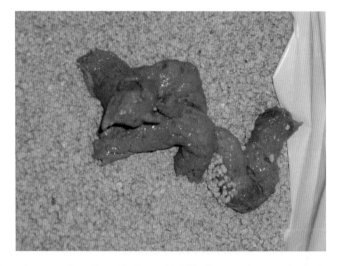

■ **Fig. 95.1.** The feces shown are from the cat in Figure 95.2. The feces are loose and voluminous. They also glisten, indicating a degree of steatorrhea.

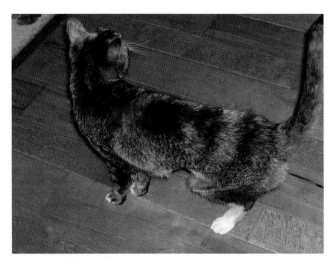

■ **Fig. 95.2.** The cat shown has been diagnosed with EPI based on a severely decreased serum fTLI concentration. The cat is thin and has a poor hair coat.

 ## CLINICAL FEATURES

- Thin body.
- Decreased muscle mass.
- Poor-quality hair coat (Figure 95.2).
- Cats with steatorrhea may have greasy "soiling" of the hair coat in the perineal area, but this is seen in a minority of cases.

 ## DIFFERENTIAL DIAGNOSES

- Secondary causes of chronic diarrhea and weight loss (e.g., hepatic failure, renal failure, hypoadrenocorticism, and hypothyroidism in dogs or hyperthyroidism in cats).
- Primary gastrointestinal disease (i.e., infectious, inflammatory, neoplastic, mechanical, or toxic).

 ## DIAGNOSTICS

Minimum Database
- The minimum database (i.e., complete blood count, chemistry profile, and urinalysis) usually does not show any abnormalities.
- Indicated in dogs and cats with suspected EPI to rule out other differential diagnoses.

Exocrine Pancreatic Function Tests
Trypsin-Like Immunoreactivity (TLI)
- Diagnostic test of choice in both dogs and cats.
- Principle of test – serum TLI can be measured by an assay that detects trypsinogen and trypsin that is directly released into the blood from the pancreatic acinar cells; serum TLI is detected in the serum of all normal dogs and cats with a functional exocrine pancreatic tissue.

- Serum TLI concentrations are dramatically reduced with EPI.
  - In dogs – cTLI ≤2.5 μg/L.
  - In cats – fTLI ≤8.0 μg/L.
- Canine and feline TLI tests are species specific.
- Indicated in any dog or cat with weight loss and/or loose stools, or any of the other clinical signs described.
- Advantages – simple, quick, single serum specimen (fasted), highly sensitive and specific for EPI in both species.

Other Exocrine Pancreatic Function Tests
- Assays of fecal proteolytic activity using casein-based substrates have been used to diagnose EPI in both dogs and cats. However, fecal proteolytic activity is associated with false-positive and false-negative test results and should only be used in exotic species for which a serum TLI test is not available.
- An assay for the measurement of fecal elastase has been described for use in dogs. However, this test is associated with a high rate of false-positive test results and cannot be recommended at this point. A positive test result, suggesting EPI, must be verified by measurement of a serum cTLI concentration.

Cobalamin and Folate
- Often run as a panel with TLI.
- Used to assess for concurrent dysbiosis or concurrent small intestinal disease (such as IBD).
- Cobalamin (vitamin B12) is frequently deficient in both dogs and cats with EPI and can lead to treatment failure or complications if not addressed.

Pathologic Findings
- Chronic pancreatitis – microscopically, acini and possibly islets are depleted and replaced by fibrous tissue. There may also be an active inflammatory infiltration.
- Pancreatic acinar atrophy – marked atrophy/absence of pancreatic acinar tissue on gross and histopathologic inspection in dogs with PAA.
- Pancreatic hypoplasia – a pancreas that is macroscopically small with normal histopathology.

THERAPEUTICS

- Treatment objective is a clinically healthy patient through digestive enzyme supplementation. However, exocrine pancreatic function does not recover in most patients. Also, digestive function does not normalize despite digestive enzyme supplementation.
- Treatment may also need to address specific nutritional deficiencies, most importantly cobalamin deficiency, secondary small intestinal dysbiosis, and/or failure to respond to enzyme supplementation alone.

Drug(s) of Choice
- Powdered pancreatic enzyme supplements are the treatment of choice.
  - Enzyme powder should be mixed directly into the food.
  - Initially a dosage of 1 teaspoon/10 kg body weight with each meal should be used, with at least two meals daily to promote weight gain.
  - Preincubation of enzymes with the food does not appear to improve the efficacy of oral enzyme therapy significantly.

- The enzyme product should contain at least 70 000 USP lipase per teaspoon of product (equals approximately 23 000 IU lipase), with less expensive products often failing to reach these levels.
- If a patient refuses to consume the enzyme supplement, the use of raw chopped pancreas from any species should be considered.
- Microencapsulated products can also be used, but tablets and capsules containing enzyme powder should be avoided.
- Most dogs and cats respond to therapy within 5–7 days. After a complete response has been achieved, the amount of pancreatic enzyme supplement may be gradually reduced to a dose that prevents return of clinical signs.

- Cobalamin supplementation is crucial if the patient is cobalamin deficient.
  - Pure injectable cyanocobalamin at 250 µg/injection in cats and 250–1500 µg/injection in dogs; once a week for six weeks, one more dose a month after that, and a recheck of serum cobalamin concentration a month after the last dose.
  - Pure cyanocobalamin for oral use at 250 µg/dose in cats and 250–1500 µg/dose in dogs; once a day for 120 days, followed by a recheck of serum cobalamin concentration two weeks after the last dose.
- Administration of a proton pump inhibitor (e.g., omeprazole at 0.7–1.0 mg/kg PO q12h) may improve the condition in nonresponsive patients.
- Oral antibiotic therapy (tylosin 25 mg/kg PO q12h) may be required for 4–6 weeks in patients with concurrent small intestinal dysbiosis, but in most patients dysbiosis resolves spontaneously upon commencement of enzyme replacement therapy.

Precautions/Interactions

- Oral bleeding may be observed in some patients receiving digestive enzyme powder. A rare coagulopathy due to vitamin K deficiency must first be excluded. In most of these patients, the dose can be decreased and oral bleeding will cease.
- Also, wetting the pet food/enzyme mix with water may help.

Alternative Drugs

- The cost of pancreatic enzyme replacement is very high. Additionally, some cats refuse to consume the pancreatic enzyme supplement. These patients can often be successfully managed by administration of raw chopped pancreas from any species.
- 1–3 oz of pancreatic tissue per 10 kg body weight with each meal.
- There is a small infectious risk with using raw pancreatic tissue.
  - Bovine: bovine spongioform encephalopathy.
  - Porcine: Aujeszky's disease.
  - Game pancreas: *Echinococcus multilocularis*.
- Raw pancreas can be kept frozen for months without losing enzymatic activity.

Diet

- The type of diet does not play a role in the management of EPI in dogs or cats.
- However, both low-fat and high-fiber diets should be avoided.
- Approximately 80% of all dogs with EPI and virtually all cats with EPI are cobalamin deficient and require cobalamin supplementation.
- Severely malnourished dogs may also require supplementation with tocopherol.
- Body stores of other fat-soluble vitamins (i.e., vitamins A and K) are probably also decreased in dogs and cats with EPI, but supplementation does not appear to be crucial.

Activity

There are no restrictions on the activity level of the patient.

Surgical Considerations

Mesenteric torsion has been reported in German shepherd dogs with EPI in Finland but not North America.

COMMENTS

Client Education

- Discuss hereditary nature in German shepherd dogs.
- Discuss expense of pancreatic enzyme supplementation and need for life-long therapy in almost all patients.
- Discuss the possibility of diabetes mellitus in patients with chronic pancreatitis.

Patient Monitoring

- Response to therapy should be verified at least by phone on a weekly basis for a few weeks.
- Diarrhea should improve markedly – fecal consistency typically normalizes within one week of initiating digestive enzyme replacement.
- Gain in body weight.
- However, serum TLI concentration does not normalize with treatment and thus does not need to be monitored.
- Patients that fail to respond after two weeks of enzyme therapy and cobalamin supplementation, if indicated, should be placed on antibiotics for concurrent intestinal dysbiosis.
- Once body weight and conditioning normalize, gradually reduce the daily dosage of enzyme supplements to a level that maintains normal fecal quality and body weight.

Prevention/Avoidance

Do not breed patients that belong to a breed predisposed to pancreatic acinar atrophy.

Possible Complications

- Approximately 20% of dogs fail to respond to pancreatic enzyme supplementation and need further evaluation and therapy.
- Most patients with EPI have cobalamin deficiency and need to be managed accordingly.
- Some dogs treated with pancreatic enzyme supplements develop oral ulcerations. In most of these dogs, the dose of pancreatic enzyme supplements can be decreased, while maintaining therapeutic response. In a few patients, the dose of pancreatic enzyme supplement needs to be adjusted frequently to avoid treatment failure and oral ulceration.

Expected Course and Prognosis

- Most cases of EPI are irreversible, and life-long therapy is required. However, there are anecdotal reports of patients that showed a spontaneous recovery.
- Patients with EPI alone have a good prognosis with appropriate enzyme supplementation and supportive management.
- Prognosis is more guarded in patients with EPI and concurrent diabetes mellitus.

Abbreviations

- cTLI = canine trypsin-like immunoreactivity
- EPI = exocrine pancreatic insufficiency
- fTLI = feline trypsin-like immunoreactivity
- IBD = idiopathic inflammatory bowel disease
- PAA = pancreatic acinar atrophy

See Also

- Cobalamin Deficiency
- Inflammatory Bowel Disease
- Intestinal Dysbiosis
- Nutritional Approach to Exocrine Pancreas Disease

Suggested Reading

Batchelor DJ, Noble PJ, Taylor RH, et al. Prognostic factors in canine exocrine pancreatic insufficiency: prolonged survival is likely if clinical remission is achieved. J Vet Intern Med 2007;21:54–60.

German AJ. Exocrine pancreatic insufficiency in the dog: breed associations, nutritional considerations, and long-term outcome. Top Compan Anim Med 2012;27:104–108.

Steiner JM. Exocrine pancreas. In: Steiner JM, ed. Small Animal Gastroenterology. Hannover: Schlütersche, 2008, pp. 283–306.

Thompson KA, Parnell NK, Hohenhaus AE, et al. Feline exocrine pancreatic insufficiency: 16 cases (1992–2007). J Feline Med Surg 2009;11:935–940.

Westermarck E, Wiberg M. Exocrine pancreatic insufficiency in the dog: historical background, diagnosis, and treatment. Top Compan Anim Med 2012;27:96–103.

Westermarck E, Saari SA, Wiberg ME. Heritability of exocrine pancreatic insufficiency in German shepherd dogs. J Vet Intern Med 2010;24:450–452.

Author: Jörg M. Steiner med.vet., Dr.med.vet., PhD, DACVIM, DECVIM-CA, AGAF

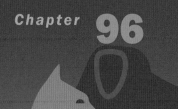
Pancreatic Abscess

DEFINITION/OVERVIEW

- Circumscribed collection of purulent material, usually containing little or no necrosis, in close proximity to the pancreas.
- Definition not well defined and universally accepted in veterinary medicine.

ETIOLOGY/PATHOPHYSIOLOGY

- Pancreatic abscess formation is an uncommon complication of acute (more commonly) or chronic pancreatitis in dogs and much less commonly in cats.
- Pancreatic abscesses have been reported to occur in 1.4–6.5% of dogs with pancreatitis.
- In contrast to humans, most reported cases (>80%) of pancreatic abscesses in dogs and cats are sterile; however, this might be the result of prior antibiotic use in many cases.

Systems Affected

Gastrointestinal.

SIGNALMENT/HISTORY

No breed or sex predisposition reported.

Risk Factors

Predisposing factors for pancreatitis (e.g., ingestion of a fatty meal, severe hypertriglyceridemia, hypercalcemia, administration of certain drugs) may be identified.

Historical Findings

- Clinical signs are nonspecific and indistinguishable from those of acute pancreatitis in most cases.
- Initial clinical signs likely reflect pancreatitis before the formation of a pancreatic abscess.
- Sudden onset of anorexia, depression, and vomiting are more commonly reported.
- Diarrhea and abdominal pain may also be present.

CLINICAL FEATURES

- Anorexia, depression, and vomiting are the most common findings.
- A mass might be identified on abdominal palpation in a small number of cases.

Blackwell's Five-Minute Veterinary Consult Clinical Companion: Small Animal Gastrointestinal Diseases,
First Edition. Edited by Jocelyn Mott and Jo Ann Morrison.
© 2019 John Wiley & Sons, Inc. Published 2019 by John Wiley & Sons, Inc.
Companion website: www.fiveminutevet.com/gastrointestinal

- Fever or hypothermia might be present.
- Ascites or icterus is identified less commonly.
- Animals are often critically ill and typically do not improve despite treatment for pancreatitis.

 ## DIFFERENTIAL DIAGNOSIS

- Clinical presentation is nonspecific.
- Pancreatic abscesses are almost always associated with pancreatitis; differential diagnosis based on clinical and clinicopathologic data is the same as for pancreatitis.
- In many animals, a diagnosis of pancreatitis might be reached but the presence of a pancreatic abscess might be missed.
- Differential diagnosis for a pancreatic mass or fluid collection includes pancreatic abscess, pancreatic pseudocyst, pancreatic phlegmon, and pancreatic neoplasia.

 ## DIAGNOSTICS

Complete Blood Count/Biochemistry/Urinalysis

- Clinicopathological findings are nonspecific and do not differ from those of pancreatitis.
- Almost any type of hematologic abnormality may be seen.
- Serum biochemistry findings are highly variable and reflect the severity of pancreatitis.

Imaging

- Abdominal radiographs may show an increased fluid pattern, loss of serosal detail, or mass effect in the proximal abdomen; sensitivity and specificity are very low.
- Abdominal ultrasonography is both useful and practical for the detection of pancreatic abscesses; sensitivity is considered to be high (dependent on operator skill level).
- Differentiation of pancreatic abscesses from other pancreatic fluid collections (e.g., pseudocyst, necrosis) or masses might be difficult based on ultrasound alone.
- Fine-needle aspiration (FNA) can be performed during ultrasound examination.

Other Diagnostics Tests

- The diagnosis is usually based on cytologic and bacteriologic analysis (culture) of material obtained through ultrasound-guided FNA or surgery.
- Histopathology may be required for a definitive diagnosis in many cases.
- Cytology typically reveals highly cellular fluid characterized by degenerate neutrophils.
- Bacteria may or may not be present; bacterial cultures are positive in 0–22% of cases, although many dogs may have received antibiotics prior to culture.

 ## THERAPEUTICS

Drug(s) of Choice

- Supportive care (e.g., fluid therapy, analgesia, antiemetics, nutrition, plasma transfusion) is required in almost all cases as indicated for the management of acute pancreatitis.
- The use of antibiotics is not routinely recommended for the management of acute pancreatitis in dogs and cats unless an infection is identified or highly possible; little is known about antibiotic use in the treatment of pancreatic abscesses but it should be kept in mind that in most cases these abscesses are sterile.

Nursing Care

Supportive care and continuous patient monitoring are required in most cases as indicated for severe acute pancreatitis cases.

Diet

Typically, a low-fat diet is recommended in dogs with pancreatitis; a moderate-fat/high-protein diet is usually recommended for cats.

Activity

The patient's activity should be restricted.

Surgical Considerations

- Surgical intervention is almost always recommended for the treatment of a pancreatic abscess; several techniques have been described.
- The goal is to debride the abscess, collect samples for culture and histopathology, and provide drainage for the abscess and peritoneal cavity if peritonitis is present.

 COMMENTS

Client Education

- Pancreatic abscess is a severe complication of pancreatitis; most patients are critically ill and require long-term and intensive hospitalization; most cases are surgically managed.
- Prognosis is guarded to poor.

Patient Monitoring

Most patients are critically ill and therefore continuous patient monitoring is required.

Possible Complications

- Ascites (septic or sterile inflammatory exudate) may be seen with rupture of the abscess and/or as a result of peritonitis.
- Extrahepatic biliary tract obstruction.
- Several other complications may be seen as a result of surgery.

Expected Course and Prognosis

Mortality rates in dogs with pancreatic abscesses range from 50% to 86%, making the presence of a pancreatic abscess a poor prognostic indicator.

Abbreviations

- FNA = fine needle aspiration

See Also

- Acute Abdomen
- Diarrhea, Acute
- Nutritional Approach to Exocrine Pancreatic Disease
- Pancreatic Neoplasia
- Pancreatic Pseudocyst
- Pancreatitis, Canine
- Pancreatitis, Feline
- Vomiting, Acute

Suggested Reading

Coleman M, Robson M. Pancreatic masses following pancreatitis: pancreatic pseudocysts, necrosis, and abscesses. Compendium 2005;27(2):147–154.

Schaer M. Abscess, necrosis, pseudocyst, phlegmon, and infection. In: Washabau RJ, Day MJ, eds. Canine and Feline Gastroenterology. St Louis: Elsevier, 2013.

Xenoulis PG, Steiner JM, Monnet E. Pancreatitis. In: Monnet E, ed. Small Animal Soft Tissue Surgery. Ames: Wiley-Blackwell, 2013.

Author: Panagiotis G. Xenoulis DVM, Dr.med.vet., PhD

Chapter 97

Pancreatic Neoplasia

DEFINITION/OVERVIEW

- Malignant tumor of ductal or acinar origin arising from the exocrine pancreas.
- Usually metastatic by the time of diagnosis, affecting regional lymph nodes and visceral abdominal organs (liver) and serosal surfaces of peritoneal cavity.

ETIOLOGY/PATHOPHYSIOLOGY

- Etiology is unknown.
- N-ethyl-N'-nitro-N-nitrosoguanidine has been used to experimentally induce pancreatic duct adenocarcinoma in dogs.

Systems Affected

- Hepatobiliary – jaundice due to bile duct obstruction.
- Gastrointestinal – anorexia (especially in cats), vomiting.
- Endocrine/metabolic – diabetes mellitus.
- Hemic/lymphatic/immune – mild anemia, hyperglycemia, neutrophilia, bilirubinemia (if bile duct occlusion is present), serum lipase and amylase increase.
- Skin/exocrine – paraneoplastic alopecia in cats.

SIGNALMENT/HISTORY

- Rare in dogs – 0.5–1.8% of all tumors.
- Rare in cats – 2.8% of all tumors.
- Older female dogs and Airedale terriers at higher risk than others.
- Median age (dogs) 9.2 years.
- Mean age (cats) 11.6 years.
- Weight loss and anorexia (especially in cats), paraneoplastic alopecia in cats, vomiting, rare associated diabetes mellitus, abdominal distension due to mass effect or abdominal effusions secondary to tumor implantation on the peritoneum (i.e., carcinomatosis; common in cats), icterus (with common bile duct obstruction), and depression are common symptoms.
- Patients may present for symptoms of metastatic disease.

Risk Factors

Older female dogs and Airedales have been described as being at higher risk.

Blackwell's Five-Minute Veterinary Consult Clinical Companion: Small Animal Gastrointestinal Diseases, First Edition. Edited by Jocelyn Mott and Jo Ann Morrison.
© 2019 John Wiley & Sons, Inc. Published 2019 by John Wiley & Sons, Inc.
Companion website: www.fiveminutevet.com/gastrointestinal

Historical Findings

The history and clinical signs of pancreatic adenocarcinoma can be vague and nonspecific and mimic those of pancreatitis.

 ## CLINICAL FEATURES

- Nonspecific – fever; vomiting; weakness; anorexia; icterus; malabsorption syndrome; weight loss (especially in cats).
- Abdominal pain – variable.
- Abdominal malignant effusion – carcinomatosis, relatively more common in cats.
- Metastasis to bone and soft tissue common.
- Pathologic fractures secondary to metastasis reported.
- Palpable abdominal mass (cats).
- Paraneoplastic syndromes of epidermal necrosis, hyperinsulinemia, and hyperglucagonemia may be present.
- Average duration of clinical signs (cats): 41 days, range 2–180 days.

 ## DIFFERENTIAL DIAGNOSIS

- Primary pancreatitis; may be concurrent and complicate or delay early diagnosis.
- Pancreatic pseudocyst.
- Pancreatic nodular hyperplasia.
- Hepatic neoplasia.
- Other causes of vomiting and icterus.
- Peritoneal carcinomatosis.
- Other causes of abdominal effusion in cats.

 ## DIAGNOSTICS

Imaging

- Abdominal radiographs may reveal a mass or loss of serosal detail associated with concurrent pancreatitis or peritoneal effusion (Figure 97.1).
- Ultrasonography (Figure 97.2) may reveal one or more masses or concurrent pancreatitis (mixed echogenicity, large pancreas, hyperechoic peripancreatic fat). Pancreatic thickening, abdominal effusion, and single to multiple nodules of varying size may be identified. Sonographic findings may be impossible to distinguish from pancreatic nodular hyperplasia. Rarely, ultrasound of the pancreas may appear normal except for dilation of the pancreatic duct.
- The utility of advanced imaging such as computed tomography (CT) and magnetic resonance imaging (MRI) has not been documented for pancreatic tumors in veterinary patients. In this author's institution, we require a contrast-enhanced CT (Figures 97.3 and 97.4) before surgery for surgical planning and informing the owners about the type of surgery required (i.e., colon resection, Billroth I or II reconstruction).

Diagnostic Procedures

- Surgical biopsy – definitive.
- Fine-needle aspirate cytology – supportive. In many cases, where the tumor is not resectable, the fine-needle aspirates may provide strong enough evidence to start medical treatment.

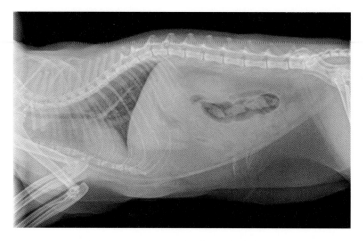

■ **Fig. 97.1.** Lateral abdominal radiograph of 13-year-old, male castrated American domestic short-haired cat, diagnosed with pancreatic adenocarcinoma. The cat had a history of 14 days of lethargy, weight loss, hiding, and decreased appetite. Plain radiography raised suspicion for a potential mass in the cranial abdomen.

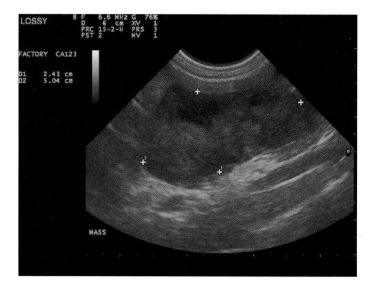

■ **Fig. 97.2.** Abdominal ultrasound revealed a 5 × 2.4 cm pancreatic mass that appeared to be at the left limb of the pancreas, with irregular borders and of mixed echogenicity.

Pathologic Findings

- Exocrine pancreatic adenocarcinoma may be derived from ductal or acinar epithelium.
- Common histologic patterns comprise tubules, acini, or solid sheets, and tumor stroma ranges from delicate to scirrhous. Although histologic subclassifications are recognized, association of subtypes with biologic behavior has not been documented.

 ## THERAPEUTICS

- Most cases of pancreatic adenocarcinoma present with metastatic disease (regional lymph nodes and liver) or are locally and extensively invasive at the time of diagnosis.
- No curative options are currently available.

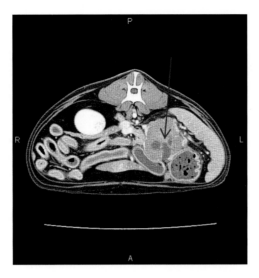

■ **Fig. 97.3.** Abdominal CT. The primary tumor arises from the left pancreatic limb and appears as a mixed iso- and hypoattenuating mass that enhances heterogeneously with central areas of nonenhancement (*red arrow*).

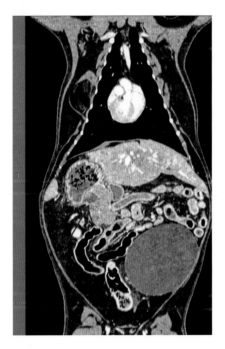

■ **Fig. 97.4.** Abdominal CT. The tumor is immediately caudal to the gastric body, causes cranial and ventral displacement and distortion of the pylorus, and does not appear to invade the colon.

- Nonmetastatic, surgically amendable tumors can be resected surgically – these cases carry the longest survival.
- Gemcitabine is used in humans for the treatment of pancreatic carcinoma, and while used in dogs with cancer, it has not been established as the standard of care for dogs with pancreatic adenocarcinoma.
- Always consult a veterinary oncologist for updates in treating this rare neoplasm and check with the AVMA for available clinical trial (https://ebusiness.avma.org/aahsd/study_search.aspx).

Drug(s) of Choice

- Palliation of pain with aggressive analgesic combinations is necessary
- Palliation for symptoms due to carcinomatosis may be attempted via intraperitoneal chemo (carboplatin), toceranib administration, or palliative abdominal irradiation.

Appropriate Health Care

Treat concurrent pancreatitis, if present.

Nursing Care

Antiemetics and supportive care (hydration and caloric requirements).

Surgical Considerations

- Surgical intervention to alleviate intestinal and biliary obstruction, if necessary. These procedures are associated with a high morbidity rate and should only be considered for referral to experienced surgical oncologists.
- Surgery is typically not a good option in many cases, due to the extent of the disease at the time of diagnosis.
- If surgery is an option, partial or total pancreatectomy may prolong survival.

   COMMENTS

Expected Course and Prognosis

- Progression to death is often rapid given the advanced disease stage on diagnosis and the lack of curative treatment.
- Despite the grave prognosis, rare individual patients treated with complete resection of their tumor and chemotherapy, in the absence of systemic metastasis, may have prolonged survival.

Synonyms

- Pancreatic adenocarcinoma
- Exocrine pancreatic carcinoma

Abbreviations

- AVMA = American Veterinary Medical Association
- CT = computed tomography
- MRI = magnetic resonance imaging

Suggested Reading

Cave T, Evans H, Hargreaves J, et al. Metabolic epidermal necrosis in a dog associated with pancreatic adenocarcinoma, hyperglucagonaemia, hyperinsulinaemia, and hypoaminoacidaemia. J Small Anim Pract 2007;48:522–526.

Hecht S, Penninck DG, Keating JH. Imaging findings in pancreatic neoplasia and nodular hyperplasia in 19 cats. Vet Radiol Ultrasound 2006;48:45–50.

Linderman MJ, Brodsky EM, de Lorimier LP, Clifford CA, Post GS. Feline exocrine pancreatic carcinoma: a retrospective study of 34 cases. Vet Comp Oncol 2013;11(3):208–218.

Withrow SJ. Exocrine pancreatic cancer. In: Withrow and MacEwen's Small Animal Clinical Oncology, 5th ed. St Louis: Elsevier Saunders, 2012.

Author: Nick Dervisis DVM, PhD, DACVIM (Oncology)

Chapter 98

Pancreatic Nodular Hyperplasia

DEFINITION/OVERVIEW

- Pancreatic nodular hyperplasia (PNH) is a nonneoplastic hyperplasia of exocrine pancreatic epithelial (acinar) cells.
- The epithelial cells maintain the architecture of the acinar arrangement and the cellular nuclei are similarly maintained in a basilar orientation.
- PNH is the most frequently detected lesion within the canine and feline pancreas.
- PNH is commonly an incidental finding at laparotomy or at necropsy.

ETIOLOGY/PATHOPHYSIOLOGY

- The cause of pancreatic nodular hyperplasia is not known.
- In general, hyperplasia tends to be a response to injury; however, PNH has been demonstrated in the pancreata of dogs both with and without concurrent pathology (e.g., inflammation, necrosis, and/or fibrosis).
- The presence and severity of PNH show a positive correlation with age in dogs, and in older dogs, >5 years of age, is considered by many to be an age-related change.
- Some have suggested that the presence of PNH in dogs <5 years of age is indicative of inflammation and scarring rather than neoplasia or hyperplasia.
- There is no evidence that PNH predisposes to neoplasia.

Systems Affected

Pancreas of dogs and cats.

SIGNALMENT/HISTORY

- Dogs and cats of any age may be found to have PNH.
- Older dogs and cats are more likely to have PNH.

Risk Factors

Previous pancreatic disease, including inflammation, necrosis, and fibrosis, may increase the likelihood of PNH. However, dogs and cats without such history may also have PNH.

CLINICAL FEATURES

There are no clinical features associated with PNH.

Blackwell's Five-Minute Veterinary Consult Clinical Companion: Small Animal Gastrointestinal Diseases,
First Edition. Edited by Jocelyn Mott and Jo Ann Morrison.
© 2019 John Wiley & Sons, Inc. Published 2019 by John Wiley & Sons, Inc.
Companion website: www.fiveminutevet.com/gastrointestinal

DIFFERENTIAL DIAGNOSIS

- Grossly pancreatic adenomas may appear similar to PNH.
- Ultrasonographically, PNH cannot be distinguished from other forms of neoplasia.

 DIAGNOSTICS

Complete Blood Count/Biochemistry/Urinalysis

No specific findings indicative of PNH.

Additional Laboratory Tests

There are no laboratory tests that identify PNH.

Imaging

- Radiographs – tend not to be very useful for detecting PNH in dogs, but in cats a cranial abdominal mass or mass effect may be observed.
- Ultrasound – there are no published studies describing the appearance of PNH in dogs. In cats, findings can include multiple small (0.3–1.0 cm) hypoechoic nodules and an enlarged pancreas (up to 2 cm in thickness). Ultrasound cannot distinguish PNH from neoplasia in dogs or cats.

Diagnostic Procedures

Biopsy and histopathology are necessary for definitive diagnosis of PNH.

Pathologic Findings

- Grossly, PNH may present as a solitary nodule, but more often it is present as multiple small nodules that are white or tan in color and measure from a few millimeters up to 1 cm in size. They are well circumscribed and may protrude from the pancreatic surface (Figure 98.1).
- Histologically, PNH nodules are not encapsulated as are adenomas, and they do not tend to compress adjacent tissue either at all or as much as adenomas. Hyperplastic nodules are larger than adjacent nodules. They consist of acinar cells of varying sizes and shapes and may either be pale or more eosinophilic than normal acinar cells. The cytoplasm may be vacuolated, but there is no cellular atypia.
- In dogs, inflammatory infiltrates of lymphocytes, fibrosis, and/or lobular atrophy may be observed in proximity to PNH.

 THERAPEUTICS

There are no therapeutics necessary or special dietary requirements for animals with PNH.

 COMMENTS

Expected Course and Prognosis

PNH is considered an incidental finding that is age related and carries an excellent prognosis.

Synonyms

- Benign nodular hyperplasia (BNH)

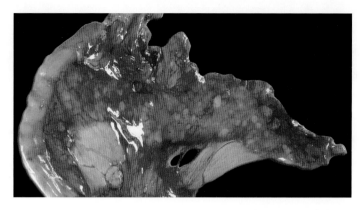

■ **Fig. 98.1.** Gross appearance of feline pancreatic nodular hyperplasia in a necropsy specimen. Source: Courtesy of Dr Matti Kiupel.

Abbreviations

- PNH = pancreatic nodular hyperplasia

See Also

- Pancreatic Neoplasia
- Pancreatitis, Canine
- Pancreatitis, Feline

Suggested Reading

Head KW, Else RW, Dubielzig RR. Tumors of the alimentary tract. In: Meuten DJ, ed. Tumors in Domestic Animals, 4th ed. Ames: Wiley-Blackwell, 2002, pp. 478–481.

Hecht S, Penninck DG, Keating JH. Imaging findings in pancreatic neoplasia and nodular hyperplasia in 19 cats. Vet Radiol Ultrasound 2007;48(1):45–50.

Newman SJ, Steiner JM, Woosley K, Barton L, Williams DA. Correlation of age and incidence of pancreatic exocrine nodular hyperplasia in the dog. Vet Pathol 2005;42:510–513.

Newman SJ, Steiner JM, Woosley K, Williams DA, Barton L. Histologic assessment and grading of the exocrine pancreas in the dog. J Vet Diagn Invest 2006;18:115–118.

Author: Kate Holan DVM, DACVIM

Chapter 99

Pancreatic Parasites

DEFINITION/OVERVIEW

- *Platynosomum fastosum* (also known as *Eurytrema fastosum*) and *Eurytrema procyonis* are two flukes that can affect the bile and pancreatic ducts of cats.

ETIOLOGY/PATHOPHYSIOLOGY

- *P. fastosum* – disease is referred to as platynosomiasis or "lizard poisoning." Cats are infected by consumption of lizards, the third intermediate or paratenic host of *P. fastosum*. After consumption of the infective form of *P. fastosum*, the parasite travels via the duodenal papilla into the biliary system or pancreatic ducts of cats. Cats or other definitive hosts shed eggs in feces that infect the first intermediate host (snails) before passing to the second intermediate host (terrestrial isopods). These terrestrial isopods infect lizards who consume them.
- *E. procyonis* – disease is referred to as eurytrematosis and is thought to be uncommon other than very few case reports of primarily pancreatic disease in cats. Cats are infected by consumption of grasshoppers or other arthropods, the second intermediate hosts of *E. procyonis*. After consumption of the infective form of *E. procyonis*, the parasite travels to the pancreatic ducts primarily to mature to the adult fluke. Cats and raccoons, the other definitive host for which the parasite is named, shed eggs in feces that infect the first intermediate host (snails). Grasshoppers and other second intermediate hosts become infected by consumption of sporocysts deposited on vegetation by the snails.

Systems Affected

- *P. fastosum* – hepatobiliary, gastrointestinal.
- *E. procyonis* – gastrointestinal, hepatobiliary.

SIGNALMENT/HISTORY

- *P. fastosum* – no definitive breed or sex predilections exist among cats with platynosomiasis. Some reports note higher number of female cats infected. Infections are most commonly reported in the south-eastern United States, Hawaii, Caribbean, and South America.
- *E. procyonis* – no breed or sex predilections exist among cats with eurytrematosis. Infections are found in the eastern half of the United States.

Risk Factors

- *P. fastosum* – cats with outdoor access that consume lizards.
- *E. procyonis* – cats with outdoor access that consume grasshoppers and other arthropods.

Blackwell's Five-Minute Veterinary Consult Clinical Companion: Small Animal Gastrointestinal Diseases, First Edition. Edited by Jocelyn Mott and Jo Ann Morrison.
© 2019 John Wiley & Sons, Inc. Published 2019 by John Wiley & Sons, Inc.
Companion website: www.fiveminutevet.com/gastrointestinal

Historical Findings

- *P. fastosum* – many cats are thought to be asymptomatic. Vague clinical signs such as lethargy and inappetence are most commonly reported. Other reported signs include weight loss, diarrhea, vomiting, depression, dull hair coat, and hair loss.
- *E. procyonis* – usually asymptomatic; noted in 10% of a stray cat population in Missouri in the 1980s. Rarely, obstruction of the pancreatic duct has been reported to cause exocrine pancreatic insufficiency and/or pancreatitis leading to gastrointestinal signs such as weight loss and vomiting.

 # CLINICAL FEATURES

- *P. fastosum* – some infected cats show no signs at all. Severely affected cats may show signs of hepatic failure, jaundice, abdominal distension, weight loss and poor body condition, or fever. There are few reports of an association with platynosomiasis and cholangiocarcinomas in cats in Brazil. Recent studies have shown pancreatitis to be very rare in cats with platynosomiasis.
- *E. procyonis* – many infected cats show no signs at all. Cats in which flukes obstruct the pancreatic ducts show signs of pancreatitis or exocrine pancreatic insufficiency, such as weight loss, poor appetite, or vomiting.

 # DIFFERENTIAL DIAGNOSIS

- *P. fastosum* – other causes of hepatobiliary disease in cats such as bacterial cholangitis, lymphocytic or neutrophilic cholangitis, hepatobiliary neoplasia, pancreatitis.
- *E. procyonis* – other causes of pancreatic disease such as pancreatitis, exocrine pancreatic insufficiency, pancreatic neoplasia, or other causes of gastrointestinal disease.

 # DIAGNOSTICS

Complete Blood Count/Biochemistry/Urinalysis

P. fastosum – complete blood count may show eosinophilia. Chemistry panel may show increased alanine aminotransferase (ALT) more commonly than increased alkaline phosphatase (ALP), increased bilirubin in advanced cases, or may be normal.

Other Laboratory Tests

- *P. fastosum.*
  - Feline pancreatic lipase immunoreactivity (fPLI): usually within normal limits.
  - Fecal: detection is difficult due to low numbers of eggs and high morphologic variation among eggs; most successful reported method of fecal evaluation is formalin-ether sedimentation, less effective are direct smear, zinc sulfate, or sucrose and modified detergent flotation. Eggs are thick-walled and embryonated, with an operculum at one end. Mature eggs measure 34–50 × 23–35 μm.
- *E. procyonis.*
  - fPLI: may be increased, as in one case report.
  - Fecal: most eggs are detected via centrifugal flotations (zinc sulfate or sucrose). Eggs are thick-walled, have one operculum, and measure 30 × 50 μm approximately.

Imaging

- *P. fastosum* – abdominal ultrasound may reveal distended bile or pancreatic ducts, thickened gallbladder wall, or the presence of flukes within the ducts or pancreatitis more rarely.
- *E. procyonis* – abdominal ultrasound: one report of mildly enlarged pancreas with an enlarged and thickened pancreatic duct containing hypoechoic material.

Pathologic Findings

- *P. fastosum.*
  - Gross pathology: flukes within bile or pancreatic ducts or gallbladder, biliary duct distension, hepatomegaly, mesenteric lymphadenopathy, ascites.
  - Histopathology: cholangitis, cholecystitis, cirrhosis, biliary duct hyperplasia, hepatic lipidosis, flukes or eggs, chronic pancreatitis, cholangiocarcinoma.
- *E. procyonis.*
  - Gross pathology: flukes within pancreatic ducts, bile ducts, or gallbladder, thickened, nodular, or discolored pancreas.
  - Histopathology: flukes or eggs, inflammation, hyperplasia, and fibrosis of the pancreatic ducts and surrounding parenchyma, eosinophilic pancreatic infiltrate, neutrophilic pancreatic infiltrate.

 # THERAPEUTICS

- *P. fastosum* – goal of therapy is elimination of adult flukes and cessation of shedding of eggs in feces. Secondary therapy may be related to hepatic dysfunction, which may not improve with fluke therapy.
- *E. procyonis* – goal of therapy is elimination of adult flukes, cessation of shedding of eggs in feces, and resolution of pancreatic inflammation (if present). Secondary therapy may be related to exocrine pancreatic insufficiency and/or pancreatitis.

Drug(s) of Choice

- *P. fastosum* – no drug is labeled for the treatment of platynosomiasis in cats. Suggested protocols include praziquantel 20 mg/kg PO once daily for 3–5 days or praziquantel 5.75 mg/kg PO once with a second single dose 3–4 weeks later.
- *E. procyonis* – no drug is labeled for the treatment of eurytrematosis in cats. One report exists of cessation of egg shedding and resolution of pancreatic changes on abdominal ultrasound after praziquantel/pyrantel/febantel therapy (Drontal Plus®, Bayer) 1.5 tablets (34 mg praziquantel, 34 mg pyrantel, and 170 mg febantel) PO once daily for five days.

Precautions/Interactions

Praziquantel – do not use in cats younger than six weeks.

Alternative Drugs

- *P. fastosum* – none currently recommended.
- *E. procyonis* – reports of the use of fenbendazole 30 mg/kg PO once daily for six days are mixed in terms of cessation of fecal egg shedding.

Appropriate Health Care

- *P. fastosum* – consider supportive care for hepatic dysfunction if present or persistent beyond fluke treatment.
- *E. procyonis* – consider supportive care for pancreatitis if present, or pancreatic enzyme supplementation if feline trypsin-like immunoreactivity (fTLI) supports diagnosis of exocrine pancreatic insufficiency.

Diet

- *P. fastosum* – patients should be prevented from further consumption of the paratenic host (lizard).
- *E. procyonis* – patients should be prevented from further consumption of grasshoppers and other arthropods.

Activity

No changes.

 COMMENTS

Patient Monitoring

- *P. fastosum* – repeat fecal examination to ensure eggs are no longer being shed.
- *E. procyonis* – repeat fecal examination to ensure eggs are no longer being shed, follow-up abdominal ultrasound, fPLI or fTLI as needed to monitor pancreatic changes (if present at diagnosis).

Prevention/Avoidance

- *P. fastosum* – prevent cat from consuming paratenic host (lizard).
- *E. procyonis* – prevent cat from consuming second intermediate host (arthropod).

Possible Complications

- *P. fastosum* – liver cirrhosis, liver failure, liver tumors, pancreatitis.
- *E. procyonis* – pancreatitis, exocrine pancreatic insufficiency.

Expected Course and Prognosis

- *P. fastosum* – many cats are asymptomatic. Fluke burden does not appear to correlate with disease. Prognosis is likely related to degree of hepatic dysfunction and cirrhosis at diagnosis.
- *E. procyonis* – many cats are asymptomatic. Cats with severe pancreatic changes may have permanent exocrine pancreas dysfunction (exocrine pancreatic insufficiency). Too few reports of disease exist to accurately predict the expected course and prognosis.

Synonyms

- *P. fastosum* – lizard poisoning

Abbreviations

- ALP = alkaline phosphatase
- ALT = alanine aminotransferase
- fPLI = feline pancreatic lipase immunoreactivity
- fTLI = feline trypsin-like immunoreactivity

See Also

- Exocrine Pancreatic Insufficiency
- Hepatic Neoplasia, Malignant
- Pancreatitis, Feline
- Vomiting, Chronic

Suggested Reading

Andrade RLFS, Dantas AFM, Pimentel LA, et al. Platynosomum fastosum-induced cholangiocarcinomas in cats. Vet Parasitol 2012;190:277–280.

Basu AK, Charles RA. A review of the cat liver fluke Platynosomum fastosum Kossack, 1910 (Trematoda: Dicrocoeliidae). Vet Parasitol 2014;200:1–7.

Hoffman DA, Piech TL, Taylor HL, Royal AB. What is your diagnosis? Pancreatic aspirate from a cat. Vet Clin Pathol 2017;46(3):540–541.

Koster LS, Shell L, Ketzis J, et al. Diagnosis of pancreatic disease in feline platynosomosis. J Feline Med Surg 2017;19(12):1192–1198.

Vyhnal KK, Barr SC, Hornbuckle WE, et al. Eurytrema procyonis and pancreatitis in a cat. J Feline Med Surg 2008;10(4):384–387.

Author: Jessica C. Pritchard VMD, MS, DACVIM (SAIM)

Chapter 100

Pancreatic Pseudocyst

DEFINITION/OVERVIEW

- Collection of enzyme-rich pancreatic fluid containing tissue debris and blood.
- It is not a true cyst because it is lined by inflammatory tissue instead of epithelium.
- Definition not well defined and universally accepted in veterinary medicine.

ETIOLOGY/PATHOPHYSIOLOGY

- Pancreatic pseudocysts result from autodigestion and liquefaction of pancreatic tissue during severe necrotizing pancreatitis.
- It is a rare complication of pancreatitis in dogs and cats.

Systems Affected

Gastrointestinal.

SIGNALMENT/HISTORY

No breed or sex predisposition reported.

Risk Factors

Predisposing factors for pancreatitis (e.g., ingestion of a fatty meal, severe hypertriglyceridemia, hypercalcemia, administration of certain drugs) may be identified.

Historical Findings

- Clinical signs are nonspecific and indistinguishable from those of acute pancreatitis in most cases.
- Initial clinical signs likely reflect pancreatitis before the formation of a pancreatic pseudocyst.
- Pancreatitis might resolve and the formation of the pseudocyst may follow days or weeks later and may cause clinical signs such as anorexia, depression, vomiting, diarrhea, and abdominal pain.

CLINICAL FEATURES

- Anorexia, depression, and vomiting are the most common findings.
- A mass might be identified on abdominal palpation.
- Animals are often critically ill and typically do not improve despite treatment for pancreatitis.

Blackwell's Five-Minute Veterinary Consult Clinical Companion: Small Animal Gastrointestinal Diseases,
First Edition. Edited by Jocelyn Mott and Jo Ann Morrison.
© 2019 John Wiley & Sons, Inc. Published 2019 by John Wiley & Sons, Inc.
Companion website: www.fiveminutevet.com/gastrointestinal

DIFFERENTIAL DIAGNOSIS

- Clinical presentation is nonspecific.
- Pancreatic pseudocysts are almost always associated with pancreatitis; differential diagnosis based on clinical and clinicopathologic data is the same as for pancreatitis.
- In many animals, a diagnosis of pancreatitis might be reached but the presence of a pancreatic pseudocyst be missed, especially if it is small and does not cause severe clinical signs.
- Differential diagnosis for a pancreatic mass or fluid collection includes pancreatic abscess, pancreatic pseudocyst, pancreatic phlegmon, and pancreatic neoplasia.

DIAGNOSTICS

Complete Blood Count/Biochemistry/Urinalysis

- Clinicopathological findings are nonspecific and do not differ from those of pancreatitis.
- Almost any type of hematologic abnormality may be seen.
- Serum biochemistry findings are highly variable and reflect the severity of pancreatitis.

Imaging

- Abdominal radiographs may show an increased fluid pattern, loss of serosal detail, or mass effect in the proximal abdomen; sensitivity and specificity are very low.
- Abdominal ultrasonography is both useful and practical for the detection of pancreatic pseudocysts; sensitivity is considered to be high.
- Differentiation of pancreatic pseudocysts from other pancreatic fluid collections (e.g., abscesses, necrosis) or masses might be difficult based on ultrasound alone.
- Fine-needle aspiration (FNA) can be performed during ultrasound examination.

Additional Diagnostic Tests

- The diagnosis is usually based on cytologic and bacteriologic analysis (culture) of material obtained through ultrasound-guided FNA or surgery.
- Cytology may reveal a hypocellular fluid or a highly cellular fluid with an inflammatory component; bacteria might be present if the pseudocyst is infected.
- Histopathology may be required for a definitive diagnosis in many cases.
- High amylase and lipase activities and possibly trypsin-like immunoreactivity (TLI) concentrations are usually present in the fluid.

THERAPEUTICS

Drug(s) of Choice

- Very few cases of pancreatic pseudocysts have been published and therefore definitive treatment recommendations cannot be made.
- Small pseudocysts may remain undiagnosed and may resolve spontaneously. Follow-up of small pseudocysts via noninvasive imaging (e.g., ultrasound) may be recommended.
- Fine-needle aspiration may be helpful in cases that are stable but require some intervention. Repeated aspirations may be needed. Such cases should be monitored closely.

■ Supportive care (e.g., fluid therapy, analgesia, antiemetics, nutrition) may be required in cases where clinical signs such as vomiting, diarrhea, and anorexia are present. Antibiotics should be used if infection is present.

Nursing Care

Supportive care and patient monitoring are required in cases with severe clinical signs or when pseudocysts are medically managed.

Diet

Typically, a low-fat diet is recommended in dogs with pancreatitis; a moderate-fat/high-protein diet is usually recommended for cats.

Activity

The patient's activity should be restricted.

Surgical Considerations

■ Surgical intervention is recommended for the treatment of large pancreatic pseudocysts or smaller pseudocysts that cause problems or that do not resolve with medical treatment or when infection is present.
■ Techniques are poorly described but are similar to those described for pancreatic abscesses.

 COMMENTS

Client Education

■ Pancreatic pseudocyst is a rare complication of pancreatitis.
■ Some cases will be managed medically but some cases are severe and may require hospitalization and surgery.
■ Prognosis is good to guarded.

Patient Monitoring

Continuous patient monitoring may be required in some severe cases, especially when medical management is chosen.

Possible Complications

■ Ascites (septic or sterile inflammatory exudate) may be seen with rupture of the cyst.
■ Extrahepatic biliary tract obstruction.
■ Several other complications may be seen as a result of surgery.

Expected Course and Prognosis

Unknown.

Abbreviations

■ FNA = fine needle aspiration
■ TLI = trypsin-like immunoreactivity

See Also

■ Nutritional Approach to Exocrine Pancreatic Disease
■ Pancreatic Abscess
■ Pancreatic Neoplasia
■ Pancreatitis, Canine
■ Pancreatitis, Feline

Suggested Reading

Coleman M, Robson M. Pancreatic masses following pancreatitis: pancreatic pseudocysts, necrosis, and abscesses. Compendium 2005;27:147–154.

Schaer M. Abscess, necrosis, pseudocyst, phlegmon, and infection. In: Washabau RJ, Day MJ, eds. Canine and Feline Gastroenterology. St Louis: Elsevier, 2013.

Xenoulis PG, Steiner JM, Monnet E. Pancreatitis. In: Monnet E, ed. Small Animal Soft Tissue Surgery. Ames: Wiley-Blackwell, 2013.

Author: Panagiotis G. Xenoulis DVM, Dr.med.vet., PhD

Chapter 101

Pancreatitis, Canine

DEFINITION/OVERVIEW

- Inflammation of the pancreas associated with a mixed inflammatory infiltrate.
- Classified as acute or chronic based on the speed of onset and severity of clinical signs as well as the presence or absence of irreversible histologic changes such as tissue fibrosis.

ETIOLOGY/PATHOPHYSIOLOGY

- Premature intrapancreatic activation of zymogens, such as trypsinogen, results in local inflammation (mainly neutrophils and macrophages), edema, and necrosis of the pancreas and peripancreatic fat.
- The release of pancreatic enzymes and inflammatory cytokines results in local (abdominal pain, anorexia, vomiting) as well as possible systemic signs (pyrexia, systemic inflammatory response syndrome (SIRS), multiple organ dysfunction syndrome (MODS), and acute kidney injury (AKI)).
- Although an autoimmune mechanism similar to that seen in humans is suspected in English cocker spaniels, this remains unproven.

Systems Affected

- Cardiovascular – loss of plasma proteins secondary to loss of endothelial cell function results in decreased oncotic pressure and hypovolemia. Circulating inflammatory cytokines as well as electrolyte abnormalities (hypocalcemia, hypokalemia) can result in cardiac arrhythmias.
- Gastrointestinal (GI) – local and/or generalized sterile peritonitis can occur secondary to increased vascular permeability. Local inflammation with mucosal breakdown can cause bacterial translocation from the GI tract.
- Hemic/lymphatic/immune – in severe cases of acute pancreatitis, circulating proinflammatory cytokines, in combination with altered endothelial cell function, can result in complications such as SIRS and/or disseminated intravascular coagulation (DIC).
- Hepatobiliary – significant hepatocellular damage can occur secondary to regional inflammation, release of pancreatic enzymes into the peritoneal cavity, and ischemic injury. Inflammation of the pancreas can also result in extrahepatic biliary duct obstruction (extrahepatic cholestasis).
- Renal/urologic – AKI can occur as a consequence of MODS.
- Respiratory – regional vasculitis can cause pulmonary edema and/or pleural effusion. In severe cases, life-threatening acute respiratory distress syndrome can develop.

Blackwell's Five-Minute Veterinary Consult Clinical Companion: Small Animal Gastrointestinal Diseases,
First Edition. Edited by Jocelyn Mott and Jo Ann Morrison.
© 2019 John Wiley & Sons, Inc. Published 2019 by John Wiley & Sons, Inc.
Companion website: www.fiveminutevet.com/gastrointestinal

SIGNALMENT/HISTORY

- Miniature schnauzers, Yorkshire terriers, and other terrier breeds appear to be predisposed to development of acute pancreatitis. Cocker and Cavalier King Charles spaniels are at increased risk of chronic pancreatitis. A possible association exists between the development of pancreatitis and missense or insertion mutations in the gene encoding pancreatic secretory trypsin inhibitor (SPINK1) in miniature schnauzers.
- No clear gender associations have been identified although females are overrepresented in some reports.
- Although most dogs with pancreatitis are middle to older aged (>7 years), dogs of any age can be affected.

Risk Factors

- Breed – miniature schnauzers, terriers.
- Dietary indiscretion – access to garbage or fatty table foods.
- Hypertriglyceridemia – while an association exists between hypertriglyceridemia and pancreatitis, a causative link remains unclear.
- Infectious – vector-borne diseases (babesiosis, ehrlichiosis, and leishmaniasis) have been identified in some cases of acute pancreatitis.
- Drugs/toxins – idiosyncratic reactions to certain drugs (l-asparaginase, azathioprine, chlorpromazine, clomipramine) have been described. Potassium bromide has been associated with the development of pancreatitis. Zinc toxicosis, mainly from ingestion of pennies minted after 1982, has also been identified as a cause of pancreatitis.
- Hypercalcemia – although not specifically documented in dogs, increased serum calcium concentrations have been shown to cause pancreatitis in multiple species.
- Surgery – possible risk factor, likely secondary to intraoperative hypoperfusion or traumatic manipulation of the pancreas.

Historical Findings

- Duration of clinical signs as well as severity can be variable, depending on the form of disease (acute vs chronic pancreatitis).
- Common manifestations can include lethargy, decreased appetite, abdominal pain, vomiting, and diarrhea +/– hematochezia.

 CLINICAL FEATURES

- Acute pancreatitis – lethargy and dehydration. Cranial abdominal pain is usually evident. Patient might display "prayer position" (kneeling) due to abdominal discomfort (Figure 101.1). Fever and icterus can occasionally be seen in severe cases.
- Chronic pancreatitis – findings can be very mild and nonspecific: lethargy, mild abdominal pain.

 DIFFERENTIAL DIAGNOSIS

- Gastrointestinal (obstruction, septic peritonitis, GI ulcer, GI neoplasia) – presence of an obstructive mass or obstructive pattern on abdominal imaging, free gas in the abdomen, abnormal intestinal wall layering, and presence of septic exudate in the abdomen.
- Hepatobiliary (cholangiohepatitis, copper hepatopathy, mucocele, neoplasia, toxicity) – abnormal fasting and/or postprandial bile acids, abdominal imaging showing significant

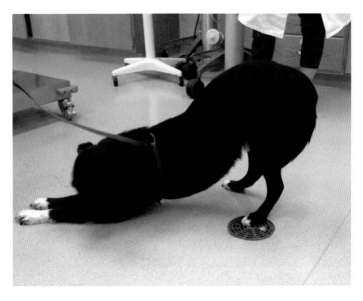

■ **Fig. 101.1.** Dog in prayer position.

gallbladder pathology, presence of neoplastic or inflammatory cells on liver histopathology, hepatic copper quantification.

■ Genitourinary (AKI, pyelonephritis, leptospirosis, uroabdomen, pyometra, prostatitis) – minimum database could reveal azotemia, hyperphosphatemia, hyperkalemia, isosthenuric urine, active urinary sediment; positive urine culture; leptospiral microscopic agglutination titers showing either a single titer of >1:1600 or convalescent titers showing a four-fold increase. Abdominal imaging showing uterine, prostatic or urinary bladder pathology.

■ Other – hypoadrenocorticism: concurrent hyponatremia and hyperkalemia, lack of a stress leukogram on minimum database, resting cortisol of less than 2 µg/dL, adrenocorticotropic hormone (ACTH) stimulation serum cortisol of <1 µg/dL; splenic torsion: finding of splenomegaly with abnormal splenic positioning on abdominal imaging.

 ## DIAGNOSTICS

Complete Blood Count/Biochemistry/Urinalysis

■ Complete blood cell count – in cases of acute pancreatitis, inflammatory leukograms with or without a left shift and toxic cellular changes can occur. In cases with DIC, thrombocytopenia might be present. Increased packed cell volume (PCV) might be noted secondary to hemoconcentration.

■ Chemistry – fluid losses secondary to vomiting and diarrhea result in a prerenal azotemia and electrolyte changes (hypokalemia, hypernatremia). Hypocalcemia, thought to be a consequence of autodigestion of mesenteric fat, is occasionally noted. Alkaline phosphatase (ALP), alanine aminotransferase (ALT), and gamma-glutamyl transferase (GGT) increases are noted secondary to focal inflammation or release of pancreatic enzymes. Hyperbilirubinemia can occur secondary to intra- or extrahepatic biliary tract obstruction. Hypercholesterolemia and hypertriglyceridemia are commonly noted.

■ Urinalysis – increased specific gravity consistent with dehydration.

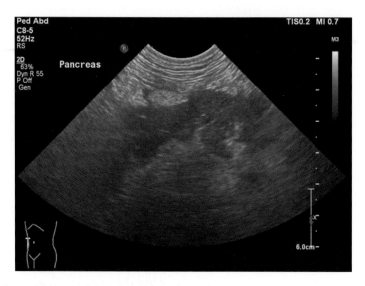

■ **Fig. 101.2.** Ultrasound image of the pancreas of a dog with acute pancreatitis. Note the diffusely hypoechoic pancreatic parenchyma and the surrounding hypeechoic mestenteric fat.

Imaging

- Radiographs – loss of serosal detail in the cranial abdomen, secondary to focal peritonitis with effusion, is seen in almost one-quarter of acute pancreatitis cases.
- Ultrasound – findings consistent with pancreatitis (hypoechoic pancreas, hyperechoic peri-pancreatic fat, focal peritonitis) are found in 60–70% of cases (Figure 101.2).

Additional Diagnostic Tests

- Pancreatic enzyme testing – amylase and lipase can be increased in cases of pancreatitis. However, since these enzymes can be produced in other tissues, their increases are not specific for pancreatitis and/or may be elevated in association with reduced glomerular filtration.
- Pancreatic lipase immunoreactivity (PLI) is the most sensitive and specific assay currently available for pancreatitis. This test is available as a quantitative (SPEC cPL, Idexx Laboratories, Westbrook, Maine) as well as a cage-side semi-quantitative (SNAP cPL, Idexx Laboratories, Westbrook, Maine) assay. The SNAP cPL assay is very effective at ruling out pancreatitis, but positive results should always be confirmed with a quantitative assay. Although renal failure can increase PLI values, they remain with reference range.
- Trypsin-like immunoreactivity (TLI) – although this assay is specific for exocrine pancreatic function, it has poor sensitivity for pancreatitis and is not recommended for diagnosis of pancreatitis.
- Pancreatic biopsy – although considered the gold standard, the sensitivity of histopathology for pancreatitis is limited due to the focal nature of the disease. In addition, canine post-mortem studies have found histopathologic pancreatic lesions consistent with pancreatitis in dogs with no clinical suspicion of the disease.

Pathologic Findings

- Acute pancreatitis – gross findings can include pancreatic hemorrhage and congestion with peripancreatic fat necrosis. Microscopic findings can include predominantly neutrophilic infiltrates with possible tissue necrosis, edema, and hemorrhage.
- Chronic pancreatitis – gross findings can include decreased size and irregular greyish appearance. Microscopic changes are characterized by predominantly lymphocytic infiltrations with periductular fibrosis.

THERAPEUTICS

- Since inciting causes of pancreatitis are rarely identified, treatment of pancreatitis is mainly supportive. However, a thorough history and diagnostic work-up are recommended in order to identify any causes that can be eliminated (drugs, toxins, infectious diseases).
- Successful treatment is based on aggressive fluid resuscitation with intravenous isotonic crystalloids (0.9% NaCl, lactated Ringer's solution) to encourage perfusion of the pancreas.
- If the patient is showing signs of hypovolemia, initial resuscitation with ¼ shock bolus (20 mL/kg) of isotonic crystalloids over 15 minutes is recommended with reassessment of the patient's condition afterwards. If the patient is dehydrated but not hypovolemic, rehydration at a slower rate (over 6–8 h) can be pursued based on estimated percentage of dehydration (volume (mL) = % dehydration × body weight (kg) × 1000).
- In cases where hypoalbuminemia is present, colloid support with synthetic colloids (Voluven®, hetastarch) or plasma might be needed (10–20 mL/kg/day).
- Hypokalemia is often present due to vomiting and diarrhea. Potassium supplementation with intravenous fluids is necessary to maintain normokalemia. Supplementation should not surpass 0.5 mEq/kg/h.

Drug(s) of Choice

- Analgesic – fentanyl as an IV constant rate infusion (2–5 μg/kg/h); buprenorphine (0.01–0.02 mg/kg 3–4 times daily IV or IM). Because some dogs will be in a compromised hemodynamic state, nonsteroidal antiinflammatory drugs (carprofen, meloxicam, deracoxib, etc.) should be avoided.
- Antiemetics – maropitant 1 mg/kg SQ once daily; ondansetron 0.5–1.0 mg/kg IV or SQ three times daily; metoclopramide as an IV constant rate infusion (2 mg/kg/day).
- Antibiotics – usually not indicated since pancreatitis is a sterile process. In cases of severe acute pancreatitis where bacterial translocation from the GI tract is suspected, broad-spectrum antibiotic therapy is recommended (ampicillin/sulbactam 30 mg/kg IV three times daily).
- Fresh frozen plasma – although controversial, some clinicians recommend the use of fresh frozen plasma to replenish alpha-2-macroglobulin, albumin, and coagulation factors.
- Glucocorticoids – use of corticosteroids has not been shown to be of any benefit in cases of pancreatitis in human or veterinary medicine. However, some clinicians do report anecdotal benefit in severe cases of chronic pancreatitis.

Precautions/Interactions

- Anticholinergics.
- Azathioprine.
- Chlorothiazide.
- L-asparaginase.
- Meglumine antimonite.
- Potassium bromide.

Appropriate Health Care

Most cases require temporary hospitalization to stabilize and control vomiting.

Nursing Care

Patients with pancreatitis can be at increased risk of aspiration pneumonia because of the concurrent presence of vomiting and lethargy. Therefore, aggressive management of vomiting (antiemetics and promotility drugs, suction of gastric contents with nasogastric tube) as well as nursing care (maintain in sternal recumbency with elevated head) should be instituted to minimize this complication.

Diet

- Food should be withheld as long as the patient has uncontrolled vomiting.
- Continued enteral feeding should be encouraged as it helps support enterocyte health, decreases chances of bacterial translocation, and decreases incidence of vomiting episodes in dogs with pancreatitis.
- Feeding cranial to the duodenum (prepyloric) has been shown to be a safe approach to feeding pancreatitis cases. Therefore, if the patient is not eating voluntarily, assisted feedings with nasoesophageal, nasogastric or esophageal feeding tubes should be used to deliver low-fat diets. High-protein/high-fat diets should be avoided since they may promote pancreatic secretions and delayed gastric emptying.

Surgical Considerations

- Elective surgical interventions should be avoided in patients with active pancreatitis due to the risk of hypoperfusion to the pancreas. Whenever possible, minimally invasive techniques (laparoscopy) or alternatives to surgery (ultrasound-guided percutaneous drainage) should be used.
- Surgical intervention may be indicated if there is suspicion of an infected necrotic area of the pancreas, pancreatic abscess, or pancreatic enlargement causing extrahepatic biliary obstruction.

 COMMENTS

Client Education

Clients should be informed about the possible complications, variable clinical severity, and risk of reoccurrence associated with pancreatitis.

Patient Monitoring

- The patient's hydration status as well as electrolyte levels should be monitored frequently. Special attention should be paid to development of systemic signs suggestive of SIRS or MODS (increased respiratory rate, decreased urine production, bleeding).
- Pancreatitis is a painful condition. The patient's need for more or less aggressive pain control should be frequently reassessed.
- Since ultrasound findings can lag behind clinical improvement and circulating PLI levels can remain increased for extended periods, the decision of when a patient is ready to be discharged from veterinary care should be based on the overall clinical disease activity.

Prevention/Avoidance

Patients with a history of pancreatitis should be fed a low-fat diet and medications known to be triggers for pancreatitis should be avoided.

Possible Complications

- Acute complications – extrahepatic biliary tract obstruction, aspiration pneumonia, SIRS, MODS.
- Chronic complications – exocrine pancreatic insufficiency, diabetes mellitus.

Expected Course and Prognosis

- Negative prognostic factors – increases in blood urea/creatinine, thrombocytopenia and marked increases in SpecPL have been associated with increased mortality. Increased ALT has been associated with extended hospitalization in dogs with acute pancreatitis.
- Prognosis is generally good for mild cases. Severe cases with development of SIRS/MODS have a more guarded prognosis.

Abbreviations

- ACTH = adrenocorticotropic hormone
- AKI = acute kidney injury
- ALP = alkaline phosphatase
- ALT = alanine aminotransferase
- DIC = disseminated intravascular coagulation
- GGT = gamma-glutamyl transferase

- GI = gastrointestinal
- MODS = multiple organ dysfunction syndrome
- PLI = pancreatic lipase immunoreactivity
- SIRS = systemic inflammatory response syndrome
- TLI = trypsin-like immunoreactivity

See Also

- Acute Abdomen
- Icterus
- Pancreatic Abscess
- Pancreatic Neoplasia
- Pancreatic Nodular Hyperplasia

- Pancreatic Parasites
- Pancreatic Pseudocysts
- Pancreatitis, Feline
- Vomiting, Acute

Suggested Reading

Thompson LJ, Seshadri R, Raffe MR. Characteristics and outcomes in surgical management of severe acute pancreatitis: 37 dogs (2001-2007). J Vet Emerg Crit Care 2009;19:165–173.

Xenoulis P. Diagnosis of pancreatitis in dogs and cats. J Small Anim Pract 2015;56:13–26.

Xenoulis PG, Steiner JM. SNAP tests for pancreatitis in dogs and cats: SNAP canine pancreatic lipase and SNAP feline pancreatic lipase. Topic Compan Anim Med 2016;31:134–139.

Authors: Jean-Sébastien Palerme DVM, MSc, DACVIM, Albert E. Jergens DVM, PhD, DACVIM

Chapter 102

Pancreatitis, Feline

DEFINITION/OVERVIEW

- Inflammation of the pancreas most often of unknown cause(s).
- Acute pancreatitis – inflammation of the pancreas that occurs abruptly with little or no permanent pathologic change.
- Chronic pancreatitis – continuing inflammatory disease that is accompanied by irreversible morphologic change such as fibrosis. Some clinicians report this form as most common.

ETIOLOGY/PATHOPHYSIOLOGY

- Host defense mechanisms normally prevent pancreatic autodigestion by pancreatic enzymes, but under select circumstances, these natural defenses fail; autodigestion occurs when these digestive enzymes are activated within acinar cells.
- Local and systemic tissue injury is due to the activity of released pancreatic enzymes and a variety of inflammatory mediators, such as kinins, free radicals, and complement factors, released by infiltrating neutrophils and macrophages. The most common pathologies involving the feline pancreas include acute necrotizing pancreatitis (ANP) and acute suppurative pancreatitis.
- Etiology is most often unknown; possibilities include the following.
  - Hepatobiliary tract disease – both inflammatory and degenerative (hepatic lipidosis).
  - Pancreatic trauma/ischemia.
  - Duodenal reflux.
  - Drugs/toxins (organophosphates).
  - Pancreatic duct obstruction.
  - Hypercalcemia.
  - Inflammatory gastrointestinal disease.
  - Nutrition – excessive lean body mass is associated with ANP.

Systems Affected

- Gastrointestinal – altered gastrointestinal (GI) motility (ileus) due to regional chemical peritonitis; local or generalized peritonitis due to enhanced vascular permeability; concurrent inflammatory bowel disease (IBD) may be seen in some cats.
- Hepatobiliary – lesions due to shock, pancreatic enzyme injury, inflammatory cellular infiltrates, hepatic lipidosis, and intra/extrahepatic cholestasis. Feline gastrointestinal inflammatory disease (concurrent cholangitis +/– inflammatory bowel disease) may be seen in some cats.
- Respiratory – pulmonary edema or pleural effusion.

Blackwell's Five-Minute Veterinary Consult Clinical Companion: Small Animal Gastrointestinal Diseases,
First Edition. Edited by Jocelyn Mott and Jo Ann Morrison.
© 2019 John Wiley & Sons, Inc. Published 2019 by John Wiley & Sons, Inc.
Companion website: www.fiveminutevet.com/gastrointestinal

- Cardiovascular – cardiac arrhythmias may result from release of myocardial depressant factor.
- Hematologic – activation of the coagulation cascade and systemic consumptive coagulopathy (DIC) may occur.

 SIGNALMENT/HISTORY

- No genetic basis for disease pathogenesis has been identified.
- True prevalence is unknown but it is a relatively common clinical disorder.
- Necropsy surveys suggest an increased prevalence in cats with cholangitis, and inflammatory bowel disease. The unique feline pancreaticobiliary anatomy and resident intestinal microbiota likely contribute to multiorgan inflammatory disease in this species.
- Cat of any age. Mean age for acute pancreatitis is 7.3 years.
- There may be breed predilection with Siamese cats and domestic shorthairs.

Risk Factors

- Breed.
- Obesity.
- Organophosphate poisoning.
- Concurrent hepatic/intestinal inflammatory disease.

Historical Findings

- Vague, nonspecific, and nonlocalizing signs. Anorexia, lethargy, and vomiting are reported most frequently.
- Lethargy/anorexia.
- Vomiting.
- Weakness.
- Abdominal pain.
- Diarrhea – small bowel and large bowel diarrhea and fever are less common in cats than dogs.

 CLINICAL FEATURES

- Severe lethargy.
- Dehydration – common; due to GI losses.
- Abdominal pain – may adopt a "prayer position" and/or resist abdominal palpation. Abdominal pain is recognized much less frequently in cats than dogs.
- Mass lesions may be palpable.
- Fever – observed in 25% of cats.

 DIFFERENTIAL DIAGNOSIS

- GI disease (obstruction, foreign body, perforation, infectious gastroenteritis, ulcer disease) – exclude with complete blood cell count/biochemistry/urinalysis, diagnostic imaging, and paracentesis. Gastrointestinal or hepatic neoplasia – exclude with tissue biopsy.
- Urogenital disease (pyelonephritis, prostatitis or abscessation, pyometra, urinary tract rupture or obstruction, acute renal failure) – exclude with complete blood cell count/biochemistry/ urinalysis, urine culture/sensitivity, and imaging.
- Hepatobiliary disease (cholangitis and extrahepatic biliary obstruction (EHBO)) – exclude with complete blood cell count/biochemistry/urinalysis, bile acids, imaging, and liver biopsy.
- Abdominal neoplasia – exclude with imaging and cytology or biopsy.

DIAGNOSTICS

Complete Blood Count/Biochemistry/Urinalysis

- Complete blood count – often reveals nonregenerative anemia (40%), leukocytosis (38%), and/or leukopenia (15%).
- Serum biochemistries – often show prerenal azotemia; liver enzyme activities (ALT, ALP) are often elevated because of hepatic ischemia or exposure to pancreatic enzymes; hyperbilirubinemia with intra/extrahepatic biliary obstruction; hyperglycemia with necrotizing pancreatitis due to hyperglucagonemia; hypoalbuminemia, hypercholesterolemia, and hypertriglyceridemia are common. Hypocalcemia is more common in cats than dogs, and a low ionized calcium concentration is a negative prognostic indicator in cats.
- Urinalysis – increased urine specific gravity associated with dehydration or can be unremarkable.

Other Laboratory Tests

- Serum pancreatic lipase immunoreactivity (fPL) is a highly sensitive and specific serologic marker of acute pancreatic inflammation. A cage-side fPL assay (SNAP fPL) has been developed as a useful screening tool.
- Elevation in SNAP fPL should be followed up by laboratory measurement of serum Spec fPL to quantitate the degree of elevation.

Imaging

- Abdominal radiographs – may include increased soft tissue opacity in the right cranial abdominal compartment; loss of visceral detail ("ground glass appearance") due to abdominal effusion; static gas pattern in the proximal duodenum.
- Abdominal ultrasound – nonhomogeneous solid or cystic mass lesions suggest pancreatic abscess; may be a pancreatic mass or altered echogenicity (hypoechoic) in the area of the pancreas; pancreas is usually enlarged with irregular borders, surrounding mesentery may be hyperechoic due to focal peritonitis, may see peritoneal effusion and extrahepatic biliary obstruction.
- fPL assay and pancreatic ultrasound in combination have the highest specificity for an antemortem diagnosis of acute pancreatitis.

Other Diagnostic Procedures

- Ultrasound-guided needle aspiration biopsy may confirm inflammation (cytology), abscess, or cyst.
- Laparoscopy with pancreatic forceps biopsy for histologic diagnosis.
- Histopathologic evaluation may miss focal or segmental pancreatic inflammation and results should be interpreted with caution.

Pathologic Findings

- Gross findings (acute pancreatitis) – mild swelling with edematous pancreatitis.
- Gross findings (chronic pancreatitis) – pancreas is reduced in size, firm, gray, and irregular; may contain extensive adhesions to surrounding viscera.
- Microscopic changes (acute pancreatitis) – include edema, parenchymal necrosis, hemorrhage, and neutrophilic cellular infiltrate with acute lesions.
- Microscopic changes (chronic pancreatitis) – pancreatic fibrosis around ducts, ductal epithelial hyperplasia, atrophy, and mononuclear cellular infiltrate.

THERAPEUTICS

Drug(s) of Choice

- Animals with intermittent vomiting should be treated with antiemetics. Maropitant (1 mg/kg SQ or PO q24h) or ondansetron (0.1–0.2 mg/kg slow IV q12h) are good first-choice options.
- Analgesics to relieve abdominal pain, e.g., butorphanol (0.1–0.4 mg/kg SQ q6h), buprenorphine (0.005–0.015 mg/kg IM or IV q6–12h) or fentanyl CRI (2–4 µg/kg/h) as needed.
- Antibiotics *only* if evidence of sepsis from bacterial translocation and to prevent pancreatic infection.

Precautions/Interactions

- Anticholinergics (e.g., atropine).
- Azathioprine.
- Chlorothiazide.
- Estrogens.
- Furosemide.
- Tetracycline.
- L-asparaginase.
- Only use antibiotics if a clear clinical condition exists, such as infection.

Appropriate Health Care

- Eliminate the inciting cause (if possible).
- Supportive care is most important.
- Aggressive IV fluid therapy. Fluid therapy goals – correct hypovolemia and maintain pancreatic microcirculation.
- An isotonic crystalloid such as lactated Ringer's solution (LRS) or Normosol-R® is the first-choice rehydration fluid.
- Correct initial dehydration (mL = % dehydration × weight in kg × 1000) and give over 4–6 h.
- May need colloids to improve pancreatic circulatory needs and prevent ischemia.
- Following replacement of deficits, give additional fluids to match maintenance requirements (2.5 × weight in kg) and ongoing losses (estimated).
- Potassium chloride (KCl) supplementation usually needed because of potassium loss in the vomitus; base potassium supplementation on measured serum levels (use 20 mEq of KCl/L of IV fluid if serum potassium levels are not known; do not administer faster than 0.5 mEq/kg/h).

Diet

- Continue to feed orally unless vomiting is intractable; feeding maintains intestinal epithelial integrity and minimizes bacterial translocation.
- Initiate enteral feeding via esophagostomy, gastrostomy enteral feeding device, or nasoesophageal tube placement.
- NPO in animals with persistent vomiting for the shortest time possible; when there has been no vomiting for 12 hours, offer small volumes of water; if tolerated, begin small, frequent feedings of a diet that does not contain excessive amounts of dietary fat. Most nutritionists agree that excessive dietary fat restriction is not necessary in cats with pancreatitis.

Activity

Restrict.

Surgical Considerations

- May need surgery to remove pseudocysts, abscesses, or devitalized tissue seen with necrotizing pancreatitis.
- May need laparotomy and pancreatic biopsy to confirm pancreatitis and/or rule out other, nonpancreatic diseases such as hepatic cholangitis, lipidosis, and/or IBD.
- Extrahepatic biliary obstruction from pancreatitis requires ductal decompression with surgical correction.

 COMMENTS

Client Education

- Discuss the need for extended hospitalization.
- Discuss the expense of diagnosis and treatment.
- Discuss possible short-term and long-term complications.

Patient Monitoring

- Evaluate hydration status closely during first 24 hours of therapy; twice-daily check including physical examination, body weight, hematocrit, total plasma protein, BUN, and urine output. Evaluate the effectiveness of fluid therapy after 24 hours and adjust flow rates and fluid composition accordingly; repeat biochemistries to assess electrolyte/acid–base status.
- Watch closely for systemic complications involving a variety of organ systems; perform appropriate diagnostic tests as needed.
- Gradually taper fluids down to maintenance requirements if possible. Maintain oral alimentation or enteral nutrition as described above, being careful to feed diets that do not contain excessive amounts of dietary fat.
- Monitor for clinical evidence of IBD and/or hepatobiliary disease and treat accordingly.
- Monitor for progression to diabetes mellitus, exocrine pancreatic insufficiency (EPI), and/or hepatic lipidosis in cats with ANP.

Prevention/Avoidance

- Weight reduction if obese.
- Avoid high-fat diets.

Possible Complications

- Failed response to supportive therapy.
- Life-threatening associated conditions such as EPI, diabetes mellitus, and hepatic lipidosis.
- Progression of acute pancreatitis to chronic pancreatitis.

Life-Threatening

- Pulmonary edema (e.g., adult respiratory distress syndrome).
- Cardiac arrhythmias.
- Peritonitis.
- DIC.

Non-Life-Threatening

- Diabetes mellitus.
- EPI.
- Chronic pancreatitis.
- Cholangitis and hepatic lipidosis.
- Inflammatory bowel disease.

Expected Course and Prognosis

- Guarded for most patients with ANP; cats with multi-organ inflammation may be less responsive to treatment.
- More guarded to poor for patients with severe necrotizing pancreatitis, decreased ionized calcium fraction, and systemic conditions.

Abbreviations

- ALP = alkaline phosphatase
- ALT = alanine aminotransferase
- ANP = acute necrotizing pancreatitis
- BUN = blood urea nitrogen
- CRI = constant rate infusion
- DIC = disseminated intravascular coagulation
- EHBO = extrahepatic biliary obstruction
- EPI = exocrine pancreatic insufficiency
- fPL = feline pancreatic lipase immunoreactivity
- GI = gastrointestinal
- IBD = inflammatory bowel disease
- NPO = nothing *per os*

See Also

- Acute Abdomen
- Cholangitis/Cholangiohepatitis Syndrome
- Exocrine Pancreatic Insufficiency
- Inflammatory Bowel Disease

Suggested Reading

Simpson KW. Pancreatitis and triaditis in cats: causes and treatment. J Small Anim Pract 2015;56:40–49.

Stockhaus C, Teske E, Schellenberger K, et al. Serial serum feline pancreatic lipase immunoreactivity concentrations and prognostic variables in 33 cats with pancreatitis. J Am Vet Med Assoc 2013; 243:1713–1718.

Author: Albert E. Jergens DVM, PhD, DACVIM

Clinical Signs of Hepatobiliary Disease

Chapter 103

Icterus

DEFINITION/OVERVIEW

- Icterus, also known as jaundice, is the yellow discoloration of the mucous membranes, skin, and sclera that occurs secondary to the presence of increased serum levels of bilirubin (hyperbilirubinemia).
- Serum bilirubin levels must exceed approximately 2 mg/dL for icterus to be clinically detectable.

ETIOLOGY/PATHOPHYSIOLOGY

- Bilirubin is the product of the degradation of heme-containing molecules such as (predominantly) hemoglobin, myoglobin, and p450 cytochrome enzymes.
- During red blood cell senescence, macrophages of the reticuloendothelial system in the bone marrow, spleen, and liver cleave hemoglobin into heme and globin. Heme is then degraded into biliverdin and iron. Biliverdin (green pigment) is subsequently converted to bilirubin (yellow pigment) by bilirubin reductase. This unconjugated bilirubin is transported to the liver bound to albumin, where it is conjugated to glucoronic acid and excreted into the bile. Conjugated bilirubin is then stored in the gallbladder before being secreted into the small intestine via the common bile duct. In the colon, bilirubin is metabolized to urobilinogen by the intestinal flora and finally oxidized to stercobilin, which imparts the characteristic brown color to stool.
- Although over 80% of the urobilinogen is excreted in the feces, 10–20% is reabsorbed via enterohepatic circulation. In addition, approximately 5% of the reabsorbed urobilinogen is renally excreted.
- Hyperbilirubinemia occurs when bilirubin production exceeds the hepatobiliary system's capacity for elimination. Since icterus is a specific consequence of hyperbilirubinemia, its causes are generally categorized based on the step at which bilirubin is accumulating: prehepatic (hemolysis), hepatic (decreased conjugation and biliary excretion of bilirubin), or posthepatic (decreased excretion of bile).

Systems Affected

- Cardiovascular – in cases of prehepatic icterus (hemolysis), decreased oxygen-carrying capacity results in increased respiratory and heart rates. Also, decreased blood viscosity from moderate to marked anemia can cause a physiologic heart murmur.
- Nervous – in cases of icterus caused by severe liver dysfunction, hepatic detoxification of neurotoxins (mainly ammonia) is compromised, causing multiple neurologic signs such as depression, nausea, cortical blindness, and seizures (hepatic encephalopathy).

Blackwell's Five-Minute Veterinary Consult Clinical Companion: Small Animal Gastrointestinal Diseases,
First Edition. Edited by Jocelyn Mott and Jo Ann Morrison.
© 2019 John Wiley & Sons, Inc. Published 2019 by John Wiley & Sons, Inc.
Companion website: www.fiveminutevet.com/gastrointestinal

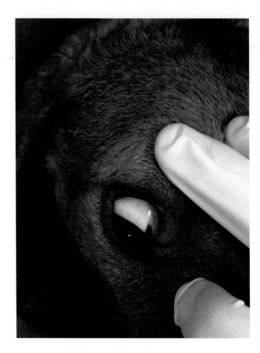

■ **Fig. 103.1.** Icteric conjunctiva in a dog with immune-mediated hemolytic anemia.

■ Ophthalmic – deposition of bilirubin in the sclera will cause their appearance to shift from white to a pale to dark yellow (Figure 103.1).
■ Renal/urologic – increased bilirubin metabolism indirectly results in increased renal bilirubin excretion, causing a yellow to brown discoloration of the urine (bilirubinuria). In severe cases of icterus, when serum bilirubin levels exceed 30 mg/dL, acute kidney injury can result from pigmentary nephropathy.
■ Skin/exocrine – deposition of bilirubin in the subcutaneous tissues results in yellow discoloration of the skin.

 ## SIGNALMENT/HISTORY

■ Since icterus can have many causes, there are no specific breed, sex or age predilections.
■ Prehepatic icterus – English springer spaniels and American cocker spaniels are known to inherit a missense mutation of the phosphofructokinase gene causing a deficiency of the enzyme, which results in severe hemolysis; Basenjis, West Highland White Terriers, and Abyssinian and Somali cats can have an aberrant expression of the fetal form (instead of adult form) of pyruvate kinase, resulting in hemolysis.
■ Hepatic icterus – Bedlington terriers, Doberman pinschers, Labrador retrievers, and Dalmatians are predisposed to copper hepatopathies.
■ Posthepatic icterus – Shetland sheepdogs, Miniature Schnauzers, and Cocker spaniels are predisposed to gallbladder mucoceles (Figure 103.2).

Risk Factors

■ Prehepatic icterus.
  • Certain dog breeds (pit bulls and Staffordshire terriers) are at increased risk for hemolysis caused by *Babesia gibsoni* infection.

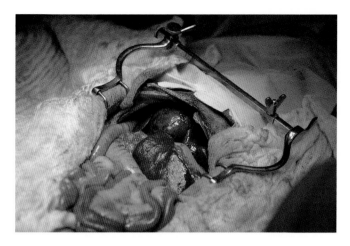

■ **Fig. 103.2.** Intraoperative picture of a gallbladder mucocele.

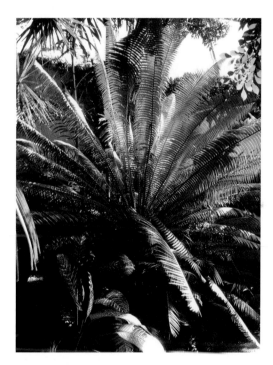

■ **Fig. 103.3.** Sago palm plant.

- Ingestion of zinc, mainly through ingestion of pennies minted after 1982, can cause hemolytic anemia.
■ Hepatic icterus.
    - Young unvaccinated dogs (infectious canine hepatitis).
    - Anorexic overweight cats (hepatic lipidosis).
    - Young purebred cats housed in catteries (feline infectious peritonitis (FIP)).
    - Exposure to toxins/drugs – voluntary (carprofen, diazepam, acetaminophen) or involuntary exposure (*Amanita* mushrooms, blue-green algae, sago palm plant (Figure 103.3), xylitol, aflatoxin) causing acute liver failure.

- Posthepatic icterus.
  - Dogs with hyperadrenocorticism and hypothyroidism are at increased risk for developing gallbladder mucoceles.
  - Ingestion of zinc, mainly through ingestion of pennies minted after 1982, can also cause pancreatitis with secondary extrahepatic biliary tract obstruction.

Historical Findings

- Pet owners will often report dark-colored urine that is sometimes confused with hematuria. In cases of severe posthepatic icterus, owners might report pale gray-colored stool (acholic feces).
- When icterus is secondary to hemolysis, owners might report a recent onset of pallor of the mucus membranes.
- With hepatic causes of icterus, owners might mention clinical signs secondary to acute or chronic liver disease such as altered mentation, abnormal bleeding, melena, polyuria and polydipsia, or abdominal distension.
- Regardless of the cause of the icterus, owners may report nonspecific clinical signs such as lethargy, weakness, anorexia or vomiting.
- Owners should be thoroughly questioned for possible exposure to hepatotoxins.

 # CLINICAL FEATURES

- Prehepatic icterus – pale mucous membranes with icterus, weakness, tachypnea, tachycardia, systolic heart murmur secondary to anemia, bounding pulse quality, hepatosplenomegaly, severe bruising.
- Hepatic and posthepatic icterus – icteric mucous membranes, hepatomegaly, palpable abdominal fluid wave (secondary to bile peritonitis or hypoalbuminemia), abdominal pain, signs of clotting abnormalities (prolonged bleeding after needle stick, melena, presence of ecchymoses and petechiae).

 # DIFFERENTIAL DIAGNOSIS

- Prehepatic icterus.
  - Immune-mediated hemolytic anemia is diagnosed with the concurrent finding of anemia with spherocytosis, autoagglutination or a positive Coombs test.
  - Infectious causes of hemolytic anemia (*Babesia* spp., *Mycoplasma hemofelis*, *Cytauxzoon felis*) can occasionally be diagnosed by light microscopy; however, polymerase chain reaction (PCR) testing is recommended due to its greater sensitivity.
  - Causes of oxidative injury should be ruled out based on a thorough history and abdominal radiographs to rule out the presence of a gastric metallic foreign body containing zinc.
  - Microangiopathic disease should be suspected if schistocytes are identified on a blood smear and should prompt investigation for hemangiosarcoma, caval syndrome, splenic torsion or disseminated intravascular coagulation (DIC).
  - Diabetic ketoacidosis (DKA) patients receiving insulin therapy and patients being fed after prolonged periods of anorexia are at increased risk of hemolytic anemia secondary to severe hypophosphatemia (refeeding syndrome).
  - Hereditary RBC defects should be considered in predisposed breeds.
- Hepatic icterus – infectious causes (bacterial cholangitis, leptospirosis, toxoplasmosis, sepsis) should be investigated with serologies as well as culture of bile and/or blood; hepatic

biopsies are required to rule out cirrhosis, copper hepatopathy, FIP or chronic hepatitis; hepatic lipidosis should be suspected with increases in ALP without concurrent gamma-glutamyl transferase (GGT) increases.

- Posthepatic icterus – abdominal imaging can allow the identification of pancreatitis, gallbladder mucocele, neoplasia (of the pancreas, biliary tract or duodenum), or cholelithiasis. The finding of free abdominal fluid in the area of the gallbladder can suggest bile peritonitis or ascites caused by hypoproteinemia.

 ## DIAGNOSTICS

Complete Blood Count/Biochemistry/Urinalysis

- Complete blood count – in cases of hemolysis, a low packed cell volume (PCV) (<25%) with concurrent normal to increased total solids is present. RBC regeneration (reticulocyte counts >60 000/μL or >40 000/μL for dogs and cats, respectively) is also common. When hemolysis is caused by immune- or infectious-mediated disease, a mild to moderate inflammatory leukogram can be present along with a mild to moderate thrombocytopenia. Blood smear review might reveal the presence of intracellular parasites or RBC morphological changes (spherocytes, schistocytes, Heinz bodies).
- Chemistry – differentiation of conjugated and unconjugated bile acids does not distinguish between causes of icterus. Moderate to severe increases in all hepatic enzymes (ALT, ALP, GGT) are common. Increases in these enzymes can be present due to primary liver disease, cholestatic disease, or hypoxemia secondary to anemia. Although ALP and GGT usually increase together, cats with hepatic lipidosis will commonly have ALP increases with a normal GGT value. In cases of hepatic synthetic failure, albumin, cholesterol, urea, and glucose serum concentrations can be decreased. Patients being treated for DKA or at risk of refeeding syndrome might have severe hypophosphatemia and hypokalemia.
- Urinalysis – bilirubinuria is an expected finding. However, mild to moderate bilirubinuria can be normal in dogs, since they have a lower renal threshold for bilirubin reabsorption than cats, and their kidneys are capable of converting heme to bilirubin and excreting it in urine. Since urinary excretion of urobilinogen is multifactorial, its absence in the urine of an icteric patient is not diagnostic for an extrahepatic bile duct obstruction.

Other Laboratory Tests

- Serum bile acids – this test is redundant in icteric patients without significant hemolysis since hyperbilirubinemia implies liver dysfunction.
- Coagulation testing – if suspicious of primary liver dysfunction, prothrombin time (PT), partial thromboplastin time (PTT), and proteins invoked by vitamin K absence (PIVKA) values should be assessed, especially if there is clinical bleeding or if fine needle aspirates or biopsies are being considered as part of the diagnostic plan.
- Leptospiral microscopic agglutination test (MAT) – since only approximately 50% of leptospirosis cases are diagnosed on a single serology, convalescent titers should be tested whenever leptospirosis is suspected.

Imaging

- Radiographs – in cases with ascites or biliary peritonitis, poor serosal detail might be present. Splenomegaly is commonly reported in cases of hemolytic disease and splenic neoplasia. Metallic foreign bodies can be detected in the stomach. Causes of extrahepatic biliary obstruction (EHBO) might be detected (abdominal mass, cholelithiasis, pancreatitis). Hepatomegaly or microhepatica can be found in cases of acute or chronic liver disease, respectively.

- Ultrasound – this can be very useful in differentiating hepatic versus posthepatic causes of icterus. A dilated biliary tree and/or bile duct, bile sludging, gallbladder mucocele, or cholelithiasis can be easily identified in cases of EHBO. Findings consistent with pancreatitis (hypoechoic pancreas with hyperechoic peripancreatic fat) can be identified. Changes in echogenicity of the liver can be present in primary liver diseases (neoplastic infiltration, hepatic lipidosis, cirrhosis, etc.). The finding of free fluid in the area of the gallbladder is suggestive of bile peritonitis.

Additional Diagnostic Tests

- Hepatic aspirates – cytology can be useful in diagnosing infiltrative neoplastic disease or hepatic lipidosis.
- Hepatic biopsies – submission for histopathology and copper quantification is required for diagnosis of chronic hepatitis, cirrhosis, cholangitis, and copper hepatopathy.
- Bile culture – more sensitive than culture of liver biopsies. Anaerobic and aerobic culture is recommended for identification of bacterial cholangitis.

 # THERAPEUTICS

Ultimately, successful treatment of icteric patients depends on correct identification and treatment of the underlying disease and the reader is directed to specific chapters about these diseases for further recommendations. However, general supportive care is indicated in all cases.

Drug(s) of Choice

- N-acetylcysteine – for acute treatment of patients with hepatotoxicities (or for those unable to take enteral medications), administer a 5% solution slowly over 20 minutes at a dose of 140 mg/kg intravenously, followed by additional doses of 70 mg/kg every 8–12 hours.
- S-adenosylmethionine (SAMe) – antioxidant therapy can be beneficial in limiting further hepatic damage. Administer 90 mg once daily PO (cats) or approximately 20 mg/kg once daily PO (dogs). SAMe should always be administered on an empty stomach.
- Silymarin – this antioxidant might also have antifibrotic effects on the liver. Administer 20–50 mg/kg/day. In cases of acute liver injury, oral bioavailability might be impaired.
- Ursodiol – this medication is proposed to enhance bile flow as well as improve the production of water-soluble bile acids. Some clinicians avoid its use in cases of EHBO due to a possible increased risk of gallbladder rupture. Administer 10–15 mg/kg once daily PO.
- Vitamin E – use of this antioxidant vitamin helps prevent lipid peroxidation in cases of liver failure and cholestasis. Administer 100–400 units once daily (dogs) or 30–50 units once daily (cats).

Precautions/Interactions

- Although rare, pigment nephropathy can occur at high serum concentrations of bilirubin (>30 mg/dL). Clinicians should monitor renal values in cases with increasing bilirubin levels and consider hemodialysis in cases where there is concern for acute kidney injury.
- When using sedatives, avoid the use of drugs that are hepatically metabolized (opioids, acepromazine, diazepam) in patients with hepatic/posthepatic icterus.

Surgical Considerations

- In all cases of hemolytic anemias where a metallic foreign body is present in the gastrointestinal tract, removal of the foreign body is indicated as any zinc-containing metal can be a trigger for the hemolysis. If endoscopic removal is not possible, gastrotomy is recommended.

- Surgical decompression (cholecystectomy, cholecystoenterotomy) is commonly required for relief of EHBO caused by gallbladder disease (mucocele, cholecystolith or neoplasia).

 ## COMMENTS

Patient Monitoring

- Prehepatic icterus – patients should have PCV and total solids monitored initially at least 2–4 times daily until values stabilize or improve. Bilirubin values should decrease as the patient's PCV increases.
- Hepatic and posthepatic icterus – failure of improvement or worsening of bilirubin values should prompt reassessment of initial diagnosis and therapeutic plan.

Possible Complications

- Prehepatic icterus – pulmonary thromboembolism is the leading cause of death of patients with immune-mediated hemolytic anemia.
- Posthepatic icterus – if EHBO cases are not managed aggressively, gallbladder rupture with bile peritonitis can occur.

Expected Course and Prognosis

While the prognosis of icterus is largely dependent on the underlying cause, the underlying diseases are often significant enough to warrant a guarded to fair prognosis.

Synonyms

- Jaundice

Abbreviations

- ALP = alkaline phosphatase
- ALT = alanine transferase
- DIC = disseminated intravascular coagulopathy
- DKA = diabetic ketoacidosis
- EHBO = extrahepatic biliary obstruction
- FIP = feline infectious peritonitis
- GGT = gamma-glutamyl transferase
- MAT = microscopic agglutination test

- PCR = polymerase chain reaction
- PCV = packed cell volume
- PIVKA = proteins invoked by vitamin K absence
- PT = prothrombin time
- PTT = partial thromboplastin time
- RBC = red blood cell
- SAMe = S-adenosylmethionine

See Also

- Bile Duct Obstruction (Extrahepatic)
- Biliary Duct or Gallbladder Rupture and Bile Peritonitis
- Biliary Neoplasia
- Cholangitis, Destructive
- Cholangitis/Cholangiohepatitis Syndrome
- Cholecystitis and Choledochitis
- Cholecystitis, Emphysematous
- Cholelithiasis
- Cirrhosis and Fibrosis of the Liver
- Copper-associated Hepatopathy
- Gallbladder Mucocele
- Hepatic Failure, Acute

- Hepatic Lipidosis
- Hepatic Neoplasia, Malignant
- Hepatitis, Chronic.
- Hepatitis, Granulomatou
- Hepatitis, Infectious (Viral) Canine
- Hepatitis, Lobular Dissecting
- Hepatitis, Nonspecific, Reactive
- Hepatitis, Suppurative and Hepatic Abscess
- Hepatopathy, Infectious
- Hepatotoxins
- Leptospirosis
- Pancreatitis, Canine
- Pancreatitis, Feline

Suggested Reading

Center SA. Metabolic, antioxidant, nutraceutical, probiotic, and herbal therapies relating to the management of hepatobiliary disorders. Vet Clin North Am Small Anim Pract 2004;34:67–172.

Mansfield C, Beths T. Management of acute pancreatitis in dogs: a critical appraisal with focus on feeding and analgesia. J Small Anim Pract 2015;56:27–39.

Watson P. Canine breed-specific hepatopathies. Vet Clin North Am Small Anim Pract 2017;47:665–682.

Acknowledgments: The author and editors acknowledge the prior contribution of Dr Sharon Center.

Author: Jean-Sébastien Palerme DVM, MSc, DACVIM

Chapter 104

Coagulopathy of Liver Disease

DEFINITION/OVERVIEW

- The liver is indispensable to formation, function, and final removal of most hemostatic factors.
- Liver or hepatobiliary disease can disrupt all phases of hemostasis, from platelet function to clot formation and breakdown. The expression of a coagulopathy is unpredictable and ranges from clinically silent test abnormalities to subclinical thrombosis or overt bleeding.

ETIOLOGY/PATHOPHYSIOLOGY

The traditional model of hepatobiliary disease causing an acquired bleeding disorder has been replaced by the concept of deficient, yet rebalanced interactions of procoagulant, antithrombotic, and fibrinolytic factors, which result in a patient that can be easily tipped towards thrombosis or hemorrhage. Processes associated with precipitating or intensifying a subclinical coagulopathy include concurrent disease, drug therapy, biopsy, or surgery. Liver diseases can have the following results.

- Hemostatic factor deficiency caused by:
  - Hepatic synthetic failure of chronic hepatitis accompanying:
    - Noninfectious hepatitis – dog: idiopathic, drugs, toxins, copper associated; cat: idiopathic, cholangitis or cholangiohepatitis.
    - Infectious hepatitis – viral, bacterial.
  - Decreased functional hepatic mass – portosystemic shunts (PSS), hepatic neoplasia (lymphoma, carcinoma, hemangiosarcoma).
- Vitamin K deficiency associated with cholestasis.
- Hypofibrinogenemia or hyperfibrinogenemia, which can be caused by hepatic synthetic failure or hepatitis, respectively.
- Disseminated intravascular coagulation (DIC) secondary to:
  - Hepatitis.
  - Decreased hepatic clearance of factors or by-products.
  - Hepatic neoplasia (lymphoma, carcinoma, hemangiosarcoma).
- Functional and quantitative platelet defects related to:
  - Defective platelet aggregation – increased bile acids, reduced hepatic clearance of factors or by-products, and increased aged, less active platelets.
  - Hyperactive platelets.
  - PSS – platelet sequestration in spleen.
  - Decreased hepatic thrombopoietin.
- Decreased anticoagulation – vitamin K deficiency, PSS, and hepatic synthetic failure.

Blackwell's Five-Minute Veterinary Consult Clinical Companion: Small Animal Gastrointestinal Diseases, First Edition. Edited by Jocelyn Mott and Jo Ann Morrison.
© 2019 John Wiley & Sons, Inc. Published 2019 by John Wiley & Sons, Inc.
Companion website: www.fiveminutevet.com/gastrointestinal

Systems Affected

Thrombosis and hemorrhage can affect every organ system, but most notable are the following.

- Vascular.
  - Microvascular thrombosis – glomerular capillary thrombosis.
  - Macrovascular thrombosis – portal vein thrombosis (cat, dog), splenic vein thrombosis (dog).
- Renal – subcapsular and renal cortical hemorrhage or infarction.
- Respiratory – pulmonary thromboembolism.

 SIGNALMENT/HISTORY

Risk Factors

- Infection – bacterial, viral, tick-borne agent.
- Endocrine disorders – hyperadrenocorticism, diabetes mellitus, hypothyroidism.
- Drugs or toxins – corticosteroids, antibiotics, nonsteroidal antiinflammatory drugs (NSAIDs).
- Neoplasia – lymphoma, hepatobiliary, splenic.
- Pancreatitis – acute necrotizing pancreatitis.
- Protein-losing enteropathy.
- Immune-mediated hemolytic anemia or thrombocytopenia.
- Protein-losing nephropathy – nephrotic syndrome.
- Cardiac disease – hypertrophic cardiomyopathy.

Historical Findings

Bleeding from nose, coughing, pigmenturia, patches of discolored skin, exercise intolerance, dark-colored stool.

 CLINICAL FEATURES

Epistaxis, hyphema, dyspnea, cyanosis, tachypnea, hemoptysis, hematemesis, hematoma, ecchymoses and petechiae, acute abdominal pain, ascites (hemoabdomen), hematuria, hematochezia, or melena.

 DIFFERENTIAL DIAGNOSIS

- DIC – secondary to other comorbid diseases, other than liver disease.
- Drug or rodenticide toxicity.
- Severe blunt force trauma.
- Severe gastrointestinal disease.
- Inherited coagulopathy.

 DIAGNOSTICS

- Minimum database for patients with hepatobiliary disease comprises a complete blood count including platelet count, clinical chemistry, urinalysis, imaging, and screening coagulation tests that include prothrombin time (PT), activated partial thromboplastin time (PTT), and thrombin time (TT) (Figure 104.1).

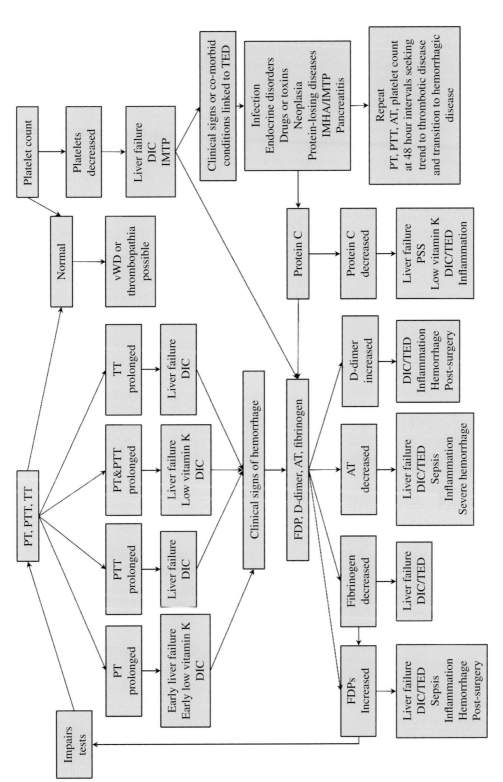

■ **Fig. 104.1.** Algorithm for diagnosis of coagulopathy of liver diseases.

- Additional coagulation testing consists of the following.
  - Testing for platelet/endothelial abnormalities comprises buccal mucosal bleeding time (BMBT), von Willebrand factor (vWf), and thromboelastography (TEG).
  - To assess fibrinolysis or risk of thrombosis, especially with comorbid risk factors (see above), add fibrinogen/fibrin degradation products (FDPs), D-dimers, antithrombin (AT), and protein C (PC).
  - TEG – bedside test that assesses function and interaction of platelets, blood cell components, procoagulant/anticoagulant factors, and fibrinolysis, by measuring kinetics of clot formation and lysis, and clot strength. Utility for pets with liver disease is limited and there is no apparent advantage over traditional coagulation testing. In humans, TEG helps detect mechanism of bleeding and evaluate response to treatment.

Significant Hemostatic Test Patterns

- Normal PT and PTT do not exclude an emerging coagulopathy or bleeding following biopsy or surgery.
- Variables that lead to PT or PTT insensitivity for predicting or detecting bleeding propensity include the following.
  - PT or PTT become prolonged when individual factors at <30% normal activity.
  - Fibrinogen less than 75 mg/dL in the dog or 50 mg/dL in the cat can prolong PT, PTT, and TT.
  - Increased FDPs can impair, PT, PTT, TT, and platelet function.
  - Not measuring interactions between platelets, endothelium or fibrinolytic, and anticoagulant system.
- PT or PTT, or both, prolonged – hepatic disease (failure or cholestasis), DIC, vitamin K deficiency, inherited factor deficiency.
- PT, PTT, and TT prolonged, and thrombocytopenia – hepatic synthetic failure and DIC. Differentiating whether a coagulopathy is caused by hepatic disease or DIC can be difficult, since these conditions can have a shared etiology and hepatic failure in itself can contribute to DIC. Coagulation testing should be expanded to include FDPs, D-dimer, fibrinogen, and AT.
- Decreased AT and PC – suggests predisposition for hypercoagulable state or thrombosis.
  - Cats – hepatic lipidosis and cholangitis.
  - Dogs – hepatic synthetic failure or congenital PSS.
- Predicting possible complication from biopsy – test <24 h before procedure.
  - Dog –fibrinogen <50% of lower reference interval or prolonged PT.
  - Cats – PTT prolonged >1.5× upper reference interval.
  - Cats and dogs – thrombocytopenia (<80,000 platelets/μL) or markedly prolonged PT or PTT (no consensus on threshold values that present increased risk).

 # THERAPEUTICS

- The objectives of treatment are to stop or minimize an ongoing coagulopathy (rescue) and prevent a procedure-induced bleed (prophylactic).
- In order to avoid iatrogenic complications, the idea of a balanced yet precarious scarcity of clotting factors and anticoagulant substances should be factored into decisions regarding therapeutic choices and postintervention testing.
- All drugs mentioned below have indications for use as both rescue and prophylactic therapies.

Drug(s) of Choice

- Fresh frozen plasma – 10–20 mL/kg IV at 4–6 mL/min up to t.i.d. until bleeding stops or coagulation times improve; may need repeating in 8–12 h.
- Fresh whole blood – 12–20 mL/kg IV.
- Vitamin K1 (phytonadione) – at least 2–3 days before surgical or biopsy procedures: 0.5–1.5 mg/kg q12h SQ with small-gauge needle up to three doses in 24-h period followed by 1 mg/kg q24h SQ or PO (provided normal enteric bile acid uptake).
- Clopidogrel – 18.75 mg/cat PO q24h or 1 mg/kg PO q24h dogs.

Precautions/Interactions

Drugs that affect any portion of the coagulation cascade (e.g., NSAIDs, corticosteroids, antibiotics, blood products) should be used with caution in patients with advanced (end-stage) chronic hepatic disease, especially in those with altered coagulation tests or decreased AT or PC activity.

Nursing Care

Patients with severe coagulopathies associated with liver disease require hospitalization for plasma and/or blood transfusions and supportive care.

Surgical Considerations

Coagulation status should be thoroughly evaluated prior to liver biopsy and/or surgical intervention.

Activity

Patients' activities should be altered to minimize conditions that can precipitate hemorrhage or thrombosis, such as blunt force trauma (e.g., exercise, rough play, falls) and heat stress.

COMMENTS

Patient Monitoring

Because hemostatic factors have half-lives as short as 6 h, changes in physical examination findings or minimum database results that forecast worsening hepatobiliary disease may signal a rapid change in coagulation status and should prompt retesting.

Possible Complications

- DIC.
- Bleeding post biopsy or with progression of liver disease
- Death.

Expected Course and Prognosis

- Prognosis depends on underlying hepatic disease.
- Patients with hepatic disease and DIC have a guarded prognosis.

Abbreviations

- AT = antithrombin
- BMBT = buccal mucosal bleeding time
- DIC = disseminated intravascular coagulation

- FDPs = fibrinogen/fibrin degradation products
- IMHA = immune-mediated hemolytic anemia

- IMTP = immune-mediated thrombocytopenia
- NSAIDs = nonsteroidal antiinflammatory drugs
- PC = protein C
- PSS = portosystemic shunts

- PT = prothrombin time
- PTT = activated partial thromboplastin time
- TED = thromboembolic disease
- TEG = thromboelastography
- TT = thrombin time
- vWD = von Willebrand's disease

See Also

- Acute Abdomen
- Bile Duct Obstruction (Extrahepatic)
- Cholangitis/Cholangiohepatitis Syndrome
- Cirrhosis and Fibrosis of the Liver
- Copper-Associated Hepatopathy
- Hematemesis
- Hematochezia
- Hepatic Lipidosis

- Hepatic Neoplasia, Malignant
- Hepatitis, Chronic
- Hepatitis, Infectious (Viral) Canine
- Hepatopathy, Infectious
- Hepatotoxins
- Melena
- Portosystemic Shunting, Acquired
- Protein-Losing Enteropathy

Suggested Reading

Hemostasis. Cornell University College of Veterinary Medicine eclinpath. Available at: www.eclinpath.com/hemostasis/

Stockham SL, Scott MA. Hemostasis. In: Stockham SL, Scott MA, eds. Fundamentals of Veterinary Clinical Pathology, 2nd ed. Ames: Blackwell Publishing, 2008.

Author: Peter J. Fernandes DVM, DACVP

Diseases of the Liver

Chapter 105

Arteriovenous Malformation of the Liver

DEFINITION/OVERVIEW

- Intrahepatic arteriovenous (AV) malformations are communications between proper hepatic arteries (high pressure) and intrahepatic portal veins (low pressure); this anatomic union results in hepatofugal (away from the liver) splanchnic circulation.
- Blood flows directly from a hepatic artery into the portal vasculature retrograde into the vena cava through multiple acquired portosystemic shunts (APSS).
- Associated with ascites, intrahepatic and extrahepatic portal hypertension, and APSS.
- Uncommon, usually congenital, but may be acquired (surgical injury, trauma, neoplasia).

ETIOLOGY/PATHOPHYSIOLOGY

- Although rare, it is typically congenital in dogs and cats.
- In most cases, a branch of the hepatic artery communicates directly with the portal vein by multiple aberrant shunting vessels within the liver. This creates a high-pressure system that results in blood flow away from the liver and arterialization of the portal vein. Due to the excessive portal hypertension that results, multiple extrahepatic shunts open to decompress the portal system.

Systems Affected

- Gastrointestinal – vomiting, diarrhea, anorexia, gastrointestinal (GI) bleeding/melena/hematemesis.
- Nervous – ataxia, unresponsiveness, pacing, circling, blindness, seizures, and coma.
- Renal/urologic – stranguria, pollakiuria, hematuria, dysuria, ammonium urate stones.

SIGNALMENT/HISTORY

- Dogs, less common in cats.
- Age-related presentation (congenital): <2 years.
- No sex or breed predilection.

Risk Factors

- Usually congenital vascular malformations (single or multiple vessels) reflecting failed differentiation of common embryologic anlage.
- Rarely secondary to abdominal trauma, inflammation, neoplasia, surgical interventions, or diagnostic procedures (e.g., liver biopsy).
- Portal hypertension.

Blackwell's Five-Minute Veterinary Consult Clinical Companion: Small Animal Gastrointestinal Diseases, First Edition. Edited by Jocelyn Mott and Jo Ann Morrison.
© 2019 John Wiley & Sons, Inc. Published 2019 by John Wiley & Sons, Inc.
Companion website: www.fiveminutevet.com/gastrointestinal

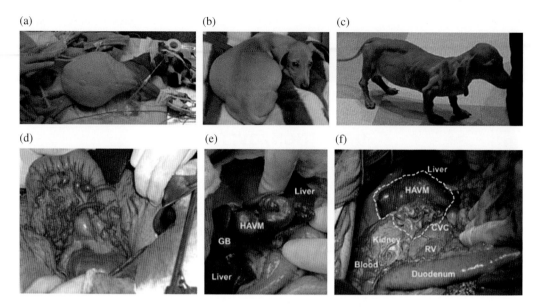

■ **Fig. 105.1.** (a) Anesthetized hepatic arteriovenous malformation (HAVM) boxer puppy with massive ascites. Dachshund puppy with HAVM prior to embolization (b) and a few weeks after embolization (c) demonstrating dramatically reduced ascites but also the often underestimated cachexia that accompanies this condition due to portal hypertension and reduced gastrointestinal absorption. (d) HAVM intraoperative picture demonstrating too numerous to count acquired extrahepatic shunts secondary to the HAVM portal hypertension. (e,f) Intraoperative pictures of HAVMs demonstrating the vascular dilation present throughout the affected liver lobes(s), multiple shunts with distended renal veins and vena cava, and often some associated bleeding.

Historical Findings

Vague or acute illness – lethargy, anorexia, vomiting, diarrhea, weight loss, polydipsia, dementia, abdominal distension, stranguria/signs of obstructive uropathy, stunted growth.

CLINICAL FEATURES

- Lethargic, poor body condition.
- Ascites in 75% of dogs (Figure 105.1a,b).
- Heart murmurs in 20% of dogs.
- Rarely, bruit auscultated over AV malformation.

DIFFERENTIAL DIAGNOSIS

- Central nervous system (CNS) signs – infectious disorders (e.g., distemper); toxicity (e.g., lead); hydrocephalus; idiopathic epilepsy; metabolic disorders (e.g., hypoglycemia, hypokalemia or hyperkalemia); hepatic encephalopathy (HE) (e.g., acquired liver disease or portosystemic vascular anomalies (PSVA)).
- Abdominal effusion.
    - Pure transudate: ascites, protein-losing nephropathy, protein-losing enteropathy, liver disease.
    - Modified transudate: congenital cardiac malformations, right-sided heart failure, pericardial tamponade, supradiaphragmatic vena caval obstruction, neoplasia, portal vein thrombosis.
    - Hemorrhage.

■ Portal hypertension – chronic hepatic disease, ductal plate malformations/congenital hepatic fibrosis, noncirrhotic or idiopathic portal hypertension, cirrhosis, portal thrombi.

DIAGNOSTICS

Complete Blood Count/Biochemistry/Urinalysis

■ Erythrocyte microcytosis (APSS), target cells, schistocytes.
■ Hypoalbuminemia with normal or low serum globulins; alkaline phosphatase (ALP) and alanine aminotransferase (ALT) activity normal or moderately increased; variable low blood urea nitrogen (BUN) and hypocholesterolemia; bilirubin typically normal (anicteric).
■ Hyposthenuria or isosthenuria.
■ Ammonium biurate crystalluria.

Other Laboratory Tests

■ Coagulation tests – variable, may be normal; low protein C activity reflects APSS.
■ Total serum bile acids – preprandial values variable, postprandial values increased; classic shunting pattern.
■ Plasma ammonia – usually increased, inferred from ammonium biurate crystalluria.
■ Peritoneal fluid – pure transudate (total protein <2.5 g/dL) or modified transudate.

Imaging

■ Radiography – abdominal effusion; microhepatia or normal-sized liver due to enlarged lobe with AV malformation; renomegaly; normal thorax.
■ Abdominal ultrasound – abdominal effusion; liver lobe with AV malformation (large compared to most other liver lobes that are atrophied due to portal hypoperfusion); tortuous anechoic tubules represent AV structure with unidirectional pulsating or turbulent flow on color flow Doppler; hepatic artery and/or portal vein branches may appear tortuous; hepatofugal portal flow (away from the liver); renomegaly; urolithiasis; rule out portal thrombosis (luminal filling defect, abrupt blood flow termination).
■ Computed tomography.
  • Gold standard.
  • Three-dimensional reconstruction illustrates AV malformation, large liver lobe, atrophied liver.
■ Echocardiography – rule out right-sided heart disease, pericardial disease, and vena caval occlusion.

Other Diagnostic Tests

■ Exploratory laparotomy
■ Liver biopsy is imperative (Figure 105.1d–f).

Pathologic Findings

■ Gross findings include vascular dilation throughout the affected liver lobes and multiple shunts.
■ Biopsies from unaffected liver lobes show similar findings to those with venovenous portosystemic shunts (PSS) (i.e., ductular proliferation, hypoplasia of intrahepatic portal tributaries, arteriolar proliferation or duplication, increased lymphatics around central veins, etc.).
■ Biopsies near the malformation often have largely dilated portal venules, marked arteriolar hyperplasia and muscular proliferation, and sinusoidal capillarization.
■ Some portal veins have evidence of thrombus formation and recanalization.

THERAPEUTICS

- Preoperative medical management is similar to that for PSS, with the goal being stabilization for surgical treatment.
- Surgical treatment for AV malformations is complicated and often considered more of a palliative option rather than a cure, as approximately 75% of dogs continued to require dietary or medical management of clinical signs.

Drug(s) of Choice

Hepatic Encephalopathy

See Hepatic Encephalopathy/Portosystemic Vascular Anomaly.

Ascites

- Restrict sodium intake.
- Furosemide (0.5–2 mg/kg PO IM or IV q12–24h) combined with spironolactone. Use furosemide with caution as it potentiates further hypokalemia.
- Spironolactone (0.5–2 mg/kg PO q12h, double initial dose as loading dose once).
- Chronic diuretic therapy that is individualized to response; 4–7-day assessment intervals should be used to titrate dose to response, avoiding dehydration, and electrolyte and HE complications.
- Diuretic-resistant ascites may require therapeutic abdominocentesis to initiate diuresis.
- Vasopressin V2 receptor antagonists (i.e., tolvaptan) may control ascites accumulation.

Bleeding Tendencies

See Coagulopathy of Liver Disease.

Gastrointestinal Hemorrhage

- Histamine type-2 receptor antagonists (famotidine 0.5–2 mg/kg PO, IV, or SQ q12h) or proton pump inhibitors (omeprazole 1.0 mg/kg PO q12–24h or pantoprazole 1 mg/kg IV q24h; omeprazole may induce p450 cytochrome-associated drug interactions and may have a 24–48h delayed onset of action; some clinicians recommend chronic treatment to minimize gastrointestinal bleeding and ulceration that may be chronic problems).
- Gastroprotectant – sucralfate 1 g/25 kg PO q8h; titrate to effect, beware of drug interactions as sucralfate may bind other medications, reducing bioavailability.
- Eliminate endoparasitism.

Precautions/Interactions

Avoid drugs dependent on hepatic biotransformation or first-pass hepatic extraction (reduced by APSS) or that react with GABA-benzodiazepine receptors because of propensity for HE.

Appropriate Health Care

Treat HE and ascites prior to surgical approach or percutaneous selective acrylamide embolization.

Nursing Care

- HE – resolve endoparasitism, electrolyte and hydration disturbances, treat infections, initiate treatments to alter enteric uptake and formation of HE toxins.
- Ascites – mobilize by restricting activity and sodium intake and instituting dual diuretic therapy (furosemide and spironolactone); reserve therapeutic abdominocentesis for tense ascites impairing ventilation, nutrition, sleep, or recumbent posture.

Diet

- Easily digestible.
- Should contain a protein source of high biologic value; restricted protein +/– supplemented milk and vegetable proteins if signs of HE noted.
- Restrict nitrogen intake to ameliorate HE and hyperammonemia.
- Restrict sodium to attenuate ascites formation.

Surgical Considerations

- Resection of liver lobe containing AV malformation is complicated by coexistence of additional hepatic vascular malformations; clinical cure possible but unlikely.
- Cyanoacrylate glue embolization; complicated by risk of thromboembolism of additional vasculature; temporary improvement but treatment may be curative (Figure 105.1c).
- Multiple microscopic vascular malformations continue portal hypertension and APSS.
- Do not ligate APSS or band the vena cava.

 COMMENTS

Patient Monitoring

Biochemistry – initially monthly until stabilized after surgery or AV malformation embolization, thereafter quarterly; monitor for hypoalbuminemia, infection, optimization of HE management, and control of ammonium biurate crystalluria.

Possible Complications

- Surgical complications include hemorrhage, portal hypertension, systemic hypotension, bradycardia, and portal or mesenteric vein thrombus formation.
- Cyanoacrylate glue embolization complications include nontarget embolization of glue and risk of thromboembolism of the portal vein.
- Historical complications associated with general anesthesia, seizures, hemorrhage, infection, etc.

Expected Course and Prognosis

- Approximately 75% of dogs continue to require dietary or medical management of clinical signs because of coexisting microscopic vascular malformations across the liver; APSS persists, requiring continued management of HE.
- Approximately 30% recurrence rate requiring future interventions.
- Long-term outcome is fair if patient survives surgical resection of AV malformation or embolization.

Synonyms

- AV fistula

Abbreviations

- ALKP = alkaline phosphatase
- ALT = alanine aminotransferase
- APSS = acquired portosystemic shunt
- BUN = blood urea nitrogen
- CNS = central nervous system
- CT = computed tomography

- GABA = gamma-aminobutyric acid
- GI = gastrointestinal
- HAVM = hepatic arteriovenous malformation
- HE = hepatic encephalopathy
- PSS = portosystemic shunts
- PSVA = portosystemic vascular anomalies

See Also

- Coagulopathy of Liver Disease
- Hepatic Encephalopathy
- Hypertension, Portal
- Nutritional Approach to Hepatic Disease
- Portosystemic Shunting, Acquired
- Portosystemic Vascular Anomaly, Congenital

Suggested Reading

Berent AC, Tobias KM. Portosystemic vascular anomalies. Vet Clin North Am Small Anim Pract 2009;39(3):513–542.

Weisse C. Hepatic arteriovenous malformations (AVMs) and fistulas. In: Weisse C, Berent A, eds. Veterinary Image-Guided Interventions. Ames: John Wiley & Sons, 2015, pp. 227–237.

Acknowledgments: The author and editors acknowledge the prior contribution of Dr Sharon Center.

Author: Ashleigh Seigneur DVM, MVSc, DACVIM

Chapter 106

Cholangitis/Cholangiohepatitis Syndrome

DEFINITION/OVERVIEW

- Cholangitis = inflammation of the bile duct.
- There are four main categories of cholangitis.
  - Neutrophilic.
  - Lymphocytic.
  - Destructive.
  - Chronic (described with liver fluke infection).
- Cholangiohepatitis = inflammation of the bile duct and surrounding, nearby hepatic parenchyma.
- Cholangitis may be the favored term. In some instances, cholangitis/cholangiohepatitis will be described as a syndrome, abbreviated CCHS.

ETIOLOGY/PATHOPHYSIOLOGY

Neutrophilic Cholangitis

- Also described as suppurative or exudative.
- More frequently identified in cats (compared to dogs).
- Suspected to result from ascending infection from the gastrointestinal (GI) tract, which may explain the feline preponderance (considering unique feline anatomy).
- Characterized by neutrophilic influx into the lumen/epithelium of the bile ducts.

Lymphocytic Cholangitis

- Also described as lymphocytic cholangiohepatitis, lymphocytic portal hepatitis, nonsuppurative cholangitis.
- More common in cats than dogs.
- Etiology is unknown but may show some characteristics/components similar to well-differentiated, malignant lymphoma. The disease is considered to be chronic and (slowly) progressive.
- Characterized by consistent infiltration of small lymphocytes in the portal area.

Destructive Cholangitis

- Described in dogs.
- Etiology is uncertain but idiosyncratic drug reaction (e.g., sulfonamides) and viral infectious diseases (e.g., canine distemper) are suspected, along with potential toxic insults.
- Characterized by destruction of the biliary epithelium and severe intrahepatic cholestasis.
- See Chapter 107 for all additional information.

Blackwell's Five-Minute Veterinary Consult Clinical Companion: Small Animal Gastrointestinal Diseases, First Edition. Edited by Jocelyn Mott and Jo Ann Morrison.
© 2019 John Wiley & Sons, Inc. Published 2019 by John Wiley & Sons, Inc.
Companion website: www.fiveminutevet.com/gastrointestinal

Chronic Cholangitis

- Associated with hepatic fluke infection.
- More common in cats but can be found in dogs in endemic areas.
- Etiology is the result of infection by Opisthorchiidae (fluke requiring two intermediate hosts for the life cycle: water snails and fish). Geographic distribution of the parasite is world-wide. In North America, species of fluke include:
  - *Amphimerus pseudofelineius.*
  - *Metorchis conjunctus.*
  - *Parametorchis complexum.*
- Parasites migrate from the GI tract to the liver via the biliary tract, resulting in thickened, dilated large bile ducts. Inflammation may be seen in the bile ducts and portal areas.

Systems Affected

- Gastrointestinal – with severe and progressive disease, portal hypertension (PH) with subsequent GI manifestations may be seen. See Chapter 130 for details. Patients with acute disease may show loss of appetite, vomiting, and diarrhea. Acholic feces may develop with severe cholestatic disease.
- Hemic/lymphatic/immune – severe hepatic disease (acute or chronic) may result in coagulation disorders.
- Hepatobiliary – hepatic and biliary insults may result in chronic and progressive damage to nearby parenchyma and tissues. Some changes (e.g., fibrosis or cirrhosis) may be permanent.
- Musculoskeletal – patients with chronic progressive disease may demonstrate loss of body weight, condition, and lean muscle mass.
- Nervous – severely affected patients may show hepatic encephalopathy (HE).
- Renal/urologic – rarely, PH may result in hepatorenal syndrome, an uncommon condition where PH and ongoing hepatic failure result in renal injury and eventual renal failure, likely as a result of changes in renal perfusion and electrolyte balance.

 SIGNALMENT/HISTORY

- Feline disease – potentially Himalayan, Persian, Siamese, Norwegian forest cat. Male cats may be predisposed to some forms.
- Neutrophilic cholangitis – primarily young to middle-aged cats.
- Lymphocytic cholangitis – primarily middle-aged to older cats.
- Canine disease – potentially increased risk for dog breeds with predisposition to hepatic toxicity (e.g., Doberman pinscher).
- Chronic disease (due to flukes) – in endemic areas to support the parasite life cycle. Any dog or cat that ingests raw fish may become infected.
- No genetic basis has been identified.

Risk Factors

Neutrophilic

- Patients with GI tract disease (e.g., inflammatory bowel disease, small intestinal bacterial overgrowth, etc.) where alterations in GI microbiome may result could be at risk for ascending bacterial infection.
- The term *triaditis* encompasses concurrent inflammation of the pancreas, GI tract, and liver, and may predispose to neutrophilic cholangitis.

- Other factors that may impede normal biliary tract anatomy and flow (e.g., cholelithiasis, pancreatitis, extrahepatic biliary duct obstruction (EHBDO), etc.) may also predispose to neutrophilic cholangitis.

Lymphocytic
Unknown.

Chronic, Fluke Associated
Environmental factors that support the parasite life cycle and lifestyle risks (where patients may have exposure to raw fish).

Historical Findings

- Depending on the diagnosis, historical signs may be acute (neutrophilic) or chronic (lymphocytic). As with many other hepatic diseases, signs may be vague and nonspecific.
  - Lethargy.
  - Changes in appetite/loss of appetite.
  - Vomiting.
  - Soft stools/diarrhea.
  - Polyuria/polydipsia.

 CLINICAL FEATURES

Neutrophilic

- Fever.
- Abdominal pain (especially cranial abdomen).
- Icterus.
- Dehydration.
- Hepatomegaly.
- Ascites.
- Potential signs of advanced disease: coagulopathy, HE, etc.
- Ptyalism may be a more consistent finding of HE in cats, compared to dogs.

Lymphocytic

Any or all of the above findings for neutrophilic disease may be seen with lymphocytic. However, fever is *not* a consistent finding.

Chronic, Fluke Associated

- Any or all of the above findings may also be seen with chronic/fluke-associated disease.
- Acute presentations may present with signs more consistent with EHBDO.
- More severe signs may be seen with heavy parasite burdens or repeat infections.

 DIFFERENTIAL DIAGNOSIS

- Hepatic differentials.
  - Hepatic lipidosis.
  - Extrahepatic biliary duct obstruction (numerous etiologies possible).
  - Cholelithiasis.
  - Hepatic neoplasia (primary or metastatic).
  - Fibrosis/cirrhosis.
  - Ductal plate malformation.

- Portal hypertension.
- Hepatotoxicity (numerous etiologies possible).
■ Extrahepatic differentials.
- Hemolytic anemia.
- Sepsis/bacteremia.
- Pancreatitis/other pancreatic disease.
- Primary GI disease.

DIAGNOSTICS

Complete Blood Count/Biochemistry/Urinalysis

Neutrophilic

■ Anemia, usually nonregenerative but poorly responsive regenerative anemia may be seen.
■ Leukocytosis.
■ Neutrophilia with or without left shift.
■ In severely affected patients (septic), leukopenia and neutropenia may be found.
■ Hyperbilirubinemia.
■ Increased alanine aminotransferase (ALT) – very consistent finding.
■ Increased alkaline phosphatase (ALP).
■ Hyperglobulinemia.
■ Azotemia (most commonly prerenal).
■ Electrolyte imbalances.
■ Bilirubinuria.

Lymphocytic

■ Anemia, usually nonregenerative but poorly responsive regenerative anemia may be seen.
■ Increased ALT.
■ Increased ALP.
■ Hyperglobulinemia.
■ Hypoalbuminemia.
■ Hyperbilirubinemia.

Chronic, Fluke Associated

■ Nonregenerative anemia.
■ Eosinophilia.
■ Lymphocytosis.
■ Hyperbilirubinemia.
■ Increased ALT.
■ Increased ALP.

Other Laboratory Tests

■ Fecal analysis (sometimes repeated tests may be needed) may show evidence of parasitic infection (flukes). Negative results do not rule out infection.
■ Feline leukemia virus/feline immunodeficiency virus (FeLV/FIV) – in cats with unknown viral status, FeLV/FIV testing should be performed to elucidate underlying or complicating disease factors.
■ Bile acids – fasting and postprandial bile acids, in the nonicteric patient, may be performed to assess degree of potential hepatic dysfunction.
■ Coagulation profile testing – at a minimum, assessment of coagulation status (prothrombin time (PT) and partial thromboplastin time (PTT)) should be assessed in patients presenting with coagulopathies and prior to any invasive diagnostics (e.g., hepatic aspirate or biopsy).

- Ammonia – fasting ammonia level may be used to assess for hyperammonemia in patients presenting with signs of HE or with clinical suspicion of HE.
- Cobalamin/folate – fasting cobalamin and folate levels may be determined in patients where primary or secondary GI disease is suspected (e.g., inflammatory bowel disease).
- Pancreatic specific lipase – species-specific lipase testing may be performed in patients where pancreatitis is suspected or may be contributing to clinical status.
- Peritoneal effusion analysis – patients with peritoneal effusion should have an abdomino-centesis performed for fluid analysis and cytology and, potentially, culture and sensitivity.

Imaging

- Radiographs may be unremarkable but may show evidence of peritoneal effusion, neoplasia, radiodense choleliths, or other disease processes. Hepatomegaly may be present.
- Ultrasound.
  - Ultrasound is a more sensitive test for detecting peritoneal effusion and may help guide aspiration of abdominal fluid.
  - Hepatic imaging can be unremarkable but does not rule out disease.
  - Potential visible lesions include changes in the gallbladder wall and biliary tree (thickening, irregularity), radiolucent choleliths, evidence of fluke infection (visible structures within biliary ducts), changes in hepatic architecture, lymphadenopathy.
  - Ultrasound appearance may also help guide method to obtain tissue samples for eventual diagnosis (histopathology, culture and sensitivity, etc.).
  - Other diseases that may be found on ultrasound include pancreatitis, GI disease, neoplasia, etc.

Additional Diagnostic Tests

Note that any invasive hepatic testing should only be performed once current coagulation status is known and it has been deemed safe to proceed.

- Hepatic cytology – may demonstrate bacteria and evidence of lipid cytoplasmic inclusions, consistent with hepatic lipidosis. Cytology alone is not sufficient to make a diagnosis of cholangiohepatitis but may provide sufficient samples for culture and sensitivity.
- Hepatic histopathology – needed to diagnosis cholangitis/cholangiohepatitis and differentiate between different types. Several methods to obtain biopsy samples exist (Table 106.1).
- Culture and sensitivity – samples of hepatic tissue and bile should always be submitted for culture and sensitivity. Samples for microbiology may be from cytology or histopathology.
- Ultrasound-guided cholecystocentesis – can be performed safely (risk of gallbladder rupture) and allows sampling for cytology, culture and sensitivity, and potentially identification of fluke eggs (sample may contain higher egg counts than fecal sample).

Pathologic Findings

- Gross findings are nonspecific and do not provide a means to differentiate between the types of cholangitis. Gross signs may include the following:
  - Changes in color of hepatic tissue and/or biliary structures.
  - Hepatomegaly.
  - Regional lymphadenopathy.
  - Enlarged, tortuous biliary ducts.
  - Evidence of bile peritonitis if biliary rupture has occurred.
- Histopathology.
  - Neutrophilic – neutrophils within biliary epithelium/lumen. Edema and neutrophils may be within portal areas. Acute, severe disease may result in hepatic abscesses when

TABLE 106.1. **Methods for obtaining hepatic biopsy samples.**

Biopsy method	Pros	Cons	Notes
Ultrasound guidance	Least invasive May be least expensive Least painful	Samples may not be sufficient quantity or quality to make diagnosis	Complications include vasovagal response, hemorrhage, nondiagnostic samples
Laparoscopy	Minimally invasive Larger sample size Able to directly visualize and sample multiple tissues	Expensive equipment Availability may be limited Not recommended in cases of EHBDO	May need to convert to open laparotomy procedure with complications/uncontrolled hemorrhage
Laparotomy	Largest sample sizes Able to collect representative tissue samples throughout abdomen	Most invasive Longest recovery time/most painful Complications may hinder incision healing	Would allow complete evaluation and ability to address EHBDO, when present

EHBDO, extrahepatic biliary duct obstruction

inflammation extends into the hepatic parenchyma. More chronic disease will show a mixed inflammatory infiltrate.

- Lymphocytic – moderate to marked small lymphocytes infiltrate into the portal areas; lymphocytes may also be seen around bile ducts or within biliary epithelium (this is not considered a hallmark of the disease); concurrent fibrosis and biliary duct proliferation may be seen.
- Chronic (fluke) – larger bile ducts become dilated and proliferative. Slight to moderate inflammatory infiltrates (neutrophils and macrophages) within the ducts and portal areas (may also include plasma cells). Eosinophils are an inconsistent finding, as are adult flukes or fluke eggs. Other findings include fibrosis and a possible development of cholangiocellular carcinoma.

THERAPEUTICS

- Specific, targeted therapies are indicated for each of the types of cholangitis.
  - Neutrophilic = antimicrobials.
  - Lymphocytic = immune modulation.
  - Chronic = antiparasitics.
- General hepatic supportive measures will be indicated, based on patient status and clinical findings. Examples of these measures include the following:
  - Coagulation support.
  - Therapy for HE.
  - Antioxidants/general hepatic support.
  - Intravenous fluid support for dehydration.
  - Nutritional support, etc.
- Readers should see details on these supportive measures in other chapters.
- Patients with comorbid conditions (e.g., pancreatitis) should undergoing therapy for those conditions concurrently.

Drug(s) of Choice

Neutrophilic

- Antimicrobial treatment.
- Base therapy on results of culture and sensitivity, especially with concerns of antibiotic resistance. While pending results, or in instances where diagnostic sampling cannot be pursued, empiric therapy choices should target GI enteric populations. When possible and when patient status warrants more aggressive treatment and hospitalization, IV antibiotics are recommended. Considerations for empiric therapy should also include biliary excretion and favorable hepatic metabolism.
- Reasonable empiric options are shown in Table 106.2.
- Ideally, duration of therapy will be based on follow-up culture and sensitivity testing. In cases where this is not pursued, a reasonable amount of time for empiric antimicrobial treatment is 4–6 weeks. Normalization of bloodwork results and return to favorable clinical status help guide treatment decisions.

Lymphocytic

- Immune modulation treatment.
- Glucocorticoids are considered the mainstay of therapy. Other medications that may also provide some degree of immune suppression may be considered (Table 106.3).

Chronic (fluke)

Anticestodal therapy is indicated (Table 106.4).

TABLE 106.2. Empiric options for antimicrobials.

Drug example	Dosage	Notes
Marbofloxacin	2 mg/kg IV, SQ, or PO q24h	GI side effects possible
Amoxicillin-clavulanate	12.5–25 mg/kg PO q8–12h	GI side effects possible
Metronidazole	10 mg/kg IV or PO q12h	May reduce dose with evidence of severe hepatic injury

IV, intravenous; PO, by mouth (*per os*); SQ, subcutaneous.

TABLE 106.3. Options for immune modulation treatment.

Medication	Dosage	Notes
Prednisolone	2 mg/kg/day (canine) or 4 mg/kg/day (feline)	Taper to lowest effective dose. Side effects common at high doses
Ursodeoxycholic acid	10–15 mg/kg PO q24h	Recommended to administer with food
Metronidazole	10 mg/kg IV or PO q12h	Use in combination with prednisolone
Chlorambucil	1–2 mg/cat PO q24h × 3 d then every 3 d	May be used in conjunction with prednisolone

IV, intravenous; PO, by mouth (*per os*).

TABLE 106.4. **Anticestodal treatment.**		
Drug	Dosage	Notes
Praziquantel	10–25 mg/kg SQ or PO q24h × 3–5 d	May be painful on injection
PO, by mouth (*per os*); SQ, subcutaneous.		

Precautions/Interactions

- Monitor for signs of hepatotoxicity, especially with medications with potential hepatotoxicity (e.g., metronidazole) or that share a common metabolic pathway (e.g., cytochrome p450 enzyme pathway).
- Long-term prednisolone use in cats may predispose to the development of diabetes mellitus, especially when higher doses are utilized.

Nursing Care

- Patients may be relatively stable or may present with severe clinical illness. Extensive hospitalization with intensive care and monitoring may be required in some cases.
- As with any hepatopathy, nutritional status should be considered and, especially in cats, placement of a feeding tube may be warranted.
- Hospitalized patients should be monitored for signs of hepatic decompensation (e.g., development of neurologic signs, hypoglycemia, coagulopathy, etc.).

Diet

- Hepatic lipidosis may be a contributing factor or may develop as a complication in a cat with cholangitis.
- Caloric intake should be monitored closely and interventions to support nutrition (e.g., placement of a feeding tube) should be pursued early rather than later in the disease process. Depending on the type of feeding tube used (e.g., esophagostomy tube), certain oral medications may be administered through the tube, facilitating therapy.
- See Chapter 132 for detailed information.

Activity

- Patients with clinical illness will usually self-restrict activity. Patients with profound clinical illness should be on cage rest until clinical status stabilizes.
- For patients with chronic (fluke)-associated disease, limiting exposure to reduce potential reinfection is recommended.

Surgical Considerations

- Anesthesia/surgery is part of the diagnostic work-up (see Histopathology above).
- Primary considerations include the following.
  - Assessment of coagulation status and ability to support coagulation when indicated.
  - Risk of precipitation of HE or hepatic failure.
- Analgesic therapy is indicated for any invasive procedure. Use of local analgesic therapy may allow reduced dosages of systemic analgesics (many of which have hepatic metabolism).
- Biliary tract rupture, causing bile peritonitis, is a surgical indication and is associated with significant morbidity and mortality.

COMMENTS

- Some patients may have multiple medications prescribed for treatment of the condition so potential medication interactions/untoward side effects may be seen.
- Diagnostic evaluation and supportive care may be extensive, but some cases will respond very well to appropriate treatment.

Client Education

- Close monitoring of clinical signs and ensuring caloric intake are paramount. Monitor patients for signs of potential drug interactions or medication side effects.
- Do not alter medication schedule without discussing with veterinarian.
- For antibiotic therapy, administer the entire course of the antibiotic.

Patient Monitoring

- Clinical status should be monitored constantly.
- Bloodwork abnormalities should be followed up as appropriate based on severity of abnormalities (e.g., hypoglycemia, ALT, neutrophilia, etc.). Note anticipated serum half-life when considering recheck schedule for tests such as hepatic enzymes.
- Patients should be monitored for body weight, body condition score, and lean muscle mass (muscle condition score).

Prevention/Avoidance

- Prevention/avoidance would be applicable to chronic (fluke) cholangitis and would include limited exposure to the environment and no ingestion of raw fish. Reinfection is possible even after successful treatment.
- Minimize potential complicating or predisposing conditions (e.g., inflammatory bowel disease, pancreatitis, hepatic lipidosis, etc.).

Possible Complications

- Feline hepatic lipidosis.
- Hepatic abscess.
- Hepatic fibrosis/cirrhosis.
- EHBDO.
- Cholangiocellular carcinoma.
- Biliary tract rupture.

Expected Course and Prognosis

- Neutrophilic cholangitis and chronic (fluke) cholangitis may be cured with successful and, in some cases aggressive, support and therapy.
- Patients presenting with advanced disease or evidence of hepatic failure have a more guarded initial prognosis.
- Lymphocytic cholangitis may not be curable but extended survival times have been reported. The development of diabetes mellitus will complicate therapy and may affect prognosis.

Abbreviations

- ALP = alkaline phosphatase
- ALT = alanine aminotransferase
- CCHS = cholangitis/cholangiohepatitis syndrome
- EHBDO = extrahepatic biliary duct obstruction
- FeLV = feline leukemia virus
- FIV = feline immunodeficiency virus

- GI = gastrointestinal
- HE = hepatic encephalopathy
- PH = portal hypertension

- PT = prothrombin time
- PTT = partial thromboplastin time

See Also

- Biliary Duct Obstruction (Extrahepatic)
- Cholecystitis, Emphysematous
- Coagulopathy of Liver Disease
- Hepatic Encephalopathy
- Hepatic Failure, Acute
- Hepatic Lipidosis

- Hepatitis, Chronic
- Hepatitis, Suppurative and Hepatic Abscess
- Hepatopathy, Infectious
- Hepatotoxins
- Icterus
- Nutritional Approach to Hepatic Disease

Suggested Reading

Boland L, Beatty J. Feline cholangitis. Vet Clin North Am Small Anim Pract 2017;47:703–724.

Bunch S, Charles J. Standards for Clinical and Histological Diagnosis of Canine and Feline Liver Diseases. St Louis: Saunders Elsevier, 2006.

Marolf AJ, Leach L, Gibbons DS, et al. Ultrasonographic findings of feline cholangitis. J Am Anim Hosp Assoc 2012;48:36–42.

Otte CM, Rothuizen J, Favier RP, et al. A morphological and immunohistochemical study of the effects of prednisolone or ursodeoxycholic acid on liver histology in feline lymphocytic cholangitis. J Feline Med Surg 2014;16:796–804.

Tamborini A, Jahns H, McAllister H, et al. Bacterial cholangitis, cholecystitis, or both in dogs. J Vet Intern Med 2016;30:1046–1055.

Acknowledgments: The author and editors acknowledge the prior contribution of Dr Sharon Center.

Author: Jo Ann Morrison DVM, MS, DACVIM

Chapter 107

Cholangitis, Destructive

DEFINITION/OVERVIEW

- Destructive cholangitis is one of four forms of cholangitis recognized in small animals. It is characterized by loss of bile ducts in the smaller portal areas with subsequent portal inflammation and eventual portal fibrosis. This condition has been reported in dogs but not to the author's knowledge in cats.
- Sclerosing cholangitis is a descriptive term used to describe cholangitis with loss of bile ducts and "onion-like" rings of fibrous tissue surrounding portal triads and is more commonly seen in cats than dogs. Sclerosing cholangitis is not recognized as a distinct form of cholangitis in either species. It likely represents an advanced stage of biliary inflammation/fibrosis that can be caused by a number of other conditions such as lymphocytic cholangitis, certain drug reactions, or chronic biliary tract obstruction (see extrahepatic biliary obstruction).
- This chapter will focus on destructive cholangitis.

ETIOLOGY/PATHOPHYSIOLOGY

- The incidence of destructive cholangitis in dogs is not known but this condition appears to be uncommon.
- The underlying cause is often not identified in dogs but the following factors have been proposed (but not proven) to cause destructive cholangitis.
  - Idiosyncratic reactions to drugs, such as sulfonamide antimicrobials. It should be emphasized that this condition is uncommon and many dogs are given this drug without developing complications.
  - Viral infections (e.g., canine distemper virus infection).
  - Toxins.
  - Immune-mediated reactions.
- Inflammation surrounding the interlobular bile ducts, characterized by pigment-laden macrophages, neutrophils, and/or eosinophils, results in their loss (with preservation of portal veins and hepatic arteries), and eventually leads to portal fibrosis. Loss of interlobular bile ducts leads to severe intrahepatic cholestasis with resultant icterus and possibly acholic feces.

Systems Affected

- Hepatobiliary.
- Gastrointestinal (acholic feces and potential malassimilation).
- Skin (icterus, or lesions associated with drug reactions).

Blackwell's Five-Minute Veterinary Consult Clinical Companion: Small Animal Gastrointestinal Diseases, First Edition. Edited by Jocelyn Mott and Jo Ann Morrison.
© 2019 John Wiley & Sons, Inc. Published 2019 by John Wiley & Sons, Inc.
Companion website: www.fiveminutevet.com/gastrointestinal

SIGNALMENT/HISTORY

- Dogs; to the author's knowledge this disease has not been reported in cats.
- This condition has been reported in a variety of dog breeds. However, it is possible that breeds of dog that are more likely to develop idiosyncratic reactions to certain drugs may be at increased risk. For example, Doberman pinschers are at increased risk of side effects when given sulfonamide antimicrobials compared to other breeds.
- Dogs with destructive cholangitis has been reported with ages ranging from nine months to 11 years. The median age at onset in one study was six years.
- No sex predisposition has been reported.

Historical Findings

Reported historical findings include (from most to least common): pigmenturia (due to bilirubinuria), anorexia/hyporexia, decreased activity/exercise intolerance, acholic feces, vomiting, and polydipsia.

CLINICAL FEATURES

- Icterus was reported in all the cases described to date.
- Abdominal palpation may elicit signs of pain and/or reveal hepatomegaly but can also be unremarkable.
- Patients may also show signs of dehydration on presentation.

DIFFERENTIAL DIAGNOSIS

- Extrahepatic bile duct obstruction.
- Hemolysis.
- Chronic hepatitis.
- Acute liver injury/failure.
- Hepatic neoplasia.
- Cholestasis associated with sepsis.

DIAGNOSTICS

Complete Blood Count/Biochemistry/Urinalysis

- The serum bilirubin concentration was increased in all the cases described to date and may be markedly increased.
- Serum liver enzyme activities, especially markers of cholestasis (ALP and GGT), are markedly increased.
- Leukocytosis characterized by neutrophilia is also possible.
- Prehepatic hyperbilirubinemia (due to hemolysis) is ruled out by assessing the patient's hematocrit, red blood cell indices with a complete blood count, and blood smear examination.
- Abnormal bilirubinuria is another consistent finding.

Other Laboratory Tests

- Serum pancreas specific lipase concentration can be measured (by Spec cPL) to help rule out pancreatitis as a cause of extrahepatic bile duct obstruction.

- There is no value in measuring serum bile acid concentrations in animals with hyperbilirubinemia, apart from rare cases where hemolysis cannot be excluded.
- Coagulation testing, including measurement of activated partial thromboplastin time and prothrombin time, is helpful to investigate the possibility of a coagulopathy secondary to cholestasis and hepatic insufficiency.

Imaging

- Survey abdominal radiographs – may reveal hepatomegaly and can also help rule out other causes of icterus such as hepatic or pancreatic neoplasia. Normal findings do not rule out destructive cholangitis.
- Ultrasonography – is essential to rule out extrahepatic bile duct obstruction. Reported ultrasound findings in dogs with destructive cholangitis include hepatomegaly, mildly dilated intrahepatic bile ducts, areas of diffuse hyperechogenicity, and areas of focal hypoechogenicity. A normal ultrasound examination does not rule this condition out.

Other Diagnostic Tests

Liver Biopsy

- Diagnosis of this disease requires biopsy and histopathologic assessment of liver tissue.
- The patient's bleeding risk should be assessed prior to biopsy. This is achieved by performing a platelet count, hematocrit, bleeding times, buccal mucosal bleeding time, and ideally measuring fibrinogen.
- Liver biopsy can be performed percutaneously with a Tru-Cut™ type needle, laparoscopically, or during a laparotomy. Laparoscopic and surgical biopsies are larger and are therefore preferred. Several liver lobes should be sampled.

Pathologic Findings

Destructive cholangitis is characterized by destruction and loss of the bile ducts in the smaller portal areas with subsequent inflammation (pigment-laden macrophages, neutrophils and/or eosinophils) and eventually portal fibrosis (Figure 107.1).

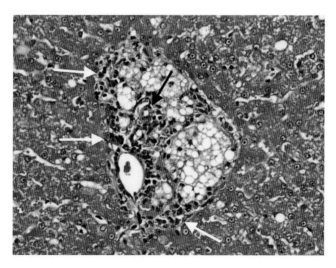

■ **Fig. 107.1.** Destructive cholangitis in a dog (hematoxylin and eosin). Note that there is only one bile duct visible (*black arrow*) in this portal tract and that there is mixed periportal infiltrate (*white arrows*). Source: Courtesy of Dr John Cullen, North Carolina State University.

THERAPEUTICS

Drug(s) of Choice

- There is insufficient information in the veterinary literature to make definitive treatment recommendations.
- Immunosuppressive drugs such as prednisolone (1 mg/kg/day PO) and cyclosporine (5–10 mg/kg/day PO) have been used to treat this disease in a small number of dogs. However, their efficacy for this purpose is not known.
- Analgesia is indicated for dogs with abdominal pain, e.g., buprenorphine (0.01–0.02 mg/kg IV, IM, or SQ q6–12h).
- There is a theoretical rationale for the use of cytoprotective agents such as S-adenosylmethionine (20 mg/kg PO q24h), silymarin (combined with phosphatidylcholine, 3–6 mg/kg PO q24h), and ursodeoxycholic acid (10–15 mg/kg PO q24h).
- Vitamin K1 (0.5–1.5 mg/kg SQ q12h for three doses) is indicated for patients with cholestasis.
- If secondary bacterial infection is confirmed or highly suspected, therapy with antimicrobials is indicated.

Precautions/Interactions

If possible, discontinue drugs implicated in causing this disease and avoid the use of other potentially hepatotoxic drugs.

Appropriate Health Care

These patients are often dehydrated and anorectic at the time of diagnosis and therefore may require hospitalization. Once the patient is stabilized, outpatient care may be possible.

Nursing Care

- If the patient is dehydrated, any balanced fluid such as lactated Ringer's solution is adequate.
- Plasma transfusion may be needed for dogs with clinically apparent coagulopathies.

Diet

- Placement of a feeding tube may be necessary for anorectic patients.
- Unless concurrent hepatic encephalopathy is present, there are no special dietary restrictions for these patients. They can therefore be fed any diet that is palatable and provides high-quality nutrition (e.g., maintenance or intestinal diets).
- Patients with concurrent hepatic encephalopathy should initially be fed a "liver support" diet which is moderately protein restricted and ideally has a nonmeat protein source.

Activity

No restrictions.

Surgical Considerations

No surgical procedures are available for relief of destructive cholangitis in veterinary patients.

COMMENTS

Client Education

It is important clients realize that destructive cholangitis carries a poor prognosis in dogs. There are no specific treatments for this disease and so supportive care is provided.

Patient Monitoring

- During hospitalization, the patient should be monitored closely. Physical examination should be performed at least once a day and it may also be necessary to check serum electrolytes, liver enzyme activities, bilirubin, and albumin on a daily basis.
- After hospitalization, during recovery the patient should be initially be examined every 1–2 weeks. A serum chemistry panel should also be checked during these visits.

Prevention/Avoidance

- The use of sulfonamides should be avoided in Doberman pinschers.
- Animals receiving sulfonamides should have their serum bilirubin concentration and liver enzyme activities checked periodically and this medication should be discontinued if sentinel signs of a drug reaction, including skin lesions, lymphadenopathy, or fever, occur.

Possible Complications

Dehydration, malnutrition, portal hypertension, ascites, acquired portosystemic collateral blood vessels, hepatic encephalopathy, hepatic insufficiency, and bleeding disorders.

Expected Course and Prognosis

- The prognosis of dogs affected by this disease is generally guarded/poor as only two of 10 that were followed up in the literature recovered.
- Dogs are often sick at the time of diagnosis and fail to respond to supportive care.

Abbreviations

- ALP = alkaline phosphatase
- GGT = gamma-glutamyl transferase

See Also

- Bile Duct Obstruction (Extrahepatic)
- Cirrhosis and Fibrosis of the Liver
- Hepatotoxins
- Nutritional Approach to Hepatic Diseases

Suggested Reading

Gabriel A, van den Ingh TS, Clercx C, Peeters D. Suspected drug-induced destructive cholangitis in a young dog. J Small Anim Pract 2006;47(6):344–348.

Kodama A, Sakai H, Kimura T, et al. Destructive cholangitis in an adult Jack Russell terrier. Case Rep Vet Med 2012, Article ID 758784.

Osumi T, Ohno K, Kanemoto H, et al. A case of recovery from canine destructive cholangitis in a miniature dachshund. J Vet Med Sci 2011;73(7):937–939.

van den Ingh TSGAM, Cullen JM, Twedt DC, et al. Morphological classification of biliary disorders of the canine and feline liver In: Rothuizen J, Bunch SE, Charles JA, et al, eds. WSAVA Standards for Clinical and Histological Diagnosis of Canine and Feline Liver Disease. St Louis: Elsevier Saunders, 2006, pp. 61–76.

van den Ingh TS, Rothuizen J, van Zinnicq Bergman HMS. Destructive cholangiolitis in seven dogs. Vet Q 1988;10:240–245.

Author: Jonathan A. Lidbury BVMS, MRCVS, PhD, DACVIM, DECVIM-CA

Chapter 108

Cirrhosis and Fibrosis of the Liver

DEFINITION/OVERVIEW

- Fibrosis – replacement of normal hepatic architecture with fibrin, collagen, and extracellular matrix.
- Cirrhosis – the end-stage of chronic liver disease, most commonly hepatitis; a diagnosis of cirrhosis includes the following: hepatic fibrosis, abnormal (regenerative) nodules, vascular anastomoses. Two forms are recognized: micronodular and macronodular. Cirrhosis is much more common in dogs than cats.

ETIOLOGY/PATHOPHYSIOLOGY

- Fibrosis is usually the result of (chronic) inflammation.
  - Hepatic injury leads to liberation of cytokines and other inflammatory mediators.
  - While the underlying pathophysiology is incompletely understood, activation of the hepatic stellate cell (HSC) appears to be a key event. The HSC is normally quiescent but upon activation, begins to produce and release large amount of collagen.
  - In the case of ductal plate malformation, fibrosis may occur without underlying inflammation.
- Cirrhosis may be considered an end-stage result of ongoing hepatic injury and fibrosis. Ongoing/extensive fibrosis negatively impacts hepatic circulation and perfusion, resulting in the vascular changes that may be noted on histopathology. The overall functional hepatic mass is reduced, resulting in the development of regenerative nodules.
- Cirrhosis and fibrosis are considered permanent changes. Antifibrotic therapy is an area of great interest and research in the human field.
- Due to the permanent and (currently) irreversible nature of these conditions, early diagnosis and intervention are paramount to prognosis.
- Fibrosis and cirrhosis are considered histopathologic diagnoses and result from hepatic insults or other hepatic diseases.

Systems Affected

- Cardiovascular – may be negatively impacted (reduced circulatory volume, electrolyte derangements) by presence of end-stage hepatic disease or portal hypertension (PH).
- Endocrine/metabolic – hypoglycemia may be a component of advanced hepatic disease. When present, hypoglycemia due to hepatic dysfunction represents an end-stage manifestation as hepatic glucose production is maintained as long as possible. Hypoglycemia may also be seen with sepsis/bacteremia due to gastrointestinal (GI) tract compromise.

Blackwell's Five-Minute Veterinary Consult Clinical Companion: Small Animal Gastrointestinal Diseases, First Edition. Edited by Jocelyn Mott and Jo Ann Morrison.
© 2019 John Wiley & Sons, Inc. Published 2019 by John Wiley & Sons, Inc.
Companion website: www.fiveminutevet.com/gastrointestinal

- Gastrointestinal – splanchnic congestion and GI edema may be seen and bacterial translocation from the GI lumen is possible. Resultant portal hypertension and ascites may negatively impact appetite.
- Hemic/lymphatic/immune – hepatic lesions may impact iron metabolism, resulting (along with potential chronic hemorrhage) in microcytic, hypochromic anemia. Reduced functional hepatic mass may result in coagulopathy.
- Hepatobiliary – with ongoing fibrosis and cirrhosis, portal hypertension and end-stage liver disease may result.
- Musculoskeletal – loss of body condition and lean body mass may be seen.
- Nervous – hepatic encephalopathy (HE) may be seen in advanced cases.
- Renal/urologic – hepatorenal syndrome may be seen in late stage of disease. Also, removal of large volume of ascites may result in dehydration/hypovolemia/hypotension. Electrolyte abnormalities may be present. Uncommonly, ammonium urate/biurate crystals or uroliths may be present.
- Respiratory – large volumes of peritoneal effusion (if present) may impair normal respirations.
- Skin/exocrine – hepatocutaneous syndrome (HCS) is a manifestation of hepatic disease that may be seen with glucagonomas/poorly regulated diabetes mellitus. Some cases will respond favorably to treatment.

 # SIGNALMENT/HISTORY

- There are multiple breed predispositions for particular hepatic diseases: copper-associated hepatopathy, chronic hepatitis, intrahepatic and extrahepatic portosystemic shunts, etc. See individual diseases for details.
- Any patient may develop fibrosis/cirrhosis with the appropriate predisposing factors.
  - Excessive dietary copper concentration or inherent copper metabolism defect.
  - Necroinflammatory hepatic disease.
  - Exposure to hepatotoxins.
  - Chronic hepatitis/cholangiohepatitis.
  - Specific parasitic infections.
  - Extrahepatic biliary obstruction (EHBO).
- Depending on the etiology, age at presentation may vary from young to geriatric.

Risk Factors

- Breed predispositions.
- Dietary copper concentration.
- Exposure to hepatotoxins (e.g., phenobarbital, nonsteroidal antiinflammatory drugs (NSAIDs)).
- Certain infectious or parasitic agents may have geographic prevalences.
- Discrete hepatotoxins may also have geographic boundaries (e.g., sago palms).

Historical Findings

- Signs may be insidious in onset and thus, some patients may present with advanced disease. Primary signs may be somewhat vague and nondescript.
  - Loss of appetite/lethargy.
  - Nausea/vomiting/diarrhea or constipation.
  - Abdominal distension due to peritoneal effusion.
  - Jaundice may be seen in some patients.

CLINICAL FEATURES

- Lethargy, depression, signs of HE.
- Dull hair coat; other cutaneous lesions if HCS present.
  - Open, crusting, oozing paw pads.
  - Difficulty/painful walking.
  - Erosions/oozing lesions around mucocutaneous junctions.
- Ascites.
- Icterus.
- Hemorrhage/evidence of thrombosis.
- Hematuria/stranguria with crystalluria/uroliths.
- Hepatic palpation may be abnormal with hepatomegaly/nodular changes. Microhepatica and large-volume ascites may preclude hepatic palpation.
- Splenomegaly may be palpable with splenic congestion and PH.

DIFFERENTIAL DIAGNOSIS

- Differential diagnoses for the etiologies of cirrhosis/fibrosis are numerous. As fibrosis and cirrhosis are histopathologic diagnoses, examples of etiologies for the potential causative agents will be described here, following the DAMNIT-PV scheme.
  - Degenerative – chronic cholangiohepatitis.
  - Anomalous – congenital portosystemic shunt or ductal plate malformation.
  - Metabolic – copper-associated hepatopathy.
  - Neoplastic – diffuse hepatocellular carcinoma.
  - Infectious/immune mediated/idiopathic – acute hepatic failure secondary to leptospirosis.
  - Toxin – xylitol intoxication or aflatoxins.
  - Parasitic – *Platynosomum fastosum* infection (feline).
  - Vascular – portal vein thrombosis.

DIAGNOSTICS

Complete Blood Count/Biochemistry/Urinalysis

- Microcytic, hypochromic anemia may be seen with chronic hemorrhage and/or abnormalities in iron metabolism. Red blood cells may show morphologic changes due to potential microangiopathic states.
- White blood cell changes may be variable depending on the disease process: stress leukogram, leukopenia, paraneoplastic changes, etc. may be seen.
- Platelet counts may be normal, elevated (e.g., with chronic hemorrhage) or decreased (e.g., paraneoplastic, disseminated intravascular coagulation (DIC) or immune-mediated destruction).
- Hepatic enzymes may be increased or within normal limits. With fibrosis or cirrhosis, it is most common for alanine aminotransferase (ALT) to be more significantly elevated than other liver enzymes. Bilirubin concentrations may be normal or elevated.
- Other values on biochemistry that may support hepatic dysfunction include hypoalbuminemia, hypocholesterolemia, hypoglycemia, and decreased blood urea nitrogen (BUN).
- Electrolyte changes may be seen with ascites (e.g., hyponatremia) or diuretic use (e.g., hypokalemia).
- Urinalysis results commonly show isosthenuria. Other potential findings include bilirubinuria or ammonium urate/biurate crystalluria.

Other Laboratory Tests

- Fasting and postprandial bile acid profile – results are expected to be significantly elevated in cases with extensive fibrosis/cirrhosis. Bile acids are not indicated in patients clinically icteric.
- Fasting ammonia testing – expected to be elevated in cases with severe hepatic dysfunction and HE; sample handing requirements reduce the clinical utility of this test.
- Ammonia tolerance testing – not recommended due to concerns about exacerbation of potential HE.
- Coagulation testing.
  - Prothrombin time (PT)/partial thromboplastin time (PTT) may be prolonged where coagulation factor production is reduced, especially vitamin K-related factors.
  - D-dimers will be elevated in cases of thrombosis/DIC.
  - Thromboelastography (TEG) – tracings may be normal or may show evidence of hypocoagulation or hypercoagulation.
  - Protein C concentrations will be reduced and have been shown to be prognostic in cases of portosystemic shunting.

Imaging

Radiographs
- Hepatic margins may be enlarged and irregular with a possible mass effect. Conversely, micro-hepatica may be present. The presence of ascites may obscure hepatic and abdominal detail.
- Splenomegaly may be present. Relative increase in renal size may be noted in patients with congenital portosystemic shunts. Ammonium (bi)urate uroliths are not typically radiodense.

Ultrasonography
- Internal hepatic architecture may be visualized and ascitic fluid may be present in between liver lobes. Irregular, mixed-echogenicity lesions that are nodular in appearance may be seen. Areas that are densely infiltrated with fibrosis/collagen may appear hyperechoic to the surrounding parenchyma.
- Other lesions that may represent an underlying etiology (e.g., neoplasia, lymphadenopathy, abnormal vasculature, etc.) may be seen in some patients.

Advanced Imaging
- Computed tomography (CT) or magnetic resonance imaging (MRI) may be pursued in some cases. Extremely large patients may be difficult to fully visualize via ultrasound and CT may provide better detail. In some cases, a CT scan may be faster than abdominal ultrasound, depending on the CT unit.
- Surgical planning may benefit from advanced imaging and CT studies with contrast may demonstrate abnormal vascular patterns. Thoracic CT scans have a higher sensitivity than three-view thoracic radiographs in the detection of pulmonary metastasis.

Additional Diagnostic Tests

- Abdominocentesis in patients should be performed with peritoneal effusion and samples submitted for fluid analysis, cytology, and, potentially, culture and sensitivity. Patients that are undergoing repeated therapeutic centesis procedures should have fluid sampled routinely to look for evidence of contamination or other complications of the procedure.
- Hepatic cytology from fine needle aspiration is unlikely to be helpful or diagnostic in cases of fibrosis or cirrhosis due to the thickened hepatic capsule and increased fibrin/collagen within the hepatic parenchyma.
- Additional testing may be warranted in cases where specific etiologies are suspected (e.g., microscopic agglutination testing or polymerase chain reaction for leptospirosis).

Pathologic Findings

- Fibrotic livers are typically smaller than normal and may appear firmly nodular with an irregular capsule. In some instances (e.g., ductal plate malformation), the overall liver size may be close to normal.
- Cirrhotic livers are typically very grossly abnormal, although gross appearance will not correlate with histopathologic diagnosis. Nodular changes are usually obvious and color may vary. Presence of ascites and abnormal vascular connections may also be seen on gross examination.
- Histopathology findings will depend upon the underlying etiology. Common findings include:
  - Bridging fibrosis.
  - Vascular anastomoses.
  - Hepatocyte loss or atrophy.
  - Regenerative nodules.
- Potential findings include:
  - Inflammatory cell infiltrates (e.g., lymphoplasmacytic) in cases of chronic hepatitis.
  - Increased concentrations of copper in cases of copper-associated hepatopathy.
  - Neoplastic cells in cases of hepatic malignancy.

 # THERAPEUTICS

- Objectives of treatment will depend upon the severity and chronicity of disease and patient status. Some patients with advanced disease, significant loss of liver function, and poor quality of life may not be candidates for therapy as many hepatic lesions are irreversible. Other patients with less severe disease or potentially more hepatic reserve may respond favorably to treatment.
- If an active underlying etiology can be identified (e.g., copper-associated hepatopathy) then therapy targeted to that etiology should be initiated. See individual disease chapters for details on treatment. Minimize use, reduce dosage, or avoid medications with potential hepatoxicity.
- Supportive and symptomatic therapy for fibrosis/cirrhosis will be discussed further.

Drug(s) of Choice

Antifibrotics

- Note that there is currently no evidence to indicate that fibrosis may be slowed or reversed with commercially available medications. Owners should be made aware that therapy is not evidence based.
  - Colchicine 0.025–0.03 mg/kg PO q24–48h. Numerous side effects exist and commercial availability may be intermittent.
  - Ursodiol 7.5 mg/kg PO q12h with food. May negatively impact appetite.

Antiinflammatory/Immune Modulation

- When an inflammatory or immune-mediated etiology is identified or suspected.
  - Prednisone/prednisolone 1–4 mg/kg PO q24h then taper to lowest effective dose while minimizing side effects. Caution for use with potential drug interactions.
  - Azathioprine (canine only) 1–2 mg/kg PO q48h after daily loading dose for three days. Combined use with prednisone has been described but may increase risk for pancreatitis.
  - The use of other immune modulators is poorly described.

Hepatoprotection

■ Efficacy of treatment is unknown but medications are generally considered safe and with minimal side effects.
- S-adenylmethionine 20 mg/kg PO q24h or per package insert on empty stomach to increase oral absorption.
- Vitamin E 10 units/kg q24h with food.
- Silybin 2–5 mg/kg PO q24h.
- Zinc 1.5–3 mg PO q24h. May also be a component of therapy for HCS.

Ascites

■ When peritoneal effusion secondary to portal hypertension is present, diuretic therapy may be prescribed.
- Furosemide 2.75–5.5 mg/kg IV (avoid IM injections in patients with decreased lean body mass or in presence of coagulopathy) q12–24h. Dose may be increased in increments of 2.2 mg/kg until therapeutic effect. Furosemide may waste potassium and serum potassium levels should be maintained so close monitoring is essential. Watch for development of azotemia with aggressive diuretic therapy.
- Spironolactone 1–2 mg/kg PO q12h. Potassium sparing but considered less potent than furosemide; more successful when used in combination with other diuretics.
- Hydrochlorothiazide 0.5–1 mg/kg PO q12h (based on spironolactone content). Available as combination product (in a 1:1 ratio; Aldactazide®) with spironolactone. Helps avoid potassium loss and dehydration that may be seen with furosemide.
- Telmisartan – dosage is uncertain but 1 mg/kg PO q24h has been reported. An angiotensin II receptor blocker which should not be used in pregnant animals. Use has not been explored in PH but it has been used in cases of proteinuria and congestive heart failure.

Coagulation Support

■ In cases where active hemorrhage is suspected or identified, therapeutics to support coagulation are indicated. See Chapter 104 for more detailed information.
- Vitamin K 0.5–1 mg/kg SQ q12–24h or 2.5 mg/kg PO q24h. Oral absorption may be increased with concurrent feeding of a fatty meal.
- Plasma (fresh or fresh frozen) 5–15 mL/kg IV. Monitor for volume overload or potential anaphylactic reaction.

Hepatic Encephalopathy Support

■ With severe hepatic dysfunction, HE may manifest in a number of ways. See Chapter 114 for more detailed information.
- Lactulose 0.25–0.5 mL/kg PO q6–8h. Adjust dose until 2–3 soft stools per day. Decrease dose if diarrhea. May be given orally or via enema if patients are not able to swallow. Rectal absorption may be increased if cleansing enemas are administered prior to usage.
- Antibiotic therapy – multiple products exist. Neomycin 20 mg/kg PO q8–12h – do not use in cases of GI hemorrhage or azotemia. Metronidazole usage has also been described for treatment of HE, but consider hepatic metabolism of medication and potential drug interactions.

Precautions/Interactions

■ Drugs with extensive hepatic metabolism should be reduced or avoided. Note common pathways for metabolism (e.g., cytochrome p450) and monitor for potential drug interactions. With drug interactions, potential exists for slowed metabolism and inadvertent increases in blood levels. Note potential signs of drug toxicity.

■ With severe hepatic disease, blood albumin levels may be decreased and alter the metabolism or distribution of drugs with extensive protein binding.

Alternative Drugs

Dexamethasone may replace other glucocorticoids.

Nursing Care

- Will depend upon the etiology and manifestation of fibrosis/cirrhosis. Some unique considerations include coagulopathies, HE, respiratory or mobility difficulties with large-volume ascites.
- Monitoring is warranted for response to therapy and/or side effects or complications of treatment and medications.

Diet

- Patients should be encouraged to eat and diet should be high quality and energy dense. Presence of ascites may diminish appetite.
- Sodium restriction may be indicated in cases with ascites.
- Protein restriction may be indicated in HE, but recent literature indicates that previous protein restriction recommendations may have been too severe. See Chapter 132 for more information.

Activity

- Patients with coagulation disorders should be restricted to cage rest/leash walking for elimination only.
- Maintenance of muscle mass should be encouraged with controlled exercise when clinically indicated.
- Restrict activity if large-volume ascites is present although many patients will self-limit activity.

Surgical Considerations

- Surgery may be considered with certain underlying etiologies (e.g., congenital portosystemic shunts) but the majority of cases are managed medically.
- Anesthesia, when indicated, should be performed with caution and with hepatic-sparing protocols (e.g., avoidance or reduced dose of medications with hepatic metabolism/excretion). The presence of large-volume ascites may compromise patient respiration during anesthesia so therapeutic abdominocentesis may be warranted.
- The procedure of abdominocentesis can be accomplished without anesthesia in the vast majority of cases. Analgesic therapy (local anesthesia) may be indicated with some patients but overall, abdominocentesis is very well tolerated.
- Consider coagulation status prior to invasive procedures (e.g., hepatic biopsy).

 COMMENTS

- Fibrosis and cirrhosis represent chronic and, presently, irreversible states.
- Patients that present with chronic hepatopathy of unknown etiology should be encouraged to pursue diagnostics prior to the development of fibrosis or cirrhosis.

Client Education

- Identifying the etiology for fibrosis or cirrhosis may require extensive and in some cases invasive diagnostics.
- In some cases, an etiology may not be identified and management will focus on supportive care.
- Monitoring for quality of life indicators as described below.

Patient Monitoring

- Body condition score and assessment of muscle mass at each veterinary visit.
- Body weight and abdominal girth measurement, especially immediately prior to and following abdominocentesis.
- Abnormalities of bloodwork (e.g., hepatic enzymes, bilirubin, hypoglycemia, hypoalbuminemia, electrolytes) should be monitored frequently as changes may precipitate health complications.
- General indicators of quality of life (e.g., appetite, respiratory effort, energy level, etc.) should be monitored continuously.

Prevention/Avoidance

- Prevention or avoidance is not feasible in most instances.
- Pursue early surgical correction, when clinically indicated, in cases with diseases that may be surgically addressed (e.g., single/congenital portosystemic shunts).
- Avoidance of hepatotoxins (especially chronic exposure).
- For patients with genetic basis for disease (e.g., Bedlington terriers), consider genetic testing/breeding practices.

Possible Complications

- Acute GI hemorrhage.
- Hepatic encephalopathy.
- Renal failure (with hepatorenal syndrome).
- Septicemia/endotoxemia.
- Thromboembolism.

Expected Course and Prognosis

- The prognosis is guarded (fibrosis) to grave (cirrhosis) without treatment, regardless of etiology.
- Major determinants of prognosis include etiology and chronicity.
- Decision for humane euthanasia based on deterioration of quality of life may be necessary.

Abbreviations

- ALT = alanine aminotransferase
- BUN = blood urea nitrogen
- CT = computed tomography
- DIC = disseminated intravascular coagulation
- EHBO = extrahepatic biliary obstruction
- GI = gastrointestinal
- HCS = hepatocutaneous syndrome
- HE = hepatic encephalopathy
- HSC = hepatic stellate cell
- MRI = magnetic resonance imaging
- NSAID = nonsteroidal antiinflammatory drug
- PH = portal hypertension
- PT = prothrombin time
- PTT = partial thromboplastin time
- TEG = thromboelastography

See Also

- Bile Duct Obstruction (Extrahepatic)
- Cholangitis/Cholangiohepatitis Syndrome
- Coagulopathy of Liver Disease
- Hepatotoxins
- Hepatic Encephalopathy
- Hypertension, Portal
- Nutritional Approach to Hepatic Disease

Suggested Reading

Bunch S, Charles J. Standards for Clinical and Histological Diagnosis of Canine and Feline Liver Diseases. St Louis: Saunders Elsevier. 2006.

Kanemoto H, Ohno K, Sakai M, et al. Expression of fibrosis-related genes in canine chronic hepatitis. Vet Pathol 2011;48:839–845.

Trepanier LA. Applying pharmacokinetics to veterinary clinical practice. Vet Clin North Am Small Anim Pract 2013;43:1013–1026.

Acknowledgments: The author and editors acknowledge the prior contribution of Drs Sharon Center and Sean McDonough.

Author: Jo Ann Morrison DVM, MS, DACVIM

Chapter 109

Copper-Associated Hepatopathy

DEFINITION/OVERVIEW

- Pathologic accumulation of copper (Cu) within hepatocytes causing hepatic injury, inflammation, and necrosis, and leading to potential cirrhosis or hepatic failure if untreated. There are two main forms of the disease.
    - Primary copper-associated hepatopathy (CAH): an inborn error of copper metabolism leading to primary copper accumulation.
    - Secondary CAH: an unrelated cholestatic disorder causing Cu to accumulate secondary to the cholestasis. Cu metabolism is likely normal in these patients, once the cholestatic condition has been treated successfully.
    - Differentiation between the two forms is primarily accomplished via identification of the zone of Cu accumulation within hepatic tissue and also Cu quantification with tissue samples (described in detail below).

ETIOLOGY/PATHOPHYSIOLOGY

- Normal Cu metabolism is complex and begins with Cu absorption from the gastrointestinal (GI) tract. In general, after absorption, copper is transported to the liver via the portal circulation and stored, metabolized, or secreted in bile. Key components in normal Cu metabolism include the following.
- Albumin: primary transport of Cu from the intestine to the liver.
- Hepatocytes: site of four main destinations for copper.
    - Incorporated into enzymatic pathways for hepatic use.
    - Bound to ceruloplasmin.
    - Stored within hepatocytes as Cu metallothionein.
    - Excreted into bile.
- Ceruloplasmin: synthesized in the liver and serves as a major copper transport protein to extrahepatic sites.
- Copper transporters: intracellular proteins that carry Cu to varying hepatocyte locations; examples include:
    - ATP7b1 – transport Cu to ceruloplasmin and bile canaliculus.
    - COX17 – transport Cu to mitochondria.
    - COMMD1 (MURR1) – transport Cu for biliary excretion.
- There are three main etiologies for excessive copper accumulation.
    - Excessive Cu ingestion (dietary or toxicity). Amount of ingested copper overwhelms the ability to maintain normal Cu concentration.

Blackwell's Five-Minute Veterinary Consult Clinical Companion: Small Animal Gastrointestinal Diseases, First Edition. Edited by Jocelyn Mott and Jo Ann Morrison.
© 2019 John Wiley & Sons, Inc. Published 2019 by John Wiley & Sons, Inc.
Companion website: www.fiveminutevet.com/gastrointestinal

- Disorders of Cu storage.
- Compromised Cu excretion.
  - An autosomal recessive, genetic defect identified in Bedlington terriers involving a loss of function of the MURR1 (COMMD1) protein.
  - A different genetic defect (involving the ATP7b gene) is responsible for Wilson's disease (humans).
- Defined genetic defects in Cu metabolism have been identified in the Bedlington terrier and are suspected but not specifically identified in multiple other breeds:
  - Doberman pinscher.
  - Labrador retriever.
  - Dalmatian.
  - Skye terrier.
  - West Highland white terrier.
  - Anatolian shepherd dog.
- A genetic test is available for the Bedlington terrier COMMD1 defect.

Systems Affected

- Gastrointestinal – signs of loss of appetite, weight loss, vomiting, and diarrhea.
- Hemic/lymphatic/immune – rarely, acute hemolytic anemia may be seen, likely due to acute exposure to high Cu levels.
- Hepatobiliary – increasing Cu concentrations will induce hepatic necrosis and inflammation with ongoing hepatic damage unless appropriate intervention is pursued. If CAH is left untreated, hepatic fibrosis, cirrhosis, and fulminant hepatic failure may result.
- Nervous – depending on the genetic defect, Cu may also accumulate in the brain, and hepatic encephalopathy (HE) may be a manifestation of profound hepatic disease.
- Ophthalmic – increased amounts of Cu may accumulate in the ocular tissues.
- Renal/urologic – some patients with abnormally increased hepatic Cu concentrations may also show a reversible proximal tubular defect, mimicking Fanconi's syndrome (e.g., glucosuria with euglycemia). Polyuria and polydipsia (likely multifactorial) have also been reported.

SIGNALMENT/HISTORY

- Theoretically, any dog or cat may develop a CAH. In reality, the condition is much more common in dogs than in cats and certain breeds have a known or suspected genetic basis for the primary condition. The role of genetics in secondary CAH, resulting from cholestasis or from dietary overload, is currently unknown.
- The following age ranges have been reported for primary CAH.
  - Bedlington terrier – Cu tends to accumulate slowly, with most affected dogs presenting with clinical signs between four and six years of age; it is important to note that dogs can show clinical signs at any age.
  - Dalmatians – reported range for chronic hepatitis in a European study was 3–12 years with a median age of four years and seven months. Another study on 10 Dalmatians showed an age range of 2–10 years of age with a mean age of six years.
  - Doberman pinschers – predominantly observed in female dogs with most presenting between four and seven years of age.
  - Labrador retrievers – reported range in 24 Labradors with chronic hepatitis and increased Cu concentrations was 3.9–14.0 years with a median age of 9.3 years.
  - Skye terrier – a report of nine Skye terriers had affected dogs ranging from 18 months to 15 years.

- West Highland white terrier – reported range in a study of hepatitis was 2–14 years, with an average age of 6.9 years.
- In a European study of chronic hepatitis, female dogs were overrepresented for Dalmatians, Doberman pinschers, and Labrador retrievers.

Risk Factors

- The Bedlington terrier is currently the only breed in which a genetic lesion that fully explains the disease process in affected patients has been identified. In other breeds, some genetic basis has been identified but those defects do not totally explain the disease in all affected patients of that breed. This likely represents incomplete identification of other, concurrent genetic lesions, or a multifactorial basis for the disease in those breeds (e.g., Labrador retriever).
- Dietary Cu concentration (including water Cu concentration) may play a role in both primary and secondary cases of CAH.
- Clinical disease of CAH may also be precipitated when another hepatic insult occurs, or with exposure to a potential hepatotoxin, including prescribed medications.

Historical Findings

- Note that depending on the breed, disease, environment, and other factors, the subclinical stage may be protracted. Clinical signs may initially be vague and nonspecific.
  - Lethargy.
  - Inappetence.
  - Vomiting.
  - Diarrhea.
- If disease has become advanced, additional signs include:
  - Polyuria/polydipsia.
  - Jaundice.
  - Abdominal distension.
  - Neurologic signs if HE.
  - Rarely, patients may present with signs consistent with an acute hemolytic crisis.

 # CLINICAL FEATURES

- Anemia.
- Evidence of coagulopathy (hemorrhage or thrombosis).
- Icterus.
- Bilirubinuria.
- Ascites.
- Potential discomfort on abdominal palpation.
- Melena may be present on rectal examination.
- Hepatic palpation may be difficult due to presence of ascites and potential microhepatica.
- Signs of HE may be present.
- Weight loss.
- Loss of body condition/cachexia with advanced disease.

 # DIFFERENTIAL DIAGNOSIS

Differential diagnoses will depend upon the clinical presentation of the patient. Differentials for specific manifestations of CAH will be presented below.

Icterus

- Pets presenting with icterus should be immediately assessed to determine if icterus is prehepatic/hepatic/posthepatic in origin. This can be done in a very step-wise manner.
    - Packed cell volume (PCV) and total protein (TP), slide agglutination test (positive agglutination), and evaluation of a peripheral blood smear (for spherocytosis) can be used to identify prehepatic/hemolytic icterus.
    - Posthepatic icterus (i.e., biliary obstruction) may be investigated via abdominal imaging (radiographs and ultrasound (US)).
    - Hepatic icterus can then be evaluated and investigated as per other hepatic diseases.
- Differentials for CAH then include:
    - Acute hepatitis.
    - Chronic hepatitis.
    - Cholangiohepatitis.
    - Neoplasia (primary or metastatic).
    - Fibrosis/cirrhosis.
    - Ductal plate malformation.
    - Infectious disease.
    - Hepatic abscess.
    - Hepatic lipidosis.
    - Cholelithiasis.
    - Hepatotoxins.
    - Congenital or acquired portosystemic shunting.
    - Portal hypertension.
    - Parasitic infection.
    - Trauma.

Coagulopathy

- Patients with CAH may have defects in primary (platelets) or secondary (coagulation factor) hemostasis. Differentials may include the following.
    - Primary hemostasis.
        - Thrombocytopenia: immune mediated (primary or secondary), infectious, toxicity, disseminated intravascular coagulation (DIC), etc.
        - Thrombocytopathia: azotemia, congenital disease (e.g., von Willebrand factor deficiency).
    - Secondary hemostasis.
        - DIC.
        - Vitamin K antagonism.
        - Hepatic failure.

Neurologic (HE)

- Patients presenting with signs consistent with HE may have intracranial or extracranial disease. Differentials include the following.
    - Intracranial: neoplasia, infarct, meningitis, encephalitis, infectious disease, etc.
    - Extracranial: hypoglycemia, hepatic disease, severe electrolyte disturbances, etc.
- Based on history, physical examination, and initial diagnostics, hepatic disease will become apparent in clinically ill patients. Patient signalment should increase the suspicion for potential primary CAH. Secondary CAH may also be present with other primary hepatic diseases.

DIAGNOSTICS

Complete Blood Count/Biochemistry/Urinalysis

Complete Blood Count

- Depending on the presentation, the complete blood count (CBC) may be within normal limits. The PCV/TP (as described above) should be immediately checked upon presentation of an icteric patient. Potential findings on the CBC include the following.
  - Anemia: strongly regenerative if immune mediated in etiology; nonregenerative if etiology is chronic disease, chronic hemorrhage, or loss of normal iron metabolism due to hepatic disease.
  - Leukocytosis: as component of stress leukogram or if infectious or inflammatory disease has triggered decompensation of CAH.
  - Platelets: thrombocytopenia, thrombocytosis, or normal.

Biochemistry

- Hyperbilirubinemia may be present with prehepatic, hepatic, or posthepatic icterus.
- Elevated alanine aminotransferase (ALT): classic finding consistent with hepatic necrosis; expect ALT to be significantly higher than alkaline phosphatase (ALP). Elevation may be present in subclinical stage in at-risk breeds and represents a possible target for prospective monitoring (described in more detail below).
- With worsening hepatic function: hypoglycemia, hypoalbuminemia, hypocholesterolemia, decreased blood urea nitrogen (BUN) may be present.

Urinalysis

- Isosthenuria.
- Bilirubinuria.
- Ammonium urate (biurate) crystalluria.
- With acquired Fanconi's syndrome, glucosuria may be noted. Additional compounds lost in urine (e.g., amino acids, electrolytes) require special testing to quantify.

Other Laboratory Tests

- Fasting and postprandial bile acid profile: results are expected to be significantly elevated in cases with extensive hepatic disease or CAH that has progressed to cirrhosis. Bile acids are not indicated in patients clinically icteric.
- Fasting ammonia testing: expected to be elevated in cases with severe hepatic dysfunction and HE; sample handing requirements reduce the clinical utility of this test.
- Ammonia tolerance testing: not recommended due to concerns about exacerbation of potential HE.
- Coagulation testing.
  - Prothrombin time (PT)/partial thromboplastin time (PTT). PT and PTT may be prolonged where coagulation factor production is reduced, especially vitamin K-related factors.
  - D-dimers will be elevated in cases of thrombosis/DIC.
  - Thromboelastography (TEG) tracings may be normal or may show evidence of hypocoagulation or hypercoagulation.

Imaging

- Abdominal radiographs may be unremarkable in cases of CAH, especially if early in the clinical course or in the subclinical phase. More advanced disease may show radiographic findings similar to cirrhosis.

- Similar to radiographs, ultrasound may be relatively unremarkable if the disease has not advanced. More advanced disease may show ultrasonographic findings similar to cirrhosis. Ultrasound may also be helpful in determining methodology for obtaining hepatic biopsy (see below).
- Computed tomography (CT) may be pursued in some cases. Extremely large patients may be difficult to fully visualize via US and CT may provide better detail. In some cases, a CT scan may be faster than abdominal US, depending on the CT unit.

Additional Diagnostic Tests

- Abdominocentesis should be performed in patients with peritoneal effusion and samples submitted for fluid analysis, cytology, and, potentially, culture and sensitivity. Patients undergoing repeated therapeutic centesis procedures should have fluid sampled routinely to look for evidence of contamination or other complications of the procedure.
- Hepatic cytology from fine needle aspiration is unlikely to be helpful or diagnostic in cases of CAH and does not provide an adequate sample for accurate diagnosis.
- Additional testing may be warranted in cases where specific etiologies for concurrent hepatic disease are suspected (e.g., microscopic agglutination testing or polymerase chain reaction for leptospirosis).
- Hepatic biopsy for histopathology and Cu quantification.
    - Histopathology.
        - Required to delineate hepatic injury, determine any additional or concurrent hepatic pathology, assess extent of necrosis, and identify affected zones.
        - Primary CAH: primary zone of hepatocellular (cytosolic) Cu accumulation is zone 3 (= centrilobular region)
        - Secondary CAH: primary zone of hepatocellular (cytosolic) Cu accumulation is zone 1 (= periportal region).
        - Note that Cu may not be visible with routine hematoxylin and eosin (H&E) stains. Therefore, if CAH is suspected, special stains must be requested: rubeanic acid. rhodanine.
        - Histopathology also allows identification of inflammatory cell infiltrates that may occur secondary to pathologic Cu retention.
    - Cu quantification.
        - Recommend contacting laboratory prior to submitting samples to ensure proper sample handling, required amount of hepatic tissue, and ability to determine and report Cu quantification in dry weight liver (DWL).
        - Normal canine liver Cu concentration is less than 400–500 mg/kg (or μg/g) DWL.
        - Patients with CAH are commonly greater than 800 mg/kg DWL although results may reach and even exceed 10 000 mg/kg DWL.

Pathologic Findings

Gross

- The end-stage of untreated CAH will be cirrhosis. Cirrhotic livers are typically very grossly abnormal, although gross appearance will not correlate with histopathologic diagnosis. Nodular changes are usually obvious and color may vary.
- Presence of ascites and abnormal vascular connections may also be seen on gross examination.

Histopathology

- Staining with rhodamine or rubeanic acid highlights Cu laden hepatocytes in zone 3 (primary CAH) or zone 1 (secondary CAH). Cu accumulates within the lysosomes in the cytosol.

- Cu retention may trigger an influx of inflammatory cells (mixed or mononuclear).
- Hepatic necrosis is a consistent finding (evidenced on biochemistry as elevated ALT).
- Other evidence of cirrhosis (e.g., hepatocyte atrophy, fibrosis, etc.) may be seen in advanced cases.
- In some cases, usually advanced or severe CAH, histopathologic Cu findings may be inconsistent and/or results may seem discordant between histopathology and Cu quantification. Consultation with specialists may be helpful in these instances.

 # THERAPEUTICS

The main objective of treatment is to produce a negative Cu balance. There are two main methods to accomplish this: Cu chelation (see Table 109.1) and dietary Cu restriction. Additional therapies may be warranted based on clinical presentation (e.g., HE, coagulopathies, portal hypertension, etc.) or results of diagnostic testing (e.g., chronic hepatitis, hypoglycemia, hepatic necrosis, etc.). See individual chapters for details on these aspects of treatment.

Drug(s) of Choice

TABLE 109.1. Copper chelators.			
Drug name	Dose	Side effects	Notes
D-Penicillamine (DPA)	10–15 mg/kg PO q12h	Vomiting, anorexia, potential dermatologic reaction	Do not give with food
Trientene	5–15 mg/kg PO q12h	Acute renal failure possible with higher dose	Do not give with food. May be prohibitively expensive
Zinc	5–10 mg/kg PO q12h. Dosing is based on elemental zinc	Vomiting, anorexia. Different forms of zinc are available (acetate, gluconate, sulfate) and individual patients may tolerate one form over another	Do not give with food. Interferes with intestinal Cu absorption so does not represent true chelation. Should not be used as sole therapy when active chelation is required

Cu, copper; PO, by mouth (*per os*).

Precautions/Interactions

- Zinc should not be administered concurrently with penicillamine or trientine as zinc may render other chelators ineffective.
- Do not administer vitamin C (ascorbic acid).
- Avoid use of other medications with potential hepatoxicity (e.g., nonsteroidal antiinflammatory drugs (NSAIDs)).
- Plasma levels of zinc may be measured to ensure recommended therapeutic range (200–300 µg/dL) is achieved and levels that may cause red blood cell hemolysis (greater than 1000 µg/dL) are avoided.
- Long-term chelation therapy, in conjunction with dietary Cu restriction, may result in Cu deficiency so therapy must be monitored.

Alternative Drugs

- In cases that are not as significantly affected and where more directed chelation therapy may not be absolutely necessary, zinc may be used in lieu of DPA or trientine.
- Dietary Cu restriction should still be a component of therapy.

Nursing Care

- Clinically ill patients will require hospitalization with appropriate supportive care based on patient status.
- Once stabilized, long-term chelation therapy is performed on an outpatient basis.

Diet

- The other cornerstone of therapy is feeding a Cu-restricted diet. Those patients with primary CAH should eat Cu-restricted diets for life.
- Commercially formulated prescription "liver diets" are Cu restricted (4 mg/kg of diet).
- Protein may be added to prescription liver diet if higher protein dietary content is desired or clinically indicated.
- Water may also contain Cu and water levels of Cu may be tested. Use another water source if Cu is greater than 0.2 parts per million.
- Treats/snacks/training treats may also contain higher levels of Cu than desired. Check all labels and nutritional analysis for Cu content.
- Consultation with a board-certified veterinary nutritionist is recommended for questions regarding Cu-restricted nutrition and for patients with complicated nutritional requirements (i.e., those with concurrent diseases).
- After successful chelation therapy, lifetime dietary Cu restriction may be sufficient to maintain normal Cu balance in some dogs with primary CAH, with or without supplemental zinc or additional chelation. Adjust therapy to individual patient.
- Dogs with primary CAH that are diagnosed in the subclinical phase (i.e., at-risk breed evaluated proactively) should be started on dietary Cu restriction immediately.

Activity

- Clinically ill patients should have activity restricted until clinical signs abate (e.g., HE, coagulopathy, lethargy, etc.).
- Once outpatient therapy has been successfully initiated, normal activity may be resumed.

Surgical Considerations

- Hepatic biopsy with Cu quantification (as described above) is required for diagnosis. Biopsy specimens may be obtained via exploratory laparotomy, laparoscopy, or US guidance. If present, ascites may be a contraindication to obtaining hepatic biopsy via US guidance. Practitioners are encouraged to contact submission laboratories prior to the procedure to ensure appropriate and adequate specimens are obtained.
- Anesthesia and surgical techniques, including anticipation of potential complications (e.g., hemorrhage, exacerbation of HE, etc.), tailored to patients with hepatic disease are recommended.
- Follow-up histopathology and Cu quantification are recommended to determine efficacy of therapy and specifically inform chelation decisions. Follow-up testing, when pursued, is recommended within a year of initiation chelation and dietary therapy. In cases where additional biopsies cannot be obtained (due to owner concerns around anesthesia risk or finances), evaluation of serum biochemical parameters for normalization may be used to inform treatment decisions.

 COMMENTS

- If diagnosed prior to the development of fibrosis/cirrhosis, the prognosis for primary CAH is good to excellent with appropriate therapy and follow-up.

■ Discuss potential risk of CAH with owners of at-risk breeds. Proactive monitoring of serum ALT may identify dogs in the subclinical phase. Monitor closely with potential hepatic insults (e.g., NSAID administration).

■ A genetic test is available for Bedlington terriers.

■ Remember that specific staining for Cu is required on histopathology samples.

Client Education

■ Chelation therapy may be prolonged initially (6–12 months may be necessary) and intermittent chelation may be needed throughout the dog's life.

■ Follow-up monitoring while on chelation therapy must be pursued as Cu deficiency is possible.

■ Dietary Cu restriction is life-long.

■ Affected Bedlington terriers should not be bred and related dogs should be tested.

Patient Monitoring

■ Follow-up hepatic histopathology and Cu quantification as described.

■ Follow-up bloodwork monitoring for normalization of CBC, serum biochemistry values. Minimum monitoring of serial serum ALT concentrations every 3–6 months.

■ Serum zinc levels may be monitored as described.

■ Long-term monitoring of body weight, body condition score, and lean muscle mass.

Prevention/Avoidance

■ Genetic testing for Bedlington terriers.

■ Proactive monitoring of serum ALT concentration in at-risk breeds (every six months with routine physical examination).

■ Avoid or minimize exposure to potential hepatotoxins in at-risk breeds.

Possible Complications

■ Rare drug side effects have been reported with chelation therapy.

■ Potential risk for Cu deficiency with aggressive or prolonged chelation therapy in conjunction with dietary Cu restriction.

Expected Course and Prognosis

■ Prognosis improves with early detection and intervention.

■ Patients presenting in fulminant hepatic failure or with advanced cirrhosis have a guarded to poor prognosis.

■ Best prognosis associated with identification of primary CAH in the subclinical phase (based on ALT monitoring and clinical suspicion) and initiation of appropriate therapy.

Abbreviations

■ ALP = alkaline phosphatase
■ ALT = alanine aminotransferase
■ BUN = blood urea nitrogen
■ CAH = copper-associated hepatopathy
■ CBC = complete blood count
■ CT = computed tomography
■ Cu = copper
■ DIC = disseminated intravascular coagulation
■ H&E = hematoxylin and eosin
■ HE = hepatic encephalopathy
■ NSAID = nonsteroidal antiinflammatory drug
■ PT = prothrombin time
■ PTT = partial thromboplastin time
■ TEG = thromboelastography
■ US = ultrasound

See Also

- Cholangitis/Cholangiohepatitis Syndrome
- Cirrhosis and Fibrosis
- Coagulopathy of Liver Disease
- Hepatic Encephalopathy
- Hepatic Failure, Acute
- Hepatitis, Chronic
- Hepatotoxins
- Icterus
- Nutritional Approach to Hepatic Disease

Suggested Reading

Bexfield NH, Buxton RJ, Vicek TJ, et al. Breed, age and gender distribution of dogs with chronic hepatitis in the United Kingdom. Vet J 2012;193:124–128.

Dirksen K, Fieten H. Canine copper-associated hepatitis. Vet Clin North Am Small Anim Pract 2017; 47:631–44.

Dirksen K, Spee B, Penning LC, et al. Gene expression patterns in the progression of canine copper-associated chronic hepatitis. PLoS One 2017;12:e0176826.

Haywood S, Rutgers HC, Christian MK. Hepatitis and copper accumulation in Skye terriers. Vet Pathol 1988;25:408–414.

Hyun C, Filippich LJ. Inherited canine copper toxicosis in Australian Bedlington Terriers. J Vet Sci 2004;5:19–28.

Shih JL, Keating JH, Freeman LM, et al. Chronic hepatitis in Labrador retrievers: clinical presentation and prognostic factors. J Vet Intern Med 2007;21:33–39.

Spee B, Arends B, van den Ingh TS, et al. Copper metabolism and oxidative stress in chronic inflammatory and cholestatic liver diseases in dogs. J Vet Intern Med 2006;20:1085–1092.

Thornburg LP. A perspective on copper and liver disease in the dog. J Vet Diagn Invest 2000;12:101–110.

Thornburg LP, Rottinghaus G, Dennis G, et al. The relationship between hepatic copper content and morphologic changes in the liver of West Highland white terriers. Vet Pathol 1996;33:656–661.

Webb CB, Twedt DC, Meyer DJ. Copper-associated liver disease in dalmatians: a review of 10 Dogs (1998-2001). J Vet Intern Med 2002;16:665–668.

Acknowledgments: The author and editors acknowledge the prior contribution of Drs Sharon Center and Sean McDonough.

Author: Jo Ann Morrison DVM, MS, DACVIM

Chapter 110

Ductal Plate Malformation

DEFINITION/OVERVIEW

- Ductal plate malformation is the current terminology used to describe complex congenital hepatobiliary (portal triad) abnormalities.
- The intrahepatic bile ducts appear to be the primary site of the developmental lesion.
- Persistence of embryonic bile ducts (potentially as a result of an embryologic maturation arrest defect) appears to be a key factor.
- Previous reports have used the term congenital hepatic fibrosis. Other terms that have been used include Caroli's disease and congenital cystic disease of the liver.
- Main components of the disorder include biliary cystic lesions, a lack of inflammatory infiltrate, and fibrosis. Some cases will be clinically silent until secondary conditions (described below) develop.
- Proposed terminology suggests to follow much of the human literature, although this is an area of potential future change, based on more extensive pathologic and inheritance studies.

ETIOLOGY/PATHOPHYSIOLOGY

- Ductal plate malformation disorders result in multiple phenotypic expressions and likely represent a complex inheritance with a complicated development. Main pathologic and histopathologic manifestations will be described here, recognizing that the clinical approach and management may not depend upon the specific genetic mutation and resultant lesion(s) encountered.
    - Caroli's disease – congenital sacculation and dilation of the extrahepatic and large intrahepatic bile ducts. Cystic lesions in the kidneys may also be seen, and may represent a related congenital condition. In humans, this has been determined to be an autosomal recessive inheritance. Maturation arrest of the medium intrahepatic bile ducts is thought to be the cause.
    - Congenital hepatic fibrosis – diffuse periportal to bridging fibrosis with numerous small or irregular bile ducts. Inflammation is minimal to absent and there is no evidence of chronic hepatitis or cirrhosis. This may also be termed juvenile polycystic disease. Maturation arrest of the small interlobular bile ducts appears to be the cause.
    - Von Meyenburg complexes – discrete fibrotic areas with small, irregular bile ducts, also called bile duct hamartoma. These complexes may be seen with particular conditions but may be clinically insignificant.
- The overall incidence of ductal plate malformation lesions is poorly understood and may be underdiagnosed.

Blackwell's Five-Minute Veterinary Consult Clinical Companion: Small Animal Gastrointestinal Diseases, First Edition. Edited by Jocelyn Mott and Jo Ann Morrison.
© 2019 John Wiley & Sons, Inc. Published 2019 by John Wiley & Sons, Inc.
Companion website: www.fiveminutevet.com/gastrointestinal

- Liver samples that are not evaluated until later in life (with acquired, chronic lesions complicating the histopathologic interpretation) may lead to a primary diagnosis of cirrhosis, chronic hepatitis, or cholangitis. The underlying congenital disease may be overlooked in these cases.
- Ductal plate malformation cases are anticipated to be clinically silent until secondary conditions arise. The abnormal biliary structures are hypothesized to increase the susceptibility to conditions such as:
  - Ascending bacterial infection.
  - Cholelithiasis.
  - Choledochitis.
  - Extrahepatic biliary duct obstruction (EHBDO).
- Early recognition, diagnosis, and institution of appropriate therapy are recommended. This requires knowledge of the potential for congenital disease, familiarity with predisposed breeds, and evaluation of patients with clinical signs or patients with potential subclinical disease based on biochemical evidence of a potential hepatopathy.

Systems Affected

- Endocrine/metabolic – hypoglycemia may result from hepatic dysfunction.
- Gastrointestinal – changes in appetite, vomiting, diarrhea, weight loss.
- Hemic/lymphatic/immune – anemia from chronic disease or potentially hemorrhage. Possibility of leukocytosis/leukopenia with bacterial complications (e.g., ascending biliary infection).
- Hepatobiliary – progressive disease from initial congenital lesion(s) may result in changes consistent with cirrhosis (fibrosis, regenerative nodules, vascular proliferation) or with secondary complicating factors (e.g., EHBDO, as described above). More advanced cases may develop acquired portosystemic shunts (APSS) or portal hypertension (PH).
- Musculoskeletal – patients with congenital disease may show poor or stunted growth with poor body condition. Loss of body weight, body condition, and lean muscle mass may be seen with progressive disease.
- Nervous – hepatic encephalopathy (HE) may be seen in advanced cases.
- Renal/urologic – cystic lesions may be identified in renal parenchyma with some congenital or acquired disorders. Advanced cases of hepatic failure may show hepatorenal syndrome.

 SIGNALMENT/HISTORY

- Sex predilections have not been identified for ductal plate malformations. However, multiple breeds are known, or suspected, to have a genetic predisposition. Note that due to the incompletely understood nature of the disorder, potential overlap with other congenital hepatic lesions (e.g., portal vein hypoplasia) cannot be ruled out.
  - Golden retrievers.
  - Boxers.
  - Skye terriers.
  - Cairn terriers.
  - West Highland white terriers.
  - Persian cats (with polycystic kidney disease).
- As ductal plate malformation is a congenital lesion, affected cases may be seen early in life. However, clinically silent cases may not be diagnosed until much later in life, when complicating factors have arisen.

- Reported age range is three months to 12 years.
- Known related patients (e.g., littermates, common ancestor) may be diagnosed with the same disease.

Risk Factors

- Genetic lesions with unknown incompletely defined specific mutations.
- Clinical manifestations may only result when additional hepatic insults arise.
  - Ascending bacterial infections, potentially due to conditions that alter the gastrointestinal (GI) microbiome. Examples may include small intestinal bacterial overgrowth or inflammatory bowel disease.
  - Cholelithiasis or other etiologies for EHBDO (e.g., pancreatitis).

Historical Findings

- Vague and nonspecific historical findings include:
  - Loss of energy/lethargy.
  - Changes in appetite, loss of appetite.
  - Soft stools/diarrhea.
  - Polyuria/polydipsia.
- Astute owners may notice changes in or slowed growth.
- More advanced cases (e.g., APSS) may show ascites, HE, or related signs.

 # CLINICAL FEATURES

Any one or combination of the following signs may be present:
- Abdominal effusion or cranial abdominal pain.
- Icterus or pale mucous membranes.
- Fever may be seen in cases with infectious component.
- Potential hepatomegaly or microhepatica.
- Melena may be found on rectal palpation.
- Neurologic signs may be seen with HE.
- Rarely, cases may have ammonium urate urolithiasis or crystalluria.

 # DIFFERENTIAL DIAGNOSIS

As ductal plate malformation is a histopathologic diagnosis, examples of etiologies for a general approach to a case presenting with primary hepatic manifestations will be described here, following the DAMNIT-PV scheme. The clinical presentation of the patient should impact the differential list (e.g., signalment, presenting signs, etc.).
- Degenerative: chronic cholangiohepatitis/cirrhosis.
- Anomalous: congenital portosystemic shunt or arteriovenous malformation.
- Metabolic: copper-associated hepatopathy.
- Neoplastic: diffuse hepatocellular carcinoma.
- Infectious/immune mediated/idiopathic: acute hepatic failure secondary to canine viral hepatitis infection.
- Toxin: xylitol intoxication or aflatoxins.
- Parasitic: *Platynosomum fastosum* infection (feline).
- Vascular: portal vein thrombosis.

DIAGNOSTICS

Complete Blood Count/Biochemistry/Urinalysis

Complete Blood Count

- Depending on the presentation, the complete blood count (CBC) may be within normal limits. Potential pathologic findings on the CBC include the following.
  - Anemia: nonregenerative if etiology is chronic disease, chronic hemorrhage, or loss of normal iron metabolism due to hepatic disease. Target cells may be seen in canine patients.
  - Leukocytosis: as component of stress leukogram or if infectious or inflammatory disease has triggered decompensation of ductal plate malformation.
  - Platelets: thrombocytopenia, thrombocytosis, or normal.

Biochemistry

- Hyperbilirubinemia may be present with hepatic or posthepatic icterus.
- Elevated alanine aminotransferase (ALT) and alkaline phosphatase (ALP): one or the other or both enzymes may be elevated and a wide range of values has been reported. Also, enzymes may be within normal limits.
- With worsening hepatic function or insult: hypoglycemia, hypoalbuminemia, hypocholesterolemia, decreased blood urea nitrogen (BUN) may be present.
- If concurrent cystic lesions are present in the kidneys, azotemia may be noted.

Urinalysis

- Isosthenuria.
- Bilirubinuria.
- Ammonium urate (biurate) crystalluria.

Other Laboratory Tests

- Fasting and postprandial bile acid profile: results are expected to be elevated in cases with extensive hepatic disease or ductal plate malformation that has progressed to cirrhosis. Bile acids are not indicated in patients clinically icteric.
- Fasting ammonia testing: expected to be elevated in cases with severe hepatic dysfunction and HE; sample handing requirements reduce the clinical utility of this test.
- Ammonia tolerance testing: not recommended due to concerns about exacerbation of potential HE.
- Coagulation testing.
  - Prothrombin time (PT)/partial thromboplastin time (PTT) may be prolonged where coagulation factor production is reduced, especially vitamin K-related factors.
  - D-dimers will be elevated in cases of thrombosis/disseminated intravascular coagulation (DIC).
  - Thromboelastography (TEG) tracings may be normal or may show evidence of hypocoagulation or hypercoagulation.

Imaging

Radiographs

- Abdominal radiographs may show a normal hepatic silhouette, microhepatica, or hepatomegaly.
- Potential evidence of additional pathology (e.g., cholelithiasis) may be noted.
- More advanced disease may show radiographic findings similar to cirrhosis and PH (e.g., ascites).

Ultrasound

- Abnormal vascular/cystic/biliary structures may be visible although imaging may be difficult / challenging. Overlying GI gas may also contribute to imaging challenges. Ultrasound (US) is safe and noninvasive, but computed tomography (CT) may be preferred (see below) for superior visualization.
- More advanced disease may show ultrasonographic hepatic findings similar to cirrhosis.
- In some cases, cystic lesions may be seen in renal tissue with certain genetic mutations and/ or evidence of urolithiasis.
- Ultrasonographic study may help inform methodology for diagnostic hepatic biopsy (discussed below).

Advanced Imaging

- Computed tomography may be pursued in some cases. Depending on availability, CT may provide a faster image study and has the advantage of concurrent contrast administration.
- Short-term anesthesia/immobilization, etc. may be necessary to complete the study.
- Extremely large patients may be difficult to fully visualize via US and CT may provide better detail.
- Contrast studies can identify abnormal vascular connections and also may allow delineation of cystic biliary structures from vascular structures, helping inform decisions for biopsy methodology and further describing and delineating the (sometimes complicated) anatomy.

Additional Diagnostic Tests

- Abdominocentesis should be performed in patients with peritoneal effusion and samples submitted for fluid analysis, cytology, and, potentially, culture and sensitivity. Patients that are undergoing repeated therapeutic centesis procedures should have fluid sampled routinely to look for evidence of contamination or other complications of the procedure.
- Hepatic cytology from fine needle aspiration is unlikely to be helpful or diagnostic in cases of ductal plate malformation and does not provide an adequate sample for accurate diagnosis. If cases are complicated by a bacterial infection, bacterial organisms may be visualized on cytology.
- Additional testing may be warranted in cases where specific etiologies for concurrent hepatic disease are suspected (e.g., microscopic agglutination testing or polymerase chain reaction for leptospirosis).
- Hepatic biopsy for histopathology.
  - Required to delineate hepatic injury, determine any additional or concurrent hepatic pathology, and assess specific biliary/cystic lesions.
  - Hepatic biopsy is required for diagnosis. Biopsy specimens may be obtained via exploratory laparotomy, laparoscopy, or US guidance. If present, ascites may be a contraindication to obtaining hepatic biopsy via US guidance. Concern may exist around the ability of US guidance to provide a sufficient sample for diagnosis. More robust diagnostic procedures (e.g., laparoscopy) may be warranted.
- Anesthesia and surgical techniques, including anticipation of potential complications (e.g., hemorrhage, exacerbation of HE, etc.), tailored to patients with hepatic disease are recommended.

Pathologic Findings

Multiple, excellent images of various gross and histopathologic lesions are available in the Suggested Reading titles at the end of this chapter.

Gross

Depends upon the particular mutation and presence or absence of complicating factors. Potential pathologic findings include the following.

- Hepatomegaly or microhepatica.
- Distended bile ducts with abnormal, thickened, or tortuous ducts.
- Potential presence or absence of a normal gallbladder.
- Evidence of fibrosis and/or cirrhosis.
- Atrophied or absent hepatic lobes.
- Fluid contained within biliary structures may be discolored and/or increased in viscosity.

Histopathology

- Detailed descriptions of pathologic findings unique to various genetic mutations may be found in the Suggested Reading titles provided below.
- Biliary hyperplasia is a key finding with ductal plate malformation but may also be seen secondary to other hepatic pathologies (fibrosis, cirrhosis, chronic hepatitis, etc.).
- The histologic finding most helpful in differentiating the biliary hyperplasia of congenital disease from secondary (acquired) biliary hyperplasia is lack of proliferation of the embryonic bile ducts.
    - Embryonic bile ducts exhibit positive uptake of Ki67. Therefore, negative staining with Ki67 indicates proliferating bile ducts not embryonic in origin but a secondary (acquired) change.
    - Other immunohistochemical stains (CK19) serve as a marker for embryologic biliary structures and can be used to bolster a diagnosis of congenital disease.
    - Practitioners should contact laboratory facilities offering histopathologic services to discuss immunohistochemistry options.

 THERAPEUTICS

- Objectives of treatment are to minimize progression of hepatic injury and avoid potential complicating or secondary factors.
- See specific chapters for treatment details of various clinical presentations.
- There is no specific, targeted medical treatment for ductal plate malformation.

Precautions/Interactions

- Drugs with extensive hepatic metabolism should be avoided or used with caution. Targeted dose reduction may be warranted.
- Be aware of common metabolic pathways (e.g., cytochrome p450) and monitor for signs of potential drug interactions, especially in patients on polypharmacy (e.g., signs of drug toxicity (e.g., vomiting, diarrhea) and potentiation of HE).

Nursing Care

- Supportive care as indicated based on clinical state and presentation.
- With early detection, most patients will be maintained on an outpatient basis.

Diet

- The role of dietary manipulation to support hepatic function (e.g., vitamin K supplementation) and potentially help avoid hepatic injury (e.g., secondary to copper accumulation) is not currently well described, but is unlikely to be harmful.
- Severe protein restriction is not recommended unless HE is present.
- See Chapter 132 for more details.

Activity

- In the subclinical phase, restricted activity is not recommended, beyond minimizing exposure to potential environmental hepatotoxins (e.g., sago palms).
- Patients with clinical illness will self-restrict activity in many cases.
- Severely ill patients should have enforced cage rest.

Surgical Considerations

- Large cystic lesions may be addressed by surgical exploration and resection. It is recommended to refer to a board-certified small animal surgeon for surgical intervention and appropriate supportive care in the perioperative period.
- Considerations for anesthesia and surgical risks for patients with ductal plate malformation and potentially complicating factors are recommended to discuss with owners.
  - Potentiation of HE.
  - Coagulation abnormalities.
  - Infection and dehiscence, etc.

 COMMENTS

- Description and understanding of this collection of congenital lesions are likely to expand and potentially change over time. Updates to the peer-reviewed literature should be followed closely.
- As with most congenital diseases, early and accurate diagnosis is recommended. The prognosis for ductal plate malformation is more favorable when diagnosis is obtained early in the disease course.

Client Education

- Monitor for potential drug side effects or untoward clinical responses. Individual patient responses may vary but prolonged survival is possible. Pursue veterinary evaluation with any changes in patient status.

Patient Monitoring

- Clinical signs and status – continuously.
- Follow-up evaluation for changes in clinical pathology tests should be tailored to the individual patient (for example, hypoglycemia should be assessed repeatedly until stabilized).
- Long-term monitoring for stable outpatients could be considered every 4–6 months or upon any clinical change.

Prevention/Avoidance

- Avoid/prevent intestinal parasitic infection.
- Pursue diagnostics quickly for clinical signs that may be attributed to GI, hepatobiliary, or urinary (renal) disease.
- If bacterial infections are diagnosed or suspected, pursue appropriate antibiotic therapy to help avoid ascending biliary infections.
- Early detection of congenital disease is ideal as this helps minimize/avoid future hepatic injury.

Possible Complications

Eventual progression to more severe hepatic disease.
- Acquired portosystemic shunts.
- Portal hypertension.

- Cirrhosis.
- Hepatic encephalopathy.
- Coagulopathies of liver disease.

Expected Course and Prognosis

- With early diagnosis, intervention, and close monitoring, long-term survival (for multiple years) post diagnosis is possible.
- Prognosis changes if patients present with advanced disease and evidence of decompensation.

Synonyms

- Caroli's disease
- Congenital cystic disease of the liver
- Congenital hepatic fibrosis
- Juvenile polycystic disease

Abbreviations

- ALP = alkaline phosphatase
- ALT = alanine aminotransferase
- APSS = acquired portosystemic shunts
- BUN = blood urea nitrogen
- CBC = complete blood count
- CT = computed tomography
- DIC = disseminated intravascular coagulation
- EHBDO = extrahepatic biliary duct obstruction
- GI = gastrointestinal
- HE = hepatic encephalopathy
- PH = portal hypertension
- PT = prothrombin time
- PTT = partial thromboplastin time
- TEG = thromboelastography
- US = ultrasound

See Also

- Cholangitis/Cholangiohepatitis Syndrome
- Cirrhosis and Fibrosis
- Coagulopathy of Liver Disease
- Copper-Associated Hepatopathy
- Hepatic Encephalopathy
- Hepatic Failure, Acute
- Hepatitis, Chronic
- Hepatotoxins
- Icterus
- Nutritional Approach to Hepatic Disease

Suggested Reading

Brown DL, van Winkle T, Cecere T, et al. Congenital hepatic fibrosis in 5 dogs. Vet Pathol 2010;47: 102–107.

Bunch S, Charles J. Standards for Clinical and Histological Diagnosis of Canine and Feline Liver Diseases. St Louis: Saunders Elsevier, 2006.

Gorlinger S, Rothuizen J, Bunch S, et al. Congenital dilatation of the bile ducts (Caroli's disease) in young dogs. J Vet Intern Med 2003;17:28–32.

Pillai S, Center SA, McDonough SP, et al. Ductal plate malformation in the liver of boxer dogs: clinical and histological features. Vet Pathol 2016;53:602–613.

Watson P. Canine breed-specific hepatopathies. Vet Clin North Am Small Anim Pract 2017;47:665–682.

Acknowledgments: The author and editors acknowledge the prior contribution of Dr Sharon Center.

Author: Jo Ann Morrison DVM, MS, DACVIM

Chapter 111

Glycogen Storage Disease

DEFINITION/OVERVIEW

Glycogen storage diseases (GSDs) are rare inherited disorders of glycogen synthesis, glycogen breakdown, or glycolysis.

ETIOLOGY/PATHOPHYSIOLOGY

- Recall that the body stores glucose as glycogen in liver and muscle cells, and when energy is needed, breaks down glycogen and then glucose through glycolysis to form adenosine triphosphate (ATP). In animals affected by GSDs enzyme deficiencies result in:
  - Glycogen accumulation in tissue: leading to organ enlargement and dysfunction as outlined below.
  - Impaired hepatic mobilization of glycogen for energy: leading to hypoglycemia.
- GSDs are classified based on the defective/deficient enzyme and tissues affected. In humans, more than a dozen GSDs exist, while four types of GSDs affect dogs and one affects cats (Table 111.1).

Systems Affected

- Hepatobiliary – hepatic enlargement, fibrosis with disease progression in GSD III.
- Endocrine/metabolic – hypoglycemia due to failure of glycolysis.
- Musculoskeletal – glycogen accumulation in muscle.
- Nervous – neuroglycopenia, weakness.
- Cardiovascular – glycogen accumulation in heart muscle.

SIGNALMENT/HISTORY

- GSDs typically manifest in juveniles, days to months after birth.
- Type Ia – young Maltese puppies with growth failure, hepatomegaly, and hypoglycemia. Autosomal recessive inheritance leads to deficient glucose-6-phosphatase.
- Type II – variable onset from six months to one year of age in Lapland and Lapphund dogs (Swedish, Finnish). Dogs show signs of megaesophagus (regurgitation, failure to thrive, dysphagia), progressive muscular weakness, panting. Autosomal recessive inheritance leads to deficiency of acid alpha-glucosidase.

Blackwell's Five-Minute Veterinary Consult Clinical Companion: Small Animal Gastrointestinal Diseases,
First Edition. Edited by Jocelyn Mott and Jo Ann Morrison.
© 2019 John Wiley & Sons, Inc. Published 2019 by John Wiley & Sons, Inc.
Companion website: www.fiveminutevet.com/gastrointestinal

TABLE 111.1. Glycogen storage diseases in dogs and cats.			
Disorder	Enzymatic defect	Breed(s) reported	Tissue involvement
Type Ia (von Gierke)	Glucose-6-phosphatase	Maltese	Liver, kidney
Type II (Pompe)	Acid alpha-glucosidase	Lapland dogs, Lapphund dogs	Heart, skeletal muscle
Type IIIa (Cori)	Glycogen debranching	Curly-coated retriever, German shepherd dog	Liver, skeletal muscle
Type IV (Andersen)	Glycogen branching	Norwegian forest cat	Skeletal muscle, neurons
Type VII (Tauri)	Phosphofructokinase	English springer spaniel, whippet, mixed breeds, American cocker spaniel	Erythrocytes, skeletal muscle

- Type IIIa – affected dogs have biochemical abnormalities by six months, but signs are often first noted by owners around one year. Reported signs include weakness, lethargy, exercise intolerance, and collapse. Autosomal recessive mutation in glycogen debranching enzyme leading to deficiency.
- Type IV – most affected kittens die at or shortly after birth secondary to hypoglycemia. If the neonatal period is survived, many kittens suffer progressive neurologic and cardiac decline at five months. Autosomal recessive inheritance leading to deficiency in glycogen branching enzyme.
- Type VII – deficiency of the muscle phosphofructokinase leads to hemolytic crises and myopathy noted in adult dogs.

Risk Factors

- Inheritance as listed above resulting in the following enzyme deficiencies.
  - Type Ia: glucose-6-phosphatase.
  - Type II: acid alpha-glucosidase.
  - Type III: glycogen debranching enzyme.
  - Type IV: glycogen branching enzyme.
  - Type VII: phosphofructokinase.

Historical Findings

- Weakness: Type Ia, II, IIIa, IV, VII.
- Failure to thrive: Type Ia, II, IV.
- Regurgitation: Type II.
- Discolored urine: Type VII.
- Collapse: Type II, IIIa, VII.

 ## CLINICAL FEATURES

- Type Ia – poor body condition, hepatomegaly and/or abdominal distension, mental dullness, death or euthanasia by two months.
- Type II – poor body condition, vomiting or regurgitation, muscle weakness, cardiac changes, death or euthanasia by two years.

- Type IIIa – depression, weakness, stunted growth, abdominal distension from hepatomegaly.
- Type IV – death shortly after birth is common; in surviving kittens, signs include tremors, muscle atrophy, weakness progressing to tetraplegia, sudden death from arrhythmias.
- Type VII – dogs present with compensated hemolytic anemia, episodic weakness, exercise-induced intravascular hemolysis, hemoglobinuria. One patient had a progressive myopathy at 11 years of age; no liver effects.

DIFFERENTIAL DIAGNOSIS

- Diagnosis is often suspected based on breed and familial history.
- Diseases causing juvenile hypoglycemia (malnutrition, hepatic vascular anomaly, endoparasites, transient fasting, sepsis, congenital hypoadrenocorticism) and muscle weakness (infectious diseases, endocrinopathy, immune-mediated disease, hypokalemia, other neuromyopathies) should be ruled out.

DIAGNOSTICS

Complete Blood Count/Biochemistry/Urinalysis

- Type Ia – hypoglycemia, lactic acidemia, increased cholesterol, triglycerides, and uric acid.
- Type II – increased alanine aminotransferase (ALT), aspartate aminotransferase (AST), and alkaline phosphatase (ALP) activities.
- Type IIIa – hypoglycemia, increased ALT, AST, ALP, and creatine kinase (CK) activities.
- Type IV – hypoglycemia.
- Type VII – anemia, reticulocytosis, pigmenturia, no hepatic effects.

Other Laboratory Tests

- Genetic testing: type I in Maltese dogs, type II in Lapland and Lapphund dogs, type III in curly-coated retrievers, type IV in Norwegian forest cats, type VII in English springer spaniels, whippets, American cocker spaniels and *in vitro* erythrocyte testing.
- Depending upon GSD, tissue enzyme analysis and glycogen determination (types Ia, II, IIIa, IV), electromyography (types IIIa, IV), and echocardiography (types II, IV) may aid in the diagnosis.

Pathologic Findings

- Type Ia – emaciation, massive hepatomegaly due to hepatocyte glycogen and lipid vacuolation and similar change in renal tubular epithelium.
- Type II – glycogen accumulation in skeletal, smooth, and cardiac muscle.
- Type IIIa – hepatomegaly due to glycogen accumulation, glycogen in skeletal muscle.
- Type IV – generalized muscle atrophy, glycogen accumulation in skeletal muscle, central nervous system, and peripheral nervous system.
- Type VII – polysaccharide deposits in skeletal muscle.

THERAPEUTICS

Drug(s) of Choice

- Glucose supplementation in animals with hypoglycemia (types Ia, IIIa, IV).
- Gene therapy has been used experimentally in dogs with GSD Ia.

Precautions/Interactions

Use caution with anesthesia and drugs metabolized by the liver in animals with hepatic dysfunction (type Ia, IIIa).

Nursing Care

Supportive care.

Diet

Control hypoglycemia (types I and III) with frequent feedings of a high-carbohydrate diet until diagnosis is confirmed; glucose solutions usually used.

Activity

- Most animals with weakness will self-regulate.
- Dogs with type VII should avoid strenuous exercise that precipitates crises.

Surgical Considerations

Monitor for hypoglycemia, cardiac instability, hepatic dysfunction, depending upon which GSD affects the animal.

 COMMENTS

Patient Monitoring

- Monitor for progressive weakness, hypoglycemia, and other specific signs dependent upon GSD diagnosed (hemolytic crises, regurgitation, etc.).
- Treat symptomatically.

Prevention/Avoidance

Avoid purchase of puppies/kittens from lines with histories of disease.

Possible Complications

- Premature death in most cases, although dogs with type VII can have a normal lifespan.
- Repeated hospitalization for hemolytic crises in type VII is possible.

Expected Course and Prognosis

- Poor prognosis with death before adulthood: type Ia, VI.
- Poor prognosis with death in early adulthood: type IIIa, II.
- Good prognosis with appropriate care: type VII.

Synonyms

- Dextrinosis
- Glycogenosis

Abbreviations

- ALP = alkaline phosphatase
- ALT = alanine aminotransferase
- AST = aspartate aminotransferase
- ATP = adenosine triphosphate
- CK = creatine kinase
- GSD = glycogen storage disease

See Also

- Portosystemic Vascular Anomaly, Congenital

Suggested Reading

Brooks ED, Koeberl DD. Large animal models and new therapies for glycogen storage disease. J Inherit Metab Dis 2015;38(3):505–509.

Fyfe JC, Kurzhals RL, Hawkins MG, et al. A complex rearrangement in GBE1 causes both perinatal hypoglycemic collapse and late-juvenile-onset neuromuscular degeneration in glycogen storage disease type IV of Norwegian forest cats. Mol Genet Metab 2007;90(4):383–392.

Gregory BL, Shelton DG, Bali DS, et al. Glycogen storage disease type IIIa in curly-coated retrievers. J Vet Intern Med 2007;21:40–46.

Seppälä EH, Reuser AJJ, Lohi H. A nonsense mutation in the acid α-glucosidase gene causes pompe disease in Finnish and Swedish Lapphunds. PLoS One 2013;8(2):e56825.

Authors: Jessica C. Pritchard VMD, MS, DACVIM (SAIM), Sharon A. Center DVM, DACVIM

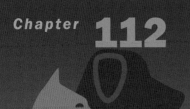

Chapter 112

Glycogen-Type Vacuolar Hepatopathy

DEFINITION/OVERVIEW

- Glycogen-type vacuolar hepatopathy (VH) – reversible hepatocellular cytosolic vacuolation.
- Reflects many primary disorders including glucocorticoid treatment, hyperadrenocorticism, atypical adrenal hyperplasia (sex hormone hyperplasia), chronic systemic illnesses (inflammatory, neoplastic), and, rarely, congenital glycogen storage disorders.
- Typified by high alkaline phosphatase (ALP) activity, usually without hyperbilirubinemia or hepatic insufficiency.
- A similar but remarkably severe VH is seen in hepatocutaneous disease; lesions may reflect chronic phenobarbital administration.
- Glycogen VH may coexist with cytosolic lipid vacuolation – comparatively rare in dogs but may be associated with idiopathic hyperlipidemia, diabetes mellitus, hypothyroidism, and rare inborn errors of glycogen/lipid metabolism.

ETIOLOGY/PATHOPHYSIOLOGY

- Approximately 55% of cases with VH are reported to be associated with endogenous or exogenous glucocorticoids.
- Glucocorticoids: induce reversible increase in hepatocyte glycogen within 2–3 days; injectable or reposital drug formulation induces most severe VH compared to PO or topical (ocular, cutaneous, aural) forms.
- Cell expansion causes hepatomegaly; ballooning degeneration leads to hepatic parenchymal collapse; with severe nodularity, the lesions may grossly be mistaken for cirrhosis.
- The variable response to glucocorticoids among dogs relates to: (1) drug type, (2) route of administration, (3) drug dose, (4) treatment duration, and (5) individual patient sensitivity; VH may follow low-dose, short-term oral treatment.
- VH may reflect:
  - Congenital glycogen storage disorders.
  - Breed-specific disorders.
  - Hepatic nodular hyperplasia.
  - Stress response.
  - Cytokines.
  - An acute-phase response.
- This may be initiated by nonhepatic systemic disorders or neoplasia (especially lymphoma), without exogenous glucocorticoid exposure or adrenal disease.
- VH is common in dogs with gallbladder mucocele.

Blackwell's Five-Minute Veterinary Consult Clinical Companion: Small Animal Gastrointestinal Diseases,
First Edition. Edited by Jocelyn Mott and Jo Ann Morrison.
© 2019 John Wiley & Sons, Inc. Published 2019 by John Wiley & Sons, Inc.
Companion website: www.fiveminutevet.com/gastrointestinal

Systems Affected

- Hepatobiliary – usually normal hepatic function is maintained; severe degenerative VH can lead to hepatic dysfunction, jaundice, ascites, and liver failure.
- All systems affected by steroid hormones or a primary systemic disease.

 # SIGNALMENT/HISTORY

- Dogs – common; often accompanies primary necroinflammatory liver disorders.
- Cat – rare; liver vacuolation with triglyceride accumulation (i.e., hepatic lipidosis) is more common.
- Breed predilections – those predisposed to hyperadrenocorticism develop glycogen VH (i.e., miniature poodles, dachshunds, boxers, Boston terriers), Scottish terriers (sex hormone adrenal hyperplasia, hyperlipidemia), and others with hyperlipidemia (miniature schnauzers, Shetland sheepdogs) may develop mixed glycogen/lipid VH.
- Mean age and range.
  - Middle-aged to old dogs: spontaneous hyperadrenocorticism (>75% older than nine years); chronic systemic inflammation or neoplasia.
  - Dogs of any age: iatrogenic VH subsequent to glucocorticoid administration.
  - Young dogs or cats: genetic glycogen storage disease.

Risk Factors

- Glucocorticoid administration.
- Hyperadrenocorticism (spontaneous) – typical or atypical.
- Underlying systemic illness provoking acute-phase response or stress. Examples: severe dental disease, inflammatory bowel disease (IBD), chronic pancreatitis, systemic neoplasia (especially lymphoma), chronic infections (urinary tract, skin), hypothyroidism, etc.
- Chronic administration of phenobarbital.
- Hyperlipidemia.

Historical Findings

- Reflect glucocorticoids or underlying systemic illness.
- Rarely, signs of hepatic disease or failure; hepatic failure can develop with severe chronic VH.
- HE observed in some dogs with hepatocutaneous syndrome.
- Glucocorticoid excess: polyuria and polydipsia; polyphagia; endocrine alopecia; abdominal distension – weak muscles, loss of elasticity; skeletal muscle weakness; excessive panting; lethargy; friable skin; bruising tendencies; urinary tract infections, may be asymptomatic; corneal ulcers.
- Adrenal sex hormone hyperplasia: may display some signs of glucocorticoid excess but often fewer and less severe; endocrine alopecia may be the only sign; some dogs remain asymptomatic except for chronic progressive marked ALP activity and degenerative VH.
- Other causes: depend on system affected; chronic phenobarbital may cause severe VH.
- Sex hormone hyperplasia causing VH may increase risk for dysplastic hepatic foci and hepatocellular carcinoma (e.g., Scottish terriers).

 # CLINICAL FEATURES

- Hepatomegaly.
- Relate to steroid hormone excess or underlying disease; depends on severity and duration.

DIFFERENTIAL DIAGNOSIS

- Other diffuse hepatopathies (especially those causing hepatomegaly and increased ALP activity); passive congestion; neoplasia (primary or metastatic to liver); necroinflammatory liver disease; anticonvulsant hepatopathy; hepatomegaly due to amyloid (rare).
- VH distinguishing features: most dogs have a 5–10-fold increase in ALP > alanine aminotransferase (ALT) or aspartate aminotransferase (AST); increased cholesterol; normal serum bilirubin; normal/mild increase in total serum bile acids (TSBA); heterogeneous or homogeneous hyperechoic hepatic parenchyma on ultrasonography (nodules or "Swiss cheese" pattern); characteristic cytology: hepatocytes engorged due to expanded "rarified" cytoplasm.

DIAGNOSTICS

Complete Blood Count/Biochemistry/Urinalysis

Complete Blood Count

- Depends on underlying disease.
- Nonregenerative anemia: anemia of chronic disease or hypothyroidism.
- Relative polycythemia from steroid excess.
- Stress leukogram: hyperadrenocorticism; glucocorticoid exposure; stress of illness.
- Thrombocytosis: neoplasia; hyperadrenocorticism; splenic disease.

Biochemistry

- ALP markedly increased: typically 5–10 times normal concentrations (ALP glucocorticoid isoenzyme cannot differentiate cause of VH because other liver disorders also induce this isoenzyme).
- Variable gamma-glutamyl transferase (GGT), ALT, AST activity.
- Serum albumin and total bilirubin are usually normal; high bilirubin usually implicates another hepatobiliary or hemolytic process.
- Hypercholesterolemia: hyperadrenocorticism, sex hormone adrenal hyperplasia.
- Breed-related hyperlipidemias.

Other Laboratory Tests

- ALP glucocorticoid isoenzyme: lacks specificity and, thus, clinical utility.
- TSBA: may be mildly increased.
- Ammonia tolerance test: usually normal.
- Pituitary adrenal axis: adrenocorticotropic hormone (ACTH) response test or low-dose dexamethasone suppression test (LDDST), ± high-dose dexamethasone suppression test (HDDST), and endogenous ACTH may help differentiate nonadrenal illness, adrenal or pituitary disorders.
- Urine cortisol:creatinine ratio: at-home urine collection helps rule out hyperadrenocorticism; high ratio may reflect stress or nonadrenal illness.
- Thyroid testing: diagnose or rule out hypothyroidism.
- Triglycerides (fasting): diagnose or rule out hyperlipidemia.
- Canine pancreatic lipase immunoreactivity: may indicate "subclinical" pancreatic inflammation or inflammatory bowel disease.
- Coagulation assessments such as prothrombin time, activated partial thromboplastin time, fibrinogen, and mucosal bleeding time: usually normal; bench assessments have low value in predicting iatrogenic hemorrhage; buccal mucosal bleeding time may be more relevant.

Imaging

- Abdominal radiography: reveals hepatomegaly or other underlying conditions.
- Thoracic radiography: may reveal lymphadenopathy, metastatic disease, cardiac or pulmonary disorders.
- Abdominal ultrasonography: discloses hepatomegaly, diffuse hyperechoic hepatic parenchyma or multifocal nodular "mottling" (Figure 112.1); multifocal lesions suggest nodules ("Swiss cheese pattern") formed by progressive hepatocellular ballooning degeneration; may disclose underlying primary visceral abnormalities (e.g., mesenteric lymphadenopathy, neoplasia) or adrenal disorders (adrenals may be large with hyperadrenocorticism, sex hormone adrenal hyperplasia, chronic stress or neoplasia).

Other Diagnostic Procedures

- Hepatic fine-needle aspiration for cytology: 22 gauge, 2.5–3.75 cm (1–1.5 in.) Ultrasonography (US)-guided needle aspiration; target nodules and normal parenchyma.
- Cytology: glycogen vacuolation is common in many primary liver disorders. Used to rule out vacuolar change; cannot definitively confirm illness caused only by VH.
  - Cytologic features.
  - Hepatocellular cytosolic distension: "rarefication" or granular appearance with increased cell fragility (Figures 112.2 and 112.3); canalicular bile casts may be observed; primary VH is not associated with inflammatory infiltrates; common association with extramedullary hematopoiesis (EMH) may be misinterpreted as suppurative inflammation.
- Tissue culture and sensitivity: if suppurative inflammation suspected, submit aerobic and anaerobic bacterial cultures.
- Hepatic biopsy: verifies VH; excludes other primary hepatic disease; pursue if a systemic disorder is not discovered explaining high ALP and VH; use of a US-guided Tru-Cut needle biopsy will confirm VH but may miss primary hepatic disease; laparoscopy (recommended) or laparotomy (if visceral inspections and biopsies indicated) are additional options to obtain hepatic biopsy specimens and to help evaluate for primary hepatic disease.

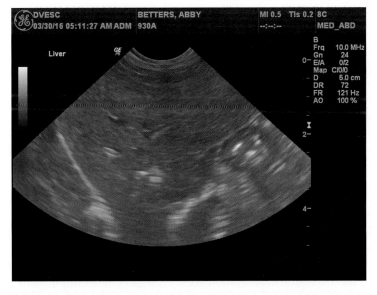

■ **Fig. 112.1.** Hepatic ultrasonographic image showing diffusely coarse architecture with nodular appearance ("mottling").

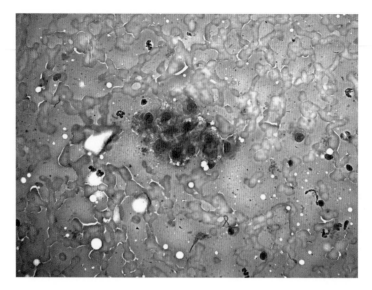

■ **Fig. 112.2.** Cytologic appearance of hepatocytes showing vacuolar changes and associated hemorrhage (50× view).

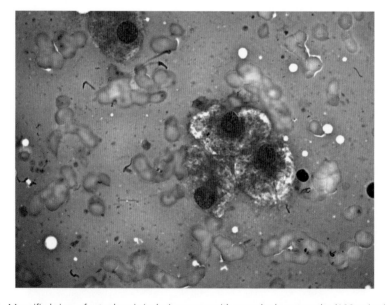

■ **Fig. 112.3.** Magnified view of cytoplasmic inclusions seen with vacuolar hepatopathy (100× view).

Pathologic Findings

- Gross: variable; normal to moderate hepatomegaly; inconsistent surface irregularity; tan or pale color; may be confused with cirrhosis if nodular severe degenerative VH.
- Microscopic: marked vacuolization and ballooning of hepatocytes; no consistent zonal distribution or foci of hepatic degeneration; focal aggregates of neutrophils due to extramedullary hematopoiesis (EMH); severe degenerative VH leads to parenchymal collapse forming nodules surrounded by a thin partition with minimal collagen deposition.

THERAPEUTICS

- Management of VH is dependent on the underlying disease process and any arising complicating factors (hypertension, proteinuria, etc.).
- If VH is suspected to be idiopathic, management is controversial and no studies have been performed to critically evaluate therapy.

Drug(s) of Choice

- Liver support therapy with SAMe (Denosyl or Denamarin), milk thistle, or other antioxidants may have some benefit but are unlikely to result in decrease of serum ALP or resolve VH.
- Pituitary-dependent hyperadrenocorticism or adrenal hyperplasia syndrome (sex hormone) is usually treated medically: op'-DDD (mitotane or Lysodren), trilostane or ketoconazole; op'-DDD preferred for sex hormone adrenal hyperplasia as trilostane augments sex hormone accumulation; l-deprenyl and melatonin have no published data to demonstrate effectiveness.
- Manage primary inflammatory disorders that necessitate immunosuppressive or antiinflammatory medications: use polypharmacy to minimize glucocorticoid exposure (see Alternative Drugs) if symptomatic or progressive VH.
- Neoplasia: tumor resection, chemotherapy or radiation, as appropriate.
- Dental disease: antibiotics and dentistry.
- IBD: hypoallergenic/hydrolyzed protein diets and immunomodulation (avoid glucocorticoids).
- Pyelonephritis, chronic dermatitis, or other infectious disorders: long-term antimicrobial treatment based on microbial culture and sensitivity tests; other appropriate medications as indicated per the primary disease.
- Hypothyroidism: supplemental levothyroxine to achieve euthyroid state.

Precautions/Interactions

- Avoid hepatotoxic drugs if severe VH.
- Beware of drug interactions if using ketoconazole for adrenal disease.
- Avoid drugs with hepatic ALP induction effects.
- Glucocorticoids: caution in VH patients; use lowest effective dose regimen (e.g. alternate-day protocol if prednisone or prednisolone); special caution in hyperlipidemia as glucocorticoids may worsen clinical signs of abdominal pain, vomiting, pancreatitis; glucocorticoid therapy increases insulin requirements in diabetes mellitus; may augment gallbladder mucocele formation; may provoke hepatic lipidosis in cats.

Alternative Drugs

Polypharmacy protocol may reduce glucocorticoid usage in management of immune mediated or inflammatory disorders (e.g. metronidazole, azathioprine, chlorambucil, cyclophosphamide, mycophenolate, or cyclosporine).

Diet

- Hyperlipidemia or pancreatitis: restrict dietary fat and fatty supplements.
- Obesity: gradual kcal restriction; treat predisposing disorder if present.

Surgical Considerations

- Depends on underlying conditions.
- Adrenal and/or liver masses may be resectable.
- Hypophyseal masses: resection only by experienced surgeons.

COMMENTS

- Before concluding that VH is idiopathic, a thorough work-up to rule out underlying diseases should be performed.
- It is prudent to monitor suspected idiopathic VH cases frequently due to possible complications of the disease (i.e., hypertension, development of clinical hyperadrenocorticism, risk for developing biliary mucocele, neoplasia, etc.).

Patient Monitoring

- Hepatomegaly: abdominal palpation; imaging.
- Normalizing enzymes: biochemistry.
- Adrenal function: ACTH stimulation tests.
- Neoplasia: physical exams and imaging.
- Control of infection: repeat cultures.
- Hyperlipidemia: assess gross plasma lipemia; measure triglycerides and cholesterol.
- Suspected idiopathic VH: ultrasound, baseline bloodwork every 6–12 months.

Prevention/Avoidance

- Limit glucocorticoid exposure.
- Use alternate-day therapy with prednisone/prednisolone; titrate to lowest effective dose; use alternative medications to control primary illness.

Possible Complications

Numerous, and related to multisystemic effects of glucocorticoids and associated conditions.

Expected Course and Prognosis

- Typically, good prognosis but does depend heavily on underlying cause; most patients are asymptomatic for VH despite high ALP; however, progressive degenerative hepatopathy leading to diffuse nodule formation and hepatic insufficiency may develop in chronic VH in dogs with high ALP activity.
- Laboratory and pathologic features reversible before degenerative parenchymal collapse.
- Dogs with sex hormone hyperplasia, VH, and dysplastic hepatocellular foci appear at risk for development of hepatocellular carcinoma.
- Associated conditions.
  - Pulmonary thromboembolism and myopathy due to hyperadrenocorticism.
  - Pancreatitis associated with hyperlipidemia.
  - Gallbladder mucocele.

Synonyms

- Corticosteroid hepatopathy
- Glucocorticoid hepatopathy
- Steroid hepatopathy
- Vacuolar change

Abbreviations

- ACTH = adrenocorticotropic hormone
- ALP = alkaline phosphatase
- ALT = alanine aminotransferase
- AST = aspartate aminotransferase
- EMH = extramedullary hematopoiesis
- GGT = gamma-glutamyl transferase
- HDDST = high-dose dexamethasone suppression test

- IBD = inflammatory bowel disease
- LDDST = low-dose dexamethasone
  suppression test

- TSBA = total serum bile acids
- US = ultrasonography
- VH = vacuolar hepatopathy

See Also

- Gallbladder Mucocele

- Pancreatitis, Canine

Suggested Reading

Cortright CC, Center SA, Randolph JF, et al. Clinical features of progressive vacuolar hepatopathy in Scottish Terriers with and without hepatocellular carcinoma: 114 cases (1980–2013). J Am Vet Med Assoc 2014;245:797–808.

Sepesy LM, Center SA, Randolph JF, et al. Vacuolar hepatopathy in dogs: 336 cases (1993–2005). J Am Vet Med Assoc 2006;229:246–252.

Twedt DC. Idiopathic vacuolar hepatopathy. In: Bonagura JD, Twedt DC, eds. Kirk's Current Veterinary Therapy, 15th ed. St Louis: Elsevier, 2014, pp. 606–608.

Acknowledgments: The author and editors acknowledge the prior contribution of Dr Sharon Center.

Author: Ashleigh Seigneur DVM, MVSc, DACVIM

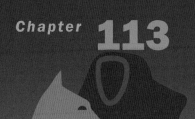
Hepatic Amyloid

DEFINITION/OVERVIEW

- Amyloidosis is the extracellular deposition of insoluble fibrillary B-pleated proteinaceous matrix (amyloid).
- Hepatic amyloid is the deposition of amyloid within the liver parenchyma.
- Amyloid has distinctive staining properties and fibrillary ultrastructure.

ETIOLOGY/PATHOPHYSIOLOGY

- Amyloidosis can be acquired, occurring secondary to inflammatory or lymphoproliferative disorders, or can be familial, the result of a genetic disorder.
- Amyloid is derived from many different proteins; certain proteins are associated with specific diseases.
- Serum amyloid A (SAA), an acute-phase protein produced by hepatocytes, is produced during inflammation and is associated with the most commonly reported generalized form of amyloidosis in small animals.
- Amyloid AL, which is a monoclonal IgG light chain and is associated with plasma cell dyscrasia, is not commonly reported in small animals and is not the form associated with hepatic amyloidosis.
- Familial amyloidosis is recognized in certain kindreds of pure-bred cats, certain breeds and kindreds of dogs, and in systemic inflammatory disorders.
- Organ rupture (liver; cats) or hepatic failure (dog) can result as a consequence of amyloid deposition.

Systems Affected

- Amyloid may accumulate focally or systemically.
- Liver and kidneys are most commonly affected; other organ systems can also be affected.
- Renal/urologic – renal amyloidosis is more common in dogs; Chinese shar-pei dogs frequently have systemic involvement that includes the liver.
- Hepatobiliary – hepatic amyloidosis is more commonly reported in cats, although renal involvement is more commonly reported in Abyssinian cats.

Blackwell's Five-Minute Veterinary Consult Clinical Companion: Small Animal Gastrointestinal Diseases, First Edition. Edited by Jocelyn Mott and Jo Ann Morrison.
© 2019 John Wiley & Sons, Inc. Published 2019 by John Wiley & Sons, Inc.
Companion website: www.fiveminutevet.com/gastrointestinal

SIGNALMENT/HISTORY

- Dogs – Chinese shar-peis with "shar-pei fever syndrome"; akitas with cyclic fever and polyarthropathy; collies with "gray collie syndrome"; beagles with juvenile polyarteritis syndrome.
- Renal signs usually develop first in dogs, although hepatic insufficiency may develop.
- Dogs are often young, <6 years of age, at time of clinical onset of disease.
- Cats – oriental shorthair, Siamese, Devon rex, domestic shorthair, Abyssinian.
- Often cats are <5 years of age when first symptomatic; most present initially for lethargy and anorexia; hepatic signs and coagulopathies predominate.
- Renal signs predominate in Abyssinians where the disease is familial.
- Cats naturally infected with feline immunodeficiency virus (FIV) have been described to have systemic amyloid deposition, with kidneys, liver, and spleen most affected.

Risk Factors

- Familial immunoregulatory disorders.
- Chronic infections – bacterial, viral, fungal.
- Chronic inflammation – immune-mediated conditions.
- Neoplasia.
- Acquired immune deficiencies – FIV infection in cats.

Historical Findings

- Episodic fever and swollen hocks – shar-pei.
- Episodic polyarthropathy, pain, signs of meningitis – akita, beagle.
- Acute lethargy, episodic in nature.
- Anorexia and vomiting, episodic in nature.
- Polyuria/polydipsia – especially if renal involvement.

 CLINICAL FEATURES

- Pallor – hepatic rupture.
- Hypothermia – cats.
- Abdominal effusion – hemorrhage or ascites.
- Hepatomegaly – amyloidosis.
- Jaundice – may or may not be present.
- Peripheral edema – due to hypoalbuminemia secondary to pathologic proteinuria.
- Joint pain or effusion – shar-pei, akita.
- Nonlocalized pain, meningeal pain, and abdominal discomfort – due to inflammatory disorders promoting amyloid.

 DIFFERENTIAL DIAGNOSIS

- Chronic hepatic inflammation.
- Infiltrative hepatic neoplasia.
- Primary or rodenticide-induced coagulopathy.
- Glomerulonephritis.
- Pyelonephritis.
- Systemic lupus erythematosus (SLE).

- Abdominal trauma.
- Peritonitis.
- Meningitis.
- Immune-mediated or infectious polyarthropathy.

DIAGNOSTICS

Complete Blood Count/Biochemistry/Urinalysis

- Anemia secondary to hepatic hemorrhage or liver lobe rupture or chronic inflammation.
- Leukocytosis with a left shift during febrile episodes in shar-pei and akita.
- Platelets may be normal or low if hepatic rupture has occurred.
- Normal or elevated: liver enzyme activities, especially alanine aminotransferase (ALT) in cats, total bilirubin, serum bile acids; these may be normal in severe hepatic amyloid deposition.
- Azotemia – due to renal interstitium amyloid deposition in cats and often in the shar-pei.
- Proteinuria – due to glomerular amyloid deposition in dogs and sometimes in the shar-pei. Note that there is a difference in renal amyloid deposition locations between primary (familial) and secondary amyloidosis.
- Hyperglycemia – common in cats, likely stress related.
- Dilute urine – renal failure.
- Feline systemic amyloidosis can involve multiple organ systems affecting multiple bloodwork parameters – thyroid, cardiac, renal, intestinal, pancreatic, bone marrow, lymph nodes, and adrenal glands.

Additional Laboratory Tests

- Coagulation profiles – normal to prolonged clotting times, hyperfibrinogenemia.
- Synovial fluid – analysis and culture; dogs with joint swelling or pain and/or fever.
- Lyme disease testing – enzyme-linked immunosorbent assay (ELISA) for C6 antibody presence in dogs with joint swelling/pain or fever.
- Cerebral spinal fluid (CSF) – if meningeal pain is present to assess for increased protein and/ or suppurative inflammation.

Imaging

- Abdominal radiography – assess for hepatomegaly; variable renal size; abdominal effusion.
- Abdominal ultrasound – assess for hepatomegaly, hypoechoic and/or heterogeneous parenchyma (diffuse amyloid), rounded or irregular liver lobe edges; variable renal size with normal or equivocally hypoechoic parenchyma (renal amyloid); inconsistent mesenteric lymphadenopathy; thickened gut wall (amyloid deposition); abdominal effusion.

Diagnostic Procedures

- Fine needle aspiration cytology – may identify the presence of amyloid (Figure 113.1).
- Liver or other tissue biopsy.
- Abdominocentesis – to assess for hemorrhage (esp. in cats) or transudative effusion (seen with diffuse hepatopathy).

Pathologic Findings

- Gross – liver may be normal to pale in color; large, firm to friable; hemorrhage may be focal (subcapsular hematomas, capsular tears) to overt hepatic rupture (Figure 113.2).
- Microscopic – diffuse acellular amorphous material in the space of Disse associated with hepatic cord atrophy; may primarily involve blood vessels in the portal triads (Abyssinian cats).

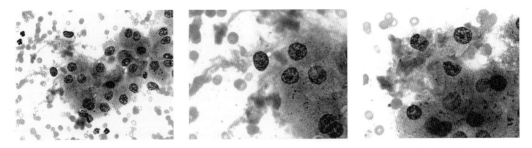

■ **Fig. 113.1.** Fine needle aspirate of liver showing hepatic amyloid. Source: Courtesy of Dr Michael A. Scott, Michigan State University.

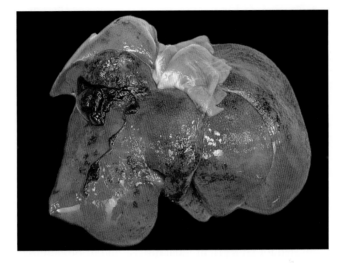

■ **Fig. 113.2.** Gross specimen of feline liver with amyloidosis. Source: Courtesy of Dr Matti Kiupel, Michigan State University.

- Staining.
  - Amyloid stains amorphous pink with routine hematoxylin and eosin.
  - May stain turquoise blue with Masson's trichrome.
  - Congo red staining with bright field: amyloid is salmon pink but with polarized light is birefringent (B-pleated sheet structure refracts polarized light) and apple green.
- Centrilobular necrosis secondary to anemia-induced hypoxia may be diagnosed in cats that present for hemoabdomen secondary to a liver lobe rupture. The presence of amyloid may be missed in these situations if special stains are not used.

 THERAPEUTICS

- Amyloid is insoluble and therefore cannot be specifically treated; guarded to poor prognosis.
- Severity of clinical signs dictates treatment options.
- There is no curative treatment; goal is to manage the underlying disease process if possible; colchicine may reduce further organ amyloid deposition but will not eliminate amyloid that is already deposited; see below.

Drug(s) of Choice

■ Colchicine – dogs: 0.03 mg/kg PO q24h; cats: no published dosages available, but anecdotal reports of use in cats at a dosage of 0.020–0.035 mg/kg PO q24h exist; may block amyloid deposition in early disease or control deposition in chronic disorders in dogs; modulates expression of adhesion molecules and chemotactic factors; causes microtubule polymerization by binding to tubulin, blocking cell mitosis in cells such as neutrophils. Effects attenuate inflammatory response triggering acute-phase protein (amyloid precursor) production. Monitor complete blood cell count for bone marrow toxicity; observe patient for enteric side effects (vomiting, diarrhea (bloody)); beware of toxicity if coadministered with p450-blocking drugs (e.g., ketoconazole, omeprazole, cimetidine). Use colchicine without added probenecid. Monitor for hypertension. Limited experience in cats.

■ Dimethyl sulfoxide (DMSO) – dogs: controversial treatment; use medical grade only; dogs: 80–90 mg/kg given as no more than a 25% solution in sterile water to help reduce injection site pain, PO or SQ, three times a week; may promote dissolution of amyloid fibrils or provide antiinflammatory or antiamyloid effect. Side effects: garlic odor, objectionable taste, nausea, and anorexia. In humans, this treatment given PO daily (3–20 g/patient) has benefit in polysytemic amyloidosis but not renal amyloidosis associated with renal failure. No experience in cats.

■ Lactulose – dogs: 2.5–15 mL PO q8–12h; cats: 2.5–5.0 mL PO q8–12 h; for patients with suspected hepatic encephalopathy. If oral administration is not tolerated, this may be given as a retention enema.

■ Nonsteroidal antiinflammatory drugs (NSAIDs) – in dogs (shar-pei fever syndrome) to reduce pain and fever if present.

■ Vitamin K1 – dogs and cats: initially at three doses of 0.5–1.5 mg/kg SQ or IM. Subsequent dosing may be necessary, especially in cats. Monitor prothrombin time (PT); dosing interval should be determined by resolution of prolongation of PT.

■ Medications as indicated for concurrent renal disease and/or proteinuria if present.

Precautions/Interactions

■ Colchicine combined with probenecid may cause vomiting as probenecid prolongs residence time of colchicine.

■ Colchicine toxicity can occur if it is administered with a p450 cytochrome-inhibiting drug.

■ Colchicine may cause/enhance bone marrow suppression if administered with antineoplastics, immunosuppressive medications, chloramphenicol, or amphotericin B.

Appropriate Health Care

■ Fluids – for dehydration.

■ Blood transfusion – for acute blood loss is necessary in cats with hepatic amyloid-induced liver lobe rupture.

Diet

■ Ensure adequate caloric intake; malnutrition contributes to morbidity and mortality in shar-peis.

■ No specific diet; may ultimately need to consider a hepatic or renal diet; case dependent.

Surgical Considerations

Hepatic lobe resection is necessary for cats presenting for emergent hepatic lobe fracture and resultant hemoabdomen.

COMMENTS

Client Education

- Familial amyloidosis is recognized in shar-pei dogs and Abyssinian cats; it is suspected in Siamese cats.
- In shar-pei dogs, amyloidosis is a known autosomal recessive trait.

Patient Monitoring

- No specific monitoring; as needed for episodic recrudescence of lethargy, anorexia or fever.
- PT will need to be monitored for patients receiving vitamin K1 therapy so that appropriate dosing intervals can be determined.

Prevention/Avoidance

- Breeding of animals with known or suspected familial hepatic amyloidosis should be avoided.
- Breedings that have produced progeny with familial hepatic amyloidosis should be discontinued.

Possible Complications

Organ rupture.

Expected Course and Prognosis

- Shar-pei – with hepatic amyloid may survive >2 years; most have episodes of fever and cholestasis; some have resolution of clinical signs and diminished hepatic amyloid with colchicine.
- Early intervention with colchicine in shar-pei dogs may decrease proteinuria and slow progression of chronic kidney disease (CKD).
- Akitas with cyclic clinical signs – grave prognosis.
- Cats surviving liver hemorrhage often have repeated episodes of hemoabdomen within weeks to months of initial presentation, although survival times of at least 30 months with few recurrences have been reported.

Abbreviations

- AL = amyloid light chain
- ALT = alanine aminotransferase
- CKD = chronic kidney disease
- CSF = cerebrospinal fluid
- DMSO = dimethyl sulfoxide
- ELISA = enzyme-linked immunosorbent assay

- FIV = feline immunodeficiency virus
- NSAID = nonsteroidal antiinflammatory drug
- PT = prothrombin time
- SAA = serum amyloid A
- SLE = systemic lupus erythematosus

See Also

- Hepatic Encephalopathy
- Icterus

Suggested Reading

Asproni P, Abramo F, Millanta F, Lorenzi D, Poli A. Amyloidosis in association with spontaneous feline immunodeficiency virus infection. J Feline Med Surg 2013;15(4):300–306.

Beatty JA, Barrs VR, Martin PA. Spontaneous hepatic rupture in six cats with systemic amyloidosis. J Small Anim Pract 2002;43:355–363.

Loevan KO. Hepatic amyloidosis in two Chinese Shar-pei dogs. J Am Vet Med Assoc 1994;204:1212–1216.

Merlini G, Bellotti V. Molecular mechanisms of amyloidosis. N Engl J Med 2003;349:583–596.

Acknowledgments: The author and editors acknowledge the prior contribution of Dr Sharon Center.

Author: Kate Holan DVM, DACVIM

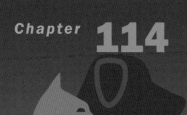
Hepatic Encephalopathy

DEFINITION/OVERVIEW

Hepatic encephalopathy (HE) is a syndrome characterized mainly by neurological abnormalities secondary to liver dysfunction and/or portosystemic shunts (PSS).

ETIOLOGY/PATHOPHYSIOLOGY

- In dogs, HE is usually the result of portosystemic shunting, either due to congenital PSS (CPSS; most common cause, >60% of cases) or the formation of multiple acquired PSS (APSS) due to portal hypertension (e.g., as a result of cirrhosis). Liver dysfunction without macroscopic shunting might account for a small percentage of HE cases.
- In cats, HE is usually associated with arginine deficiency due to hepatic lipidosis or CPSS.
- Less commonly, HE can be the result of acute liver failure without preexisting liver disease.
- Rarely, urea cycle enzyme deficiencies can lead to hyperammonemia and HE.
- Multifactorial origin – result of multiple compounds and predisposing factors that act synergistically to cause neurological dysfunction.
- Ammonia dysmetabolism plays a central role. Ammonia derived mainly from the breakdown of dietary proteins and other nitrogenous substances by colonic bacteria is absorbed by the intestine and bypasses the liver (PSS) or escapes detoxification by the liver in liver failure, therefore accumulating in the blood. Hyperammonemia has inhibitory effects on the central nervous system (CNS) due to altered amino acid membrane transport, blockade of gamma-aminobutyric acid (GABA) receptors, inhibition of Na/K-dependent ATPase, glutamine depletion, altered glutamine receptors, and impaired cerebral energy metabolism. Ammonia also causes astrocyte swelling mainly through excessive glutamine production by astrocytes, which acts as an osmolyte. This results in cerebral edema, increased intracranial pressure, and eventually death.
- Other factors that may play a role in the pathogenesis of HE in dogs and cats include altered balance of inhibitory (GABA) and excitatory (L-glutamate) amino acid neurotransmitters, increased brain concentration of endogenous benzodiazepines, concurrent systemic inflammatory response syndrome (SIRS), and amino acid imbalances.

Systems Affected

- Nervous – altered behavior; disorientation, aimless wandering, head pressing, depression, lethargy, seizures; more likely in cats.
- Gastrointestinal – vomiting, anorexia, and diarrhea.
- Renal/urologic – severe glomerular and/or tubular injury due to inadequate clearance of high concentrations of ammonia or ammonia metabolites from the systemic circulation, ammonium biurate urolithiasis.

Blackwell's Five-Minute Veterinary Consult Clinical Companion: Small Animal Gastrointestinal Diseases,
First Edition. Edited by Jocelyn Mott and Jo Ann Morrison.
© 2019 John Wiley & Sons, Inc. Published 2019 by John Wiley & Sons, Inc.
Companion website: www.fiveminutevet.com/gastrointestinal

SIGNALMENT/HISTORY

- Pure-bred small and toy-breed dogs with extra-hepatic CPSS (Yorkshire terriers, Jack Russell Terriers, Dachshunds, Havanese, Maltese, Dandie Dinmont Terriers, Pugs and Miniature Schnauzers).
- Large-breed dogs with intrahepatic CPSS (Irish wolfhounds, Labrador and golden retrievers, Australian cattle dogs, Australian shepherds, and Old English sheepdogs).
- Dog breeds predisposed to chronic hepatitis and copper-associated hepatopathy (e.g., Doberman pinschers, Dalmatians, Labradors, West Highland white terriers, and others).
- Cats with extrahepatic CPSS (domestic shorthair and longhair, Persian, Siamese, Himalayan, Burmese, Birman, British shorthair, British blue, ragdoll, and Tonkinese).
- No sex predilections.
- CPSS – most commonly, but not exclusively, in animals less than 1–2 years old.
- Chronic liver disease with extrahepatic APSS in animals of any age.

Genetics

- Disrupted closure of ductus venosus – WEE1 gene overexpression in hepatocytes of dogs with intrahepatic CPSS.
- Development of extrahepatic portal vascularization – VCAM1 gene underexpression in hepatocytes of dogs with extrahepatic CPSS.
- Undetermined polygenic inheritance of extrahepatic PSS in certain small-breed dogs.

Risk Factors

- There are several risk factors reported for HE in dogs and cats but for most of them there is limited scientific evidence to support their role in HE.
- High-protein meal; constipation; dehydration; uremia; gastrointestinal bleeding; bowel obstruction; metabolic alkalosis; hypokalemia; hypoglycemia; drugs (benzodiazepines, diuretics); sepsis; inflammation; estrus.

Historical Findings

- Wide range of clinical abnormalities ranging from mild depression and weakness to seizures, coma, and death.
- Clinical signs in the early course of HE are often nonspecific, subtle, and episodic, and are frequently undetected by owners and/or clinicians.
- Many animals have minimal and nonspecific clinical signs throughout their lives that are not detected by owners and/or clinicians. In other cases, clinical signs progress in intensity and frequency.
- Common clinical signs – altered behavior and neurologic signs (e.g., head pressing, ataxia, seizures, blindness); depression and lethargy; vomiting; ptyalism; shaking.
- Clinical signs (especially neurologic signs) may or may not be exacerbated by meal ingestion (particularly high-protein meal).
- Dysuria due to ammonium biurate urolithiasis in dogs.
- Prolonged recovery after sedation or general anesthesia – impaired hepatic metabolism.
- Episodic lethargy and depression.
- Learning disabilities.
- "Odd" behavior.
- Disorientation, aimless wandering, head pressing.
- Amaurotic blindness.
- Weight loss, failure to gain weight, anorexia and/or vomiting; hypersalivation especially in cats.

- Polyuria and polydipsia (PU/PD).
- Seizures; more frequent in cats than in dogs.
- Nonresponsiveness to external stimuli and coma; usually end-stage HE.
- Signs more frequent in cats than in dogs – hypersalivation, seizures, aggressive behavior, disorientation, ataxic stupor.
- Signs more frequent in dogs than in cats – compulsive behavior (head pressing, disorientation, aimless wandering), vomiting, diarrhea, PU/PD, hematuria, pollakiuria, and dysuria.

CLINICAL FEATURES

- Signs of cerebral disease – obtundation, ataxia, weakness, conscious proprioceptive and cranial nerve deficits, seizures; can be the presenting complaint in some dogs.
- Signs associated with underlying liver disease – ascites, pleural effusion, and subcutaneous edema; associated with severe hypoalbuminemia.
- CPSS – dogs may have normal size but are usually stunted; microhepatica. Cats are usually well grown and in good body condition; microhepatica and golden or copper-colored irises.
- Signs of lower urinary tract disease – obstructive uropathy due to ammonium biurate urolithiasis; imparts orange/brown color to urine.

DIFFERENTIAL DIAGNOSIS

- Uremic encephalopathy.
- Sepsis.
- Hypoglycemia.
- Primary gastrointestinal disease.
- Urinary tract infection.
- Ketoacidosis.
- CNS neoplasia.
- CNS malformations – hydrocephalus, storage disease.
- Brain abscess.
- Cerebral edema.
- Infectious meningoencephalitides – canine distemper, feline infectious peritonitis (FIP), feline leukemia virus (FeLV), feline immunodeficiency virus (FIV).
- Toxoplasmosis; especially in cats.
- Intracranial hemorrhage.
- Idiopathic epilepsy.
- Cobalamin deficiency (dogs).
- Thiamine deficiency (cats).
- Ethylene glycol or xylitol and lead toxicosis.

DIAGNOSTICS

Complete Blood Count/Biochemistry/Urinalysis

- PSS – red blood cell microcytosis; not always associated with concurrent anemia, poikilocytosis (cats), target cells (dogs), Heinz body formation (cats).
- Blood urea nitrogen (BUN) and creatinine – low concentrations due to PU/PD, high glomerular filtration rate (GFR), and reduced hepatic synthesis.

- Liver enzymes – variable increases and combinations in APSS depending on the cause; may be within normal range, especially in cats; usually increased alkaline phosphatase (ALP) in cats with hepatic lipidosis.
- Albumin – low serum concentration common in APSS; less common with CPSS.
- Cholesterol – low concentration common in PSS and fulminant hepatic failure.
- Bilirubin – high concentration may be seen in APSS depending on cause; usually normal in CPSS; usually high in cats with hepatic lipidosis.
- Glucose – hypoglycemia contributes to generalized weakness and seizures; sporadically seen in PSS (especially toy breeds), cirrhosis or fulminant hepatic failure.
- Ammonium biurate crystalluria – may lead to urolithiasis causing hematuria, pyuria, and proteinuria due to mechanical inflammation and infection.
- Low urine specific gravity – common in CPSS.

Other Laboratory Tests

- Blood ammonia – fasting hyperammonemia is a relatively sensitive and very specific indicator for HE; however, there are cases with HE with normal plasma concentration of ammonia; ammonium anions are very unstable in plasma; immediate measurement of serum ammonia and appropriate handling of blood samples after collection are crucial; ammonia tolerance testing (administration of NH_4Cl solution rectally) – most useful diagnostic method assessing ammonia intolerance (caution: may induce HE).
- Serum bile acids – pre- and postprandial serum bile acids extremely sensitive and specific for hepatic insufficiency or PSS associated with HE; more reliable test than blood ammonia.
- Plasma protein C – low activity in dogs with substantial shunting.
- Abdominal fluid analysis – pure or modified transudate; acquired liver disease.
- Coagulation tests – abnormalities (increased prothrombin time (PT), activated partial thromboplastin time (APTT), proteins invoked by vitamin K absence or antagonism (PIVKA), low fibrinogen) are relatively commonly seen due to liver dysfunction, disseminated intravascular coagulation (DIC), vitamin K deficiency, especially in APSS; usually not associated with spontaneous bleeding; caution when scheduling biopsies or other surgery.

Imaging

- Imaging is crucial and almost always necessary for the definitive diagnosis of PSS.
- Plain abdominal radiographs – small liver size, renomegaly with or without uroliths usually indicates the presence of CPSS in young dogs; does not allow visualization of the shunt(s).
- Ultrasonography – detection of possible underlying disorder, portal vasculature evaluation, visualization of single or multiple PSS; operator and machine dependent.
- Computed tomography (CT) – liver size determination; visualization of PSS; visualization and quantification of cerebral edema; exclusion of brain tumors and/or hemorrhage; requires general anesthesia which constitutes major disadvantage.
- CT angiography – commonly used for the detection of CPSS; more valuable than abdominal ultrasound examination.
- Angiography, magnetic resonance imaging (MRI) angiography, and portal scintigraphy may also be used.

Other Diagnostic Procedures

- Exploratory laparotomy may be needed in some cases for shunting visualization.
- Histologic examination of hepatic tissue is often required for diagnosis of the underlying cause in animals with acquired liver disease.

Pathologic Findings

- Gross – liver changes reflect underlying disorder; rare brain herniation in acute HE.
- Microscopic – liver lesions: define causal hepatic disorders and identify portal hypoperfusion associated with PSS; CNS lesions: polymicrocavitation and Alzheimer type II astrocyte changes – inconsistent in dogs.

 THERAPEUTICS

Drug(s) of Choice

- Antimicrobials – altering intestinal microbiota and reducing protein degradation and production of ammonia by colonic bacteria; empiric antimicrobial selection: metronidazole (7.5 mg/kg q8–12h) or neomycin (10–20 mg/kg PO q8–12h; use with caution for ototoxicity and nephrotoxicity with chronic administration) can be used; amoxicillin (12.5–25 mg/kg PO q12h) can also be used, especially in cats; ampicillin (20 mg/kg IV q6–8h) can be given intravenously in animals that cannot receive oral medications; combine above antimicrobial treatments with lactulose; for rifaximin (semi-synthetic rifamycin derivate), although very effective in humans, safety and efficacy data for the treatment of HE in dogs and cats are not well established.
- Nonabsorbable fermented carbohydrates – lactulose (more commonly used); reduced ammonia production/absorption; starting dose in chronic HE is 0.1–1 mL/kg PO q6–8h; dose is then adjusted until the patient passes 3–4 soft stools/day; administration of the above dose rectally as enema (after warm water enemas for cleansing the rectum) diluted with 30% warm water and retained for at least 30 minutes is used for the emergency treatment of acute HE.
- Anticonvulsants – used in animals with HE if seizures occur and in animals that seizure after or preventively before surgical treatment of CPSS; levetiracetam is recommended because it is fast acting, the primary excretion route is renal and can be administered orally (20 mg/kg q8h) and intravenously in emergency situations (20 mg/kg bolus; repeated if necessary up to 60 mg/kg). Zonisamide or potassium bromide (KBr) may be used as secondary choices. Benzodiazepines and phenobarbital should ideally be avoided.
- Mannitol – relief of symptoms associated with cerebral edema (forebrain deficits, increased systemic pressure with reflex bradycardia); administration over 30 minutes, at a dose of 1 g/kg diluted in saline; reduction of intracranial pressure by light head lifting (15–20° incline).
- Warm water enemas – cleansing enemas mechanically clear colon (10–15 mL/kg rectally, until return of clear fluid) prior to administration of lactulose per rectum.

Precautions/Interactions

- Ampicillin – acute anaphylaxis after intravenous administration; diarrhea in higher than recommended doses given orally.
- Lactulose – may cause fluid and electrolyte imbalances; avoid excessive use.
- Levetiracetam – occasional inappetence and lethargy; simultaneous administration of phenobarbital may enhance clearance of levetiracetam.
- Mannitol – excessive fluid loss and dehydration due to profound diuresis; contraindicated in dehydrated patients.
- Metronidazole – CNS toxicity (depression, ataxia, seizures, vomiting) using dose that exceeds 30 mg/kg/day.
- Neomycin – ototoxicity, nephrotoxicity, and diarrhea.

- Diazepam – prolonged sedation (dog and cat); ataxia, increased appetite (dogs) and paradoxical excitement and hepatic necrosis (cats); contraindicated in patients with impaired liver function.
- Phenobarbital – polyphagia, sedation, ataxia, and lethargy; dose-dependent adverse effects; hepatotoxicity in high doses; shortens the half-life of levetiracetam; chronic administration is contraindicated in animals with liver disease/failure.

Nursing Care

- Identification and elimination of any possible precipitating factor promoting HE.
- Balanced crystalloid fluids – avoidance of dehydration and electrolyte abnormalities; supplement fluids with 2.5–5% dextrose in hypoglycemic patients; provide 20–30 mEq/L potassium chloride (do not exceed 0.5 mEq/kg/h); sodium-restricted fluids with acquired liver disease associated with ascites, and/or marked hypoalbuminemia.
- Prevention of aspiration pneumonia in comatose patients – endotracheal intubation.

Diet

- Dietary protein restriction is the mainstay of medical management.
- Ideal diet formulation has not been established; low- or moderate-protein diets (12–18% on a dry matter basis) containing high-quality proteins are commonly used; diets designed for liver or, less ideally, renal disease are preferred; severe protein restriction is no longer recommended.
- Nonmeat protein sources are likely more beneficial in dogs than meat proteins.
- Diets with moderate levels (24–31%) of high-quality proteins are preferred in cats because of higher dietary protein requirements compared to dogs; commercial feline liver support diets are commonly used; nonmeat protein sources not recommended in cats.
- Animals with liver disease but no signs of HE likely do not benefit from dietary protein restriction.
- Ensure thiamin repletion – administer 50–100 mg daily for three days in cats, then in water-soluble vitamins in fluids (anaphylactoid reactions may occur with injectable thiamin).
- Feeding tubes – may be used in animals with severe and prolonged anorexia (especially in cats).

Activity

In general, animals with HE should be kept inactive or allowed only gentle activity when clinical signs are mild.

Surgical Considerations

- CPSS – complete closure of the shunting vein is often recommended; various techniques have been described.
- APSS – generally impossible to correct surgically because of their multiple nature; surgery contraindicated.

 COMMENTS

Client Education

- HE can relapse if underlying disorder cannot be identified and eliminated.
- Owners may be trained to make minor adjustments in doses of certain medications used (e.g., lactulose) and for appropriate administration of enemas when necessary.
- CPSS – surgical closure is the treatment of choice, but there might be adverse complications; postsurgical clinical signs (i.e., seizures) may persist, requiring chronic medical management.

Patient Monitoring

Frequent patient reevaluations focusing on behavior, body condition and weight, hydration status, serum concentration of certain biochemical parameters such as glucose, BUN, creatinine, albumin, and potassium.

Prevention/Avoidance

If possible, avoid all the risk factors listed above.

Expected Course and Prognosis

- Depends on the underlying cause of HE.
- CPSS – some mild cases may have a good prognosis when managed with medical treatment alone; in more severe cases, prognosis is guarded to poor without surgical closure of shunts.
- APSS – depends on the underlying disorder.
  - Acute hepatic failure: may be fully or partially reversible.
  - Chronic hepatic failure: usually not reversible.

Synonyms

- Hepatic coma
- Portosystemic encephalopathy

Abbreviations

- ALP = alkaline phosphatase
- APSS = acquired portosystemic shunts
- APTT = activated partial thromboplastin time
- BUN = blood urea nitrogen
- CNS = central nervous system.
- CPSS = congenital portosystemic shunts.
- CT = computed tomography
- DIC = disseminated intravascular coagulation
- FeLV = feline leukemia virus.
- FIP = feline infectious peritonitis.
- FIV = feline immunodeficiency virus.
- GABA = gamma-aminobutyric acid
- GFR = glomerular filtration rate
- HE = hepatic encephalopathy
- MRI = magnetic resonance imaging
- PIVKA = proteins invoked by vitamin K absence or antagonism
- PSS = portosystemic shunts.
- PT = prothrombin time.
- PU/PD = polyuria/polydipsia
- SIRS = systemic inflammatory response syndrome

See Also

- Cirrhosis and Fibrosis of the Liver
- Coagulopathy of Liver Disease
- Hepatic Failure, Acute
- Hepatic Lipidosis
- Hepatitis, Chronic
- Hypertension, Portal
- Nutritional Approach to Hepatic Disease
- Portosystemic Shunting, Acquired
- Portosystemic Vascular Anomaly, Congenital

Suggested Reading

Cocker S, Richter K. Diagnostic evaluation of the liver. In: Ettinger SJ, Feldman EC, Cote E, eds. Textbook of Veterinary Internal Medicine, Expert Consult, 8th ed. St Louis: Saunders, 2017.

Gow AG. Hepatic encephalopathy. Vet Clin North Am Small Anim Pract 2017;47(3):585–599.

Lidbury JA, Cook AK, Steiner JM. Hepatic encephalopathy in dogs and cats. J Vet Emerg Crit Care 2016;26(4):471–487.

Acknowledgments: The author and editors acknowledge the prior contribution of Dr Sharon Center.

Authors: Manolis K. Chatzis DVM, PhD, Panagiotis G. Xenoulis DVM, Dr.med.vet., PhD

Chapter 115

Hepatic Failure, Acute

DEFINITION/OVERVIEW

- Liver dysfunction occurring in the absence of known preexisting liver disease in the presence of encephalopathy and coagulopathy.
- Occurs when over 70% of hepatocellular mass is lost so that insufficient hepatic parenchyma remains to maintain synthetic and excretory homeostasis.

ETIOLOGY/PATHOPHYSIOLOGY

- Necrosis – secondary to insufficient perfusion, hypoxia, hepatotoxins or their adducts (drugs, other xenobiotics, toxins), heat excess, or infectious agents.
- Severity of hepatic dysfunction depends on insult type and lobular (zonal) distribution.
- Reduced perfusion or hypoxia usually affects zone 3 (pericentral or centrilobular region).
- Toxins – affect zone where toxin is metabolized or adducts formed, or where there is specific organelle tropism or propensity for oxidative injury (e.g., copper accumulation increases zone 3 vulnerability).
- Accompanied by enzyme leakage and markers of impaired liver function, hyperbilirubinemia, and acute-onset splanchnic hypertension due to sinusoidal or centrilobular collapse.
- Hepatic failure – associated with a variety of metabolic derangements, i.e., altered glucose homeostasis, protein synthesis (albumin, transport proteins, procoagulants, and anticoagulants), and detoxification capabilities.

Systems Affected

- Hepatobiliary – hepatocellular necrosis; hepatic failure and jaundice.
- Nervous – hepatic encephalopathy (HE); cerebral edema.
- Gastrointestinal – vomiting; diarrhea; melena; hematochezia due to acute splanchnic hypertension ± coagulopathy.
- Hemic/lymphatic/immune – pro- and anticoagulant factor imbalances; disseminated intravascular coagulation (DIC).
- Renal/urologic – renal tubular damage from specific toxins or physiologic vasoconstriction; tubular injury, i.e., copper-associated hepatopathy, leptospirosis, xylitol toxicity, nonsteroidal antiinflammatory drug (NSAID) toxicity.
- Hyperdynamic circulatory status: low systemic and pulmonary vascular resistance, increased cardiac output and metabolic rate, systemic hypotension and splanchnic hypertension.

Blackwell's Five-Minute Veterinary Consult Clinical Companion: Small Animal Gastrointestinal Diseases, First Edition. Edited by Jocelyn Mott and Jo Ann Morrison.
© 2019 John Wiley & Sons, Inc. Published 2019 by John Wiley & Sons, Inc.
Companion website: www.fiveminutevet.com/gastrointestinal

SIGNALMENT/HISTORY

- More common in dog than in cat.
- Breeds with apparent predisposition to chronic hepatitis and copper-associated hepatopathy (e.g., Labrador retriever, Doberman pinscher) may have higher risk, e.g., Labrador retrievers and NSAID toxicity enhanced by copper-associated hepatopathy.
- No age predilection.
- No sex predilection.

Risk Factors

- Administration of any potentially hepatotoxic substance or any drug.
- Exposure to environmental toxins (e.g., *Amanita* mushroom, food-borne aflatoxin, cycad (sago palm) ingestion, blue-green algae, artificial sweetener xylitol (gum, candy) – dogs.
- Enzyme inducers (e.g., phenobarbital) – may increase risk for certain toxicities by enhancing xenobiotic toxin formation, e.g., acetaminophen toxicity is greatly enhanced by phenobarbital.
- Subcutaneous administration of intranasal *Bordetella* vaccine.

Historical Findings

- Acute-onset nonspecific clinical signs; lethargy, abdominal distension (i.e., effusion, organomegaly), abdominal discomfort/pain.
- Neurologic signs (seizures, head pressing) can occur if HE is present.
- Gastrointestinal signs; inappetence, anorexia, vomiting, and diarrhea are common.
- Renal signs: polyuria/polydipsia (PU/PD), pigmenturia are common.
- Icterus.

CLINICAL FEATURES

- Physical examination findings can vary significantly based on disease severity and may be normal in early disease.
- Cranial abdominal organomegaly.
- Abdominal effusion.
- Abdominal pain.
- Coagulopathy – melena, hematochezia, hematemesis.
- Icterus.
- Hepatic encephalopathy.
- Seizures.

DIFFERENTIAL DIAGNOSIS

- Severe acute pancreatitis – differentiated via laboratory tests and imaging.
- Severe acute gastroenteritis – differentiated via laboratory tests and imaging.
- Protein-losing enteropathy – differentiated via laboratory tests and imaging.
- Hypoadrenocorticism – differentiated via adrenocorticotropic hormone stimulation test.
- Acutely decompensated chronic liver disease – distinguished by review of medical records, blood tests, abdominal ultrasonography, and liver biopsy.

DIAGNOSTICS

Complete Blood Count/Biochemistry/Urinalysis

- Anemia and panhypoproteinemia – bleeding, marrow toxicity, direct enteric toxicity.
- Thrombocytopenia – bleeding, DIC, or portal hypertension.
- Liver enzyme activity – high acute ALT and AST; smaller increases in ALP and GGT.
- Hypoglycemia – grave prognosis.
- Hypocholesterolemia – impaired synthesis or enteric loss with hemorrhage.
- Normal to low BUN concentration: reduced urea cycle function, PU/PD.
- Hyperbilirubinemia – may be absent initially.
- Bilirubinuria may precede hyperbilirubinemia – always abnormal in cats.
- Ammonium urate crystalluria signifies hyperammonemia, hepatic insufficiency or portosystemic shunting.
- Acquired Fanconi's syndrome – granular casts and renal glucosuria indicate proximal tubule injury (e.g., carprofen, copper, leptospirosis, other toxicities, especially in dogs).

Additional Laboratory Tests

- Total serum bile acid testing (TSBA) – high values indicate hepatic dysfunction, cholestasis, or portosystemic shunting.
- Plasma ammonia concentration – high values coincide with high TSBA, confirm hepatic insufficiency; hyperammonemia inconsistent but reflected by ammonium biurate crystalluria; hyperammonemia may reflect concurrent myonecrosis.
- Coagulation tests – coagulation factor deficiencies, platelet dysfunction, low fibrinogen, low antithrombin or protein C activity, and DIC suggest severe liver failure, decompensated DIC, or enteric losses with hemorrhage.

Imaging

- Abdominal radiography – may observe a normal to slightly large liver ± effusion.
- Abdominal ultrasonography – may observe extrahepatic disorders (e.g., pancreatitis), altered circulation (ratio of hepatic vein:portal vein), altered liver echogenicity or surface contour reflecting chronic injury (e.g., remodeling implicated by heterogeneous liver texture, nodularity, or hepatofugal portal blood flow); rule out biliary obstruction as source of hyperbilirubinemia.

Other Diagnostic Procedures

- Liver biopsy – confirms necrosis and characterize lesion zonal distribution.
- Fine-needle liver aspirate – screening for lymphoma or other round cell neoplasia, mycoses, feline hepatic lipidosis, or abscesses. Accuracy is poor for many liver diseases.
- Bacterial cultures – aerobic and anaerobic liver and bile cultures.
- Serology – infectious disease titers (i.e., leptospirosis, mycoses, toxoplasmosis).

Pathologic Findings

- Gross – slightly large, mottled liver.
- Microscopic – confirms necrosis; zonal involvement; may assist in determining underlying cause: hypoxia leading to zone 3; certain toxins cause zone 1 or 3 necrosis; reticulin staining confirms zonal involvement, confirms retention or loss of reticulin substructure that orchestrates organized regeneration (Figures 115.1 and 115.2).

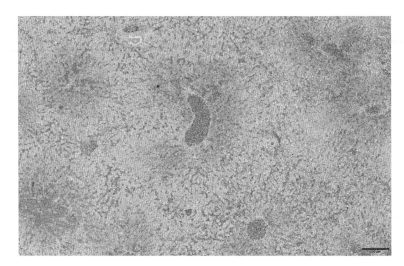

■ **Fig. 115.1.** Liver of an eight-year-old, spayed female, black Labrador retriever with suspected toxicosis (hematoxylin and eosin, 4×) Marked diffuse, acute centrilobular to midzonal hepatopathy. Source: Courtesy of Dr Randi Gold.

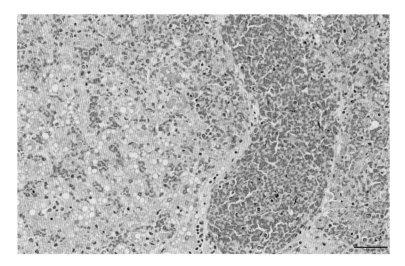

■ **Fig. 115.2.** Liver of an eight-year-old, spayed female, black Labrador retriever with suspected toxicosis (hematoxylin and eosin, 60×). This closer view highlights centrilobular to midzonal hepatocellular cytoplasmic vacuolation (lipid type) and necrosis. Source: Courtesy of Dr Randi Gold.

 THERAPEUTICS

Etiology-specific treatment is not always possible and hospitalization for aggressive supportive care is critical.

Drug(s) of Choice

- Blood component therapy – plasma and other blood products may be indicated in coagulopathic patients. Correction of coagulopathies in humans is reserved for patients with evidence of spontaneous hemorrhage. Additional research is needed before this recommendation can be widely adopted in veterinary patients. Ammonia concentrations can increase significantly during red blood cell storage so care must be exercised during administration.

- Fluid therapy – often required, and correction of dehydration, acid–base abnormalities, and electrolyte abnormalities should be prioritized as these disturbances can precipitate HE. The lactate in lactated Ringer's solution is the salt form of the compound and cannot cause lactic acidosis alone. The majority of animals with lactic acidosis suffer from decreased tissue perfusion and reestablishment of perfusion by fluid therapy helps resolve the lactic acidosis.

- Synthetic colloids – are an appropriate choice in patients with low oncotic pressure due to hypoalbuminemia (secondary to bleeding, protein loss, or decreased production). The use of hydroxyethyl starches has been questioned in human patients due to various adverse reactions reported in randomized clinical trials that include coagulation abnormalities, immunologic reactions, and an increased incidence of acute kidney injury. There are no studies in dogs or cats documenting acute kidney injury, with limited clinical information on coagulation adverse effects. Clinicians are cautioned not to extrapolate these findings but exercise caution as appropriate.

- Cerebral edema – is a common complication of acute liver failure in humans and is associated with HE. Patients presenting with forebrain signs should be treated. Common interventions include mannitol, hypertonic saline, and slight elevation of the head to facilitate venous drainage.

- Antimicrobial therapy – patients in acute liver failure are susceptible to sepsis due to infection from enteric bacterial translocation. Sepsis/systemic inflammatory response syndrome (SIRS) is a major risk for cerebral edema. These patients should be carefully evaluated for evidence of infection and broad-spectrum antimicrobial therapy started in cases where bacterial infection is suspected.

- Early administration of N-acetylcysteine may improve microvascular perfusion and tissue oxygenation, and mitigate oxidative damage.

- Antiemetic drug therapy – patients often present with anorexia or vomiting. Antiemetic therapy is indicated in these cases. Choices include maropitant (1 mg/kg IV/SQ q24h), ondansetron (0.1–1 mg/kg I, q12h), metoclopramide (1–2 mg/kg/24h, IV constant rate infusion (CRI)).

- Hepatic encephalopathy – patients with sign of HE can be treated with lactulose (0.5–2.0 mL/kg PO q8h or rectally if PO hazardous, adjusted to achieve soft fecal consistency), metronidazole (7.5 mg/kg PO q12h or rectally if PO hazardous), rifaximin (5–10 mg/kg PO or rectally q12h), neomycin (22 mg/kg PO or rectally q12h; **caution:** may be ototoxic and renal toxic if increased absorption as a result of reduced intestinal mucosal integrity), amoxicillin-clavulanate (15 mg/kg, PO, q12h).

- Hepatoprotective antioxidant drug therapy – patients in liver failure have decreased glutathione (GSH) levels resulting in oxidative damage and may benefit from hepatoprotective therapy including vitamin E (10 IU/kg PO q24h), N-acetylcysteine (140 mg/kg IV or PO; IV use 10% solution diluted 1:2 in saline, administer via 0.25 μm nonpyrogenic filter; follow with 70 mg/kg q6–12h), S-adenosylmethionine (SAMe) (20 mg/kg PO q24h), silibinin (milk thistle) efficacy reported for *Amanita* toxicity and certain other toxins; use product complexed with polyunsaturated phosphatidylcholine (PPC) (2–5 mg/kg PO q24h), ursodeoxycholic acid (10–15 mg/kg divided q12h PO).

- Decreasing enterohepatic circulation – cholestyramine 30–40 mg/kg mixed with water PO q24h; bile acid-binding resin that can absorb certain toxins in the alimentary canal that undergo enterohepatic circulation diminishing their systemic availability, e.g., anecdotal, sago palm (cycad toxin).

- Coagulopathies – vitamin K1 (0.5–1.5 mg/kg SQ or IM, three doses at 12 h intervals, then once to twice weekly) and fresh frozen plasma.

■ Gastrointestinal bleeding – omeprazole (1.0–2.0 mg/kg PO q12–24h) or pantoprazole (may induce p450 cytochrome-associated drug interactions).

Precautions/Interactions

■ Drugs biotransformed primarily in the liver, altering liver perfusion, or metabolizing enzyme activity should be avoided; may be difficult as many drugs are metabolized in hepatic pathways or eliminated in bile.
■ Vitamin C – 100–500 mg q24h, *avoid* if high liver iron or copper concentrations; ascorbate may augment transition metal-associated oxidative injury; no evidence for vitamin C administration in liver failure.
■ Neomycin – ototoxic and renal toxic if increased absorption with reduced gut integrity.
■ Administration of stored whole blood or packed RBCs may precipitate or exacerbate HE in dogs with hepatic failure because of spontaneously generated ammonia during storage.

Appropriate Health Care

■ **Caution**: delay inserting central catheters until bleeding diatheses controlled with vitamin K1, fresh frozen plasma, or fresh whole blood.
■ Maintenance of adequate enteral nutrition and hydration is essential during treatment.

Nursing Care

Colloids (hetastarch, Voluven®, plasma) should be given if severe hypoalbuminemia is present.

Diet

■ Enteral feeding – small-volume, frequent meals to optimize digestion and assimilation.
■ Protracted vomiting – withhold food PO until controlled with antiemetic therapy.
■ Parenteral nutrition – consider when enteric nutrition is contraindicated (i.e., somnolent patient or intractable vomiting).
■ Diet composition – use normal protein (nitrogen) content in tolerant patients; moderate protein restriction if encephalopathic (2.5 g protein/kg body weight) but strive to maintain a positive nitrogen balance for hepatic regeneration.
■ Supplemental vitamins are important – water soluble (two-fold normal); vitamin E (10 IU/kg PO or by injection q24h).
■ Probiotic/prebiotic yogurt – may protect against enteric bacterial translocation; tolerated dairy protein source if HE; controversial.

Activity

Allow patients to limit their own activity.

Surgical Considerations

■ Coagulation abnormalities should be aggressively treated prior to surgical intervention (liver biopsy, esophageal tube) even if they do not normalize.
■ Hepatic encephalopathy should be treated prior to a surgical intervention.
■ Abdominal effusion should be partially evacuated prior to a surgical intervention to decrease anesthetic risk.
■ Placement of an esophageal tube should be considered if patient is anorexic at time of anesthetic procedure.

COMMENTS

Client Education

Patience is required to determine response to therapy.

Patient Monitoring

- Temperature, pulse, respiration, and mental status q1–2h until stable.
- Maintain vigilance for infection, especially catheter induced.
- Body weight – twice daily guides fluid therapy; body weight and condition used to assess nitrogen and energy allowances.
- Acid–base, electrolyte balances (especially potassium and phosphate), and glucose – q12–24h for the first 72 h.
- Sequential measurements of liver enzymes, bilirubin, cholesterol, and coagulation status q2–3 days provide evidence of recovery.

Prevention/Avoidance

- Vaccinate dogs against infectious canine hepatitis virus.
- Avoid indiscriminate ingestion of hepatotoxins and environmental exposure.
- Consider all drugs as potential toxins.

Possible Complications

- Hypoglycemia.
- Uncontrolled gastrointestinal bleeding and DIC.
- Hepatic encephalopathy, cerebral edema, brain herniation.
- Chronic hepatic insufficiency, cirrhosis, fibrosis from postnecrotic scarring.
- Acute renal failure.
- Death.

Expected Course and Prognosis

- Acute liver failure is associated with multiple etiologies and a high mortality rate approaching 90%.
- The extent of liver injury, etiopathogenesis, and supportive nursing care impacts prognosis.
- Cats with hepatic lipidosis can have a good prognosis based on the etiology.

Synonyms

- Acute liver failure
- Fulminant hepatic failure

Abbreviations

- ALP = alkaline phosphatase
- ALT = alanine aminotransferase
- AST = aspartate aminotransferase
- BUN = blood urea nitrogen
- CRI = constant rate infusion
- DIC = disseminated intravascular coagulation
- GGT = gamma-glutamyl transferase
- GSH = glutathione
- HE = hepatic encephalopathy
- NSAID = nonsteroidal antiinflammatory drug
- PU/PD = polyuria, polydipsia
- SIRS = systemic inflammatory response syndrome
- TSBA = total serum bile acids

See Also

- Coagulopathy of Liver Disease
- Hepatic Encephalopathy
- Hepatitis, Infectious (Viral) Canine
- Hepatotoxins
- Icterus
- Nutritional Approach to Hepatobiliary Disease

Suggested Reading

Center SA. Acute hepatic injury: hepatic necrosis and fulminant hepatic failure. In: Guilford GW, Center SA, Strombeck DR, et al, eds. Small Animal Gastroenterology. Philadelphia: Saunders, 1996a, pp. 654–704.

Center SA, Elston TH, Rowland PH, et al. Fulminant hepatic failure associated with oral administration of diazepam in 11 cats. J Am Vet Med Assoc 1996b;209:618–625.

Dunayer EK, Gwaltney-Brant SM. Acute hepatic failure and coagulopathy associated with xylitol ingestion in eight dogs. J Am Vet Med Assoc 2006;229:1113–1117.

Hughes D, King LG. The diagnosis and management of acute liver failure in dogs and cats. Vet Clin North Am Small Anim Pract 1995;25:437–460.

Kavanaugh CL, Cooper JC, Peters RM, Webster CR. Retrospective evaluation of acute liver failure in dogs (1995–2012): 49 cases. J Vet Emerg Crit Care 2016;26(4):559–567.

Acknowledgments: The author and editors acknowledge the prior contribution of Dr Sharon Center.

Author: Yuri A. Lawrence DVM, MS, MA, PhD, DACVIM (SAIM)

Chapter 116

Hepatic Lipidosis

DEFINITION/OVERVIEW

- Feline hepatic lipidosis (HL) is one of the most common hepatobiliary diseases in cats.
- Characterized by excessive accumulation of triglycerides in >80% of hepatocytes leading to distension of the cytosolic compartment, canalicular compression, severe intrahepatic cholestasis, and impairment of liver function.
- Usually develops secondary to a primary condition causing negative energy balance as a result of anorexia or catabolism.
- If left untreated, it leads to progressive metabolic dysregulation and death.

ETIOLOGY/PATHOPHYSIOLOGY

- Cats, as strict carnivores, have developed unique adaptations of lipid and protein metabolism; they have limited ability to synthesize fatty acids (FA) and essential amino acids. They also have a unique tendency to accumulate triglycerides in hepatocytes. This predisposes them to the development of HL.
- The pathogenesis of feline HL is poorly understood but involves the following: increased influx in the hepatocyte of free FA from peripheral fat stores (increased fat mobilization); increased *de novo* triglyceride synthesis; impaired hepatic beta-oxidation of fatty acids; decreased dispersal of hepatic triglycerides in the form of very low-density lipoproteins (VLDLs).
- The excessive accumulation of triglycerides in the hepatocyte leads to displacement of the organelles to the periphery of the cell, resulting in organelle dysfunction and canalicular compression.

Idiopathic or Primary Hepatic Lipidosis

- It is currently debatable whether idiopathic HL truly exists. In the vast majority of cases (>85%), antecedent health problems causing anorexia or malassimilation are present, thus predisposing to HL.
- In the remaining cases, the underlying cause of HL may simply remain undiagnosed or HL might be caused by food deprivation (e.g., nonpalatable food, stressful events leading to decreased food intake, extreme weight loss programs).

Blackwell's Five-Minute Veterinary Consult Clinical Companion: Small Animal Gastrointestinal Diseases, First Edition. Edited by Jocelyn Mott and Jo Ann Morrison.
© 2019 John Wiley & Sons, Inc. Published 2019 by John Wiley & Sons, Inc.
Companion website: www.fiveminutevet.com/gastrointestinal

Secondary Hepatic Lipidosis

Practically any disease or condition that causes prolonged anorexia and/or catabolism may lead to HL. Most common causes include the following.

- Primary liver disease – cholangitis; portosystemic shunts (PSS); extrahepatic biliary obstruction (EHBO); cholelithiasis; neoplasia.
- Gastrointestinal – inflammatory bowel disease (IBD); intestinal lymphoma; obstruction; pancreatitis.
- Urogenital disease – chronic kidney disease; feline lower urinary tract disease (FLUTD).
- Infectious diseases – feline infectious peritonitis (FIP); feline immunodeficiency (FIV); feline leukemia virus (FeLV); toxoplasmosis.
- Neoplasia.
- Rapid weight loss protocol.

Systems Affected

- Hepatobiliary – severe intrahepatic cholestasis, hepatic dysfunction or failure.
- Gastrointestinal – anorexia; vomiting, diarrhea.
- Nervous – hepatic encephalopathy (HE), ptyalism.
- Musculoskeletal – sarcopenia, weakness.
- Hematology – abnormal red blood cell shapes (poikilocytes), Heinz body hemolysis.
- Renal/urologic – potassium loss.

SIGNALMENT/HISTORY

- Hepatic lipidosis is seen very commonly in cats; very rarely, it can also affect dogs.
- There is no breed or sex predilection.
- Most cats are middle aged but age of affected cats ranges from one to 16 years.

Risk Factors

- Obesity.
- Anorexia.
- Catabolism or rapid weight loss.
- Vitamin B12 deficiency.

Historical Findings

- Hyporexia or anorexia.
- Weight loss.
- Lethargy/depression.
- Jaundice.
- Vomiting.
- Diarrhea or constipation.
- Ptyalism (usually due to hepatic encephalopathy).
- Neck ventroflexion (as a result of weakness, hypokalemia, and/or thiamin deficiency).
- Abnormalities due to underlying disease leading to HL.

CLINICAL FEATURES

- Lethargy or severe depression.
- Jaundice.
- Dehydration.

- Weakness – neck ventroflexion, recumbency.
- Ptyalism.
- Neurologic signs (due to hepatic encephalopathy).
- Hepatomegaly.
- Others, depending on underlying or primary disease.

 ## DIFFERENTIAL DIAGNOSIS

- It is important to recognize that the diseases listed below, including primary hepatic disease, can coexist with HL and findings might reflect both conditions and confuse the clinician.
- Infectious diseases affecting the liver – hepatic toxoplasmosis, FIP.
- Primary liver disease – cholangitis, cholelithiasis, EHBO, neoplasia, PSS.
- Pancreatitis.
- Gastrointestinal disease – IBD, intestinal lymphoma, obstruction.
- Toxicities.

 ## DIAGNOSTICS

Complete Blood Count/Biochemistry/Urinalysis

- Complete blood cell count – often normal; mild nonregenerative anemia is common; poikilocytes and Heinz bodies are common; inflammatory leukogram is common and usually reflects an inflammatory, infectious, or neoplastic underlying disorder.
- Biochemistry – most consistent findings include hyperbilirubinemia and increased ALP and ALT activities; GGT activity is normal or mildly increased (unless underlying cholangitis is present); low BUN concentrations are relatively common due to impaired urea cycle function; glucose concentrations can be normal, increased (usually as a result of insulin resistance), or decreased (uncommon; indicates severe liver dysfunction); hypoalbuminemia is relatively common due to anorexia and/or liver dysfunction; hyperglobulinemia may be present due to underlying inflammatory disease; common electrolyte abnormalities include hypokalemia, hypophosphatemia (<2 mg/dL), and hypomagnesemia. The first two are associated with increased mortality in feline HL and are often related to refeeding syndrome.
- Urinalysis – often normal; lipiduria and low urine specific gravity may be seen.

Other Laboratory Tests

- Coagulation testing – coagulation abnormalities (increased prothrombin time (PT), activated partial thromboplastin time (APTT), activated clotting time (ACT), proteins invoked by vitamin K absence or antagonism (PIVKA)) are common in cats with HL (45–77% of cases); clinical bleeding tendencies (e.g., following venipuncture or liver biopsy) can also be commonly seen; abnormalities correct with parenteral vitamin K1 therapy.
- Serum bile acids – increased in most cases; redundant test if jaundice is present.
- Hyperammonemia – uncommon.
- B12 deficiency – relatively common finding; replacement may have therapeutic significance.

Imaging
Radiography
- Nondiagnostic.
- Hepatomegaly is seen in most cases.
- May show findings of underlying disorder.

Abdominal Ultrasonography

- Hepatomegaly and diffuse hyperechoic hepatic parenchyma are consistent findings and reflect hepatic lipid accumulation.
- Accuracy for diagnosing feline HL was 70% in one study; similar findings may be seen in other conditions, including healthy obese cats.
- Useful for identifying primary disease causing HL.

Additional Diagnostic Tests

- Presumptive diagnosis is based on history, clinical findings, increased ALP activity, and diffuse hyperechoic hepatic parenchyma.
- Fine-needle aspiration (FNA) cytology of the liver: usually confirms diagnosis; >80% of hepatocytes show severe cytosolic vacuolation (Figure 116.1); cannot rule out underlying primary hepatic disorders (e.g., cholangitis, EHBO, neoplasia).
- Liver biopsy – rarely needed or recommended to confirm HL; useful for definitive diagnosis of underlying hepatic disorders leading to HL; associated with more complications than aspiration such as anesthetic complications and risk of bleeding; usually done only if there is poor response to initial treatment or if history and clinical and clinicopathologic findings suggest a possible underlying hepatic disease (e.g., increased GGT).
- **Caution**: if biopsy, FNA, feeding tube placement, or any invasive procedure is to be performed, (a) patient needs to be stabilized before anesthesia to reduce risk of death; (b) vitamin K1 needs to be administered to reduce risk of hemorrhage (0.5–1.5 mg/kg SQ or IM; three doses at 12 h intervals, last dose at least 12 h before the procedure).

Pathologic Findings

- Gross – hepatomegaly, yellow/pale color with reticulated appearance, friable/greasy consistency.
- Microscopic – diffuse, severe hepatocellular vacuolation (>80% of hepatocytes); large (macrovesicular) or small (microvesicular) vacuolation.

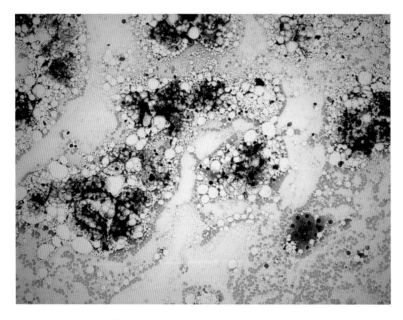

■ **Fig. 116.1.** Fine needle aspirate of feline liver showing hepatic lipidosis.

THERAPEUTICS

Feeding an appropriate diet in adequate amounts, via feeding tube, and correction of hypoperfusion and electrolyte disturbances are the cornerstones of treatment.

Drug(s) of Choice

- Antiemetics – most cats with HL vomit and/or have nausea; maropitant (1 mg/kg IV, SQ, PO q24h), ondansetron (0.1–0.5 mg/kg IV 2–3 times per day), and metoclopramide (0.2 mg/kg IV q4–6h or 1 mg/kg/d IV as a CRI) can be used alone or in combination as needed. Metoclopramide is a weak antiemetic in cats and may be more useful for its prokinetic effects.
- Antacid medications – may be needed to reduce the risk of reflux esophagitis; omeprazole (1 mg/kg PO q12h) is usually preferred; famotidine (0.5–1.0 mg/kg q12–24h) may also be used although the effectiveness of H2-blockers in cats for increasing gastric pH has been questioned by recent studies.
- Vitamin K1 – recommended for all cats with suspected HL; needs to be administered to reduce risk of hemorrhage (0.5–1.5 mg/kg SQ or IM; three doses at 12 h intervals; last dose at least 12 h before a planed invasive procedure).
- Other medications may be needed depending on the underlying condition (e.g., antibiotics with concurrent infections).

Precautions/Interactions

- Benzodiazepines and barbiturates should be avoided because they interact with neuro-receptors and may provoke HE.
- Propofol should be avoided because it may provoke hemolysis in cats with Heinz body anemia.
- Ursodeoxycholic acid is unlikely to be beneficial and may be harmful in HL; therefore, it should probably be avoided.
- Dose adjustments of medications may be needed due to the possibility of liver dysfunction.

Alternative Drugs

The following drugs may be helpful when used in conjunction with the main treatment modalities of HL (i.e., mainly feeding, fluid therapy, and supportive care). However, the clinical benefits from their use in cats with HL have not been adequately demonstrated and definitive recommendations cannot be made.

- S-adenosylmethionine (SAMe): 200 mg/cat PO q24h; may help correct hepatic glutathione (GSH) depletion, which is known to occur in cats with HL and increases risk for oxidative injury; need for dosing on empty stomach complicates use.
- L-carnitine: 250–500 mg/cat/day Carnitine increases fatty acid beta-oxidation and decreases triglyceride accumulation in the liver in overweight cats.
- Taurine: 250–500 mg/cat/day.
- Thiamin: 50–100 mg/cat/day.
- Vitamin B12: 250 µg/cat, once a week for 4–6 weeks and then determine chronic vitamin B12 needs by sequential B12 concentration measurements.
- Vitamin E: 10 IU/kg/day PO.

Appropriate Health Care

- The vast majority of cats with HL need to be hospitalized for some period of time, especially those with severe clinical signs (e.g., if recumbent or with neck ventroflexion); when stabilized, cats can be discharged for home care.
- Some cats with HL and mild clinical signs may be managed as outpatients.

Nursing Care

- Fluid therapy – most cats are dehydrated and/or hypovolemic; 0.9% NaCl solutions are preferred; solutions containing lactate are not recommended by some authors because liver dysfunction leads to delayed lactate clearance and hyperlactatemia, although this is controversial; solutions containing dextrose should be avoided because they can worsen glucose intolerance and hyperglycemia and may promote hepatic triglyceride accumulation.
- Electrolyte abnormalities should be corrected as soon as possible and before feeding is initiated because postprandial insulin release can worsen hypokalemia and hypophosphatemia.
- Hypokalemia – treated with potassium chloride supplementation.
- Hypophosphatemia – potassium phosphate supplementation usually needed if hypophosphatemia is severe (<2 mg/dL; especially at initial feeding (refeeding syndrome)). Reduction of potassium chloride administration may be needed with concurrent potassium phosphate supplementation to avoid hyperkalemia.
- Hypomagnesemia – magnesium supplementation is rarely needed; however, hypomagnesemia can worsen renal wasting of potassium and worsen hypokalemia or make it difficult to correct.

Diet

- Appropriate nutritional support as described below is the cornerstone of HL treatment.
- Enteral nutrition is preferred over parenteral nutrition unless intractable vomiting is present; in most cases, food should be provided through a feeding tube.
- The initial feeding tube of choice is the nasoesophageal tube because it does not require general anesthesia and is not invasive; most cats with HL are unstable at admission due to severe electrolyte abnormalities and may also have coagulation abnormalities; once the cat is stable and coagulopathies have been corrected, the nasoesophageal tube may be replaced by an esophagostomy tube if necessary; laparotomy for gastrostomy tube placement is not recommended due to increased risk of death.
- Force feeding should be avoided because it is stressful for the cat, rarely provides adequate calorie intake, and might lead to food aversion.
- Appetite stimulants (e.g., mirtazapine, cyproheptadine, midazolam) should not be used instead of feeding tubes because they are highly unlikely to provide adequate energy intake; some produce sedation and some may be harmful to the liver.
- Feeding of a high-protein (30–40% of metabolizable energy), high-calorie diet is essential. Most commercially available high-protein recovery veterinary diets are usually adequate.
- Energy requirements: 50–60 kcal/kg of ideal weight/day; begin by administering about one-third of the total amount of food required per day on the first day and gradually increase the amount of food over the following 3–4 days; this decreases the risk of refeeding syndrome. Refeeding syndrome often develops as a result of rapid caloric administration to a starved patient causing hyperglycemia and rapid insulin release, leading to severe hypophosphatemia, hypokalemia, and hypomagnesemia.
- Cats with HL cannot tolerate large volumes of food and therefore several small meals per day (e.g., 6–8) should be offered and administered slowly over 10–15 minutes.
- Once the cat is stabilized and starts feeling better, food should be offered daily PO to assess interest in food; feeding tubes should be removed only when adequate amounts of food are consumed by the cat; this might take several weeks in some cases.

Activity

Mild activity is desirable in most cats and may enhance gastrointestinal motility in cats that develop dysmotility of the gastrointestinal tract; however, most cats are initially too weak for any activity.

Surgical Considerations

- Surgery is almost never indicated for HL unless a liver biopsy or exploratory laparotomy for investigation of underlying disorders is deemed necessary.
- Surgery should not be performed until hydration, electrolyte depletions, and vitamin K1 deficiency have been corrected.

 COMMENTS

Client Education

- Long-term and initially intensive hospitalization is needed for most cats.
- Feeding tubes may be retained for several weeks or months even when cats are discharged.
- Most cats will fully recover with appropriate treatment.

Patient Monitoring

- Body weight, hydration status, and electrolytes should initially be assessed or measured 1–2 times per day in order to appropriately adjust treatment.
- Serum bilirubin concentration should be measured every 1–3 days; it may take 1–2 weeks or even longer to normalize and predicts recovery.
- Liver enzyme activities usually take weeks to normalize and do not predict recovery.
- Cats can be discharged when dehydration and electrolyte abnormalities have been corrected, vomiting is controlled, gastroparesis is resolved, serum bilirubin is declining, and activity is increased. Treatment is continued at home in most cases.

Prevention/Avoidance

- Avoid prolonged food deprivation in cats (e.g., avoid prolonged fasting; prioritize placement of feeding tubes in cats with prolonged anorexia).
- Warn owners of all cats that even short-term anorexia in cats (2–3 days) is important and should prompt seeking veterinary advice.
- Prevent obesity because it is a known risk factor for HL.
- Planned weight reduction in obese cats should not exceed 2% bodyweight per week.

Possible Complications

- Refeeding syndrome after initiation of feeding through feeding tubes.
- HE after initiation of dietary support (rarely).
- Hepatic failure can lead to death.

Expected Course and Prognosis

- Complete recovery usually takes up to 3–6 weeks.
- With appropriate and rapidly introduced treatment as described above, the majority of cats (>80%) will recover; however, the underlying disease can influence the outcome (e.g., neoplasia).
- Once the cat has recovered, HL rarely recurs.
- HL does not cause chronic liver dysfunction.

Synonyms

- Fatty liver syndrome
- Hepatic steatosis

Abbreviations

- ALP = alkaline phosphatase
- ALT = alanine aminotransferase
- CRI = constant rate infusion
- EHBO = extrahepatic biliary obstruction
- FA = fatty acids
- FeLV = feline leukemia virus
- FIP = feline infectious peritonitis
- FIV = feline immunodeficiency
- FLUTD = feline lower urinary tract disease
- FNA = fine needle aspiration

- GGT = gamma-glutamyl transferase
- GSH = glutathione
- HE = hepatic encephalopathy
- HL = hepatic lipidosis
- IBD = inflammatory bowel disease
- PIVKA = proteins invoked by vitamin K absence or antagonism
- PSS = portosystemic shunts
- SAMe = S-adenosylmethionine
- VLDL = very low-density lipoprotein

See Also

- Cobalamin Deficiency
- Hepatic Encephalopathy
- Icterus
- Inflammatory Bowel Disease

- Nutritional Approach to Hepatic Disease
- Pancreatitis, Feline
- Portosystemic Shunts
- Ptyalism.

Suggested Reading

Armstrong PJ, Blanchard G. Hepatic lipidosis in cats. Vet Clin North Am Small Anim Pract 2009;39:599–616.

Center SA. Feline hepatic lipidosis. Vet Clin North Am Small Anim Pract 2005;35:225–269.

Valtolina C, Favier RP. Feline hepatic lipidosis. Vet Clin North Am Small Anim Pract 2017;47:683–702.

Acknowledgments: The author and editors acknowledge the prior contribution of Dr Sharon Center.

Author: Panagiotis G. Xenoulis DVM, Dr.med.vet., PhD

Chapter 117

Hepatic Neoplasia, Benign

DEFINITION/OVERVIEW

- A benign liver tumor of epithelial origin.
- May be more common than primary malignant liver tumors.

Systems Affected

- Hepatobiliary – hepatomegaly, liver mass.
- Gastrointestinal – vomiting, anorexia.
- Hemic/lymphatic/immune – chronic mild anemia, acute blood loss-associated anemia.

SIGNALMENT/HISTORY

- Rare in dog and very rare in cat.
- Affected dogs commonly >10 years of age.
- Breed predispositions unknown.

Risk Factors

Definitive cause or risk factors for tumor development are unknown.

Historical Findings

- Usually asymptomatic; however, when clinical signs present, symptoms may be nonspecific. Typically incidental finding.
- Acute tumor rupture may cause hemoperitoneum with resultant weakness and hypovolemic shock-like symptoms.
- Occasionally, large tumors may cause cranial abdominal pain, vomiting, and inappetence.

CLINICAL FEATURES

- Physical examination may be normal.
- Hepatomegaly (asymmetric).
- Sometimes abdominal hemorrhage is present.

DIFFERENTIAL DIAGNOSIS

- Hepatocellular carcinoma.
- Hepatic nodular hyperplasia.

Blackwell's Five-Minute Veterinary Consult Clinical Companion: Small Animal Gastrointestinal Diseases, First Edition. Edited by Jocelyn Mott and Jo Ann Morrison.
© 2019 John Wiley & Sons, Inc. Published 2019 by John Wiley & Sons, Inc.
Companion website: www.fiveminutevet.com/gastrointestinal

- Hepatic abscess.
- Abdominal mass.
- Splenomegaly.

DIAGNOSTICS

Complete Blood Count/Biochemistry/Urinalysis

- Complete blood count.
  - Usually unremarkable.
  - Anemia – regenerative anemia if tumor is bleeding, or anemia of chronic disease.
  - Leukocytosis with a left shift – large tumors with necrotic centers (rare).
- Biochemistry.
  - Liver enzymes variable.
  - Alkaline phosphatase (ALP), alanine aminotransferase (ALT), aspartate aminotransferase (AST) – normal or mild to markedly high.
  - Serum total bilirubin values – usually normal.
- Urinalysis is unremarkable.

Other Laboratory Tests

- Serum bile acids are usually normal unless tumor growth compromises hepatic perfusion and biliary flow.
- Coagulation abnormalities consistent with disseminated intravascular coagulation (DIC) occur rarely with large necrotic or hemorrhagic tumors.

Imaging

Radiography

- May demonstrate a single mass lesion or apparent asymmetry of hepatic silhouette.
- Rarely, gas in necrotic center of tumor.

Abdominal Ultrasonography

- May identify discrete mass effect with variable echogenicity, ranging from normal liver echogenicity to mixed echogenicity, presence of multiple nodules, or cystic mass appearance.

Abdominal Computed Tomography

- May allow for improved assessment regarding surgical feasibility, especially for large tumors, or tumors associated with critical structures, such as the gallbladder.
- May detect additional lesions, depending on the contrast enhancement protocol.

Diagnostic Procedures

- Hepatic aspiration cytology with ultrasonographic guidance may allow the identification of normal hepatocytes or cells with mild atypia. This diagnostic procedure will not be useful to differentiate between benign and low-grade malignant hepatic tumors, but may help to exclude other neoplastic diseases, such as lymphoma.
- Hepatic biopsy with Tru-Cut needle; several core biopsies are necessary to provide enough tissue for histopathologic characterization. Due to the overlap between the hepatocellular adenoma and the low-grade hepatocellular carcinoma, it may be difficult to obtain a definitive diagnosis.
- Hepatic biopsy via laparoscopy.
- Abdominal exploratory surgery followed by mass resection (liver lobectomy) and histopathology is the best way to concurrently obtain a definitive diagnosis and treat the disease.

Pathologic Findings

Gross Pathology

- Usually well-circumscribed single nodules <10 cm in diameter.
- May be yellow-brown.
- Often soft, highly vascular, and friable.
- Occasionally multiple.
- Occasionally very large (>20 cm).

Microscopic Findings

- May be difficult to distinguish from nodular hyperplasia, normal liver tissue, or low-grade hepatocellular carcinoma.
- Usually well-defined trabecular pattern; not necessarily encapsulated.
- Compression of adjacent hepatic parenchyma common.
- Mitotic figures infrequent.
- Affected liver cells resemble normal hepatocytes but often are larger and have a clear cytosol.

 # THERAPEUTICS

- Surgical resection for large tumors, or tumors that cause clinical signs or organ dysfunction.
- Transarterial embolization or chemoembolization is an experimental option for large, non-resectable tumors. In such cases, referral to an oncologic surgeon or experienced board-certified surgeon is strongly advised, as many large tumors are actually resectable.

Appropriate Health Care

Bleeding tumor – requires immediate emergency care: hemodynamic stabilization, blood transfusion, and exploratory surgery.

Surgical Considerations

- Excision recommended for large, single-mass lesions.
- Between 60% and 70% of the liver can be resected if the patient is healthy, and appropriate postoperative supportive care is available.
- Biopsy of local lymph nodes, normal-appearing liver, and any abnormal tissue identified during the exploratory surgery is of paramount importance.

 # COMMENTS

Patient Monitoring

- Liver enzymes – sequential evaluation, especially if they were elevated at the time of diagnosis.
- Abdominal ultrasonography – every 3–4 months for the first year; preferred method of reevaluation.

Possible Complications

Risk of tumor necrosis and massive abdominal hemorrhage if not resected.

Expected Course and Prognosis

Excellent.

Synonyms

Hepatoma – a confusing term that should be avoided; refers to hepatocellular carcinoma in human medicine and hepatocellular adenoma in veterinary medicine.

Abbreviations

- ALP = alkaline phosphatase
- ALT = alanine aminotransferase
- AST = aspartate aminotransferase
- DIC = disseminated intravascular coagulation

See Also

- Hepatic Neoplasia, Malignant

Suggested Reading

Cave TA, Johnson V, Beths T, et al. Treatment of unresectable hepatocellular adenoma in dogs with transarterial iodized oil and chemotherapy with and without an embolic agent: a report of two cases. J Vet Comp Oncol 2004;1:191–199.

Warren-Smith CM, Andrew S, Mantis P, Lamb CR. Lack of associations between ultrasonographic appearance of parenchymal lesions of the canine liver and histological diagnosis. J Small Anim Pract 2012;53(3):168–173.

Author: Nick Dervisis DVM, PhD, DACVIM (Oncology)

Chapter 118

Hepatic Neoplasia, Malignant

DEFINITION/OVERVIEW

- Malignant epithelial liver tumor.
- Accounts for about 50% of malignant hepatic tumors in dogs and is the second most common primary liver tumor in cats.
- Can present in three forms: massive, nodular, and diffuse.
  - Massive liver carcinomas are defined as a large, solitary mass confined to a single liver lobe.
  - Nodular carcinomas are defined as multifocal and involve two or more liver lobes.
  - Diffuse involvement may represent the progression of the disease or an aggressive form of the disease, with multifocal or coalescing nodules in all liver lobes or diffuse effacement of the hepatic parenchyma.
- Metastasis to regional lymph nodes, lungs, and peritoneal cavity in dogs is associated with the nodular and diffuse forms of hepatocellular carcinoma.
- The metastatic rate varies from 0% to 37% for dogs diagnosed with massive hepatocellular carcinoma (HCC) and 93–100% for dogs with nodular and diffuse HCCs.

ETIOLOGY/PATHOPHYSIOLOGY

Systems Affected

- Hepatobiliary – hepatomegaly, liver mass.
- Gastrointestinal – vomiting, diarrhea, anorexia.
- Endocrine/metabolic – hypoglycemia.
- Hemic/lymphatic/immune – chronic mild anemia, acute blood loss-associated anemia.

SIGNALMENT/HISTORY

- Uncommon in dogs and rare in cats.
- Affected dogs commonly >10 years of age.
- No breed predispositions, although golden retrievers, miniature schnauzers, and male dogs are overrepresented in some studies.

Risk Factors

- Unknown.
- May be associated with chronic inflammation or hepatotoxicity.
- 20% of dogs with HCC may be diagnosed with additional tumors (most were benign and endocrine in origin in a single study).

Blackwell's Five-Minute Veterinary Consult Clinical Companion: Small Animal Gastrointestinal Diseases, First Edition. Edited by Jocelyn Mott and Jo Ann Morrison.
© 2019 John Wiley & Sons, Inc. Published 2019 by John Wiley & Sons, Inc.
Companion website: www.fiveminutevet.com/gastrointestinal

Historical Findings

- Vomiting.
- Diarrhea.
- Anorexia.
- Cranial abdominal organomegaly.

 ## CLINICAL FEATURES

- Typically absent until disease is advanced, unless it causes biliary obstruction.
- Often an incidental finding.
- Lethargy.
- Weakness.
- Anorexia.
- Weight loss.
- Polydipsia.
- Diarrhea.
- Vomiting.
- Hepatomegaly (asymmetric) – consistent; precedes development of overt clinical signs.
- Abdominal hemorrhage.

 ## DIFFERENTIAL DIAGNOSIS

- Hepatic adenoma.
- Nodular hyperplasia.
- Biliary cystadenoma.
- Bile duct adenoma/carcinoma.
- Metastatic neoplasia.
- Polycystic liver disease – less common form; fibrous stroma hyperplasia with anaplastic duct cells; few cysts.
- Hepatic lymphoma.
- Hepatic hemangiosarcoma.
- Hepatic carcinoid.

 ## DIAGNOSTICS

Imaging

Radiography (Figure 118.1)

- May demonstrate a single mass lesion, apparent asymmetry of hepatic silhouette, or hepatomegaly.
- Rarely, gas in necrotic center of tumor.
- Loss of serosal detail in case of hemoabdomen.

Abdominal Ultrasonography (Figure 118.2)

- Discrete mass lesion with variable echogenicity, depending on the presence of intratumoral necrosis, hemorrhage, gas, or cystic cavities.
- Massive enlargement of a single liver lobe is occasionally observed.
- Mixed echogenic pattern – most common.
- Nodular pattern of lesions.

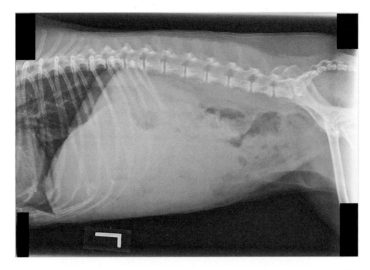

■ **Fig. 118.1.** Left lateral abdominal radiograph. A 14-year-old, spayed female Jack Russell terrier is diagnosed with recurrent hepatocellular carcinoma. The dog presented to the emergency service with a history of straining to defecate for the past week and a bout of vomiting. The previous surgery was performed two years before the current visit. On plain abdominal radiography, a large cranial abdominal mass is appreciated to be associated with the liver.

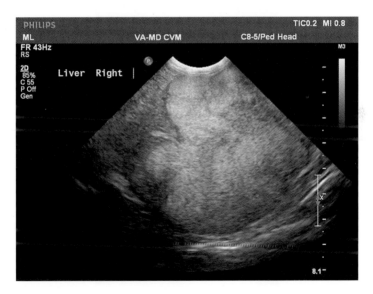

■ **Fig. 118.2.** Abdominal ultrasound. Abdominal ultrasonography revealed a large (5.5 × 8 cm) lobulated hyperechoic mass in the caudate/right lateral lobe of the liver.

Computed Tomography (CT)/Magnetic Resonance Imaging (MRI) (Figures 118.3 and 118.4)

- May be indicated when the tumor is suspected to involve critical anatomical structures, (major vessels, bile duct), and may help plan the surgical approach and inform owners on the risk associated with surgery.
- At the author's institution, contrast-enhanced CT is routinely used for surgical planning.

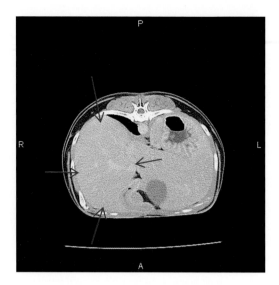

■ Fig. 118.3. Abdominal CT. Contrast-enhanced CT revealed a large, heterogeneously enhancing mass in the right lateral liver lobe (*red arrows*).

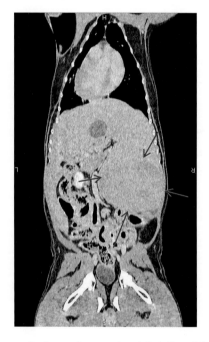

■ Fig. 118.4. Abdominal CT. The mass (*red arrows*) causes dorsal deviation of the right kidney and left sided deviation of the caudal vena cava, gallbladder, duodenum, and pancreas.

Diagnostic Procedures

- Aspiration cytology – to exclude other types of neoplasia (lymphoma, sarcoma, etc.). Aspirate cytology cannot reliably differentiate between hepatocellular carcinoma and benign hepatocellular proliferation (adenoma, hyperplasia).
- Surgical hepatic biopsy for confirmation.
- If tumor is not surgically resectable, ultrasound-guided needle biopsy may be useful in obtaining definitive diagnosis.

Pathologic Findings

- Three clinical subtypes of this tumor are described – massive, nodular, and diffuse.
- Nodular forms account for 30% and diffuse types account for 10% of all reported hepatocellular carcinomas in dogs, and both types involve multiple liver lobes.
- Massive form that is confined to one lobe accounts for about 60% of canine hepatocellular carcinoma cases.
- Color varies from almost white to normal liver color.
- Presence of necrotic center is common in large tumors.
- Diffusely infiltrated tumors may not be grossly apparent other than hepatomegaly.

 THERAPEUTICS

Consult a veterinary oncologist for updates in treating the nodular and diffuse forms of this neoplasm and check with the American Veterinary Medical Association (AVMA) for available clinical trials (https://ebusiness.avma.org/aahsd/study_search.aspx).

Drug(s) of Choice

No medical treatment options have been successful in reducing tumor recurrence or risk for metastasis.

Appropriate Health Care

- Abdominal ultrasonography: two weeks postoperative for baseline and every 3–4 months for the first year.
- Abdominal CT and/or MRI are more sensitive than ultrasonography for detection of small, recurrent lesions.
- Monitor liver enzymes serially, if they were elevated on diagnosis.

Surgical Considerations

- Complete excision (liver lobectomy) recommended when possible. Excision with microscopically dirty margins can still afford durable tumor control and long survival times.
- Massive form is often amenable to surgical resection.
- Nodular and diffuse forms are often not amenable to surgery.
- Between 60% and 70% of the liver lobes can be resected if the patient is healthy and is given appropriate postoperative care.

 COMMENTS

Expected Course and Prognosis

- Prognosis is variable; histologic classification is not prognostic.
- Massive forms treated with surgery have a better prognosis than do the nodular or diffuse forms.
- Median survival of dogs with massive form treated with surgery may be >1460 days.
- Local tumor recurrence or *de novo* tumor growth is not uncommon.
- Right-sided liver tumors (right lateral lobe or caudate process of the caudate lobe) may have a poorer prognosis due to potential caudal vena cava trauma during surgical dissection.
- Increased alanine aminotransferase (ALT) and aspartate aminotransferase (AST) are associated with a poor prognosis.

Synonyms

- Hepatic carcinoma
- Liver carcinoma

Abbreviations

- ALT = alanine aminotransferase
- AST = aspartate aminotransferase
- CT = computed tomography
- HCC = hepatocellular carcinoma
- MRI = magnetic resonance imaging

Suggested Reading

Liptak, JM. Hepatobiliary tumors. In: Withrow and MacEwen's Small Animal Clinical Oncology, 5th ed. St Louis: Elsevier Saunders, 2012.

Liptak JM, Dernell WS, Monnet E, et al. Massive hepatocellular carcinoma in dogs: 48 cases (1992–2002). J Am Vet Med Assoc 2004a;225(8):1225–1230.

Liptak JM, Dernell WS, Withrow SJ. Liver tumors in cats and dogs. Compend Contin Educ Pract Vet 2004b;26:50–56.

Author: Nick Dervisis DVM, PhD, DACVIM (Oncology)

Chapter 119

Hepatic Nodular Hyperplasia and Dysplastic Hyperplasia

 DEFINITION/OVERVIEW

Hepatic Nodular Hyperplasia (HNH)

- Benign parenchymal feature in middle-aged to older dogs.
- Nonencapsulated, ≤2 cm (rarely up to 5 cm), expansile nodule of hepatocellular hyperplasia, maintaining a modified lobular architecture with recognizable central and portal elements that are irregularly spaced, organized hepatic cord structure one cell wide, without marginal parenchymal collapse or fibrosis (is not a regenerative nodule), smooth margins.
- Hepatocyte phenotype may be similar to surrounding parenchyma but may contain glycogen or lipid vacuoles.
- May associate with increased liver enzymes in elderly dogs, especially alkaline phosphatase (ALP).
- Clinical concern derives from association with increased liver enzyme activity and ultrasound (US) detection of hepatic nodules or hepatic nodularity during exploratory surgery.
- Variable US appearance.
- Biopsy specimens must include affected and unaffected liver for appropriate interpretation.
- Nodular hyperplasia may be mistaken for regeneration secondary to chronic hepatitis or hepatocellular neoplasia (adenoma) with needle core biopsies or when only nodular tissue without normal hepatic tissue is sampled.

Hepatocellular Dysplastic Hyperplasia (HDH)

- Potentially preneoplastic proliferative hepatocellular foci in dogs with glycogen-type vacuolar hepatopathy (VH).
- Nonencapsulated, variably sized, reduced reticulin substructure, expansile nodules of non-vacuolated hepatocytes forming wide (two cells wide, normal = one cell wide) disorganized hepatic cords, an irregular (serrated) margin interfacing with adjacent "normal VH"-affected hepatocytes, and lacking remodeled marginal lesions (fibrosis, parenchymal collapse).
- Associated with VH-related increased liver enzymes, dominated by increased ALP activity.
- Recognized as an antecedent hepatic lesion in dogs developing hepatocellular carcinoma (e.g., Scottish terriers, also other breeds) and is seemingly associated with increased sex hormone concentrations (androgens, progestins).
- Variable US appearance depending on size, number, distribution.
- May be mistaken for nodular regeneration without special stains to detail reticulin substructure and collagen fibril deposition.

Blackwell's Five-Minute Veterinary Consult Clinical Companion: Small Animal Gastrointestinal Diseases, First Edition. Edited by Jocelyn Mott and Jo Ann Morrison.
© 2019 John Wiley & Sons, Inc. Published 2019 by John Wiley & Sons, Inc.
Companion website: www.fiveminutevet.com/gastrointestinal

ETIOLOGY/PATHOPHYSIOLOGY

- HNH etiology unknown; metabolic factors, prior injurious events. In humans, associated with infarcts but no evidence of this in dogs.
- HDH etiology may represent hormonal influence promoting neoplastic transformation (sex hormone-related adrenal hyperplasia).

Systems Affected

- HNH – hepatobiliary nodules.
- HDH – hepatobiliary foci and adrenal hyperplasia.

SIGNALMENT/HISTORY

HNH

- Age-related lesion.
- Nodules develop by 6–8 years of age; one study documented lesions in all geriatric dogs >14 years of age.

HDH

- Associated with glycogen-type VH.
- Reflects adrenal hyperplasia syndromes.

CLINICAL FEATURES

- HNH does not cause clinical illness.
- Large nodules that rupture and bleed or nodules impairing hepatic sinusoidal perfusion likely represent misdiagnosed hepatic adenomas or well-differentiated hepatocellular carcinoma.
- HDH is associated with glycogen-type VH syndromes (see Chapter 112).

DIFFERENTIAL DIAGNOSIS

- Necroinflammatory liver disease.
- Regenerative nodular hyperplasia involves the entire liver.
- Formation of irregular nodules of variable size that are segregated by parenchymal collapse, often marginated by fibrous connective tissue.
- Demonstrated loss of lobular architecture, sinusoidal fibrosis, reduced reticulin substructure, and wide disorganized hepatic cords.
- Neoplasia.
- Hepatic adenoma – mass lesions with margins reflecting expansile compression on normal adjacent liver, encapsulated, hepatic cords double wide, disorganized, reduced reticulin substructure, and minimal atypia.
- Hepatocellular carcinoma – single or multiple confluent or separate mass lesions, margins reflecting irregular expansile compression on normal adjacent liver, partially encapsulated, variable width of disorganized hepatic cords >2 cells, multiple phenotypes differing from adjacent normal tissue, variable atypia (may be well differentiated), may display pseudoglandular pattern associated with giant canaliculi, well vascularized with arterial twigs; retention of some normal lobular elements possible (primarily at the periphery).

DIAGNOSTICS

Complete Blood Count/Biochemistry/Urinalysis

- Complete blood cell count – no association with HNH; HDH (see Chapter 112).
- Biochemistry profile – increased serum ALP activity may be encountered with HNH and HDH; may range 2.5–16-fold normal; higher with HDH and VH syndrome (see Chapter 112); usually normal total protein, albumin, bilirubin, and cholesterol.
- Urinalysis – no consistent findings.

Other Laboratory Tests

Total serum bile acids (TSBA) usually normal, unless lesions are diffuse and severe.

Imaging

- Abdominal radiography – no abnormalities except hepatomegaly with HDH due to VH.
- Abdominal US – variable echogenicity relating to histologic features, nodule number and size, and associated VH. HNH often not noted until liver grossly inspected at surgery or laparoscopy.

Other Diagnostic Procedures

- Aspiration cytology – may yield normal hepatocytes, hepatocytes with cytosolic rarefaction and fragility consistent with VH (glycogen retention), or cells with discrete lipid (triglyceride) vacuoles (HNH); occasional binucleated hepatocytes may reflect cell proliferation or other concurrent disease (common in portosystemic vascular anomaly/hepatoportal microvascular dysplasia); hepatocytes may be small with size variation in HDH.
- Liver biopsy – collection of a needle biopsy specimen may not clearly differentiate HNH lesion because of small specimen size; definitive diagnosis requires targeted sampling of a large enough tissue specimen to include lesion and adjacent normal hepatic tissue. HDH may be recognized on needle samples.
- Recommended biopsy methods – laparoscopy, open wedge biopsy during laparotomy, or multiple 14 G needle samples.
- Special stains – reticulin, Masson's trichrome, periodic acid–Schiff (PAS) with and without amylase predigestion.

Pathologic Findings

- HNH gross – single or multiple mass lesions, rarely >2 cm in diameter; color similar to adjacent normal hepatic tissue or paler if vacuolated with glycogen or lipid.
- HNH microscopic – unevenly spaced and sized hepatic lobules with preservation of hepatic veins and portal tracts. Nodules are typically only mildly compressive without peripheral zones of parenchymal collapse or mantling fibrosis. Variable vacuolization of hepatocytes.
- HDH gross – single or multiple lesions, usually small, may appear darker colored compared to adjacent tissue.
- HDH microscopic – unencapsulated areas of proliferative hepatocytes with irregular margins and no compression of adjacent parenchyma. Hepatic cords highly disorganized, one to two hepatocytes wide. PAS staining with and without amylase predigestion confirms excess glycogen in vacuolated hepatocytes (see Chapter 112). Up to a third of affected dogs develop hepatocellular carcinoma.

THERAPEUTICS

- HNH – usually none required; rupture of large nodules indicates hepatocellular carcinoma misdiagnosis; may necessitate blood transfusion and emergency mass excision. Palliate or alleviate underlying cause of VH.
- HDH – recommend biochemical assessments for rising ALP or alanine aminotransferase (ALT) that may indicate transformation of mass lesion to a neoplastic phenotype; US inspection of adrenal glands for adrenomegaly or nodules, US surveillance for expanding mass lesions that should be surgically removed; assess pituitary adrenal axis for typical or atypical hyperadrenocorticism; if increased sex hormones >2.5× upper reference interval, consider adrenal modulation with agent that does not increase sex hormones.

Drug(s) of Choice

- HDH – if increased sex hormones, progressive VH, nodule formation, increasing ALP, or confirmed hepatocellular carcinoma (after mass resection), consider adrenal modulation with a drug that does not increase sex hormone concentrations (Lysodren or mitotane); trilostane increases sex hormone concentrations and would be inappropriate.
- Scottish terrier syndrome does not respond to adrenal modulation; instead use surveillance to detect emerging hepatocellular carcinoma.

Precautions/Interactions

- HDH – trilostane increases sex hormone concentrations and would be inappropriate.

COMMENTS

Client Education

- HNH – incidental age-associated lesion.
- HDH – association with adrenal hyperplasia syndromes. Periodic monitoring for emergence of progressively enlarging mass suggestive of hepatocellular carcinoma advised.

Patient Monitoring

- Quarterly biochemical profiles.
- Sequential abdominal US to evaluate progression of hepatic nodules.
- See Chapter 112 for related disorders.

Possible Complications

- HNH – incidental age-associated lesion.
- HDH – up to one-third of affected dogs develop hepatocellular carcinoma.

Expected Course and Prognosis

- More extensive numbers of nodules may develop in some dogs with HNH and HDH.
- HDH predicts risk for primary hepatocellular neoplasia which requires surveillance and surgical treatment.

Abbreviations

- ALP = alkaline phosphatase
- ALT = alanine aminotransferase
- HDH = hepatic dysplastic hyperplasia
- HNH = hepatic nodular hyperplasia
- PAS = periodic acid–Schiff
- TSBA = total serum bile acids
- US = ultrasound
- VH = vacuolar hepatopathy

See Also

- Cirrhosis and Fibrosis of the Liver
- Chronic Hepatitis
- Glycogen-Type Vacuolar Hepatopathy
- Hepatic Neoplasia, Benign
- Hepatic Neoplasia, Malignant

Suggested Reading

Cortright CC, Center SA, Randolph JF, et al. Clinical features of progressive vacuolar hepatopathy in Scottish Terriers with and without hepatocellular carcinoma: 114 cases (1980–2013). J Am Vet Med Assoc 2014;245:797–808.

Sepesy LM, Center SA, Randolph JF, et al. Vacuolar hepatopathy in dogs: 336 cases (1993–2005). J Am Vet Med Assoc 2006;229:246–252.

Stowater JL, Lamb CR, Schelling SH. Ultrasonographic features of canine hepatic nodular hyperplasia. Vet Radiol 1990;31:268–272.

Warren-Smith CM, Andrew S, Mantis P, Lamb CR. Lack of associations between ultrasonagraphic appearance of parenchymal lesions of the canine liver and histological diagnosis. J Small Anim Pract 2012;53(3):168–173.

Authors: Sean P. McDonough DVM, PhD, DACVP, Sharon A. Center DVM, DACVIM

Chapter 120

Hepatitis, Chronic

DEFINITION/OVERVIEW

- Hepatic injury associated with active necroinflammatory liver injury.
- Nonsuppurative inflammation – most common; lymphocytes, plasma cells, macrophages, occasional neutrophils.
- Chronicity – progressive remodeling, regenerative nodule formation, fibrosis, eventuating in cirrhosis (see Chapter 108).

ETIOLOGY/PATHOPHYSIOLOGY

- Multitude of initiating events cause hepatic injury that alters hepatic architecture, damages membranes and/or organelles, and activates cytokine and cell-mediated immune responses; hepatic components become targeted foci.
- Initial injury may include infectious agents, toxins, or therapeutic agents but cause often remains undetermined.
- Inflammatory cells, including predominantly lymphocytes (T cells, NK T cells), Kupffer cells (hepatic macrophages resident in the lumen of sinusoids), and neutrophils are initial effector cells; INF-gamma, TNF-alpha, FasL, IL-4, and numerous chemokines and oxidative free radicals are commonly involved.
- Oxidant injury is an important pathomechanism of membrane and organelle injury.
- Initial zone of injury demarcates area of necroinflammatory response – zone 1 (periportal) common in many forms of idiopathic hepatitis whereas zone 3 incriminates copper (Cu)-associated injury, nonsteroidal antiinflammatory drugs (NSAID) and other toxins, or repeated ischemic/hypoxic insult.
- Lesion progression is variable and may include portal and periportal lymphoplasmacytic infiltrates, interface hepatitis with piecemeal necrosis of the limiting plate and variable lobular necroinflammatory activity. Chronic inflammation – progressive fibrosis with bridging between involved zones.
- Bridging fibrosis and regenerative nodules distort lobular architecture, leading to cirrhosis.
- Progressive development of cholestasis.
- Cirrhosis and hepatic failure – late stage.
  - Cirrhosis – consequence of chronic fibrogenesis and hepatic regenerative response; typified by regenerative nodules; reduced functional hepatic mass; collagen deposition along sinusoids and/or around portal triads that compromises sinusoidal perfusion.
  - Fibrosis – usually reflects chronic injury; associated with release of cytokines/mediators that stimulate extracellular matrix (ECM) production or accumulation.

Blackwell's Five-Minute Veterinary Consult Clinical Companion: Small Animal Gastrointestinal Diseases, First Edition. Edited by Jocelyn Mott and Jo Ann Morrison.
© 2019 John Wiley & Sons, Inc. Published 2019 by John Wiley & Sons, Inc.
Companion website: www.fiveminutevet.com/gastrointestinal

- Cirrhosis/fibrosis – leads to hepatic dysfunction, sinusoidal hypertension; intrahepatic shunting in collagenized sinusoids or through recanalized vascular pathways within fibrotic partitions between regenerative nodules.
- Sinusoidal hypertension – leads to (1) hepatofugal portal venous flow (away from the liver), (2) mesenteric splanchnic hypertension, (3) formation of acquired portosystemic shunts (APSS), (4) episodic hepatic encephalopathy (HE), (5) splanchnic pooling of blood, decreased effective blood volume, renal sodium and water retention that culminate in ascites formation, (6) portal hypertensive enteric vasculopathy predisposing to enteric bleeding.

Systems Affected

- Hepatobiliary – inflammation; necrosis; cholestasis; fibrosis.
- Gastrointestinal (GI) – emesis; diarrhea; anorexia, portal hypertension leads to ascites formation and propensity for enteric bleeding (portal hypertensive gastroenteric vasculopathy).
- Neurologic – HE (advanced stage).
- Hemic – red blood cell microcytosis reflecting APSS; bleeding tendencies: failed factor synthesis or activation or thrombocytopenia; coagulopathy (advanced stage).
- Renal/urologic – polyuria/polydipsia; isosthenuria; ammonium biurate crystalluria (advanced stage).
- Endocrine/metabolic – hypoglycemia if end-stage liver failure (provoked by prolonged inappetence).
- Respiratory – tachypnea if tense ascites; bicavity effusion (leakage across diaphragm (rare), pulmonary edema (rare).

 # SIGNALMENT/HISTORY

- Occurs in dogs.
- Breed or familial predisposition for chronic hepatitis – Doberman pinscher, Labrador retriever, West Highland white terrier, and Dalmatian may develop chronic hepatitis related to low tolerance to Cu levels in commercial diets; cocker spaniel, standard poodle, Maltese, Skye terrier, others.
- Inherited copper-associated hepatopathy only proven in the Bedlington terrier – autosomal recessive, genetic test available.
- Average age 6–8 years (range 2–14 years).
- Inconsistency among reports for any breed of a predominant gender.

Risk Factors

- Immunostimulants (unknown role of agents such as vaccinations) and molecular mimicry of cell epitopes by infectious agents or infection of sinusoidal endothelium may promote inflammatory reactions associated with chronic hepatitis.
- Cu-associated hepatopathy – neoepitope formation from oxidant injury.
- Hepatic iron accumulation – may result from supplementation.
- Drugs – inducers or inhibitors of microsomal enzymes or conditions diminishing hepatic antioxidant status may augment liver damage from certain toxins.

Historical Findings

- May be no signs in early disease.
- Lethargy.
- Anorexia, weight loss, vomiting, reduced body condition.
- Polyuria and polydipsia.

CLINICAL FEATURES

- May be no signs in early disease.
- Lethargy, poor coat, declining body condition.
- Variable jaundice.
- Liver size – normal to small, depends on chronicity.

Late-Stage Physical Findings

- Ascites.
- Hepatic encephalopathy.
- Obstructive uropathy: ammonium biurate cystoliths.
- Bleeding tendencies – variable, uncommon.

DIFFERENTIAL DIAGNOSIS

- Acute hepatitis – history; liver biopsy.
- Congenital portosystemic shunt (PSVA) – abdominal ultrasonography; radiographic or multisector computed tomography contrast venography (latter preferred); colorectal scintigraphy; liver biopsy.
- Primary hepatic neoplasia – radiography or ultrasonography; cytology; biopsy.
- Metastatic neoplasia or carcinomatosis.
- Chronic pancreatitis.
- Causes of abdominal effusion – hypoalbuminemia; right heart failure; carcinomatosis; bile peritonitis.
- Other causes of portal hypertension.
- Jaundice – extrahepatic biliary duct obstruction (EHBDO); bile peritonitis, hemolysis.

DIAGNOSTICS

Complete Blood Count/Biochemistry/Urinalysis

- Complete blood cell count – nonregenerative anemia; red blood cell microcytosis if APSS; variable leukogram, thrombocytopenia; low total protein if chronic disease.
- Biochemistry – high liver enzymes; variable total bilirubin, albumin, blood urea nitrogen (BUN), glucose, and cholesterol; hepatic failure suggested by low values of albumin, BUN, glucose, and cholesterol, in the absence of other explanations.
- Urinalysis – variable urine concentration; bilirubinuria; ammonium biurate crystalluria if APSS.

Other Laboratory Tests

- Total serum bile acids (TSBA) – variable depending on extent of hepatic remodeling, sinusoidal hypertension, and cholestasis.
- Ammonia intolerance – reflects APSS; insensitive to cholestatic changes.
- Coagulation tests – reflect panlobular injury and/or chronicity; early disease has no abnormalities but perhaps high fibrinogen; advanced stage or severe panlobular injury may note prolonged prothrombin time (PT), activated partial thromboplastin time (APTT), proteins invoked by vitamin K absence or antagonism (PIVKA), low fibrinogen, increased fibrin degradation products (FDP) or D-dimers (**note:** some D-dimer tests are too sensitive for differential diagnostic utility); coagulation tests reflect severity of liver dysfunction, synthetic failure, disseminated intravascular coagulation (DIC), and vitamin K adequacy; low protein C activity suggests APSS or hepatic failure.

- Abdominal effusion – chronic liver disease or portal hypertension: pure or modified transudate.
- Liver zinc values – low with chronic disease and especially if APSS.
- Serologic tests – for possible infectious agents, e.g., leptospirosis, rickettsial diseases, *Borrelia*, *Bartonella*, endemic fungal agents.
- Antinuclear antibody (ANA) titer –for potential autoimmune-mediated disease; **note:** low-level positive titers are nonspecific.
- Immunohistochemical staining of liver sample – confirms infectious agent or origin of infiltrative cells.

Imaging
Abdominal Radiography
- Microhepatia – suggests late-stage disease.
- Abdominal effusion – obscures image.
- Ammonium biurate calculi – radiolucent unless combined with radiodense minerals.

Ultrasonography (US)
- Liver size depends on disease stage; microhepatia in late stage.
- Normal to variable parenchymal and biliary tract echogenicity; may note nodularity and irregular liver margins.
- APSS – tortuous vessels caudal to left kidney or near splenic vein with Doppler color flow interrogation.
- Abdominal effusion – visualize small pockets; US facilitates sampling.
- Uroliths (tiny to large) – renal pelvis or urinary bladder; may signify ammonium biurate urolithiasis.
- Rule out EHBDO (jaundice, high enzymes); identify mass lesions, cholelithiasis; gallbladder mucocele; cholecystitis, choledochitis; cystic lesions (abscess). Enables fine needle aspiration – cytology and cholecystocentesis for bile collection.

Colorectal/Splenoportal Scintigraphy
- 99 M-Technetium pertechnetate isotope time activity curve displays first isotope distribution: delivery to liver = no shunting, delivery to heart = shunting.
- Colorectal scintigraphy (CRS) – sensitive and noninvasive, detects portosystemic shunting but cannot differentiate PSVA from APSS.
- Splenoportal scintigraphy – offers no diagnostic advantage, is invasive and requires US-guided splenic injection.

Other Diagnostic Procedures
Aspiration Cytology
- Fine-needle aspiration cytology – *cannot define* fibrosis or nonsuppurative inflammation; *cannot* lead to a definitive recommendation for therapy. May identify hepatic vacuolation and canalicular cholestasis: common changes observed in canine liver disorders; neoplasia; infectious agents.
- Cannot definitively diagnose chronic hepatitis, hepatic fibrosis, or copper-associated hepatopathy with cytology.

Liver Biopsy
- Liver biopsy – needed for definitive diagnosis; acquire biopsies from multiple lobes.
- Tru-Cut needle biopsy – 18 G needle core too small for accuracy; use 14–16 G.
- Laparoscopy – best biopsy method; permits gross visualization, documents APSS, provides biopsy access to multiple liver lobes and focal lesions.

Bacterial Culture

- Aerobic and anaerobic cultures and sensitivity of liver and bile; use bile containing particulate debris for best sample – bacteria are found tangled with biliary precipitates.

Metal Analyses

- Determine copper, iron, and zinc concentrations (dry matter basis).
- Low zinc commonly associated with portosystemic shunting; high iron common in necroinflammatory disorders, contributes to oxidative injury; copper analysis results may reflect sampling of regenerative nodules or fibrotic regions or regions of parenchymal extinction, leading to low measurements compared to intact parenchyma.
- Digital scanning of biopsy slide stained with rhodanine can accurately quantify liver copper concentration.

Pathologic Findings

- Gross – early: no gross change; late stage: microhepatia with irregular surface or margins (fine or coarse nodules), tortuous APSS.
- Microscopic – nonsuppurative inflammation involving zone of necroinflammatory injury; variable cholestasis and biliary hyperplasia; piecemeal and/or bridging necrosis; interface hepatitis; disruption of limiting plate in zone 1 lesions; in late-stage disease: bridging between or within zones; regenerative nodules, and transition to cirrhosis.
- Histopathology.
  - Immune-mediated hepatitis – periportal, lobular, or centrilobular lymphoplasmacytic infiltrates, hepatic cord disorganization, sinusoidal fibrosis (space of Disse), biliary hyperplasia (ductular reaction).
  - Cu hepatopathy – initially centrilobular, may evolve to immune-mediated hepatitis.
  - Cirrhosis – diffuse lesion; fibrosis associated with nodular regeneration and hepatic lobule distortion; periportal/sinusoidal fibrosis.

 THERAPEUTICS

Drug(s) of Choice

- Treatments for specific etiologies: chelate Cu if copper-associated hepatopathy; withdraw potentially hepatotoxic drugs.
- No clinical trials prove efficacy of specific regimens to date.
- Copper chelation – see Chapter 109.
- Immunomodulation.
  - Prednisolone/prednisone – 2–4 mg/kg daily PO; taper to lowest effective dose (e.g., 0.25–0.5 mg/kg PO q48h); for data on survival effect see Suggested Reading. If ascites, use dexamethasone to avoid mineralocorticoid effect (to account for increased potency, divide prednisone dose by 8–10 for dexamethasone dose); for data on canine survival influence, see Suggested Reading.
  - Azathioprine – in dogs: 1–2 mg/kg PO q24h; use loading q24h dose for 3–5 days *then* titrate to q48h; contraindicated in cats (toxic); in dogs: combined with prednisone, antioxidants, antifibrotics (polyunsaturated phosphatidylcholine), and possibly cyclosporine. During chronic therapy, titrate dose by 25–50% reduction after 2–6 months based on sequential biochemistries showing improvements (e.g., declining total bilirubin and liver enzyme activity); monitor complete blood cell count and biochemistry profile q7–10 days for first month to ensure absence of hematopoietic, hepatic, and pancreatic toxicity; if acute hematopoietic toxicity,

stop therapy, allow recovery, then reintroduce at 25% dose reduction; if insidious chronic hematopoietic toxicity (after months) or acute cholestatic liver or pancreatic injury, discontinue therapy.

- Mycophenolate mofetil – similar mechanism of effect as azathioprine; dose: 10–15 mg/kg PO q12h; eliminated by hepatic glucuronidation and renal excretion; monitor as for azathioprine and titrate dose similarly. May have fewer side effects than azathioprine.
- Microemulsified cyclosporine – 5 mg/kg PO q24h; limited long-term experience; variable response.

■ Ursodeoxycholic acid – immunomodulatory, hepatoprotectant, antifibrotic, choleretic, antiendotoxic, antioxidant; dose 7.5 mg/kg PO q12h; administered with food for best assimilation; tablets have best bioavailability; may prepare aqueous solution; safe; maintain indefinitely.

■ Antifibrotics.
- Immunomodulators, SAMe, silibinin, vitamin E: also considered as antifibrotics as they interrupt signaling processes, promoting activation of sinusoidal myofibrocytes and collagen production.
- Polyunsaturated phosphatidylcholine (PPC) – antifibrotic, immunomodulatory, antioxidant, hepatoprotectant effects; dose: 25 mg/kg/day PO with food. Use PhosChol® form (preformed active ingredient: dilinolylphosphatidylcholine); beneficial in some forms of liver disease (humans, animal models); may provide a corticosteroid-sparing effect allowing reduced glucocorticoid dosing; safely prescribed without liver biopsy.
- Colchicine – imparts antiinflammatory, antifibrotic, and immunomodulatory effects; 0.025–0.03 mg/kg PO q24–48 h; controversial evidence for benefit in reducing fibrosis in human liver disorders; mechanism of action is via polymerization of microtubules curtailing collagen formation; metaphase arrest may provoke GI and bone marrow toxicity; neurologic adverse effects described in humans; avoid form complexed with probenecid (prolongs drug retention time); used when fibroplasia is the overriding histologic feature but not in ductal plate malformations.
- Silibinin with PPC – hepatoprotectant (studied against numerous toxins), antifibrotic, and antioxidant effects, may also promote hepatocellular regeneration; no metaanalysis in humans confirms beneficial influence in chronic hepatitis that does not have a viral cause. 2–5 mg/kg/day PO (PPC complexed form only). May alter glucuronidation of some drugs, unclear if causes drug interactions.

■ Antioxidants.
- Vitamin E – alpha-tocopherol, 10 IU/kg PO q24h.
- S-Adenosylmethionine (SAMe) – use bioavailable proven GSH donor; 20 mg/kg/day enteric-coated tablet PO given on empty stomach for best absorption.
- Avoid vitamin C (ascorbate) – if high tissue copper or iron concentration, augments oxidant injury associated with transition metals.
- Zinc (zinc acetate) – antioxidant; antifibrotic, blocks enteric copper uptake, required for urea cycle enzymes. Elemental zinc 1.5–3 mg/kg PO daily supplement if low liver zinc concentration (<120 μg/g dry weight liver); adjust dose using sequential plasma zinc concentrations (avoid plasma ≥800 μg/dL).

■ Hepatoprotectants.
- Ursodeoxycholate, vitamin E, SAMe provide hepatoprotectant effects in addition to other benefits.
- Silibinin – efficacy unclear, use PPC complexed form (bioavailable), 2–5 mg/kg PO q24h.

■ Bleeding tendencies – see Chapter 104.
■ Gastrointestinal signs/hemorrhage.

- Histamine type-2 receptor antagonists – famotidine 0.5–2 mg/kg PO, IV, SQ q12–24 h.
- Proton pump inhibitors – omeprazole 1.0 mg/kg q24h PO or pantoprazole 1 mg/kg q24h IV. Omeprazole may induce p450 cytochrome-associated drug interactions and may have a 24–48 h delayed onset of action.
- Some clinicians recommend chronic treatment with proton pump inhibitors to minimize gastrointestinal bleeding and ulceration that may become a chronic problem.
- Sucralfate – gastroprotectants 0.25–1.0 g/10 kg PO q8–12 h; titrate to effect, beware of drug interactions as sucralfate may bind other medications, reducing bioavailability.
- Eliminate endoparasitism.

Specific Conditions
Ascites
- Restrict activity and sodium intake; combine with diuretic therapy.
- Dietary sodium restriction (0.2% dry matter basis or <100 mg/100 kcal).
- Diuretics – slowly mobilize effusion with combination of furosemide (0.5–2 mg/kg IV, SQ, PO q12h) and spironolactone (0.5–2 mg/kg PO q12h; loading spironolactone is important, use doubled dose once); recheck and adjust dose at 4–7-day intervals by 25–50%. Titrate dose to response, may use q48h or intermittently to mobilize recurrent ascites.
- Therapeutic large-volume abdominocentesis – if ascites is nonresponsive to mobilization in 7–14 days with concurrent diuretics and sodium restriction; may require fluid support as a result of intravascular to abdominal fluid shift causing postcentesis hypotension syndrome and acute renal failure.
- Consider vasopressin V2 antagonists (aquaretics) with low-dose diuretics for treatment of resistant ascites; tolvaptan has been used experimentally in dogs at 10 mg/kg without adverse effects to mobilize water.

HE
See Chapter 114.

Precautions/Interactions
- Diuretics – dehydration, hypokalemia, alkalosis worsen HE.
- Glucocorticoids – increased susceptibility to infection, enteric bleeding, sodium and water retention, protein catabolism, and HE.
- Avoid drugs or reduce dose if first-pass hepatic extraction; if require hepatic conjugation or biotransformation, e.g., metronidazole – reduce conventional dose to 7.5 mg/kg PO q12h (often used for HE).
- Zinc overdose may cause hemolysis.
- NSAIDs – avoid; potentiate enteric bleeding; may worsen ascites; potentially centrilobular hepatic necrosis-hepatotoxic metabolites.
- Avoid drugs requiring hepatic metabolism whenever possible.
- Avoid medications that alter hepatic biotransformation or excretion pathways (e.g., cimetidine, quinidine, ketoconazole).
- Avoid concurrent treatment with metoclopramide if spironolactone used for diuresis (causes aldosterone release).

Alternative Drugs
- Dexamethasone – if ascites, replace prednisone or prednisolone with dexamethasone (to remove mineralocorticoid effect); divide prednisone or prednisolone dose by 7–10; taper dose to observed efficacy.
- Mycophenolate: alternative for azathioprine.

Appropriate Health Care

- Inpatient – for diagnostic testing and therapy in overtly ill dogs.
- Outpatient – if condition is stable at diagnosis; slowly titrated onto medical therapy.

Nursing Care

- Depends on underlying condition.
- Fluid therapy – balanced polyionic fluids supplemented to correct electrolyte aberrations or hypoglycemia; restrict sodium if ascites.
- Water-soluble vitamins.
- Ascites: managed with sodium-restricted diet, enforced rest, diuretics (furosemide combined with spironolactone).
- Therapeutic abdominocentesis – aseptic procedure for removing large-volume symptomatic ascites compromising food intake, ventilation, or sleep; if diuretics and sodium restriction ineffectual.
- For diuretic-resistant ascites: calculate sodium intake against measured renal sodium excretion (collect urine over 12 h, measure sodium and creatinine in well-mixed sample, and in sera); guides adjustments in management (i.e., increase sodium restriction vs increase diuretic).

Diet

- Adequate calories and protein – avoid catabolism to maintain muscle mass (attenuates hyperammonemia); monitor body condition.
- Dietary protein – restrict quantity *only* if signs of HE or observed ammonium biurate crystalluria; feed balanced diet; if HE, avoid fish and red meat source protein (dogs).
- Meal frequency – feed several small meals per day to optimize nutrient assimilation.
- Sodium restriction – with ascites or severe hypoalbuminemia: <100 mg/100 kcal or <0.2% dry matter basis formula.
- Good-quality vitamin supplement – vitamin metabolism perturbed with liver disease and losses in urine; avoid copper supplements if copper-associated hepatopathy.
- Thiamin – ensure repletion to avoid Wernicke's encephalopathy; 50–100 mg PO q24h; **caution**: anaphylactoid reactions may occur with injectable thiamin.
- Partial parenteral nutrition – may consider, if short-term inappetence to minimize catabolism.
- Total parenteral nutrition – if inappetence lasts >7 days; branched-chain amino acids remain controversial in dogs with liver dysfunction.
- Fat restriction rarely needed.

Activity

Keep patient warm, inactive, and hydrated; inactivity may promote hepatic regeneration, euglycemia, and ascites mobilization.

Surgical Considerations

- APSS – do not ligate nor band the vena cava.
- Cirrhosis – high anesthetic risk; gas anesthesia preferred – isoflurane or sevoflurane.

 COMMENTS

Zoonotic Potential

- Dogs with leptospirosis-associated chronic liver disease (rare) may shed organisms.
- *Bartonella*; rickettsial agents (via endemic vectors).

Client Education

- Control rather than cure is the expected goal; medications usually will be required for life; disease is cyclic; quarterly evaluations important.
- Inform client of the lack of long-term veterinary studies proving efficacy of single or polypharmacy approaches; recommendations derived from clinical experience, studies in humans, and animal disease models.
- Antifibrotics may reduce fibrosis but limited evidence; fibrosis diminished by control of inflammation and underlying primary process.
- Attenuate factors provoking HE – dehydration; azotemia, infection; catabolism; hypokalemia; alkalemia; high-protein meals; endoparasitism; enteric bleeding; certain drugs.

Patient Monitoring

- At-home behavior, body condition, muscle mass, weight – adjust protein and energy intake to nitrogen tolerance and apparent energy needs.
- Complete blood cell count, biochemistry, and urinalysis – monthly or quarterly, depends on patient status; look for signs of drug toxicity, disease remission, synthetic function, ammonium biurate urolithiasis, and urinary tract infections.
- Serial monitoring of TSBA – usually does not add prognostic or diagnostic information.
- Abdominal girth; reflects ascites volume.
- Azathioprine, mycophenolate, colchicine – monitor for possible bone marrow toxicity (serial complete blood cell counts), GI toxicity, and other effects.

Possible Complications

- HE, septicemia, bleeding – may be life-threatening.
- DIC – may be a terminal event.

Expected Course and Prognosis

- Chronic hepatitis can be a cyclic disease with occasional flare-ups indicated by sequential assessment of liver enzymes.
- Some dogs achieve solid long-term remission.
- Some dogs with Cu-associated hepatopathy can achieve permanent remission of apparent "immune-mediated" inflammation upon effective Cu chelation and appropriate nutritional management.
- Presence of ascites indicates severe disease with shorter survival.
- Severe disease complicated by development of APSS, HE, and ascites may require occasional hospitalizations for adjustment of nutritional and medical interventions.
- Sodium restriction and diuretics may require titration to achieve optimal control of ascites.

Abbreviations

- ACT = activated clotting time
- ANA = antinuclear antibodies
- APSS = acquired portosystemic shunt(s)
- APTT = activated partial thromboplastin time
- ARF = acute renal failure
- CRS = colorectal scintigraphy
- Cu = copper
- DIC = disseminated intravascular coagulation
- ECM = extracellular matrix
- EHBDO = extrahepatic bile duct occlusion
- FasL = fas-ligand
- FDP = fibrin degradation products
- GI = gastrointestinal
- HE = hepatic encephalopathy
- IL-4 = interleukin 4
- INF = interferon
- NSAID = nonsteroidal antiinflammatory drug

- PIVKA = proteins invoked by vitamin K absence or antagonism
- PPC = polyunsaturated phosphatidylcholine
- PSVA = portosystemic vascular anomaly

- PT = prothrombin time
- TNF = tumor necrosis factor
- TSBA = total serum bile acids
- US = ultrasound

See Also

- Cirrhosis and Fibrosis of Liver
- Coagulopathy of Liver Disease
- Copper-Associated Hepatopathy
- Diabetic Hepatopathy
- Hepatic Encephalopathy

- Hepatic Failure, Acute
- Hypertension, Portal
- Nutritional Approach to Hepatic Disease
- Portosystemic Shunting, Acquired

Suggested Reading

Center SA. Metabolic, antioxidant, nutraceutical, probiotic, and herbal therapies relating to the management of hepatobiliary disorders. Vet Clin North Am Small Anim Pract 2004;34:67–172.

Raffan E, McCallum A, Scase TJ. Ascites is a negative prognostic indicator in chronic hepatitis in dogs. J Vet Intern Med 2009;23:63–66.

Strombeck DR, Miller LM, Harrold D. Effects of corticosteroid treatment on survival time in dogs with chronic hepatitis: 151 cases (1977–1985). J Am Vet Med Assoc 1988;193:1109–1113.

Authors: Sean P. McDonough DVM, PhD, DACVP, Sharon A. Center DVM, DACVIM

121

Hepatitis, Granulomatous

DEFINITION/OVERVIEW

- Granulomatous hepatitis is an uncommon disease in which granulomas (often multifocal) are found in the liver. Granulomatous hepatitis may occur secondary to systemic disease or be confined to the liver.

ETIOLOGY/PATHOPHYSIOLOGY

- Granulomatous hepatitis has many infectious and noninfectious causes.
- Infectious causes include the following.
    - Bacterial (*Bartonella*, *Borrelia*, *Brucella*, *Leptospira*, *Helicobacter*, *Mycobacterium*, *Nocardia*).
    - Fungal (histoplasmosis, coccidioidomycosis, aspergillosis, cryptococcosis).
    - Parasites (schistosomiasis, visceral *Toxocara* larval migrans, dirofilariasis, *Capillaria hepatica*, hepatozoonosis). Aberrant migration of *Angiostrongylus vasorum* has been documented as a cause of granulomatous hepatitis with severe liver dysfunction in a dog.
    - Protozoal (leishmaniasis, toxoplasmosis, cytauxzoonosis).
    - Viral (feline infectious peritonitis).
    - Protothecosis.
- Noninfectious causes include the following.
    - Idiopathic.
    - Adverse reaction to drugs, herbal or holistic remedies.
    - Neoplasia (lymphosarcoma).
    - Histiocytosis (neoplasia or histiocytic syndrome).
    - Lymphangiectasia.
    - Immune-mediated inflammation.
    - Copper-associated hepatic necrosis.

Systems Affected

- Hepatobiliary.
- Gastrointestinal – intestinal lymphangiectasia has been associated with hepatic lipogranulomas.

Blackwell's Five-Minute Veterinary Consult Clinical Companion: Small Animal Gastrointestinal Diseases,
First Edition. Edited by Jocelyn Mott and Jo Ann Morrison.
© 2019 John Wiley & Sons, Inc. Published 2019 by John Wiley & Sons, Inc.
Companion website: www.fiveminutevet.com/gastrointestinal

SIGNALMENT/HISTORY

- No breed or age predisposition.
- More common in dogs than cats.

Risk Factors

- Exposure to infectious agents.
- Exposure to drugs, holistic or herbal remedies.

Historical Findings

- Lethargy.
- Anorexia.
- Pyrexia.
- Abdominal pain.
- Polyuria/polydipsia.

CLINICAL FEATURES

- Physical examination may be normal.
- Abnormalities can include icterus, abdominal distension with ascites and/or hepatomegaly and pyrexia.

DIFFERENTIAL DIAGNOSIS

- Other diseases of the liver such as chronic hepatitis, copper-associated hepatopathy, neoplasia, toxic hepatopathy, and infectious hepatopathy can present similarly to granulomatous hepatopathy.
- Sometimes clinical signs and diagnostics may predominantly show involvement of other organs besides the liver such as lymphadenopathy, splenomegaly, pulmonary signs, etc.

DIAGNOSTICS

Complete Blood Count/Biochemistry/Urinalysis

- Neutrophilia and/or thrombocytopenia may be present.
- Hypoalbuminemia, hyperglobulinemia, and alkaline phosphatase (ALP) and alanine aminotransferase (ALT) elevations. ALP is often elevated more than ALT and indicates underlying cholestasis.

Other Laboratory Tests

- Culture of liver and bile. Bile yields positive cultures more frequently than liver tissue.
- Fecal flotation to identify ova and parasites. Fecal polymerase chain reaction (PCR) can be performed for schistosomiasis.
- Bile acids may be elevated and indicate concurrent liver dysfunction.
- Serology and PCR tests for infectious agents should be pursued.

Imaging

- Abdominal radiographs may reveal hepatomegaly, masses, and/or ascites. Thoracic radiographs may reveal lymphadenopathy or pulmonary changes consistent with infectious diseases or neoplasia.

■ Abdominal ultrasound may reveal variable hepatic parenchymal echogenicity (diffuse or focal), involvement of other abdominal organs such as lymphadenopathy or splenomegaly, and effusion.

Additional Diagnostic Tests

■ Liver biopsy is required for diagnosis of granulomatous hepatitis. Biopsies may be obtained laparoscopically, via ultrasound guidance or by surgery. Biopsy multiple liver lobes.
■ Use 14–16 gauge Tru-Cut for ultrasound-guided liver biopsy.
■ Once liver biopsy is obtained, special tests to identify infectious agents may be necessary.
  • Fluorescence *in situ* hybridization (FISH) of histopathological samples is more sensitive than standard histopathology for identifying bacteria as part of etiology.
  • Fungal stains such as Grocott-Gomori methenamine-silver nitrate stain may be necessary to identify fungal elements in liver biopsies.
  • PCR can be used on hepatic biopsies to detect DNA of some infectious agents.
■ Hepatic copper quantification may be evaluated as excessive hepatic copper accumulation has been reported in some dogs with granulomatous hepatitis.

Pathologic Findings

■ Gross – liver may be enlarged; may have nodules or irregularities on surface.
■ Histopathology findings include hepatic inflammation characterized by macrophages, often with epithelioid appearance and presence of lymphocytes, plasma cells, and fibroblasts.

 ## THERAPEUTICS

■ Treatment for the specific cause of granulomatous hepatitis should be initiated. However, the specific etiology is not always evident.

Drug(s) of Choice

■ If an infectious disease is identified, then treatment with appropriate antibiotics, antifungals or anthelmintics is recommended.
■ If no infectious cause is determined, then trial treatment for bartonellosis (doxycycline 10–15 mg/kg PO q12h; enrofloxacin 5 mg/kg PO q12h; azithromycin 5–10 mg/kg PO q24h) or empirical treatment for possible bacterial infection (enrofloxacin 10 mg/kg PO q24h; cephalexin 22 mg/kg PO q12h) may be pursued, prior to initiating immunosuppressive therapy.
■ Discontinue any drugs, including holistic or herbal remedies, to which the pet may be having an adverse reaction.
■ Idiopathic or immune-mediated causes of granulomatous hepatitis may require immunosuppressive therapy with corticosteroids (prednisolone/prednisone 2–4 mg/kg daily PO; taper to lowest effective dose) +/– azathioprine (in dogs: 1–2 mg/kg PO q24h; use loading q24h dose for 3–5 days then titrate to q48h) or mycophenolate mofetil (10–15 mg/kg PO q12h).
■ If copper-associated hepatic necrosis is present, pet may benefit from chelation therapy with penicillamine (7–15 mg/kg PO q12h) or zinc acetate (elemental zinc 1.5–3 mg/kg PO daily supplement).

Precautions/Interactions

■ Immunosuppression may exacerbate an infectious disease.
■ Avoid drugs that require hepatic biotransformation or lower drug dosage.
■ Azathioprine is contraindicated in cats.

Appropriate Health Care

- Some pets may be treated as outpatients.

Nursing Care

- Some pets may require hospitalization with intravenous fluids and supportive care.
- Nutritional support may be necessary.

Diet

- A copper-restricted diet may be needed with copper-associated hepatopathy.

Surgical Considerations

- Surgical or laparoscopic liver biopsies may be recommended.
- Exploratory surgery may be required for biopsies if there is involvement of additional abdominal organs, including the liver.

 COMMENTS

Client Education

- Cirrhosis or end-stage liver disease may result, depending on response of liver to treatment.
- Holistic or herbal remedies should only be given to pets on the advice of a veterinarian familiar with that mode of therapy.

Patient Monitoring

- Hospitalized patients may require hematologic and biochemistry profiles, imaging and clotting profiles every day to every few days until their condition stabilizes and to monitor for progression to liver failure.
- Outpatients under treatment may require regular follow-up hematologic and biochemistry profiles, convalescent serological tests, imaging, and physical examinations.

Prevention/Avoidance

- Anthelmintic use can prevent some parasitic causes of granulomatous hepatitis.

Possible Complications

- Cirrhosis and fibrosis.
- Chronic hepatitis.
- Liver failure.
- Coagulopathy.
- Multiple acquired portosystemic shunts.

Expected Course and Prognosis

- Prognosis depends on underlying cause of granulomatous hepatitis.

Abbreviations

- ALP = alkaline phosphatase
- ALT = alanine aminotransferase
- FISH = fluorescence *in situ* hybridization
- PCR = polymerase chain reaction

See Also

- Copper-Associated Hepatopathy
- Hepatitis, Chronic
- Hepatopathy, Infectious
- Leptospirosis
- Nutritional Approach to Hepatic Disease

Suggested Reading

Chapman BL, Hendrick MJ, Washabau RJ Granulomatous hepatitis in dogs: nine cases (1987–1990). J Am Vet Med Assoc 1993;203:680.

Cook S, Preistnall SL, Blake D, et al. Angiostrongylus vasorum causing severe granulomatous hepatitis with concurrent multiple acquired PSS. J Am Anim Hosp Assoc 2015;51(5):320–324.

Hutchins RG, Breitschwerdt EB, Cullen JM, et al. Limited yield of diagnoses of intrahepatic infectious causes of canine granulomatous hepatitis from archival liver tissue. J Vet Diagn Invest 2012;24:888–894.

Im J, Burney DP, McDonough SP, et al. Canine hepatitis associated with intrahepatic bacteria in three dogs. J Am Anim Hosp Assoc 2018;54(1):65–70.

Johnson SE. Parenchymal disorders. In: Washabau RJ, Day MJ, eds. Canine and Feline Gastroenterology. St Louis: Saunders Elsevier, 2013.

Willard MD. Inflammatory canine hepatic disease. In: Ettinger SJ, Feldman EC, eds. Textbook of Veterinary Internal Medicine, 7th ed. St Louis: Saunders Elsevier, 2010.

Author: Jocelyn Mott DVM, DACVIM (SAIM)

Chapter 122

Hepatitis, Infectious (Viral) Canine

DEFINITION/OVERVIEW

- Infectious canine hepatitis (ICH) is a relatively rare disease of dogs caused by canine adenovirus type 1 (CAV-1).
- CAV-1 has worldwide geographic distribution and also causes disease in wolves, coyotes, skunks, and bears. It causes encephalitis in foxes.
- It has also been called Rubarth's disease after the veterinarian Dr Carl Sven Rubarth who first described the disease in the late 1940s.
- CAV-1 is antigenically related to CAV-2, the causative agent of canine infectious laryngotracheitis.

ETIOLOGY/PATHOPHYSIOLOGY

- CAV-1 is spread via direct dog-to-dog oronasal contact or via contact of contaminated fomites. Air-borne transmission is not an important means of contracting the virus.
- CAV-1 is shed in saliva, feces, and urine.
- After initial infection, the virus replicates in the tonsils, then spreads to the regional lymph nodes and bloodstream via lymphatics.
- The virus targets hepatocytes and vascular endothelial cells of multiple organs, including the eyes, causing hemorrhage, necrosis, and inflammation of affected organs; corneal edema causes the classic "blue eye." Initially, Kupffer cells within the liver are infected; when cellular lysis occurs, adjacent hepatocytes are damaged.
- The virus replicates in the nucleus of host cells and inclusion bodies are formed. Cellular lysis results in massive viremia and tissue damage; disseminated intravascular coagulation (DIC) can ensue.
- Clinical signs tend to manifest after an initial incubation period of 4–9 days, although some dogs may show no signs of illness.
- Antibody response occurs seven days after infection and limits tissue damage.
- The virus can persist in the renal glomeruli, iris, ciliary body, and cornea.
- Glomerulonephritis can develop 1–2 weeks after acute signs resolve and produce proteinuria and interstitial nephritis, but chronic renal failure has not been described.
- Anterior uveitis and corneal edema may persist and lead to glaucoma.
- Viral shedding in the urine can persist for up to 6–9 months after infection.
- Chronic hepatitis with fibrosis has been described in dogs experimentally infected with CAV-1 that survived acute infection.

Blackwell's Five-Minute Veterinary Consult Clinical Companion: Small Animal Gastrointestinal Diseases,
First Edition. Edited by Jocelyn Mott and Jo Ann Morrison.
© 2019 John Wiley & Sons, Inc. Published 2019 by John Wiley & Sons, Inc.
Companion website: www.fiveminutevet.com/gastrointestinal

Systems Affected

- Hepatobiliary.
- Ophthalmic.
- Respiratory – lungs.
- Hemic/lymphatic/immune – spleen.
- Renal/urologic – kidneys.
- Nervous – brain.

 SIGNALMENT/HISTORY

- Most common in dogs <1 year of age.
- Any dog that is not vaccinated is susceptible.
- No breed or sex predilection.

Risk Factors

- Unvaccinated dogs.
- Dogs having contact with other species capable of shedding the virus (see above).

Historical Findings

- Dogs of <1 year of age with no history of vaccination or unknown vaccination history that present with clinical signs including fever, respiratory, gastrointestinal, and/or hepatic disease.
- Dogs of <1 year of age with corneal edema.

 CLINICAL FEATURES

- Depend on the immunologic status of the dog and the degree of cytotoxic injury.
- Three clinical disease syndromes are recognized.
    - Peracute – initial illness lasts for 24–48 h before circulatory collapse, coma, and death occur. Fever and central nervous system signs predominate.
    - Acute – most commonly observed. Dogs with acute disease either recover or die within a two-week period. High morbidity and mortality rates of 10–30% are reported. Clinical signs can include fever, anorexia, lethargy, weakness, tonsillitis, conjunctivitis, inappetence, lymphadenitis, coughing, tachypnea, hepatomegaly, vomiting, hematemesis, diarrhea, and icterus. Corneal edema is also common. Neurologic signs occur rarely.
    - Chronic – this occurs in dogs with partial immunity. After initial infection, death is ultimately due to hepatic failure in weeks (subacute) or months (chronic).

 DIFFERENTIAL DIAGNOSIS

- Other canine viral diseases – parvovirus, canine distemper, canine herpes virus (neonatal).
- Other infectious hepatopathies – leptospirosis, granulomatous hepatitis.
- Toxic hepatitis.

 DIAGNOSTICS

Complete Blood Count/Biochemistry/Urinalysis

- Complete blood cell count – findings can be variable and can include:
    - Red blood cells – schizocytes, anemia, nucleated red blood cells.

- White blood cells – leukopenia (in early disease), leukocytosis, band neutrophils, toxic changes.
- Platelets – thrombocytopenia.
- Lymphocytes – lymphopenia (initially), lymphocytosis (during recovery).

■ Biochemistry profile – liver enzyme activity is high initially, can decline within 14 days; hypoglycemia and hypalbuminemia reflect hepatic failure and/or vasculitis and endotoxemia; hyponatremia and hypokalemia due to gastrointestinal losses; hyperbilirubinemia if survival past acute infection.

■ Urinalysis – proteinuria (glomerular injury), granular and/or hyaline casts (renal tubular damage), bilirubinuria.

Additional Laboratory Tests

■ Fasting serum ammonia levels if hepatic encephalopathy (HE) is suspected in dogs with neurologic signs.

■ Coagulation profile – to assess for DIC, hepatic failure.

■ Platelet function test may reveal reduced platelet adhesion.

■ Serology for antibodies to CAV-1 – may be negative in acutely infected dogs; recent vaccine history can complicate interpretation of titers; in unvaccinated dogs, a four-fold rise in titers over a 2–3-week period with compatible clinical signs is diagnostic for ICH.

■ Polymerase chain reaction (PCR) – real-time PCR not currently available; conventional PCR is able to differentiate between virulent CAV-1 and vaccine virus, which is CAV-2 in all current vaccines; this is a rapid antemortem test; positive results from urine can be difficult to interpret relative to other sites due to the potential shedding of virus in the urine of asymptomatic dogs. Nasal, rectal or ocular swabs or blood as well as tissue obtained at necropsy can be submitted.

■ Virus isolation – CAV-1 is usually present in quantities sufficient for detection in animals with acute disease. Any body fluid or tissue can be submitted; anterior segment of the eye, kidney, tonsil, and urine are ideal; parenchymal organs may not yield as much unless it is early in the course of infection (first week). This is not offered by many commercial laboratories.

Imaging

■ Abdominal radiographs – normal or enlarged liver, poor detail due to effusion.

■ Abdominal ultrasonography – may identify hepatomegaly with a hypoechoic parenchyma, abdominal effusion, and lymphadenopathy.

Diagnostic Procedures

■ Liver aspiration for cytology – may identify intranuclear hepatocyte inclusions.

■ Liver biopsies – if cytology is not diagnostic, biopsy can be obtained for histopathology and PCR.

■ Necropsy – for postmortem diagnosis.

Pathologic Findings

■ Gross – acute changes include ascites or hemoabdomen, an enlarged liver with a dark or mottled appearance, enlarged and/or edematous lymph nodes, mild splenomegaly, fibrin deposition on many organs, thickened gallbladder wall, renal infarcts. Perivascular necrosis of the liver and other organs, petechial and ecchymotic subserosal hemorrhages, and bloody fluid within the intestinal tract are also commonly observed.

■ Histopathology – findings can be variable based on the clinical syndrome present. Hepatic changes are most characteristic and include centrilobular to panlobular hepatic necrosis and intranuclear inclusion bodies within Kupffer cells and hepatocytes with a mixed inflammatory infiltrate. Fibrosis may be present in dogs with chronic disease. Renal changes can include interstitial nephritis, hemorrhage, and thrombosis. Neurologic findings include spongiosis, neuronal necrosis, hemorrhage, and perivascular cuffing with mononuclear cells. Viral inclusion bodies are present within the endothelial cells of meningeal vessels, cornea, renal glomeruli, and tonsils. Immunohistochemistry can confirm the presence of virus in tissues.

 THERAPEUTICS

Drug(s) of Choice

There are no specific drugs for ICH. Therapy is supportive and can include the following aspects.

- Fluids.
  - Crystalloids – balanced polyionic fluids; avoid lactate if fulminant hepatic failure is present; monitor closely and avoid overhydration due to increased vascular permeability and hypoalbuminemia.
  - Electrolytes – supplementation if necessary; depletion can exacerbate HE.
  - Dextrose – supplement as necessary to maintain normal blood glucose levels.
  - Whole blood or plasma – as needed for coagulopathy; these products are preferred over colloidal support for maintenance of oncotic pressure as colloids are contraindicated in patients with coagulopathies and thrombocytopenia.
- Antiemetics.
  - Ondansetron (0.1–0.2 mg/kg IVq6–12 h or 0.1–1 mg/kg PO q12–24 h).
  - Maropitant (1 mg/kg q24 h SQ).
  - Metoclopramide (0.2–0.5 mg/kg PO or SQ q6–8 h or 0.01–0.02 mg/kg/h CRI).
- Gastroprotectants.
  - Antacids – pantoprazole (0.7–1 mg/kg IV q12–24 h), omeprazole (0.5–1 mg/kg PO q12–24 h).
  - Sucralfate (0.5–1 g PO q8h).
- Antibiotics – ticarcillin (33–50 mg/kg q6–8 h IV) combined with metronidazole (reduce conventional dose to 7.5 mg/kg IV q8–12 h) and a fluoroquinolone (e.g., enrofloxacin 11 mg/kg q12h IV, PO).
- Hepatoprotectants – ursodeoxycholic acid (10–15 mg/kg PO once daily or divided, with food).
- Antioxidants.
  - N-acetylcysteine (140 mg/kg load, then 70 mg/kg q8h).
  - Vitamin E (10 IU/kg/day PO).
  - S-adenosylmethionine (SAMe) – once oral medications are possible (20 mg/kg/day PO).
- Management of HE – see Chapter 114.
- Ocular medications as needed for possible corneal ulceration and/or prevention of glaucoma.

Precautions/Interactions

Make appropriate drug dosage adjustments for severe liver failure, age of patient, and/or protein levels if they are low.

Nursing Care

- Monitor hydration status, electrolytes, albumin levels, packed cell volume/total solids (PCV/TS), acid–base and coagulation status regularly (once to twice daily) as dictated by degree of illness and trends in changes in these parameters.
- Monitor for acute renal failure.

Diet

- There are no specific dietary recommendations for ICH.
- Placement of a feeding tube may be necessary for dogs that will not eat on their own.
- Partial or total parenteral nutrition may be necessary for severely affected dogs that do not tolerate enteral nutrition.

Activity

No specific restrictions.

 ## COMMENTS

Client Education

- There is no evidence that CAV-1 infects humans.
- The current vaccine (since 1980) is an attenuated live vaccine with CAV-2 which provides strong protection against CAV-1.
- Puppies should be vaccinated every 3–4 weeks starting at six weeks of age. The last vaccine should be given NO EARLIER than 16 weeks of age due to the presence of maternal antibody.
- Maternal antibody persists until puppies are 12 weeks of age; this can interfere with immunization and necessitates vaccination up until 16 weeks of age.
- Immunity with the current available vaccine lasts for at least three years, possibly longer.
- If the vaccine is accidentally inhaled, transient tonsillitis and respiratory signs might develop.
- Immunity to natural infection is probably lifelong.

Patient Monitoring

- Monitor fluid, electrolyte, acid–base, and coagulation status to adjust supportive measures.
- Monitor for acute renal failure.

Prevention/Avoidance

- The best way to prevent ICH is through appropriate vaccination practices.
- Proper disinfection of areas that have the potential for outbreaks, e.g., shelters, is important.
- The virus can survive for months at room temperature but is inactivated by disinfectants capable of inactivating canine parvovirus (CPV).
- The prevention of overcrowding and isolation of any sick animals that may carry ICH or any other infectious disease are key.
- Preventing contact between domestic dogs and species which could possibly be shedding the virus, such as coyotes, wolves, and foxes, can help prevent infection.

Possible Complications

- Fulminant hepatic failure.
- Hepatic encephalopathy.
- Septicemia.
- Acute renal failure.
- DIC.
- Glaucoma.
- Chronic hepatitis.

Expected Course and Prognosis

Prognosis depends on the severity of the disease and the immune status of the dog.
- Peracute – poor prognosis; death within 24–48 h.
- Acute – variable; guarded to good prognosis.
- Poor antibody response (titer 1:16–1:50) – chronic hepatitis may develop.
- Good antibody response (titer >1:500 IgG) – complete recovery in 5–7 days is possible.
- Recovered patients – may develop chronic liver or renal disease.

Abbreviations

- CAV = canine adenovirus
- CPV = canine parvovirus
- CRI = constant rate infusion
- DIC = disseminated intravascular coagulation
- HE = hepatic encephalopathy
- ICH = infectious canine hepatitis
- PCR = polymerase chain reaction
- PCV/TS = packed cell volume/total solids
- SAMe = S-adenosylmethionine

See Also

- Coagulopathy of Liver Disease
- Hepatic Encephalopathy
- Hepatic Failure, Acute
- Hepatitis, Chronic
- Hepatopathy, Infectious
- Nutritional Approach to Hepatic Disease

Suggested Reading

Gocke DJ, Preisig R, Morris TQ, et al. Experimental viral hepatitis in the dog: production of persistent disease in partially immune animals. J Clin Invest 1967;46:1506–1517.

Greene CE. Infectious canine hepatitis. In: Greene CE, ed. Infectious Disease of the Dog and Cat, 3rd ed. Philadelphia: Saunders, 2012, pp. 42–47.

Sykes JE. Infectious canine hepatitis. In: Sykes JE, ed. Canine and Feline Infectious Diseases. St Louis: Elsevier Saunders, 2014, pp. 182–186.

Wong M, Woolford L, Hasan NH, Hemmatzadeh F. A Novel recombinant canine adenovirus type 1 detected from acute lethal cases of infectious canine hepatitis. Viral Immunol 2017;30(4):258–263.

Acknowledgments: The author and editors acknowledge the prior contribution of Dr Sharon Center.

Author: Kate Holan DVM, DACVIM

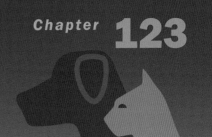

Chapter 123

Hepatitis, Lobular Dissecting

DEFINITION/OVERVIEW

- Lobular dissecting hepatitis (LDH) is a form of chronic hepatitis that has been reported to occur mainly in young dogs which may be siblings or come from the same kennel.
- It is not known whether LDH is just a unique pattern of liver injury or whether it is a distinct disease process.
- Lobular dissecting hepatitis is histologically characterized by bands of myofibrocytes and thin strands of extracellular matrix between individual and small groups of hepatocytes, which cause dissection of the original lobular architecture.

ETIOLOGY/PATHOPHYSIOLOGY

- Lobular dissecting hepatitis is an uncommon form of hepatitis in dogs and in one study represented 7/101 (7%) of cases. Most cases have been reported in the Netherlands and Japan but the disease's distribution is worldwide.
- The etiology of LDH is unknown and it may be a pattern of injury rather than a distinct disease. It probably has more than one cause.
  - It has been postulated that because multiple sometimes unrelated dogs from the same kennel were affected without evidence of exposure to a toxin, an infectious cause of LDH is possible. However, there is no direct evidence to support this and individual dogs can also be affected.
  - Hepatic copper accumulation is an important cause of hepatitis in dogs and some dogs with LDH have been reported to have increased hepatic copper content based on histology. However, it is not known if this was a primary cause of liver injury in these dogs.
  - Other potential causes of LDH include toxins and autoimmunity.
- The pathogenesis of LDH has not been well defined but it is likely that hepatic injury leads to a predominantly sinusoidal infiltrate (usually of mononuclear cells) and activation of hepatic stellate cells. This leads to an increased rate of extracellular matrix deposition and eventually panlobular sinusoidal hepatic fibrosis. Hepatic fibrosis contributes to the development of hepatic portal hypertension, which in turn can cause ascites and the development of acquired portosystemic collateral blood vessels. Portosystemic shunting results in ammonia dysmetabolism and can lead to hepatic encephalopathy. Loss of hepatocytes can lead to hepatic synthetic failure with hypoalbuminemia, which further contributes to the development of ascites.

Systems Affected

- Hepatobiliary.
- Central nervous (with hepatic encephalopathy).

Blackwell's Five-Minute Veterinary Consult Clinical Companion: Small Animal Gastrointestinal Diseases, First Edition. Edited by Jocelyn Mott and Jo Ann Morrison.
© 2019 John Wiley & Sons, Inc. Published 2019 by John Wiley & Sons, Inc.
Companion website: www.fiveminutevet.com/gastrointestinal

SIGNALMENT/HISTORY

- Dogs.
- Breed predilections – uncertain; early cases series were composed of standard poodles and American cocker spaniels but other breeds of dogs can also be affected.
- The median age and range is 20 months (3–72 months).
- No sex predilection has been reported.

Historical Findings

- Because the disease progresses quickly, most dogs have relatively advanced disease at the time of diagnosis. They present with a subacute to chronic illness of 2–6 weeks' duration.
- The following findings are commonly reported (from most to least frequently): abdominal distension, weight loss, anorexia, decreased activity levels, diarrhea, polydipsia, and vomiting.

CLINICAL FEATURES

- The most common physical examination findings are ascites and icterus.
- Patients with hepatic encephalopathy may be ataxic and have altered mentation.

DIFFERENTIAL DIAGNOSIS

Other differential diagnoses for dogs with ascites and icterus include acute liver injury/failure, chronic copper-associated hepatitis, idiopathic chronic hepatitis, granulomatous hepatitis, hepatobiliary neoplasia, pancreatitis, and pancreatic neoplasia.

DIAGNOSTICS

Complete Blood Count/Biochemistry/Urinalysis

- Neutrophilia has been reported in dogs with LDH but its absence does not rule out this disease.
- There are no serum chemistry panel changes that are pathognomonic for LDH. In most dogs, serum liver enzyme activities (ALT, ALP, GGT, and AST) are increased. Other common serum chemistry panel changes include hyperbilirubinemia and hypoalbuminemia.
- Urinalysis may reveal a low specific gravity (in dogs with polyuria) and abnormal bilirubinuria.

Other Laboratory Tests

- Serum pancreas specific lipase concentration can be measured (by Spec cPL) to help rule out pancreatitis as a cause of extrahepatic bile duct obstruction.
- The abdominal effusion produced by portal hypertension is a transudate.
- There is no value in measuring serum bile acid concentrations in animals with hyperbilirubinemia apart from rare cases where hemolysis cannot be excluded.
- Coagulation testing, including measurement of activated partial thromboplastin time and prothrombin time, is helpful to investigate the possibility of a coagulopathy secondary to cholestasis and hepatic insufficiency.

Imaging

- Survey abdominal radiographs – may reveal microhepatica or reduced abdominal detail due to free fluid, and can also help rule out other causes of icterus such as hepatic or pancreatic neoplasia. Normal findings do not rule out LDH.
- Ultrasonography – is helpful to rule out extrahepatic bile duct obstruction and hepatic masses. Changes consistent with LDH include microhepatica and the presence of multiple nodules within the hepatic parenchyma. Secondary changes such as ascites and acquired portosystemic collateral may also be appreciated. It is possible for dogs with LDH to have no significant ultrasound findings.

Liver Biopsy

- Diagnosis of this disease requires biopsy and histopathologic assessment of liver tissue.
- The patient's bleeding risk should be assessed prior to biopsy. This is achieved by performing a platelet count, hematocrit, clotting times, buccal mucosal bleeding time, and ideally measuring fibrinogen.
- Liver biopsy can be performed percutaneously with a Tru-Cut type needle, laparoscopically, or during a laparotomy. Laparoscopic and surgical biopsies are larger and are therefore preferred. Several liver lobes should be sampled.
- Samples of liver should be submitted for bacterial culture and copper quantification. Histologic staining for copper and connective tissue should be requested.

Pathologic Findings

- The liver of affected dogs is usually small and pale, with a smooth surface but occasionally hyperplastic nodules (Figure 123.1).
- Lobular dissecting hepatitis is histologically characterized by bands of myofibrocytes and thin strands of extracellular matrix between individual and small groups of hepatocytes, which cause dissection of the original lobular architecture.
- There is an associated mixed inflammatory cell infiltrate, which is predominantly composed of lymphocytes and plasma cells (Figure 123.2).

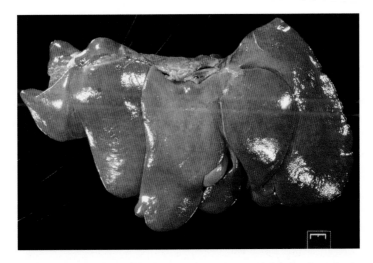

■ **Fig. 123.1.** Liver of eight-month-old male intact Labrador retriever with lobular dissecting hepatitis. The liver is diffusely small (microhepatica) with a coarse surface. The ventral borders of the right and left medial lobes are mildly rounded. Source: Courtesy of Dr Aline Rodrigues Hoffman and Dr Randi Gold, Texas A&M University.

■ **Fig. 123.2.** Liver of a dog with lobular dissecting hepatitis (hematoxylin and eosin). Severe, diffuse, chronic, interstitial and bridging fibrosis with hepatocellular individualization; with mild multifocal, random, chronic, lymphoplasmacytic hepatitis with necrosis. Source: Courtesy of Dr Aline Rodrigues Hoffmann and Dr Randi Gold, Texas A&M University.

 THERAPEUTICS

Drug(s) of Choice

- No drugs have been proven to be effective at preventing the progression of this disease so most treatments are supportive.
- Immunosuppressive/antiinflammatory drugs such as prednisolone (1 mg/kg/day PO) have been used to treat this disease in a small number of dogs and are used by some clinicians to treat idiopathic chronic hepatitis. However, their efficacy for treating LDH is not proven.
- There is a theoretical rationale for the use of cytoprotective agents such as S-adenosylmethionine (20 mg/kg PO q24h), silymarin (combined with phosphatidylcholine; 3–6 mg/kg PO q24h), ursodeoxycholic acid (10–15 mg/kg PO q24h), and vitamin E (10–15 IU/kg PO q24h).
- Vitamin K1 (0.5–1.5 mg/kg SQ q12h for three doses) is indicated for patients with cholestasis.
- The antifibrotic efficacy of colchicine is questionable and this drug is associated with a high rate of adverse effects. Therefore, the author does not recommend its use in dogs.
- Patients with known or suspected gastric ulceration should be treated with omeprazole (0.5–1 mg/kg q12h).
- Dogs with ascites should initially be treated with spironolactone (2 mg/kg PO q24h, increased to 2 mg/kg PO q12h if needed).
- Dogs may require treatment for hepatic encephalopathy.

Precautions/Interactions

Avoid potentially hepatoxic drugs if possible.

Appropriate Health Care

Outpatient, unless the patient is debilitated from dehydration, hypoproteinemia, or cachexia.

Nursing Care

- If the patient is dehydrated, any balanced fluid such as lactated Ringer's solution is adequate.
- Plasma transfusion may be needed for dogs with clinically apparent coagulopathies.

Diet

- Placement of a feeding tube may be necessary for anorectic patients.
- Patients with ascites may benefit from a sodium-restricted diet, such as a commercial "hepatic support" diet.
- Patients with hepatic copper accumulation should be fed a copper-restricted diet, such as a commercial "hepatic support" diet.
- Patients with concurrent hepatic encephalopathy should initially be fed a commercial "hepatic support" diet which is moderately protein restricted and ideally has a nonmeat protein source.

Activity

No restrictions.

Surgical Considerations

No surgical procedures are available for relief of LDH in veterinary patients.

 COMMENTS

Client Education

Clients should be made aware that LDH carries a less favorable prognosis than other forms of chronic hepatitis and usually progresses quickly.

Patient Monitoring

- Hospitalized patients should be monitored closely. Physical examination should be performed at least once a day and it may also be necessary to check serum electrolytes, liver enzyme activities, bilirubin, and albumin on a daily basis.
- Outpatients have varying needs in terms of the frequency of recheck appointments; dogs that are in end-stage liver disease may need weekly examinations whereas stable dogs may only need to be examined every 2–3 months. During these visits, the dogs' general physical condition, e.g., body weight and the presence of ascites, should be checked. Serum biochemistry panels are also helpful.

Possible Complications

Dehydration, malnutrition, portal hypertension, ascites, acquired portosystemic collateral blood vessels, hepatic encephalopathy, hepatic insufficiency, gastrointestinal bleeding, portal vein thrombosis, and hemostatic disorders.

Expected Course and Prognosis

- The prognosis of dogs affected by this disease is generally guarded/poor as many have advanced disease at the time of diagnosis and it rapidly progresses to cirrhosis.
- In one study, the median survival time of seven dogs with LDH was only 0.4 months.

Abbreviations

- ALP = alkaline phosphatase
- ALT = alanine aminotransferase
- AST = aspartate transaminase
- GGT = gamma glutamyl transferase
- LDH = lobular dissecting hepatitis

See Also

- Copper-associated Hepatopathy
- Hepatic Encephalopathy
- Hepatitis, Chronic
- Hypertension, Portal
- Nutritional Approach to Hepatic Diseases

Suggested Reading

Kanemoto H, Sakai M, Sakamoto Y, et al. American Cocker Spaniel chronic hepatitis in Japan. J Vet Intern Med 2013;27:1041–1048.

Poldervaart JH, Favier RP, Penning LC, van den Ingh TS, Rothuizen J. Primary hepatitis in dogs: a retrospective review (2002–2006). J Vet Intern Med 2009;23:72–80.

van den Ingh TS, Rothuizen J. Lobular dissecting hepatitis in juvenile and young adult dogs. J Vet Intern Med 1994;8:217–220.

van den Ingh TSGAM, Cullen JM, Twedt DC et al. Morphological classification of parenchymal disorders of the canine and feline liver: 2. Hepatocellular death, hepatitis and cirrhosis. In: Rothuizen J, Bunch SE, Charles JA, et al, eds. WSAVA Standards for Clinical and Histological Diagnosis of Canine and Feline Liver Disease. St Louis: Elsevier Saunders, 2006, pp. 85–101.

Author: Jonathan A. Lidbury BVMS, MRCVS, PhD, DACVIM, DECVIM-CA

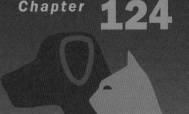

Chapter 124

Hepatitis, Nonspecific, Reactive

DEFINITION/OVERVIEW

- Nonspecific reactive hepatitis (NSRH) is a nonspecific response of the liver to a variety of extrahepatic disease processes or a residual lesion from previous hepatic inflammation.
- It is histologically characterized by an inflammatory infiltrate in portal areas and in the hepatic parenchyma without hepatocellular necrosis.

ETIOLOGY/PATHOPHYSIOLOGY

- This lesion is a relatively common finding in liver tissue collected during necropsy and is likely to be a common cause of increased liver enzyme activities in dogs and cats. However, it is less common to definitively diagnose this condition by antemortem liver biopsy.
- A wide variety of inflammatory/febrile conditions, especially those of the gastrointestinal tract, can cause NSRH. Therefore, the following list is not exhaustive.
  - Gastrointestinal disease – infectious disease (viral, protozoal, fungal, nematodes, bacterial), nonspecific gastroenteritis, inflammatory bowel disease, diet-responsive enteropathy, antibiotic-responsive enteropathy, and neoplasia.
  - Pancreatitis.
  - Febrile illnesses, e.g., arthropod-borne infections.
- The liver may be secondarily affected by extrahepatic disease for a variety of reasons. First, the liver has a unique blood supply of which a large proportion comes via the hepatic portal vein. Consequently, NSRH can be caused by bacteria, cytokines, drugs, toxins, and other substances derived from organs in the splanchnic bed. The liver also contains a relatively large population of resident macrophages (Kupffer cells) and is therefore susceptible to oxidative injury. Whatever the trigger, for acute conditions a predominantly neutrophilic infiltrate is typical, whereas with chronic conditions a mononuclear inflammation is more common. These inflammatory cells may further contribute to tissue injury, e.g., due to oxidative burst activity of neutrophils.

Systems Affected
- Hepatobiliary.
- Gastrointestinal.

SIGNALMENT/HISTORY

- Dog and cat.
- There are no breed predilections.

Blackwell's Five-Minute Veterinary Consult Clinical Companion: Small Animal Gastrointestinal Diseases, First Edition. Edited by Jocelyn Mott and Jo Ann Morrison.
© 2019 John Wiley & Sons, Inc. Published 2019 by John Wiley & Sons, Inc.
Companion website: www.fiveminutevet.com/gastrointestinal

- Dogs and cats of any age can be affected.
- No sex predilection has been reported.

Historical Findings

- Historical findings are due to the underlying disease and are therefore very variable.
- It is possible for patients to have NSRH in the absence of clinical signs.

CLINICAL FINDINGS

- Physical examination findings are due to the underlying disease and are therefore very variable.
- It is possible for patients with NSRH to have no significant findings upon physical examination.

DIFFERENTIAL DIAGNOSIS

A wide range of diseases can cause increased serum liver enzyme activities including chronic hepatitis (dogs), acute liver injury/failure, hepatic lipidosis (cats), hepatobiliary neoplasia, vacuolar hepatopathy, cholangitis, endocrinopathies, and biliary tract disease.

DIAGNOSTICS

Complete Blood Count/Biochemistry/Urinalysis

- Serum liver enzyme activities are often mildly to moderately increased (ALT up to 2 times the upper limit of normal, ALP up to 3–4 times the upper limit of normal).
- Bilirubin and markers of hepatic synthetic capacity (albumin, cholesterol, BUN, and glucose) are not affected by NSRH (although they could be affected by its underlying cause).
- Other laboratory abnormalities are related to the underlying disease process.

Other Laboratory Tests

- Patients with NSRH have normal preprandial and postprandial bile acid concentrations.
- Other laboratory tests may be required to rule out underlying causes of NSHR, e.g., measurement of pancreas specific lipase concentrations to diagnose pancreatitis.
- Other laboratory tests can also help to rule out other causes of increased liver enzyme activities, e.g., measuring serum total T4 +/– free T4 concentrations to rule out hyperthyroidism in a cat.

Imaging

Survey abdominal radiographs and ultrasonography are usually unremarkable but could be useful in documenting abnormalities in organs outside the alimentary tract that may be the cause of NSRH.

Liver Biopsy

- Diagnosis of this disease requires biopsy and histopathological assessment of liver tissue. However, when working up a dog or cat with increased liver enzyme activities, it is important to rule out and address extrahepatic disease before performing liver biopsy. Consequently, it is not common to definitively diagnose this condition antemortem.
- It is more common to make a presumptive diagnosis or to diagnose NSRH as an incidental postmortem finding.

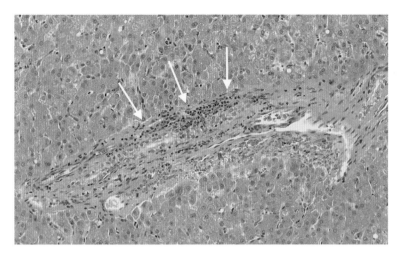

■ **Fig. 124.1.** Liver of a five-year-old female spayed mixed-breed dog with nonspecific reactive hepatitis (hematoxylin and eosin). There is a mild mononuclear cell infiltrate in the portal tract (*arrows*) but no evidence of hepatocyte apoptosis/necrosis or significant fibrosis. This dog had recovered from a previous hepatic injury but had persistently elevated liver enzyme activities. Source: Courtesy of Dr John Cullen, North Carolina State University.

Pathologic Findings

- NSRH is characterized by an inflammatory infiltrate in portal areas and the hepatic parenchyma without hepatocellular necrosis/apoptosis.
- With acute extrahepatic diseases, there is a mild/moderate predominantly neutrophilic infiltrate in the stroma of the portal areas. With chronic extrahepatic disease or with residual hepatic disease, the inflammatory infiltrate is predominantly mononuclear (Figure 124.1).
- It is differentiated from chronic hepatitis by the absence of hepatocellular necrosis/apoptosis and fibrosis.

      # THERAPEUTICS

Drug(s) of Choice

See recommendations for specific underlying conditions.

Precautions/Interactions

See recommendations for specific underlying conditions.

Alternative Drugs

See recommendations for specific underlying conditions.

Appropriate Health Care

Outpatient, unless the patient is debilitated from dehydration, hypoproteinemia, or cachexia.

Nursing Care

See recommendations for underlying condition.

Diet

See dietary recommendations for underlying condition.

Activity

No restrictions.

Surgical Considerations

See recommendations for underlying condition.

 COMMENTS

Client Education

Emphasize that there is usually an underlying cause for NSRH and that this should be identified and addressed.

Patient Monitoring

- See recommendations for specific underlying conditions.
- Serum liver enzyme activities (ALT and ALP) can be periodically rechecked (usually every 2–4 weeks).
- Normalization of serum liver enzyme activities suggests resolution of NSRH.

Prevention/Avoidance

See specific underlying conditions.

Possible Complications

See specific underlying conditions.

Expected Course and Prognosis

The prognosis depends upon the underlying condition; if that is successfully treated, NSRH is also expected to resolve.

Synonyms

- Nonspecific reactive hepatopathy
- Reactive hepatitis
- Reactive hepatopathy

Abbreviations

- ALP = alkaline phosphatase
- ALT = alanine aminotransferase
- BUN = blood urea nitrogen
- NSRH = nonspecific reactive hepatitis
- T4 = thyroxine

Suggested Reading

Cullen JM, Stalker MJ. Liver and biliary system. In: Maxie MG, ed. Jubb, Kennedy and Palmer's Pathology of Domestic Animals, 6th ed. St Louis: Elsevier Saunders, 2015, pp. 258–352.

Johnston SE. Liver – parenchymal disorders. In: Washabau RJ, Day MJ, eds. Canine and Feline Gastroenterology. St Louis: Elsevier Saunders, 2013, pp. 879–904.

van den Ingh TSGAM, Cullen JM, Twedt DC, et al. Morphological classification of parenchymal disorders of the canine and feline liver: 2. Hepatocellular death, hepatitis and cirrhosis. In: Rothuizen J, Bunch SE, Charles JA, et al, eds. WSAVA Standards for Clinical and Histological Diagnosis of Canine and Feline Liver Disease. St Louis: Elsevier Saunders, 2006, pp. 85–101.

Author: Jonathan A. Lidbury BVMS, MRCVS, PhD, DACVIM, DECVIM-CA

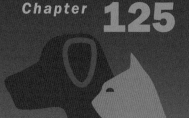

Chapter 125

Hepatitis, Suppurative and Hepatic Abscess

DEFINITION/OVERVIEW

- Bacterial infection involving the hepatobiliary system; variable in size and distribution.
- Distribution and lobular involvement are variable. Forms include multifocal microabscessation; diffuse suppurative cholangitis/cholangiohepatitis; cholecystitis; choledochitis, or discrete focal necrosuppurative lesions; lesions associated with pyogenic bacteria.
- Large abscesses are commonly associated with hepatocellular carcinoma (HCA) in dogs where opportunistic organisms populate necrotic regions.

ETIOLOGY/PATHOPHYSIOLOGY

Enteric aerobes and anaerobes are the most common organisms isolated; therefore, any disorder that alters gut wall permeability can permit these organisms to enter the liver via the portal circulation.

Systems Affected

- Hepatobiliary – impaired function, icterus.
- Renal/urologic – polyuria, polydipsia, proteinuria.

SIGNALMENT/HISTORY

- Dog and cat.
- No breed predilection.
- Hepatic abscesses – most common in old dogs with HCA and necrotic foci; may also be secondary to immunosuppression or diabetes mellitus; in neonates, hepatic abscesses may develop subsequent to omphalitis.
- Suppurative septic cholangitis/cholangiohepatitis: most common in young to middle-aged male cats secondary to retrograde bile duct infection or hematogenous distribution of translocated enteric bacteria via the portal vein.
- Cholestatic disorders (e.g., extrahepatic biliary duct obstruction (EHBDO), gallbladder (GB) mucocele) predispose to enteric bacterial translocation due to reduced delivery of bile acids and secretory IgA (normally regulate the enteric bacterial population and reduce enteric bacterial translocation); cholestasis also impairs canalicular bacterial egress from the liver.

Risk Factors

- Hematogenous infection via the portal vein, hepatic artery, or umbilical vein.
- Biliary tree obstruction, preexisting hepatobiliary or pancreatic disease, and inflammatory bowel disease: predispose to enteric bacterial translocation.

Blackwell's Five-Minute Veterinary Consult Clinical Companion: Small Animal Gastrointestinal Diseases, First Edition. Edited by Jocelyn Mott and Jo Ann Morrison.
© 2019 John Wiley & Sons, Inc. Published 2019 by John Wiley & Sons, Inc.
Companion website: www.fiveminutevet.com/gastrointestinal

- Ascending biliary tract infection.
- Cholecystoenterostomy.
- HCA with necrotic foci.
- Compromised immune responses: diabetes mellitus, glucocorticoid administration, hyper-adrenocorticism, hypothyroidism, chemotherapy, immune-mediated disorders managed with immunosuppressives.
- Recurrent urinary tract infections; pyelonephritis.
- Penetrating wounds.
- Complication of hepatic biopsy or other surgery.

Historical Findings

- Anorexia.
- Lethargy.
- Gastrointestinal signs: vomiting, diarrhea.
- Weight loss.
- Polyuria and polydipsia.
- Trembling.
- Fever.
- May become jaundiced.

 CLINICAL FEATURES

- Fever or hypothermia (cats).
- Abdominal pain: cranial abdomen.
- Dehydration.
- Hepatomegaly: focal, with large abscess or mass.
- Coagulopathy (i.e., petechiae/ecchymoses).
- Effusion: abdominal distension or fluid wave.
- May develop jaundice.
- Endotoxemia: tachycardia, tachypnea, hypotension, hypoglycemic collapse.

 DIFFERENTIAL DIAGNOSIS

- Infectious or necroinflammatory disease – most patients are febrile.
- Hepatic abscess – fever, abdominal pain, and/or hepatomegaly (especially if risk factors).
- Pancreatitis or pancreatic abscess.
- Hepatobiliary neoplasia.
- Hematoma.
- Metastatic neoplasia.
- Biliary cystadenoma.
- Gastrointestinal obstruction or perforation.
- Peritonitis or other intraabdominal abscess.
- Cholecystitis, choledochitis, cholelithiasis.

 DIAGNOSTICS

Complete Blood Count/Biochemistry/Urinalysis

Complete Blood Count
- Neutrophilic leukocytosis with a left shift and toxic white blood cell changes.
- Monocytosis.

- Thrombocytopenia.
- Nonregenerative anemia.

Chemistry
- Variably increased ALT > ALP activity.
- Increased AST.
- Hypoalbuminemia.
- Hyperglobulinemia.
- Inconsistent hyperbilirubinemia.
- Inconsistent hypoglycemia.
- Inconsistent hypocalcemia (cats).
- Features reflecting endotoxemia (gram-negative bacterial infection).

Urinalysis
- Usually normal.
- Bilirubinuria.
- Proteinuria.
- Hematuria (cats).
- Culture may or may not disclose hematogenously dispersed organisms.

Other Laboratory Tests
- Total serum bile acids (TSBA) – may be high; depends on the extent or zonal location of hepatic involvement, cholestasis, or may reflect sepsis-related cholestasis.
- Coagulation tests and red blood cell morphology (schistocytes) – consistent with disseminated intravascular coagulation (DIC).

Imaging
Radiography
- Hepatomegaly, irregular or rounded liver margins: single lobe if isolated abscess, diffuse organomegaly with suppurative cholangiohepatitis or hepatitis.
- Hepatic mass effect if large abscess or abscessed primary hepatic neoplasia.
- Reduced abdominal detail (focal or diffuse) if effusion or peritonitis.
- Gas in hepatic parenchyma or biliary tree (gas-producing bacteria): emphysematous.
- Thoracic radiographs may be consistent with pneumonia, suggestive of chronic bronchitis, or normal.

Abdominal Ultrasonography
- Best noninvasive method of abscess detection (>0.5 cm lesions); solitary, variably echogenic, cavitated lesions with hyperechoic rim.
- Dystrophic tissue mineralization or entrapped gas appears hyperechoic.
- Highly echogenic interface with cavitated mass: may be gas; combination with an abdominal effusion and hyperechoic perilesional effect supports an abscess.
- Multiple masses: some appear complex.
- Miliary abscesses: cannot discern from other parenchymal hepatic disorders.
- Suppurative septic cholangitis/cholangiohepatitis syndrome (CCHS): image not unique from nonsuppurative CCHS.
- Inconsistent regional lymphadenopathy.

Other Diagnostic Procedures
Cytology
- Cytologic evaluations are essential; histologic specimens may not reveal bacterial organisms.
- Samples.

(a)   (b)

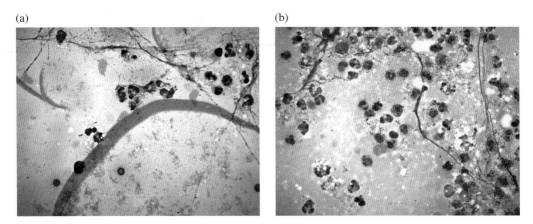

■ **Fig. 125.1.** (a,b) Fine needle aspirate of hepatic abscess in a 13-year-old female spayed Cavalier King Charles spaniel. Degenerate and nondegenerate neutrophils, vacuolated, pigment-laden macrophages, cell debris, and intracellular and extracellular bacterial rods are present.

- Effusion.
- Aspirate hepatic parenchyma and discrete lesions with ultrasound guidance.
- Cholecystocentesis: transhepatic approach, collect liquid bile and biliary debris (particulates).
- Stains: Wright-Giemsa for cytologic bacterial detection; gram stain for morphology.
- Look for bacteria within biliary debris, in white blood cells (Figure 125.1), and for signs of a primary or predisposing disease (e.g., neoplasia, vacuolar hepatopathy (VH) reflecting adrenal disease or diabetes mellitus).

Culture and Sensitivity Testing

- If suppurative or pyogranulomatous reaction (cytology): culture for aerobic and anaerobic bacteria and fungal organisms.
- Blood (aerobic and anaerobic cultures): more likely to be positive if multiple abscesses.
- Polymicrobial infections in ~30% of cases.
- Gram-negative bacteria are most common isolates: *E. coli* (most common); *Klebsiella* spp.; *Pseudomonas* spp., *Enterobacter* spp.; *Proteus* spp.; *Serratia marcescens*; *Citrobacter* spp.
- Gram-positive bacteria: *Enterococcus* spp. (most common); *Staphylococcus* spp.; *Streptococcus* spp.
- Anaerobic organisms are least common isolates: *Clostridium* spp. (most common of these); *Propionibacterium acnes*; *Bacteroides* spp. suggests polymicrobial infection and facilitates growth of other bacteria.

Pathologic Findings

Histopathology is consistent with degenerative neutrophilic inflammation and may or may not identify the inciting cause of an abscess (i.e., necrotic area which later became an abscess, presence of adenoma or neoplasia).

 THERAPEUTICS

- Inpatient if signs of sepsis.
- Intravenous fluids and antibiotics are essential.
- Fluid support: correct dehydration; rectify acid–base and electrolyte disturbances.

- Abscess: drain via hepatic lobectomy during laparotomy or under ultrasound guidance before surgery; in some patients (e.g., endotoxic shock), ultrasound-facilitated drainage is best; after drainage, monitor body temperature, liver enzymes, white blood cell count, and sequentially image with ultrasound (monitor abscess size, focal or diffuse peritonitis); judiciously repeat drainage (may require insertion of an indwelling catheter for short-term continuous drainage); consider alcoholization of abscess after drainage.
- In middle-aged/older dogs, be prepared for liver lobectomy for abscess removal and possible wide-margin resection of an HCA.
- If EHBDO, biliary decompression is essential; antimicrobials must be administered intravenously before surgical manipulations (biliary decompression) to avoid septicemia.

Drug(s) of Choice

- Antibiotics – initially based on cytology and gram stain, then adjusted based on culture and sensitivity results; continue for 2–4 months, perhaps longer.
- Initial treatment – combine antimicrobials to cover possible polymicrobial infection (common aerobic and anaerobic pathogens); common effective empirical combination includes ticarcillin (25–50 mg/kg over 15 min CRI) or amoxicillin clavulanate (13.75–20 mg/kg PO q12h), enrofloxacin (5–10 mg/kg PO, IV, or SQ q24h dogs or cats), and metronidazole (15 mg/kg IV q12h; reduce dose by 50% if hepatic dysfunction or severe cholestasis) or clindamycin (10–16 mg/kg IV or SQ per day; reduce dose if hepatic dysfunction or severe cholestasis to 5 mg/kg IV or SQ per day).
- Choleretics advised if biliary tree involved, but *not until* biliary decompression if EHBDO is present.
- Antioxidants advised.

Precautions/Interactions

- Aminoglycosides – do not use until normal hydration because of potential for renal injury; also, may not penetrate abscess capsule.
- Avoid drugs metabolized or excreted by the liver or those known to be hepatotoxic if compromised liver function; adjust dosages or frequency of drugs if reduced hepatic elimination, cholestasis, or hepatic dysfunction is suspected.

Appropriate Health Care

Treat patient aggressively for sepsis if present.

Diet

Depends upon the presence of inciting causes (i.e., inflammatory bowel disease (IBD), diabetes mellitus, etc.).

Surgical Considerations

- Depends on underlying conditions.
- Hepatic masses or abscesses may be resectable.
- Liver biopsies are warranted to determine a definitive diagnosis and look for possible inciting causes.

Patient Monitoring

- Assess vital signs, labwork abnormalities, and physical condition.
- Sequential ultrasound examinations: monitor for abscess recrudescence or suppurative peritonitis.
- If percutaneous drainage and alcoholization of an abscess is performed, ultrasound monitoring at 24 and 48 hours post procedure, as well as 15, 30, 60, and 120 days, is recommended.

Possible Complications

- DIC.
- Septicemia/endotoxemia.
- Fulminant hepatic failure.
- Septic peritonitis.
- Acute renal failure.

Expected Course and Prognosis

- Favorable prognosis with early detection and aggressive antimicrobial treatment, with judicious surgical intervention.
- Guarded prognosis if concurrent disorders, especially unresectable primary hepatic neoplasia.

Abbreviations

- CCHS = cholangitis/cholangiohepatitis syndrome
- CRI = constant rate infusion
- DIC = disseminated intravascular coagulation
- EHBDO = extrahepatic bile duct obstruction
- GB = gallbladder
- HCA = hepatocellular carcinoma
- IBD = inflammatory bowel disease
- TSBA = total serum bile acids
- VH – vacuolar hepatopathy

See Also

- Bile Duct Obstruction
- Biliary Duct or Gallbladder Rupture and Bile Peritonitis
- Biliary Neoplasia
- Cholangitis/Cholangiohepatitis Syndrome
- Coagulopathy of Liver Disease
- Hepatic Neoplasia, Benign
- Hepatic Neoplasia, Malignant
- Hepatitis, Chronic

Suggested Reading

Center SA. Hepatobiliary infections. In: Greene CA, ed. Infectious Diseases of the Dog and Cat, 4th ed. St Louis: Elsevier, 2010.

Schwarz LA, Penninck DG, Leveille-Webster C. Hepatic abscesses in 13 dogs: a review of the ultrasonographic findings, clinical data, and therapeutic options. Vet Radiol Ultrasound 1998;39:357–365.

Sergeeff JS, Armstrong PJ, Bunch SE. Hepatic abscesses in cats: 14 cases (1985–2002). J Vet Intern Med 2004;18:295–300.

Zatelli A, Bonfanti U, Zini E, et al. Percutaneous drainage and alcoholization of hepatic abscesses in five dogs and a cat. J Am Anim Hosp Assoc 2005;41:34–38.

Acknowledgments: The author and editors acknowledge the prior contribution of Dr Sharon Center.

Author: Ashleigh Seigneur DVM, MVSc, DACVIM

Chapter 126

Hepatopathy, Hyperthyroidism – Feline

DEFINITION/OVERVEIW

The hepatopathy associated with feline hyperthyroidism is a collection of liver-related biochemical abnormalities and ill-defined nonspecific hepatic histopathologic changes observed in cats with untreated or poorly controlled hyperthyroidism.

ETIOLOGY/PATHOPHYSIOLOGY

- Increased serum activities of both ALT and ALP occur in about 75% of cats with hyperthyroidism and more than 90% of cats will have increases in one of these liver enzyme activities. Increases in serum ALP activity may be due in part to increases in the contribution of bone-derived ALP and thus may not entirely be due to hepatopathy. As hepatic biopsy is rarely performed in cats with uncomplicated hyperthyroidism, the prevalence of histologic lesions is not known.
- The pathogenesis of the hepatopathy associated with feline hyperthyroidism has not been well defined. The presence of a lipid-type vacuolar hepatopathy could reflect an early step in the development of feline hepatic lipidosis due to an increased peripheral lipolysis. The hyperammonemia occasionally observed in these cats is probably due to their increased protein catabolism. Other mechanisms that have been speculated but not proven to cause hepatic injury in these patients include hypoxia (the oxygen consumption of the splanchnic bed is increased but blood flow remains constant), congestive cardiac failure in some cats, and direct toxic effects of thyroid hormones on the liver.

Systems Affected

Hepatobiliary.

SIGNALMENT/HISTORY

- Cat.
- No breed predilections.
- Hyperthyroidism is more prevalent in older cats; the median age at diagnosis is 13 years with a range of 4–22 years.
- No sex predilection has been reported.

Blackwell's Five-Minute Veterinary Consult Clinical Companion: Small Animal Gastrointestinal Diseases, First Edition. Edited by Jocelyn Mott and Jo Ann Morrison.
© 2019 John Wiley & Sons, Inc. Published 2019 by John Wiley & Sons, Inc.
Companion website: www.fiveminutevet.com/gastrointestinal

Risk Factors

Various risk factors/putative causes for feline hyperthyroidism have been reported in the literature.

- Mutations of the thyroid-stimulating hormone (TSH) receptor gene.
- Breed – nonpure-bred cats seem to be at increased risk.
- Nutritional factors – canned food, certain flavors of canned food, iodide deficiency or excess soy isoflavanoids.
- Exposure to thyroid disruptors – bisphenol A or polybrominated diphenyl ether flame retardants.

Historical Findings

Historical findings are attributable to hyperthyroidism and include (from most to least common) weight loss, polyphagia, polyuria/polydipsia, increased activity, diarrhea, vomiting, skin changes, respiratory signs, decreased appetite, decreased activity, and weakness.

 # CLINICAL FEATURES

Physical examination findings are attributable to hyperthyroidism and include (from most to least common) palpable thyroid gland, poor body condition, tachycardia, hyperactivity, heart murmur, skin changes, increased rectal temperature, cardiac gallop rhythm, and dehydrated cachexic appearance.

 # DIFFERENTIAL DIAGNOSIS

Differential diagnoses for cats with increased serum liver enzyme activities include cholangitis, feline hepatic lipidosis, hepatobiliary neoplasia, pancreatitis, intestinal disease, diabetes mellitus, toxoplasmosis, and feline infectious peritonitis (FIP).

 # DIAGNOSTICS

Complete Blood Count/Biochemistry/Urinalysis

- Serum liver enzyme activities (ALT, ALP, and AST) are often mildly to moderately increased. Four of nine cats in one study had a serum ALT activity >500 U/L. Cats with hyperthyroidism had lower serum cholesterol and glucose concentration before treatment with iodine-131 than after, but these results were usually still within the respective reference intervals for these tests.
- Cats with hyperthyroidism can also have other abnormalities such as increased serum concentrations of BUN, creatinine, and phosphate, electrolyte abnormalities, erythrocytosis, often with an increased mean cell volume, lymphopenia, and neutrophilia.

Other Laboratory Tests

- Feline hyperthyroidism is diagnosed by elevated total T4 or if total T4 is not elevated and hyperthyroidism still suspected, additional testing such as free T4 by ED, T3 suppression test, thyroid-stimulating response test, thyrotropin-releasing hormone response test, and/or thyroid scintigraphy.
- Cats with hyperthyroidism had significantly higher fasting serum ammonia concentrations than age-matched euthyroid cats and this increase resolved with successful treatment. This may reflect an increased rate of protein catabolism.

■ Preprandial and postprandial serum bile acid concentrations are not increased in cats with hyperthyroidism, indicating preservation of liver function.

Imaging

■ Ultrasonography – in 19 cats with hyperthyroidism, no abnormalities were detected before or after treatment with iodine-131.
■ This indicates that structural changes of the liver are uncommon with hepatopathy associated with feline hyperthyroidism.

Other Factors

■ A presumptive diagnosis of hepatopathy associated with feline hyperthyroidism is made based on the finding of increased serum liver enzyme activities in a cat with hyperthyroidism in the absence of other signs of hepatobiliary disease, especially if these increases resolve when euthyroidism is restored.
■ Liver biopsy is not indicated unless there is evidence to support the presence of another hepatobiliary disease process (e.g., icterus or changes consistent with cholangitis on ultrasound) or if liver enzyme activities fail to improve when the hyperthyroidism is successfully controlled.

Pathologic Findings

■ A number of nonspecific (and possibly incidental) histologic findings have been reported in the liver of cats with hyperthyroidism.
  • Pigment within hepatocytes and aggregates of mixed inflammatory cells can be found in the periportal zones of the liver (Figure 126.1).
  • Areas of lipid type vacuolation can also be seen.
  • Some cats had mild hepatic necrosis and in severe cases, centrilobular lipid-type vacuolar change and portal fibrosis have been observed.

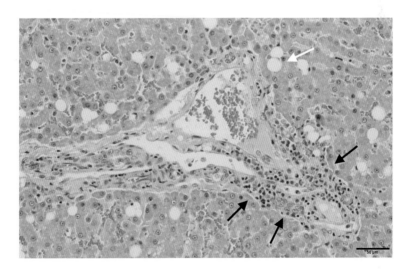

■ **Fig. 126.1.** Liver from a cat with hyperthyroidism (hematoxylin and eosin). Note the periportal histiocytic and lymphoplasmacytic inflammation (*black arrows*) and Ito cell hyperplasia (*white arrow*). Mild lipid-type vacuolation is also present. These are nonspecific changes of unknown importance. Source: Courtesy of Dr Aline Rodrigues Hoffmann and Dr Randi Gold, Texas A&M University.

THERAPEUTICS

Drug(s) of Choice

- This hepatopathy resolves with successful treatment of hyperthyroidism and therefore treatments aimed to protect or specifically treat the liver are not needed.
- Treatment of feline hyperthyroidism.
    - Methimazole (initial dose of 1.25 mg or 2.5 mg per cat PO or TD q12–24 h) is a commonly used treatment for feline hyperthyroidism.
    - Radioactive iodine-131 is another treatment option.
    - Surgical thyroidectomy may be performed, especially in rare cases of malignant thyroid disease.
    - Dietary therapy with iodine-restricted food (e.g., Hill's Y/d® diet).

Precautions/Interactions

- Methimazole can cause a hepatopathy characterized by anorexia and increased serum activities of ALT and/or ALP. This is uncommon (<2% of cats) and resolves with discontinuation of the drug and symptomatic treatment.
- Care should be taken when contemplating thyroidectomy or iodine-131 treatment in azotemic cats as restoration of a euthyroid state can result in worsening of their azotemia.

Appropriate Health Care

Hepatopathy associated with feline hyperthyroidism resolves with successful treatment of hyperthyroidism.

Diet

- Most cats with hyperthyroidism are polyphagic but a minority have a decreased appetite. Nutritional support, possibly including placement of a feeding tube, for these cats is required. Hyperthyroidism is an underlying cause of feline hepatic lipidosis.
- One option for treating feline hyperthyroidism is nutritional management with a low-iodine diet (e.g., Hill's Y/d®).

Activity

No restrictions.

Surgical Considerations

Thyroidectomy is a treatment option for feline hyperthyroidism.

COMMENTS

Client Education

Emphasize that hepatopathy associated with feline hyperthyroidism resolves with successful treatment of hyperthyroidism.

Patient Monitoring

- For cats started on methimazole, it is usual to check a serum total T4 concentration, CBC, and chemistry panel every 2–3 weeks while the dose is gradually escalated until euthyroidism is restored.
- The clinician should pay attention to the cat's serum liver enzyme activities as these should decrease during this time, suggesting resolution of hepatopathy.

Expected Course and Prognosis

The prognosis is excellent/good if euthyroidism is restored.

Abbreviations

- ALP = alkaline phosphatase
- ALT = alanine aminotransferase
- AST = aspartate transaminase
- BUN = blood urea nitrogen
- CBC = complete blood count
- ED = equilibrium dialysis
- FIP = feline infectious peritonitis
- T4 = thyroxine
- TD = transdermal
- TSH = thyroid-stimulating hormone

Suggested Reading

Berent AC, Drobatz KJ, Ziemer L, Johnson VS, Ward CR. Liver function in cats with hyperthyroidism before and after ^{131}I therapy. J Vet Intern Med 2007;21:1217–1223.

Feldman EC, Nelson RW. Feline hyperthyroidism (thyrotoxicosis). In: Feldman ED, Nelson RW, eds. Canine and Feline Endocrinology and Reproduction. Philadelphia: WB Saunders, 2004, pp. 152–215.

Scott-Moncrieff JC. Feline hyperthyroidism. In: Feldman ED, Nelson RW, Reusch CE, Scott-Moncrieff. Canine and Feline Endocrinology. St Louis: Saunders Elsevier, 2015, pp. 136–195.

Author: Jonathan A. Lidbury BVMS, MRCVS, PhD, DACVIM, DECVIM-CA

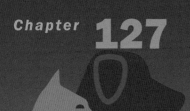

Chapter 127

Hepatopathy, Infectious

DEFINITION/OVERVIEW

Several infectious organisms (i.e., viral, bacterial, fungal, protozoal, and parasitic) can infect the hepatobiliary system as a primary or secondary target, resulting in an infectious hepatopathy.

ETIOLOGY/PATHOPHYSIOLOGY

- Causes of an infectious hepatopathy in the dog and cat include viral (canine adenovirus 1, canine herpesvirus, feline infectious peritonitis, virulent systemic calicivirus), bacterial (*Leptospira* spp., *Escherichia* spp., *Bartonella* spp., *Salmonella* spp., *Mycobacteria* spp., *Clostridium piliforme*), protozoal (coccidiosis, *Toxoplasma* spp., *Cytauxzoon* spp., *Leishmania* spp.), fungal (*Histoplasma* spp., *Cryptococcus* spp., *Aspergillus* spp., *Prototheca* spp., *Coccidioides* spp.), and parasitic (schistosomiasis, *Opisthorchis* spp., *Alaria* spp.).
- The inadvertent parenteral injection of an intranasal *Bordetella bronchiseptica* vaccine in dogs can result in an infectious hepatitis.
- Routes of infection vary based on the infecting organism but agents are transported to the hepatobiliary system through the common bile duct (gastrointestinal tract), hepatic portal vein, or hepatic artery.
- Infectious hepatopathies are not uncommon, with the incidence and geographic distribution varying based on etiology.
- Dogs are more commonly affected.

Systems Affected

- Hepatobiliary – the composition of the inflammatory infiltrate varies based on the etiologic agent. The main hallmark of an infectious hepatitis is random distribution of the lesions. This means that the inflammation and/or necrosis can affect all regions of the lobule (centrilobular, midzonal, and periportal) while toxic lesions are usually restricted to one lobular region. Certain phytotoxins affect the entire lobule.
- Gastrointestinal – weight loss, hyporexia, anorexia, vomiting, diarrhea, melena, hematochezia.
- Hemic/lymphatic/immune – coagulopathies (pro/anticoagulant factor imbalances), disseminated intravascular coagulation (DIC).
- Nervous – hepatic encephalopathy, cerebral edema.
- Renal/urologic – renal tubular damage from specific infectious agents (i.e., leptospirosis) or physiologic vasoconstriction.

Blackwell's Five-Minute Veterinary Consult Clinical Companion: Small Animal Gastrointestinal Diseases, First Edition. Edited by Jocelyn Mott and Jo Ann Morrison.
© 2019 John Wiley & Sons, Inc. Published 2019 by John Wiley & Sons, Inc.
Companion website: www.fiveminutevet.com/gastrointestinal

- Respiratory – acute respiratory distress syndrome, acute lung injury.
- Endocrine/metabolic – systemic inflammatory response syndrome.
- Cardiovascular – systemic hypotension, DIC.
- Skin/exocrine – subcutaneous edema (vasculitis).
- Ophthalmic – uveitis.

 # SIGNALMENT/HISTORY

- There is no apparent sex or breed predisposition collectively; however, specific etiologies affect different species (i.e., leptospirosis) and populations.
- Canine herpes virus affects neonatal puppies.
- Virulent systemic feline calicivirus affects adult cats more severely.
- Leishmaniasis is occasionally encountered in dogs, particularly foxhounds in the United States of America.
- Systemic *Aspergillus terreus* is often seen in German shepherd dogs (possible genetic mucosal immunity defect).

Risk Factors

- Risk factors vary with etiology but general mechanisms include an immunocompromised state, immunosuppressive drug therapy, trauma, extrahepatic infection, sepsis, altered blood flow, and neoplasia.
- Lack of immunization places dogs at risk for infectious canine hepatitis.
- Cattery and shelter populations are at risk for virulent systemic calicivirus.
- Immunocompromised state is a risk factor for *Clostridium piliforme*.
- Risk factors associated with biliary tract infection include advanced age, recent episodes of cholangitis, acute cholecystitis, choledocholithiasis, and obstructive jaundice.

Historical Findings

- Clinical signs are nonspecific and dogs and cats may be asymptomatic.
- Possible clinical signs include inappetence, anorexia, vomiting, diarrhea, lethargy, weight loss, pyrexia, polyuria, polydipsia, bleeding diathesis, abdominal effusion, and icterus.

 # CLINICAL FEATURES

- Physical examination is often unremarkable unless icterus is noted.
- Patients may exhibit abdominal discomfort, poor body condition, and lethargy.
- Evidence of systemic inflammatory response syndrome may be noted.

 # DIFFERENTIAL DIAGNOSIS

Primary Hepatobiliary Disease

- Gallbladder mucocele – distinguished on abdominal ultrasound.
- Hepatic neoplasia (i.e., hepatocellular carcinoma, hepatic lymphoma) – distinguished based on hepatic histology and occasionally cytology (lymphoma).
- Acute hepatitis – distinguished based on hepatic histology.
- Chronic hepatitis – distinguished based on hepatic histology.
- Hepatic lipidosis (cats) – may occur concurrently and can be distinguished on hepatic histology definitively although hepatic cytology often adequate.

Extrahepatic Biliary Disease

- Pancreatitis – distinguished based on abdominal sonogram and serologic testing.
- Hemolysis – distinguished based on complete blood count.
- Gastrointestinal disease – distinguished based on intestinal biopsy and gastrointestinal function testing.
- Right-sided congestive heart failure – distinguished based on echocardiography in cases of hepatic enlargement with abdominal effusion.

 DIAGNOSTICS

Minimum database would include a complete blood count, biochemical panel, and a urinalysis.

Complete Blood Count/Biochemistry/Urinalysis

- Complete blood count results are variable depending on disease severity and systemic involvement. There may be evidence of systemic inflammatory response syndrome >18 000 WBC/µL (dogs), >19 000 WBC/µL (cats) or <5000 WBC/µL if present.
- Serum biochemical panel may demonstrated increased liver enzyme concentrations (ALT, AST, GGT, ALKP) and rarely evidence of synthetic failure (hypocholesterolemia, decreased blood urea nitrogen, hypoglycemia, hypoalbuminemia). Additionally, cholesterol and bilirubin may also be increased particularly if significant extrahepatic biliary obstruction is present.
- Urinalysis may denote bilirubinuria and crystalluria, and assist in determination of hydration status.

Additional Laboratory Tests

- Bile acid testing in an icteric patient may be warranted to confirm hepatic involvement in cases that are equivocal, although this is considered controversial and of questionable value.
- Assessment of coagulation status should be performed particularly prior to any surgical intervention or procedure and should include clotting times (prothrombin time/partial thromboplastin time), platelet count, and buccal mucosal bleeding time. Other tests of coagulation can be utilized (i.e., thromboelastography) if available.
- Serology and polymerase chain reaction (PCR) analysis should be considered in cases with nondiagnostic cytology/histopathology samples and are more reliable than cytology or histology for certain organisms (i.e., leptospirosis, toxoplasmosis, schistosomiasis, histoplasmosis).
- Diagnosis of leptospirosis depends on demonstrating a rise in convalescent titer or PCR detection of leptospiral DNA in blood or urine because the identification of organisms in stained liver specimens is difficult.
- Special stains are needed to identify *Clostridium piliforme* in liver tissue because organisms do not grow in routine bacterial culture media.
- Diagnosis of *Mycobacterium* can be difficult because many are slow-growing, acid-fast organisms which may not be found in tissue sections, and PCR from formalin-fixed tissue may be falsely negative. *Mycobacterium* spp. have been detected by both histologic staining and PCR from formalin-fixed liver specimens from dogs with pyogranulomatous hepatitis.
- Diagnosis of toxoplasmosis can be difficult; while a positive IgM titer indicates active clinical disease, IgG titers may be found in chronic infections and in animals lacking clinical disease.
- Fecal analysis may be indicated for parasitism.

Imaging

- Survey abdominal radiographs are often normal but a large or small liver and abdominal effusion may be observed.
- Abdominal sonogram is recommended for assessment of the hepatobiliary system, to rule out extrahepatobiliary disease, and lesion identification.

Diagnostic Procedures

- Fine needle aspirates of liver should be acquired even in a sonographically normal liver for cytologic evaluation.
- Percutaneous ultrasound-guided cholecystocentesis should be routinely performed and submitted for cytology, aerobic/anaerobic culture and sensitivity.
- Definitive diagnosis in most cases requires laparoscopic or surgical liver biopsy and samples submitted for histopathologic evaluation, aerobic and anaerobic culture and sensitivity, and copper quantification.
- Additional fresh samples of the liver should be saved for atypical bacterial infections such as mycobacteria and *Bartonella*, special stains, and fluorescence *in situ* hybridization.

Pathologic Findings

- The main hallmark of an infectious hepatitis is random distribution of the lesions. This means that the inflammation and/or necrosis can affect all regions of the lobule (centrilobular, midzonal, and periportal) while toxic lesions are usually restricted to one lobular region or in certain phytotoxins (i.e., blue-green algae, toxic mushrooms) the entire lobule. There are exceptions to this rule. A few viral infections will have a centrilobular distribution (i.e., canine infectious hepatitis).
- Virulent systemic calicivirus results in hepatocyte necrosis ranging from focal to extensive necrosis associated with neutrophilic inflammatory foci and intrasinusoidal fibrin deposits.
- No specific histologic lesions are pathognomonic for leptospirosis. Lesions following acute experimental infection in dogs have included mixed perivascular periportal infiltrates of neutrophils, lymphocytes, and plasma cells with mild hepatic lipidosis, hepatocyte dissociation, and intracanalicular bile plugs. Chronic lesions can have lymphocytic inflammation and fibrosis.
- Fungi (*Histoplasma*, *Cryptococcus*, *Coccidioides*, *Aspergillus*, *Prototheca*) and *Mycobacterium* spp. infection in the liver are associated with granulomatous inflammation. Some are visible on hematoxylin and eosin (H&E) stain but often a special stain (Gomori methenamine-silver, periodic acid–Schiff) is required for diagnostic confirmation (Figures 127.1 and 127.2).
- Histologic findings consistent with protozoal infections such as *Toxoplasma* and *Neospora* can be random multifocal areas of necrosis while *Hepatozoon* and *Leishmania* are characterized by a granulomatous hepatitis. All can have phagocytized organisms (zoites, amastigotes) seen within macrophages.
- Acute lesions caused by wandering nematodes and flukes often result in a traumatic hepatitis. Aberrant migration of eggs can provoke an eosinophilic and granulomatous inflammation with fibrosis.

 # THERAPEUTICS

- The treatment for an infectious hepatopathy is organism-specific antimicrobial therapy.
- Antimicrobial choice should be based on the results of culture and sensitivity testing in cases of bacterial infections or known susceptibility in the case of leptosporosis.
- Cases of extrahepatic biliary obstruction, hepatic abscessation, and bacterial cholecystitis may require surgery.
- Supportive care should be provided as indicated.

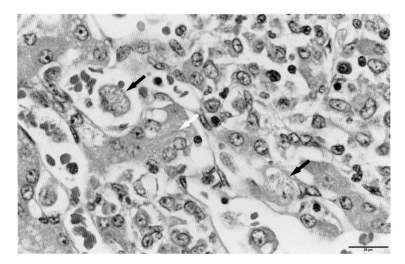

■ **Fig. 127.1.** Liver of an eight-month-old, female spayed, blue merle Australian heeler dog with hepatic histoplasmosis (hematoxylin and eosin, 60×). Granulomatous hepatitis with bile casts (cholestasis; *white arrow*), hepatocellular vacuolation (glycogen type), and intrahistiocytic fungal yeast (*black arrows*). Source: Courtesy of Dr Randi Gold.

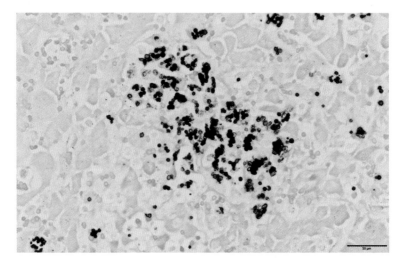

■ **Fig. 127.2.** Liver of an eight-month-old, female, domestic longhair cat with hepatic histoplasmosis (Gomori methenamine-silver, 60×). Special stains demonstrate numerous *Histoplasma capsulatum* yeasts. Source: Courtesy of Dr Randi Gold.

Drug(s) of Choice

- Acute treatment is limited to symptomatic therapy with withholding of antimicrobials until samples for culture and sensitivity testing have been acquired in cases of bacterial infection or a definitive diagnosis determined in other infectious causes, unless signs of systemic inflammatory response syndrome are observed and empirical definitive therapy becomes warranted. Empiric therapy should have activity against opportunistic enteric bacteria. A combination of a beta-lactamase-resistant penicillin, metronidazole (8.0 mg/kg PO q12h), and enrofloxacin (2.5–5 mg/kg PO, IM, or IV q12h) may be beneficial.
- Drugs that have good tissue penetration and are -cidal are preferred.
- Viral hepatopathies are treated symptomatically.

- Doxycycline (5 mg/kg PO q12h) for four weeks is recommended to treat both the active and carrier phases of leptospirosis. Penicillins can be used for the acute phase if doxycycline is not tolerated.
- Diagnosis of *Mycobacterium* spp. in an animal should be reported to local health officials. Six to nine months of a multidrug treatment regimen is advised; single-agent treatment is not advised owing to concern for emergence of resistant strains.
- Coccidioidomycosis and histoplasmosis can be treated successfully with several antifungal medications (itraconazole and fluconazole are preferred to ketoconazole), including the new azoles voriconazole and posaconazole.
- Clindamycin (12.5 mg/kg PO or IM q12h for four weeks) is the drug of choice for the treatment of toxoplasmosis. Dose reduction may be necessary in severe hepatic insufficiency due to extensive hepatic metabolism.
- The most common treatment recommended for canine leishmaniasis is allopurinol (7–20 mg/kg PO q8–24h) given for 3–24 months or indefinitely.

Precautions/Interactions

Pharmacokinetics may be affected by altered liver function.

Alternative Drugs

An extended antimicrobial spectrum may be indicated in cases of multidrug-resistant infection.

Appropriate Health Care

- Vitamin K1 supplementation is indicated if defects in clotting function are identified.
- The role of nutraceutical therapy in infectious hepatopathies is largely theoretical. Choleretics, such as ursodeoxycholic acid and cholestyramine, are of value in promoting bile flow and this is indicated if extrahepatic biliary obstruction is not present.
- Antioxidant therapy with S-adenosyl-L-methionine (SAMe), N-acetylcysteine, or silymarin is believed to restore glutathione levels that are reduced in liver disease, leading to increased oxidative damage and disease potentiation.

Nursing Care

Patients without surgical disease or systemic involvement can be managed as an outpatient.

Diet

- A nutritional plan should be considered at three days of anorexia and instituted by five days.
- Protein restriction is only indicated if there are signs of hepatic encephalopathy.

Activity

Patients should be allowed to limit their own activity.

Surgical Considerations

- Surgical resection is the preferred treatment for hepatic abscesses and immediate surgical intervention may be indicated in cases of a compromised gallbladder or severe extrahepatic biliary obstruction.
- A complete assessment of coagulation status is a requirement for any patient with hepatic disease undergoing a surgical intervention or procedure.
- Placement of an esophageal tube should be considered if the patient is anorexic at time of anesthetic procedure.

COMMENTS

Client Education

- Long-term follow-up is often necessary so patience and a financial commitment are required.
- Recurrence or relapse can occur so vigilance is necessary.
- Etiology-specific chronic (>6 months) therapy may be necessary in some cases (i.e., coccidioidomycosis).

Patient Monitoring

- Patient should be evaluated at two-week intervals initially with lesion assessment/measurement if present and assessment of any drug adverse effects and then every 3–4 weeks chronically until resolution.
- Serologic assessment (titers, polymerase chain reaction) should be serially performed until undetectable on consecutive evaluations.
- Treatment should be continued until organism is undetectable.

Prevention/Avoidance

Prevention and avoidance will vary based on the etiology.

Possible Complications

- Systemic inflammatory response syndrome.
- Sepsis.
- Disseminated intravascular coagulation.
- Acute respiratory distress syndrome.
- Acute lung injury.
- Multiple drug-resistant organisms.

Expected Course and Prognosis

- Generally, infectious hepatitis has a fair prognosis with effective treatment of the etiologic agent.
- Patients that present in acute liver failure have a poor to grave prognosis (see Chapter 115).

Synonyms

Infectious hepatitis or hepatopathy is a general term referring to primary hepatic disease with an infectious etiology that can include various genera.

Abbreviations

- ALKP = alkaline phosphatase
- ALT = alanine aminotransferase
- AST = aspartate aminotransferase
- DIC = disseminated intravascular coagulation
- GGT = gamma-glutamyl transferase
- H&E = hematoxylin and eosin
- PCR = polymerase chain reaction

See Also

- Cholecystitis, Emphysematous
- Cholecystitis and Choledochitis
- Coagulopathy of Liver Disease
- Leptospirosis
- Hepatitis, Infectious (Viral) Canine
- Hepatitis, Suppurative and Hepatic Abscess
- Hepatitis, Granulomatous

Suggested Reading

Center SA. Infectious diseases of the liver in small animals. Merck Veterinary Manual. Available at: www.merckvetmanual.com/digestive-system/hepatic-disease-in-small-animals/infectious-diseases-of-the-liver-in-small-animals

Cullen JM, Stalker MJ. Liver and biliary system. In: Maxie MG, ed. Jubb, Kennedy, and Palmer's Pathology of Domestic Animals, 6th ed. St Louis: Elsevier, 2016, pp. 258–352.

Lawrence YA, Ruaux CG, Nemanic S, Milovancev M. Clinical findings, sonographic features, bacterial isolates, treatment, and outcome of bacterial cholecystitis and bactibilia in dogs: 10 cases (2010–2014). J Am Vet Med Assoc 2015;246 (9):982–989.

Webb CB. Canine inflammatory/infectious hepatic disease. In: Ettinger SJ, ed. Textbook of Veterinary Internal Medicine, 8th ed. St Louis: Saunders, 2016.

Authors: Yuri A. Lawrence DVM, MS, MA, PhD, DACVIM (SAIM), Randi Gold VMD, PhD

Chapter 128

Hepatoportal Microvascular Dysplasia

DEFINITION/OVERVIEW

- Hepatoportal microvascular dysplasia (MVD) describes intrahepatic microscopic vascular malformations with decreased hepatic perfusion in tertiary branches of the portal vein; this is accommodated by the compensatory increase in hepatic arterial perfusion; MVD lacks macroscopic portosystemic shunting but genetically associates with congenital portosystemic vascular anomalies (portosystemic vascular anomaly (PSVA), shunts) as a component of a complex polygenic autosomal syndrome.
- Occurs as an isolated malformation or in association with PSVA.
- Clinically distinct from intrahepatic portal vein atresia which has numerous acquired portosystemic shunts (APSS).
- Histologic features in all conditions that impair hepatopetal portal circulation (forward flow of splanchnic blood toward the liver) overlap; histopathology cannot distinguish between congenital PSVA and MVD.
- Clinicopathologic hallmark – increased total serum bile acid (TSBA) concentrations.
- Coexistence of MVD with PSVA explains: (1) failure of TSBA to normalize after complete PSVA occlusion (some dogs); and (2) inability to fully attenuate PSVA (some dogs).
- MVD diagnosis is confused by inappropriate terminology where "portal vein hypoplasia" has been proposed to describe features of portal venous hypoperfusion. "Hypoplasia" defines lack of development – impossible to ascertain from liver biopsy without clinical features and vascular imaging details; MVD is one of many causes of portal venous hypoperfusion.

ETIOLOGY/PATHOPHYSIOLOGY

- Malformations impairing intrahepatic portal venous perfusion deprive hepatocytes of hepatotropic factors, causing lobular atrophy and impairment of rapid extraction of bile acids from the enterohepatic circulation.
- Compensatory increase in hepatic arterial perfusion (hepatic arterial buffer response) maintains liver viability. Increased hepatic arterial perfusion causes coiling of hepatic arterioles which is recognized histologically as increased numbers of arteriolar profiles in portal tracts and a plexiform pattern of arterioles as they wrap around mildly hyperplastic bile ducts.
- Absence of macroscopic portosystemic shunting directly into the systemic circulation explains the lack of clinical signs and hepatic encephalopathy (HE) in dogs with MVD.
- Finding signs consistent with HE in a dog thought to have MVD strongly indicates PSVA or APSS; in a young dog, APSS develop with portal venous atresia, ductal plate malformation (DPM, with congenital hepatic fibrosis (CHF) phenotype), noncirrhotic portal hypertension (NCPH), or splanchnic portal venous thromboembolism (TE).

Blackwell's Five-Minute Veterinary Consult Clinical Companion: Small Animal Gastrointestinal Diseases,
First Edition. Edited by Jocelyn Mott and Jo Ann Morrison.
© 2019 John Wiley & Sons, Inc. Published 2019 by John Wiley & Sons, Inc.
Companion website: www.fiveminutevet.com/gastrointestinal

- Prevalence of PSVA/MVD trait in small pure-breed dogs: 30–80%, varies with breed.
- Genetic association of MVD and PSVA in kindreds of certain breeds confirms that MVD is most common with a ratio of 10–30:1 for MVD:PSVA.

Systems Affected

- Hepatobiliary – usually asymptomatic.
- Renal/urologic – MVD dogs *do not* develop ammonium biurate crystalluria/urolithiasis; if such is discovered, consider mistaken MVD diagnosis in a dog with PSVA, APSS, rare inborn errors of ammonia detoxification, or uric acid membrane transporter mutations (bulldogs, black Russian terriers, Dalmatians, some cats).

 SIGNALMENT/HISTORY

- Occurs in dogs; not identified in cats.
- Small breeds.
- Commonly affected breeds: Yorkshire terriers, Maltese, Cairn terriers, Tibetan spaniels, Shih tzus, Havanese, miniature schnauzers, pugs, papillons, Norfolk terriers, bichon frise, West Highland white terriers.
- Not identified in large-breed dogs.
- MVD usually tested at 4–6 months of age using paired TSBA tests (collected before and 2 h after a meal); neonatal testing not advised; more reliable results at four months of age or older.

Risk Factors

- Pure-bred small dog breeds and mixes of these breeds.
- Compelling evidence supports inheritance of PSVA/MVD as a complex polygenic autosomal trait in many small pure-breed dogs.
- TSBA >25 μM/L designates phenotype (affected/not affected) PSVA/MVD trait (Cornell University).
- Unaffected parents may produce affected progeny due to suspected polygenic inheritance.

Historical Findings

- Asymptomatic – unremarkable history; occasionally delayed anesthetic recovery or drug intolerance reported.
- Symptomatic dogs represent misclassified diagnosis: PSVA or disorders causing APSS.
- MVD dogs are not hyperbilirubinemic.
- MVD dogs do not develop ascites.
- MVD is often recognized serendipitously during routine screening tests or diagnostic evaluations for unrelated health problems, or during TSBA testing in breeds with high PSVA/MVD prevalence.
- Important to consider and rule out other causes of increased TSBA; concurrent illnesses may complicate TSBA interpretation (e.g., gastrointestinal malabsorption causes low TSBA values).

 CLINICAL FEATURES

- Unremarkable.
- No HE in MVD – if HE identified, suspect PSVA or disorders causing APSS.

- If concurrent inflammatory bowel disease – vomiting, diarrhea, inappetence, increased liver enzymes; may lead to centrilobular and/or portal tract inflammation; most severe in eosinophilic IBD.
- HE, jaundice, or ascites – do not occur.

 # DIFFERENTIAL DIAGNOSIS

- PSVA – suspected in symptomatic young dogs with increased TSBA or HE; however, 20% of PSVA dogs are asymptomatic.
- Symptomatic dogs >2 years of age – may have APSS caused by inflammatory, infiltrative, neoplastic, or toxic hepatopathies; DPM with CHF phenotype; rare PSVA dogs show late-onset signs (e.g., miniature schnauzers; dogs with portoazygous shunts) reflecting small relative shunt fraction; portal vein atresia (true intrahepatic portal hypoplasia) and NCPH (acquired loss of tertiary branches of the intrahepatic portal vein) associate with portal hypertension, ascites, and APSS.
- Histopathologic features of all disorders causing portal hypoperfusion are similar.

 # DIAGNOSTICS

Complete Blood Count/Biochemistry/Urinalysis

- Complete blood cell count – normal.
- Biochemistry – generally unremarkable; hepatic enzyme activities normal (expect high alkaline phosphatase (ALP) in young patients due to bone growth) or cyclically increased alanine aminotransferase (ALT) if coexistent inflammatory bowel disease or degenerative/inflammatory centrilobular lesions; mild hypoglobulinemia or hypoalbuminemia noted in ~50% of young dogs.
- Urinalysis – specific gravity within normal range, no ammonium biurate crystalluria.
- Hyperammonemia is not documented in dogs with MVD, without concurrent portal atresia or PSVA.

Other Laboratory Tests

- TSBA – paired pre- and postprandial TSBA; recommended diagnostic test; values >25 μmol/L confirm abnormal liver function or perfusion; "shunting pattern" common.
- Shunting pattern – postprandial TSBA concentrations 0.5–3-fold > preprandial TSBA occurs with MVD, PSVA, APSS; ~15–20% of dogs and ~10% of cats have fasting > postprandial TSBA; thus, random single TSBA in the "normal range" must be followed up by paired TSBA testing.
- >25 μM/L – cutoff for TSBA in dogs.
- No need to fast patient before meal-provoked enterohepatic bile acid challenge because of physiologic variables influencing fasting values; do not use "fasting" value ranges.
- Important TSBA testing strategy: food-initiated enterohepatic bile acid challenge is essential; verify meal consumption; feed typical size and meal type for that patient.
- Magnitude of TSBA increase: typically lower for MVD vs PSVA but wide overlap in values impairs utility of TSBA as a stand-alone test to distinguish MVD.
- Quantitative abnormal TSBA values cannot discriminate "severity" of MVD between dogs; sequential testing shows vacillating abnormal values (reflect physiologic variables).
- Clearance studies – Cairn terriers with MVD had reduced clearance of an organic anion indicator dye (ICG), confirming reduced liver perfusion; this test has low clinical utility.

- Protein C reflects severity of portosystemic shunting in dogs; is not validated in cats.
- General considerations for laboratory testing:
  - MVD: protein C usually ≥70%.
  - Symptomatic PSVA: protein C <70%.
  - Asymptomatic PSVA protein C may be ≥70%; more common in portoazygous PSVA.

Imaging

- Abdominal radiography – lack microhepatica and renomegaly observed in PSVA.
- Abdominal ultrasonography – no macroscopic shunting vessel; liver size subjectively normal or "slightly" small; experienced operator may suspect portal hypoperfusion that may vary among lobes.
- Mesenteric portovenography – subtle abnormalities of blunted small portal vein branches, protracted contrast "blush" due to truncation of tertiary portal branches that trap contrast. **Caution:** PSVA may be overlooked if radiographic portography only completed in a single recumbent posture.
- Colorectal (CRS) or splenoportal scintigraphy – normal or slightly increased shunt fraction in MVD; rules out macroscopic shunt (PSVA, APSS); CRS may demonstrate irregular liver lobe perfusion in MVD.

Diagnostic Procedures

- Liver biopsy – sample several liver lobes as MVD does not uniformly affect all liver lobes; *avoid sampling* caudate lobe as this receives perfusion from the first portal vein branch; is often the best perfused liver lobe.
- Histologic evaluation – required for definitive diagnosis of portal hypoperfusion but must be considered in context of clinical, clinicopathologic, and imaging details; rules out most acquired hepatobiliary disorders causing increased TSBA except portal TE and NCPH.
- US-guided needle biopsies – may not sample enough tissue for definitive diagnosis; limits sampling to one or two left-sided liver lobes.
- Surgical wedge or laparoscopic liver biopsies – reliably diagnostic if biopsies of several lobes obtained.

Pathologic Findings

Gross

- Normal appearance and liver size.
- Some liver lobes may appear small.

Microscopic

- *Cannot* discriminate MVD, PSVA, NCPH or extrahepatic portal venous TE/occlusion without history, clinical findings, and imaging details.
- Hepatic histopathology reflects portal venous hypoperfusion: (1) lobular atrophy with small hepatocytes and inconsistent close spacing of portal tracts and centrilobular regions without parenchymal collapse, predominantly small-sized portal tracts with an increased proportion of "miniaturized" portal tracts (monads, solitary small bile ducts and dyads, bile duct and hepatic arteriole); (2) increased arteriolar profiles in portal tracts and orphaned arterioles without other portal tract elements in parenchyma – physiologic compensatory increase in arteriolar perfusion likely involves the biliary arterial plexus, arteries are coiled in response to increased pressure and flow with formation of new arterial twigs; (3) lymphatic distension – in portal tracts, adjacent to hepatic veins, and variably, beneath the liver capsule; reflects increased ultralymph formation from arterialized sinusoidal perfusion.

- Unique MVD features: (1) maldevelopment of tertiary portal vein branches – inconsistent perfused portal veins in portal tracts, portal veins may demonstrate dilated, thin-walled unusual appearance, (2) malposition of hepatic venules adjacent to portal triads sharing borders = "fusion complexes"; (3) prominent constriction of the spiral smooth muscle of hepatic venules (influences transhepatic perfusion) suggests physiologic hypertrophy or constriction, perhaps reflecting increased pressure; (4) increased numbers of binucleated hepatocytes (esp. near portal tracts); (5) randomly distributed but mildly disorganized hepatic cords with occasional, irregularly widened sinusoids (random distribution); (6) inconsistent involvement of hepatic lobes: normal, mild to severe.
- Note: liver biopsy in any dog ≤4 months of age demonstrates juvenile portal triads (small).

 THERAPEUTICS

Precautions/Interactions

May observe slow recovery from injectable anesthetics and apparent adverse drug reactions with medications undergoing first-pass hepatic extraction or hepatic metabolism.

Appropriate Health Care

- Asymptomatic – requires no medical interventions except avoidance of drugs dependent on hepatic first-pass extraction, conjugation, metabolism.
- *Do not need*: ursodeoxycholic acid, S-adenosylmethionine (SAMe, unless chronically increased liver enzymes), silibinin (milk thistle) or dietary protein restriction.
- Suspected HE and/or protracted vomiting or diarrhea – hospitalize for supportive care and diagnostic evaluations; these dogs have other disorders that may complicate MVD (hepatic encephalopathy, PSVA, congenital disease, inflammatory bowel disease).
- Rarely, dogs with zone 3 degenerative changes develop a chronic progressive hepatopathy which leads to hepatic dysfunction, portal hypertension, and ascites; diagnosis requires hepatic imaging and liver biopsy; may require management for hepatic insufficiency and ascites; more common in Maltese, Shih tzu, bichon frise, Yorkshire terrier.
- Confirmed MVD associated with nonsuppurative zone 3 inflammation (especially involving eosinophils) and inflammatory bowel disease: usually managed with low-dose dexamethasone (0.05 mg/kg PO q48–72 h, rather than prednisone to avoid mineralocorticoid supplementation which may provoke ascites), hypoallergenic diet (protein restriction if HE) or a hydrolyzed protein diet, and low-dose metronidazole 7.5 mg/kg PO q12h; if low protein C, add mini-dose aspirin 0.5 mg/kg PO q12–24 h or clopidogrel. *Must have liver biopsy* to confirm need for glucocorticoid and anticoagulants.

Diet

- Dogs with MVD do not require a protein-restricted diet.
- Dogs with HE do not have simple MVD; these have complicated illnesses or PSVA.

Activity

Normal activity.

 COMMENTS

Client Education

- MVD cannot be culled from a kindred based on TSBA testing; parents with normal TSBA may produce progeny with MVD or PSVA; examination of TSBA in F1 and F2 progeny is the only method of defining optimal breeding strategy, at present.

- Counsel clients that TSBA values cannot be used to grade severity of MVD.
- TSBA testing should be used to identify MVD in juvenile dogs to avoid future diagnostic confusion, e.g., adult with nonhepatic illnesses.
- Protein C – *should not be used* as a screening test without TSBA. Asymptomatic PSVA may have normal protein C. TSBA are *always* abnormal in PSVA unless testing is inadequate (lack of provocative tolerance test, or compromised enteric fat absorption).

Patient Monitoring

- Asymptomatic dogs – no specific treatment/long-term follow-up; has confirmed normal lifespan, no chronic illness, no progressive hepatic degeneration.
- Repeated TSBA tests are not advised as values remain abnormal and fluctuate due to physiologic variables that clients find difficult to understand.

Prevention/Avoidance

- Specific recommendations to eliminate MVD from a particular genetic line or breed are not possible at present.
- Based on information derived from large pedigrees of multiple dog breeds, simply breeding unaffected parents does not eliminate MVD from a kindred.
- In high-incidence kindreds, remain vigilant for vaguely ill dogs that may have PSVA; surgical exploration can miss PSVA as can portovenography if only a single recumbency is evaluated; CRS can definitively detect hepatofugal blood flow (portosystemic shunting), providing a quick YES/NO test for portosystemic shunting; protein C activity assists in differentiating dogs with PSVA from MVD to advise further expensive imaging but is not definitive as a stand-alone test.

Expected Course and Prognosis

- Most dogs with MVD remain asymptomatic and have a normal lifespan.
- Progressive increase in magnitude of TSBA values with age (juvenile to adult) has been documented in MVD.
- Generally, TSBA tests in MVD dogs are not quantitatively related to histologic severity.
- Dogs with zone 3 degenerative lesions (described above) may develop progressive hepatopathy leading to HE, portal hypertension, APSS, ascites, and rarely portal venous thromboembolism; this is a *rare* syndrome.

Synonyms

- Congenital portal hypoperfusion
- Hepatic microvascular dysplasia
- Microscopic portovascular dysplasia
- Intrahepatic portal venous atresia is not a synonym for MVD
- Portal venous hypoplasia is not a synonym for MVD

Abbreviations

- ALP = alkaline phosphatase
- ALT = alanine aminotransferase
- APSS = acquired portosystemic shunt
- CHF = congenital hepatic fibrosis
- CRS = colorectal scintigraphy
- DPM = ductal plate malformation
- HE = hepatic encephalopathy
- ICG = indocyanine green
- MVD = hepatoportal microvascular dysplasia
- NCPH = noncirrhotic portal hypertension
- PSVA = portosystemic vascular anomaly
- TE = thromboembolism

See Also

- Ductal Plate Malformation (Congenital Hepatic Fibrosis)
- Hepatic Encephalopathy
- Hypertension, Portal
- Nutritional Approach to Hepatic Diseases
- Portosystemic Shunting, Acquired
- Portosystemic Vascular Anomaly, Congenital

Suggested Reading

Allen L, Stobie D, Mauldin GN, Baer KE. Clinicopathological features of dogs with hepatic microvascular dysplasia with and without portosystemic shunts: 42 cases (1991–1996). J Am Vet Med Assoc 1999;214:218–220.

Christiansen JS, Hottinger HA, Allen L, et al. Hepatic microvascular dysplasia in dogs: a retrospective study of 24 cases (1987–1995). J Am Anim Hosp Assoc 2000;36:385–389.

Schermerhorn, T, Center SA, Dykes NL, et al. Characterization of hepatoportal microvascular dysplasia in a kindred of Cairn terriers. J Vet Intern Med 1996;10:219–230.

Toulza O, Center SA, Brooks MB, et al. Protein C deficiency in dogs with liver disease. J Am Vet Med Assoc 2006;229:1761–1771.

Authors: Sean P. McDonough DVM, PhD, DACVP, Sharon A. Center DVM, DACVIM

Chapter 129

Hepatotoxins

DEFINITION/OVERVIEW

- Hepatotoxin refers to endogenous or exogenous substances (drugs, xenobiotics, toxins) that cause hepatocyte injury.
- Direct – ("dose dependent") causes predictable injury.
- Idiosyncratic – ("dose independent" or "type II") causes unpredictable injury.

ETIOLOGY/PATHOPHYSIOLOGY

- The liver is highly susceptible because of its location (i.e., portal blood supply from intestines) and central role in metabolic and detoxification pathways. The liver is most commonly reported organ associated with true adverse drug reactions.
- Mechanisms of damage are direct (active metabolic by-products) or indirect (oxidative processes from free radical metabolites).
- May cause hepatocellular or cytolytic injury (necrosis and apoptosis), cholestasis, immunologic (innocent bystander or hapten-mediated), or mixed histopathologic patterns of injury.
- Susceptibility and severity of injury – depends upon age, species, nutritional status, concurrent drug administration, antecedent disease, antioxidant status, hepatic copper accumulation, hereditary factors, and/or current or prior exposure to the same or similar compounds.

Systems Affected

- Hepatobiliary.
- Nervous – hepatic encephalopathy (HE).
- Renal – proximal tubular necrosis or renal tubular acidosis/Fanconi syndrome; hepatorenal syndrome (rare).

Causes

Any drug, toxin, or xenobiotic may cause hepatotoxicity, with variable severity, in any individual.

Select Drugs (Dogs and Cats Unless Otherwise Noted)

- Acetaminophen.
- Anabolic steroids.
- Amiodarone.
- Azathioprine.
- Cimetadine.
- Diazepam (cats).

Blackwell's Five-Minute Veterinary Consult Clinical Companion: Small Animal Gastrointestinal Diseases, First Edition. Edited by Jocelyn Mott and Jo Ann Morrison.
© 2019 John Wiley & Sons, Inc. Published 2019 by John Wiley & Sons, Inc.
Companion website: www.fiveminutevet.com/gastrointestinal

- Doxycycline.
- Fluconazole.
- Glucosamine-based joint supplements (dogs).
- Griseofulvin (cats).
- Itraconazole.
- Ketoconazole.
- Lomustine (CCNU) (dogs).
- Mebendazole (dogs).
- Methimazole (cats).
- Mitotane (dogs).
- Nonsteroidal antiinflammatory drug (NSAIDs) (dogs).
- Oxibendazole (dogs).
- Phenytoin (dogs).
- Primidone (dogs).
- Phenobarbital (dogs).
- Stanozolol (cats).
- Sulfa drugs (dogs).
- Tetracyclines.
- Thiacetarsamide.
- Trimethoprim-sulfadiazine (dogs).
- Zonisamide.

Environmental Toxins
- *Amanita* mushrooms (amanitin-containing mushrooms).
- Aflatoxins/mycotoxins.
- Blue-green algae (*Cyanobacteria*).
- Chlorinated compounds.
- Cycad (sago palm nuts).
- Heavy metals (Pb, Zn, Mn, Ar, Fe, Cu).
- Phenolic chemicals (especially cats).
- Gossypol from cottonseed.

Endotoxins
- Enteric organisms – *Clostridium perfringens*, gram-negative bacteria.
- Food poisoning – *Staphylococcus*, *E. coli*, *Salmonella*.

Nutritional/Herbal
- *Atractylis gummifera*.
- Black cohosh.
- *Callilepis laureola*.
- Chaparral.
- Comfrey extracts (pyrrolizidine alkaloids).
- Chinese herbal medicines (certain constituents, contents difficult to characterize).
- Germander.
- Greater celandine.
- Green tea extract.
- Lipoic acid (cats).
- Kava kava (dogs).
- Licorice.
- Mistletoe.
- Pennyroyal.

- Senna.
- Usnic acid.
- Valerian.
- Xylitol (dogs).

SIGNALMENT/HISTORY

- Dog and cat.
- Cats have lower endogenous detoxification abilities; are susceptible to glutathione (GSH) depletion; dogs have higher risk for hepatotoxicity to some agents (e.g., acetaminophen, aflatoxins) due to comparatively lower hepatic GSH.
- Siamese cats – some lines have high risk (reduced glucuronide formation).
- Some dog breeds have high risk for selected drug toxicity.
    - Dobermans, Dalmatians, Samoyeds – trimethoprim sulfa.
    - Dobermans – oxibendazole.
    - Labrador retrievers – NSAIDs.
    - Cocker spaniels and German shepherds – phenobarbital.
    - Herding breeds – multidrug resistant (MDR)1 polymorphisms (deranged P-glycoprotein production) affecting various drugs or other pharmacogenetic factors.
- Any age.
- Young animals (<16 weeks of age) – immature hepatic metabolic and excretory pathways, greater exposure and risk for toxin ingestions; less discriminating eating habits.
- Older animals – may have diseases requiring drug therapy that increases risk of toxicity (e.g., cimetidine, phenobarbital, NSAIDs).
- No predominant sex.

Risk Factors

- Some dog breeds seem predisposed to select drug-associated hepatotoxicities.
- Medications influencing hepatic metabolism (enzyme inducers and p450 inhibitors).
- Antecedent hepatic disease.

Historical Findings

- Extremely variable; may see any, all or none of the following.
    - Malaise to moribund.
    - Hyporexia, vomiting, diarrhea, jaundice.
    - Signs may reflect chronic exposure or single acute exposure.
- Detailed history essential – environmental, drug, and past medical history.

CLINICAL FEATURES

- Extremely variable; may see any, all or none of the following.
    - Hypothermic to febrile body temperature, vomiting, diarrhea, weakness.
    - Icterus – overt or progressive (48–96 hours post exposure).
    - Ascites – rare (grave sign).
    - HE or coma.
    - Disseminated intravascular coagulation (DIC) secondary to liver necrosis – hemorrhage, petechiae, ecchymosis.

DIFFERENTIAL DIAGNOSIS

- Infectious disorders affecting liver/biliary tract – leptospirosis, cholecystitis, feline infectious peritonitis (FIP), toxoplasmosis, rickettsial diseases (e.g., Rocky Mountain spotted fever (RMSF), ehrlichiosis).
- Acute necrotizing pancreatitis.
- Traumatic or hypoxic liver injury.
- Hepatic neoplasia.
- Diagnosis of hepatotoxicity requires historic integration of environment, diet, medications, toxin exposure, and temporal relationship(s) of each to the other.

DIAGNOSTICS

Complete Blood Count/Biochemistry/Urinalysis

- Packed cell volume (PCV) and total solids – often normal or high in acute hepatotoxicosis (shock or dehydration).
- Alanine aminotransferase (ALT) reflects cellular membrane damage; this enzyme is often 10–100-fold normal; monitor for subsequent decline over 3–40 days; prognosis not correlated with magnitude of increase. Increased ALT may precede increases in bilirubin and alkaline phosphatase (ALP).
- Aspartate aminotransferase (AST) may reflect more severe injury (mitochondrial) than ALT; also increased in myonecrosis.
- ALP usually continues to rise for days/weeks while ALT falls.
- Creatine kinase (CK) high activity associated with myonecrosis; some hepatotoxins also damage muscle (e.g., feline diazepam toxicity); high AST with normal CK confirms hepatic damage.
- Bilirubin, albumin, blood urea nitrogen (BUN), and glucose are variable.
- Glucosuria and granular casts if proximal renal tubular injury (e.g., carprofen, copper).
- Some toxins suppress hepatic enzyme synthesis, impairing clinical recognition of hepatic injury (e.g., blue-green algae, aflatoxin).

Other Laboratory Tests

- Coagulation profile – prothrombin time (PT), activated partial thromboplastin time (APTT), fibrinogen degradation products (FDP), platelets, and antithrombin (AT) variable; monitor for DIC. Buccal mucosal bleeding time best reflects potential for hemorrhage.
- Low protein C activity – biomarker for blocked protein transcription in aflatoxicosis.
- Paired serum bile acids (SBA) (pre- and post-meal) assess hepatic function if nonicteric.
- Blood ammonia increased with severe hepatic insufficiency.

Imaging

- Abdominal radiography – acute toxicity: normal to large liver; chronic injury: variable liver size.
- Abdominal ultrasonography – variable echogenicity, hepatic size, and margins.

Other Diagnostic Procedures

- Hepatic biopsy – seldom indicated in acute toxicity (excessive risk/unnecessary for diagnosis or treatment); more helpful in confusing chronic hepatic injury; laparoscopic sampling more dependable than core needle biopsy; if performing core needle biopsies, obtain multiple samples from 14–16 gauge biopsy needle.

- Fine needle aspiration helpful to find neoplasia or etiologic agents; many toxins induce hepatocyte lipid vacuolation; variable dysplastic cell morphology in aflatoxin and cycad toxicity.

Pathologic Findings

Variable; depends on toxin's mechanism of injury (i.e., acinar zone of metabolism, product accumulation, vascular injury, and chronicity).

 # THERAPEUTICS

Objectives are to mitigate ongoing damage, support hepatic functions while reparative processes are ongoing, and provide specific antidote(s) when possible.

Drug(s) of Choice

- Electrolyte supplementation – potassium chloride (KCl): must monitor serum potassium.
- Short-acting glucocorticoids for endotoxic shock (prednisolone sodium succinate) – controversial.
- Omeprazole (1 mg/ kg PO q12h dogs and cats) or pantoprazole (1 mg/ kg IV q12–24 h dogs and cats) lessens gastric ulceration/erosion.
- Ampicillin or metronidazole theoretically protect against transmural migration of enteric flora (controversial).
- Antioxidant therapy – crisis intervention: N-acetylcysteine for acute or fulminant hepatic necrosis (140 mg/kg IV load, followed by 70 mg/kg IV q6–8 h; give over 20 min not by constant rate infusion (CRI), dilute in saline, administer with nonpyrogenic 0.25 μm filter – dogs and cats); when patient can accept oral medications and condition stabilizes, change to oral S-adenosylmethionine (SAMe; 20 mg/kg enteric-coated tablet PO q24h, on an empty stomach – dogs and cats); d-alpha-tocopherol acetate (10 IU/kg q24h PO, no evidence of beneficial effect).
- B-complex vitamins – parenteral; cofactors for hepatic metabolism.
- Silybin (active component of silymarin – milk thistle extract) – prefer form complexed with phosphatidylcholine (2–5 mg/kg q24h PO); may augment liver regeneration and provide antioxidant, hepatoprotective, and antifibrotic effects.
- Ursodeoxycholic acid (15 mg/kg/day PO dogs and cats), give with food.
- Taurine supplementation in anorectic cats (obligate taurine bile acid conjugation).

Precautions/Interactions

Avoid known hepatotoxic drugs and those that require or inhibit hepatic metabolism.

Appropriate Health Care

Inpatient; consider referral, as clinically indicated, for intensive hospitalization, supportive measures, and monitoring.

Nursing Care

- Prevention/correction of shock is imperative.
- Fluid therapy – maintain hepatic perfusion to improve oxygenation and toxin removal; administer maintenance requirements – monitor oncotic pressure and ongoing losses/hydration status; administer colloid or plasma if albumin <2.0 g/dL; fluid therapy – avoid lactate-containing fluids in fulminant hepatic failure.
- Colloid administration – plasma preferred (i.e., provides clotting and anticoagulant precursor proteins); may be followed by cautious use of synthetic colloid, if warranted.

- Bleeding tendencies – provide vitamin K1 (0.5–1.5 mg/kg SQ q12–24 h); administer fresh whole blood or fresh frozen plasma as needed. (**Caution:** stored blood products may have high ammonia concentration and cause HE.)
- Nasal oxygen – if compromised peripheral perfusion (hypotension) or pulmonary edema; may improve oxygen delivery to hepatic tissue.
- Oxidant damage likely involved with most hepatotoxins – administer thiol or GSH donors (see below); GSH important for direct conjugation of certain toxins, may facilitate detoxification of some metabolites, enhances antioxidant protection, helps correct cell redox status conferring resistance to apoptosis, promoting cell membrane repair, and cell regeneration.
- Monitor urine output – diuretics if appropriate.
- Hypoglycemia – administer dextrose (2.5–5%) to maintain euglycemia as needed.

Diet

- Protein – normal, unless overt HE.
- Nutritional support – antiemetics (maropitant) lessen nausea/promote appetite. If normal body condition score and acute disease, can wait up to 48 h for patient to voluntarily ingest food. If not eating within 48 h, first preference is nasoesophageal (NE) tube enteral nutrition.
- Energy – strict calculation cumbersome. Initial starting points are body weight kg × 50 (dogs) and body weight kg × 45 (cats), modified based upon size, body condition, and monitoring; begin with 10–20% of calculated requirement and gradually increase to full requirement over 3–5 days. Partial parenteral nutrition (PPN) only if unable to feed enterally (very rare). PPN/total parenteral nutrition (TPN) can cause severe complications – only use if trained and competent with techniques/complications.

Activity

Patients with acute hepatic failure require cage rest while hospitalized.

Surgical Considerations

Exercise caution when placing intravenous catheter or doing fine needle aspirates/biopsies.

 COMMENTS

Aggressive inpatient treatment in a critical care setting recommended to maximize therapeutic options and allow for close monitoring.

Client Education

- Potential for 3–10 days of intensive care.
- Many recover, but postnecrotic cirrhosis, acquired shunting, and chronic hepatitis sometimes develop later.

Patient Monitoring

- Prevent hypothermia.
- Monitor blood glucose, electrolytes, and PCV frequently; fluctuations may occur rapidly in critically ill patients.
- Complete blood count (CBC)/platelet, serum biochemical analyses, coagulation tests – typically monitor q48h or as warranted.
- Monitor urine output.

Prevention/Avoidance

Close scrutiny of environment and future medications.

Possible Complications
- DIC or hemorrhage.
- Gastrointestinal (GI) bleeding from gastric ulceration/erosion.
- Hepatic encephalopathy.
- Progressive hepatic failure.
- Postnecrotic cirrhosis with acquired shunting/ascites.

Expected Course and Prognosis
- Usually need 2–5 days to estimate prognosis.
- Negative indicators: intractable emesis, persistent hematemesis, intolerance to supportive treatments, oliguria, DIC, HE, decline of ALT with increasing bilirubin and/or lowering of serum albumin, decreasing serum cholesterol.
- Positive indicator: ALT declining by 20–30% or more every 48–72 h, with other evidence of improvement
- Postnecrotic cirrhosis – possible in 2–6 months.

Abbreviations
- ALP = alkaline phosphatase
- ALT = alanine aminotransferase
- AST = aspartate aminotransferase
- AT = antithrombin
- BUN = blood urea nitrogen
- CBC = complete blood count
- CCNU = chloroethylcyclohexylnitrosourea
- CK = creatine kinase
- CRI = constant rate infusion
- DIC = disseminated intravascular coagulation
- FDP = fibrin degradation products
- FIP = feline infectious peritonitis
- GGT = gamma-glutamyl transferase
- GI = gastrointestinal
- GSH = glutathione
- HE = hepatic encephalopathy
- KCl = potassium chloride
- MDR1 = multidrug resistance gene 1
- NE = nasoesophageal
- NSAID = nonsteroidal antiinflammatory drug
- PCV = packed cell volume
- PPN = partial parenteral nutrition
- PT = prothrombin time
- PTT = partial thromboplastin time
- RMSF = Rocky Mountain spotted fever
- SBA = serum bile acids
- TPN = total parenteral nutrition

See Also
- Cirrhosis and Fibrosis of the Liver
- Coagulopathy of Liver Disease
- Hepatic Encephalopathy
- Hepatic Failure, Acute

Suggested Reading
Devarbhavi H, Andrade RJ. Drug-induced liver injury due to antimicrobials, central nervous system agents, and nonsteroidal anti-inflammatory drugs, Semin Liver Dis 2014;34:145–161.

Imatoh T, Sai K, Fukazawa C, et al. Association between infection and severe drug adverse reactions: an analysis using data from the Japanese Adverse Drug Event Report datbase, Eur J Clin Pharmacol 2017;73:1643–1653.

Singh D, Cho WC, Upadhyay G. Drug-induced liver toxicity and prevention by herbal antioxidants: an overview, Front Physiol 2016;6: article 363.

Thawley V. Acute liver injury and failure, Vet Clin North Am Small Anim Pract 2017;47:617.

Trepanier LA. Idiosyncratic drug toxicity affecting the liver, skin, and bone marrow in dogs and cats, Vet Clin North Am Small Anim Pract 2013;43:1055.

Author: Michael D. Willard DVM, MS, DACVIM

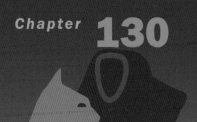
Hypertension, Portal

DEFINITION/OVERVIEW

- Increase in the pressure within the portal system; pressure greater than 13 cmH$_2$O or greater than 10 mmHg.
- Typically described based on location of etiology: prehepatic, hepatic, or posthepatic.

ETIOLOGY/PATHOPHYSIOLOGY

- Conditions that lead to increased portal pressure and resultant effects: ascites, splanchnic congestion, splenic congestion, and increased hepatic resistance.
- Prehepatic etiologies include thrombus/thromboembolic event in abdominal portal vein, trauma, neoplasia, etc.
- Hepatic etiologies include fibrosis, cirrhosis, diffuse hepatic neoplasia, uncorrected congenital portosystemic shunts, etc. Hepatic etiologies may be further divided into presinusoidal, sinusoidal, and postsinusoidal.
- Posthepatic etiologies include pericardial effusion, right auricular hemangiosarcoma, advanced heartworm disease, etc.
- As resultant pressures within the portal circulation increase, a cascade of events may be seen. Increasing pressures may result in the development of:
  - Multiple, acquired portosystemic shunts.
  - Worsening congestion in the splanchnic vasculature, resulting in gastrointestinal edema and potentially hemorrhage and bacterial translocation.
  - Distension and engorgement of the spleen.
  - Development of ascites.
    - Ascites is typically characterized as a modified transudate (protein content between 2.5 and 5.0 g/dL and cell count between 1000 and 7000 cells/µL).
    - Ascites classification (e.g., pure transudate, modified transudate, exudate) will be dependent on etiology for portal hypertension and serum albumin concentrations.

Systems Affected

- Cardiovascular – vascular components (portal, splanchnic circulation, etc.) impacted and potential development of multiple, acquired portosystemic shunts (APSS).
- Gastrointestinal – edema of gastrointestinal (GI) tract with possible complications of hemorrhage, bacterial translocation, erosions and/or ulcers, and malabsorption.
- Hemic/lymphatic/immune – hemorrhagic complications due to physical vascular changes or acquired coagulopathies due to hepatic dysfunction.

Blackwell's Five-Minute Veterinary Consult Clinical Companion: Small Animal Gastrointestinal Diseases,
First Edition. Edited by Jocelyn Mott and Jo Ann Morrison.
© 2019 John Wiley & Sons, Inc. Published 2019 by John Wiley & Sons, Inc.
Companion website: www.fiveminutevet.com/gastrointestinal

- Hepatobiliary – etiology of portal hypertension (PH) commonly arises from intrinsic hepatic disease; hepatobiliary tissue may be negatively impacted by PH due to passive congestion, hypoxic damage, and diversion of portal blood around hepatocytes.
- Musculoskeletal – loss of lean body mass and cachexic state may be seen with advanced disease.
- Nervous – hepatic encephalopathy (HE) may develop and may be associated with a poor prognosis.
- Renal/urologic – hepatorenal syndrome is a rarely described complication of late-stage/severe PH characterized by acute worsening of renal function and may be refractory to treatment.
- Skin – characteristic skin lesions (hepatocutaneous syndrome) may be seen with specific, advanced hepatic disease.

 SIGNALMENT/HISTORY

- Numerous breeds have a predisposition for congenital portosystemic shunts or other congenital hepatic lesions (e.g., Irish wolfhounds, Yorkshire terriers, etc.), and some specific genetic defects in congenital hepatic diseases have been identified (e.g., Bedlington terriers, etc.).
- Congenital lesions are more likely to present clinically in younger patients.
- Congenital disease may or may not result in PH, and some diseases may be more likely to cause PH than others (e.g., arteriovenous malformation).
- Diseases resulting in PH may be seen in any age patient, although acquired diseases are more commonly noted in older patients (e.g., neoplasia, cirrhosis resulting from chronic hepatitis, etc.).
- Dogs are much more likely to be diagnosed with PH compared to cats.

Risk Factors

- Specific genetic defects.
- Breed predispositions.
- Exposure to hepatotoxins (e.g., chemotherapy agents).

Historical Findings

- Clinical onset may be slow/insidious and some patients may present initially with advanced disease.
- Initial signs may be vague and nonspecific: lethargy, inappetence, soft stools or diarrhea, changes in water consumption.
- Astute owners may notice jaundice but icterus is not a consistent finding in PH.
- Depending on the etiology, acute episodes of collapse may be present.

 CLINICAL FEATURES

Note that clinical features will be dependent upon location/etiology of the PH.
- Ascites.
- Hepatomegaly.
- Splenomegaly.
- Abdominal discomfort/pain on palpation.
- Loss of lean body mass/cachexia.
- Muffled heart sounds/poor peripheral pulse quality.

- Icterus.
- Distended jugular veins.
- Bruit (hepatic).
- Melena may be noted on rectal examination.
- Large-volume ascites may impact ability to ambulate or ventilate normally.
- Signs of HE:
  - Blindness.
  - Tremors.
  - Confusion/stupor.
  - Seizures.
  - Behavioral changes
  - Obtunded state.

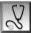

DIFFERENTIAL DIAGNOSIS

- Initial differential list is extensive and depends upon presentation, signalment, history, and physical examination findings.
- If the patient is stable upon presentation, collection of a sample of the peritoneal effusion for fluid analysis, cytology, and potentially culture and sensitivity should be initiated as quickly as possible.
- Classification of the fluid helps guide the development of differential diagnoses and additional testing.
  - Pure transudate – severe hypoalbuminemia consistent with protein-losing enteropathy (PLE) or protein-losing nephropathy (PLN).
  - Exudate – septic peritonitis, neoplasia, etc.
  - Hemorrhage – hemangiosarcoma, congenital or acquired coagulopathy, etc.
  - Urine – uroabdomen.
  - Modified transudate – differential diagnoses for PH as listed above.

DIAGNOSTICS

Complete Blood Count/Biochemistry/Urinalysis

- Complete blood count (CBC) may show thrombocytopenia (with immune-mediated disease or consumption as with thrombosis or disseminated intravascular coagulation (DIC)) or thrombocytosis (as with chronic hemorrhage).
- Stress leukogram with mature neutrophilia may be seen. In cases of bacterial translocation or other infectious complications, evidence of sepsis may be seen on the CBC.
- Red cells may show the following changes.
  - Microcytic, hypochromic anemia consistent with chronic hemorrhage/iron deficiency.
  - Schistocytes due to trauma to the red cell membrane.
  - Strongly regenerative anemia if acute hemorrhage has occurred.
  - Autoagglutination/spherocytosis if immune-mediated disease is present.
- Serum biochemistry may show decreased, normal, or increased hepatic enzyme concentrations, depending on the etiology and chronicity of disease.
- Other signs of hepatic disease include:
  - Hypoglycemia.
  - Hypoalbuminemia.
  - Decreased blood urea nitrogen (BUN).

- Decreased cholesterol.
- Bilirubin may be normal or increased.
- Electrolyte abnormalities may be present and may mimic hypoadrenocorticism (hyponatremia).
- Urinalysis changes include:
  - Hyposthenuria or isosthenuria.
  - Ammonium urate/biurate crystalluria.
  - Bilirubinuria.
  - Proteinuria, primary or secondary (depending on etiology).

Other Laboratory Tests

- Fasting and postprandial bile acid profile – not indicated in the face of clinical icterus.
- Fasting blood ammonia test – may be used to determine presence or extent of HE; sample handling and test requirements result in this test being available on a limited basis.
- Coagulation profile testing – indicated with clinical evidence of coagulopathy and prior to invasive testing (e.g., hepatic biopsy).
- Abdominal effusion testing – as listed above.

Imaging

Radiographs

- Abdominal radiographs may show peritoneal effusion, which may obscure other tissues.
- However, potential findings include hepatomegaly or microhepatica, splenomegaly or other mass effect, organ displacement, abnormal soft tissue calcification, and potentially, evidence of pulmonary metastasis or cardiac disease (depending on technique and patient positioning).

Ultrasonography

- Abdominal ultrasound is more sensitive than radiography for identifying small amounts of peritoneal effusion.
- Ultrasonography allows evaluation of the internal architecture of abdominal organs, blood flow patterns, abdominal lymph nodes, and identification and evaluation of abnormal tissue/mass effect.
- Ultrasound-guided sampling may be considered to obtain fluid samples or collect samples from solid tissues for cytology/histopathology.
- The presence of ascites may increase the risk of hemorrhage from tissues after sample collection.
- Echocardiography – may be indicated in some cases of posthepatic PH.

Computed Tomography (CT) or Magnetic Resonance Imaging (MRI)

- May be useful to elucidate vascular structures and contrast enhancement is recommended to better identify portosystemic shunts.
- Advanced imaging may be helpful in surgical planning, where surgical conditions exist.

Pathologic Findings

- Pathology findings will depend on extent and chronicity of disease and etiology of PH.
- Consistent gross findings may include the following.
  - Presence of peritoneal effusion (transparent to opaque to hemorrhagic).
  - Edematous abdominal viscera (especially GI tract).
  - Liver may appear grossly enlarged and irregular (e.g., neoplasia) or may appear small and fibrotic (e.g., end-stage cirrhosis).
  - Abnormal vasculature may be visible as multiple, tortuous vessels in the case of APSS.
  - Evidence of hemorrhage or thrombosis may be present.

- Histopathology findings will depend upon the etiology of PH. Hepatic histopathology is required for the diagnosis of disease originating from the hepatobiliary system.
- Consistent findings of hepatic parenchyma may include the following.
  - Bile duct proliferation.
  - Arteriolar hyperplasia or tortuosity.
  - Hepatocellular atrophy.
- Certain cases may show chronic hepatitis (inflammatory infiltrates) with bridging fibrosis and cirrhosis or evidence of abnormal copper accumulation.

 THERAPEUTICS

- Many cases may have advanced disease at the time of diagnosis and control of clinical signs, versus reversal of disease or cure, may be the primary objective of treatment.
- Negative prognostic indicators may include evidence of HE or coagulopathy.
- Drug therapy should be tailored to the patient, focused on the etiology/manifestation of PH.
- Primary goals of therapy include:
  - Patient comfort (includes mobilization of ascites).
  - Reduce/prevent signs of HE.
  - Maintain GI health and function.
  - Address, when possible, complicating factors and underlying etiology for PH.

Drug(s) of Choice

Diuretic Support

- Furosemide 2.75–5.5 mg/kg IV (avoid IM injections in patients with decreased lean body mass or in presence of coagulopathy) q12–24 h. Dose may be increased in increments of 2.2 mg/kg until therapeutic effect. Furosemide may waste potassium and serum potassium levels should be maintained so close monitoring is essential. Watch for development of azotemia with aggressive diuretic therapy.
- Spironolactone 1–2 mg/kg PO q12h. Potassium sparing but considered less potent than furosemide; more successful when used in combination with other diuretics.
- Hydrochlorothiazide 0.5–1 mg/kg PO q12h (based on spironolactone content). Available as combination product (in a 1:1 ratio; Aldactazide®) with spironolactone. Helps avoid potassium loss and dehydration that may be seen with furosemide.
- Telmisartan – dosage is uncertain but 1 mg/kg PO q24h has been reported. An angiotensin II receptor blocker which should not be used in pregnant animals. Usage has not been explored in PH but it has been used in cases of proteinuria and congestive heart failure.

Coagulation Support

- Vitamin K 0.5–1 mg/kg SQ q12–24 h or 2.5 mg/kg PO q24h. Oral absorption may be increased with concurrent feeding of a fatty meal.
- Plasma (fresh or fresh frozen) 5–15 mL/kg IV. Monitor for volume overload or potential anaphylactic reaction.

Hepatic Encephalopathy Support

- Lactulose 0.25–0.5 mL/kg PO q6–8h. Adjust dose until 2–3 soft stools per day. Decrease dose if diarrhea. May be given orally or via enema if patients are not able to swallow. Rectal absorption may be increased if cleansing enemas are administered prior to usage.
- Antibiotic therapy – multiple products exist: neomycin 20 mg/kg PO q8–12 h – do not use in cases of GI hemorrhage or azotemia. Metronidazole has also been described for treatment of HE, but consider hepatic metabolism of medication and potential drug interactions.

Thromboembolic Support

- Heparin 150–300 units/kg SQ q6–8 h. Loading dose of 100 units/kg SQ followed by a constant rate infusion (CRI) at 20–50 units/kg/h may be indicated for critically ill patients. Monitoring coagulation status to ensure proper dosage is recommended: antifactor Xa activity or partial thromboplastin time (PTT).
- Low molecular weight heparin – multiple products exist: dalteparin (150 units/kg SQ q8h) or enoxaparin (0.8 mg/kg SQ q8h).
- Aspirin 0.5–1 mg/kg PO q24h. Ideal dose is unknown.
- Clopidogrel 2 mg/kg PO q24h. Usage is not well documented in dogs.

General Hepatic Support

- Glucose – intravenous dextrose support, as needed to effect, in cases of hypoglycemia.
- Hepatoprotectant – multiple products exist. S-adenylmethionine at roughly 18 mg/kg or per package insert.
- Ursodeoxycholic acid 10 mg/kg PO q24h, or divided q12h, with food.

General Gastrointestinal Support

- Antinausea/antiemetics – multiple products exist. Maropitant 1 mg/kg SQ q24h. Refrigerating product may reduce pain upon injection. Caution around drug interactions.
- Antacid therapy – multiple products exist. Omeprazole 0.5–1 mg/kg PO q24h.

Precautions/Interactions

- Hypokalemia – diuretic use and decreased oral intake may lead to hypokalemia, which can precipitate an HE crisis.
- Dehydration – furosemide is a potent diuretic and can lead to dehydration and azotemia. Chronic or multimodal diuretic use may also predispose to dehydration which can lead to acute kidney injury.
- Protein depletion – higher protein content abdominal effusions and poor nutritional state may predispose to total body protein depletion. Changing blood protein levels may also impact medications that are extensively protein bound.

Alternative Drugs

Therapeutic Abdominocentesis

- Consider with refractory ascites, not amenable to medical management and in cases of patient discomfort (impairing mobility or causing respiratory embarrassment).
- Assess protein content of fluid prior to large-volume removal as removal of high-protein fluid may precipitate crisis. Consider IV replacement with colloids (10 mL/kg) to help avoid hypovolemia, circulatory collapse with large fluid shifts.
- Objective assessment of abdominal girth is recommended (e.g., measuring girth with a measuring tape at L2) and patients should have an accurate weight recorded before and after therapeutic abdominocentesis.
- Record the protein content and volume of fluid removed with each tap. Over time, with changes in disease state or complications of repeated taps, additional fluid testing may include packed cell volume (PCV) and total solids (TS), culture and sensitivity, cytology, and cell count.
- Procedure is usually well tolerated and may be performed with the patient standing or gently restrained in lateral recumbency. The use of local anesthesia at the site of abdominocentesis may facilitate the procedure.

Nursing Care

- Will depend upon the etiology and manifestation of PH. Some unique considerations include coagulopathies, HE, respiratory or mobility difficulties with large-volume ascites.

- Monitoring for response to therapy and/or side effects or complications of treatment and medications is warranted.

Diet

- Patients should be encouraged to eat and diet should be high quality and energy dense. Presence of ascites may diminish appetite.
- Sodium restriction may be indicated in cases with ascites.
- Protein restriction may be indicated in HE, but recent literature indicates that previous protein restriction recommendations may have been too severe. See Chapter 132 for more information.

Activity

- Patients with coagulation disorders should be restricted to cage rest/leash walking for elimination only.
- Maintenance of muscle mass should be encouraged with controlled exercise when clinically indicated.
- Restrict activity if large-volume ascites is present although many patients will self-limit activity.

Surgical Considerations

- Surgery may be considered with certain underlying etiologies (e.g., congenital portosystemic shunts) but the majority of cases are managed medically.
- Anesthesia, when indicated, should be performed with caution and with hepatic-sparing protocols (e.g., avoidance or reduced dose of medications with hepatic metabolism/excretion). The presence of large-volume ascites may compromise patient respiration during anesthesia so therapeutic abdominocentesis may be warranted.
- The procedure of abdominocentesis can be accomplished without anesthesia in the vast majority of cases. Analgesic therapy (local anesthesia) may be indicated with some patients but overall, abdominocentesis is very well tolerated.

 COMMENTS

- Portal hypertension represents an end-stage condition for the majority of cases/etiologies.
- Consider likely differentials and patient ability to withstand invasive or aggressive diagnostics.

Client Education

- Identifying the etiology for PH may require extensive and in some cases invasive diagnostics.
- The possibility of a cure or successful reversal of the condition is slim in most cases.
- Monitoring for quality of life indicators as described below.
- While PH is a chronic condition in many cases, acute decompensation may occur with hemorrhagic, thromboembolic, or neurologic manifestations.

Patient Monitoring

- Body condition score and assessment of muscle mass at each veterinary visit.
- Body weight and abdominal girth measurement, especially immediately prior to and following abdominocentesis.
- Abnormalities of bloodwork (e.g., hypoglycemia, hypoalbuminemia, electrolytes) should be monitored frequently as changes may precipitate health complications.
- General indicators of quality of life (e.g., appetite, respiratory effort, energy level, etc.) should be monitored continuously.

Prevention/Avoidance

- Prevention or avoidance is not feasible in most instances.
- Pursue early surgical correction, when clinically indicated, in cases with diseases that may be surgically addressed (e.g., single/congenital portosystemic shunts).
- Avoidance of hepatotoxins (especially chronic exposure).

Possible Complications

- Acute GI hemorrhage.
- Hepatic encephalopathy.
- Renal failure (with hepatorenal syndrome).
- Septicemia/endotoxemia.
- Thromboembolism.

Expected Course and Prognosis

- The prognosis is grave without treatment, regardless of etiology.
- Depending on the etiology, some cases of PH may be associated with a fair prognosis (e.g., idiopathic pericardial effusion). Other cases may demonstrate a temporary response to therapy, but the overall prognosis remains guarded to grave (e.g., cirrhosis, APSS).
- Major determinants of prognosis include etiology and chronicity.
- Decision for humane euthanasia based on deterioration of quality of life may be necessary.

Abbreviations

- APSS = acquired portosystemic shunt
- BUN = blood urea nitrogen
- CBC = complete blood count
- CRI = constant rate infusion
- CT = computed tomography
- DIC = disseminated intravascular coagulation
- GI = gastrointestinal
- HE = hepatic encephalopathy
- MRI = magnetic resonance imaging
- PCV = packed cell volume
- PH = portal hypertension
- PLE = protein-losing enteropathy
- PLN = protein-losing nephropathy
- PTT = partial thromboplastin time
- TS = total solids

See Also

- Arteriovenous Malformation of the Liver
- Cirrhosis and Fibrosis of the Liver
- Coagulopathy of Liver Disease
- Hepatic Encephalopathy
- Hepatitis, Chronic
- Nutritional Approach to Hepatic Disease
- Portosystemic Shunting, Acquired

Suggested Reading

Bunch S, Charles J. Standards for Clinical and Histological Diagnosis of Canine and Feline Liver Diseases. St Louis: Saunders Elsevier, 2006.

Buob S, Johnston AN, Webster CR. Portal hypertension: pathophysiology, diagnosis, and treatment. J Vet Intern Med 2011;25:169–186.

Lidbury JA. Hepatology. Vet Clin North Am Small Anim Pract 2017;47(3):i.

Acknowledgments: The author and editors acknowledge the prior contribution of D. Sharon Center.

Author: Jo Ann Morrison DVM, MS, DACVIM

Chapter 131

Leptospirosis

DEFINITION/OVERVIEW

- Leptospirosis is a worldwide zoonotic disease caused by pathogenic spirochetes.
- More than 150 mammalian species are affected, including dogs, cats, and humans.

ETIOLOGY/PATHOPHYSIOLOGY

- Leptospirosis is caused primarily by the species *Leptospira interrogans* and *L. kirschneri*.
- Major serovars thought to infect dogs in the past were *L. icterohaemorrhagiae* and *canicola*. Other serovars or serogroups have recently been documented in canine leptospirosis in many geographic areas, including *grippotyphosa, pomona, bratislava, australis, sejroe, ballum* and *autumnalis*.
- Cats are commonly exposed to a range of serovars or serogroups, including *icterohaemorrhagiae, canicola, grippotyphosa, pomona, hardjo, autumnalis, ballum* and *bratislava*, but clinical disease has rarely been reported.
- Animals are infected by mucosal or cutaneous contact with infected urine or urine-contaminated soil, water, food or bedding. Transmission may also occur via bite wound inoculation, ingestion of infected tissues or raw meat, and venereal or placental transfer.
- The incubation period for leptospirosis may be relatively short (seven days in experimental studies) and the organisms replicate rapidly within the blood, as early as one day after infection, before invading tissues.
- Acute kidney injury (AKI), manifested by severe interstitial nephritis, tubular epithelial cell necrosis and possibly a mild glomerular component, is a key pathogenetic fact of leptospirosis, leading to acute kidney dysfunction and leptospiruria.
- Moderate-to-severe cholestatic liver disease with concurrent hepatocellular necrosis occurs frequently in leptospirosis.
- Leptospiral pulmonary hemorrhage syndrome (LPHS) has been increasingly recognized in dogs and other species (including humans). LPHS manifests as a severe intraalveolar hemorrhage, in the absence of hemostatic impairment, vasculitis or high spirochetal load in the lung tissues.
- Vasculitis may uncommonly be a feature in leptospirosis.
- AKI with resultant oligoanuria, LPHS, and disseminated intravascular coagulation (DIC) are associated with high mortality rate.
- There is currently no clear association between infecting serovar/serogroup and clinical presentation or outcome.

Blackwell's Five-Minute Veterinary Consult Clinical Companion: Small Animal Gastrointestinal Diseases, First Edition. Edited by Jocelyn Mott and Jo Ann Morrison.
© 2019 John Wiley & Sons, Inc. Published 2019 by John Wiley & Sons, Inc.
Companion website: www.fiveminutevet.com/gastrointestinal

Systems Affected

- Renal – AKI with azotemia or (less commonly) nonazotemic polyuria.
- Hepatobiliary – cholestatic disease, hepatocellular necrosis.
- Respiratory – acute respiratory distress syndrome or LPHS.
- Ophthalmic – anterior uveitis, conjunctivitis, retinal hemorrhage/detachment.
- Gastrointestinal – acute pancreatitis, intestinal intussusception.
- Cardiovascular – myocardial damage with ventricular arrhythmias and troponin elevation.
- Hemic – bleeding tendencies.
- Musculoskeletal – myositis.
- Reproductive – abortions.
- The potential development of residual chronic liver or kidney disease in dogs recovering from leptospirosis has yet to be clarified.

 # SIGNALMENT/HISTORY

- Dog and rarely cat.
- Dogs of any breed, age, and sex may be affected.
- Signalment may change over time, and in recent North American studies, dogs 2–9.9 years old, male dogs, dogs weighing less than 15 pounds, and herding or hound breeds had the highest odds of being diagnosed with leptospirosis.

Risk Factors

- Warm and humid environments (marshy, muddy, irrigated areas) and high rainfall and flooding seasons.
- Water: leptospires survive better in stagnant than flowing water and in neutral or slightly alkaline pH.
- Swimming in or drinking water from outdoor water collections.
- Dense animal populations (kennels/shelter settings) increase chances of urine exposure.
- In developing countries, access to sewage increases exposure chances.
- Living in proximity with urbanized wild animals or rodents.
- High hydrographic density close to dogs' homes.

Historical Findings

- Fever.
- Depression.
- Anorexia.
- Weakness.
- Vomiting.
- Diarrhea.
- Dehydration.
- Icterus.
- Respiratory distress.
- Oliguria, anuria or polyuria-polydipsia.
- Bleeding tendencies.
- Stiffness.
- Sudden death.

CLINICAL FEATURES

- Weakness.
- Dehydration/hypoperfusion.
- Abdominal pain (acute abdomen).
- Jaundice.
- Bleeding tendency (petechiae and ecchymoses, melena, hematuria, hematochezia, hemoptysis).
- Fever or hypothermia.
- Weight loss.
- Respiratory distress.
- Reluctance to move, stiff gait.

DIFFERENTIAL DIAGNOSIS

Dog

- Nephrotoxicoses due to nonsteroidal antiinflammatory drugs, raisins, grapes, ethylene glycol.
- Acute hepatic injury associated with drug reactions, environmental or plant toxin exposure, other infectious agents or, rarely, neoplastic diseases.
- Respiratory distress and hemoptysis due to neoplastic and nonneoplastic pulmonary disease, dirofilariosis, angiostrongylosis, rodenticide toxicity, and cardiogenic pulmonary edema.
- Other infectious diseases including monocytic ehrlichiosis, babesiosis, infectious canine hepatitis, leishmaniosis, borreliosis, bacterial septicemia or pyelonephritis.

Cat

- In addition to the kidney-affecting intoxications listed above for dogs, ornamental house plants such as lilies may cause severe acute kidney failure.

DIAGNOSTICS

Complete Blood Count/Biochemistry/Urinalysis

- Mild-to-moderate, nonregenerative anemia. Hemolysis is not a typical feature of canine leptospirosis, as opposed to cattle.
- Neutrophilic leukocytosis with a left shift. Occasionally, a leukemoid reaction or transient leukopenia may occur.
- Mild-to-moderate thrombocytopenia, not usually associated with bleeding tendency.
- Increased fibrin degradation products and D-dimers, low antithrombin III concentrations and prolonged prothrombin time and partial thromboplastin time (liver disease and/ or DIC).
- Renal azotemia (highly increased concentrations of blood urea nitrogen and creatinine) occurs in over 80% of clinical cases (in half of the cases without concurrent hyperbilirubinemia).
- Hyperbilirubinemia and/or elevated liver enzyme activities (alanine aminotransferase, alkaline phosphatase) occur in approximately 50% of dogs (almost always in combination with azotemia). Liver biochemistry profile is more consistent with a cholestatic hepatopathy.
- Acute azotemia and elevated liver enzyme activity, especially in the presence of thrombocytopenia, should raise suspicion for canine leptospirosis.

- Electrolyte alterations: depend on degree of renal and gastrointestinal dysfunction.
- Hypo (hyper) natremia.
- Hypochloremia.
- Hypokalemia (hyperkalemia with oliguria-anuria).
- Hyper (hypo) phosphatemia.
- Hypoalbuminemia.
- Metabolic acidosis: serum bicarbonate decreased.
- Moderately to markedly elevated activity of serum creatine kinase.
- Decreased urine specific gravity, isosthenuria and rarely hyposthenuria.
- Nonhyperglycemic glycosuria.
- Cylindruria (>1 granular casts/10× objective lens).
- Hematuria (>5 red blood cells/40× objective lens).
- Pyuria (>5 white blood cells/40× objective lens).
- Leptospires are not usually visible under optical microscopy.

Other Laboratory Tests

- Increased concentrations of positive acute-phase proteins (C-reactive protein, haptoglobin).
- Increased troponin I concentration.
- Proteinuria (urine protein to creatinine ratio >0.5).

Serologic Diagnosis

Microscopic Agglutination Test (MAT)
- Currently the diagnostic test of choice.
- MAT cannot accurately predict the infecting serovar or serogroup in more than 50% of dogs.
- In a dog with compatible clinical and laboratory findings, a single titer equal to or higher than 1:800 is strongly suggestive of leptospirosis.
- Single titers may be falsely negative early in the course of infection (sensitivity 30–70%), or falsely positive due to postvaccinal or residual titers from past exposure (specificity 70–100%).
- Seroconversion (at least 1:800) or a four-fold increase in paired titers measured 2–4 weeks apart are highly suggestive of recent infection.

Point-of-Care (POC) Serologic Assays
- Low-cost, rapid serologic assays are currently available as POC tests in the clinical setting. They detect IgM antibodies (immunochromatography) or antibodies for the *lipL32* leptospiral antigen (enzyme-linked immunosorbent assay–- ELISA).
- The diagnostic sensitivity of rapid diagnostic tests, especially those detecting IgM antibodies, is similar to or higher than that of MAT in the early phase of leptospirosis. False-positive results may still occur in dogs vaccinated within the previous three months.

Polymerase Chain Reaction (PCR) Diagnosis
- Conventional and real-time PCR assays may be used to detect the DNA of pathogenic leptospires.
- Sensitivity and specificity have yet to be thoroughly assessed and are subject to interlaboratory and interassay variation.
- Blood and urine should be concurrently tested prior to initiation of antimicrobials in the antemortem setting; a range of tissues (e.g., kidney, liver, spleen) may be tested post mortem.
- May be more sensitive than MAT in the early phase of the infection.

- PCR-positive blood in a dog with clinical and clinicopathologic compatibility implies acute disease. A positive urine may indicate renal shedding in an acutely infected dog or a chronic carrier.
- A negative PCR result does not rule out leptospirosis.
- Prior vaccination does not interfere with the PCR result.
- PCR does not usually identify the implicated serovar.

Culture

- Labor-intensive and technically demanding method.
- Growth of leptospires from various specimens (e.g., blood, urine, kidney, liver) is very slow, requiring up to six months, which minimizes the clinical utility of this diagnostic method.
- More useful as a tool for the genetic typing of the implicated serovars.

Imaging

- Thoracic radiography – caudodorsal or generalized interstitial pattern with patchy alveolar consolidations (may be seen in dogs admitted with respiratory distress). Mild pleural effusion seen occasionally.
- Thoracic computed tomography may better assess the severity of pulmonary lesions.
- Abdominal ultrasonography – hepatomegaly, splenomegaly, renomegaly with pyelectasia and cortical or medullary hyperechogenicity.

Pathologic Findings

- Gross pathology– jaundice and petechial and ecchymotic lesions throughout the body (Figure 131.1). Lungs of dogs with LPHS appear wet and heavy with diffuse, severe pulmonary hemorrhage and alveolar edema. The kidneys of acutely infected dogs may be enlarged, pale or petechiated and infarcted (Figure 131.2).
- Histopathology – interstitial nephritis, acute tubular necrosis, mild hepatic necrosis, neutrophilic periportal hepatitis, and cholestasis are typical features. Lung lesions in LPHS reflect intraalveolar hemorrhage, pneumocyte necrosis, and hyaline membrane formation. Organisms may be visualized with silver stains, immunohistochemistry, or fluorescence *in situ* hybridization.

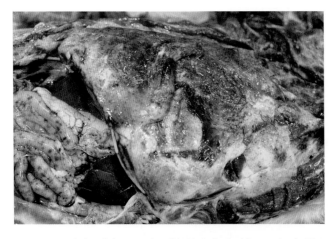

■ **Fig. 131.1.** Gross appearance of the abdomen of a dog that died of leptospirosis. Generalized jaundice and numerous petechial and ecchymotic hemorrhages are seen throughout. Source: Courtesy of V. Psychas, School of Veterinary Medicine, Aristotle University of Thessaloniki, Greece.

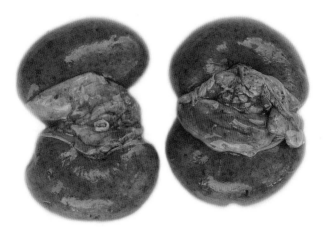

■ **Fig. 131.2.** Gross appearance of kidneys in a dog with leptospirosis. Note the numerous petechial and ecchymotic hemorrhages. Source: Courtesy of V. Psychas, School of Veterinary Medicine, Aristotle University of Thessaloniki, Greece.

 THERAPEUTICS

Primary treatment goals in canine leptospirosis include the elimination of leptospiremia and leptospiruria by means of antimicrobials, supportive care to correct dehydration, electrolyte and acid–base disturbances, and reversal of any multiorgan dysfunction/failure.

Drug(s) of Choice

- Doxycycline, 5 mg/kg PO or IV, q12h, for 2–3 weeks.
- Doxycycline is the drug of choice for the clearance of leptospiremia and leptospiruria.

Alternative Drugs

- Amoxicillin or ampicillin, 20–30 mg/kg IV, q6–8 h, for 2–3 weeks.
- Procaine penicillin G, 25 000–40 000 U/kg, IM, IV, q12h, for 2–3 weeks.
- If the dog is intolerant to oral doxycycline, an alternative drug is given parenterally and oral doxycycline is started as soon as the gastrointestinal upset abates.
- Treatment should be initiated as soon as possible and before the results of the specific diagnostics become available, and ideally should include all dogs in contact with the affected case.

Precautions/Interactions

Penicillins (dogs): adjust doses with renal insufficiency.

Nursing Care

Oliguria/Anuria

- Intravenous administration of isotonic crystalloids (lactated Ringer's or 0.9% NaCl), ideally via a jugular catheter (optimization of fluid therapy, based on central venous pressure measurement).
- Daily fluid volume should match the maintenance requirements (40–60 mL/kg), the current fluid deficits (body weight (kg) × % dehydration = volume (L) to correct) and the ongoing losses (subjectively estimated to 250–500 mL).
- If crystalloids are ineffective, furosemide (1–2 mg/kg, IV, and subsequently 1 mg/kg/h, constant rate infusion) may be considered.

- If furosemide is ineffective within 60 min, mannitol (0.5–1 g/kg, IV (15 min), subsequently 0.25–0.5 g/kg/4–6 h) may be infused.
- Fenoldopam (0.8 μg/kg/min, constant rate infusion) may be superior to dopamine in sustaining urine production.
- Urine output should be closely monitored by means of a closed indwelling catheter and collection bag system. Measuring "ins and outs" may help with fluid replacement rate calculations and may help prevent overhydration in cases of anuria/oliguria.
- Intermittent hemodialysis or continuous renal replacement therapy can be life-saving for many dogs with anuric leptospirosis refractory to medical management.

LPHS
- Oxygen therapy.
- Mechanical ventilation.
- Bronchodilators (e.g., aminophylline, theophylline).
- The potential efficacy of glucocorticoids and/or cyclophosphamide has yet to be evaluated in the dog.

COMMENTS

Client Education
- Inform client of the zoonotic potential from contaminated urine of affected dogs and their environment.
- Strict kennel hygiene and disinfection of premises (kennels or households) with iodine-based or bleach-based disinfectants.

Prevention/Avoidance
Vaccinations
- Inactivated bacterin vaccines containing 2–4 serovars (most commonly *icterohaemorrhagiae*, *canicola*, *grippotyphosa*, *pomona*) are available in most areas of the world.
- For the primary puppy vaccination schedule, vaccinations start at eight weeks of age and then a booster vaccine is administered in 2–4 weeks. For initial adult vaccination, two doses 2–4 weeks apart are recommended.
- Postvaccination immunity is serovar/serogroup specific.
- Current vaccines minimize leptospiremia and leptospiruria and effectively prevent disease.
- Duration of immunity is at least one year; revaccinations are recommended annually.

Exposure Avoidance
- Kennels: strict sanitation to avoid contact with infected urine, control rodents, monitor/remove carrier dogs until treated, isolate infected animals during treatment.
- Activity: limit access to marshy/muddy areas, ponds, areas with stagnant surface water, heavily irrigated pastures, access to wildlife or farm animals.
- Environmental contamination: *Leptospira* shedding in urine is intermittent; *Leptospira* survive in urine in the environment but do not multiply; cells survive until either drying, UV light exposure or freeze-thaw has killed the *Leptospira*.

Expected Course and Prognosis
Favorable if:
- Antimicrobial and supportive treatment is implemented early in the course of the disease.
- No anuria or severe respiratory distress occur.
- Renal replacement therapy is available in case of anuria.

Abbreviations

- AKI = acute kidney injury
- DIC = disseminated intravascular coagulation
- ELISA = enzyme-linked immunosorbent assay
- LPHS = leptospiral pulmonary hemorrhage syndrome
- MAT = microscopic agglutination test
- PCR = polymerase chain reaction
- POC = point of care

Suggested Reading

Fraune CK, Schweighauser A, Francey T. Evaluation of the diagnostic value of serologic microagglutination testing and a polymerase chain reaction assay for diagnosis of acute leptospirosis in dogs in a referral center. J Am Vet Med Assoc 2013;242:1373–1380.

Kohn B, Steinicke K, Arndt G. Pulmonary abnormalities in dogs with leptospirosis. J Vet Intern Med 2010;24:1277–1282.

Miller MD, Annis KM, Lappin MR, et al. Variability in results of the microscopic agglutination test in dogs with clinical leptospirosis and dogs vaccinated against leptospirosis. J Vet Intern Med 2011;25:426–432.

Schuller S, Francey T, Hartmann K, et al. European consensus statement on leptospirosis in dogs and cats. J Small Anim Pract 2015;56:159–179.

Sykes JE, Hartmann K, Lunn KF, et al. 2010 ACVIM small animal consensus statement on leptospirosis: diagnosis, epidemiology, treatment, and prevention. J Vet Intern Med 2011;25:1–13.

Acknowledgments: The authors and editors acknowledge the prior contribution of Dr Patrick L. McDonough.

Author: Mathios E. Mylonakis DVM, PhD

Chapter 132

Nutritional Approach to Hepatobiliary Diseases

The liver is the second largest organ in the body, which is unsurprising considering the number of vital roles it plays in food digestion and metabolism. As the first port of call for nutrient-rich blood draining from the gastrointestinal tract, the liver removes numerous toxins and pathogens, and takes up absorbed nutritional compounds for modification or storage. In addition, the liver performs *de novo* synthesis of nonessential amino acids, stores extra dietary energy in the form of glycogen and fats, and liberates stored energy, in the form of glucose, from glycogen or synthesizes glucose from other stored precursor molecules. Bile, produced in the gallbladder of the liver, is essential for digestion and absorption of fat and thus fat-soluble nutrients such as vitamins A, D, E, and K. Not only does the liver play an integral role in the uptake, storage, and utilization of nutritional compounds, it is also a key location of synthesis in the body, responsible for production of serum proteins, enzymes, glucose, and coagulation factors.

A critical consideration for nutritional therapy of patients with hepatic compromise is the unique ability of the liver to repair from most insults. Not only does the liver have incredible regenerative capacity, it also has a very large functional reserve. However, this means that impaired liver function may not be detected until 70% of functional capacity is lost. That being said, the liver can actually recover both parenchymal tissue and physiologic function even after such significant losses. Optimal nutritional support is therefore crucial to support liver function and recovery in patients with hepatic dysfunction. The underlying cause must be addressed, where possible, by following key nutritional factors, but the liver may also need additional nutritional support to promote healing and return of function.

Common hepatobiliary diseases in companion animals may typically be divided into four categories: inflammatory diseases, storage disorders, circulatory disorders, and neoplasia. The causes and types of liver diseases in dogs and cats are remarkably different. In cats, hepatobiliary disease and acute lipidosis predominate, whereas in dogs, vascular anomalies and chronic hepatitis or cirrhosis are more commonly recognized. Regardless of inciting cause, most animals with diseases affecting the liver present with similar nonspecific syndromes: decreased appetite, lethargy, weight loss, vomiting and/or diarrhea, icterus, ascites, steatorrhea, and hepatic encephalopathy (HE). General recommendations for nutritional approaches to hepatobiliary disease are sufficient for most patients (Table 132.1), although specific nutritional recommendations for the most commonly encountered hepatopathies are covered as well.

OVERALL NUTRITIONAL CONSIDERATIONS

Energy

Adequate energy intake is a critical factor for all patients with liver disease. Sufficient provision of energy ensures that dietary and body stores of protein are spared from catabolism for energy production and are instead utilized to regenerate damaged hepatocytes (Center 1998). This is

Blackwell's Five-Minute Veterinary Consult Clinical Companion: Small Animal Gastrointestinal Diseases, First Edition. Edited by Jocelyn Mott and Jo Ann Morrison.
© 2019 John Wiley & Sons, Inc. Published 2019 by John Wiley & Sons, Inc.
Companion website: www.fiveminutevet.com/gastrointestinal

TABLE 132.1. Recommended components for nutritional support in hepatobiliary disease.

Key nutritional factor	Requirement	Cats (DM basis)	Dogs (DM basis)
Energy density	High	>4200 kcal/kg	>4000 kcal/kg
Protein	Highly digestible	30–40%*	20–25%*
Carbohydrates	Complex>simple	<40%	<60%
Fat	Normal†	20–35%	15–30%

*May need to be reduced in cases with HE.
†May need to be reduced in cases with biliary obstruction and/or cholestasis.
DM, dry matter.

particularly critical in cats, whose protein utilization and thus requirements are higher than in dogs due to the peculiarities of their carnivorous metabolism (Morris 2002). It is important that sufficient nonprotein calories from easily digested sources are provided to maintain, or achieve, an optimal body condition.

Protein

Unrestricted dietary protein, within the normal recommended ranges, is often indicated, in order to provide enough amino acids for recovery and regeneration of affected tissues and to prevent protein-calorie malnutrition to which any animal with liver disease may be considered susceptible. Protein quality and digestibility must also be high, as deamination of amino acids from poor-quality sources and bacterial degradation of undigested amino acids may increase ammonia burden and contribute to or exacerbate HE (Lidbury et al. 2016). Vegetable protein sources, particularly soybean meal (Proot et al. 2009), have been proven to be beneficial in cases with HE and are recommended for many patients with liver disease. In instances where HE persists despite treatment, protein restriction may be necessary.

Carbohydrates and Fats

Provision of ample nonprotein calories is essential to reduce amino acid catabolism for energy, so high levels of carbohydrates, particularly complex carbohydrates, and moderate to high levels of fat are indicated. Calories derived from fat also increase palatability, which is beneficial to optimize voluntary intake. Thus, restriction of fat is not indicated except in cases with biliary obstruction where high levels of fat may stimulate undesired gallbladder contraction and may cause steatorrhea in cases with impaired lipid absorption due to cholestasis (Center 2009). Complex carbohydrates are preferred to simple sugars due to potential compromise of hepatic glucose tolerance in these patients.

Additional Nutritional Considerations (Table 132.2)

Oxidative stress contributes to hepatocyte apoptosis and fibrosis (Vince et al. 2014). Hepatocellular protection may thus be afforded with dietary provision of extra antioxidants, such as *vitamin E*, which attenuates lipid peroxidation and thus mitigates mitochondrial and hepatocellular membrane injury. *Vitamin C* reduces oxidized vitamin E back to its active form and dietary inclusion should be increased to support vitamin E activity. Synthesis of *taurine*, a conditionally essential amino acid in dogs and an essential amino acid in cats, may be decreased in patients with hepatic compromise, impairing bile acid conjugation. Provision of extra dietary taurine also promotes choleresis, which is beneficial in patients without

TABLE 132.2. Recommended components for additional nutritional support in hepatobiliary disease.			
Key nutritional factor	Requirement	Cats (DM basis)	Dogs (DM basis)
Taurine	Increased	≥0.3%	≥0.1%
Zinc	Increased	≥200 mg/kg	≥200 mg/kg
B vitamin complex	Increased	50–100 mg/day	50–100 mg/day
Vitamin E	Increased	≥500 IU/kg	≥400 IU/kg
Vitamin C	Increased	100–200 mg/kg	>100 mg/kg
DM, dry matter.			

biliary obstruction. *Ursodeoxycholic acid* is commonly used in treatment of liver diseases for humans (Buryova et al. 2013) and may also be supplemented for choleretic support at 15–20 mg/kg/day in patients without obstructive cholestasis. Dietary *zinc* is beneficial in reducing copper absorption in patients with copper hepatotoxicity and also has antifibrotic and hepatoprotective properties. *Water-soluble B vitamins* are stored within the liver and reduced levels may be present in patients with hepatic disease (Center 1998; Reed et al. 2007). Supplementation with nutraceuticals *S-adenosylmethionine* (SAMe), *polyenylphosphatidylcholine* (PEP) and *silymarin* or *silybin*, naturally occurring compounds with antioxidant and hepatoregenerative effects, may also be beneficial to suppress free radical damage, conserve protective glutathione concentrations, and mitigate hepatocellular fibrosis (Au et al. 2013; Mosallenejad et al. 2012). SAMe may be dosed at 20 mg/kg/day for both dogs and cats, PEP at 25 mg/kg/day for both dogs and cats, and silymarin at 40–50 mg/kg/day.

General Feeding Recommendations

All patients with liver disease benefit from multiple small meals spaced over the course of the day. This is especially relevant for patients with, or at high risk of developing, HE. If voluntary intake is insufficient, placement of a tube for assisted enteral nutritional support is indicated. Placement of a nasoesophageal tube may be required if the patient is unfit for anesthesia or only very short-term (3–5 days) support is anticipated. Nasoesophageal tubes are well tolerated in the short term by many patients, but only liquid diets may be provided due to the small luminal diameter of the tube. Longer term support may be provided through use of an esophagostomy or gastrostomy (surgically or percutaneously placed) tube, which are typically well tolerated both in hospital and after discharge, and allow administration of homogenized canned diets (Yam and Cave 2003).

Key Points

- Small frequent meals.
- High energy density.
- Highly digestible, high-quality protein source.
- Supplementation with arginine and taurine if required.
- Antioxidant and antiinflammatory support.
- If HE present: increase carbohydrates, supplement with soluble fiber +/– lactulose, vegetable protein.
- If biliary obstruction present: decrease fat.

INFLAMMATORY DISEASES

Hepatitis represents one of if not the most commonly recognized liver diseases in companion animals (Edwards 2004; Watson 2004). In cats, the inflammation is more centered on the biliary tree, and cholangiohepatitis is the most frequently diagnosed (Edwards 2004). In dogs, chronic hepatitis or cirrhosis are most commonly recognized (Watson 2004).

Cholangiohepatitis

In cats, infection with enteric bacteria, particularly *Escherichia coli*, thought to ascend from the common entrance of the bile and pancreatic ducts at the major duodenal papilla in the duodenum, is the most common cause of acute (neutrophilic) cholangiohepatitis (Cox 2006). Concurrent cholecystitis, pancreatitis, and inflammatory bowel disease are common. Chronic (mostly lymphocytic) cholangiohepatitis is also recognized in cats, either due to primary immunologic mechanisms or as a sequel to unresolved neutrophilic cholangitis, but is less common. Regardless of the etiology, cholangitis often leads to cholestasis with biliary sludge or even inspissated bile which may partially or completely obstruct biliary drainage (Box 132.1).

BOX 132.1. Cholestasis

Cholestasis frequently occurs in patients with inflammatory liver disease either due to extra- or intraluminal biliary obstruction, deficiency of choleretic factors, inspissation of bile contents within the gallbladder or a combination of the above. Clinically, this may be indicated by steatorrhea due to lipid malabsorption, and serum biochemistry may reveal hypercholesterolemia. Nutritional considerations for patients with nonobstructive cholestasis include use of choleretic agents, such as taurine and ursodeoxycholic acid, mild to moderate fat restriction if lipid malabsorption occurs, and parenteral supplementation with fat-soluble vitamin K. Cholecystoliths causing biliary obstruction often require surgical removal, although improved choleresis may be sufficient in cases of sludging or inspissation where full obstruction has not yet occurred.

Specific Nutritional Considerations

Cats with cholangiohepatitis may be inappetent, and foods with very high energy and protein density are indicated in order to reduce the volume required to meet daily nutritional needs and avoid concurrent development of hepatic lipidosis (HL) (Edwards 2004) (Table 132.3).

Additional Nutritional Considerations

Choleretic, antiinflammatory, and antioxidant support, as per general hepatic disease recommendations, is strongly indicated. Antibiotic therapy, a requirement of therapy for acute infectious cholangitis, may hinder vitamin K synthesis by destroying gut flora. Thus dietary

---

TABLE 132.3. Recommended components for nutritional support in cholangiohepatitis.

Key nutritional factor	Requirement	Amount (DM basis)
Energy density	High	>4400 kcal/kg
Protein	Increased	40–55%
Fat	Decreased*	<15%

*Only if biliary obstruction or lipid malabsorption are present.
DM, dry matter.

supplementation of vitamin K may also be beneficial, although parenteral vitamin K administration may be required in cases with cholestasis and lipid malabsorption (Edwards 2004).

Feeding Recommendations

In all cases, follow recommendation for small, frequent meals as per general hepatic disease. Tube feeding may be required in cases when inappetence and anorexia are marked and persistent in order to avoid secondary HL.

Key Points

- High energy density.
- High protein.
- Choleretic support.

Chronic Hepatitis

In dogs, chronic hepatitis describes a condition of progressive parenchymal necrosis, typically associated with lymphoplasmacytic inflammation. While the involvement of inflammatory cells suggests an immunomodulatory disorder and autoantibodies have been recognized, the underlying cause may actually be a primary disorder such as a storage hepatopathy, infectious hepatitis, iatrogenic (drug associated), autoimmune disease, or undeterminable (Favier 2009).

Certain breeds of dog are at greater risk, including cocker spaniels, cairn terriers, Doberman pinschers, springer spaniels, Great Danes, Labrador retrievers, samoyeds, and West Highland white terriers. Furthermore, dogs with copper storage disease, such as Bedlington terriers, Dalmatians and Skye terriers, often progress to chronic hepatitis. Long-standing inflammation progressing to fibrosis not only reduces the functional capacity of the hepatic parenchyma but may also cause portal hypertension and/or extrahepatic biliary obstruction. Portal hypertension is typically associated with ascites, gastrointestinal ulceration, and HE from development of portosystemic shunts (PSS). Often, chronic hepatitis progresses to cirrhosis, resulting eventually in complete liver failure.

Specific Nutritional Considerations

Veterinary diets formulated for liver disease are ideal, except for the reduced protein levels, so supplemental vegetable-derived protein is recommended, especially if the dog is underweight or muscle loss occurs. Moderation of dietary carbohydrate is recommended as glucose intolerance often occurs secondary to cirrhosis (Table 132.4).

Additional Nutritional Considerations

Dietary restriction of sodium is indicated in cases with ascites, and additional zinc provision may be beneficial for its antifibrotic and hepatoprotective properties (Table 132.5).

Feeding Recommendations

Follow general feeding recommendations for hepatic disease, as described above.

TABLE 132.4. Recommended components for nutritional support in canine chronic hepatitis.

Key nutritional factor	Requirement	Amount (DM basis)
Protein	Increased*	25–30%
Carbohydrates	Moderate	<45%
Fat	Decreased†	<10%

*If HE present, decrease until clinical signs are abated, ideally no lower than 20%.
†If biliary obstruction or lipid malabsorption are present.
DM, dry matter.

TABLE 132.5. Recommended components for additional nutritional support in canine chronic hepatitis.

Key nutritional factors	Requirement	Amount (DM basis)
Sodium	Restricted	0.08–0.2%
Zinc	Increased	>300 mg/kg

DM, dry matter.

Key Points
- High-quality, highly digestible vegetable protein.
- Unrestricted Protein unless HE develops.
- Choleretic support.
- Sodium restriction.
- Zinc supplementation.
- Antioxidant and antiinflammatory support.

STORAGE DISORDERS

Feline Hepatic Lipidosis

Hepatic lipidosis is an acquired hepatopathy which arises from the culmination of lipid dysregulation in the liver, triglyceride accumulation within the hepatocytes and subsequent cholestasis and hepatic dysfunction. HL may occur secondary to diabetes mellitus, pancreatitis, IBD or other diseases causing anorexia, or it may occur as an idiopathic disorder. Risk of primary or idiopathic HL are increased by obesity and anorexia (Armstrong and Blanchard 2009).

Insufficient dietary intake during periods of fasting, energy restriction, or starvation causes the body to mobilize lipids stored in fatty tissue for beta-oxidation to produce energy. However, the compromised liver of the obese cat may be overwhelmed by the influx of fatty acids, resulting in HL. Furthermore, protein malnutrition can rapidly result in deficiency of essential amino acids in the starved cat due to their unique carnivorous metabolism, including those required for the production of L-carnitine, essential for fatty acid oxidation, and very low-density lipoproteins (VLDLs) neeeded for exportation of triglycerides from the liver (Verbrugghe and Bakovic 2013). In this way, starvation not only reduces the liver's ability to oxidize the fatty acids delivered to it for energy metabolism, but also impairs its ability to clear these excess fatty acids from its parenchyma, resulting in intracellular lipid accumulation and HL.

Specific Nutritional Considerations

Considering the pathogenesis, the nutritional considerations of primary concern are energy and protein. Sufficient energy is critical to prevent further lipolysis and protein catabolism, yet must be controlled as excess energy consumption would contribute to hepatic triglyceride accumulation. Thus, an energy-dense diet fed to meet resting energy requirements (RER) is recommended. Perhaps counterintuitively, fat restriction is not indicated in cases of HL, and moderate inclusion of dietary fats provides energy, spares further catabolism of amino acids, and provides fat-soluble vitamins and essential fatty acids. Protein is required not only to promote production of VLDLs and L-carnitine, but also to attain an anabolic state where the cat's liver may undergo regeneration. Cats with HL rarely exhibit HE, and so protein restriction is rarely indicated (Table 132.6).

TABLE 132.6. Recommended components for nutritional support in feline hepatic lipidosis.

Key nutritional factors	Requirement	Amount (DM basis)
Energy density	High	>4400 kcal/kg
Protein	High quality	40–55%*
Fat	Moderate	15–25%

*May need to be reduced if HE present.
DM, dry matter.

Additional Nutritional Considerations

Supplementation with *L-carnitine* stimulates fatty acid oxidation by enhancing influx of fatty acids in mitochondria and has been shown to be protective against development of ketosis and HL in fasting cats (Blanchard et al. 2002). While it is unknown how beneficial supplementation is for cats already afflicted with HL, inclusion of L-carnitine over 0.02% DM is recommended. Supplementation of *SAMe* (20 mg/kg/day) is particularly indicated for support of phospholipid and lipoprotein synthesis, especially VLDLs, and L-carnitine production. Adequate provision of essential amino acids, in particular the sulfur-amino acids *methionine*, *cysteine*, and *taurine*, is crucial for endogenous SAMe and L-carnitine production. *Vitamin C* is required for L-carnitine synthesis, so inclusion of 100–200 mg is similarly recommended. The water soluble *B-vitamins* can be rapidly lost and deficiency can occur rapidly when intake is reduced. Furthermore, pyridoxine (B6), folate (B9), cobalamin (B12), and choline are all involved in liver lipid metabolism. Inadequate synthesis of long-chain polyunsaturated fatty acids, including *eicosapentanoic acid* (EPA) and *docosahexaenoic acid* (DHA), has been suggested to contribute to the development of HL (Verbrugghe and Bakovic 2013). In particular, EPA has been shown to be beneficial in rats and humans with fatty liver disease (Tanaka et al. 2008, 2010) and dietary supplementation for afflicted cats may also be indicated, though dose rates must be extrapolated from other species (Table 132.7).

Feeding Recommendations

Affected cats are almost exclusively anorectic, so placement of a tube for assisted nutritional therapy is required. Nasogastric tubes are least invasive but are not without complications, only accommodate liquid diets, and are not indicated for long-term nutritional support. Esophageal

TABLE 132.7. Recommended components for additional nutritional support in feline hepatic lipidosis.

Key nutritional factor	Requirement	Amount (DM basis)
L-carnitine	Increased	1000 mg/kg
Methionine	Increased	>0.17%
Methionine + cysteine	Increased	>0.34%
Taurine	Increased	≥0.3%
B vitamin complex	Increased	50–100 mg/day
EPA	Increased	>1%

DM, dry matter.

and percutaneous endoscopic gastrostomy (PEG) tubes are preferred, which also allow delivery of blended canned diets and may be left *in situ* once the cat is discharged from hospital if voluntary intake has not yet met requirements. Reintroduction of nutrition to the starved cat must be conservative and instigated only once the patient is hemodynamically stable and fluid electrolyte and acid–base imbalances have been corrected to avoid refeeding syndrome and metabolic complications (Brenner et al. 2011).

Initial tube feeding should provide only one-third of the cat's calculated RER over the first 24-h period, gradually increasing by one-third daily, provided no complications arise, until full RER is achieved. These feedings should be as small, frequent meals at least four times daily. Assisted nutritional support may be required for a number of weeks to months until voluntary food intake is adequate. As obesity is a predisposing factor, weight loss is a long-term strategy for prevention of recurrence. However, weight loss plans should not be implemented until the cat is fully recovered, and when initiated, careful follow-up is essential to ensure weight loss is at a suitable rate (maximum 2% of initial body weight per week) and the cat does not become inappetent.

Key Points
- Fluid therapy to correct electrolyte imbalances.
- Early nutritional therapy.
  - Tube feeding – nasogastric if required then esophagostomy or gastrostomy.
  - Start with one-third of RER and slowly increase.
- High-protein, energy-dense diet, unless HE present.
- Long-term nutritional support.

Canine Copper Storage Hepatopathy

Increased accumulation of copper within the liver can be due to a primary hereditary copper metabolism defect or secondary to chronic cholestatic liver disease (Hoffman 2009). Quantification of hepatic copper may help in differentiating between the two, with concentrations of 750–2000 μg/g dry weight being attributable to either, but concentrations in excess of 2000 μg/g being strongly suggestive of primary inherited storage disease. Copper storage disease with autosomal recessive inheritance has been described only in the Bedlington terrier, but other dog breeds recognized to suffer from primary copper storage disorders include Skye terriers, West Highland white terriers, Dalmatians, Doberman pinschers, and Labrador retrievers.

Specific Considerations

Copper restriction is the hallmark of nutritional management of copper storage diseases. Copper chelation is often indicated in patients with primary copper storage disease; common drugs used include D-penicillamine and trientine. Veterinary therapeutic liver diets are copper restricted but are also lower than ideal in protein, so supplementation with a low-copper protein source is recommended, especially if the dog is underweight or when muscle loss is present (Table 132.8). Additionally, therapeutic diets using plant-based protein sources may have copper restriction adequate for these patients.

TABLE 132.8. Recommended components for nutritional support in canine copper storage hepatopathy.

Key nutritional factors	Requirement	Amount (DM basis)
Copper	Restricted	<0.5%

DM, dry matter.

TABLE 132.9. Recommended components for additional nutritional support in canine copper storage hepatopathy.

Key nutritional factor	Requirement	Amount (DM basis)
Zinc	Increased	>300 mg/kg

DM, dry matter.

Additional Nutritional Considerations

Dietary supplementation with *zinc* (inclusion at >300 mg/kg DM or supplementation with Zn gluconate 3 mg/kg/day) is important to block copper absorption. Zinc has been shown to induce intestinal metallothionein synthesis, trapping copper within enterocytes and preventing systemic absorption. In addition, zinc has antifibrotic and hepatocytoprotective effects. Antioxidant support is also strongly indicated as excessive copper is associated with oxidative damage to hepatocytes (Hoffman 2009) (Table 132.9).

Feeding Recommendations

Follow general feeding recommendations for hepatic disease, as described above.

Key Points

- Copper restriction.
- Zinc supplementation.
- Antioxidant support.

CIRCULATORY DISORDERS

Portosystemic Shunts

Portosystemic shunts are more common in dogs than in cats. These may be congenital shunts or secondary to portal hypertension. Congenital shunts may be intrahepatic, which occur more frequently in large-breed dogs, or extrahepatic, which occur most often in small-breed dogs and cats (Berent and Tobias 2009). Intrahepatic shunts are functional remnants of the ductus venosus, while extrahepatic shunts are anomalous embryonic vessels. The hereditary nature has been established in the Irish wolfhound and is suspected in a number of other breeds.

Acquired PSS most commonly develop secondary to portal hypertension from other primary liver diseases such as cirrhosis and neoplasia, or as a sequel to other disorders. Clinically, patients with PSS typically display signs of HE, with or without polyuria/polydipsia. Stunted growth is common in cases with congenital shunts. Urocystoliths characterized by ammonium urate or purines are common due to increased urinary excretion of ammonia and uric acid.

Specific Considerations

In the absence of HE, standard nutritional management for general hepatic disease is often sufficient to meet the key nutritional factors for portosystemic shunts (Box 132.2).

Table 132.10 shows requirements for patients with HE.

Additional Nutritional Considerations (Table 132.11)

Vascular Dysplasia

Microvascular dysplasia (MVD) and primary portal vein hypoplasia (PVH) are congenital vascular anomalies recognized most commonly in small-breed dogs, particularly cairn terriers, Yorkshire terriers, and Maltese. Both conditions commonly lead to hepatic arterialization in the portal triad and development of microscopic intrahepatic shunts (Berent and Tobias 2009).

BOX 132.2. Hepatic encephalopathy

Hepatic encephalopathy most frequently occurs in patients with PSS (Lidbury et al. 2016). Strict dietary protein restriction, to reduce ammonia generation from undigested protein by gut bacteria, was traditionally the cornerstone of HE management. Recently, however, it has been discovered that the main source of postprandial ammonia generation is not in fact dietary derived but is from enterocyte metabolism. Furthermore, it has been suggested that dogs with either congenital or acquired PSS have higher dietary protein requirements than healthy dogs. Protein-calorie malnutrition may result from strict protein restriction, and decreased dietary protein leads to increased body protein catabolism, further contributing to circulating ammonia levels. Low-protein veterinary diets designed for chronic renal failure were recommended for patients with HE, although this is not ideal, due not only to the unnecessary protein restriction but also to the source of the protein, which was typically from nitrogen and heme iron-rich organ meats. Now, normal to only slightly reduced protein levels are recommended, with *vegetable proteins* associated with improved clinical outcomes (Lidbury et al. 2016; Proot et al. 2009).

When protein restriction is required to control clinical signs, protein should be offered at the minimum requirement (18% for dogs, 26% for cats) then the protein level should be titrated up to the highest tolerable level. *Dairy proteins* may also be of use for home-made diets for dogs, but only if supplemental *arginine* is provided. For cats, dairy protein is relatively deficient in arginine and poorly tolerated by many cats, and protein restriction is strongly contraindicated, so management of HE by alternative methods (fiber supplementation, vegetable protein, medical management) is required. *SAMe*, a nutritional supplement with valuable applications in many hepatic pathologies, is contraindicated in cases with HE as it is a source of methionine, a sulfur-amino acid which can exacerbate blood ammonia levels. Easily digestible *complex carbohydrates* may attenuate clinical signs. Moreover, indigestible carbohydrate components or *total dietary fiber* may help to decrease nitrogenous load and improve frequency and character of fecal excretion. *Insoluble fiber* can decrease ingesta transit time, thus decreasing absorption of noxious bile acids, endotoxins, and other bacterial products. Fermentable *soluble fiber* (e.g., psyllium husk, lactulose) may help reduce ammonia absorption from the colon and ameliorate toxic effects by providing a substrate for colonic acidophilic bacteria. These bacteria ferment soluble fiber and produce short chain fatty acids which both nourish enterocytes and decrease luminal pH, thus ion trapping ammonia as NH^{4+} within the colonic lumen for fecal excretion (Center 1998). Furthermore, bacterial growth requires incorporation of nitrogen into their cell walls, further reducing colonic nitrogen content. Dietary supplementation with psyllium husk (1 tsp per 5–10 kg BW) or lactulose (0.25–0.5 mg/kg, titrated to production of 2–3 loose stools per day) is recommended. *Zinc* supplementation may also increase ammonia metabolism.

TABLE 132.10. Recommended components for nutritional support in hepatic encephalopathy.

Key nutritional factor	Requirement	Cats (DM basis)	Dogs (DM basis)
Protein	Vegetable	26–35%	15–20%*
Carbohydrates	Increased	45–55%	30–40%
Total dietary fiber	Increased	3–8%	3–8%
Soluble fiber	Increased	>1.5%	>1.5%

*Protein restriction below 18% DM is not ideal for long-term maintenance; titrate increasing protein against signs of HE to establish ideal total protein intake for the patient.
DM, dry matter.

TABLE 132.11. Recommended components for additional nutritional support in hepatic encephalopathy.

Nutritional factor	Requirement	Cats (DM basis)	Dogs (DM basis)
Zinc	Increased	>300 mg/kg	>300 mg/kg
SAMe	Contraindicated*	0	0

*SAMe is a source of methionine and is contraindicated in patients with HE.
DM, dry matter.

TABLE 132.12. Recommended components for nutritional support in vascular dysplasia.		
Key nutritional factors	**Requirement**	**Amount (DM basis)**
Sodium	Restricted	0.08–0.2%
Vitamin K	Increased	>1.63 mg/kg
DM, dry matter.		

Signs of MVD are mostly related to the acquired PSS and may be difficult to differentiate from congenital PSS, particularly as the breed predispositions for the conditions overlap and some dogs may have both congenital PSS and MVD or PVH. In dogs with PVH, clinical signs of portal hypertension predominate, so associated signs such as ascites and GI ulceration may help to distinguish from congenital PSS.

Specific Considerations

Standard nutritional management of hepatic disease is often sufficient to meet the key nutritional factors for both MVD and PVH. Veterinary diets formulated for liver disease are ideal, although for patients with PVH and no evidence of HE, supplemental vegetable-derived protein is recommended.

Additional Nutritional Considerations

Dietary restriction of *sodium* is absolutely indicated to minimize hypertension and decrease risk of ascites. Due to the risk of GI ulceration, *vitamin K* supplementation is advised – as there is no issue with cholestatic disease, dietary vitamin K supplementation may be sufficient, or else parenteral administration is advised (Table 132.12).

Feeding Recommendations

No specific feeding recommendations; follow general feeding recommendations for hepatic disease.

Key Points

- Sodium restriction to minimize hypertension.
- Protein restriction if HE present.

References

Armstrong PJ, Blanchard G. Hepatic lipidosis in cats. Vet Clin North Am Small Anim Pract 2009;39:599–616.

Au AY, Hasenwinkel JM, Frondoza CG. Hepatoprotective effects of S-adenosylmethionine and silybin on canine hepatocytes in vitro. J Anim Physiol Anim Nutr 2013;97:331–341.

Berent AC, Tobias KM. Portosystemic vascular anomalies. Vet Clin North Am Small Anim Pract 2009;39:513–541.

Blanchard G, Paragon BM, Milliat F, Lutton C. Dietary L-carnitine supplementation in obese cats alters carnitine metabolism and decreases ketosis during fasting and induced hepatic lipidosis. J Nutr 2002;132:204–210.

Brenner K, KuKanich KS, Smee NM. Refeeding syndrome in a cat with hepatic lipidosis. J Feline Med Surg 2011;13(8):614–617.

Buryova H, Chalupsky K, Zbodakoca O, et al. Liver protective effect of ursodeoxycholic acid includes regulation of ADAM17 activity. BMC Gastroenterol 2013;13(155);1–12.

Center SA. Nutritional support for dogs and cats with hepatobiliary disease. J Nutr 1998;128(12):2733S–2746S.

Center SA. Diseases of the gallbladder and biliary tree. Vet Clin North Am Small Anim Pract 2009;39:543–598.

Cox M. Unravelling the mystery of feline cholangiohepatitis. Vet Tech 2006;27(9):538–541.

Edwards M. Feline cholangiohepatitis. Compendium 2004;26(11):855–861.

Favier RP. Idiopathic hepatitis and cirrhosis in dogs. Vet Clin North Am Small Anim Pract 2009;39:481–488.

Hoffman G. Copper-associated liver diseases. Vet Clin North Am Small Anim Pract 2009;39:489–511.

Lidbury JA, Cook AK, Steiner JM. Hepatic encephalopathy in dogs and cats. J Vet Emerg Crit Care 2016;26(4):471–487.

Morris JG. Idiosyncratic nutrient requirements of cats appear to be diet-induced evolutionary adaptations. Nutr Res Rev 2002;15:153–168.

Mosallanejad B, Avizeh R, Varzi NH, Pourmadhi M. Evaluation of prophylactic and therapeutic effects of silymarin on acute toxicity due to tetracycline severe overdose in cats: a preliminary study. Iran J Vet Res 2012;13(1):16–22.

Proot S, Biourge V, Teske E, Rothuizen J. Soy protein isolate versus meat-based low-protein diet for dogs with congenital portosystemic shunts. J Vet Intern Med 2009;23:794–800.

Reed N, Gunn-Moore D, Simpson K. Cobalamin, folate and inorganic phosphate abnormalities in ill cats. J Feline Med Surg 2007;9:278–288.

Tanaka N, Sano K, Horiuchi A, Tanaka E, Kiyosawa K, Aoyama T. Highly purified eicosapentaenoic acid treatment improves nonalcoholic steatohepatitis. J Clin Gastroenterol 2008;42(4):413–418.

Tanaka N, Zhang X, Sugiyama E, et al. Eicosapentaenoic acid improves hepatic steatosis independent of PPARα activation through inhibition of SREBP-1 maturation in mice. Biochem Pharmacol 2010;80:1601–1612.

Verbrugghe A, Bakovic M. Peculiarities of one-carbon metabolism in the strict carnivorous cat and the role in feline hepatic lipidosis. Nutrients 2013;5:2811–2835.

Vince AR, Hayes MA, Jefferson BJ, Stalker MJ. Hepatic injury correlates with apoptosis, regeneration, and nitric oxide synthase expression in canine chronic liver disease. Vet Pathol 2014;51(5):932–945.

Watson PJ. Chronic hepatitis in dogs: a review of current understanding of the aetiology, progression, and treatment. Vet J 2004;167:228–241.

Yam P, Cave C. Enteral nutrition: options and feeding protocols. In Practice 2003;25(3):118–159.

Suggested Reading

Decaro N, Capolo M, Elia G, et al. Infections canine hepatitis: An "old" disease reemerging in Italy. Res Vet Sci 2007;83:269–273.

Wang B, Lumin L, Jing F, et al. Effects of long-chain and medium-chain fatty acids on apoptosis and oxidative stress in human liver cells with steatosis. J Food Sci 2016;81(3):H794–H800.

Authors: Sarah Dodd DVM, BSc, Caitlin Grant DVM, BSc, Adronie Verbrugghe DVM, PhD, Dip ECVCN

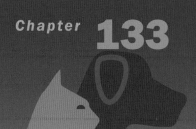

Chapter 133

Portosystemic Shunting, Acquired

DEFINITION/OVERVIEW

Acquired portosystemic shunts (PSS) are vascular connections between the portal vein and systemic venous circulation which develop in response to portal hypertension (PH). These vessels are embryonic remnants that connect the portal vasculature and the vena cava. Once opened, they divert blood flow from the splanchnic veins directly to the central venous circulation instead of allowing the blood to filter through the liver first. This leads to clinical signs associated with resulting hepatic encephalopathy.

ETIOLOGY/PATHOPHYISIOLOGY

Portal hypertension and secondary acquired PSS fall into three categories of origin.

- Prehepatic – the abdominal portion of the portal vein is either too small or is occluded, including portal vein hypoplasia, portal vein atresia, portal vein thrombosis, or neoplastic or granulomatous occlusion or infiltration into the portal vein. This category includes surgical correction of a congenital portosystemic shunt if the patient's portal vein is too underdeveloped to accept the new blood flow.
- Hepatic.
  - Presinusoidal – occlusion or thrombosis of the intrahepatic portion of portal vein or several of its tributaries, including idiopathic noncirrhotic portal hypertension, hepatic arteriovenous (AV) fistula, and ductal plate abnormalities (Caroli's disease).
  - Sinusoidal – hepatic parenchymal diseases causing fibrosis and thus increased resistance to blood flow through the liver (most often chronic inflammatory or toxic diseases with resulting cirrhosis). Also includes congenital hepatic fibrosis.
  - Postsinusoidal – increased pressure within or occlusion of intrahepatic tributaries to the hepatic vein; rare "sinusoidal obstruction syndrome."
- Posthepatic – increased pressure anterior to the hepatic vein, including any cause of increased central venous pressure (right-sided congestive heart failure, pericardial effusion, Budd–Chiari syndrome, caval thrombosis, occlusive thoracic neoplasm, caval syndrome from *Dirofilaria immitis* infestation,etc.).

Generally, the above causes of resistance to portal flow need to be present for weeks to months to elicit the development of acquired PSS. The portal hypertension itself often leads to development of ascites due to increased hydrostatic pressure and congestion of the splanchnic circulation. Gastrointestinal (GI) ulceration and bleeding are also possible. Clinical signs of hepatic encephalopathy also often occur, as can bacteremia, as a result of loss of hepatic filtration and processing of blood flowing out of the gastrointestinal tract.

Blackwell's Five-Minute Veterinary Consult Clinical Companion: Small Animal Gastrointestinal Diseases, First Edition. Edited by Jocelyn Mott and Jo Ann Morrison.
© 2019 John Wiley & Sons, Inc. Published 2019 by John Wiley & Sons, Inc.
Companion website: www.fiveminutevet.com/gastrointestinal

Acquired PSS are uncommon in patients with chronic hepatopathies unless they have progressed to cirrhosis. They are an uncommon complication of surgical correction of a congenital portosystemic shunt.

Systems Affected

- Gastrointestinal – ulceration and bleeding.
- Hepatobiliary – organ of origin.
- Nervous – hepatic encephalopathy.

 # SIGNALMENT/HISTORY

- Breed – ductal plate malformation; increased incidence in Persian and Himalayan cats and boxer dogs. Congenital PSS – Yorkshire terrier, pug, Maltese, and others.
- No sex predilection.
- Age – young dogs and cats <1 year for portal vein atresia, idiopathic noncirrhotic portal hypertension, or congenital PSS. Middle-aged to older dogs and cats have increased risk for inflammatory hepatopathy such as chronic active hepatitis.
- The genetics of these conditions have not been precisely determined.
- Clinical signs.
  - Ascites due to portal hypertension is common but variable in severity.
  - GI ulceration due to hypertensive splanchnic vasculopathy. May cause profound hemorrhage, anorexia, vomiting, diarrhea, melena, abdominal pain, and anemia.
  - Hepatic encephalopathy signs are common, including anorexia, lethargy, stupor, polyuria, polydipsia, blindness, ptyalism (especially in cats), disorientation, seizures.
  - Hematuria or urethral obstruction due to urate calculi; uncommon.

Risk Factors

- Chronic untreated or advanced inflammatory hepatopathy.
- Young pet suspected to have congenital PSS that presents with ascites is likely to have portal hypertension and may already have developed acquired PSS.
- High-protein foods or GI bleed may precipitate hepatic encephalopathy, which may be the first signs to alert owners to a problem.

Historical Findings

- Abdominal distension.
- Lethargy, poor appetite, vomiting, diarrhea, melena.
- Hepatic encephalopathy – dull mentation, postprandial sleepiness, bizarre behaviors, stupor or seizures, drooling (cats > dogs); this may be worse after a meal.
- Hematuria, pollakiuria, polyuria/polydipsia.
- Jaundice.

 # CLINICAL FEATURES

- Thin body condition.
- Abdominal distension with fluid wave/ascites.
- Pallor of mucous membranes and melena on rectal exam if GI bleeding.
- Obtundation, absent or delayed menace reflex, ataxia, paresis.
- Icterus if chronic hepatopathy or chronic biliary occlusion.

DIFFERENTIAL DIAGNOSIS

- Congenital PSS typically are single vessels, whereas acquired PSS are typically multiple.
- Ascites has dozens of other differentials, including cardiovascular failure, hypoproteinemia, neoplastic, parasitic, inflammatory, and infectious etiologies.
- Hepatic encephalopathy could be mistaken for hypoglycemia, a variety of neurotoxins, or primary brain diseases.

DIAGNOSTICS

Complete Blood Count/Biochemistry/Urinalysis

- Complete blood cell count – microcytosis, mild to severe anemia due to chronic disease and GI losses, thrombocytopenia if concurrent disseminated intravascular coagulation or if consumed in severe GI bleed, thrombocytosis if chronic GI bleed.
- Serum biochemistry profile – reduced tests of liver production (blood urea nitrogen (BUN), glucose, albumin, cholesterol), possibly elevated hepatocellular and biliary enzymes (alanine aminotransferase (ALT), aspartate aminotransferase (AST), alkaline phosphatase (ALKP), gamma-glutamyl transferase (GGT), total bilirubin).
- Electrolytes – may have hyponatremia secondary to decreased effective circulating volume.
- Urinalysis – dilute urine, possible urate crystalluria.

Other Laboratory Tests

- Serum bile acids – usually moderate to severe elevation; the magnitude of elevation is not predictive of acquired versus congenital shunting, and in rare cases may be normal due to inherent test idiosyncrasies.
- Prothrombin time and partial thromboplastin time – may be prolonged if hepatocellular failure.
- Protein C activity – not discriminatory for congenital versus acquired PSS, but is helpful to discern hepatic microvascular dysplasia (portal vein hypoplasia) from PSS. Canine patients with low protein C activity <70% have a high chance of having a PSS. This has not been assessed in cats.

Imaging

- Radiographs – usually microhepatica (unless posthepatic cause for PH – will see hepatomegaly), +/– poor serosal detail, +/– ascites.
- Ultrasound – hepatomegaly may be seen if there is posthepatic origin to the portal hypertension. Otherwise there will be a small liver with diminished portal vascular markings; aberrant tortuous vessels may be seen, especially between the spleen and the left gonadal veins, in the left dorsal perirenal area. There may be ascites, +/– urolithiasis. The portal vein may be enlarged or tortuous, or may be small if portal vein hypoplasia exists. The biliary tract can also be assessed, as it may be a contributor to chronic hepatopathy.
- Scintigraphy – colonic-portal scintigraphy, or transsplenic portal scintigraphy with ^{99}Tc-pertechnetate (^{99m}TcO$_4^-$) will determine the percent of blood shunting past the liver and to the heart. Normal values are <15%. This is accurate for determination of shunt presence but not as accurate for determination of shunt anatomy, or acquired versus congenital PSS. Requires sedation.
- Computed tomography or magnetic resonance imaging contrast angiography – preferred for the most accurate noninvasive identification of acquired PSS and their anatomy. Requires sedation or anesthesia.

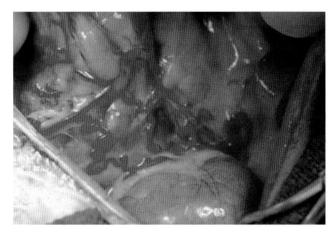

■ **Fig. 133.1.** The acquired PSS can be seen in this patient as tortuous engorged vessels entering the left renal and gonadal veins.

Other Diagnostic Tests

■ Ascites fluid analysis – typically pure or modified transudate. Postsinusoidal and posthepatic causes of PH will have higher protein content (>3.0) whereas sinusoidal, presinusoidal, and prehepatic causes of PH will have a low protein content (<2.5).
■ Hepatic biopsy – surgical, laparoscopic, or ultrasound-guided samples can be obtained. For most causes of PH and acquired PSS, the liver is often small and fibrotic, so ultrasound-guided samples may be difficult to obtain and possibly too small for thorough assessment. The acquired PSS can be seen upon exploratory laparotomy (Figure 133.1).

Pathologic Findings

■ Gross pathologic findings most often include a small, lobulated, firm liver with mild to moderate clear ascitic fluid, and multiple tortuous vessels connecting the splanchnic vessels to systemic venous circulation (often splenic to renal or gonadal veins).
■ Histopathology will determine if PH and subsequent acquired PSS are due to congenital, inflammatory, fibrotic or vascular etiology.
■ Ductal plate abnormalities: characteristic patterns of bile duct proliferation and fibrosis.
■ Portal hypoperfusion (AV fistula, noncirrhotic portal hypertension, portal vein obstruction/atresia/stenosis): loss or reduction in portal vasculature; arteriolar hyperplasia, tortuosity, or reduplication; hepatocellular atrophy.
■ Chronic hepatic inflammation as cause of PH: inflammatory cells (often lymphoplasmacytic +/– neutrophilic) centered in the periportal region, +/– bile canalicular plugging, hepatocyte degeneration and apoptosis, and bridging fibrosis.
■ Posthepatic PH: congestion of centrilobular or perivenular areas, centrilobular hepatocyte degeneration. Fibrosis may occur and bridge between central veins with chronicity.
■ Prehepatic PH: histopathology of the liver may be normal or may have mild hepatocyte degeneration.

 # THERAPEUTICS

Objectives of treatment.
■ Control and prevent signs of hepatic encephalopathy.
■ Control ascites accumulation.

- Prevent GI ulceration, vomiting, and diarrhea.
- Slow or stop progression of the underlying condition which led to development of the acquired PSS in the first place.

Drug(s) of choice

- Lactulose – acidifies colonic lumen, traps ammonia as ammonium ions in the lumen, and prevents absorption into portal vein. Dose varies by patient size and severity of symptoms 1–10 mL PO q8–12 h; may also be given as a retention enema for encephalopathic crisis.
- Neomycin – aminoglycoside that limits urease-producing bacteria in the GI lumen; typically has very low oral bioavailability, so effects are only on luminal bacteria. Dose is 20 mg/kg PO q8–12 h (dogs and cats).
- Amoxicillin (10 mg/kg PO q8–12 h dogs and cats) or metronidazole (7.5 mg PO q8–12 h dogs and cats) – systemic antibiotics for the same purpose as neomycin.
- Spironolactone (1–2 mg/kg PO q12h dogs) – blocks aldosterone action in the renal collecting ducts (renin-angiotensin-aldosterone system is upregulated with the loss of effective circulating volume in acquired PSS). This is also potassium sparing, which is important because hypokalemia can worsen hepatic encephalopathy.
- A low dose of furosemide (1–2 mg/kg PO q12h) is often added to enhance natriuresis.
- Famotidine (1 mg/kg PO q12h dogs and cats) or omeprazole (1 mg/kg PO q12–24 h dogs and cats) – very important to reduce the chance of GI ulceration and bleeding from portal hypertension and splanchnic vasculopathy.
- Glucocorticoids – if indicated by hepatic biopsy showing chronic inflammation (example: methlyprednisolone 0.4 mg/kg PO q12h).
- Aspirin (0.5–1 mg/kg PO daily for dogs, 5 mg PO q3 days for cats), clopidogrel (1 mg/kg daily in dogs, 18.75 mg/day in cats), heparin (200–400 IU/kg SQ q8h), or dalteparin (low molecular weight heparin, 150 units/kg SQ q8–12 h for dogs) – only if needed to address portal vein thrombosis or caval thrombosis. Often used in combination to shift the vascular balance from hypercoagulable to hypocoagulable.

Precautions/Interactions

- Neomycin – may become absorbed systemically if there is GI ulceration; systemic absorption can cause nephrotoxicity, as this is an aminoglycoside antibiotic.
- Metronidazole – is metabolized and cleared by the liver, so dose should be kept below 10 mg/kg q12h. Side effects may include neurotoxicity/ataxia.
- Diuretics may cause electrolyte imbalances and prerenal azotemia; electrolytes and renal parameters should be monitored periodically. Hypokalemia should be avoided, as it may worsen hepatic encephalopathy.
- Glucocorticoid doses should be kept conservative to reduce risk of GI ulceration. Preferably the glucocorticoid chosen should have limited mineralocorticoid effects (i.e., dexamethasone, methylprednisolone or triamcinolone) to reduce side effects of sodium and fluid retention.

Alternative Drugs

- Rifaximin – antibiotic, alternative to neomycin, improved safety margin, very expensive.
- Losartan – angiotensin II receptor blocker; used in humans with PH, reduces PH, reduces splanchnic endothelial dysfunction, attenuates hepatic fibrosis; limited experience in dogs/cats.
- Bosentan – endothelin-1 receptor antagonist; also used in people with PH, limited experience in dogs/cats.

Appropriate Health Care

Patients with acquired PSS and PH should be monitored closely by their veterinarian, with strict adherence to diet and medications to improve outcomes.

Nursing Care

Patients may need more attention to their medication and diet needs than a healthy pet, such as efforts to hand feed the pet and keeping a close watch for hematochezia or melena, watching for ascites, and monitoring for signs of hepatic encephalopathy.

Diet

- To reduce risk of hepatic encephalopathy, a reduced-protein diet or a diet based around dairy or vegetable protein is recommended.
- Potassium should be higher in the diet (hypokalemia exacerbates hepatic encephalopathy).
- Sodium should be limited to reduce ascites.
- Multiple smaller meals are more readily assimilated than two larger meals and less likely to cause an encephalopathic event.

Activity

Exercise restriction is not required, but a pet with significant ascites and/or encephalopathy may not want to be very active.

Surgical Considerations

There is no surgery available to correct multiple acquired portosystemic shunts, although these shunts may be the undesired result of ligation of a congenital portosystemic shunt if the existing portal system was too hypoplastic to accept increased blood flow.

 COMMENTS

Client Education

- Advise clients to watch for abdominal distension, inappetence, vomiting, diarrhea, blood in the stool, or neurologic symptoms.
- The prognosis is guarded to poor for many of these pets, so if anything unusual is noted it should be brought to the attention of a veterinarian.
- Dietary management is important but can be difficult as these pets may have a poor appetite owing to their underlying liver disease.

Patient Monitoring

- Frequency of veterinary visits depends on the underlying cause of the shunting.
- Stable patients with idiopathic noncirrhotic portal hypertension or related disorders should have a complete blood count, chemistry panel, urinalysis, possibly ammonia levels and other diagnostics as needed about every 4–6 months.
- Patients in overt hepatic failure from chronic hepatopathy may need weekly veterinary visits to try to support the various needs of the patient.

Prevention/Avoidance

- The only scenario in which acquired PSS could be prevented is when it results from a chronic inflammatory hepatopathy; early detection and treatment of chronic hepatitis can prevent development of fibrosis and hence acquired PSS.
- Avoiding clinical signs related to acquired PSS is mostly reliant on following guidelines for proper diet and medication regimen.

Possible Complications

- Severe gastrointestinal bleeding.
- Hepatic encephalopathy to include seizures.
- Severe ascites.
- Hepatic failure – anorexia, weakness/lethargy, vomiting, diarrhea.

Expected Course and Prognosis

- Acquired PSS occur as a result of severe hepatic, portal, or other vascular pathology.
- Other than idiopathic noncirrhotic portal hypertension, most of the inciting conditions have a guarded to poor long-term prognosis.
- Eventually most patients will die from complications of hepatic failure.

Synonyms

Acquired portosystemic shunt is also referred to as multiple portosystemic shunt.

Abbreviations

- ALKP = alkaline phosphatase
- ALT = alanine aminotransferase
- AST = aspartate aminotransferase
- AV = arteriovenous
- BUN = blood urea nitrogen
- GGT = gamma-glutamyl transferase
- GI = gastrointestinal
- PH = portal hypertension
- PSS = portosystemic shunt

See Also

- Arteriovenous Malformation of the Liver
- Cirrhosis and Fibrosis of the Liver
- Ductal Plate Malformation
- Hepatic Encephalopathy
- Hepatitis, Chronic
- Hepatoportal Microvascular Dysplasia
- Hypertension, Portal
- Portosystemic Vascular Anomaly

Suggested Reading

Adam FH, German AJ, McConnell JF, et al. Clinical and clinicopathologic abnormalities in young dogs with acquired and congenital portosystemic shunts: 93 cases (2003-2008). J Am Vet Med Assoc 2012;241:760–765.

Bertolini G. Acquired portal collateral circulation in the dog and cat. Vet Radio Ultrasound 2010;51:25–33.

Bunch SE, Johnson SE, McCullen JM. Idiopathic noncirrhotic portal hypertension in dogs: 33 cases (1982-1998). J Am Vet Med Assoc 2000;218:392–399.

Buob S, Johnston AN, Webster CRL. Review article: portal hypertension: pathophysiology, diagnosis and treatment. J Vet Intern Med 2011;25:169–186.

Acknowledgments: The author and editors acknowledge the prior contribution of Dr Sharon Center.

Author: Julie Stegeman DVM, DACVIM (SAIM)

Chapter 134

Portosystemic Vascular Anomaly, Congenital

DEFINITION/OVERVIEW

- The portal vein drains blood from the gastrointestinal tract (GIT), pancreas, and spleen and supplies 75% of blood flow to the liver.
- A congenital portosystemic shunt (CPSS) is a macroscopic vessel that connects portal vasculature to systemic venous vasculature.
- Portal blood will bypass the liver: it flows away from the liver, also referred to as centrifugal flow.
- Simple classifications: congenital versus acquired, extrahepatic versus intrahepatic, single versus multiple.
- Shunt morphologies are classified based on shunt origin and insertion (Figure 134.1).
- Most CPSS are single vessels when they insert into the venous vasculature.
- Extrahepatic CPSS tends to affect small-breed dogs and cats.
- Intrahepatic CPSS tends to affect large-breed dogs and cats.

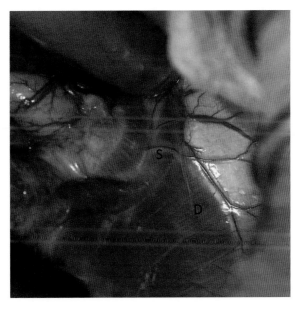

■ **Fig. 134.1.** Intraoperative view of a portosystemic shunt (splenophrenic morphology). D, diaphragm; S, shunt.

Blackwell's Five-Minute Veterinary Consult Clinical Companion: Small Animal Gastrointestinal Diseases, First Edition. Edited by Jocelyn Mott and Jo Ann Morrison.
© 2019 John Wiley & Sons, Inc. Published 2019 by John Wiley & Sons, Inc.
Companion website: www.fiveminutevet.com/gastrointestinal

ETIOLOGY/PATHOPHYSIOLOGY

- Shunt vessel allows blood from GIT, pancreas, and spleen to bypass the liver and enter systemic circulation.
- In young animals, portal blood carries tropic factors to the liver for hepatic development and growth; shunting results in a small liver that is hypoperfused and has intrahepatic microvascular abnormalities.
- The liver is meant to detoxify/cleanse the portal blood. The portal blood contains enteric toxins, nitrogenous toxins, and bacteria that enter into systemic circulation without being cleared by the liver. These toxins lead to the clinical signs and changes seen in patients with CPSS.
- Amount of shunting blood may correlate with the degree of clinical signs.

Systems Affected

- Nervous – up to 95% of patients can have varying degrees of hepatic encephalopathy (HE). Ammonia is produced by GIT bacterial metabolism of nitrogen-containing products such as protein. Central nervous system metabolism is altered by ammonia along with other neuro-toxic substances such as benzodiazepine-like compounds, aromatic amino acids, bile acids, glutamate gamma-aminobutyric acid (GABA), mercaptans, and phenols.
  - Clinical signs of HE include abnormal behavior, vocalization, ataxia, head pressing, stargazing, lethargy, pacing, circling, blindness, drooling (cats), and unresponsiveness.
  - Neurologic clinical signs may also include seizures.
- Gastrointestinal – patients may have GIT clinical signs and gastric ulceration from altered blood flow, increased gastric acid secretion, decreased prostaglandins, abnormal mucous production, and poor mucosal integrity.
  - Clinical signs tend to be intermittent. Include hyporexia to anorexia, diarrhea (occasional melena), vomiting, and pica. Cats may have ptyalism.
  - Bleeding ulcers can lead to HE clinical signs; this is more common with intrahepatic shunts.
  - Patients may have retained deciduous teeth.
- Renal/urogenital – ammonium urate or biurate stones may form in the kidneys, ureters, and/or bladder in ~35% of dogs. Hyperammonuria and impaired transformation of uric acid to water soluble allantoin lead to formation of stones. Poor medullary concentration gradient, increased kidney blood flow, increased adrenocorticotropic hormone, and psychogenic polydipsia from HE may contribute to polyuria/polydipsia (PU/PD).
  - Some patients may present with only lower urinary tract clinical signs (stranguria, pollakiuria, hematuria, obstruction).
  - Stones may cause secondary urinary tract infection.
  - Patients may be cryptorchid.
  - Patients may have large kidneys noted on palpation or imaging and a history of PU/PD.
- Asymptomatic – up to 20% of dogs have clinicopathologic abnormalities noted on routine or preanesthetic bloodwork.

SIGNALMENT/HISTORY

- Yorkshire terriers, Havanese, Maltese, Dandie Dinmont terriers, pugs, and miniature schnauzers have an odds ratio of 20 or more for occurrence of extrahepatic portosystemic shunts (EHPSS).
- Other small breeds overrepresented include shih tzu, Lhasa apso, Chihuahua, dachshunds, bichon frise, Tibetan spaniel.

- Irish wolfhounds, Labrador retrievers, golden retrievers, Australian cattle dogs, and Australian shepherds are overrepresented large-breed dogs with intrahepatic portosystemic shunts (IHPSS).
- Small-breed dogs can have IHPSS and large-breed dogs can have EHPSS.
- Hereditary patterns have been found in Maltese, cairn terriers, Yorkshire terriers, Irish wolfhounds, and Australian cattle dogs.
- Domestic shorthair, Persians, Siamese, Himalayans, Burmese are feline breeds more commonly affected.
  - Most patients with clinical signs are <2 years of age, although they can be >10 years.

Risk Factors

- Clinical signs may be episodic or exacerbated.
- Drugs such as nonsteroidal antiinflammatory drugs (NSAIDs) or steroids may increase the risk of GIT bleeding and HE.
- High-protein meals increase risk of HE.
- Drugs metabolized by the liver may have a prolonged effect. Drugs such as benzodiazepines and antihistamines may increase risk of HE.
- Blood transfusions can increase risk of HE.
- Constipation and small intestinal bacterial overgrowth can increase risk of HE.

Historical Findings

- Small or "runt" of litter: common.
- Hepatic encephalopathy: 40–95%.
- Abnormal behavior: lethargy, head pressing, pacing, stargazing, ataxia, aggression, circling, blindness.
- Seizures.
- Gastrointestinal signs: common.
- Weight loss or failure to gain weight.
- Vomiting, diarrhea, inappetence, pica.
- Hematemesis, hematochezia.
- Ptyalism in cats.
- PU/PD: common.
- Clinical signs of lower urinary tract disease: 20–53%.
- Hematuria, stranguria, pollakiuria, obstruction.
- Older male dogs are more likely to have urolithiasis.
- Slow recovery from anesthesia.
- May have other congenital abnormalities.
- Cryptorchidism in up to 30% male cats and up to 50% male dogs.
- Heart murmurs.
- Retained deciduous teeth.
- Asymptomatic: 20%.
- Copper-colored irises in cats.

CLINICAL FEATURES

- Physical exam may be normal.
- Patient may be small in size for breed.
- Quiet or have abnormal mentation for age.
- Patient may present with seizures.

- HE signs may be pronounced with abnormal neurologic exam.
  - Altered mentation.
  - Conscious proprioception deficits.
  - Lateralizing signs such as head tilt, nystagmus, anisocoria.
- Comatose or laterally recumbent.
- Copper iris in cats.
- Ptyalism in cats.
- Other congenital abnormalities.
  - Cryptorchidism.
  - Heart murmur.
  - Retained deciduous teeth.

DIFFERENTIAL DIAGNOSIS

- Portal vein hypoplasia (PVH) (previously referred to as microvascular dysplasia – MVD). Similar presentation to CPSS, typically slightly older with milder clinical signs.
- Multiple acquired extrahepatic portosystemic shunts (Figure 134.2). Occur secondary to causes of chronic portal hypertension such as hepatic cirrhosis, PVH with portal hypertension and hepatic arteriovenous malformation (HAVM). May also have ascites.
- HAVM – usually young animals with moderate to severe clinical signs.
- HE – can be caused by primary liver disease. Usually older with chronic history.
- Neurologic diseases – developmental (e.g., hydrocephalus, atlantoaxial malformations, idiopathic epilepsy, enzyme deficiencies), infectious/inflammatory (e.g., encephalitis, distemper, toxoplasmosis, feline infectious peritonitis, feline leukemia virus, feline immunodeficiency virus), ischemic, metabolic (e.g., hypoglycemia, hypokalemia, hypocalcemia), toxin (e.g., lead, recreational drugs), trauma.
- Seizures – hypoglycemia, central nervous system (CNS) disorders.
- GIT – mechanical obstruction, gastroenteritis (e.g., dietary indiscretion), parasites, inflammatory diseases.
- PU/PD – urine concentration disorders (e.g., diabetes insipidus).
- Lower urinary tract disease – infection, urolithiasis.

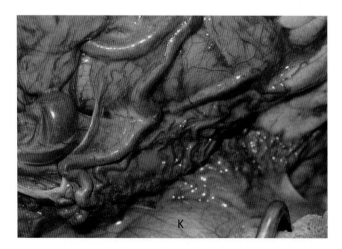

■ **Fig. 134.2.** Multiple acquired shunts near the kidney of a dog. K, kidney.

DIAGNOSTICS

Complete Blood Count/Biochemistry/Urinalysis

- CBC – microcytosis, hypochromasia, mild nonregenerative anemia, leukocytosis, target cells (dogs), poikilocytes (cat).
- Biochemistry profile – decreased albumin, cholesterol, blood urea nitrogen (BUN), glucose, decreased creatinine, increased alkaline phosphatase (ALKP) (young animal – bone isoenzyme activity), variable elevated hepatocellular enzymes (usually no more than 2–3 times reference range).
- Urinalysis – isosthenuria, hyposthenuria, ammonium biurate crystalluria, active sediment if urolithiasis (hematuria, pyuria, proteinuria), bacteria if secondary urinary tract infection (UTI).

Other Laboratory Tests

- Paired bile acids (liver function test) – fasting or baseline may be normal or elevated, 2-h postprandial usually markedly high (>100 μmol/L); always use paired samples around meal ingestion, no need to fast. Preference is to have paired sample and to obtain quantitative value.
- Ammonia (liver function test) – basal ammonia may be normal or elevated; elevated ammonia with ammonia tolerance test. Need in-house ammonia analyzer.
- Coagulation tests – normal to prolonged.
- Protein C – <70% with PSVA, >70% with PVH, MVD.

Imaging

- Radiographs: findings not specific for disease. Microhepatica, renomegaly, urolithiasis (ammonium urate stones are radiolucent, but may combine with other radiodense mineral stones such as struvite or calcium oxalate).
- Ultrasound (US): user-sensitive imaging modality.
  - Microhepatica, urolithiasis (kidney, ureter, bladder). Findings supportive of a shunt: anomalous vessel connecting to portal vein, turbulent flow in vena cava. Shunt localization possible, easier with intrahepatic shunts (Figure 134.3).
  - Microbubble injection can be used to identify shunt (splenic injection of heparinized blood with microbubbles with hepatic US observation for hepatopetal delivery).

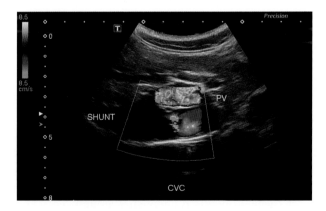

■ **Fig. 134.3.** Abdominal ultrasound image of an intrahepatic shunt. CVC, caudal vena cava; PV, portal vein.

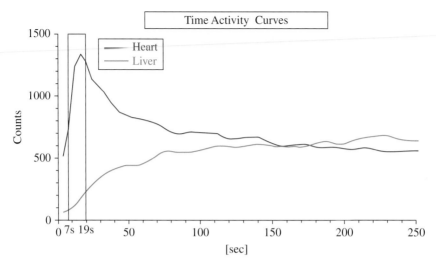

■ **Fig. 134.4.** Transplenic nuclear scintigraphy demonstrating time activity curve with increased uptake of the radionucleotide in the heart before the liver which indicates a portosystemic shunt.

- Scintigraphy: use of radioisotopes requires approved facilities. Gamma-camera acquires dynamic images of radiopharmaceutical uptake in heart and liver, with appearance in the heart first indicative of a shunt. Shunt fraction ≤15% = normal; shunt fraction >60% consistent with shunt with 100% sensitivity.
  - Transcolonic: radiopharmaceutical given per rectum. Can detect presence of a shunt but cannot determine shunt number, termination, or classify as intra- or extrahepatic.
  - Transplenic: radiopharmaceutical given into spleen with ultrasound guidance. Requires less radiopharmaceutical so faster clearance. Can detect presence of a shunt, can determine shunt number, termination (portoazygous, portocaval, multiple acquired), but cannot classify as intra- or extrahepatic (Figure 134.4).
- Computed tomography (CT) angiography: dual-phase to evaluate portal, venous, and arterial vasculature (Figure 134.5). Considered gold standard in people. Noninvasive, cross-sectional, with additional processing options such as three-dimensional (3D) reconstruction (Figure 134.6). Can detect presence of shunt, determine shunt number, termination and can classify as intra- or extrahepatic. Can be performed with heavy sedation or general anesthesia.
- Magnetic resonance imaging (MRI) angiography: cross-sectional, additional processing options (3D reconstruction), noninvasive. Increased time and cost compared to CT angiography.
- Portography: operative technique, requiring portable fluoroscopy or temporary closure of abdomen to make images.
  - Most commonly performed with jejunal or splenic vein catheterized for contrast injection.
  - Percutaneous ultrasound-guided splenic injection.
  - Retrograde transjugular or transfemoral vein.

Pathologic Findings

- Necropsy: small liver, presence of shunt or multiple acquired shunts.
- Histopathology of liver biopsy: hypoplasia of intrahepatic portal tributaries, hepatocellular lobular atrophy, arterial proliferation or duplication, bile duct proliferation, lipogranulomas, cytoplasmic vacuolar changes, increased lymphatics around central veins, smooth muscle hypertrophy, Kupffer cell hypertrophy.

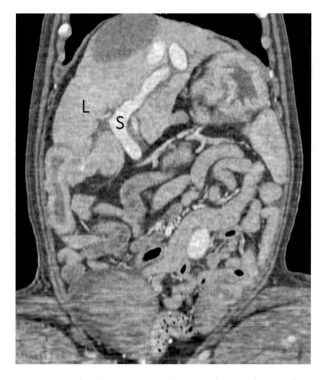

■ **Fig. 134.5.** Dorsal reconstruction of a CT angiogram with an intrahepatic shunt. L, liver parenchyma; S, shunt.

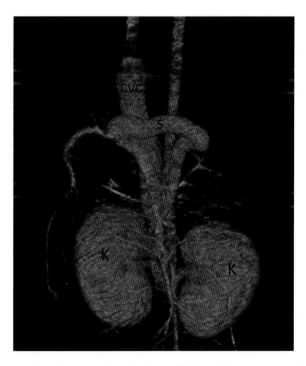

■ **Fig. 134.6.** 3D reconstruction of an extrahepatic shunt. CVC, caudal vena cava; K, kidney; PV, portal vein; S, shunt.

THERAPEUTICS

- Attenuation of shunt vessel is treatment of choice for patients with CPSS.
- Prior to intervention, patients should receive medical management for 2–4 weeks to reduce circulating levels of ammonia and other neurotoxins.
- Medical management is indicated for long-term management when surgery is not possible or declined.
- Multiple acquired shunts are only managed medically.
- Goals are to decrease absorption of ammonia or neurotoxins from GIT, increase removal of ammonia from circulation, and improve ammonia conversion through urea cycle.
- Emergency medical management may be needed for patients with severe HE or hypoglycemia.

Drug(s) of Choice

- Lactulose: traps ammonia as ammonium and is expelled with feces. Laxative to decrease GIT transit time for reduced ammonia absorption. Can be administered orally 0.5–1.0 mL/kg q6–8h to effect or per rectum 5–10 mL/kg.
- Antibiotic: change or decrease urease-producing bacteria in the GIT. Commonly used drugs with low systemic absorption include neomycin 22 mg/kg q8h, metronidazole 7–10 mg/kg q12h, ampicillin 22 mg/kg q6–8h. Caution with neomycin if kidney disease present.
- Levetiracetam (20 mg/kg q8h): used in patients that have had nonhypoglycemic seizures or severe neurologic clinical signs. May have protective effect for postintervention seizure formation.
- Antacids: proton pump inhibitors (omeprazole 1 mg/kg q24h) or H2 blockers (famotidine 1 mg/kg q24h) should be used especially for intrahepatic shunts where GIT bleeding is more common.
- Emergency medications.
  - Lactulose enema.
  - Plasma if coagulopathy.
  - Mannitol if suspect cerebral edema.
  - Dextrose if hypoglycemic seizures.
  - Seizures: midazolam and/or propofol. Caution with use of diazepam especially if seizure is HE induced. Once seizure is controlled, loading doses of levetiracetam, potassium bromide, sodium bromide, or phenobarbital can be considered.

Precautions/Interactions

- Caution when using NSAIDs, steroids or medications that increase risk of GIT hemorrhage.
- Avoid high dietary protein.
- Sedatives and anesthesia may have prolonged effects due to decreased liver metabolism and interactions with GABA receptors.

Alternative Drugs

- Hepatoprotective medications: can be used especially if underlying liver disease is present. SAMe 17–22 mg/kg q24h. Milk thistle 8–20 mg/kg q8h, vitamin E 15 IU/kg q24h, ursodeoxycholic acid 10–15 mg/kg q24h.
- Probiotic cultures, acarbose, L-ornithine,-L-aspartate: have been used to manage HE in people.

Appropriate Health Care

- Attenuation of the CPSS will improve survival times and quality of life.
- Long-term medical management should be instituted when surgery is not possible or declined.
- Avoid breeding.

Nursing Care

No specific recommendations beyond expected care for hospitalized patients.

Diet

- Balanced, readily digestible diet that has some protein restriction. Commercial liver diets can be used and supplemented.
- Diet must contain protein to avoid muscle catabolism. Consider working with a nutritionist to establish the ideal protein quantity.
- Milk, plant or soy-based protein is favored over meat-based protein.

Activity

Normal.

Surgical Considerations

- Gradual attenuation of a CPSS is recommended to reduce complications. Gradual occluder devices (ameroid, cellophane) take weeks to close.
- Surgical procedures are most common for attenuation of EHPSS.
- Interventional vascular procedures or surgery for attenuation of IHPSS.
- Acute complete occlusion of the shunt is rarely tolerated and may result in death or severe complications.
- Liver biopsy of at least two lobes is recommended at the time of shunt attenuation.

Surgery

- Ameroid constrictor: device made of outer ring of stainless steel and inner ring of casein that will absorb fluid and expand inward and induce fibrosis. Device placed around shunt close to systemic insertion (Figure 134.7).
- Cellophane: placed around shunt vessel close to systemic insertion (Figure 134.8). Induces fibrosis. May be less effective in cats.
- Hydraulic occluder device: device that is inflatable via a subcutaneous placed injection port (Figure 134.9). Rarely used.
- Suture ligation: silk suture placed around shunt and tightened to tolerable reduction in flow. Typically done in conjunction with portal pressure measurement. Rarely used.

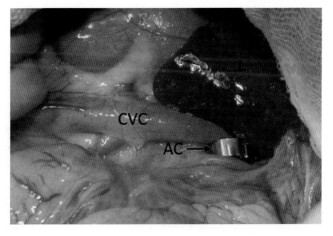

■ **Fig. 134.7.** Intraoperative view of an ameroid constrictor placed around extrahepatic shunt vessel as it terminates in caudal vena cava. AC, ameroid constrictor; CVC, caudal vena cava; L, liver.

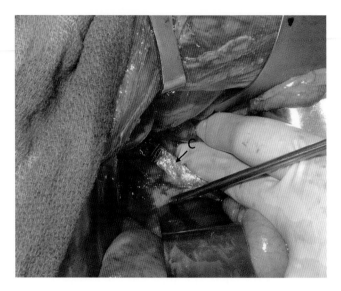

■ **Fig. 134.8.** Intraoperative view of cellophane placed around extrahepatic portosystemic shunt. C, cellophane with hemoclips placed across.

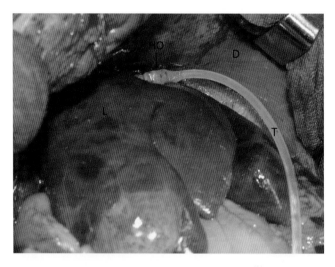

■ **Fig. 134.9.** Intraoperative view of hydraulic occluder placed around intrahepatic portosystemic shunt. D, diaphragm; HO, hydraulic occluder; L, liver; T, tubing.

Interventional Vascular Procedures

- Percutaneous transjugular coil embolization (PTCE) is minimally invasive and can be performed for both extra- and intrahepatic shunts.
- Used more commonly for intrahepatic shunts.
- Requires fluoroscopy and endovascular equipment and expertise.
- Stent placed into vena cava at level of shunt and coils are placed into shunt while monitoring portal pressures.
- May require multiple procedures.
- Reduced complications compared to surgery for intrahepatic shunts.

COMMENTS

Client Education

- Immediately after surgery, patients must remain on medical management because the shunt is still patent.
- Patients are hospitalized for 1–2 days after surgery for monitoring.
- Patients with bladder stones should have them removed at the time of shunt surgery.

Patient Monitoring

- Clinical signs and bile acids are most commonly used to assess outcome. Imaging modalities can be used to further evaluate patients that have elevated bile acids or continued or recurrent clinical signs.
- Clinical signs: patients should have a reduction in clinical signs on medical management alone. Following surgery, the clinical signs should continue to improve until normal.
- Bile acids: paired samples are monitored every 6–8 weeks until normal or stable. Should be improved compared to preoperative samples. Bile acids commonly stay mildly elevated due to microvascular changes in the liver.
- Complete blood count and biochemistry profile: can be monitored for improvement in any abnormalities noted.
- Scintigraphy: can be performed at 8–12 weeks after surgery to assess for shunting. If shunting is identified, need additional imaging to determine if abnormal flow is persistent through shunt or from multiple acquired shunts secondary to surgery.
- CT: can be performed to evaluate portal, venous, and arterial hepatic vasculature and determine if there is persistent shunting or formation of multiple acquired shunts.

Prevention/Avoidance

Ask about family history when acquiring breeds that are overrepresented.

Possible Complications

Acute

- Acute portal hypertension: can range in severity from mild ascites to hypovolemic shock, hemorrhagic diarrhea, abdominal pain, vomiting, and death. Uncommon when performing gradual occlusion using cellophane or ameroid or PTCE. Mild ascites is self-limiting and will resolve. Can monitor abdominal girth after surgery.
- Hemorrhage: bleeding is uncommon complication from surgery. Patients may have coagulation abnormalities but rarely clinical. Hetastarch, long anesthesia, and hypothermia may increase the risk of bleeding
- Hypoglycemia: most common in young and toy breeds. Fairly common and blood glucose should be monitored during anesthesia and after surgery. Treat with dextrose until eating and blood glucose levels are maintained.
- Seizures: may be mild or can be intractable and may be more common in cats. See above treatment recommendations. If intractable, may consider mechanical ventilation for 12–24 h with medical management. Patients treated with levetiracetam prior to surgery may have reduced rates of postoperative seizures.

Long Term

- Chronic portal hypertension: patients may be at risk of developing multiple acquired shunts.
- Persistence or recurrence of clinical signs: may indicate persistent shunting through vessel, additional congenital shunt vessel not detected initially, or formation of multiple acquired shunts.

Expected Course and Prognosis

- Mortality rates for dogs with EHPSS.
  - 7% with ameroid constrictor placement.
  - 6–9% with cellophane banding.
  - 2–32% with suture placement.
- Mortality rates for dogs with IHPSS.
  - 1% with PTCE.
  - 0–9% with ameroid constrictor.
  - 27% with cellophane banding.
  - 6–23% with suture placement.
- Mortality rates for cats.
  - 0–4% with ameroid constrictor or suture.
  - 0–23% with cellophane banding.
- Outcome for dogs with EHPSS – good to excellent in 78–94%.
- Outcome for dogs with IHPSS – good to excellent in 81%.
- Outcome for cats.
  - Postoperative complications more common.
  - Good to excellent outcome in 56–80%.

Synonyms

- Liver shunt
- Patent ductus venosus
- Portoazygous shunt
- Portocaval shunt

Abbreviations

- 3D = three-dimensional
- ALKP = alkaline phosphatase
- BUN = blood urea nitrogen
- CNS = central nervous system
- CPSS = congenital portosystemic shunt
- CT = computed tomography
- EHPSS = extrahepatic portosystemic shunts
- GABA = gamma-aminobutyric acid
- GIT = gastrointestinal tract
- HAVM = hepatic arteriovenous malformation
- HE = hepatic encephalopathy
- IHPSS = intrahepatic portosystemic shunt
- MRI = magnetic resonance imaging
- MVD = microvascular dysplasia
- NSAID = nonsteroidal antiinflammatory drug
- PTCE = percutaneous coil embolization
- PU/PD = polyuria/polydipsia
- PVH = portal vein hypoplasia
- SAMe = S-adenosylmethionine
- UTI = urinary tract infection

See Also

- Arteriovenous Malformation of the Liver
- Hepatic Encephalopathy
- Hepatoportal Microvascular Dysplasia
- Nutritional Approach to Hepatobiliary Diseases
- Portosystemic Shunting, Acquired
- Ptyalism

Suggested Reading

Berent AC, Tobias KM. Hepatic vascular anomalies. In: Johnston SA, Tobias KM, eds. Veterinary Surgery Small Animal, 2nd ed. St Louis: Elsevier Saunders, 2017, pp. 1852–1886.

Greenhalgh SN, Reeve JA. Long-term survival and quality of life in dogs with clinical signs associated with a congenital portosystemic shunt after surgical or medical treatment. J Am Vet Med Assoc 2014;245:527–533.

Klopp L, Marolf AJ. Portosystemic shunts. In: Monet E, ed. Small Animal Soft Tissue Surgery. Ames: John Wiley & Sons, 2013.

Thieman Mankin KM. Current concepts in congenital portosystemic shunts. Vet Clin North Am 2015;45:477–487.

Weisse C, Berent AC. Endovascular evaluation and treatment of intrahepatic posrtosystemic shunts in dogs: 100 cases (2001–2011). J Am Vet Med Assoc 2014;244:78–94.

Acknowledgments: The authors and editors acknowledge the prior contribution of Dr Sharon Center.

Authors: Kathleen L. Ham DVM, MS, DACVS-SA, James Howard DVM, MS, Amy N. Zide DVM, Nina R. Kieves DVM, DACVS-SA, DACVSMR

Diseases of the Biliary Tract

Chapter 135

Bile Duct Obstruction (Extrahepatic)

DEFINITION/OVERVIEW

Any pathologic process that impairs bile flow from liver and gallbladder (GB) to duodenum can result in extrahepatic biliary duct obstruction (EHBDO).

ETIOLOGY/PATHOPHYSIOLOGY

- Cholestasis caused by biliary tree obstruction at the level of the common bile duct (CBD) causing extrahepatic bile duct obstruction or at the level of the hepatic ducts. Obstruction at the level of the hepatic duct(s) may involve one, several, or all hepatic ducts. EHBDO may result from intraluminal obstruction (cholelithiasis, inspissated bile, liver flukes), extraluminal compression (pancreatitis, neoplasia, diaphragmatic hernia) or mural thickening (biliary neoplasia, cholecystitis, cholangitis, stricture).
- In dogs, pancreatitis and neoplasia are most common causes of EHBDO.
- In cats, neoplasia, pancreatitis, cholelithiasis, liver flukes (*Platynosomum concinnum*), and foreign bodies are most common causes of EHBDO.
- Serious hepatobiliary injury may follow within weeks of duct obstruction secondary to accumulation of inflammatory mediators, neutrophils, noxious bile acids and other bile constituents accumulating in the periductal area; mechanical effect of duct distension (hydrostatic pressure); and oxidative injury.
- Absence of bile salts in small intestines can lead to absorption of endotoxins and subsequent endotoxemia, hypotension, sepsis, and death.
- Biliary cirrhosis, portal hypertension, and acquired portosystemic shunts may develop with EHBO of a duration of six weeks or more.

Systems Affected

- Hepatobiliary – cholelithiasis; cholangiohepatitis; biliary neoplasia; biliary foreign bodies; congenital abnormalities of extrahepatic biliary tract; gallbladder mucocele.
- Gastrointestinal – duodenal foreign body or neoplasia; pancreatitis, pancreatic neoplasia, pancreatic pseudocyst.
- Cardiovascular – perioperative and postoperative hypotension.
- Hemic/lymphatic/immune – thrombosis or coagulopathy.
- Renal/urologic – postoperative renal failure.
- Respiratory – postoperative biliary surgery complications can include pulmonary thromboembolism, acute respiratory distress syndrome, aspiration pneumonia, and overhydration.

Blackwell's Five-Minute Veterinary Consult Clinical Companion: Small Animal Gastrointestinal Diseases, First Edition. Edited by Jocelyn Mott and Jo Ann Morrison.
© 2019 John Wiley & Sons, Inc. Published 2019 by John Wiley & Sons, Inc.
Companion website: www.fiveminutevet.com/gastrointestinal

SIGNALMENT/HISTORY

- EHBDO occurs in dogs and cats.
- Animals predisposed to pancreatitis and choleliths, e.g., GB mucocele (GBM) –hyperlipidemic breeds (e.g., miniature schnauzer, Shetland sheepdog).
- Animals with large duct ductal plate malformation (DPM) phenotype (Caroli's malformation) predisposed to infection and cholelithiasis.
- Siamese have a higher prevalence of cholangiohepatitis and pancreatitis which may progress to EHBDO.
- Choleliths appear more common in small-breed dogs and cats.
- Middle-aged to older animals with acquired diseases; younger animals with DPM.
- No sex predominance is reported.

Risk Factors

- Cholelithiasis.
- Choledochitis.
- Neoplasia.
- Gallbladder mucocele.
- Obstructive biliary sludge and inspissated bile.
- Bile duct malformations: choledochal cysts, polycystic hepatobiliary disease, DPM, Caroli's malformation, cystadenoma encroaching on porta hepatis (cats).
- Parasitic infestation: flukes (cats).
- Extrinsic compression: lymph nodes, neoplasia, pancreatitis, CBD entrapment in diaphragmatic hernia; foreign body obstruction of sphincter of Oddi in duodenum.
- Duct fibrosis: trauma, peritonitis, pancreatitis; major duct involvement in feline cholangitis/cholangiohepatitis.
- Duct stricture: blunt trauma, iatrogenic surgical manipulations.

Historical Findings

- Depend on underlying disorder and "completeness" of EHBDO.
- Progressive lethargy and vague illness.
- Progressive jaundice.
- Weight loss.
- Intermittent vomiting.
- Anorexia.
- Pale (acholic) stools: complete EHBDO.
- Polyphagia: complete EHBDO causes nutrient malassimilation (fat).
- Bleeding tendencies: within 10 days of complete EHBDO, more severe/overt in cats.
- Gastrointestinal ulceration is most common at pyloric–duodenal junction and can result in gastrointestinal bleeding.

CLINICAL FEATURES

- Depend on underlying cause.
- Weight loss.
- Severe jaundice.
- Hepatomegaly unless biliary cirrhosis.
- Cranial mass effect – extrahepatic biliary structures (small dogs and cats).
- Vague cranial abdominal discomfort.

- Bleeding tendencies – chronic EHBDO.
- Orange urine: severe bilirubinuria.
- Dehydration.
- +/– Intermittent fever.

DIFFERENTIAL DIAGNOSIS

- Mass lesions – primary or metastatic hepatobiliary neoplasia.
- Diffuse infiltrative liver disease – neoplastic, inflammatory, hepatic lipidosis, amyloid (rare).
- Infectious hepatitis – bacterial, viral, flukes.
- Decompensated chronic hepatitis.
- Copper-associated hepatopathy.
- Severe hepatic fibrosis/cirrhosis.
- Fulminant hepatic failure.
- Biliary cysts – choledochal (cats), cystadenoma, polycystic liver disease (cats) compressing CBD at porta hepatis, DPM.
- Pancreatitis – CBD stenosis, stricture.
- Hepatic lipidosis (HL) – cats: canalicular collapse causes jaundice.
- Cholangitis/cholangiohepatitis – cats, especially sclerosing or destructive cholangitis form.

DIAGNOSTICS

Complete Blood Count/Biochemistry/Urinalysis

- Anemia – mild nonregenerative (chronic disease) or regenerative (enteric bleeding due to hypertensive splanchnic vasculopathy, ulcerations, coagulopathy due to portal hypertension).
- Leukogram – variable, neutrophilic leukocytosis, left-shifted leukogram with sepsis.
- Liver enzymes – variable; marked increases in alkaline phosphatase (ALP) and gamma-glutamyl transferase (GGT) reflect ductal injury; high alanine aminotransferase (ALT) and aspartate aminotransferase (AST) reflect hepatocyte injury.
- High GGT may indicate severe cholestasis and increased risk of infection and sepsis.
- Hyperbilirubinemia is present in all cases of EHBDO. Total bilirubin may be moderate to markedly high.
- Albumin – variable, usually normal except with EHBDO duration >6 weeks (biliary cirrhosis)
- Globulins – normal or increased.
- Hypercholesterolemia – common.
- Bilirubinuria and bilirubin crystals.
- Absence of urobilinogen – unless enteric bleeding; unreliable definitive test for EHBDO.

Other Laboratory Tests

- Serum bile acids – always markedly increased; superfluous test if hepatobiliary jaundice already suspected.
- Coagulation abnormalities – within 10 days of EHBDO, affected patients develop vitamin K deficiency (prothrombin time (PT) most sensitive); may develop disseminated intravascular coagulation (DIC).
- Fecal examination – acholic stools suggest EHBDO; may be masked by small-volume melena; trematode eggs if fluke infestation.
- Thromboelastography is consistent with hypercoagulability in dogs with EHBDO.

Imaging

- Abdominal radiography – hepatomegaly; variable mass lesion in area of gallbladder, pancreatitis pattern, mineralized cholelith(s) (Figures 135.1, 135.2).
- Abdominal ultrasonography – evidence of obstruction within 72–96 h (distended, tortuous CBD, cystic duct, and intrahepatic bile ducts); may disclose underlying or primary disorder (e.g., pancreatitis, cystic lesions, mass lesions, choleliths).
- Distended common bile duct (greater than 5 mm in cats, 3 mm in dogs) is a useful indicator of EHBDO. The degree of CBD dilation is most affected by duration of biliary obstruction rather than cause.
- Gallbladder wall thickening may be present (feline gallbladder wall thickness >1 mm, canine >3 mm).

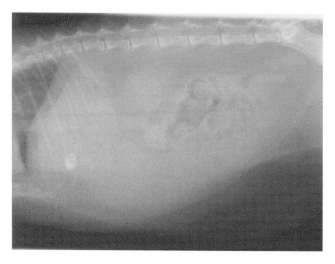

■ **Fig. 135.1.** Lateral abdominal radiograph of a dog with choleliths visible in the cranial ventral aspect. Source: Courtesy of Dr Jim Hoskinson.

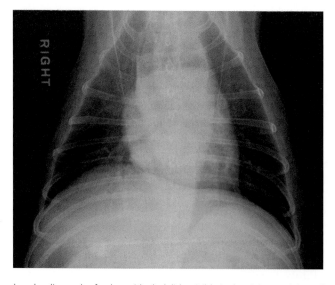

■ **Fig. 135.2.** Ventrodorsal radiograph of a dog with choleliths visible in the right cranial quadrant. Source: Courtesy of Dr Jim Hoskinson.

- The hepatic ducts are usually not seen on ultrasound in cats. Distended intrahepatic ducts often appear tortuous and tubular close to porta hepatis. Although not pathognomonic for EHBDO, dilation of intrahepatic and/or extrahepatic ducts is common in EHBDO in cats. In dogs, dilation of intrahepatic ducts can be an early sign of EHBDO.
- Doppler interrogation may be used to differentiate distended intrahepatic bile ducts from blood vessels.
- Gallbladder may not be distended in EHBDO.
- Common bile duct may remain distended with resolution of EHBDO.
- Hepatobiliary scintigraphy can be used to help determine patency of the bile duct (i.e., complete EHBDO or partial EHBDO).

Diagnostic Procedures

- Hepatic aspiration cytology – used to rule in HL (cats) or sample mass lesions; avoid aspiration of obstructed biliary structures as this may cause bile leakage and peritonitis.
- Laparotomy – allows tissue biopsy; biliary decompression; mass excision: cholelith or inspissated bile removal; creation of biliary–enteric anastomosis; stent insertion.
- Always submit liver and biliary tree biopsies for histology; submit representative samples from all tissues and bile for bacterial culture (aerobic, anaerobic).

Pathologic Findings

- Gross – distended, tortuous bile duct, distended GB: cause often grossly apparent; when obstruction has been present >2 weeks: large, dark green or mahogany-colored liver; chronic complete obstruction of cystic duct associated with white or clear GB bile.
- Microscopic – early: biliary epithelial hyperplasia and bile ductule proliferation and dilation with intraluminal biliary debris (mucin, inflammatory cells, usually neutrophils) and periductular edema, and early fibrosis; chronic distension of biliary structures: leads to devitalized biliary epithelium with necrotic debris, intraluminal suppurative debris, mixed periportal inflammatory infiltrates, periductal edema with thick laminating circumferential fibrosis, multifocal parenchymal necrosis.

 # THERAPEUTICS

Treat underlying condition and achieve biliary decompression.

Drug(s) of Choice

- Antibiotics (depending on underlying cause) may be recommended before and after surgery. Broad-spectrum antimicrobials for potential biliary infections as surgical manipulations may disseminate bacteremia; initially use antibiotics with wide spectrum as follows – triad of: ticarcillin 25 mg/kg IV q8h, metronidazole 7.5 mg/kg IV or PO q12h, enrofloxacin 5 mg/kg PO q12–24h (24-h dose in cats no greater than 5 mg/kg/24h to avoid retinopathy). Postoperative antibiotics may be based on liver and bile cultures.
- *Without biliary decompression, antibiotics are unable to effectively penetrate biliary tract.*
- Vitamin K1: provide 12–36 h before surgery (0.5–1.5 mg/kg IM or SQ), three doses at 12-h intervals. **Caution**: avoid IV administration, may cause anaphylaxis. If chronic EHBDO irresolvable, parenteral vitamin K1 given chronically with frequency titrated using PT; too much vitamin K1 causes hemolytic (Heinz body) anemia in cats.
- Vitamin E (alpha-tocopherol acetate) – 10–100 IU/kg; a larger than normal (normal = 10 IU/kg/day) oral dose needed in chronic EHBDO because of fat malabsorption (lack of enteric bile acids). If chronic EHBDO irresolvable (rare), use polyethylene glycol alpha-tocopherol succinate (TPGS-vitamin E) 10 U/kg/day PO.

- S-adenosylmethionine (SAMe) with proven bioavailability and efficacy as glutathione (GSH) donor – 20 mg/kg/day PO enteric-coated tablet 1–2 h before feeding; provides numerous additional metabolic benefits.
- Ursodeoxycholic acid – 10–15 mg/kg PO per day *after* biliary decompression as a choleretic; ensure adequate hydration to achieve choleresis; *inappropriate before biliary decompression*: can accelerate liver injury in EHBDO. Does not facilitate fat assimilation in chronic EHBDO. Beneficial effects: antifibrotic, antiendotoxic, hepatoprotectant, antiapoptotic, immunomodulator.
- Gastrointestinal protectants – omeprazole (1 mg/kg PO q12h) or pantoprazole (1 mg/kg IV q12h) combined with sucralfate (250 mg–1 g PO q6–8h) for local cytoprotection; stagger sucralfate administration from other oral medications to avoid drug interactions.
- Praziquantel (20–40 mg/kg SQ for three days) to treat liver flukes.

Precautions/Interactions

- Provide biliary decompression before institution of ursodeoxycholic acid.
- Take care to reduce drug dosages for medications eliminated in bile if EHBDO.
- Anticipate possible perioperative complications including hypotension with decreased vasopressor response, reduced myocardial contractility, coagulopathies, decreased wound healing, acute renal failure, hemorrhage, vasovagal reflex, and increased susceptibility to endotoxemia during anesthesia or surgery.

Appropriate Health Care

Inpatient – surgical intervention for EHBDO unless the cause is pancreatitis with prospect for resolution with supportive care.

Nursing Care

- Fluid therapy – depends on underlying conditions; rehydrate and provide maintenance fluids before general anesthesia and surgical interventions; supplement polyionic fluids with potassium chloride and phosphate, judicious electrolyte adjustments based on electrolyte status.
- Water-soluble vitamins – in intravenous fluids; B complex (2 mL/L polyionic fluids).
- Initiate antibiotic therapy before surgery.
- Vitamin K1 – parenteral administration if EHBDO >5–7 days.

Diet

- Maintain nitrogen balance – avoid protein restriction.
- Restrict fat – if overt fat malassimilation caused by lack of enteric bile acids in chronic EHBDO – rare incidence.
- Supplement fat-soluble vitamins – vitamins E and K most urgent; supplementing vitamins D and A can lead to toxicity.
- Water-soluble vitamin E – necessary in chronic EHBDO.

Activity

Depends on patient status and coagulopathy.

Surgical Considerations

- Increasing hyperbilirubinemia with evidence of EHBDO on ultrasound are indications for surgery and decompression of biliary tract. There are many decompressive surgical techniques including cholecystoenterostomy, choledochoenterostomy, cholecystostomy tube placement or choledochal stenting. If choledocholithiasis can be flushed normograde or retrograde, surgical decompression procedures may be avoided.

- Excise masses, remove choleliths and inspissated bile; ensure common duct patency.
- Resect GB – if necrotizing cholecystitis or GB mucocele.
- Biliary–enteric anastomosis – if irresolvable occlusion, fibrosing pancreatitis, or neoplasia; anastomotic stoma at least 2.5 cm wide. Chronic recurrent infection likely after biliary–enteric anastomosis. Temporary stent instead of biliary enteric anastomosis may be complicated by infection and stent obstruction, esp. in cats.
- Refractory hypotension, hemorrhage and bradycardia (vasovagal reflex) – may develop during biliary tree manipulation; ensure availability of emergency drugs (anticholinergics) and ventilatory support for rescue endeavors.
- Ensure IV catheter access and volume expansion – use colloids when necessary, plasma preferred; be prepared for hemorrhage (have blood available for transfusions).
- Sclerosing or destructive feline cholangitis (intrahepatic ductopenia) may clinically emulate EHBDO; does not respond to biliary tree decompression; liver biopsy necessary.

 # COMMENTS

Client Education

- Inform client that surgical biliary decompression is essential (unless resolvable pancreatitis or cholelith obstruction); EHBDO progresses to biliary cirrhosis within six weeks; exception is pancreatitis causing EHBDO that may self-resolve within 2–3 weeks.
- Warn client that surgical success is contingent on underlying cause, results of liver biopsy, infection, and individual variables.
- Inform client that there is high perioperative and postoperative morbidity and mortality with EHBDO dogs and cats.
- Inform client of possible postoperative complications including ascending cholangiohepatitis, hepatic abscesses, stricture/stenosis and/or reobstruction.

Patient Monitoring

- Depends on underlying condition.
- Total bilirubin values acutely reflect biliary decompression; values normalize within days of relief of obstruction.
- Liver enzyme activities – decline slowly.
- Complete blood cell count – repeat q2–3 days initially if septic.
- Bile peritonitis – evaluate abdominal girth, body weight, and fluid accumulation (e.g., by palpation, ultrasonography preferred, abdominocentesis).
- Determine necessity for pancreatic enzyme supplementation based on site of biliary–enteric anastomosis; patients with cholecystojejunostomies may benefit from enzyme supplementation; cannot rely on trypsin-like immunoreactivity (TLI) to estimate pancreatic exocrine adequacy in this circumstance; evaluate body weight and condition; check feces for steatorrhea (fat malassimilation; suspend feces in water and microscopically examine for lipid globules – only relevant if animal is fed a normal fat-containing diet; if steatorrheic after biliary–enteric anastomosis and nonicteric, reduce dietary fat and supplement with pancreatic enzymes). Pancreatic enzymes can induce oral or esophageal ulcers, especially in cats; must be mixed in food and followed by liquid or food to prevent mucosal injury.

Possible Complications

- Bile peritonitis.
- Postoperative ascending cholangiohepatitis +/– hepatic abscesses.
- Restenosis of bile duct – if not bypassed.

- Stenosis of biliary–enteric anastomosis.
- Severe enteric hemorrhage with EHBDO – hypertensive enteric vasculopathy with coagulopathy (vitamin K deficiency).
- Biliary hemorrhage during surgery.
- Septic bacteremia or systemic inflammatory response syndrome during or after surgery.
- Unresponsive hypotension during surgery.
- Vasovagal reflex – biliary tree manipulation.
- Chronic weight loss.
- Chronic vomiting and diarrhea secondary to exocrine pancreatic insufficiency.
- Enterotomy dehiscence.
- Postoperative renal failure.
- Gastrointestinal ulceration.

Expected Course and Prognosis

- Depends on underlying disease.
- Perioperative morbidity and mortality in cats with EHBDO are high and prognosis is guarded.
- Mortality is high in cats with neoplasia as cause of EHBDO.
- Mortality is approximately 40% with nonneoplastic causes of EHBDO in cats.
- Mortality rates for extrahepatic biliary tract surgery are reported between 22% and 64% for dogs and cats.
- Prognosis good if fibrosing pancreatitis and pancreatic inflammation resolve; bile duct patency may return.
- Be aware: biliary tree may appear distended on subsequent ultrasounds.
- Permanent peribiliary fibrosis from EHBDO may occur.
- Cats with sclerosing cholangitis can appear to have EHBDO but show no response to biliary decompression; liver biopsy essential for diagnosis.

Synonyms

- Extrahepatic biliary obstruction

Abbreviations

- ALP = alkaline phosphatase
- ALT = alanine aminotransferase
- AST = aspartate aminotransferase
- CBD = common bile duct
- DIC = disseminated intravascular coagulation
- DPM = ductal plate malformation
- EHBDO = extrahepatic bile duct obstruction
- GB = gallbladder
- GBM = gallbladder mucocele
- GGT = gamma-glutamyl transferase
- GSH = glutathione
- HL = hepatic lipidosis
- PT = prothrombin time
- TLI = trypsin-like immunoreactivity
- TPGS-vitamin E = d-alpha-tocopheryl polyethylene glycol succinate

See Also

- Biliary Neoplasia.
- Biliary Duct or Gallbladder Rupture and Bile Peritonitis
- Cholangitis/Cholangiohepatitis Syndrome
- Cholangitis, Destructive
- Cholecystitis and Choledochitis
- Cholelithiasis
- Coagulopathy of Liver Disease
- Gallbladder Mucocele
- Hepatic Neoplasia, Benign
- Hepatic Neoplasia, Malignant
- Icterus
- Liver Fluke Infestation
- Nutritional Approach to Hepatobiliary Diseases
- Pancreatic Neoplasia
- Pancreatitis, Canine
- Pancreatitis, Feline

Suggested Reading

Bacon NJ, White RA. Extrahepatic biliary tract surgery in the cat: a case series and review. J Small Anim Pract 2003;44(5):231–235.

Baker SG, Mayhew PD, Mehler SJ. Choledochotomy and primary repair of extrahepatic biliary duct rupture in seven dogs and two cats. J Small Anim Pract 2011;52:32–37.

Center SA. Interpretation of liver enzymes. Vet Clin North Am Small Anim Pract 2007;37(2):297–333.

Center SA. Diseases of the gallbladder and biliary tree. Vet Clin North Am Small Anim Pract 2009;39(3):543–598.

Gaillot HA, Penninck DG, Webster CRL, et al. Ultrasonographic features of extrahepatic biliary obstruction in 30 cats. Vet Radiol Ultrasound 2007;48(5):439–447.

Head LL, Daniel GB. Correlation between hepatobiliary scintigraphy and surgery or postmortem examination findings in dogs and cats with extrahepatic biliary obstruction, partial obstruction or patency of the biliary system: 18 cases (1995–2004). J Am Vet Med Assoc 2005;227(10):1618–1624.

Leveille R, Biller DS, Shiroma JT. Sonographic evaluation of the common bile duct in cats. J Vet Intern Med 1996;10(5):296–299.

Mayhew PD, Weisse CW. Treatment of pancreatitis-associated extrahepatic biliary tract obstruction by choledochal stenting in seven cats. J Small Anim Pract 2008;49(3):133–138.

Mayhew PD, Holt DE, McLear RC, et al. Pathogenesis and outcome of extrahepatic biliary obstruction in cats. J Small Anim Pract 2002;43(6):247–253.

Mayhew PD, Savigny MR, Otto CM, et al. Evaluation of coagulation in dogs with partial or complete extrahepatic biliary tract obstruction by means of thromboelastography. J Am Vet Med 2013;242(6):778–785.

Morrison S, Prostredny J, Roa D. Retrospective study of 28 cases of cholecystoduodenostomy performed using endoscopic gastrointestinal anastomosis stapling equipment. J Am Anim Hosp Assoc 2008;44(1):10–18.

Papazoglou LG, Mann FA, Wagner-Mann C, et al. Long-term survival of dogs after cholecystectomy: a retrospective study of 15 cases (1981–2005). J Am Anim Hosp Assoc 2008;44(2):67–74.

Spain HN, Penninck DG, Webster CR, et al. Ultrasonographic and clinicopathologic features of segmental dilatations of the common bile duct in four cats. J Fel Med Surg Open Rep 2017;3(1):1–9.

Acknowledgments: The author and editors acknowledge the prior contribution of Dr Sharon Center.

Author: Jocelyn Mott DVM, DACVIM (SAIM)

Biliary Duct or Gallbladder Rupture and Bile Peritonitis

DEFINITION/OVERVIEW

- Bile peritonitis is the inflammatory response to generalized or localized leakage of bile into the peritoneal cavity.
- Bile in the peritoneal cavity results in severe chemical peritonitis and requires immediate surgical intervention.
- Septic bile peritonitis is associated with a less favorable prognosis and outcome.

ETIOLOGY/PATHOPHYSIOLOGY

- Rupture or leakage of the gallbladder or biliary tract may result from blunt or penetrating abdominal trauma, obstruction, inflammation or infection of the biliary tract.
- Trauma more commonly results in rupture of the common bile duct due to rapid gallbladder emptying and shearing forces.
  - Gallbladder rupture is most commonly associated with necrotizing cholecystitis, with the poorly vascularized fundus being the most common site of rupture.
  - Gallbladder mucocele may result in complete biliary obstruction and bile peritonitis.
- Gallbladder perforations have been classified according to onset and distribution of peritonitis
  - Acute perforation with generalized peritonitis.
  - Subacute perforation with pericholecystic abscess and adhesion formation.
  - Chronic perforation with cholecystoenteric fistula formation.
- Bile salts are toxic to tissues and result in increased tissue permeability of vasculature within the peritoneal membrane and tissue necrosis.
- Bile salts encourage bacterial growth, with most common sources including endogenous anaerobic bacteria from the liver and intestinal tract.
  - The presence of bacteria within the peritoneal cavity results in impaired local host defense mechanisms, reduced phagocytic activity, and increased lipopolysaccharide levels.
- Chemical peritonitis secondary to bile peritonitis can result in severe fluid losses into the peritoneal cavity and resulting hypovolemic shock.
- High morbidity and mortality associated with bile peritonitis are proposed to be due to:
  - Toxic effect of bile salts.
  - Loss of fluid in the peritoneal cavity.
  - Bacterial peritonitis.

Blackwell's Five-Minute Veterinary Consult Clinical Companion: Small Animal Gastrointestinal Diseases, First Edition. Edited by Jocelyn Mott and Jo Ann Morrison.
© 2019 John Wiley & Sons, Inc. Published 2019 by John Wiley & Sons, Inc.
Companion website: www.fiveminutevet.com/gastrointestinal

Systems Affected

- Hepatobiliary – bile peritonitis may result secondary to extrahepatic biliary obstruction secondary to cholecystitis, cholelithiasis, gallbladder mucocele or neoplasia.
- Gastrointestinal – biliary obstruction and bile peritonitis may result in severe peritonitis, pancreatitis, and gastrointestinal hemorrhage.
- Cardiovascular – may result in evidence of hypovolemic shock and hypotension secondary to third space fluid loss. Septic bile peritonitis may result in systemic inflammatory response and septic shock.
- Hematologic – biliary obstruction and lack of bile secretion into the gastrointestinal tract lead to decreased intestinal absorption of vitamin K and a resulting coagulopathy. Systemic inflammation may also result in consumption of coagulation factors and the development of disseminated intravascular coagulopathy.
- Renal – acute tubular necrosis may occur secondary to severe peritonitis and systemic inflammation.
- Respiratory – dyspnea and respiratory complications may occur secondary to bile peritonitis due to pulmonary thromboembolism, aspiration pneumonia or acute respiratory distress syndrome.

 SIGNALMENT/HISTORY

- No breed predilection noted.
- No sex predilection.
- Median age of dogs with biliary rupture secondary to gallbladder disease was 8.1 years.
- Median age of dogs with biliary rupture secondary to trauma was significantly younger at 2.8 years.
- More common in the dog than the cat.

Risk Factors

- Cholecystitis.
- Gallbladder mucocele.
- Cholelithiasis.
- Neoplasia.
- Trauma.

Historical Findings

- Nonspecific findings.
- Vomiting.
- Icterus.
- Inappetence/anorexia.
- Abdominal discomfort.
- Abdominal distension.
- Diarrhea.
- Weight loss.
- Lethargy.

 CLINICAL FEATURES

- Clinical signs can range from mild to severe.
- Icterus.

- Abdominal pain.
- Fever.
- Abdominal distension/fluid wave.
- Cardiovascular shock.
- Tachycardia.
- Hypotension.
- Poor pulse quality.
- Cold extremities.
- Pale mucous membranes.
- Prolonged capillary refill time.
- Septic bile peritonitis was often associated with a shorter duration of clinical signs.
- Chronic signs have been reported and are often associated with a nonseptic effusion.

 DIFFERENTIAL DIAGNOSIS

- Abdominal effusion.
  - Septic peritonitis.
  - Hemoabdomen.
  - Uroabdomen.
  - Pancreatitis.
  - Chylous effusion.
  - Neoplastic effusion.
  - Right-sided congestive heart failure.
- Icterus.
  - Hemolysis.
  - Hepatic disease.
  - Extrahepatic biliary obstruction.
- Abdominal pain.
  - Gastrointestinal obstruction.
  - Peritonitis.
  - Pancreatitis.
  - Torsion/volvulus.

 DIAGNOSTICS

Complete Blood Count/Biochemistry/Urinalysis

- Inflammatory leukogram characterized by neutrophilia and left shift.
- Mild anemia.
- Hemoconcentration.
- Increased alanine aminotransferase (ALT).
- Increased alkaline phosphatase (ALP).
- Hyperbilirubinemia.
- Hypoalbuminemia.
- Hyponatremia.
- Hypokalemia.
- Hypochloremia.
- Azotemia.
- Hypercholesterolemia.
- Bilirubinuria.

Other Laboratory Tests

■ Coagulation panel –prolongation of prothrombin time and partial thromboplastin time.

Imaging

■ Abdominal radiography.
  • Generalized poor serosal detail.
  • Mass effect in the region of the liver.
  • Cholelithiasis.
  • Gas present in the biliary tract.
■ Thoracic radiography.
  • Pleural effusion.
  • Other signs consistent with trauma.
■ Ultrasound.
  • Abdominal effusion.
  • Distended gallbladder.
  • Hyperechoic bile sediment.
  • Distended common bile duct.
  • Perihepatic/pancreatic mass effect.
  • Choleliths.
  • Gas present in the gallbladder.
  • Peritonitis.
  • Gallbladder mucocele (Figure 136.1).
  • Not specific for bile leakage.

Other Diagnostic Tests

■ Abdominocentesis.
  • Most helpful in the diagnosis of bile peritonitis.
  • Abdominal fluid should be collected for cytology and culture.

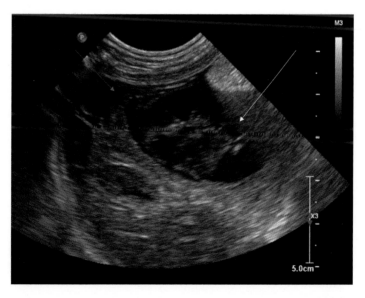

■ **Fig. 136.1.** Abdominal ultrasound of gallbladder mucocele. Red arrow – free peritoneal effusion; white arrow – gallbladder mucocele.

- If a small volume of effusion is present, a four-quadrant paracentesis technique can be utilized.
- If paracentesis is unsuccessful, diagnostic peritoneal lavage can be performed for fluid collection.
- Bilirubin concentration has not been evaluated in samples obtained via diagnostic peritoneal lavage.
- Cytology.
  - Modified transudate that can progress to an exudate later in the disease process.
  - Protein and cellularity increase with time secondary to chemical peritonitis.
  - Grossly, the effusion may appear greenish to yellow-orange.
  - Predominant cell type: neutrophils.
  - Bile pigment or bilirubin crystals may be seen free in the background or engulfed in macrophages.
  - White bile – acellular, amorphous, and fibrillary blue extracellular material may be observed on cytologic analysis.
  - Abdominal fluid to serum bilirubin ratio >2:1
  - 100% sensitivity of bile peritonitis in dogs.
- Culture and sensitivity.
  - Most common bacterial isolate: *Escherichia coli*.
  - Other organisms:
    - *Enterococcus*.
    - *Enterobacter*.
    - *Klebsiella*.
    - *Streptococcus*.
    - *Pseudomonas*.
    - *Bacteroides*.
    - *Actinobacter*.

Pathologic Findings

- Cholecystitis.
- Cystic mucinous hyperplasia.
- Gallbladder necrosis.

 THERAPEUTICS

- Cardiovascular resuscitation.
  - Fluid resuscitation.
    - Crystalloids.
    - Consider fresh frozen plasma for colloidal support.
  - Heat support.
- Correction of electrolyte abnormalities.
- Correction of acid–base abnormalities.
- Pain control.
- Antimicrobial therapy.
- Surgical intervention: bile peritonitis constitutes a surgical emergency. Surgical treatment options include:
  - Primary repair.
  - Biliary diversion.
  - Cholecystectomy.

- Liver biopsy should be considered at the time of surgical intervention.
- Copious abdominal lavage should be performed during surgical management.
- Closed abdominal drainage techniques are often utilized in the postoperative period.
- Jackson–Pratt drains may be used in the postoperative period.

Drug(s) of Choice

- Antimicrobial therapy.
  - Broad-spectrum antibiotic therapy should be initiated pending culture and sensitivity.
  - Sensitivity results demonstrate that bacterial isolates are most commonly sensitive to:
    - Enrofloxacin.
    - Amikacin.
    - Chloramphenicol.
- Pain control. Consider multimodal analgesia.
  - Fentanyl 3 µg/kg IV bolus followed by 3–5 µg/kg/h continuous rate infusion (dogs and cats).
  - Hydromorphone 0.05–0.1 mg/kg IV q4h.
  - Oxymorphone 0.1 mg/kg IV q4–6h (dogs and cats).
  - Methadone 0.1–0.3 mg/kg IV q4h (dogs and cats).
  - Ketamine 0.1–0.2 mg/kg/h (dogs and cats).
  - Lidocaine 30–50 µg/kg/min.
  - Epidural analgesia can be considered for ongoing pain control.
- Antiemetics.
  - Maropitant 1 mg/kg SQ q24h (dogs and cats).
  - Ondansetron 0.1–1 mg/kg IV q8h (dogs and cats).
- Vitamin K1 0.1–1.5 mg/kg SQ/IM q24h for three doses (dogs and cats).
- Pantoprazole 1 mg/kg IV q12h (dogs and cats).
- Metoclopramide 0.3 mg/kg IV bolus considered for prokinetic effects prior to surgical intervention in cases of severe ileus.

Appropriate Health Care

- Bile peritonitis is a surgical emergency.
- Cardiovascular stabilization is essential prior to surgical intervention.
  - Fluid therapy.
  - Vasopressor support.

Nursing Care

- Hospitalization and intensive monitoring are essential postoperatively to optimize successful outcome.
- Patients should be hospitalized and receive 24-h care.
- Cardiovascular status should be monitored closely in the perioperative and postoperative period.
  - Vital signs should be monitored frequently.
  - Blood pressure should be monitored.
  - Hypotension should be treated with fluid therapy and vasopressor support.
  - Electrocardiogram monitoring. Monitor for any arrhythmias.
- Bloodwork and coagulation status should be routinely monitored in the postoperative period.
  - Monitor blood glucose.
  - Monitor packed cell volume and total solids.

Diet

- Feeding tube placement should be highly considered at the time of surgical intervention (esophagostomy or gastrostomy tube).
- Enteral feeding should be initiated once the patient has achieved cardiovascular stability.

Activity

- Patients often have a prolonged recovery and critical postoperative period.
- Activity should be restricted for a minimum of two weeks to allow for recovery and incisional healing.

Surgical Considerations

- Bile peritonitis is a surgical emergency.
- Several surgical techniques can be utilized in the management of bile peritonitis.

 # COMMENTS

Client Education

Bile peritonitis requires immediate intervention.

Patient Monitoring

- Patients should be monitored very closely in the immediate postoperative period.
- Cardiovascular status should be closely monitored.
- Enteral nutrition should be provided early in the postoperative period.

Possible Complications

- Postoperative complications are common.
- Complications often include:
  - Anemia.
  - Hypoproteinemia.
  - Disseminated intravascular coagulopathy.
  - Pancreatitis.
  - Hypotension.
  - Surgical site dehiscence.
  - Arrhythmias.
  - Hepatic encephalopathy.

Expected Course and Prognosis

- Overall mortality for dogs and cats with bile peritonitis is 50%.
- The most common cause of death is euthanasia.
- Most significant factor affecting survival is the presence or absence of bacteria.
  - Up to 73% mortality for septic bile peritonitis reported.
  - One report showed 27% survival with septic bile peritonitis vs 100% survival in animals with a negative culture.
- Increased creatinine prior to surgery associated with higher mortality.
- Increased blood urea nitrogen was not associated with outcome.
- Elevated partial thromboplastin time prior to surgery associated with higher mortality.
- Survivors have been reported to have lower white blood cell counts in comparison to nonsurvivors.

- Postoperative hypotension associated with higher mortality (mean arterial pressure less than 70 mmHg).
- Dogs with positive cultures often had a shorter duration of clinical signs.
- Traumatic bile peritonitis has a reportedly better prognosis.

See Also

- Bile Duct Obstruction (Extrahepatic)
- Cholecystitis and Choledochitis
- Gallbladder Mucocele
- Icterus

Suggested Reading

Amsellem PM, Seim HB, MacPhail CM, et al. Long-term survival and risk factors associated with biliary surgery in dogs: 34 cases (1994–2004). J Am Vet Med Assoc 2006;229:1451–1457.

Ludwig LL, McLoughlin MA, Graves TK, et al. Surgical treatment of bile peritonitis in 24 dogs and 2 cats: a retrospective study (1987–1994). Vet Surg 1997;26:90–98.

Mehler SJ. Complications of the extrahepatic biliary surgery in companion animals. Vet Clin North Am Small Anim Pract 2011;41:949–967.

Mehler SJ, Mayhew PD, Drobatz KJ, et al. Variables associated with outcome in dogs undergoing extrahepatic biliary surgery: 60 cases (1988–2002). Vet Surg 2004;33:644–649.

Owens SD, Gossett R, McElhaney MR, et al. Three cases of canine bile peritonitis with mucinous material in abdominal fluid as the prominent cytologic finding. Vet Clin Pathol 2003;32:114–120.

Author: Rebecca A.L. Walton DVM, DACVECC

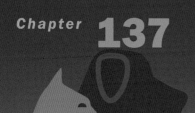

Chapter**137**

Biliary Neoplasia

DEFINITION/OVERVIEW

- Uncommon tumor in dogs and cats.
- Arises from the epithelial cells lining the intra- or extrahepatic bile ducts or gallbladder; less commonly, neuroendocrine carcinoma (carcinoid) has been reported to arise within the biliary system.
- May be benign (more common in cats) or malignant (more common in dogs).
- Dogs.
    - Most common primary biliary neoplasm is bile duct carcinoma (cholangiocarcinoma).
    - Malignant neoplasm arising from the epithelial cells lining the biliary ducts and/or gallbladder.
    - Cholangiocarcinoma is the second most common malignant hepatobiliary tumor in dogs after hepatocellular carcinoma.
    - More likely to be intrahepatic.
- Cats.
    - Most common primary hepatobiliary neoplasm is bile duct adenoma (biliary cystadenoma).
    - Benign epithelial neoplasia arising from the cells lining the biliary ducts or gallbladder.
    - May undergo malignant transformation into cystadenocarcinoma.
    - Most common malignant hepatobiliary tumor in cats is cholangiocarcinoma.
- Biliary neoplasia presents as a single tumor (massive form) in 37–46% of cases, multifocal (nodular form) in up to 54%, or diffuse in 17–54%.
- Cholangiocarcinoma is highly metastatic in both species, with metastasis occurring in up to 88% of dogs and 67–80% of cats.
- Common metastatic sites for malignant biliary neoplasms include the regional lymph nodes, lungs, and peritoneum (carcinomatosis).
- Other metastatic sites include intestine, pancreas, heart, spleen, kidney, spinal cord, urinary bladder, and bone.
- Hepatobiliary neuroendocrine carcinoma (carcinoid) has an aggressive biologic behavior with a metastatic risk of 93% in dogs.

ETIOLOGY/PATHOPHYSIOLOGY

- The development of a mass effect and/or neoplastic infiltration within the biliary system may cause a variety of clinical problems in dogs and cats. However, in some cases, there may be no clinical signs and the tumor is found incidentally when the patient is being evaluated routinely or for an unrelated problem.

Blackwell's Five-Minute Veterinary Consult Clinical Companion: Small Animal Gastrointestinal Diseases, First Edition. Edited by Jocelyn Mott and Jo Ann Morrison.
© 2019 John Wiley & Sons, Inc. Published 2019 by John Wiley & Sons, Inc.
Companion website: www.fiveminutevet.com/gastrointestinal

- For some patients, laboratory abnormalities may be noted on routine screening, leading to additional diagnostics that ultimately identify the tumor(s).
- In severe cases, biliary neoplasia can lead to both intra- and extrahepatic biliary obstruction(s), which can secondarily lead to hepatic dysfunction, pancreatitis, and gastrointestinal distress.

Systems Affected

- Hepatobiliary – mass effect and/or infiltration of the liver, gallbladder, and associated biliary tree.
- Exocrine – pancreatitis secondary to direct compression/infiltration and/or mechanical extrahepatic biliary obstruction.
- Gastrointestinal – anorexia and vomiting secondary to pancreatitis and/or biliary obstruction.
- Respiratory – pulmonary metastasis.
- Metabolic – weight loss (cancer cachexia).
- Hemic – coagulopathy secondary to hepatic dysfunction.
- Renal – acute kidney injury secondary to systemic inflammation seen with pancreatitis and/or bile peritonitis.
- Skin – paraneoplastic alopecia along the ventral abdomen in cats with biliary carcinoma.

SIGNALMENT/HISTORY

- Dogs and cats both affected.
- Affected animals typically >10 years of age.
- Possible predilection for Labrador retrievers.
- Possible predisposition for female dogs.
- Male cats may be predisposed.

Risk Factors

- Potential association between cholangiocarcinoma and trematode (hookworms, whipworms) infection.
- Carcinoma of the canine biliary tract has been experimentally induced by N-ethyl-N′-nitro-N-nitrosoguanidine.

Historical Findings

- Anorexia.
- Lethargy.
- Weight loss.
- Vomiting.
- Polydipsia and polyuria.
- Icterus.
- Abdominal distension.

CLINICAL FEATURES

- Hepatomegaly +/– discretely palpable abdominal mass or mass effect.
- Icterus.
- Abdominal distension due to ascites.

- Abdominal pain.
- Cachexia.
- Paraneoplastic alopecia may be present in cats with biliary carcinoma.

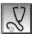

DIFFERENTIAL DIAGNOSIS

- Hepatocellular adenoma (hepatoma).
- Hepatocellular carcinoma.
- Biliary cystadenoma.
- Hepatic nodular hyperplasia.
- Cirrhosis.
- Chronic active hepatitis.
- Hepatic abscess.
- Gallbladder mucocele.

DIAGNOSTICS

The following laboratory tests are part of routine evaluation of sick patients and may show significant abnormalities as listed below; however, these changes are not necessarily specific for neoplastic disease and simply indicate insult to or insufficiency within the biliary system.

Complete Blood Count/Biochemistry/Urinalysis

- Complete blood cell count – anemia, leukocytosis.
- Serum biochemical profile.
  - Elevated hepatic enzyme (e.g., ALP, GGT, ALT, AST) activity.
  - Hyperbilirubinemia.
  - Hypoalbuminemia.
  - Azotemia (especially cats).
- Urinalysis – bilirubinuria may be present in cats.

Other Laboratory Tests

- Coagulation profile.
  - Prolongation of prothrombin (PT) and partial thromboplastin time (PTT).
  - Elevation in D-dimers and fibrinogen.
- Bile acid assay.
  - Elevation in pre- and (most importantly) postprandial bile acids.
- Alpha-fetoprotein (an oncofetal glycoprotein): elevated in 55% of dogs with bile duct carcinoma and may help differentiate neoplastic from nonneoplastic lesions in dogs.

Imaging

The following imaging tests are commonly performed once a pathologic process involving the abdominal cavity has been recognized.

Abdominal Radiography

- May localize a mass or mass effect to the hepatobiliary region.
- May demonstrate loss of detail in patients with ascites.
- May demonstrate caudal and lateral displacement of the stomach.
- May demonstrate mineralization of the biliary tree.

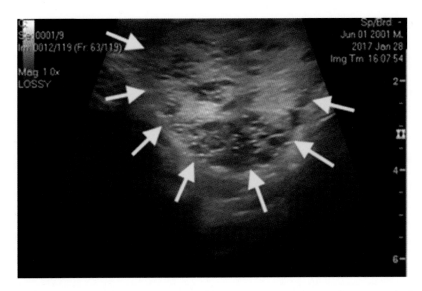

■ **Fig. 137.1.** Biliary cystadenoma in a cat. Note the fairly well-circumscribed mass effect within the liver (arrow). Both solid and characteristic cystic components are noted within this mass.

Abdominal Ultrasonography
- Will identify peritoneal effusion.
- May identify location of lesions.
- Aids in characterization of lesions.
  - Massive, nodular, or diffuse.
  - Cystic (Figure 137.1) or solid.
  - Dilated and tortuous biliary tract.
  - Dilated and/or thickened gallbladder.
- Helps assess for intraabdominal metastasis.
- Used to guide fine needle aspirate cytology or biopsy of lesion(s).

Thoracic Radiography (Three Views)
Used to screen for pulmonary metastasis.

Computed Tomography (CT) and Magnetic Resonance Imaging (MRI)
- More sensitive and specific in characterization of lesion(s).
- Can detect smaller lesions not visible on ultrasound.
- May provide indication of tumor type (especially for feline biliary cystadenomas).
- Can better assess relationship of tumor(s) to other structures for surgical planning.
- More sensitive indicator of pulmonary metastasis than radiography.

Other Diagnostic Tests
- Abdominocentesis and cytologic evaluation of peritoneal fluid, if present. May confirm carcinomatosis.
- Ultrasound-guided fine needle aspirate cytology or Tru-Cut™ biopsy.
  - Agreement between cytology and histopathology varies amongst studies.
  - There is greater likelihood of correct diagnosis (up to 90%) with biopsy.
  - Coagulation prolife is recommended prior to such procedures, as moderate to severe bleeding is a complication that may occur in ~5% of cases.
- Laparoscopy or laparotomy may be used to obtain larger sample for definitive diagnosis.

Pathologic Findings

- Gross findings.
  - Morphologic types of hepatobiliary tumors include massive, nodular, or diffuse.
  - Can be intrahepatic (most common in dogs), extrahepatic, or within the gallbladder (rare).
  - Malignant lesions often involve multiple lobes, whereas benign lesions (adenomas/cystadenomas) tend to be solitary.
- Histopathologic findings.
  - Histologic subtypes of bile duct carcinoma include solid (cholangiocarcinoma) and cystic (biliary cystadenocarcinoma) forms.
  - Histologic classification (solid vs cystic) is not prognostic.
  - Immunohistochemistry for hepatocyte paraffin-1 and claudin-7 may be needed to distinguish between hepatocellular and biliary neoplasms, respectively.
  - Immunohistochemical staining for neuron-specific enolase (NSE) can help confirm neuroendocrine etiology.

 # THERAPEUTICS

- Patients should first be stabilized with general supportive care in order to correct dehydration and manage pain.
- Once deemed stable, complete surgical excision of the tumor is the treatment of choice. Up to 80% of the liver can be resected if the remaining liver tissue is functional.
- If a biliary cystadenoma (cats) is identified and the tumor is confined to one or two lobes, long-term local control and survival is likely after complete surgical removal.
- If a biliary or neuroendocrine carcinoma is identified, liver lobectomy can be performed if the tumor is localized to a single liver lobe (i.e., massive form).
- More often, these are multifocal or diffuse morphologies for which no effective surgical treatment exists.

Drug(s) of Choice

- Chemotherapy – no effective protocol identified.
- There are anecdotal reports of the use of Palladia® (toceranib phosphate) and metronomic chemotherapy for advanced hepatobiliary neoplasia, but no published data exist.

Precautions/Interactions

Medications requiring metabolism by the liver or relying upon enterohepatic circulation should be used with caution (i.e., avoid altogether or significantly reduce dose) if evidence of hepatic dysfunction.

Alternative Drugs

It is unknown whether the use of hepatoprotective nutraceuticals provides any therapeutic benefit for biliary neoplasms.

Appropriate Health Care

- General supportive measures include the following.
  - Intravenous fluids.
  - Antiemetics.
  - Analgesics.
  - Appetite stimulants.

- Antiinflammatories.
- Nutrition (enteral or parenteral).

Diet

- Low-protein diet may be instituted for patients with hepatic insufficiency.
- Low-fat diet can be considered for patients with evidence of secondary pancreatitis.

Surgical Considerations

- Hepatic dysfunction may alter the metabolism of some anesthetic drugs, so such agents should be used with caution and the use of lower doses or alternative drugs considered (ideally under the guidance of a board-certified internist or anesthesiologist).
- Coagulopathies secondary to hepatic dysfunction may be present and thus special attention should be paid to hemostasis.
- Blood products such as plasma should be considered as indicated based on laboratory test results, ideally under the guidance of a board-certified surgeon or critical care specialist.

 COMMENTS

Client Education

As above.

Patient Monitoring

Physical examination, lab work (especially liver enzymes), abdominal ultrasonography, and thoracic radiography should be performed periodically after tumor resection in order to screen for tumor recurrence and/or metastasis.

Prevention/Avoidance

Anthelmintic therapy is warranted due to the potential association between bile duct carcinoma and infection with trematodes.

Possible Complications

- Tumor rupture and/or hemorrhage.
- Biliary obstruction.
- Pancreatitis.
- Hepatic dysfunction leading to hepatic encephalopathy and/or coagulopathy.

Expected Course and Prognosis

- Excellent prognosis following complete resection of benign biliary tumors in cats.
- Biliary carcinoma is an aggressive cancer with a high rate of metastasis in both dogs and cats.
- Widespread intraperitoneal carcinomatosis is common in cats.
- Guarded to poor prognosis for patient with nonresectable and/or advanced disease at the time of diagnosis.
- Even with surgical resection, most patients die within six months of surgery due to local recurrence and/or metastasis.
- Biliary neuroendocrine carcinoma (carcinoid) is also very aggressive with a high metastatic rate and associated poor prognosis.

Abbreviations

- ALP = alkaline phosphatase
- ALT = alanine aminotransferase
- AST = aspartate aminotransferase
- CT = computed tomography
- GGT = gamma-glutamyl transferase

- MRI = magnetic resonance imaging
- NSE = neuron-specific enolase
- PT = prothrombin time
- PTT = partial thromboplastin time

Suggested Reading

Liptak JM. Hepatobiliary tumors. In: Withrow SJ, Vail DM, eds. Small Animal Clinical Oncology, 5th ed. St Louis: Saunders Elsevier, 2013, pp. 405–410.

Patnaik AK, Lieberman PH, Erlandson RA, Antonescu C. Hepatobiliary neuroendocrine carcinoma in cats: a clinicopathologic, immunohistochemial, and ultrastructural study of 17 cases. Vet Pathol 2005;42:331–337.

Selmic LE. Hepatobiliary neoplasia. Vet Clin Small Anim 2017;47:725–735.

Van Sprundel R, van den Ingh T, Guscetti F, et al. Classification of primary hepatic tumors in the dog. Vet J 2013;197:596–606.

Van Sprundel R, van den Ingh T, Guscetti F, et al. Classification of primary hepatic tumors in the cat. Vet J 2014;202:255–266.

Authors: Christine Mullin VMD, DACVIM (Oncology), Craig A. Clifford DVM, MS, DACVIM (Oncology)

Chapter 138

Cholecystitis and Choledochitis

DEFINITION/OVERVIEW

- Cholecystitis = an inflammatory infiltrate in the gallbladder (GB) wall.
- Choledochitis = an inflammatory infiltrate in the large bile duct.

ETIOLOGY/PATHOPHYSIOLOGY

- Necrotizing cholecystitis may develop secondary to thromboembolism, blunt abdominal trauma, bacterial infection, extrahepatic biliary obstruction (cystic duct obstruction or distal duct obstruction by choleliths, stricture, or neoplasia), or a mature gallbladder mucocele (causing tense gallbladder distension). Extension of an inflammatory or neoplastic process from adjacent hepatic tissue also may be an underlying cause. Necrotizing cholecystitis can present with or without gallbladder rupture, or as a chronic syndrome associated with adhesions between the gallbladder, omentum, and adjacent viscera. Bacteria are commonly cultured from the gallbladder wall.
- A nonnecrotizing cholecystitis, inflammation of the gallbladder may involve nonsuppurative inflammation; may be associated with infectious agents, systemic disease, or neoplasia; or may reflect blunt abdominal trauma or gallbladder obstruction by occlusion of the cystic duct (e.g., cholelithiasis, neoplasia, or choledochitis). Cystic duct occlusion incites gallbladder inflammation secondary to bile stasis; this process is augmented by mechanical irritation of a cholelith. The gallbladder wall thickens, and the lumen distends with a white, viscid, mucin-laden bile (white bile).
- Gastrointestinal disease can result in enteric bacteria transmigrating the bowel wall, passing into the portal circulation, entering the liver, GB, and bile, dispersing endotoxins and bacteria initiating sepsis, and in some cases, bile and/or septic peritonitis.

Systems Affected

- Hepatobiliary – can result in hepatitis and gallbladder rupture.
- Gastrointestinal – weight loss, hyporexia, anorexia, vomiting, diarrhea, melena, hematochezia.
- Hemic/lymphatic/immune – coagulopathies (pro/anticoagulant factor imbalances), disseminated intravascular coagulation (DIC).

Blackwell's Five-Minute Veterinary Consult Clinical Companion: Small Animal Gastrointestinal Diseases, First Edition. Edited by Jocelyn Mott and Jo Ann Morrison.
© 2019 John Wiley & Sons, Inc. Published 2019 by John Wiley & Sons, Inc.
Companion website: www.fiveminutevet.com/gastrointestinal

- Nervous – hepatic encephalopathy, cerebral edema.
- Renal/urologic – renal tubular damage from specific infectious agents (i.e., leptospirosis) or physiologic vasoconstriction.
- Respiratory – acute respiratory distress syndrome, acute lung injury.
- Endocrine/metabolic – systemic inflammatory response syndrome.
- Cardiovascular – systemic hypotension.

SIGNALMENT/HISTORY

- Dog and cat.
- No breed or sex predilection.
- Necrotizing cholecystitis (dogs) – usually middle-aged or older animals.

Risk Factors

- Impaired bile flow at cystic duct or GB, GB dysmotility, or ischemic insult to the GB wall may precede cholecystitis.
- Irritants in sludged bile (e.g., lysolecithin, prostaglandins, choleliths, liver flukes) or retrograde flow of pancreatic enzymes (cats) may initiate/augment GB or duct inflammation.
- Previous enteric disorders, trauma, abdominal surgery – may be contributing factors.
- Anomalous GB or duct development: choledochal cyst (rare, cats > dogs).
- Bacterial infection – common; retrograde invasion via ducts from intestine or hematogenous dispersal from splanchnic circulation.
- Toxoplasmosis and biliary coccidiosis – rare.
- Necrotizing cholecystitis (dogs) – ruptured GB (common) and complicating cholelithiasis; *E. coli* and *Enterococcus* spp. common isolates.
- Emphysematous cholecystitis/choledochitis – rare, associations with diabetes mellitus, traumatic GB ischemia, acute cholecystitis (with or without cholelithiasis); common gas-forming organisms – *Clostridia* spp. and *E. coli* often cultured.

Historical Findings

- Clinical signs are nonspecific and include variable icterus, inappetence, anorexia, lethargy, vomiting, diarrhea, vague abdominal pain (may be postprandial with cholecystitis or gallbladder mucocele).
- Pyrexia.
- Postprandial discomfort/distress.
- Patients may be asymptomatic.

CLINICAL FEATURES

- Physical examination may vary significantly depending on severity of disease.
- Patient may be icteric if hyperbilirubinemic.
- Diarrhea may be noted on rectal examination.
- Abdominal pain.
- Abdominal distension if effusion present.
- Pyrexia.
- Examination may be normal.

DIFFERENTIAL DIAGNOSIS

- Pancreatitis.
- Focal or diffuse peritonitis.
- Bile peritonitis.
- Gastroenteritis causing biliary involvement.
- Cholelithiasis.
- Cholangiohepatitis.
- Hepatic necrosis or abscessation.
- Extrahepatic biliary obstruction (EHBO).
- Gallbladder mucocele (GBM).
- Septicemia.
- Hepatitis (chronic, acute).

DIAGNOSTICS

Complete Blood Count/Biochemistry/Urinalysis

- Variable leukocytosis with toxic neutrophils and inconsistent left shift.
- High bilirubin; bilirubinuria.
- High ALT, AST, ALP, and GGT activities.
- High cholesterol and bilirubin if EHBO.
- Hypercholesterolemia and/or hyperlipidemia (triglycerides): breed-related, endocrine, pancreatitis, nephrotic syndrome.

Additional Laboratory Tests

- Abdominocentesis – inflammatory effusion.
- Bile culture – *E. coli*, *Enterococcus* spp., *Klebsiella* spp., *Pseudomonas* spp., *Clostridium* spp., others.
- Bile cytology – bactibilia with or without concurrent inflammatory infiltrate.
- Coagulation tests – abnormal if chronic EHBO (vitamin K deficiency) or DIC in severe conditions with sepsis.

Imaging

- Abdominal radiography – may reveal loss of cranial abdominal detail with focal or diffuse peritonitis or effusion; ileus; radiodense choleliths; gas in biliary structures; radiodense GB (dystrophic mineralization due to chronic inflammation, porcelain GB, rare).
- Ultrasonography – fluid interface surrounding GB enhances wall image; diffusely thick GB wall, segmental hyperechogenicity and/or laminated wall in necrotizing cholecystitis; double-rimmed GB wall.
- Choledochitis involving common bile duct (CBD): thick wall, intraluminal debris, extends into hepatic ducts.
- GB rupture implicated by discontinuous GB wall, pericholecystic fluid or generalized effusion, and hyperechogenicity of surrounding tissue; failure to image GB: may implicate rupture or agenesis.
- GB rupture considered a surgical emergency.

- Detection of gas within the biliary tree or gallbladder heralds an emphysematous process associated with sepsis and should prompt antibiotic administration before surgical intervention.
- Ultrasound may be normal.

Pathologic Findings

- Gross appearance – erythematous GB; may appear green-black if necrotizing lesion; tenacious "inspissated" biliary material common with GBM; pigmented choleliths if infection; blood with hemobilia; CBD with thick wall, variable intraductal debris (e.g., biliary particulates, suppurative inflammation).
- Microscopic – inflammatory infiltrate in the gallbladder or biliary mucosa (Figures 138.1, 138.2).

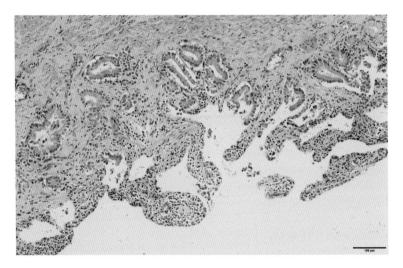

■ **Fig. 138.1.** Gallbladder of a nine-year-old, male castrated Persian cat with cholangiohepatitis (hematoxylin and eosin, 10×). Mild, multifocal, chronic, lymphoplasmacytic cholecystitis. Source: Courtesy of Dr Randi Gold.

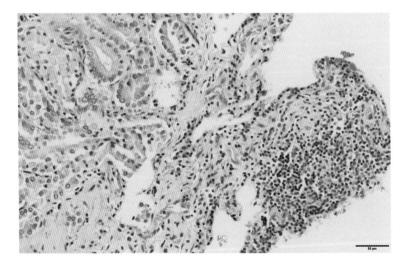

■ **Fig. 138.2.** Gallbladder of a nine-year-old, male castrated Persian cat with cholangiohepatitis (hematoxylin and eosin, 20×). Closer view highlighting bile ducts and lymphoplasmacytic inflammation. Source: Courtesy of Dr Randi Gold.

THERAPEUTICS

- Etiology-specific therapy based on the results of culture and sensitivity if applicable.
- Consider cholecystectomy for clinical cases, cases that fail to respond to medical management or cases with compromised gallbladder wall.

Drug(s) of Choice

- Antibiotics – withhold until samples have been acquired for aerobic and anaerobic culture and sensitivity testing unless there is evidence of systemic inflammatory response syndrome or sepsis. An empiric choice should include coverage for enteric gram-negative and anaerobic flora. Antibiotic drug therapy should be continued for 4–6 weeks and based on the results of aerobic and anaerobic culture and sensitivity.
- Ursodeoxycholic acid: 10–15 mg/kg PO daily divided q12h with food.
- Antioxidants: vitamin E (alpha-tocopherol acetate) 10 IU/kg PO q24h; S-adenosylmethionine (SAMe) (20 mg/kg PO q24h), silybin (5 mg/kg PO q12h).
- Vitamin K1 0.5–1.5 mg/kg SQ or IM q12h for three doses; treat early to allow response before surgical manipulations.

Precautions/Interactions

- Ursodeoxycholic acid – contraindicated in uncorrected EHBO or bile peritonitis.
- Vitamin K1 – **caution:** never administer IV (anaphylactoid reaction).

Appropriate Health Care

Maintenance of adequate enteral nutrition and hydration is essential during treatment.

Nursing Care

Remain vigilant for vasovagal reflex (abrupt pathologic bradycardia, hypotension, cardiac arrest) when biliary structures manipulated or during cholecystocentesis; be prepared with anticholinergics (atropine).

Diet

- There are no specific dietary considerations.
- Protein restriction should only be prescribed if there is evidence of hepatic encephalopathy.

Activity

Allow the patient to limit their own activity.

Surgical Considerations

- Consider cholecystectomy for cases that fail to respond to medical management or cases with compromised gallbladder wall.
- Samples of bile, gallbladder wall, choleliths, and liver tissue should be submitted for aerobic and anaerobic culture. Cytologic evaluations of tissue imprints and bile help initial selection of antimicrobials (based on bacterial morphology and gram staining).
- Assessment of coagulation status recommended particularly if there is any evidence of cholestasis.
- Vitamin K1 should be administered (0.5–1.5 mg/kg IM or SQ, three doses q12h) before surgery to avert hemorrhagic complications.
- If emergency surgery is necessary, fresh frozen plasma should be given judiciously based on coagulation tests and a buccal mucosal bleeding time.

COMMENTS

Client Education

- Patience is required for long-term antibiotic administration.
- Reevaluation of treatment efficacy required to ensure resolution of infection if present.
- Surgery may be indicated in cases that fail medical management.

Patient Monitoring

- Physical examination and pertinent diagnostic testing – repeat every 2–4 weeks until abnormalities resolve.
- Antimicrobial therapy should be continued for a minimum of four weeks and two weeks beyond a negative bacterial culture and normal bile cytology.

Prevention/Avoidance

Antimicrobial therapy should be continued until disease resolution (negative culture) to prevent recurrence.

Possible Complications

- Sepsis.
- Systemic inflammatory response syndrome.
- Gallbladder rupture.
- Peritonitis.
- Multidrug-resistant infections.

Expected Course and Prognosis

- The prognosis is generally good with medical and surgical management.
- Septic peritonitis and gallbladder rupture are generally associated with a more guarded prognosis.

Synonyms

The etiology, if known, may precede the name, i.e., bacterial cholecystitis, necrotizing cholecystitis, nonnecrotizing cholecystitis, emphysematous cholecystitis.

Abbreviations

- ALP = alkaline phosphatase
- ALT = alanine aminotransferase
- AST = aspartate aminotransferase
- CBD = common bile duct
- DIC = disseminated intravascular coagulation
- EHBO = extrahepatic biliary obstruction
- GB = gallbladder
- GBM = gallbladder mucocele
- GGT = gamma-glutamyl transferase
- GSH = glutathione

See Also

- Bile Duct Obstruction (Extrahepatic)
- Biliary Duct or Gallbladder Rupture and Bile Peritonitis
- Cholangitis/Cholangiohepatitis Syndrome
- Cholelithiasis
- Coagulopathy of Liver Disease
- Gallbladder Mucocele
- Nutritional Approach to Hepatobiliary Diseases

Suggested Reading

Center SA. Diseases of the gallbladder and biliary tree. Vet Clin North Am Small Anim Pract 2009;39(3):543–598.

Lawrence YA, Ruaux CG, Nemanic S, Milovancev M. Clinical findings, sonographic features, bacterial isolates, treatment, and outcome of bacterial cholecystitis and bactibilia in dogs: 10 cases (2010–2014). J Am Vet Med Assoc 2015;246(9):982–989.

Acknowledgments: The author and editors acknowledge the prior contribution of Dr Sharon Center.

Author: Yuri A. Lawrence DVM, MS, MA, PhD, DACVIM (SAIM)

Chapter 139

Cholecystitis, Emphysematous

DEFINITION/OVERVIEW

- Necrotizing inflammation of the gallbladder caused by a gas-forming bacterial infection damaging the gallbladder wall.
- Associated with cholecystitis, cholelithiasis, traumatic ischemia, mature gallbladder mucocele formation, diabetes mellitus, and neoplasia.
- Severe gallbladder inflammation can lead to gallbladder rupture leading to bile peritonitis, which will need emergency medical and surgical treatments.

ETIOLOGY/PATHOPHYSIOLOGY

- Ascending infection from the small intestine.
- Hematogenous spread of an infection occurring elsewhere in the body.
- Cholelithiasis.
- Incompetent sphincter of the gallbladder duct.
- Occlusion of the cystic artery.
- Gallbladder mass.

Systems Affected

- Gastrointestinal – vomiting, diarrhea, hyporexia, anorexia, and abdominal pain.
- Hepatobiliary – cholangiohepatitis and extrahepatic biliary obstruction.

SIGNALMENT/HISTORY

- Rare in dogs.
- Not reported in cats.
- Due to the paucity of reported cases, risk factors for developing emphysematous cystitis have not been identified.
- In a review of 23 dogs with necrotizing cholecystitis, there was a male-to-female ratio of 65:35 and an average age of 9.5 years. Of the 11 dogs reported to have emphysematous cholecystitis, two were diabetic.

Blackwell's Five-Minute Veterinary Consult Clinical Companion: Small Animal Gastrointestinal Diseases,
First Edition. Edited by Jocelyn Mott and Jo Ann Morrison.
© 2019 John Wiley & Sons, Inc. Published 2019 by John Wiley & Sons, Inc.
Companion website: www.fiveminutevet.com/gastrointestinal

CLINICAL FEATURES

- Vomiting.
- Lethargy.
- Hyporexia to anorexia.
- Abdominal pain.
- Fever.
- Icteric.
- Shock from endotoxemia and bacteremia can occur in severe cases.

 ## DIFFERENTIAL DIAGNOSIS

- Cholangiohepatitis.
- Cholelithiasis.
- Extrahepatic biliary obstruction.
- Gallbladder mucocele.
- Liver lobe torsion and entrapment.
- Hepatic or perihepatic abscess.
- Pancreatitis.
- Peritonitis.
- Septicemia.

 ## DIAGNOSTICS

Complete Blood Count/Biochemistry/Urinalysis

- Neutrophilic leukocytosis with inconsistent toxic changes and left shift.
- Mild anemia.
- Severe thrombocytopenia with disseminated intravascular coagulopathy (DIC).
- Hyperbilirubinemia.
- Elevation of alkaline phosphatase (ALP), gamma-glutamyl transferase (GGT), alanine aminotransferase (ALT), and aspartate aminotransferase (AST).
- Hypoalbuminemia.
- Bilirubinuria.

Other Laboratory Tests

- Prothrombin time and activated partial thromboplastin time – prolonged if there is chronic extrahepatic biliary obstruction (vitamin K deficiency) or in DIC.
- Bile culture – *Clostridium perfringens*, *Escherichia coli*.

Imaging

- Abdominal radiography – a spherically shaped, gas-filled opacity corresponding in shape and position to the gallbladder will be seen (Figure 139.1).
- Ultrasonography – gas shadows in the area of the gallbladder.

Pathologic Findings

Gross appearance of gallbladder – large and distended; partially black and friable gallbladder wall.

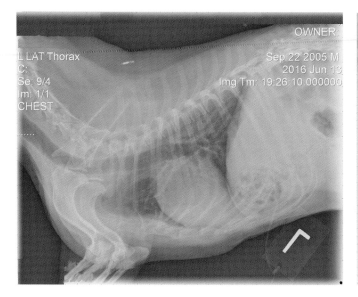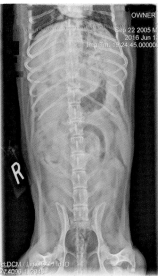

■ **Fig. 139.1.** Lateral and ventrodorsal abdominal radiographs of a dog with emphysematous cholecystitis. Source: Courtesy of Pasadena Veterinary Specialists.

 ## THERAPEUTICS

- Requires inpatient treatments for stabilization for diagnostic testing and preoperative evaluation.
- Intravenous fluid therapy to restore fluid and electrolytes.
- Cholecystectomy to remove diseased gallbladder.

Drug(s) of Choice

- Antibiotics – broad-spectrum antibiotics should be instituted preoperatively; combination of metronidazole (15 mg/kg IV q12h; 7.5 mg/kg IV q12h in cases with extrahepatic biliary obstruction), potentiated ampicillin (22–30 mg/kg IV q8h) and fluoroquinolone (enrofloxacin 10 mg/kg IV q24h) is recommended; use of antibiotics can be adjusted based on bile culture and sensitivity results post operation.
- Vitamin K – 0.5 mg/kg SQ q12h if suspect extrahepatic biliary obstruction.
- Vitamin E – 10 IU/kg as antioxidant.
- S-adenosylmethionine – 20 mg/kg PO q24h as antioxidant.
- Antiemetic – maropitant 0.5 mg IV q24h; ondansetron 0.2–0.5 mg/kg IV q12h.
- H2-receptor antagonist – famotidine 0.5 mg/kg IV q12h.
- Proton pump inhibitor – pantoprazole 1 mg/kg IV q24h over 15 min.

Precautions/Interactions

- Ursodeoxycholic acid – do not use if there is bile peritonitis or evidence of extrahepatic biliary duct obstruction.

Nursing Care

- Perioperative intravenous fluid, antibiotics, and antiemetic.
- Pain management is crucial.
- Monitor caloric intake through enteral nutrition.

Diet

- Trickle feeding may be necessary postoperatively.
- Low-fat diet is recommended post-cholecystectomy.

Activity

- Restricted activity for two weeks postoperatively.

Surgical Considerations

- Surgery for cholecystectomy is the only treatment.
- During surgery, obtaining liver biopsy and bile culture is crucial.
- Duodenal biopsy is recommended in case of underlying gastrointestinal (GI) disease causing secondary emphysematous cholecystitis.

 COMMENTS

Client Education

- Monitor caloric intake.
- Monitor water consumption and urine output.
- Monitor for jaundice.
- Report any diarrhea and/or vomiting.
- Use pain medication as directed.
- Continue the use of antibiotics as directed.

Patient Monitoring

- Physical examination with follow-up complete blood count and chemistry panel is recommended every 2–4 weeks until all abnormalities are resolved.
- Routine recheck is recommended every 3–4 months once patient is fully recovered.

Prevention / Avoidance

- Early diagnosis and aggressive surgical and medical treatment are the key for recovery.

Possible Complications

- Bile peritonitis can occur if not treated appropriately.

Expected Course and Prognosis

- Survival time is influenced by the age and condition of the patient.
- Prognosis is usually poor without early surgical intervention.
- Reported mortality rate of 39% is likely due to delayed diagnosis.

Abbreviations

- ALP = alkaline phosphatase
- ALT = alanine aminotransferase
- AST = aspartate aminotransferase
- DIC = disseminated intravascular coagulation
- GGT = gamma-glutamyl transferase
- GI = gastrointestinal

See Also

- Biliary Duct or Gallbladder Rupture and Bile Peritonitis
- Cholecystitis and Choledochitis
- Cholelithiasis
- Coagulopathy of Liver Disease
- Gallbladder Mucocele
- Nutritional Approach to Hepatobiliary Diseases

Suggested Reading

Armstrong JA, Taylor SM, Tryon KA, et al. Emphysematous cholecystitis in a Siberian husky. Brief communications. Can Vet J 2000;41:60–62.

Avgeris S, Hoskinson JJ. Emphysematous cholecystitis in a dog: a radiographic diagnosis. J Am Anim Hosp Assoc 1992;28:344–346.

Burk RL, Johnson GF. Emphysematous cholecystitis in the nondiabetic dogs: three case histories. Vet Radiol 1980;21:242–245.

Martin RA, Lanz OI, Tobias KM. Liver and biliary system. In: Slatter D, ed. Textbook of Small Animal Surgery, 3rd ed. Philadelphia: WB Saunders, 2002, pp. 708–726.

Author: Vivian K. Yau DVM, DACVIM (SAIM)

Cholelithiasis

DEFINITION/OVERVIEW

- Choleliths form when supersaturation of bile with calcium-based salts and/or cholesterol occurs with a nidus for crystallization.
- Bile pigments, bile mucoproteins, bacteria, and refluxed intestinal contents can act as a nidus.
- Gallbladder stasis, mucus hypersecretion, and increased water absorption from bile are also necessary for cholelith formation.

ETIOLOGY/PATHOPHYSIOLOGY

- Cholelithiasis in dogs and cats is uncommon.
- Gallbladder is most common location for cholelithiasis. Choledocholiths occur in the biliary ducts.
- Choleliths rarely cause extrahepatic biliary obstruction (EHBO).
- Feline choleliths often form secondary to cholecystitis and/or cholangiohepatitis. The hepatobiliary disease may predispose to cholelithiasis by altered gallbladder motility, excess mucin production, and ascending infections.
- Cholelith composition in dogs and cats is usually pigment based (cats are usually calcium carbonate; dogs usually calcium bilirubinate). Cholesterol and mixed choleliths have also been described in dogs.
- Bilirubin cholelithiasis has been reported in cats and humans with hemolysis.

Systems Affected

- Hepatobiliary.
- Gastrointestinal.
- Hemic/lymphatic/immune – pyruvate kinase deficiency-induced hemolysis in cats can lead to bilirubin cholelithiasis.

SIGNALMENT/HISTORY

- Dogs and cats with cholelithiasis may be asymptomatic or may be clinical with signs of extrahepatic biliary obstruction.
- Can occur in dogs and cats. Small-breed dogs more commonly affected.
- Miniature schnauzers and miniature poodles have increased incidence.
- Animals usually middle aged to older.

Blackwell's Five-Minute Veterinary Consult Clinical Companion: Small Animal Gastrointestinal Diseases, First Edition. Edited by Jocelyn Mott and Jo Ann Morrison.
© 2019 John Wiley & Sons, Inc. Published 2019 by John Wiley & Sons, Inc.
Companion website: www.fiveminutevet.com/gastrointestinal

Risk Factors

- Hypercholesterolemia or hypertriglyceridemia may be risk factors for canine cholelithiasis.
- Gallbladder dysmotility may be risk factor.
- Lithogenic diet (low protein, high cholesterol, low methionine, low taurine) in dogs.
- Cholecystitis or inflammatory liver disease.

Historical Findings

- Clinical signs may wax and wane.
- Asymptomatic.
- Vomiting, intermittent abdominal pain, anorexia, lethargy, icterus, fever, and diarrhea associated with extrahepatic biliary obstruction.

CLINICAL FEATURES

- Physical examination usually normal in asymptomatic patients.
- Patients with EHBO may be jaundiced, dehydrated, exhibit abdominal pain and/or fever.

DIFFERENTIAL DIAGNOSIS

- Other diseases causing EHBO including inflammatory or infectious disease, neoplasia, and pancreatitis.
- Cholecystitis.
- Cholangiohepatitis.
- Gallbladder mucocele.
- Bile peritonitis.

DIAGNOSTICS

Complete Blood Count/Biochemistry/Urinalysis

- May or may not include neutrophilia with left shift and/or nonregenerative anemia.
- Biochemistry abnormalities are indicative of obstructive cholelithiasis and may include elevated alanine aminotransferase (ALT), alkaline phosphatase (ALP), gamma-glutamyl transferase (GGT), hyperbilirubinemia, and hypercholesterolemia.
- Bilirubinuria may be the first sign of obstructive cholelithiasis.

Other Laboratory Tests

- Cytology and aerobic and anaerobic culture of bile collected by cholecystocentesis may detect presence of inflammation and bactibilia.
- Most common isolates are of enteric origin.
- Healthy canine bile can have enteric bacteria whereas healthy feline bile is sterile.
- Serum leptin may be a useful biomarker of disease in dogs in future.

Imaging

- Abdominal radiographs may reveal radiopaque choleliths (Figures 140.1 and 140.2). Cholesterol choleliths are radiolucent.
- Abdominal ultrasound can often identify choleliths. Choleliths are echogenic focal structures in the gallbladder which usually produce acoustic shadowing on ultrasound.

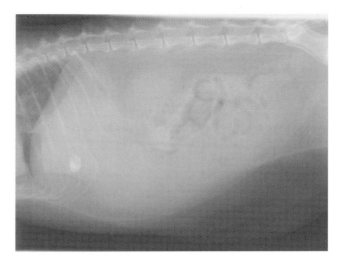

■ **Fig. 140.1.** Lateral abdominal radiograph of a dog with choleliths visible in the cranial ventral aspect. Source: Courtesy of Dr Jim Hoskinson.

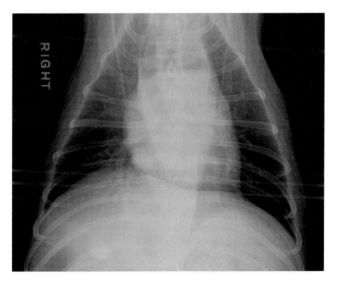

■ **Fig. 140.2.** Ventrodorsal radiograph of a dog with choleliths visible in the right cranial quadrant. Source: Courtesy of Dr Jim Hoskinson.

Gallbladder wall thickening and/or surrounding fluid may be present. The first change with extrahepatic biliary obstruction is common bile duct (CBD) dilation (CBD will exceed 5 mm) followed by dilation of the intrahepatic biliary tract 5–7 days later.
■ Computed tomographic cholangiography in select cases can be used for better visualization and to evaluate patency and integrity of biliary tract.

Additional Diagnostic Tests

In surgical cases, histopathology and culture of liver, gallbladder, bile, and choleliths should be performed. Cholelith analysis is also recommended.

THERAPEUTICS

Drug(s) of Choice

- Choleliths in humans are largely cholesterol based and thus often responsive to cholelith dissolution with ursodeoxycholate (UDCA). Due to the different cholelith composition found in dogs and cats, it is not likely that UDCA administration results in cholelith dissolution in these species. If therapy is attempted, recommended dosage is UDCA 10–15 mg/kg/day PO, given with food.
- S-adenosylmethionine (sAMe) has a choleretic effect at 40–60 mg/kg/day in cats.
- Management of concurrent cholecystitis with antibiotics which penetrate bile and reach high concentrations may be indicated. Enrofloxacin, ampicillin or cephalosporins are appropriate.
- Pulsatile antibiotic therapy for cholecystoenterostomy cases may be needed to control infections secondary to retrograde movement of intestinal contents into the biliary system.
- Concurrent hepatitis or cholangiohepatitis may necessitate the use of immunomodulatory drugs.

Precautions/Interactions

UDCA not recommended in cases of EHBO.

Nursing Care

Patients with obstructive cholelithiasis may require hospitalization to correct dehydration and electrolyte abnormalities prior to surgical intervention.

Diet

Patients with hypertriglyceridemia or hypercholesterolemia may benefit from fat-restricted diets.

Surgical Considerations

- Surgical intervention is necessary with complete extrahepatic biliary tract obstruction and cholecystitis.
- Cholecystectomy is thought to prevent further bile stasis and cholelithiasis formation. A low mortality and morbidity rate has been reported in dogs and cats.
- Choledochotomy may in some cases be performed to remove stones from the CBD.
- Cholecystoenterostomy is deemed appropriate when biliary bypass is necessary. These procedures have been associated with recurrence of cholelithiasis and higher postoperative morbidity and mortality rates. Hypotension is a serious perianesthetic risk.

COMMENTS

Client Education

- Choleliths may be asymptomatic and incidental in their pets.
- Cholelithiasis can also occur concurrently with infectious, inflammatory and neoplastic diseases of the hepatobiliary system or pancreas. These concurrent diseases need to be identified and treated.
- Cholelithiasis can reoccur.

Patient Monitoring

- In asymptomatic patients, periodic ultrasound may be beneficial to monitor cholelithiasis and possible progression of disease.
- Postoperative patients may need more regular monitoring (biochemistry panel, complete blood counts, physical examination, urinalysis +/– ultrasound) dependent on surgical procedure and response.

Prevention/Avoidance

- Avoid lithogenic diets (marginal-protein, high-carbohydrate, high-cholesterol diet).
- Treat underlying hepatobiliary diseases that may contribute to environment for cholelithiasis formation.

Possible Complications

- Gallbladder rupture.
- Cholecystocutaneous fistula (rare).
- Retrograde cholangitis and stoma stricture can occur with cholecystoenterostomy patients.

Expected Course and Prognosis

- The majority of patients may remain asymptomatic for cholelithiasis.
- Patients that require surgical intervention may have low morbidity and mortality rates with cholecystectomy or choledochotomy.
- Cholecystoenterostomy patients have a more guarded prognosis.

Abbreviations

- CBD = common bile duct
- EHBO = extrahepatic biliary obstruction
- UDCA = ursodeoxycholate

See Also

- Bile Duct Obstruction (Extrahepatic)
- Biliary Duct or Gallbladder Rupture or Bile Peritonitis
- Biliary Neoplasia
- Cholangitis/Cholangiohepatitis Syndrome
- Cholecystitis and Choledochitis
- Gallbladder Mucocele
- Nutritional Approach to Hepatobiliary Diseases

Suggested Reading

Center SA. Diseases of the gallbladder and biliary tree. Vet Clin North Am Small Anim Pract 2009;39(3):543–598.

Christian JS, Rege RV. Methionine, but not taurine, protects against formation of canine pigment gallstones. J Surg Res 1996;61:275–281.

Eich CS, Ludwig LL. The surgical treatment of cholelithiasis in cats: a study of nine cases. J Am Anim Hosp Assoc 2002;38:290–296.

Elwood CM, White RN, Freeman K, et al. Cholelithiasis and hyperthyroidism in a cat. J Feline Med Surg 2001;3(4):247–252.

Fabbi M, Volta A, Quintavalla F, et al. Cholecystocutaneous fistula containing multiple gallstones in a dog. Can Vet J 2014;55:1163–1166.

Harvey AM, Holt PE, Barr FJ, et al. Treatment and long term follow up of extrahepatic biliary obstruction with bilirubin cholelithiasis in a Somali cat with pyruvate kinase deficiency. J Feline Med Surg 2007;9(5):424–431.

Lee S, Kweon O, Kim WH. Associations between serum leptin levels, hyperlipidemia, and cholelithiasis in dogs. PLoS One 2017;12(10):e0187315.

Moore AL, Gregory SP. Duplex gall bladder associated with choledocholithiasis, cholecystitis, gall bladder rupture and septic peritonitis in a cat. J Small Anim Pract 2007;48(7);404–409.

Pashmakova MB, Piccione J, Bishop MA, et al. Agreement between microscopic examination and bacterial culture of bile samples for detection of bactibilia in dogs and cats with hepatobiliary disease. J Am Vet Med Assoc 2017;250(9):1007–1013.

Ward R. Obstructive cholelithiasis and cholecystitis in a keeshond. Can Vet J 2006;47:1119–1121.

Author: Jocelyn Mott DVM, DACVIM (SAIM)

Gallbladder Mucocele

DEFINITION/OVERVIEW

- Gallbladder (GB) distension with abnormal inspissated or gelatinous mucoid bile reducing bile storage (Figure 141.1).
- Gallbladder and cystic duct most commonly affected; hepatic and common bile duct occlusions may be present leading to extrahepatic biliary obstruction (EHBO).
- Gallbladder may rupture, leading to bile peritonitis.

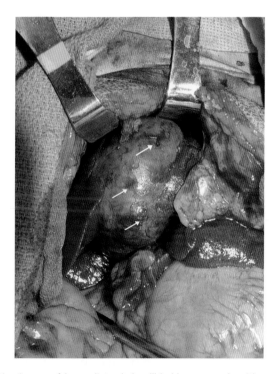

■ **Fig. 141.1.** Intraoperative image of large distended gallbladder mucocele with omental adhesions dissected away from gallbladder (*white arrows*).

Blackwell's Five-Minute Veterinary Consult Clinical Companion: Small Animal Gastrointestinal Diseases, First Edition. Edited by Jocelyn Mott and Jo Ann Morrison.
© 2019 John Wiley & Sons, Inc. Published 2019 by John Wiley & Sons, Inc.
Companion website: www.fiveminutevet.com/gastrointestinal

ETIOLOGY/PATHOPHYSIOLOGY

- Etiology remains poorly defined.
- Cystic mucosal hyperplasia leading to hypersecretion of mucus and subsequent bile hyperviscosity.
- Progressive organization of bile over weeks to months leads to increased intraluminal gallbladder wall pressure followed by mural necrosis and concurrent biliary tract obstruction.
- Approximately 50% of patients with gallbladder mucocele (GBM) present with ruptured GB.

Systems Affected

- Hepatobiliary – sludge formation within the bile ducts may cause obstruction. Bile that cannot flow from the liver will lead to hepatic bile congestion. Bacterial overgrowth in the intestine can occur when bile is not present. Those bacteria can ascend into the common bile duct and liver, leading to cholangiohepatitis. As the GB distends, inflammation of the GB can occur. The GB wall may undergo necrosis from intraluminal pressure leading to rupture.
- Gastrointestinal – gastrointestinal clinical signs are common secondary to adjacent hepatic biliary inflammation or bile peritonitis with GB rupture; vomiting causes electrolyte abnormalities; prerenal azotemia secondary to dehydration from vomiting.
- Cardiovascular – bradycardia may result from vagal stimulation (especially with cholecystocentesis); systemic shock and hypotension may occur in the course of the disease.
- Endocrine/exocrine – pancreatitis is a potential sequela of GBM and biliary disease.
- Hemic – patients are commonly hypercoagulable as evidenced by thromboelastography (TEG); patients will routinely have normal prothrombin time (PT) and activated partial thromboplastin time (APTT) profiles; hypocoagulability was traditionally suspected based on pathophysiologic models that EHBO reduced biliary salt release into the small intestine – this resulted in impaired vitamin K absorption and decreases in vitamin K-activated coagulation factors II, VII, IX, X; recent TEG research suggests that the cellular-based coagulation model is a more appropriate representation of hematologic abnormalities and patients are hypercoagulable; definitive causes have not been defined although increased platelet activation, endotoxemia, and hyperfibrinogenemia are possible contributors.

SIGNALMENT/HISTORY

- Canine patients, rare in cats.
- No sex predilection.
- Middle aged to older (average nine years).
- Small- to medium-sized breeds.
- Shetland sheepdogs are predisposed to general gallbladder disease (not only mucoceles). Associated with mutation in the canine ABCB4 gene that codes for a hepatocyte phospholipid translocator present on canalicular membranes.
- Cocker spaniels and miniature schnauzers overrepresented.

Risk Factors

- Concurrent endocrinopathies.
  - Hyperadrenocorticism (HAC): 29 times more likely to have a GBM than dogs without hyperadrenocorticism (causal relationship not defined).
  - Hypothyroidism: three times more likely to have a GBM than dogs without hypothyroidism (causal relationship not defined).

- Decreased gallbladder and biliary tract fluid absorption predisposes to sludge formation.
- Decreased gallbladder motility and biliary stasis.
- Dyslipidemias.
- Typical or atypical (sex hormone) adrenal hyperplasia.
- Glucocorticoid therapy.

Historical Findings

- Patients may be asymptomatic (30% cases).
- Vomiting (70%).
- Anorexia (65%).
- Lethargy (65%).
- Polyuria/polydipsia (PU/PD) (30%).
- Diarrhea (12.5%).

 ## CLINICAL FEATURES

- Physical exam may be normal.
- Abdominal pain (20%).
- Icteric (16%).
- Febrile (most common with ruptured GBM and bile peritonitis).
- May have physical exam findings consistent with endocrinopathy – found incidentally on abdominal ultrasound.
    - Polyuria.
    - Polyphagia.
    - Polydipsia.
- Severe cases.
    - Shock.
    - Tachycardia.
    - Weakness.
    - Recumbency.

 ## DIFFERENTIAL DIAGNOSIS

Conditions causing bile stasis or EHBO.
- Pancreatic disease.
    - Pancreatitis.
    - Pancreatic pseudocyst.
    - Pancreatic neoplasia.
    - Pancreatic abscess.
- Intestinal disease.
    - Duodenal foreign body.
    - Duodenal neoplasia.
    - Duodenal hematoma.
    - Duodenal adhesions.
    - Papillary fibrosis or damage.
    - Pyloric neoplasia.
- Biliary disease.
    - Gallbladder neoplasia.
    - Bile duct neoplasia.

- Bile duct stricture.
- Cholecystitis.
- GB dysmotility.
- Cholelithiasis.
- Choledocholithiasis.
- Biliary tract rupture.
- Biliary atresia.
- Biliary cysts.
  - Hepatic disease.
    - Cholangiohepatitis.
    - Hepatic neoplasia.
    - Hepatic abscess.
    - Hepatic congestion.
    - Diaphragmatic hernia.

DIAGNOSTICS

Complete Blood Count/Biochemistry/Urinalysis

- Inflammatory leukogram (~50% cases).
- Nonregenerative anemia.
- Alkaline phosphatase (ALP) elevation (98%). May be associated with HAC or extrahepatic biliary tract (EHBT) obstruction.
- Alanine aminotransferase (ALT) elevation (87%).
- Aspartate aminotransferase (AST) elevation (62%).
- Gamma-glutamyl transferase (GGT) elevation (85%).
- Hyperbilirubinemia (83%).
- Hypoalbuminemia with biliary tract rupture and bile peritonitis.
- Hyperlactatemia.
- Urinalysis often unremarkable. PU/PD from endocrine disease may lead to isosthenuria and hyposthenuria.

Other Laboratory Tests

- Coagulation panel is usually normal (baseline for postsurgical complications).
- Coagulation panel values can be increased or decreased.
- Coagulation panel values can be prolonged with chronic EHBT obstruction, GB rupture, bile peritonitis, sepsis, or disseminated intravascular coagulation.
- Coagulation panel values may be decreased (indicating a hypercoagulable state) in patients secondary to concurrent hyperadrenocorticism or EHBT.
- Empirical vitamin K injections are no longer recommended without performing a diagnostic coagulation panel.

Imaging

- Radiographs are nonspecific.
- Hepatomegaly.
- Gallbladder enlargement.
- Gallbladder mineralization.
- Decreased peritoneal detail secondary to focal or diffuse peritonitis.
- Intrahepatic or gallbladder emphysema secondary to septic inflammation from ascending gas-producing bacteria (rare).

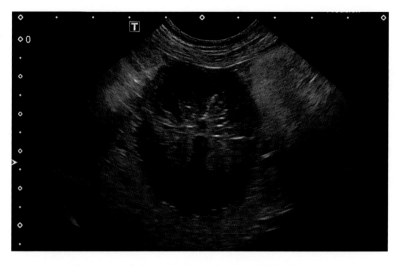

■ **Fig. 141.2.** Ultrasonographic image of classic "kiwi appearance" gallbladder mucocele. Notice the centralized echogenicity and hypoechoic margins.

- Ultrasound has 100% specificity and 86% sensitivity for detecting GBM.
- Nonspecific enlarged liver with rounded margins.
- Distended GB +/– distended common bile duct (<3 mm normal in dogs; <1 mm normal in cats).
- Heterogeneous intraluminal GB material.
  - Be aware of false diagnosis of GBM due to incidental sludge accumulation.
  - Lack of gravity-dependent intraluminal sludge.
  - Stellate or striated pattern with increased centralized echogenicity and hypoechoic margins commonly referred to as the "kiwi" appearance (Figure 141.2).
- Thickened GB wall (<3 mm normal in dogs; <1 mm normal in cats) and laminated or double-walled appearance.
- Hyperechoic gallbladder fossa region.
- Gallbladder rupture suspected with GB wall discontinuity, pericholecystic fluid, echogenic peritoneal fluid.
- Ruptured GBM may lead to false-negative diagnosis due to omental adhesions and hepatic fossa collapse.
- Gallbladder rupture can result in "free-floating mucocele mass" in abdomen.

Other Diagnostic Procedures

- Cholecystocentesis is recommended for medically managed patients with early GBM organization.
  - Unrewarding late in disease due to thick mucoid bile – risk of rupture.
  - Perform with caution.
  - Complications include bile leakage, bradycardia due to vagal stimulation, hemorrhage, and bacteremia.
  - Insert aspiration needle through liver parenchyma and into GB to help create seal of aspirate site.
- Gallbladder culture and sensitivity should be performed.
  - Anaerobic positive cultures: 9–75% of cases.
  - Aerobic positive cultures: 0–25% of cases.

Pathologic Findings

- Gross.
  - Distended GB with focal areas of erythema or hemorrhage.
  - Mural defect.
  - Focal peritonitis may be evident with adjacent omental adhesions.
  - Liver and extrahepatic biliary structures often appear normal.
  - GB contents: light green to black firm cohesive material (Figures 141.3, 141.4).
- Microscopic.
  - Mixed inflammatory infiltrate and mural fibrosis.
  - Focal areas of transmural ischemic necrosis.
  - Gallbladder cystic and papillary mucosal hyperplasia and cholecystitis.
  - Liver and extrahepatic biliary structures may be normal.

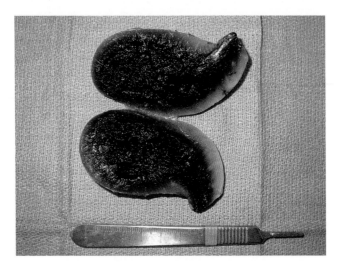

■ **Fig. 141.3.** Cross-sectional image of highly organized and inspissated bile within the lumen of a gallbladder mucocele. This was rubbery and firm when incised.

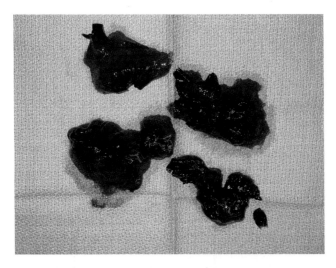

■ **Fig. 141.4.** Intraluminal contents of a gallbladder mucocele. Notice the difference in color and texture versus Figure 141.3. This material was gelatinous and soft on cross-sectional incision.

- Vacuolar hepatopathy (glycogen and/or lipid inclusions) with underlying endocrinopathy possible.
- Asymptomatic GBM removed early in disease may show only mild GB cystic mucosal hyperplasia.

THERAPEUTICS

- Surgery is standard of care.
- Surgery is emergent with EHBO and signs of rupture.
- Successful medical resolution of GBM is rare and not recommended as first-line therapy.
- Encourage hydration and allow free access to water.
- Goals are to increase bile flow and water content.
- Low-fat diet for patients with dyslipidemia.

Drug(s) of Choice

- Cholerectics and hepatoprotectants.
  - Ursodeoxycholic acid: hydrophilic bile acid used to increase biliary secretion and flow and reduce amount of hepatic cholesterol production; antiinflammatory, antiendotoxemic.
  - May cause diarrhea, vomiting, and anorexia.
  - 15 mg/kg/day PO divided twice daily with food; continue treatment after resolution of GBM.
  - S-adenosylmethionine (SAMe): increases cellular phospholipid membrane fluidity leading to cholerectic effect; antioxidant; antiinflammatory effect. May cause serotonergic effects when given concurrently with tramadol, amitriptyline, serotonin reuptake inhibitors. 20–40 mg/kg/day PO once daily on empty stomach 1 h prior to feeding. Higher dose is for choleresis.
- Antiemetics, antacids, and gastroprotectants may also be recommended.
  - Metoclopramide 0.2–0.5 mg/kg PO, IV, SQ q6–8h or 1–2 mg/kg/day by constant rate infusion (CRI).
  - Ondansetron 0.5–1.0 mg/kg PO 30 min before feeding, maximum q8h or 0.1–0.5 mg/kg slow IV push q6–12h if vomiting or nauseous.
  - Famotidine 0.5 mg/kg PO, IV, SQ q12–24h; may need to increase dose for efficacy.
  - Omeprazole or pantoprazole 1 mg/kg PO/IV q12h may induce p450 cytochrome-associated drug interactions; 24–48 h delay in onset of action.
  - Sucralfate 0.25–1.0 g PO q8–12h for upper gastrointestinal bleeding.
- Broad-spectrum antimicrobials at the time of general anesthetic induction (ampicillin/sulbactam (Unasyn™) 30 mg/kg IV once at induction).
  - Enteric gram-negative and anaerobic organisms most likely opportunists.
  - Continue treatment postoperatively if any gross contamination during surgery (amoxicillin/clavulanic acid (Clavamox™) 13.75 mg/kg PO q12h).
  - Modify antimicrobial plan based on culture and sensitivity results. Continue for four weeks postoperatively with positive cultures.

Precautions/Interactions

Cholerectics are contraindicated with EHBT obstruction.

Nursing Care

- Postoperative nursing care should be tailored to treating the patient's current systemic condition.
- Fluid support, analgesics, and patient monitoring (i.e., blood pressure, packed cell volume and total solids (PCV/TS), pain status, drain production).

- Postoperative antibiotics should be continued if gross biliary or gastrointestinal contamination was present at the time of surgery.
- Gastroprotectants are generally continued for 5–7 days following surgery.

Diet

- Patients with dyslipidemia should be fed a fat-restricted diet.
- Concurrent comorbidities should be managed appropriately with specific diets as needed (i.e., chronic kidney disease).

Activity

Patients should be strictly activity restricted postoperatively with routine monitoring and management similar to routine celiotomy recovery.

Surgical Considerations

- Cholecystectomy is the treatment of choice for GBM.
- Cholecystotomy and cholecystoenteric anastomosis not generally recommended due to recurrence and GB wall necrosis.
- Ensure patency of common bile duct prior to cholecystectomy.
- Asymptomatic patients or incidental GBM may be medically managed but will progress, necessitating surgical treatment; incidental or "premucocele" patients should be recommended for cholecystectomy at the time of diagnosis.
- Due to potential common bile duct blockage, all common bile ducts should be flushed either antegrade through the transected stump of the cystic duct into the small intestine (5 or 8 Fr red rubber) or retrograde through a small duodenotomy with a red rubber catheter (1/2 diameter of the major papilla) placed into the major papilla (Figure 141.5).
  - Retrograde flushing in cats is extremely challenging due to shared papilla with common bile duct and pancreatic dust.

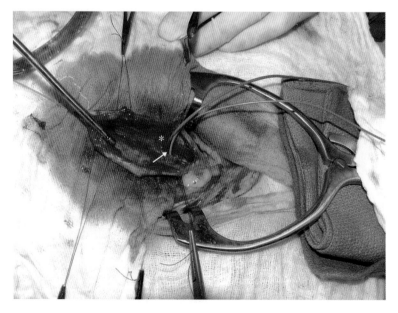

■ **Fig. 141.5.** Intraoperative duodenotomy with red rubber catheters placed into the major and minor papillas for illustration purposes. Cranial is towards the right side of the image. The major papilla is delineated with a white arrow and the minor papilla is marked by an asterisk.

- Use caution when retrograde flushing feline CBD; may cause edema in pancreas with inadvertent flushing into pancreatic duct; this may lead to severe pancreatitis.
- Laparoscopic cholecystectomy with early diagnosed GBM has excellent outcomes.
- Bile peritonitis warrants copious abdominal lavage and placement of intraperitoneal closed suction Jackson–Pratt drains.
- Liver biopsy indicated in all cases to evaluate for hepatic comorbidities.
- Submit GB for histopathology and culture with sensitivity.

 ## COMMENTS

Client Education

- Medically managed GBM is rarely successful and not recommended as patients can acutely decompensate at home.
- Surgery is the treatment of choice with rare recurrence of the disease.
- Outcome is excellent if patient survives immediate postoperative recovery.

Patient Monitoring

- Medically managed patients should be ultrasonographically monitored every four weeks with surgical intervention if no improvement.
- Postoperative patients should be reevaluated in two weeks at the time of suture removal.
- Bloodwork every 2–4 weeks until normalization of hepatic values. Postoperative bloodwork generally normalizes in two weeks to three months but clinically normal patients may have persistently elevated liver values.

Prevention/Avoidance

- Early surgical intervention provides better outcomes and decreased complications.
- Patients should be recommended for surgery at initial diagnosis of GBM.

Possible Complications

- Rupture of GBM causing bile peritonitis.
- Septic peritonitis with ruptured infected GBM.
- Hepatic duct occlusion with mucoid bile secondary to retrograde flushing against ligated cystic duct after cholecystectomy (reason for small-diameter red rubber tube with retrograde flushing).
- Shock.
- Sepsis.
- Surgical site dehiscence.
- Cholecystitis.
- Pancreatitis.
- Biliary tract leakage postoperatively.
- Reobstruction of common bile duct with gelatinous bile material.
- Hypotension.
- Disseminated intravascular coagulation.

Expected Course and Prognosis

- Excellent if the patient survives the perioperative period and there is no biliary tract rupture.
- Mortality rate 20–39%. Majority occur within first two weeks after surgery.
- Hypotension, decreased PCV, and elevated lactate associated with poorer outcomes.
- Reported overall survival rates not affected by GB rupture or positive GB cultures.

Abbreviations

- APTT = activated partial thromboplastin time
- EHBO = extrahepatic biliary obstruction
- EHBT = extrahepatic biliary tract
- GB = gallbladder
- GBM = gallbladder mucocele

- HAC = hyperadrenocorticism
- PCV = packed cell volume
- PT = prothrombin time
- PU/PD = polyuria/polydipsia
- TEG = thromboelastography
- TS = total solids

See Also

- Biliary Duct or Gallbladder Rupture and Bile Peritonitis
- Cholecystitis and Choledochitis
- Cholelithiasis

- Cholecystitis
- Hepatitis
- Bile Duct Obstruction (Extrahepatic)

Suggested Reading

Aguirre AL, Center SA, Randolph JF. Gallbladder disease in Shetland Sheepdogs: 38 cases (1995–2005). J Am Vet Med Assoc 2007;231:79–88.

Malek S, Sinclair E, Hosgood G, et al. Clinical findings and prognostic factors for dogs undergoing cholecystectomy for gallbladder mucocele. Vet Surg 2013;42:418–426.

Mayhew PD, Weisse C. Liver and biliary system. In: Tobias KM, Johnston SA, eds. Veterinary Surgery Small Animal. St Louis: Elsevier, 2012.

Mehler SJ, Mayhew PD. Gallbladder mucocele. In: Monnet E, ed. Small Animal Soft Tissue Surgery. Oxford: Wiley-Blackwell, 2013.

Smalle TM, Cahalane AK, Köster LS. Gallbladder mucocele: a review. J S Afr Vet Assoc 2015;86:1318.

Acknowledgments: The authors and editors acknowledge the prior contribution of Dr Sharon Center.

Authors: James Howard DVM, MS, Kathleen L. Ham DVM, MS, DACVS-SA, Amy N. Zide DVM, Nina R. Kieves DVM, DACVS-SA, DACVSMR

Index

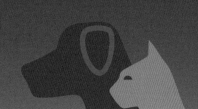

abdomen
  acute *see* acute abdomen
abdominal effusion
  AVMs of liver *vs.*, 682
  bile peritonitis *vs.*, 912
abdominal neoplasia
  feline pancreatitis *vs.*, 657
abdominal pain
  bile peritonitis *vs.*, 912
abscess(es)
  cervical
    vs. salivary mucocele, 166
  hepatic, 817–22, *820 see also* hepatic
    abscess(es)
  pancreatic, 628–31 *see also* pancreatic
    abscess(es)
  perineal
    vs. perineal hernia, 589
achalasia
  cricopharyngeal, 189–94, *192 see also*
    cricopharyngeal achalasia (CPA)
acid suppression
  in esophagitis management, 225–6
acquired portosystemic shunts (PSS), 878–84,
    881. see also portosystemic shunts (PSS),
    acquired
acute abdomen, 3–9
  clinical features, 4
  comments, 9
  definition/overview, 3
  diagnostics, 5–7
  differential diagnosis, 4–5
  etiology/pathophysiology, 3
  signalment/history, 4
  therapeutics, 7–8
acute gastritis, 289–95, *290–2,* **293**
acute gastroenteritis, 84–7, **85**
  nutritional approach to, 84–7, **85**
    fat in, **85,** 86
    feeding recommendations, 86–7

fiber in, **85,** 86
  overall considerations, 84–6, **85**
  protein in, 85, **85**
  water in, 85
  severe
    vs. acute hepatic failure, 756
acute hemorrhagic diarrhea syndrome (AHDS),
    402–8. *see also* hemorrhagic gastroenteritis
acute hepatic failure, 755–62, *758. see also* hepatic
    failure, acute
acute hepatic injury
  leptospirosis *vs.*, 860
acute hepatitis
  infectious hepatopathy *vs.*, 829
acutely decompensated chronic liver disease
  acute hepatic failure *vs.*, 756
acute pancreatitis
  necrotizing
    vs. hepatotoxins, 846
  nutritional approach to, 616–19, **617**
  severe
    vs. acute hepatic failure, 756
adenocarcinoma
  rectal
    rectal prolapse and, 45, *46*
    tenesmus due to, 45, *46*
  rectoanal polyps *vs.*, 602
adenoma(s)
  hepatic
    vs. HNH and HDH, 782
  malignant colonic neoplasia *vs.*, 565
adenomatous polyps
  colonic, 559, *560*
  definition/overview, 460, *460*
adverse food reactions, 384–8
  clinical features, 385
  comments, 388
  definition/overview, 384
  diagnostics, 385–7
  differential diagnosis, 385

Blackwell's Five-Minute Veterinary Consult Clinical Companion: Small Animal Gastrointestinal Diseases,
First Edition. Edited by Jocelyn Mott and Jo Ann Morrison.
© 2019 John Wiley & Sons, Inc. Published 2019 by John Wiley & Sons, Inc.
Companion website: www.fiveminutevet.com/gastrointestinal

adverse food reactions (*cont'd*)
etiology/pathophysiology, 384
in nutritional approach to chronic
enteropathies, 493–6, **494**, **495** *see also*
under chronic enteropathy(ies), nutritional
approach to
signalment/history, 385
therapeutics, 387–8
AHDS. *see* acute hemorrhagic diarrhea syndrome
(AHDS)
allergen(s)
dietary
in nutritional approach to chronic
enteropathies, 493–6, **494**, **495**
alveolar mucositis
definition/overview, 179
amyloid
hepatic, 742–7, *745 see also* hepatic amyloid
amyloidosis
definition/overview, 742
anal prolapse, 95–102, *96–101*
clinical features, 96, *96*
comments, 101–2
definition/overview, 95
diagnostics, 96, 98
differential diagnosis, 96, *97*
etiology/pathophysiology, 95
signalment/history, 95–6
therapeutics, 98–101, *98–101*
diet, 99
drugs of choice, 98
nursing care, 99
surgical considerations, 99–101, *99–101*
ancylostomiasis
signalment/history, 507
anorectal stricture, 593
anthelmintics
for feline chronic diarrhea, 39, **39**
antibiotic(s)
for feline chronic diarrhea, 40
antibiotic-responsive diarrhea (ARD), 354–9
clinical features, 355
comments, 358–9
definition/overview, 354, 454
diagnostics, 356–7
differential diagnosis, 355–6
etiology/pathophysiology, 354
signalment/history, 354–55
therapeutics, 357–8
anticestodal treatment
for CCHS, 693, **694**
antiemetics
for feline chronic diarrhea, 40
in nutritional approach to acute and chronic
pancreatitis, 618

antimicrobial agents
for CCHS, 693, **693**
antiprotozoal agents
for feline chronic diarrhea, 39, **39**
appetite stimulants
for feline chronic diarrhea, 40
ARD. *see* antibiotic-responsive diarrhea (ARD)
arteriovenous malformations (AVMs)
hepatic
vs. congenital portosystemic vascular
anomaly, 888
intrahepatic
definition/overview, 681
of liver, 681–6, *682*
clinical features, 682, *682*
comments, 685–6
definition/overview, 681
diagnostics, 682, 683
differential diagnosis, 682–3
etiology/pathophysiology, 681
signalment/history, 681–2
therapeutics, 684–5
ascariasis
etiology/pathophysiology, 506–7
signalment/history, 507
ascarid(s)
definition/overview, 506
ascites
acquired PSS *vs.*, 880
atresia ani, 533–8, *534–6*
clinical features, 534, *535*, *534*
comments, 537–8
definition/overview, 533
diagnostics, 535, *536*
differential diagnosis, 534
etiology/pathophysiology, 533
signalment/history, 533–4
therapeutics, 535–7, *536*
atrophic gastritis, 296–9. *see also* gastritis,
atrophic
atypical hypoadrenocorticism
BVS *vs.*, 332
AVMs. *see* arteriovenous malformations (AVMs)

bacterial enteritis, 360–9
Campylobacter, 360–5, 367, 368 *see also*
Campylobacter, bacterial enteritis due to
clinical features, 363
comments, 368–9
definition/overview, 360
diagnostics, 364–6
differential diagnosis, 364
Escherichia coli, 361–7, 369 *see also Escherichia*
coli, bacterial enteritis due to
etiology/pathophysiology, 360–2

signalment/history, 362–3
therapeutics, 366–7
Basenjis
immunoproliferative enteropathy of, 444–8
see also immunoproliferative enteropathy,
of Basenjis
bile duct obstruction
extrahepatic, 901–9, *904 see also* extrahepatic
biliary duct obstruction (EHBDO)
bile peritonitis, 910–17, *913*
clinical features, 911–12
comments, 916–17
definition/overview, 910
diagnostics, 912–14, *913*
etiology/pathophysiology, 910–11
signalment/history, 911
therapeutics, 914–16
biliary cyst(s)
EHBDO *vs.*, 903
biliary disease(s)
gallbladder mucocele *vs.*, 945–6
biliary duct rupture, 910–17, *913*
clinical features, 911–12
comments, 916–17
diagnostics, 912–14, *913*
differential diagnosis, 912
etiology/pathophysiology, 910–11
signalment/history, 911
therapeutics, 914–16
biliary neoplasia, 918–24, *921*
clinical features, 919–20
comments, 923–4
definition/overview, 918
diagnostics, 920–2, *921*
differential diagnosis, 920
etiology/pathophysiology, 918–19
signalment/history, 919
therapeutics, 922–3
biliary tract
diseases of, 899–952 *see also specific types and
biliary tract disease(s)*
biliary tract disease(s), 899–952. *see also specific
types*
bile peritonitis, 910–17, *913*
biliary duct rupture, 910–17, *913*
biliary neoplasia, 918–24, *921*
cholecystitis, 925–31, *928*
emphysematous, 932–6, *934*
choledochitis, 925–31, *928*
cholelithiasis, 937–42, *939*
EHBDO, 901–9, *904*
extrahepatic
vs. infectious hepatopathy, 830
gallbladder mucocele, 943–52, *943, 947, 948, 950*
gallbladder rupture, 910–17, *913*

bilious vomiting syndrome (BVS), 331–6, *333*, **334**
clinical features, 332
comments, 335–6
definition/overview, 331
diagnostics, 332–4, *333*
differential diagnosis, 332
etiology/pathophysiology, 331
signalment/history, 331–2
therapeutics, 334–5, **334**
brachycephalic dogs
esophagitis in, 224
BVS. *see* bilious vomiting syndrome (BVS)

CAH. *see* copper-associated hepatopathy (CAH)
calvarial hyperostosis
craniomandibular osteopathy *vs.*, 128
Campylobacter
bacterial enteritis due to, 360–5, 367, 368
clinical features, 363
comments, 368
diagnostics, 365
differential diagnosis, 364
etiology/pathophysiology, 361
signalment/history, 362–3
therapeutics, 367
canine adenovirus type 1 (CAV-1). *see also*
infectious canine hepatitis (ICH)
ICH due to, 801
canine parvovirus (CPV)-2 infection, 337–44
clinical features, 339
comments, 343–4
definition/overview, 337
diagnostics, 340–1
differential diagnosis, 339
etiology/pathophysiology, 337–8
signalment/history, 338–9
therapeutics, 341–3
carbohydrate(s)
in nutritional approach to chronic
enteropathies, 491–2, **491**
in nutritional approach to EPI, 614, **614**
in nutritional approach to hepatobiliary
diseases, 867, **867**
carcinoma(s)
hepatocellular
vs. HNH and HDH, 782
carcinoma in situ
malignant colonic neoplasia *vs.*, 565
rectoanal polyps *vs.*, 602
Caroli's disease, 721
cat(s). *see also under* feline
caudal stomatitis in, 179–85, *180, 182, 183*
see also stomatitis, caudal–feline
chronic diarrhea in, 28–44, *29, 32,* 36–7, *39,*
41, 42, *42 see also* diarrhea, chronic–feline

cat(s). *see also under* feline (*cont'd*)
  GI lymphoma in, 431–7, *433, 434 see also*
    gastrointestinal (GI) lymphoma–feline
  HL in, 763–70, *766 see also* hepatic
    lipidosis (HL)
  hyperthyroidism in, 823–7, *825 see also*
    hyperthyroidism, feline
  IBD in
    differential diagnosis, 450
  megacolon in
    vs. malignant colonic neoplasia, 565
  pancreatitis in, 656–61 *see also* pancreatitis,
    feline
  viral enterides in, 378–83, *379 see also* feline
    viral enterides
caudal mucositis
  definition/overview, 179
CAV-1. *see* canine adenovirus type 1
  (CAV-1)
CCHS. *see* cholangitis/cholangiohepatitis
  syndrome (CCHS)
central nervous system (CNS) signs
  AVMs of liver *vs.*, 682
cervical abscess(es)
  salivary mucocele *vs.*, 166
cheilitis
  definition/overview, 179
cholangiohepatitis
  definition/overview, 687
  nutritional approach to, 869–70, **869**
cholangitis, 687–96, **692–4**. *see also*
  cholangitis/cholangiohepatitis
  syndrome (CCHS)
  categories of, 687
  clinical features, 689
  comments, 695–6
  definition/overview, 687
  destructive, 697–701, *699*
    clinical features, 698
    comments, 700–1
    definition/overview, 697
    diagnostics, 698–9, *699*
    differential diagnosis, 698
    etiology/pathophysiology, 687, 698
    signalment/history, 698
    therapeutics, 700
  diagnostics, 690–2, **692**
  differential diagnosis, 689–90
  etiology/pathophysiology, 687–8
  lymphocytic, 687–96, **692–4**
  neutrophilic, 687–96, **692–4**
  sclerosing
    definition/overview, 697
  signalment/history, 688–9
  therapeutics, 692–4, **693, 694**

cholangitis/cholangiohepatitis syndrome (CCHS),
  687–96, **692–4**. *see also* cholangitis
  clinical features, 689
  comments, 695–6
  definition/overview, 687
  diagnostics, 690–2, **692**
  differential diagnosis, 689–90
  EHBDO *vs.*, 903
  etiology/pathophysiology, 687–8
  signalment/history, 688–9
  therapeutics, 692–4, **693, 694**
cholecystitis, 925–31, *928*
  clinical features, 926
  comments, 930
  definition/overview, 925
  diagnostics, 927–8, *928*
  differential diagnosis, 927
  emphysematous, 932–6, *934*
    clinical features, 933
    comments, 935
    definition/overview, 932
    diagnostics, 933, *934*
    differential diagnosis, 933
    etiology/pathophysiology, 932
    signalment/history, 932
    therapeutics, 934–5
  etiology/pathophysiology, 925–6
  signalment/history, 926
  therapeutics, 929
choledochitis, 925–31, *928*
  clinical features, 926
  comments, 930
  definition/overview, 925
  diagnostics, 927–8, *928*
  differential diagnosis, 927
  etiology/pathophysiology, 925–6
  signalment/history, 926
  therapeutics, 929
cholelithiasis, 937–42, *939*
  clinical features, 938
  comments, 940–1
  definition/overview, 937
  diagnostics, 938–9, *939*
  differential diagnosis, 938
  etiology/pathophysiology, 937
  signalment/history, 937–8
  therapeutics, 940
CHPG. *see* chronic hypertrophic pyloric
  gastropathy (CHPG)
chronic cholangitis, 687–96, **692–4**. *see also*
  cholangitis; cholangitis/cholangiohepatitis
  syndrome (CCHS)
chronic enteropathy(ies)
  diet-responsive
    definition/overview, 384

nutritional approach to, 490–505
  adverse food reactions, 493–6, **494, 495**
  altered GI microbiome, 502–3, **502**
  carbohydrates in, 491–2, **491**
  constipation, 500–2, **501, 500**
  energy in, 490–1, **491**
  fats in, **491**, 492
  fiber in, 491–2, **491**
  food intolerances, 493
  functional, 498–503, **498–502**
  IBD–related, 496–7, **497**
  IBS–related, 499–500, **500**
  lymphangiectasia, 498–9, **499, 498**
  omega-3 fatty acids in, 494–5, **495**
  overall considerations, 490–2, **491**
  PLE–related, 498, **498**
  protein in, 491, **491**
chronic gastritis, 300–5. *see also* gastritis, chronic
chronic hepatitis. *see* hepatitis, chronic
chronic hypertrophic pyloric gastropathy (CHPG),
    324–7
  clinical features, 325
  comments, 327
  definition/overview, 324
  diagnostics, 325–6
  differential diagnosis, 325
  etiology/pathophysiology, 324
  signalment/history, 324–5
  therapeutics, 326–7
chronic idiopathic large bowel diarrhea (CILBD),
    478–83, *480, 481*
  clinical features, 479
  comments, 483
  definition/overview, 478
  diagnostics, 479–81, *480, 481*
  differential diagnosis, 479
  etiology/pathophysiology, 478
  fiber-responsive, 568–72, *570, 571 see also*
    fiber-responsive large bowel diarrhea
  prevalence of, 478
  signalment/history, 478
  therapeutics, 481–3
chronic liver disease
  acutely decompensated
    vs. acute hepatic failure, 756
chronic pancreatitis
  BVS *vs.*, 332
  nutritional approach to, 616–19, **617**
CILBD. *see* chronic idiopathic large bowel
    diarrhea (CILBD)
circulatory disorders
  nutritional approach to, 874–6, **875, 876**
cirrhosis of liver, 702–10
  clinical features, 704
  comments, 708–9

definition/overview, 702
  diagnostics, 704–6
  differential diagnosis, 704
  EHBDO *vs.*, 903
  etiology/pathophysiology, 702–3
  signalment/history, 703
  therapeutics, 706–8
clostridial enterotoxicosis, 539–45, *541, 542*
  clinical features, 540
  comments, 544
  definition/overview, 539
  diagnostics, 541–3, *542, 541*
  differential diagnosis, 540
  etiology/pathophysiology, 539–40
  signalment/history, 540
  therapeutics, 543
Clostridium difficile
  clostridial enterotoxicosis related to, 539–45,
    541, 542 see also clostridial enterotoxicosis
Clostridium perfringens
  clostridial enterotoxicosis related to, 539–545,
    542 see also clostridial enterotoxicosis
CNS. *see* central nervous system (CNS)
coagulopathy of liver disease, 673–8, *675*
  CAH *vs.*, 714
  clinical features, 674
  comments, 677–8
  definition/overview, 673
  diagnostics, 674–6, *675*
  differential diagnosis, 674
  etiology/pathophysiology, 673–4
  signalment/history, 674
  therapeutics, 676–7
cobalamin
  absorption of, 345
  in nutritional approach to acute and chronic
    pancreatitis, 618
  in nutritional approach to EPI, 615, **616**
cobalamin deficiency, 345–9
  clinical features, 347
  comments, 349
  definition/overview, 345
  diagnostics, 347–8
  differential diagnosis, 347
  etiology/pathophysiology, 345–6
  signalment/history, 347
  therapeutics, 348–9
coccidia
  clinical features, 508
  etiology/pathophysiology, 507
  therapeutics, 510
colitis, 546–53
  clinical features, 547
  comments, 551–2
  definition/overview, 546

colitis (*cont'd*)
 diagnostics, 548–9
 differential diagnosis, 548
 etiology/pathophysiology, 546–7
 histiocytic ulcerative, 554–8 *see also* histiocytic
  ulcerative colitis (HUC)
 signalment/history, 547
 therapeutics, 549–51
colon
 diseases of, 531–610 *see also specific types and*
  colon disease(s)
 neoplasia of
  benign, 559–63, *560 see also* colonic
   neoplasia–benign
  malignant, 564–7, *566 see also* colonic
   neoplasia–malignant
colon disease(s), 531–610. *see also specific types*
 atresia ani, 533–8, *534–6*
 clostridial enterotoxicosis, 539–45, *541, 542*
 colitis, 546–53
 colonic neoplasia
  benign, 559–63, *560 see also* colonic
   neoplasia–benign
  malignant, 564–7, *566 see also* colonic
   neoplasia–malignant
 fiber-responsive large bowel diarrhea, 568–72,
  570, 571
 HUC, 554–8
 megacolon, 573–80, *575, 576, 579*
 perianal fistula, 581–7, *582–4*
 perineal hernia, 588–92, *591*
 proctitis, 546–53
 rectal stricture, 593–600, *596–9*
 rectoanal polyps, 601–7, *604–6*
 trichomoniasis, 608–10
colonic neoplasia–benign, 559–63, *560*
 clinical features, 561
 comments, 562–3
 definition/overview, 559
 diagnostics, 561
 differential diagnosis, 561
 etiology/pathophysiology, 559, *560*
 signalment/history, 561
 therapeutics, 562
colonic neoplasia–malignant, 564–7, *566*
 clinical features, 565
 comments, 567
 definition/overview, 564
 diagnostics, 565, *566*
 differential diagnosis, 565
 etiology/pathophysiology, 564
 signalment/history, 564–5
 therapeutics, 566–7
congenital hepatic fibrosis, 721

congenital portosystemic shunt (CPSS)
 definition/overview, 885
congenital portosystemic vascular anomaly,
  885–97, *885, 888–91, 893, 894*. *see also*
  portosystemic vascular anomaly, congenital
congestive heart failure
 right-sided
  vs. infectious hepatopathy, 830
constipation, 10–14
 clinical features, 11
 comments, 14
 definition/overview, 10
 diagnostics, 12–13
 differential diagnosis, 11–12
 etiology/pathophysiology, 10
 nutritional approach to, 500–2, **500–1**
 signalment/history, 10–11
 therapeutics, 13–14
copper-associated hepatopathy (CAH),
  711–20, **717**
 clinical features, 713
 comments, 718–20
 definition/overview, 711
 diagnostics, 715–17
 differential diagnosis, 713–14
 EHBDO *vs.*, 903
 etiology/pathophysiology, 711–12
 nutritional approach to, 873–4, **874, 873**
 signalment/history, 712–13
 therapeutics, 717–18, **717**
 types of, 711
copper chelators, 717, **717**
CPA. *see* cricopharyngeal achalasia (CPA)
CPSS. *see* congenital portosystemic shunt (CPSS)
CPV-2 infection. *see* canine parvovirus (CPV)-2
  infection
craniomandibular osteopathy, 127–33, *128–31*
 clinical features, 128, *128*
 comments, 132
 definition/overview, 127
 diagnostics, 129, *129–31*
 differential diagnosis, 128
 etiology/pathophysiology, 127
 signalment/history, 127–8
 therapeutics, 131–2
cricopharyngeal achalasia (CPA), 189–94, *192*
 clinical features, 190
 comments, 193–4
 definition/overview, 189
 diagnostics, 191, *192*
 differential diagnosis, 190
 etiology/pathophysiology, 189
 signalment/history, 190
 therapeutics, 192–3

cricopharyngeal dysphagia
  differential diagnosis, 53–4, *54*
  etiology/pathophysiology, 51
cryptosporidiosis, 350–3
  clinical features, 351
  comments, 352–3
  definition/overview, 350
  diagnostics, 351
  differential diagnosis, 351
  etiology/pathophysiology, 350
  signalment/history, 350–1
  therapeutics, 351–2
Cryptosporidium spp.
  definition/overview, 350
cyst(s)
  biliary
    vs. EHBDO, 903
  thyroglossal
    vs. salivary mucocele, 166
  tonsil
    vs. salivary mucocele, 166
Cystoisospora spp.
  etiology/pathophysiology, 507
cystoisosporiasis/coccidiosis
  signalment/history, 507–8

dermatitis
  eosinophilic
    feline, 134–40, *135–8 see also* feline
      eosinophilic dermatitis
destructive cholangitis, 697–701, *699. see also*
    cholangitis, destructive
diarrhea
  acute, 15–19
    clinical features, 16
    comments, 19
    definition/overview, 15
    diagnostics, 16–17
    differential diagnosis, 16
    etiology/pathophysiology, 15
    signalment/history, 15–16
    therapeutics, 17–18
  antibiotic-responsive, 354–9 *see also*
    antibiotic-responsive diarrhea
    (ARD)
  chronic–canine, 20–7, **20**, 22
    clinical features, 21–2
    comments, 25–6
    definition/overview, 20
    diagnostics, 22–4, *22*
    differential diagnosis, 22
    etiology/pathophysiology, 20–1, **20**
    signalment/history, 21
    therapeutics, 24–5

  chronic–feline, 28–44, **29**, *32*, 36–7, 39, **41**,
    42, *42*
    clinical features, 30
    comments, 43–4
    definition/overview, 28
    diagnostics, 31–8, *32*, 36–7
    diet, 41–2, **42**
    differential diagnosis, 30–1
    etiology/pathophysiology, 28–9
    nursing care, 41, *42*
    signalment/history, 29–30, **29**
    therapeutics, 39–42, **39**, **41**, **42**, *42*
  large bowel
    chronic idiopathic, 478–83, *480, 481 see also*
      chronic idiopathic large bowel diarrhea
      (CILBD)
    fiber-responsive, 568–72, *570, 571 see also*
      fiber-responsive large bowel diarrhea
    tylosin-responsive
      definition/overview, 454
diet
  for anal and rectal prolapse, 99
  for esophagitis, 228
  for feline chronic diarrhea, 41–2, **42**
dietary hypersensitivity
  in nutritional approach to chronic
    enteropathies, 493–6, **494**, **495**
diet-responsive chronic enteropathy
  definition/overview, 384
diffuse hepatopathy(ies)
  glycogen-type VH vs., 736
diffuse infiltrative liver disease
  EHBDO vs., 903
diverticulum(a)
  esophageal
    vs. esophagitis, 224
  gastroesophageal, 195–7 *see also*
    gastroesophageal diverticula
dog(s)
  brachycephalic
    esophagitis in, 224
  chronic diarrhea in, 20–7, **20**, 22 *see also*
    diarrhea, chronic–canine
  GI lymphoma in, 425–30 *see also*
    gastrointestinal (GI) lymphoma–canine
  GSE in Irish Setters, 441–3 *see also* gluten-
    sensitive enteropathy (GSE), in Irish Setters
  immunoproliferative enteropathy of Basenjis,
    444–8 *see also* immunoproliferative
    enteropathy, of Basenjis
  infectious hepatitis in, 801–6 *see also* infectious
    canine hepatitis (ICH)
  pancreatitis in, 649–55, *651, 652 see also*
    pancreatitis, canine

drug(s)
  administration of
    vs. megacolon, 574
ductal plate malformation, 721–8
  clinical features, 723
  comments, 727–8
  definition/overview, 721
  diagnostics, 724–6
  differential diagnosis, 723
  etiology/pathophysiology, 721–2
  signalment/history, 722–3
  therapeutics, 726–7
dysbiosis
  intestinal, 454–9, *457 see also* intestinal
    dysbiosis
dyschezia, 45–50, *46*
  clinical features, 46
  comments, 49–50
  constipation *vs.*, 11, 12
  definition/overview, 45
  diagnostics, 47–8
  differential diagnosis, 47
  etiology/pathophysiology, 45, *46*
  signalment/history, 45–6
  therapeutics, 48–9
dysmotility
  gastric and intestinal, 259–65, **263** *see also*
    gastric motility disorders; intestinal
    motility disorders
dysphagia(s), 51–7, *54, 56*
  clinical features, 53
  comments, 56–7
  definition/overview, 51
  diagnostics, 54–5
  differential diagnosis, 53–4, *54*
  etiology/pathophysiology, 51–2
  oropharyngeal
    vs. esophagitis, 224
  phases of, 51–4, *54*
  signalment/history, 52
  therapeutics, 55–6, *56*
  types of, 51–4, *54*
dysplasia(s)
  microvascular
    hepatoportal, 836–42 *see also* hepatoportal
    microvascular dysplasia (MVD)
  vascular
    nutritional approach to, 874, 876, **876**

effusion(s)
  abdominal
    vs. AVMs of liver, 682
    vs. bile peritonitis, 912
EGC. *see* eosinophilic granuloma complex (EGC)

EHBDO. *see* extrahepatic biliary duct obstruction
  (EHBDO)
emphysematous cholecystitis, 932–6, *934. see also*
  cholecystitis, emphysematous
encephalopathy(ies)
  hepatic, 748–54 *see also* hepatic
    encephalopathy (HE)
endocrine disease(s)
  megacolon *vs.*, 574
energy
  in nutritional approach to chronic
    enteropathies, 490–1, **491**
  in nutritional approach to hepatobiliary
    diseases, 866–7, **867**
enteritides
  fungal, 389–95, *390, 392 see also* fungal
    enteritides
enteritis
  bacterial, 360–9 *see also* bacterial enteritis
  intussusception *vs.*, 472
  lymphocytic-plasmacytic
    chronic vomiting associated with, 118, *118*
enterocolitis
  granulomatous, 370–7, *371, 372, 375 see also*
    granulomatous enterocolitis
enteropathy(ies)
  chronic *see* chronic enteropathy(ies)
  gluten-sensitive
    in Irish Setters, 441–3 *see also* gluten-sensitive
    enteropathy (GSE), in Irish Setters
  immunoproliferative
    of Basenjis, 444–8 *see also*
      immunoproliferative enteropathy, of
      Basenjis
  protein-losing, 513–20, *516, 518 see also*
    protein-losing enteropathy (PLE)
enterotoxicosis
  clostridial, 539–45, *541, 542 see also* clostridial
    enterotoxicosis
eosinophilic dermatitis
  feline, 134–40, *135–8 see also* feline
    eosinophilic dermatitis
eosinophilic gastroenteritis, 396–401
  clinical features, 397
  comments, 400–1
  definition/overview, 396
  diagnostics, 397–8
  differential diagnosis, 397
  etiology/pathophysiology, 396
  signalment/history, 396–7
  therapeutics, 398–400
eosinophilic granuloma complex (EGC), 134–40,
  135–8. see also feline eosinophilic
  dermatitis

EPI. *see* exocrine pancreatic insufficiency (EPI)
Escherichia coli
   bacterial enteritis due to, 361–7, 369
      clinical features, 363
      comments, 369
      diagnostics, 366–7
      differential diagnosis, 363
      etiology/pathophysiology, 361–2
      signalment/history, 363
      therapeutics, 367
esophageal disease(s), 185–256. *see also specific*
      types
   chronic vomiting associated with, 117
   CPA, 189–94, *192*
   esophageal fistula, 198–204, *200, 201*
   esophageal foreign bodies, 205–8, *206*
   esophageal neoplasia, 209–13, *211*
   esophageal stricture, 214–19, *216*
   esophagitis, 220–30, *221–3*
   gastroesophageal diverticula, 195–7
   hiatal hernia, 231–7, *232, 234, 236, 237*
   megaesophagus, 238–46, *241, 242, 244*
   nutritional approach to GERD and
      megaesophagus, 247–50, **248**
   Spirocerca lupi, 251–6, *253*
esophageal diverticula
   esophagitis *vs.*, 224
esophageal dysphagia
   differential diagnosis, 54
esophageal fistula, 198–204, *200, 201*
   clinical features, 199
   comments, 203–4
   definition/overview, 198
   diagnostics, 199–202, *200, 201*
   differential diagnosis, 199
   etiology/pathophysiology, 198
   signalment/history, 199
   therapeutics, 202–3
   types of, 198
esophageal foreign bodies, 205–8, *206*
   clinical features, 205
   comments, 208
   definition/overview, 205
   diagnostics, 206–7, *206*
   differential diagnosis, 206
   esophagitis *vs.*, 224
   etiology/pathophysiology, 205
   signalment/history, 205
   therapeutics, 207
esophageal neoplasia, 209–13, *211*
   clinical features, 210
   comments, 212–13
   definition/overview, 209
   diagnostics, 210–11, *211*

   differential diagnosis, 210
   esophagitis *vs.*, 224
   etiology/pathophysiology, 209
   signalment/history, 209–10
   therapeutics, 211–12
esophageal stricture, 214–19, *216*
   clinical features, 215
   comments, 218–19
   definition/overview, 214
   diagnostics, 215–16, *216*
   differential diagnosis, 215
   esophagitis *vs.*, 224
   etiology/pathophysiology, 214
   signalment/history, 215
   therapeutics, 217–18
esophagitis, 220–30, *221–3*
   in brachycephalic dogs, 224
   clinical features, 224
   comments, 228–9
   definition/overview, 220
   diagnostics, 224–5
   differential diagnosis, 224
   etiology/pathophysiology, 220–2, *221–3*
   GER and, 220
   signalment/history, 223
   therapeutics, 225–8
      acid suppression, 225–6
      alternative agents, 227
      diet, 228
      GI prokinetics, 226–7
      mucosal protectants, 227
esophagus
   diseases of, 185–256 *see also specific diseases*
      and esophageal disease(s)
   foreign bodies of, 205–8, *206 see also*
      esophageal foreign bodies
Eurytrema procyonis, 640–4
exocrine pancreatic insufficiency (EPI), 621–7,
      622, 623
   clinical features, *622, 623*
   comments, 626–7
   definition/overview, 621
   diagnostics, 623–4
   differential diagnosis, 623
   etiology/pathophysiology, 621
   GSE in Irish Setters *vs.*, 442
   nutritional approach to, 613–16, **614, 616**
      carbohydrates in, 614, **614**
      cobalamin in, 615, **616**
      fats in, 614–15, **614**
      feeding recommendations, 616
      fiber in, **614**, 615
      main considerations, 614–15, **614**
      protein in, 614, **614**

exocrine pancreatic insufficiency (EPI) (*cont'd*)
SIBO and, 613
signalment/history, 621–2, *622*
therapeutics, 624–6
extrahepatic biliary disease
infectious hepatopathy *vs.*, 830
extrahepatic biliary duct obstruction (EHBDO),
901–9, *904*
clinical features, 902–3
comments, 907–8
definition/overview, 901
diagnostics, 903–5, *904*
differential diagnosis, 903
etiology/pathophysiology, 901
signalment/history, 902
therapeutics, 905–7

fat(s)
in nutritional approach to acute and chronic
pancreatitis, **617**, 618
in nutritional approach to acute gastroenteritis,
85, 86
in nutritional approach to chronic
enteropathies, **491**, 492
in nutritional approach to EPI,
614–15, **614**
in nutritional approach to GERD and
megaesophagus, 248, **248**
in nutritional approach to hepatobiliary
diseases, 867, **867**
feline eosinophilic dermatitis, 134–40, *135–8*
clinical features, 135–6, *135–7*
comments, 139–40
definition/overview, 134
diagnostics, 137–8, *138*
differential diagnosis, 136
etiology/pathophysiology, 134
signalment/history, 135
therapeutics, 138–9
feline hepatic lipidosis (HL). *see* hepatic
lipidosis (HL)
feline hyperthyroidism, 823–7, *825*. *see also*
hyperthyroidism, feline
feline pancreatitis, 656–61. *see also* pancreatitis,
feline
feline viral enterides, 378–83, *379*
clinical features, 380
comments, 382–3
definition/overview, 378
diagnostics, 380–1
differential diagnosis, 380
etiology/pathophysiology, 378–80, *379*
signalment/history, 380
therapeutics, 381

fiber
in nutritional approach to acute and chronic
pancreatitis, **617**, 618
in nutritional approach to acute gastroenteritis,
85, 86
in nutritional approach to chronic
enteropathies, 491–2, **491**
in nutritional approach to GERD and
megaesophagus, 248, **248**
fiber-responsive large bowel diarrhea, 568–72,
570, 571
clinical features, 569
comments, 572
definition/overview, 568
diagnostics, 569–71, *570, 571*
differential diagnosis, 569
etiology/pathophysiology, 568
signalment/history, 569
therapeutics, 571–2
fibrosis of liver, 702–10
clinical features, 704
comments, 708–9
congenital, 721
definition/overview, 702
diagnostics, 704–6
differential diagnosis, 704
EHBDO *vs.*, 903
etiology/pathophysiology, 702–3
signalment/history, 703
therapeutics, 706–8
fistula(s)
esophageal, 198–204, *200, 201 see also*
esophageal fistula
perianal, 581–7, *582–4 see also* perianal fistula
flatulence, 58–62, *60*
clinical features, 59
comments, 62
definition/overview, 58
diagnostics, 60–1, *60*
differential diagnosis, 59–60
etiology/pathophysiology, 58
signalment/history, 58–9
therapeutics, 61–2
food intolerances
in nutritional approach to chronic
enteropathies, 493
food reactions
adverse *see* adverse food reactions
foreign body(ies)
esophageal, 205–8, *206 see also* esophageal
foreign bodies
salivary mucocele *vs.*, 166
fulminant hepatic failure
EHBDO *vs.*, 903

fungal enteritides, 389–95, *390, 392*
  clinical features, 391
  comments, 394–5
  definition/overview, 389
  diagnostics, 391–3, *392*
  differential diagnosis, 391
  etiology/pathophysiology, 389–90, *390*
  signalment/history, 390
  therapeutics, 393–4

gallbladder mucocele, 943–52, *943, 947, 948, 950*
  clinical features, 945
  comments, 951–2
  definition/overview, 943, *943*
  diagnostics, 946–9, *947, 948*
  differential diagnosis, 945–6
  etiology/pathophysiology, 944
  infectious hepatopathy *vs.*, 829
  signalment/history, 944–5
  therapeutics, 949–51, *950*
gallbladder rupture, 910–17, *913*
  clinical features, 911–12
  comments, 916–17
  diagnostics, 912–14, *913*
  etiology/pathophysiology, 910–11
  signalment/history, 911
  therapeutics, 914–16
ganglioneuromatosis
  definition/overview, 460
gastric dilation-volvulus (GDV), 266–72, *269*
  clinical features, 267–8
  comments, 271–2
  definition/overview, 266
  diagnostics, 268–9, *269*
  differential diagnosis, 267–8
  etiology/pathophysiology, 266–7
  signalment/history, 267
  therapeutics, 269–71
gastric helicobacteriosis
  Helicobacter-associated gastritis *vs.*, 319
gastric motility disorders, 259–65, **263**
  clinical features, 260–1
  definition/overview, 259
  diagnostics, 261–2
  differential diagnosis, 261
  etiology/pathophysiology, 259–60
  signalment/history, 260
  therapeutics, 262–4, **263**
gastric neoplasia
  BVS *vs.*, 332
gastric neoplasia–benign, 273–7, *275, 276*
  clinical features, 274
  comments, 276–7
  definition/overview, 273

diagnostics, 274–5, *275, 276*
  differential diagnosis, 274
  etiology/pathophysiology, 273
  signalment/history, 273
  therapeutics, 275–6
gastric neoplasia–malignant, 278–84, *280–2*
  clinical features, 279
  comments, 283–4
  definition/overview, 278
  diagnostics, 279–81, *280–2*
  differential diagnosis, 279
  etiology/pathophysiology, 278
  signalment/history, 279
  therapeutics, 282–3
gastric parasites, 285–8. *see also specific types, e.g.,*
    Physaloptera spp.
  clinical features, 286
  comments, 287
  definition/overview, 285
  diagnostics, 286
  differential diagnosis, 286
  etiology/pathophysiology, 285
  signalment/history, 285–6
  therapeutics, 287
gastritis
  acute, 289–95, *290–2*, **293**
    clinical features, 290
    comments, 294–5
    definition/overview, 289
    diagnostics, 291–2, *292, 291*
    differential diagnosis, 290
    etiology/pathophysiology, 289
    signalment/history, 289–90, *290*
    therapeutics, 292–4, **293**
  atrophic, 296–9
    clinical features, 296
    comments, 299
    definition/overview, 296
    diagnostics, 297–8
    differential diagnosis, 297
    etiology/pathophysiology, 296
    signalment/history, 296
    therapeutics, 298–9
  chronic, 300–5
    clinical features, 301
    comments, 304–5
    definition/overview, 300
    diagnostics, 302–3
    differential diagnosis, 301–2
    etiology/pathophysiology, 300
    signalment/history, 300–1
    therapeutics, 303–4
  Helicobacter-associated, 317–23, *318 see also*
    Helicobacter-associated gastritis

gastroduodenal ulceration/erosion, 306–12, *309*
  clinical features, 308
  comments, 311–12
  definition/overview, 306
  diagnostics, 308–10, *309*
  differential diagnosis, 308
  etiology/pathophysiology, 306–7
  signalment/history, 307
  therapeutics, 310–11
gastroenteritis
  acute, 84–7, **85** *see also* acute gastroenteritis
  eosinophilic, 396–401 *see also* eosinophilic
    gastroenteritis
  hemorrhagic, 402–8 *see also* hemorrhagic
    gastroenteritis
  lymphocytic-plasmacytic, 409–17, *412–14*
    see also lymphocytic-plasmacytic
    gastroenteritis
gastroesophageal diverticula, 195–7
  clinical features, 196
  comments, 197
  definition/overview, 195
  diagnostics, 196
  differential diagnosis, 196
  etiology/pathophysiology, 195
  signalment/history, 195
  therapeutics, 196–7
gastroesophageal reflux (GER), 313–16
  causes of, 247
  clinical features, 314
  comments, 315–16
  definition/overview, 313
  diagnostics, 314
  differential diagnosis, 314
  esophagitis due to, 220
  etiology/pathophysiology, 313
  signalment/history, 313–14
  therapeutics, 314–15
gastroesophageal reflux disease (GERD)
  definition/overview, 247
  nutritional approach to, 247–50, **248**
gastrointestinal (GI) disease(s)
  BVS vs., 332
  canine pancreatitis vs., 650
  clinical signs of, 1–124 *see also specific signs,*
    e.g., constipation
    acute abdomen, 3–9
    acute diarrhea, 15–19
    acute gastroenteritis, 84–7, **85**
    acute vomiting, 110–15
    anal prolapse, 95–102, *96–101*
    chronic diarrhea–canine, 20–7, **20**, 22
    chronic diarrhea–feline, 28–44, **29**, *32*, 36–7,
      39, **41**, **42**, *42*
    chronic vomiting, 116–24, *118–20*

    constipation, 10–14
    dyschezia, 45–50, *46*
    dysphagia, 51–7, *54*, *56*
    flatulence, 58–62, *60*
    hematemesis, 63–9, *63*
    hematochezia, 70–5, *71*, *72*
    melena, 76–83, *77*, *80*
    obstipation, 10–14
    ptyalism, 88–94, *89*
    rectal prolapse, 95–102, *96–101*
    regurgitation, 103–9, *104–6*, *108*
    tenesmus, 45–50, *46*
  congenital portosystemic vascular anomaly
    vs., 888
  EPI *vs.*, 623
  feline pancreatitis *vs.*, 657
  HL *vs.*, 765
  infectious hepatopathy *vs.*, 830
  obstructed
    chronic vomiting associated with, 119, *119*
gastrointestinal (GI) lymphoma–canine, 425–30
  clinical features, 426
  comments, 429–30
  definition/overview, 425
  diagnostics, 427–8
  differential diagnosis, 427
  etiology/pathophysiology, 425–6
  signalment/history, 426
  therapeutics, 428–9
gastrointestinal (GI) lymphoma–feline, 431–7,
  433, *434*
  clinical features, 432
  comments, 435–7
  definition/overview, 431
  diagnostics, 432–3, *433*, *434*
  differential diagnosis, 432
  etiology/pathophysiology, 431
  signalment/history, 431–2
  therapeutics, 434–5
gastrointestinal (GI) microbiome
  altered
    nutritional approach to, 502–3, **502**
gastrointestinal (GI) obstruction, 418–24,
  420–2
  clinical features, 419
  comments, 423–4
  definition/overview, 418
  diagnostics, 419–20, *420*, *421*
  differential diagnosis, 419
  etiology/pathophysiology, 418
  signalment/history, 418–19
  therapeutics, 420–2, *422*
gastrointestinal (GI) parasites, 506–12
  clinical features, 508
  comments, 511–12

definition/overview, 506
diagnostics, 509
differential diagnosis, 508–9
etiology/pathophysiology, 506–7
signalment/history, 507–8
therapeutics, 510–11
gastrointestinal (GI) prokinetics
in esophagitis management, 226–7
gastrointestinal reflux disease (GERD)
nutritional approach to
fat in, 248, **248**
feeding recommendations, 248–9
fiber in, 248, **248**
main considerations, 247–8, **248**
protein in, 247, **248**
gastropathy
chronic hypertrophic pyloric, 324–7 *see also*
chronic hypertrophic pyloric gastropathy
(CHPG)
GDV. *see* gastric dilation-volvulus (GDV)
genitourinary disease(s)
canine pancreatitis *vs.*, 651
GER. *see* gastroesophageal reflux (GER)
GERD. *see* gastroesophageal reflux disease
(GERD)
GI. *see under* gastrointestinal (GI)
Giardia
definition/overview, 438
giardiasis, 438–40
clinical features, 439
comments, 440
definition/overview, 438
diagnostics, 439
differential diagnosis, 439
etiology/pathophysiology, 438
signalment/history, 438
therapeutics, 439–40
gingivitis
definition/overview, 179
glossitis
definition/overview, 179
gluten-sensitive enteropathy (GSE)
in Irish Setters, 441–3
clinical features, 442
comments, 443
definition/overview, 441
diagnostics, 442
differential diagnosis, 442
etiology/pathophysiology, 441
signalment/history, 441–2
therapeutics, 442
glycogen storage diseases (GSDs), 729–33, **730**
clinical features, 730–1
comments, 732
definition/overview, 729

diagnostics, 731
differential diagnosis, 731
etiology/pathophysiology, 729, **730**
signalment/history, 729–30
therapeutics, 731–2
types of, 729–32, **730**
glycogen-type vacuolar hepatopathy (VH),
734–41, *737, 738*
clinical features, 735
comments, 740–1
definition/overview, 734
diagnostics, 736–8, *737, 738*
differential diagnosis, 736
etiology/pathophysiology, 734–35
signalment/history, 735
therapeutics, 739
granulomatous enterocolitis, 370–7, *371,
372, 375*
clinical features, 372
comments, 376–7
definition/overview, 370
diagnostics, 373–4, *375*
differential diagnosis, 373
etiology/pathophysiology, 370
signalment/history, 371–2, *372, 371*
therapeutics, 374–6
granulomatous hepatitis, 796–800. *see also*
hepatitis, granulomatous
GSDs. *see* glycogen storage diseases (GSDs)
GSE. *see* gluten-sensitive enteropathy (GSE)

hamartoma(s)
definition/overview, 460
HAVM. *see* hepatic arteriovenous malformation
(HAVM)
HDH. *see* hepatocellular dysplastic hyperplasia
(HDH)
HE. *see* hepatic encephalopathy (HE)
Helicobacter-associated gastritis, 317–23, *318*
clinical features, 319
comments, 321–2
definition/overview, 317, *318*
diagnostics, 319–20
differential diagnosis, 319
etiology/pathophysiology, 317–18
signalment/history, 319
therapeutics, 320–1
helicobacteriosis
gastric/hepatic/intestinal
vs. Helicobacter-associated gastritis, 319
Helicobacter spp.
definition/overview, 317, *318*
helminthiasis
intestinal
definition/overview, 506

hematemesis, 63–9, *63*
  clinical features, 65
  comments, 68–9
  definition/overview, 63, *63*
  diagnostics, 66–7
  differential diagnosis, 66
  etiology/pathophysiology, 63
  signalment/history, 64–5
  therapeutics, 67–8
hematochezia, 70–5, *71*, *72*
  clinical features, 71–2, *72*
  comments, 74–5
  definition/overview, 45, 70
  diagnostics, 72–3
  differential diagnosis, 72
  etiology/pathophysiology, 70
  melena *vs.*, 78
  signalment/history, 70–1, *71*
  therapeutics, 73–4
hematoma(s)
  salivary mucocele *vs.*, 166
hemolysis
  infectious hepatopathy *vs.*, 830
hemoptysis
  hematemesis *vs.*, 66
  leptospirosis *vs.*, 860
hemorrhagic gastroenteritis, 402–8
  clinical features, 404
  comments, 407–8
  definition/overview, 402
  diagnostics, 404–5
  differential diagnosis, 404
  etiology/pathophysiology, 402–3
  signalment/history, 403–4
  therapeutics, 406–7
hepatic abscess(es), 817–22, *820*
  clinical features, 818
  comments, 822
  definition/overview, 817
  diagnostics, 818–20, *820*
  differential diagnosis, 818
  etiology/pathophysiology, 817
  signalment/history, 817–18
  therapeutics, 820–2
hepatic adenoma(s)
  HNH and HDH *vs.*, 782
hepatic amyloid, 742–7, *745*
  clinical features, 743
  comments, 747
  definition/overview, 742
  diagnostics, 744–5, *745*
  differential diagnosis, 743–4
  etiology/pathophysiology, 742
  signalment/history, 743
  therapeutics, 745–6

hepatic arteriovenous malformation (HAVM)
  congenital portosystemic vascular anomaly
    vs., 888
hepatic encephalopathy (HE), 748–54
  acquired PSS *vs.*, 880
  CAH *vs.*, 714
  clinical features, 750
  comments, 753–4
  congenital portosystemic vascular anomaly
    vs., 888
  definition/overview, 748
  diagnostics, 750–2
  differential diagnosis, 750
  etiology/pathophysiology, 748
  nutritional approach to, 874, **875**
  signalment/history, 749–50
  therapeutics, 752–3
hepatic failure
  acute, 755–62, *758*
    clinical features, 756
    comments, 761–2
    definition/overview, 755
    diagnostics, 757, *758*
    differential diagnosis, 756
    etiology/pathophysiology, 755
    signalment/history, 756
    therapeutics, 758–60
  fulminant
    vs. EHBDO, 903
hepatic fibrosis
  congenital, 721
hepatic helicobacteriosis
  Helicobacter-associated gastritis *vs.*, 319
hepatic injury(ies)
  acute
    vs. leptospirosis, 860
hepatic lipidosis (HL), 763–70, *766*
  clinical features, 764–5
  comments, 769–70
  definition/overview, 763
  diagnostics, 765–6, *766*
  differential diagnosis, 765
  EHBDO *vs.*, 903
  etiology/pathophysiology, 763–4
  infectious hepatopathy *vs.*, 829
  nutritional approach to, 871–3, **872**
  signalment/history, 764
  therapeutics, 767–9
hepatic neoplasia(s)
  benign, 771–4
    clinical features, 771
    comments, 773–4
    definition/overview, 771
    diagnostics, 772–3
    differential diagnosis, 771–2

signalment/history, 771
therapeutics, 773
hepatotoxins vs., 846
infectious hepatopathy vs., 829
malignant, 775–80, *777, 778*
clinical features, 776
comments, 779–80
definition/overview, 775
diagnostics, 776–9, *777, 778*
differential diagnosis, 776
etiology/pathophysiology, 775
signalment/history, 775–6
therapeutics, 779
hepatic nodular hyperplasia (HNH), 781–5
clinical features, 782
comments, 784–5
definition/overview, 781
diagnostics, 783
differential diagnosis, 782
etiology/pathophysiology, 782
signalment/history, 782
therapeutics, 784
hepatitis
acute
vs. infectious hepatopathy, 829
chronic, 786–95
clinical features, 788
comments, 793–5
definition/overview, 786
diagnostics, 788–90
differential diagnosis, 788
etiology/pathophysiology, 786–7
nutritional approach to, 870–1, **871, 870**
signalment/history, 787
therapeutics, 790–3
vs. EHBDO, 903
vs. infectious hepatopathy, 829
granulomatous, 796–800
clinical features, 797
comments, 799–800
definition/overview, 796
diagnostics, 797–8
differential diagnosis, 797
etiology/pathophysiology, 796
signalment/history, 797
therapeutics, 798–9
infectious–canine, 801–6 *see also* infectious
canine hepatitis (ICH)
lobular dissecting, 807–12, *809, 810 see also*
lobular dissecting hepatitis (LDH)
nonspecific reactive, 813–16, *815 see also*
nonspecific reactive hepatitis (NSRH)
suppurative, 817–22, *820*
clinical features, 818
comments, 822

definition/overview, 817
diagnostics, 818–20
differential diagnosis, 818
etiology/pathophysiology, 817
signalment/history, 817–18
therapeutics, 820–2
hepatobiliary disease(s)
canine pancreatitis vs., 650–1
clinical signs of, 663–78 *see also specific signs,*
e.g., icterus
coagulopathy of liver disease, 673–8, *675*
icterus, 665–72, *666, 667*
feline pancreatitis vs., 657
nutritional approach to, 866–77, **867–76** *see*
also specific diseases
CAH, 873–4, **874, 873**
carbohydrates in, 867, **867**
cholangiohepatitis, 869–70, **869**
chronic hepatitis, 870–1, **871, 870**
circulatory disorders, 874–6, **875, 876**
energy in, 866–7, **867**
fats in, 867, **867**
feline HL, 871–3, **872**
general feeding recommendations, 868
inflammatory diseases, 869–71, **869–71**
overall considerations, 866–8, **867, 868**
protein in, 867, **867**
storage diseases, 871–4, **872–4**
primary
vs. infectious hepatopathy, 829
hepatocellular carcinoma
HNH and HDH vs., 782
hepatocellular dysplastic hyperplasia (HDH),
781–5
clinical features, 782
comments, 784–5
definition/overview, 781
diagnostics, 783
differential diagnosis, 782
etiology/pathophysiology, 782
signalment/history, 782
therapeutics, 784
hepatopathy(ies)
copper-associated, 711–20, **717** *see also*
copper-associated hepatopathy (CAH)
diffuse
vs. glycogen-type VH, 736
hyperthyroidism
feline, 823–7, *825 see also* hyperthyroidism,
feline
infectious, 828–35, *832*
clinical features, 829
comments, 834
definition/overview, 828
diagnostics, 830–1, *832*

hepatopathy(ies) (*cont'd*)
  differential diagnosis, 829–30
  etiology/pathophysiology, 828–9
  signalment/history, 829
  therapeutics, 831–3
  vacuolar
    glycogen-type, 734–41, *737, 738 see also*
      glycogen-type vacuolar hepatopathy (VH)
hepatoportal microvascular dysplasia (MVD),
    836–42
  clinical features, 837–8
  comments, 840–2
  definition/overview, 836
  diagnostics, 838–40
  differential diagnosis, 838
  etiology/pathophysiology, 836–7
  signalment/history, 837
  therapeutics, 840
hepatotoxin(s), 843–9
  clinical features, 845
  comments, 848–9
  definition/overview, 843
  diagnostics, 846–7
  differential diagnosis, 846
  etiology/pathophysiology, 843–5
  signalment/history, 845
  therapeutics, 847–8
  types of, 843–5
hernia(s)
  hiatal *see* hiatal hernia
  perineal, 588–92, *591 see also* perineal hernia
hiatal hernia, 231–7, *232, 234, 236, 237*
  clinical features, 233
  comments, 236–7
  definition/overview, 231
  diagnostics, 233–4, *234*
  differential diagnosis, 233
  esophagitis *vs.,* 224
  etiology/pathophysiology, 231, *232*
  signalment/history, 231–3
  therapeutics, 234–6, *236, 237*
histiocytic ulcerative colitis (HUC), 554–8
  clinical features, 555
  comments, 557–8
  definition/overview, 554
  diagnostics, 555–6
  differential diagnosis, 555
  etiology/pathophysiology, 554
  signalment/history, 554–5
  therapeutics, 556–7
HL. *see* hepatic lipidosis (HL)
HNH. *see* hepatic nodular hyperplasia (HNH)
hookworm(s)
  clinical features, 508
  definition/overview, 506

  etiology/pathophysiology, 506
  therapeutics, 510
HUC. *see* histiocytic ulcerative colitis (HUC)
hyperostosis
  calvarial
    vs. craniomandibular osteopathy, 128
hyperplasia(s)
  hepatic nodular, 781–5 *see also* hepatic nodular
    hyperplasia (HNH)
  hepatocellular dysplastic, 781–5 *see also*
    hepatocellular dysplastic hyperplasia
    (HDH)
  pancreatic nodular, 637–9, *639 see also*
    pancreatic nodular hyperplasia (PNH)
hypersensitivity
  dietary
    in nutritional approach to chronic
      enteropathies, 493–6, *494, 495*
hypertension
  portal, 683, 850–7 *see also* portal hypertension
hyperthyroidism
  feline, 823–7, *825*
    clinical features, 824
    comments, 826–7
    definition/overview, 823
    diagnostics, 824–5, *825*
    differential diagnosis, 824
    etiology/pathophysiology, 823
    signalment/history, 823–4
    therapeutics, 826
hypoadrenocorticism
  acute hepatic failure *vs.,* 756
  atypical
    vs. BVS, 332
  canine pancreatitis *vs.,* 651
hypoalbuminemia
  PLE–related
    vs. hypoalbuminemia from other causes,
      514–15
hypoallergenic diet
  for feline chronic diarrhea, 41–2, **42**
hypoplasia(s)
  primary portal vein
    nutritional approach to, 874, 876, **876**
hypoxic liver injury
  hepatotoxins *vs.,* 846

IBD. *see* inflammatory bowel disease (IBD)
IBS. *see* irritable bowel syndrome (IBS)
ICH. *see* infectious canine hepatitis (ICH)
icterus, 665–72, *666, 667*
  bile peritonitis *vs.,* 912
  CAH *vs.,* 714
  clinical features, 668
  comments, 671

definition/overview, 665
diagnostics, 669–70
differential diagnosis, 668–9
etiology/pathophysiology, 665–6, *666*
signalment/history, 666–8, *667*
therapeutics, 670–1
types of, *666, 666–71, 667*
idiopathic bowel syndrome
nutritional approach to, 499–500, **500**
idiopathic inflammatory bowel disease
BVS *vs.*, 332
immune modulation therapy
for CCHS, 693, **693**
immunoproliferative enteropathy
of Basenjis, 444–8
clinical features, 445
comments, 447
definition/overview, 444
diagnostics, 445–6
differential diagnosis, 445
etiology/pathophysiology, 444
signalment/history, 444–5
therapeutics, 446–7
immunosuppressive therapy
for feline chronic diarrhea, 40, **41**
infection(s). *see also specific types, e.g.,* canine
parvovirus (CPV)-2 infection
parasitic
vs. colonic neoplasia–malignant, 565
infectious canine hepatitis (ICH), 801–6
clinical features, 802
comments, 805–6
definition/overview, 801
diagnostics, 802–4
differential diagnosis, 802
EHBDO *vs.*, 903
etiology/pathophysiology, 801–2
signalment/history, 802
therapeutics, 804–5
infectious disease(s)
chronic vomiting associated with, 117, *118*
fungal enteritides *vs.*, 391
hepatotoxins *vs.*, 846
leptospirosis *vs.*, 860
liver-affected
vs. HL, 765
infectious hepatopathy, 828–35, *832. see also*
hepatopathy, infectious
inflammatory bowel disease (IBD), 449–53
chronic vomiting associated with, 118, *118*
clinical features, 450
comments, 452–3
definition/overview, 449
diagnostics, 450–1
differential diagnosis, 332, 450

etiology/pathophysiology, 449
idiopathic
vs. BVS, 332
malignant colonic neoplasia *vs.*, 565
nutritional approach to chronic enteropathies
related to, 496–7, **497**
signalment/history, 449–50
therapeutics, 451–2
inflammatory disease(s)
fungal enteritides *vs.*, 391
nutritional approach to, 869–71, **869–71**
see also specific diseases
inflammatory polyp(s)
rectoanal polyps *vs.*, 602
intestinal disease(s), 329–530. *see also specific*
diseases
adverse food reactions, 384–8
AHDS, 402–8 *see also* hemorrhagic
gastroenteritis
ARD, 354–9
bacterial enteritis, 360–9
BVS, 331–6, *333*, **334**
CILBD, 478–83, *480, 481*
cobalamin deficiency, 345–9
CPV-2 infection, 337–44
cryptosporidiosis, 350–3
eosinophilic gastroenteritis, 396–401
feline viral enterides, 378–83, *379*
fungal enteritides, 389–95, *390, 392*
gallbladder mucocele *vs.*, 945
giardiasis, 438–40
GI lymphoma–canine, 425–30
GI lymphoma–feline, 431–7, *433, 434*
GI obstruction, 418–24, *420–2*
GI parasites, 506–12
granulomatous enterocolitis, 370–7, *371,
372, 375*
GSE
in Irish Setters, 441–3
hemorrhagic gastroenteritis, 402–8
IBD, 118, *118*, 449–53
immunoproliferative enteropathy
of Basenjis, 444–8
intestinal dysbiosis, 454–9, *457*
intestinal neoplasia
benign, 460–3, *460 see also* intestinal
neoplasia–benign
malignant *see also*
intestinal neoplasia–malignant
intestinal neoplasia–malignant, 464–9, *465–8*
intussusception, 470–7, *473–5*
irritable bowel syndrome, 478–83, *480, 481*
see also chronic idiopathic large bowel
diarrhea (CILBD)
lymphangiectasia, 484–9, *487*

intestinal disease(s) (*cont'd*)
  lymphocytic-plasmacytic gastroenteritis, 409–17, *412–14*
  nutritional approach to chronic enteropathies, 490–505 *see also* chronic enteropathy(ies), nutritional approach to
  PLE, 513–20, *516, 518*
  SBS, 526–30
  SPD, 521–5, *523, 524*
intestinal dysbiosis, 454–9, *457*
  clinical features, 456
  definition/overview, 454
  diagnostics, 456–7, *457*
  differential diagnosis, 456
  etiology/pathophysiology, 454–5
  signalment/history, 455–6
  therapeutics, 457–8
intestinal helicobacteriosis
  Helicobacter-associated gastritis *vs.*, 319
intestinal helminthiasis
  definition/overview, 506
intestinal motility disorders, 259–65, **263**
  clinical features, 260–1
  comments, 264–5
  definition/overview, 259
  diagnostics, 261–2
  differential diagnosis, 261
  etiology/pathophysiology, 259–60
  signalment/history, 260
  therapeutics, 262–4, **263**
intestinal neoplasia–benign, 460–3, *460*
  clinical features, 461
  comments, 463
  definition/overview, *460*, 4601
  diagnostics, 462
  differential diagnosis, 461–2
  etiology/pathophysiology, 461
  signalment/history, 461
  therapeutics, 462
intestinal neoplasia–malignant, 464–9, *465–8*
  clinical features, 466, *466*
  comments, 468–9
  definition/overview, 464
  diagnostics, 466–7, *467, 468*
  differential diagnosis, 466
  etiology/pathophysiology, 464–5
  signalment/history, 465, *465*
  therapeutics, 467–8
intestinal obstruction
  BVS *vs.*, 332
  intussusception *vs.*, 472
intestine(s)
  disease *see also specific diseases and* intestinal disease(s)
  diseases of, 329–530

intrahepatic arteriovenous malformations (AVMs), 681
intussusception, 470–7, *473–5*
  clinical features, 471
  comments, 476–7
  definition/overview, 470
  diagnostics, 472, *473, 474*
  differential diagnosis, 472
  etiology/pathophysiology, 470
  prolapsed
    vs. rectal prolapse, 96, *97*
  signalment/history, 471
  therapeutics, 474–6, *475*
Irish Setters
  GSE in, 441–3 *see also* gluten-sensitive enteropathy (GSE), in Irish Setters
irritable bowel syndrome (IBS), 478–83, *480, 481.* *see also* chronic idiopathic large bowel diarrhea (CILBD)
  nutritional approach to, 499–500, **500**

jaundice, 665–72, *666, 667. see also* icterus

labial/buccal mucositis
  definition/overview, 179
large bowel diarrhea
  chronic idiopathic, 478–83, *480, 481 see also* chronic idiopathic large bowel diarrhea (CILBD)
  fiber-responsive, 568–72, *570, 571 see also* fiber-responsive large bowel diarrhea
LDH. *see* lobular dissecting hepatitis (LDH)
leptospirosis, 858–65, *862, 863*
  clinical features, 860
  comments, 864–5
  definition/overview, 858
  diagnostics, 860–2, *862, 863*
  differential diagnosis, 860
  etiology/pathophysiology, 858–9
  signalment/history, 859
  therapeutics, 863–4
lesion(s)
  mass
    vs. EHBDO, 903
lipidosis
  hepatic, 763–70, *766 see also* hepatic lipidosis (HL)
lipoma(s)
  colonic, 559, *560*
  definition/overview, 460
liver
  AVMs of, 681–6, *682 see also* arteriovenous malformations (AVMs), of liver
  cirrhosis of, 702–10 *see also* cirrhosis of liver
  fibrosis of, 702–10 *see also* fibrosis of liver

liver abscess(s), 812–22, *820. see also* hepatic
    abscess(es)
liver disease(s), 679–897. *see also specific*
    types
  acquired PSS, 878–84, *881*
  acutely decompensated chronic, 756
  CAH, 711–20, **717**
  CCHS, 687–96, **692–4**
  cirrhosis, 702–10 *see also* cirrhosis of liver
  coagulopathy of, 673–8, *675 see also*
    coagulopathy of liver disease
  congenital portosystemic vascular anomaly,
    885–97, *885, 888–91, 893, 894*
  destructive cholangitis, 697–701, *699*
  diffuse infiltrative
    vs. EHBDO, 903
  ductal plate malformation, 721–8
  feline hyperthyroidism, 823–7, *825*
  fibrosis, 702–10 *see also* fibrosis of liver
  gallbladder mucocele *vs.*, 946
  glycogen-type VH, 734–41, *737, 738*
  GSDs, 729–33, **730**
  HDH, 781–5
  HE, 748–54
  hepatic abscesses, 817–22, *820*
  hepatic amyloid, 742–7, *745*
  hepatic failure
    acute, 755–62, *758*
  hepatic neoplasia
    benign, 771–4 *see also* hepatic neoplasia(s),
      benign
    malignant, 775–80, *777, 778 see also* hepatic
      neoplasia(s), malignant
  hepatitis
    chronic, 786–95
    granulomatous, 796–800
    suppurative, 817–22
  hepatopathy
    infectious, 828–35, *832*
  hepatoportal MVD, 836–42
  hepatotoxins, 843–9
  HL, 763–70, *766*
  HNH, 781–5
  ICH, 801–6
  LDH, 807–12, *809, 810*
  leptospirosis, 858–65, *862, 863*
  NSRH, 813–16, *815*
  nutritional approach to hepatobiliary diseases,
    866–77, **867–76**
  portal hypertension, 850–7
  primary
    vs. HL, 765
liver failure
  acute, 755–62, *758 see also* hepatic failure,
    acute

liver injury(ies)
  acute
    vs. leptospirosis, 860
    hepatotoxins *vs.*, 846
lobular dissecting hepatitis (LDH), 807–12, *809, 810*
  clinical features, 808
  comments, 811–12
  definition/overview, 807
  diagnostics, 808–9, *809, 810*
  differential diagnosis, 808
  etiology/pathophysiology, 807
  signalment/history, 808
  therapeutics, 810–11
lymphadenopathy
  sublumbar
    vs. perineal hernia, 589
lymphangiectasia, 484–9, *487*
  clinical features, 485
  comments, 488
  definition/overview, 484
  diagnostics, 485–6, *487*
  differential diagnosis, 485
  etiology/pathophysiology, 484
  nutritional approach to, 498–9, **499, 498**
  signalment/history, 484–5
  therapeutics, 486–8
lymphocytic cholangitis, 687–96, **692–4.** *see also*
    cholangitis; cholangitis/cholangiohepatitis
    syndrome (CCHS)
lymphocytic-plasmacytic enteritis
  chronic vomiting associated with, 118, *118*
lymphocytic-plasmacytic gastroenteritis, 409–17,
    412–14
  clinical features, 410
  comments, 416–17
  definition/overview, 409
  diagnostics, 411–14, *412–14*
  differential diagnosis, 410–11
  etiology/pathophysiology, 409
  signalment/history, 409–10
  therapeutics, 414–16
lymphoma(s)
  GI
    in cats, 431–7, *433, 434 see also*
      gastrointestinal (GI) lymphoma–feline
    in dogs, 425–30 *see also* gastrointestinal (GI)
      lymphoma–canine

malformation(s)
  arteriovenous *see* arteriovenous malformations
    (AVMs)
  ductal plate, 721–8 *see also* ductal plate
    malformation
mass lesions
  EHBDO *vs.*, 903

mechanical obstruction
    megacolon vs., 574
megacolon, 573–80, *575, 576, 579*
    clinical features, **574**
    comments, 578–80
    definition/overview, 500–2, **500–1**, 573
    diagnostics, 575–6, *576, 575*
    differential diagnosis, 574
    etiology/pathophysiology, 573
    feline
        vs. malignant colonic neoplasia, 565
    perineal hernia vs., 589
    signalment/history, 574
    therapeutics, 577–8, *579*
megaesophagus, 238–46, *241, 242, 244*
    clinical features, 239–40
    comments, 245–6
    definition/overview, 238, 249
    diagnostics, 240–2, *241, 242*
    differential diagnosis, 240
    esophagitis vs., 224
    etiology/pathophysiology, 238–9, 249
    nutritional approach to, 247–50, **248**
        fat in, 248, **248**
        feeding recommendations, 248–9
        fiber in, 248, **248**
        main considerations, 247–8, **248**
        protein in, 247, **248**
    signalment/history, 239
    therapeutics, 243–5, *244*
melena, 76–83, *77, 80*
    clinical features, 78
    comments, 82–3
    definition/overview, 76, 77
    diagnostics, 78–80, *80*
    differential diagnosis, 78
    etiology/pathophysiology, 76, 77
    signalment/history, 76–8
    therapeutics, 80–2
metabolic abnormalities
    GSE in Irish Setters vs., 442
    megacolon vs., 574
metabolic disease(s)
    bone
        vs. craniomandibular osteopathy, 128
    chronic vomiting associated with, 118
microbiome(s)
    GI
        altered, 502–3, **502**
microvascular dysplasia (MVD)
    hepatoportal, 836–42 *see also* hepatoportal
        microvascular dysplasia (MVD)
    nutritional approach to, 874, 876, **876**
motility disorder(s)
    chronic vomiting associated with, 120

mucocele(s)
    gallbladder, 943–52, *943, 947, 948, 950 see also*
        gallbladder mucocele
    salivary, 164–71, *165, 168–70 see also* salivary
        mucocele
mucosal protectants
    in esophagitis management, 227
mucositis
    alveolar
        definition/overview, 179
    caudal
        definition/overview, 179
    labial/buccal
        definition/overview, 179
    sublingual
        definition/overview, 179
MVD. *see* microvascular dysplasia (MVD)

necrotizing pancreatitis
    acute
        vs. hepatotoxins, 846
necrotizing sialometaplasia (NSM)
    salivary mucocele vs., 166
neoplasia(s)
    abdominal
        vs. feline pancreatitis, 657
    biliary, 918–24, *921 see also* biliary neoplasia
    colitis vs., 548
    colonic
        benign, 559–63, *560 see also* colonic
            neoplasia–benign
        malignant, 564–7, *566 see also* colonic
            neoplasia–malignant
    craniomandibular osteopathy vs., 128
    esophageal, 209–13, *211 see also* esophageal
        neoplasia
    fungal enteritides vs., 391
    gastric
        benign, 273–7, *275, 276 see also* gastric
            neoplasia–benign
        malignant, 278–84, *280–2 see also* gastric
            neoplasia–malignant
        vs. BVS, 332
    hepatic
        benign, 771–4 *see also* hepatic neoplasia(s),
            benign
        malignant, 775–80, *777, 778 see also* hepatic
            neoplasia(s), malignant
        vs. infectious hepatopathy, 829
    HNH and HDH vs., 782
    intestinal
        benign, 460–3, *460 see also* intestinal
            neoplasia–benign
        malignant, 464–9, *465–8 see also* intestinal
            neoplasia–malignant

oral
    benign, 141–6, *142, 144, 146 see also* oral
        neoplasia–benign
    malignant, 147–54, *148, 149, 152 see also* oral
        neoplasia–malignant
    pancreatic, 632–6, *634, 635 see also* pancreatic
        neoplasia
    perineal
        vs. perineal hernia, 589
    rectal prolapse *vs.*, 96, 97
    rectoanal polyps *vs.*, 602
    salivary
        vs. salivary mucocele, 166
neoplastic disease(s)
    chronic vomiting associated with, 119, *120, 119*
nephrotoxicosis(es)
    leptospirosis *vs.*, 860
neurologic disease(s)
    chronic vomiting associated with, 119–20
    congenital portosystemic vascular anomaly
        vs., 888
    megacolon *vs.*, 574
neutrophilic cholangitis, 687–96, **692–4**. *see also*
        cholangitis; cholangitis/cholangiohepatitis
        syndrome (CCHS)
nongastrointestinal diseases
    BVS *vs.*, 332
nonspecific reactive hepatitis (NSRH), 813–16, *815*
    clinical features, 814
    comments, 816
    definition/overview, 813
    diagnostics, 814–15, *815*
    differential diagnosis, 814
    etiology/pathophysiology, 813
    signalment/history, 813–14
    therapeutics, 815–16
NSM. *see* necrotizing sialometaplasia (NSM)
NSRH. *see* nonspecific reactive hepatitis (NSRH)

obstipation, 10–14
    clinical features, 11
    comments, 14
    definition/overview, 10
    diagnostics, 12–13
    differential diagnosis, 11–12
    etiology/pathophysiology, 10
    signalment/history, 10–11
    therapeutics, 13–14
obstruction(s). *see* intestinal obstruction; *specific
        types, e.g.,* gastrointestinal (GI) obstruction
odynophagia
    definition/overview, 51
Ollulanus
    clinical features, 286
    comments, 287

definition/overview, 285
diagnostics, 286
differential diagnosis, 286
etiology/pathophysiology, 285
signalment/history, 285–6
therapeutics, 287
omega-3 fatty acids
    in nutritional approach to chronic
        enteropathies, 494–5, **495**
oral cavity diseases, 125–85
    craniomandibular osteopathy, 127–33, *128–31*
    feline eosinophilic dermatitis, 134–40, *135–8*
    oral neoplasia–benign, 141–6, *142, 144, 146*
    oral neoplasia–malignant, 147–54, *148,
        149, 152*
    phenobarbital-responsive sialadenosis, 155–8
    salivary mucocele, 164–71, *165, 168–70*
    sialadenitis, 159–63
    stomatitis, 172–8, *173–6*
        caudal–feline, 179–85, *180, 182, 183*
oral dysphagia
    differential diagnosis, 53
    etiology/pathophysiology, 51
oral neoplasia–benign, 141–6, *142, 144, 146*
    clinical features, 142–3, *142, 144*
    comments, 145–6
    definition/overview, 141
    diagnostics, 144
    differential diagnosis, 144
    etiology/pathophysiology, 141
    signalment/history, 141–2
    therapeutics, 145, *146*
oral neoplasia–malignant, 147–54, *148, 149, 152*
    clinical features, 148–9, *149*
    comments, 152–3
    definition/overview, 147
    diagnostics, 149–50
    differential diagnosis, 149
    etiology/pathophysiology, 147
    signalment/history, 147–8, *148*
    therapeutics, 150–2, *152*
oropharyngeal dysphagia
    esophagitis *vs.*, 224
osteomyelitis
    craniomandibular osteopathy *vs.*, 128
    definition/overview, 179
osteopathy
    craniomandibular, 127–33, *128–31 see also*
        craniomandibular osteopathy

pain
    abdominal
        vs. bile peritonitis, 912
palatitis
    definition/overview, 179

pancreas
  diseases of, 611–61 *see also specific types and pancreatic disease(s)*
pancreatic abscess(es), 628–31
  clinical features, 628–9
  comments, 630
  definition/overview, 628
  diagnostics, 629
  differential diagnosis, 629
  etiology/pathophysiology, 628
  signalment/history, 628
  therapeutics, 629–30
pancreatic disease(s), 611–61. *see also specific types*
  EPI, 621–7, 622, 623
    nutritional approach to, 613–16, **614, 616**
  exocrine
    nutritional approach to, 613–20, **614, 616, 617**
  gallbladder mucocele *vs.*, 945
  nutritional approach to, 613–20, **614, 616, 617**
    acute and chronic pancreatitis, 616–19, **617**
    EPI, 613–16, **614, 616**
  pancreatic abscess, 628–31
  pancreatic neoplasia, 632–6, *634, 635*
  pancreatic parasites, 640–4
  pancreatic pseudocysts, 645–8
  pancreatitis
    canine, 649–55, *651, 652*
    feline, 656–61
  PNH, 637–9, *639*
pancreatic neoplasia, 632–6, *634, 635*
  clinical features, 633
  comments, 636
  definition/overview, 632
  diagnostics, 633–4, *634, 635*
  differential diagnosis, 633
  etiology/pathophysiology, 632
  signalment/history, 632–3
  therapeutics, 634–6
pancreatic nodular hyperplasia (PNH), 637–9, *639*
  clinical features, 637
  comments, 638–9
  definition/overview, 637
  diagnostics, 638, *639*
  differential diagnosis, 638
  etiology/pathophysiology, 637
  signalment/history, 637
  therapeutics, 638
pancreatic parasites, 640–4. *see also specific types*
  clinical features, 641
  comments, 643
  definition/overview, 640
  diagnostics, 641–2
  differential diagnosis, 641

etiology/pathophysiology, 640
  signalment/history, 640–1
  therapeutics, 642–3
pancreatic pseudocysts, 645–8
  clinical features, 645
  comments, 647
  definition/overview, 645
  diagnostics, 646
  differential diagnosis, 646
  etiology/pathophysiology, 645
  signalment/history, 645
  therapeutics, 646–7
pancreatitis
  acute
    nutritional approach to, 616–19, **617**
    vs. acute hepatic failure, 756
  acute necrotizing
    vs. hepatotoxins, 846
  canine, 649–55, *651, 652*
    clinical features, 650, *651*
    comments, 654–5
    definition/overview, 649
    diagnostics, 651–2, *652*
    differential diagnosis, 650–1
    etiology/pathophysiology, 649
    signalment/history, 650
    therapeutics, 653–4
  chronic
    nutritional approach to, 616–19, **617**
    vs. BVS, 332
  EHBDO *vs.*, 903
  feline, 656–61
    clinical features, 657
    comments, 660–1
    definition/overview, 656
    diagnostics, 658
    differential diagnosis, 657
    etiology/pathophysiology, 656–7
    signalment/history, 657
    therapeutics, 659–60
  HL *vs.*, 765
  infectious hepatopathy *vs.*, 830
parasite(s)
  gastric, 285–8 *see also* gastric parasites
  GI, 506–12 *see also specific types and* gastrointestinal (GI) parasites
  pancreatic, 640–4 *see also specific types and* pancreatic parasites
parasitic infections
  colonic neoplasia–malignant *vs.*, 565
Pentatrichomonas spp., 608
perianal fistula, 581–7, *582–4*
  clinical features, 582, *583, 584*
  comments, 586–7

definition/overview, 581
diagnostics, 584
differential diagnosis, 583
etiology/pathophysiology, 581, *582*
signalment/history, 581–2
therapeutics, 584–6
perineal abscess(es)
perineal hernia *vs.,* 589
perineal hernia, 588–92, *591*
clinical features, 589
comments, 592
definition/overview, 588
diagnostics, 589
differential diagnosis, 589
etiology/pathophysiology, 588
signalment/history, 588–9
therapeutics, 589–91, *591*
perineal neoplasia
perineal hernia *vs.,* 589
periodontitis
definition/overview, 179
peristalsis
definition/overview, 259
peritonitis
bile, 910–17, *913 see also* bile peritonitis
pharyngeal dysphagia
etiology/pathophysiology, 51
pharyngitis
definition/overview, 179
phenobarbital-responsive sialadenosis, 155–8
clinical features, 155–6
comments, 157–8
definition/overview, 155
diagnostics, 156
differential diagnosis, 156
etiology/pathophysiology, 155
signalment/history, 155
therapeutics, 157
Physaloptera spp.
chronic vomiting associated with, 117, *118*
clinical features, 286
comments, 287
definition/overview, 285
diagnostics, 286
differential diagnosis, 286
etiology/pathophysiology, 285
signalment/history, 285–6
Spirocerca vs., 286
therapeutics, 287
Platynosomum fastosum, 640–4
PLE. *see* protein-losing enteropathy (PLE)
PNH. *see* pancreatic nodular hyperplasia (PNH)
polyp(s)
adenomatous

colonic, 559, *560*
definition/overview, 460, *460*
inflammatory
vs. rectoanal polyps, 602
rectoanal, 601–7, *604–6 see also* rectoanal
polyp(s)
polyuria/polydipsia (PU/PD)
congenital portosystemic vascular anomaly
vs., 888
portal hypertension, 850–7
AVMs of liver *vs.,* 682
categories of, 878
clinical features, 851–2
comments, 856–7
definition/overview, 850
diagnostics, 852–4
differential diagnosis, 852
etiology/pathophysiology, 850–1
signalment/history, 851
therapeutics, 854–6
portal vein hypoplasia (PVH)
congenital portosystemic vascular anomaly
vs., 888
primary
nutritional approach to, 874, 876, *876*
portosystemic shunts (PSS)
acquired, 878–84, *881*
categories of, 878
clinical features, 879
comments, 883
definition/overview, 878
diagnostics, 880–1, *881*
differential diagnosis, 880
etiology/pathophysiology, 878–8
signalment/history, 879
therapeutics, 881–3
congenital
definition/overview, 885
nutritional approach to, 874, **875**
portosystemic vascular anomaly
congenital, 885–97, *885, 888–91,*
893, 894
clinical features, 887–8
comments, 895–6
definition/overview, 885, *885*
diagnostics, 889–90, *889–91*
differential diagnosis, 888, *888*
etiology/pathophysiology, 886
signalment/history, 886–7
therapeutics, 892–4, *893, 894*
portosystemic vascular anomaly (PSVA)
hepatoportal MVD *vs.,* 838
prebiotics
for feline chronic diarrhea, 40

primary hepatobiliary disease
   infectious hepatopathy *vs.*, 829
primary liver disease
   HL *vs.*, 765
probiotics
   for feline chronic diarrhea, 40
proctitis, 546–53
   clinical features, 547
   comments, 551–2
   definition/overview, 546
   diagnostics, 548–9
   differential diagnosis, 548
   etiology/pathophysiology, 546–7
   rectoanal polyps *vs.*, 602
   signalment/history, 547
   therapeutics, 549–51
prokinetics
   GI
      in esophagitis management, 226–7
prolapse
   anal, 95–102, *96–101 see also* anal prolapse
   rectal, 95–102, *96–101 see also* rectal prolapse
prolapsed intussusception
   rectal prolapse *vs.*, 96, 97
prostatomegaly
   perineal hernia *vs.*, 589
protein
   in nutritional approach to acute and chronic
      pancreatitis, 617–18, **617**
   in nutritional approach to acute gastroenteritis,
      85, **85**
   in nutritional approach to chronic
      enteropathies, 491, **491**
   in nutritional approach to EPI, 614, **614**
   in nutritional approach to GERD and
      megaesophagus, 247, **248**
   in nutritional approach to hepatobiliary
      diseases, 867, **867**
protein-losing enteropathy (PLE), 513–20, *516,*
   518
   acute hepatic failure *vs.*, 756
   clinical features, 514
   comments, 519–20
   definition/overview, 498, **498**, 513
   diagnostics, 515–17, *516*
   differential diagnosis, 514–15
   etiology/pathophysiology, 513–14
   signalment/history, 514
   therapeutics, 517–19, *518*
protozoan parasites
   in cats
      treatment of, 39, **39**
pseudocyst(s)
   pancreatic, 645–8 *see also* pancreatic
      pseudocysts

PSS. *see* portosystemic shunts (PSS)
PSVA. *see* portosystemic vascular anomaly
      (PSVA)
ptyalism, 88–94, *89*
   clinical features, 91
   comments, 94
   definition/overview, 88, *89*
   diagnostics, 92–3
   differential diagnosis, 92
   etiology/pathophysiology, 88–90
   signalment/history, 90–1
   therapeutics, 93
PU/PD. *see* polyuria/polydipsia (PU/PD)
PVH. *see* portal vein hypoplasia (PVH)
pythiosis
   rectoanal polyps *vs.*, 602

rectal adenocarinoma
   rectal prolapse secondary to, 45, *46*
   tenesmus due to, 45, *46*
rectal prolapse, 95–102, *96–101*
   clinical features, 96, *96*
   comments, 101–2
   definition/overview, 95
   diagnostics, 96, 98
   differential diagnosis, 96, *97*
   etiology/pathophysiology, 95
   rectal adenocarinoma and, 45, *46*
   signalment/history, 95–6
   therapeutics, 98–101, *98–101*
      diet, 99
      drugs of choice, 98
      nursing care, 99
      surgical considerations, 99–101, *99–101*
rectal stricture, 593–600, *596–9*
   clinical features, 593–4
   comments, 599–600
   definition/overview, 593
   diagnostics, 594
   differential diagnosis, 594
   etiology/pathophysiology, 593
   signalment/history, 593
   therapeutics, 594–6, *596–9*
rectoanal polyp(s), 601–7, *604–6*
   clinical features, 601–2
   comments, 606–7, *606*
   definition/overview, 601
   diagnostics, 602–3
   differential diagnosis, 602
   etiology/pathophysiology, 601
   signalment/history, 601
   therapeutics, 603–5, *604, 605*
regurgitation, 103–9, *104–6, 108*
   clinical features, 105
   comments, 108–9

definition/overview, 103
diagnostics, 105–6, *105, 106*
differential diagnosis, 105
etiology/pathophysiology, 103–4
hematemesis *vs.*, 66
signalment/history, 104–5, *104*
therapeutics, 107
vomiting *vs.*, 117, 240
respiratory distress
leptospirosis *vs.*, 860
right-sided congestive heart failure
infectious hepatopathy *vs.*, 830
roundworm(s)
clinical features, 508
etiology/pathophysiology, 506–7
therapeutics, 510

salivary mucocele, 164–71, *165, 168–70*
clinical features, 165–6, *165*
comments, 170–1
definition/overview, 164
diagnostics, 166–7
differential diagnosis, 166
etiology/pathophysiology, 164
signalment/history, 165
therapeutics, 167–70, *168–70*
salivary neoplasia
salivary mucocele *vs.*, 166
Salmonella
bacterial enteritis due to, 360–6, 368
clinical features, 363
comments, 368
diagnostics, 364–5
differential diagnosis, 364
etiology/pathophysiology, 360–1
signalment/history, 362
therapeutics, 366–7
salmon-poisoning disease (SPD), 521–5,
523, 524
clinical features, 522
comments, 524–5
definition/overview, 521
diagnostics, 522–3, *523, 524*
differential diagnosis, 522
etiology/pathophysiology, 521–2
signalment/history, 522
therapeutics, 524
SBS. *see* short bowel syndrome (SBS)
sclerosing cholangitis
definition/overview, 697
seizure(s)
congenital portosystemic vascular anomaly
vs., 888
severe acute gastroenteritis
acute hepatic failure *vs.*, 756

severe acute pancreatitis
acute hepatic failure *vs.*, 756
short bowel syndrome (SBS), 526–30
clinical features, 527
comments, 529–30
definition/overview, 526
diagnostics, 527–8
etiology/pathophysiology, 526–7
signalment/history, 527
therapeutics, 528–9
shunt(s)
multiple acquired
vs. congenital portosystemic vascular
anomaly, 888, *888*
portosystemic *see* portosystemic shunts (PSS)
sialadenitis, 159–63
clinical features, 160
comments, 162–3
definition/overview, 159
diagnostics, 160–1
differential diagnosis, 160
etiology/pathophysiology, 159
signalment/history, 159–60
therapeutics, 161–2
sialadenosis
phenobarbital-responsive, 155–8 *see also*
phenobarbital-responsive sialadenosis
salivary mucocele *vs.*, 166
sialoadenitis
salivary mucocele *vs.*, 166
sialolith(s)
salivary mucocele *vs.*, 166
sialometaplasia
necrotizing
vs. salivary mucocele, 166
SIBO. *see* small intestinal bacterial overgrowth
(SIBO)
SID. *see* small intestinal dysbiosis (SID)
skin/subcutaneous neoplasm(s)
salivary mucocele *vs.*, 166
small intestinal bacterial overgrowth (SIBO)
definition/overview, 454
EPI and, 613
small intestinal dysbiosis (SID), 454–9, *457.*
see also intestinal dysbiosis
clinical features, 456
definition/overview, 454
diagnostics, 456–7, *457*
differential diagnosis, 456
etiology/pathophysiology, 454–5
signalment/history, 455–6
therapeutics, 457–8
space-occupying processes
rectal stricture *vs.*, 594
SPD. *see* salmon-poisoning disease (SPD)

Spirocerca lupi, 251–6, *253*
    clinical features, 252
    comments, 254–5
    definition/overview, 251
    diagnostics, 253–4, *253*
    differential diagnosis, 252
    etiology/pathophysiology, 251–2
    Physaloptera vs., 286
    signalment/history, 252
    therapeutics, 254
stomach
    diseases of, 257–327 *see also specific diseases and* stomach disease(s)
stomach disease(s), 257–327. *see also specific diseases*
    CHPG, 324–7
    gastric motility disorders, 259–65, **263**
    gastric neoplasia–benign, 273–7, *275, 276*
    gastric neoplasia–malignant, 278–84, *280–2*
    gastric parasites, 285–8
    gastritis
        acute, 289–95, *290–2,* **293**
        atrophic, 296–9
        chronic, 300–5
    gastroduodenal ulceration/erosion, 306–12, *309*
    GDV, 266–72, *269*
    GER, 313–16
    Helicobacter-associated gastritis, 317–23, *318*
    intestinal motility disorders, 259–65, **263**
stomatitis, 172–8, *173–6*
    caudal–feline, 179–85, *180, 182, 183*
        clinical features, 180, *180*
        comments, 184
        definition/overview, 179
        diagnostics, 181
        differential diagnosis, 181
        etiology/pathophysiology, 179–80
        signalment/history, 180
        therapeutics, 181–3, *182–4*
    clinical features, 173–4, *174, 175*
    comments, 177–8
    definition/overview, 172, 179
    diagnostics, 176, *176*
    differential diagnosis, 174–6
    etiology/pathophysiology, 172, *173*
    signalment/history, 172–3
    therapeutics, 177
storage diseases
    nutritional approach to, 871–4, **872–4**
stranguria
    constipation *vs.,* 11

stricture(s)
    anorectal, 593
    esophageal, 214–19, *216 see also* esophageal stricture
    rectal, 593–600, *596–9 see also* rectal stricture
sublingual mucositis
    definition/overview, 179
sublumbar lymphadenopathy
    perineal hernia *vs.,* 589
suppurative hepatitis, 817–22, *820. see also* hepatitis, suppurative
systemic disease(s)
    colonic neoplasia–malignant *vs.,* 565

tenesmus, 45–50, *46*
    clinical features, 46
    comments, 49–50
    constipation *vs.,* 11
    definition/overview, 45
    diagnostics, 47–8
    differential diagnosis, 47
    etiology/pathophysiology, 45, *46*
    signalment/history, 45–6
    therapeutics, 48–9
thyroglossal cyst(s)
    salivary mucocele *vs.,* 166
tonsil cyst(s)
    salivary mucocele *vs.,* 166
tonsillitis
    definition/overview, 179
toxicity(ies)
    HL *vs.,* 765
toxocariasis
    signalment/history, 507
traumatic liver injury
    hepatotoxins *vs.,* 846
TRD. *see* tylosin-responsive diarrhea (TRD)
Trichomonas spp., 608–10
    T. blagburni, 608–10
    T. foetus, 608–10
trichomoniasis, 608–10
    clinical features, 609
    comments, 610
    definition/overview, 608
    diagnostics, 609
    differential diagnosis, 609
    etiology/pathophysiology, 608
    signalment/history, 608–9
    therapeutics, 610
trichuriasis
    signalment/history, 507
tylosin-responsive diarrhea (TRD)
    definition/overview, 454

ulcer(s)
  definition/overview, 306
ulcerative colitis
  histiocytic, 554–8 *see also* histiocytic ulcerative
    colitis (HUC)
urinary tract disease(s)
  lower
    vs. congenital portosystemic vascular
      anomaly, 888
urogenital disease(s)
  feline pancreatitis *vs.*, 657

vacuolar hepatopathy (VH)
  glycogen-type, 734–41, *737, 738 see also*
    glycogen-type vacuolar hepatopathy (VH)
vascular anomaly
  portosystemic
    congenital, 885–97, *888–91, 893, 894 see also*
      portosystemic vascular anomaly,
      congenital
vascular dysplasia
  nutritional approach to, 874, 876, **876**
vascular ring anomaly
  esophagitis *vs.*, 224
VH. *see* vacuolar hepatopathy (VH)
vitamin B deficiency
  feline chronic diarrhea and
    treatment of, 40
vitamin B12 deficiency, 345–9. *see also* cobalamin
    deficiency
vomiting
  acute, 110–15

clinical features, 111
comments, 114–15
definition/overview, 110
diagnostics, 112–13
differential diagnosis, 112
etiology/pathophysiology, 110–11
signalment/history, 111
therapeutics, 113–14
chronic, 116–24, *118–20*
  causes of, 117–20, *118–20*
  clinical features, 117
  comments, 124
  definition/overview, 116
  diagnostics, 120–2
  differential diagnosis, 117–20, *118–20*
  etiology/pathophysiology, 116
  signalment/history, 116–17
  therapeutics, 122–3
hematemesis *vs.*, 66
regurgitation *vs.*, 117, 240
Von Meyenburg complexes, 721

water
  in nutritional approach to acute and chronic
    pancreatitis, 617
  in nutritional approach to acute
    gastroenteritis, 85
whipworm(s)
  clinical features, 508
  definition/overview, 506
  etiology/pathophysiology, 507
  therapeutics, 510